Core Procedures in Plastic Surgery

Content Strategist: Belinda Kuhn
Content Development Specialist: Poppy Garraway
Content Coordinator: Trinity Hutton
Project Manager: Caroline Jones
Design: Miles Hitchen
Illustration Manager: Jennifer Rose
Illustrator: Antbits
Marketing Manager(s) (UK/USA): Katie Alexo

Core Procedures in Plastic Surgery

Peter C. Neligan
MB, FRCS(I), FRCSC, FACS
Professor of Surgery
Department of Surgery, Division of Plastic Surgery
University of Washington
Seattle, WA, USA

Donald W. Buck II
MD
Assistant Professor of Surgery
Division of Plastic & Reconstructive Surgery
Washington University School of Medicine
St. Louis, MO, USA

For additional online content visit expertconsult

ELSEVIER
SAUNDERS
London, New York, Oxford, Philadelphia, St Louis, Sydney, Toronto

ELSEVIER
SAUNDERS

SAUNDERS an imprint of Elsevier Inc

Notices

Knowledge and best practice in this field are constantly changing. As new research and experience broaden our understanding, changes in research methods, professional practices, or medical treatment may become necessary.

Practitioners and researchers must always rely on their own experience and knowledge in evaluating and using any information, methods, compounds, or experiments described herein. In using such information or methods they should be mindful of their own safety and the safety of others, including parties for whom they have a professional responsibility.

With respect to any drug or pharmaceutical products identified, readers are advised to check the most current information provided (i) on procedures featured or (ii) by the manufacturer of each product to be administered, to verify the recommended dose or formula, the method and duration of administration, and contraindications. It is the responsibility of practitioners, relying on their own experience and knowledge of their patients, to make diagnoses, to determine dosages and the best treatment for each individual patient, and to take all appropriate safety precautions.

To the fullest extent of the law, neither the Publisher nor the authors, contributors, or editors, assume any liability for any injury and/or damage to persons or property as a matter of products liability, negligence or otherwise, or from any use or operation of any methods, products, instructions, or ideas contained in the material herein.

ISBN: 978-0-323-24399-5
e-book ISBN: 978-1-4557-2637-0

Printed in China
Last digit is the print number: 9 8 7 6 5 4 3 2 1

Contents

Preface

Time is a precious commodity and much as we would all love to be able to take the time to sit back and read the full chapter of a given topic before doing the case, life is not that generous. *Plastic Surgery 3rd Edition*, published earlier this year, is an encyclopedia of Plastic Surgery that contains detailed descriptions of both the common and the uncommon conditions in our specialty, as well as technical chapters on anatomy, operative technique etc. However, it is 6 volumes, and the online version, though comprehensive, is even bigger. For that reason, we put together this book, *Core Procedures in Plastic Surgery*, which is condensed from the 6 Volume Textbook, *Plastic Surgery 3rd Edition*. We chose the table of contents based on feedback from focus groups containing residents and attendings. It was evident these individuals wanted a quick reference resource for some of the most common things they see in day to day practice. They did not want a lot of words, but they did want a lot of pictures and videos. We hope you like the result.

In this book, we have compiled the 24 top procedures in both aesthetic and reconstructive plastic surgery. Reference is made to the chapters from which the content is extracted. There is generous use of illustrations, schematic diagrams, photographs, as well as videos extracted from the main text. A short annotated bibliography is at the end of each chapter. In addition, the book is littered with bulleted pearls of wisdom highlighting key concepts of anatomy, technique, complications and outcomes, and pre- and post-operative considerations. An icon appears beside the text or illustration to indicate video content. We hope you will find this a useful addition to your library. We have tried to design it to be intuitive and user friendly and we hope that you will appreciate the condensed format that makes for quick review in the OR or Clinic.

Peter C. Neligan
Donald W. Buck II

List of Contributors

Jamil Ahmad, MD, FRCSC
Staff Plastic Surgeon
The Plastic Surgery Clinic
Mississauga, ON, Canada

Robert J. Allen, MD
Clinical Professor of Plastic Surgery
Department of Plastic Surgery
New York University Medical Centre
Charleston, SC, USA

Sérgio Fernando Dantas de Azevedo, MD
Member
Brazilian Society of Plastic Surgery
Volunteer Professor of Plastic Surgery
Department of Plastic Surgery
Federal University of Pernambuco
Permambuco, Brazil

Daniel C. Baker, MD
Professor of Surgery
Insitiute of Reconstructive Plastic Surgery
New York University Medical Center
Department of Plastic Surgery
New York, NY, USA

Jonathan Bank, MD
Resident, Section of Plastic and Reconstructive Surgery
Department of Surgery
Pritzker School of Medicine
University of Chicago Medical Center
Chicago, IL, USA

Fritz E. Barton Jr, MD
Clinical Professor
Department of Plastic Surgery
University of Texas Southwestern Medical Center
Dallas, TX, USA

Miles G. Berry, MS, FRCS(Plast)
Consultant Plastic and Aesthetic Surgeon
Institute of Cosmetic and Reconstructive Surgery
London, UK

Phillip N. Blondeel, MD, PhD, FCCP
Professor of Plastic Surgery
Department of Plastic and Reconstructive Surgery
University Hospital Gent
Gent, Belgium

Kirsty U. Boyd, MD, FRCSC
Clinical Fellow – Hand Surgery
Department of Surgery – Division of Plastic Surgery
Washington University School of Medicine
Saint Louis, MO, USA

Donald W. Buck II, MD
Assistant Professor of Surgery
Division of Plastic & Reconstructive Surgery
Washington University School of Medicine
St. Louis, MO, USA

Giuseppe Catanuto, MD, PhD
Research Fellow
The School of Oncological Reconstructive Surgery
Milan, Italy

James Chang, MD
Professor and Chief
Division of Plastic and Reconstructive Surgery
Stanford University Medical Center
Stanford, CA, USA

Robert A. Chase, MD
Holman Professor of Surgery – Emeritus
Stanford University Medical Center
Stanford, CA, USA

Philip Kuo-Ting Chen, MD
Director
Department of Plastic and Reconstructive Surgery
Chang Gung Memorial Hospital and Chang Gung University
Taipei, Taiwan, The People's Republic of China

Mark W. Clemens, MD
Assistant Professor
Department of Plastic Surgery
Anderson Cancer Center University of Texas
Houston, TX, USA

Mark B. Constantian, MD, FACS
Active Staff
Saint Joseph Hospital
Nashua, NH (private practice)
Assistant Clinical Professor of Plastic Surgery
Division of Plastic Surgery
Department of Surgery
University of Wisconsin
Madison, WI, USA

Dai M. Davies, FRCS
Consultant and Institute Director
Institute of Cosmetic and Reconstructive Surgery
London, UK

Michael R. Davis, MD, FACS, LtCol, USAF, MC
Chief
Reconstructive Surgery and Regenerative Medicine
Plastic and Reconstructive Surgeon
San Antonio Military Medical Center
Houston, TX, USA

Jorge I. de la Torre, MD
Professor and Chief
Division of Plastic Surgery
University of Alabama at Birmingham
Birmingham, AL, USA

Amir H. Dorafshar, MBChB
Assistant Professor
Department of Plastic and Reconstructive Surgery
John Hopkins Medical Institute
John Hopkins Outpatient Center
Baltimore, MD, USA

Gregory A. Dumanian, MD, FACS
Chief of Plastic Surgery
Division of Plastic Surgery, Department of Surgery
Northwestern Feinberg School of Medicine
Chicago, IL, USA

L. Franklyn Elliott, MD
Assistant Clinical Professor
Emory Section of Plastic Surgery
Emory University
Atlanta, GA, USA

Marco F. Ellis, MD
Chief Resident
Division of Plastic Surgery
Northwestern Memorial Hospital
Northwestern University, Feinberg School of Medicine
Chicago, IL, USA

Julius W. Few Jr, MD
Director
The Few Institute for Aesthetic Plastic Surgery
Clinical Associate
Division of Plastic Surgery
University of Chicago
Chicago, IL, USA

David M. Fisher, MB, BCh, FRCSC, FACS
Medical Director, Cleft Lip and Palate Program
Division of Plastic and Reconstructive Surgery
The Hospital for Sick Children
Toronto, ON, Canada

Jack Fisher, MD
Department of Plastic Surgery
Vanderbilt University
Nashville, TN, USA

Neil A Fine, MD
Associate Professor of Clinical Surgery
Department of Surgery
Northwestern University
Chicago, IL, USA

Joshua Fosnot, MD
Resident
Division of Plastic Surgery
The University of Pennsylvania Health System
Philadelphia, PA, USA

Ida K. Fox, MD
Assistant Professor of Plastic Surgery
Department of Surgery
Washington University School of Medicine
Saint Louis, MO, USA

Allen Gabriel, MD
Assitant Professor
Department of Plastic Surgery
Loma Linda University Medical Center
Chief of Plastic Surgery
Southwest Washington Medical Center
Vancouver, WA, USA

Günter Germann, MD, PhD
Professor of Plastic Surgery
Clinic for Plastic and Reconstructive Surgery
Heidelberg University Hospital
Heidelberg, Germany

Barry H. Grayson, DDS
Associate Professor of Surgery (Craniofacial Orthodontics)
New York University Langone Medical Centre
Institute of Reconstructive Plastic Surgery
New York, NY, USA

James C. Grotting, MD, FACS
Clinical Professor of Plastic Surgery
University of Alabama at Birmingham;
The University of Wisconsin, Madison, WI;
Grotting and Cohn Plastic Surgery
Birmingham, AL, USA

Dennis C. Hammond, MD
Clinical Assistant Professor
Department of Surgery
Michigan State University College of Human Medicine
East Lansing
Associate Program Director
Plastic and Reconstructive Surgery
Grand Rapids Medical Education and Research Center for Health Professions
Grand Rapids, MI, USA

Vincent R. Hentz, MD
Emeritus Professor of Surgery and Orthopedic Surgery (by courtesy)
Stanford University
Stanford, CA, USA

Kent K. Higdon, MD
Former Aesthetic Fellow
Grotting and Cohn Plastic Surgery;
Current Assistant Professor
Vanderbilt University
Nashville, TN, USA

William Y. Hoffman, MD
Professor and Chief
Division of Plastic and Reconstructive Surgery
University of California, San Francisco
San Francisco, CA, USA

Joon Pio Hong, MD, PhD, MMM
Chief and Associate Professor
Department of Plastic Surgery
Asian Medical Center University of Ulsan School of Medicine
Seoul, Korea

Ian T. Jackson, MD, DSc(Hon), FRCS, FACS, FRACS (Hon)
Emeritus Surgeon
Surgical Services Administration
William Beaumont Hospitals
Royal Oak, MI, USA

Mark Laurence Jewell, MD
Assistant Clinical Professor of Plastic Surgery
Oregon Health Science University
Jewell Plastic Surgery Center
Eugene, OR, USA

Neil F. Jones, MD, FRCS
Chief of Hand Surgery
University of California Medical Center
Professor of Orthopedic Surgery
Professor of Plastic and Reconstructive Surgery
University of California Irvine
Irvine, CA, USA

Ryosuke Kakinoki, MD, PhD
Associate Professor
Chief of the Hand Surgery and Microsurgery Unit
Department of Orthopedic Surgery and Rehabilitation Medicine
Graduate School of Medicine
Kyoto University
Kyoto, Japan

Alex Kane, MD
Associate Professor of Surgery
Washington University School of Medicine
Saint Louis, WO, USA

Marwan R. Khalifeh, MD
Instructor of Plastic Surgery
Department of Plastic Surgery
Johns Hopkins University School of Medicine
Washington, DC, USA

Susan E. Mackinnon, MD
Sydney M. Shoenberg, Jr and Robert H. Shoenberg Professor
Department of Surgery, Division of Plastic and Reconstructive Surgery
Washington University School of Medicine
Saint Louis, MO, USA

Paul N. Manson, MD
Professor of Plastic Surgery
University of Maryland Shock Trauma Unit
University of Maryland and Johns Hopkins School of Medicine
Baltimore, MD, USA

G. Patrick Maxwell, MD, FACS
Clinical Professor of Surgery
Department of Plastic Surgery
Loma Linda University Medical Center
Loma Linda, CA, USA

Kai Megerle, MD
Research Fellow
Division of Plastic and Reconstructive Surgery
Stanford Medical Center
Stanford, CA, USA

Luis Humberto Uribe Morelli, MD
Resident of Plastic Surgery
Unisanta Plastic Surgery Department
Sao Paulo, Brazil

Colin M. Morrison, MSc (Hons), FRCSI (Plast)
Consultant Plastic Surgeon
Department of Plastic and Reconstructive Surgery
Saint Vincent's University Hospital
Dublin, Ireland

Hunter R. Moyer, MD
Fellow
Department of Plastic and Reconstructive Surgery
Emory University, Atlanta, GA, USA

John B. Mulliken, MD
Director, Craniofacial Centre
Department of Plastic and Oral Surgery
Children's Hospital
Boston, MA, USA

Maurizio B. Nava, MD
Chief of Plastic Surgery Unit
Istituto Nazionale dei Tumori
Milano, Italy

Peter C. Neligan, MB, FRCS(I), FRCSC, FACS
Professor of Surgery
Department of Surgery, Division of Plastic Surgery
University of Washington
Seattle, WA, USA

Jonas A Nelson, MD
Integrated General/Plastic Surgery Resident
Department of Surgery
Division of Plastic Surgery
Perelman School of Medicine
University of Pennsylvania
Philadelphia, PA, USA

M. Samuel Noordhoff, MD, FACS
Emeritus Superintendent
Chang Gung Memorial Hospitals
Taipei, Taiwan, The People's Republic of China

Angela Pennati, MD
Assistant Plastic Surgeon
Unit of Plastic Surgery
Istituto Nazionale dei Tumori
Milano, Italy

Oscar M. Ramirez, MD, FACS
Adjunct Clinical Faculty
Plastic Surgery Division
Cleveland Clinic Florida
Boca Raton, FL, USA

Dirk F. Richter, MD, PhD
Clinical Director
Department of Plastic Surgery
Dreifaltigkeits-Hospital Wesseling
Wesseling, Germany

Eduardo D. Rodriguez, MD, DDS
Chief, Plastic Reconstructive and Maxillofacial Surgery, R Adams Cowley Shock Trauma Center
Professor of Surgery
University of Maryland School of Medicine
Baltimore, MD, USA

Rod J. Rohrich, MD, FACS
Professor and Chairman Crystal Charity Ball
Distinguished Chair in Plastic Surgery
Department of Plastic Surgery;
Professor and Chairman Betty and Warren
Woodward Chair in Plastic and Reconstructive
Surgery
University of Texas Southwestern Medical
Center at Dallas
Dallas, TX, USA

Michelle C. Roughton, MD
Chief Resident
Section of Plastic and Reconstructive Surgery
University of Chicago Medical Center
Chicago, IL, USA

Michel Saint-Cyr, MD, FRCSC
Associate Professor Plastic Surgery
Department of Plastic Surgery
University of Texas Southwestern Medical
Center
Dallas, TX, USA

Cristianna Bonneto Saldanha, MD
Resident
General Surgery Department
Santa Casa of Santos Hospital
São Paulo, Brazil

Osvaldo Ribeiro Saldanha, MD
Chairman of Plastic Surgery
Unisanta
Santos
Past President of the Brazilian Society of
Plastic Surgery (SBCP)
International Associate Editor of Plastic and
Reconstructive Surgery
São Paulo, Brazil

Osvaldo Ribeiro Saldanha Filho, MD
São Paulo, Brazil

J. Peter Rubin, MD, FACS
Chief of Plastic Surgery
Director, Life After Weight Loss Body
Contouring Program
University of Pittsburgh
Pittsburgh, PA, USA

Joseph M. Serletti, MD, FACS
Henry Royster-William Maul Measey
Professor of Surgery; Chief
Division of Plastic Surgery
Vice Chair (Finance)
Department of Surgery
University of Pennsylvania
Philadelphia, PA, USA

Kenneth C. Shestak, MD
Professor of Plastic Surgery
Division of Plastic Surgery
University of Pittsburgh
Pittsburgh, PA, USA

Navin K. Singh, MD, MSc
Assistant Professor of Plastic Surgery
Department of Plastic Surgery
Johns Hopkins University School of Medicine
Washington, DC, USA

David H. Song, MD, MBA, FACS
Cynthia Chow Professor of Surgery
Chief, Section of Plastic and Reconstructive
Surgery
Vice-Chairman, Department of Surgery
The University of Chicago Medicine & Biological
Sciences
Chicago, IL, USA

Andrea Spano, MD
Senior Assistant Plastic Surgeon
Unit of Plastic Surgery
Istituto Nazionale dei Tumori
Milano, Italy

Scott L. Spear, MD, FACS
Professor and Chairman
Department of Plastic Surgery
Georgetown University Hospital
Georgetown, WA, USA

Alexander Stoff, MD, PhD
Senior Fellow
Department of Plastic Surgery
Dreifaltigkeits-Hospital Wesseling
Wesseling, Germany

John D. Symbas, MD
Plastic and Reconstructive Surgeon
Private Practice
Marietta Plastic Surgery
Marietta, GA, USA

Jin Bo Tang, MD
Professor and Chair
Department of Hand Surgery;
Chair
The Hand Surgery Research Center
Affiliated Hospital of Nantong University
Nantong, The People's Republic of China

Patrick L. Tonnard, MD
Coupure Centrum Voor Plastische Chirurgie
Ghent, Belgium

Charles H. Thorne, MD
Associate Professor of Plastic Surgery
Department of Plastic Surgery
NYU School of Medicine
New York, NY, USA

Francisco Valero-Cuevas, PhD
Director
Brain-Body Dynamics Laboratory
Professor of Biomedical Engineering
Professor of Biokinesiology and Physical
Therapy
By courtesy Professor of Computer Science
and Aerospace and Mechanical Engineering
The University of Southern California
Los Angeles, CA, USA

Allen L. Van Beek, MD, FACS
Adjunct Professor
University Minnesota School of Medicine
Division Plastic Surgery
Minneapolis, MN, USA

Valentina Visintini Cividin, MD
Assistant Plastic Surgeon
Unit of Plastic Surgery
Istituto Nazionale dei Tumori
Milano, Italy

Richard J. Warren, MD, FRCSC
Clinical Professor
Division of Plastic Surgery
University of British Columbia
Vancouver, BC, Canada

Acknowledgments

This work was the brainchild of Donnie Buck and the details were fleshed out by the core editorial team at Elsevier who worked with me on the big book, Plastic Surgery 3e, Belinda Kuhn, Louise Cook, ALexanrda Mortimer and Poppy Garraway. Poppy has run with it and made it a reality. Donnie has condensed the chapters from the big book to compile this collection and Caroline Jones has made sure that it is fit for press. I am grateful to all of them for their hard work and dedication. I am forever grateful to my partners at the University of Washington under the leadership of Nick Vedder, for their support. Finally, none of this would be possible without the unwavering love and support of my wife Gabrielle and my family.

PCN

I must first thank Sue Hodgson and Peter Neligan for believing in, and trusting, a young plastic surgery resident with this incredible opportunity. Working on this book has been a tremendous honor and I cannot thank Dr. Neligan enough for his mentorship and guidance throughout the process. I owe a debt of gratitude to the wonderful team at Elseiver, especially Poppy Garraway, Belinda Kuhn, and Caroline Jones who kept me on target and were responsible for making this book a reality. I would also like to thank the authors, all masters of their craft, for contributing the wonderful text, illustrations, photographs, and videos that comprise this book. Finally, I would like to thank my family, especially my children, Benjamin and Brooke, for inspiring me daily, and my beautiful wife Jennifer for her love, encouragement, and support – without her none of this would have been possible.

DWB

Video Contents

Chapter 1

Blepharoplasty

This chapter was created using content from Neligan & Warren, Plastic Surgery 3rd edition, Volume 2, Aesthetic, Chapter 8, Blepharoplasty, Julius W. Few Jr. and Marco F. Ellis.

SYNOPSIS

- Blepharoplasty is a vital part of facial rejuvenation. The traditional removal of tissue may or may not be the preferred approach when assessed in relation to modern cosmetic goals.
- A thorough understanding of orbital and eyelid anatomy is necessary to understand aging in the periorbital region, and to devise appropriate surgical strategies.
- Preoperative assessment includes a review of the patient's perceptions, assessment of the patient's anatomy, and an appropriate medical and ophthalmologic examination.
- Surgical techniques in blepharoplasty are numerous and should be tailored to the patient's own unique anatomy and aesthetic diagnosis.
- Interrelated anatomic structures including the brow and the infraorbital rim may need to be surgically addressed for an optimal outcome.

Brief introduction

- The eyelids are vital, irreplaceable structures that serve to protect the globes. Their shutter-like mechanism is essential to clean, lubricate, and protect the cornea. Any disruption or restriction of eyelid closure will have significant consequences for both the patient and the surgeon.
- Instead of the common practice of excising precious upper and, to a somewhat lesser degree, lower eyelid tissue, it is preferable to focus on restoration of attractive, youthful anatomy.
- One should first conceptualize the desired outcome, then select and execute procedures accurately designed to achieve those specific goals.
- Several important principles are advocated (Box 1.1).

Anatomical pearls

Osteology and periorbita

- The orbits are pyramids formed by the frontal, sphenoid, maxillary, zygomatic, lacrimal, palatine, and ethmoid bones ***(Fig. 1.1)***.
- The periosteal covering or periorbita is most firmly attached at the suture lines and the circumferential anterior orbital rim.
- The investing orbital septum in turn attaches to the periorbita of the orbital rim, forming a thickened perimeter known as the arcus marginalis.
- This structure reduces the perimeter and diameter of the orbital aperture and is thickest in the superior and lateral aspects of the orbital rim.
- Certain structures must be avoided during upper lid surgery.
  - The lacrimal gland, located in the superolateral orbit deep to its anterior rim, often descends beneath the orbital rim, prolapsing into the postseptal upper lid in many persons.
  - The trochlea is located 5 mm posterior to the superonasal orbital rim and is attached to the periorbita. Disruption of this structure can cause motility problems.

Lateral retinaculum

- Anchored to the lateral orbit is a labyrinth of connective tissues, known as the lateral retinaculum, that are crucial

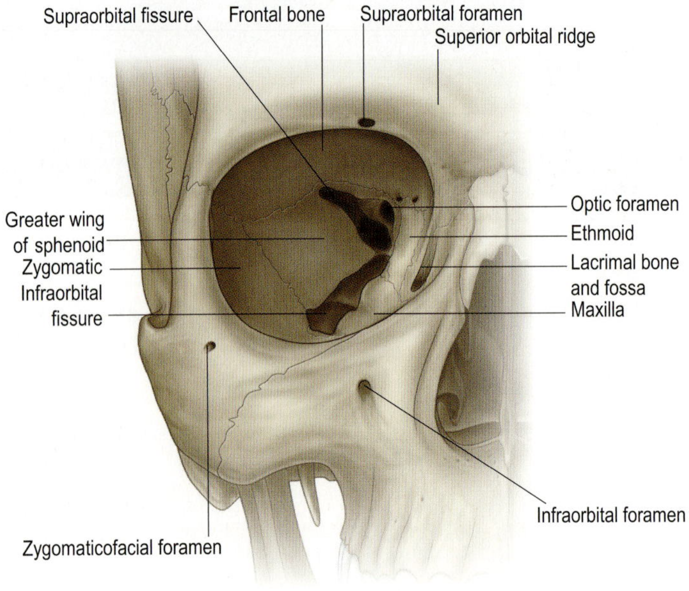

Figure 1.1 Orbital bones. Frontal view of the orbit with foramina.

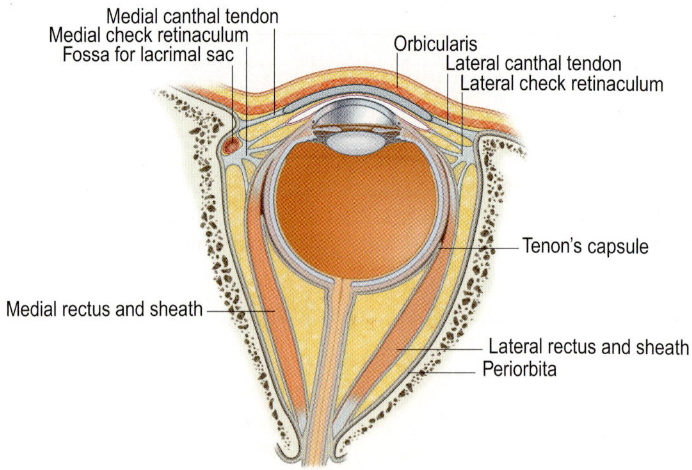

Figure 1.2 Horizontal section of the orbit showing the lateral retinaculum formed by the lateral horn of the levator, lateral canthal tendon, tarsal strap, the Lockwood suspensory ligament, and lateral rectus check ligaments.

BOX 1.1 **Principles for restoration of youthful eyes**

- Control of periorbital aesthetics by proper brow positioning, corrugator muscle removal, and lid fold invagination when beneficial.
- Restoration of tone and position of the lateral canthus and, along with it, restoration of a youthful and attractive intercanthal axis tilt.
- Restoration of the tone and posture of the lower lids.
- Preservation of maximal lid skin and muscle (so essential to lid function and aesthetics) as well as orbital fat.
- Lifting of the midface through reinforced canthopexy, preferably enhanced by composite malar advancement.
- Correction of suborbital malar grooves with tear trough (or suborbital malar) implants, obliterating the deforming tear trough (bony) depressions that angle down diagonally across the cheek, which begin below the inner canthus.
- Control of orbital fat by septal restraint or quantity reduction.
- Removal of only that tissue (skin, muscle, fat) that is truly excessive on the upper and lower lids, sometimes resorting to unconventional excision patterns.
- Modification of skin to remove prominent wrinkling and excision of small growths and blemishes.

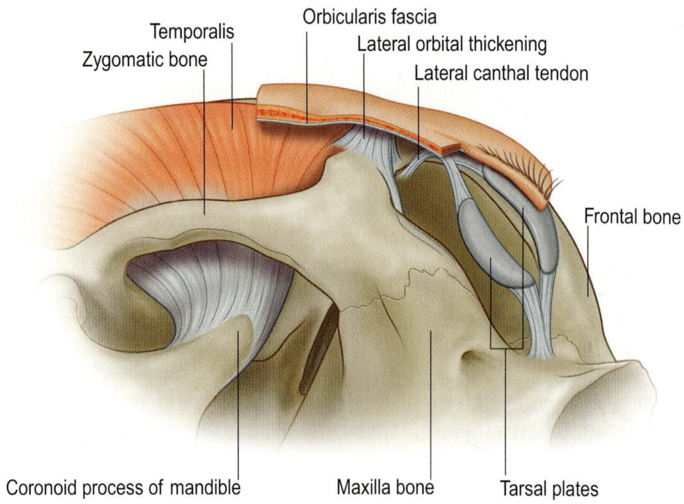

Figure 1.3 Lateral canthal tendon has separate superficial and deep components. The deep component attaches inside the orbital rim at Whitnall's tubercle. The superficial component passes from the tarsal plates to the periosteum of the lateral orbital rim and lateral orbital thickening. Both components are continuous with both superior and inferior lid tarsal plates. (Adapted from Muzaffar AR, Mendelson BC, Adams Jr WP. Surgical anatomy of the ligamentous attachments of the lower lid and lateral canthus. *Plast Reconstr Surg*. 2002;110(3):873–884.)

to maintenance of the integrity, position, and function of the globe and periorbital.

- These structures coalesce at the lateral orbit and support the globe and eyelids like a hammock ***(Fig. 1.2)***.
- The lateral retinaculum consists of the lateral canthal tendon, tarsal strap, lateral horn of the levator aponeurosis, the Lockwood suspensory ligament, Whitnall's ligament, and check ligaments of the lateral rectus muscle.
- They converge and insert securely into the thickened periosteum overlying the Whitnall tubercle.
- Controversy exists surrounding the naming of the components of the lateral canthal tendon.
- A superficial component is continuous with the orbicularis oculi fascia and attaches to the lateral orbital rim and deep temporal fascia by means of the lateral orbital thickening.
- A deep component connects directly to the Whitnall tubercle and is classically known as the lateral canthal tendon ***(Fig. 1.3)***.
- The tarsal strap is a distinct anatomic structure that inserts into the tarsus medial and inferior to the lateral canthal tendon.
- The tarsal strap attaches approximately 3 mm inferiorly and 1 mm posteriorly to the deep lateral canthal tendon, approximately 4–5 mm from the anterior orbital rim.
- It shortens in response to lid laxity, benefiting from release during surgery to help achieve a long-lasting restoration or elevation canthopexy ***(Fig. 1.4)***.

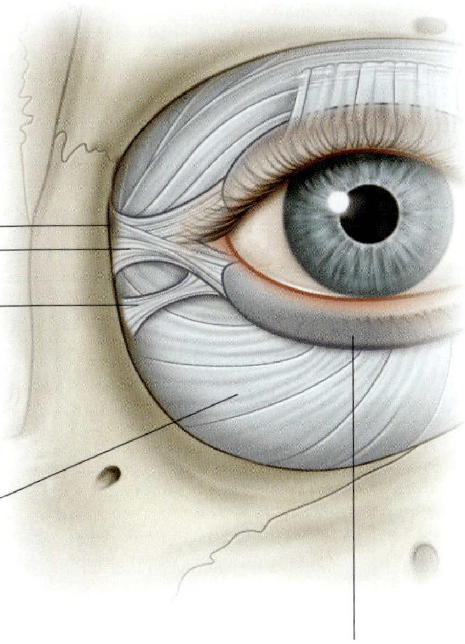

Figure 1.4 The lateral canthal tendon inserts securely into the thickened periosteum overlying Whitnall's tubercle. The tarsal strap is a distinct anatomic structure that suspends the tarsus medial and inferior to the lateral canthal tendon to lateral orbital wall, approximately 4–5 mm from the orbital rim.

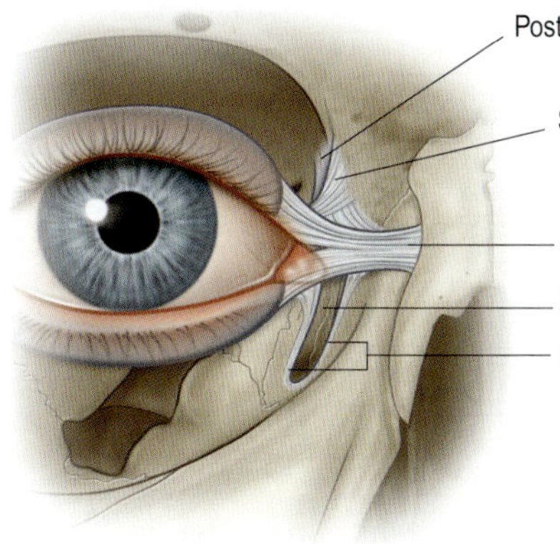

Figure 1.5 The medial canthal tendon envelops the lacrimal sac. It is tripartite, with anterior, posterior and superior limbs. Like the lateral canthal tendon, its limbs are continuous with tarsal plates. The components of this tendon along with its lateral counterpart are enveloped by deep and superficial aspects of the orbicularis muscle. (Adapted from Spinelli HM. *Atlas of Aesthetic Eyelid and Periocular Surgery*. Philadelphia: Saunders; 2004:13.)

- Adequate release of the tarsal strap permits a tension-free canthopexy, minimizing the downward tethering force of this fibrous condensation.
- This release along with a superior reattachment of the lateral canthal tendon is key to a successful canthopexy.

Medial orbital vault

- A hammock of fibrous condensations suspends the globe above the orbital floor. The medial components of the apparatus include medial canthal tendon, the Lockwood suspensory ligament and check ligaments of the medial rectus.
- The medial canthal tendon, like the lateral canthal tendon, has separate limbs that attach the tarsal plates to the ethmoid and lacrimal bones.
- Each limb inserts onto the periorbital of the apex of the lacrimal fossa. The anterior limb provides the bulk of the medial globe support ***(Fig. 1.5)***.

Forehead and temporal region

- The forehead and brow consist of four layers: skin, subcutaneous tissue, muscle, and galea.
- There are four distinct brow muscles: frontalis, procerus, corrugator superciliaris, and orbicularis oculi ***(Fig. 1.6)***.
- The frontalis muscle inserts predominately into the medial half or two-thirds of the eyebrow ***(Fig. 1.7)***, allowing the lateral brow to drop hopelessly ptotic from aging, while the medial brow responds to frontalis activation and elevates, often excessively in its drive to clear the lateral overhand. Constant contraction of the frontalis will give the appearance of deep horizontal creases in the forehead ***(Fig. 1.8)***.
- The vertically oriented procerus is a medial muscle, often continuous with the frontalis, arising from the nasal bones and inserting into the subcutaneous tissue of the glabellar region. It pulls the medial brow inferiorly and contributes to the horizontal wrinkles at the root of the nose. More commonly, these wrinkles result from brow ptosis and correct spontaneously with brow elevation.
- The obliquely oriented corrugators muscle arises from the frontal bone and inserts into the brow tissue laterally, with some extensions into orbicularis and frontalis musculature, forming vertical glabellar furrows during contraction.

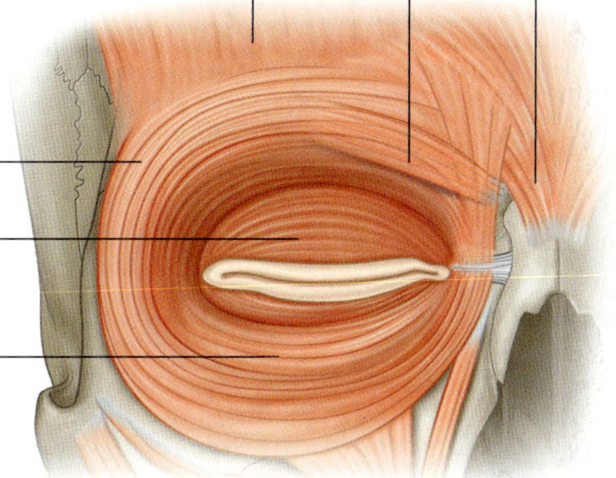

Figure 1.6 Facial muscles of the orbital region. Note that the preseptal and pretarsal orbicularis muscles fuse with the medial and lateral canthal tendons.

Eyelids

- There is much similarity between upper and lower eyelid anatomy. Each consists of an anterior lamella of skin and

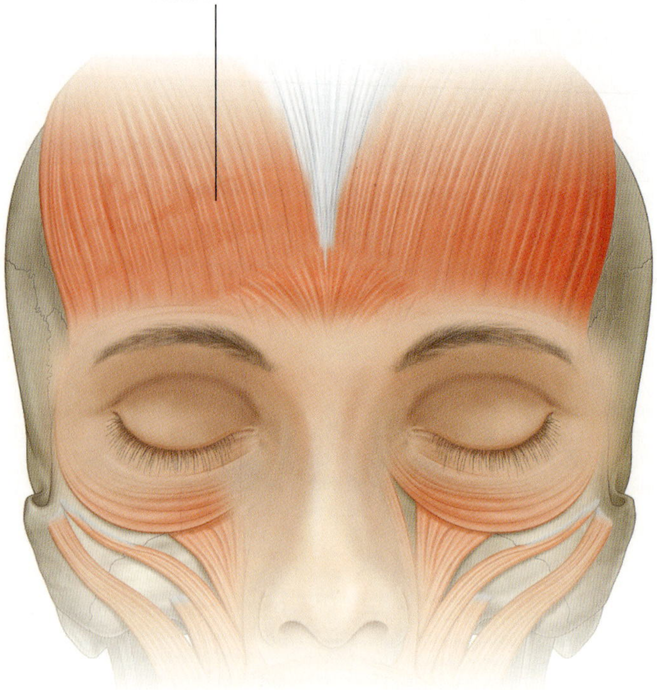

Figure 1.7 The frontalis muscle inserts predominantly into the medial half or two-thirds of the eyebrow. The medial brow responds to frontalis activation and elevates, often excessively, in its drive to clear lateral overhang.

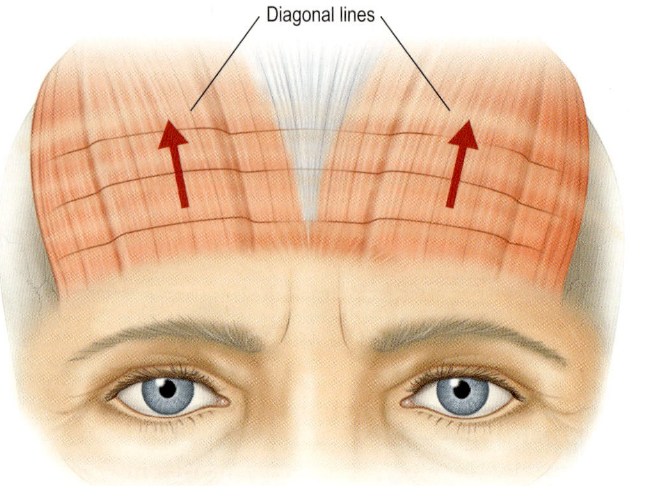

Figure 1.8 Frontalis action. The frontalis muscle inserts into the medial two thirds of the brow. Exaggerated medial brow elevation is required to clear the lateral overhang and to eliminate visual obstruction. Constant contraction of the frontalis will give the appearance of deep horizontal creases in the forehead. This necessarily means that when the lateral skin is elevated or excised, the over-elevated and distorted medial brow drops profoundly.

orbicularis muscle and a posterior lamella of tarsus and conjunctiva ***(Fig. 1.9)***.

- The orbicularis muscle, which acts as a sphincter for the eyelids, consists of orbital, preseptal, and pretarsal segments.
- The pretarsal muscle segment fuses with the lateral canthal tendon and attaches laterally to Whitnall tubercle. Medially it forms two heads, which insert into the anterior and posterior lacrimal crests (see Fig. 1.6).

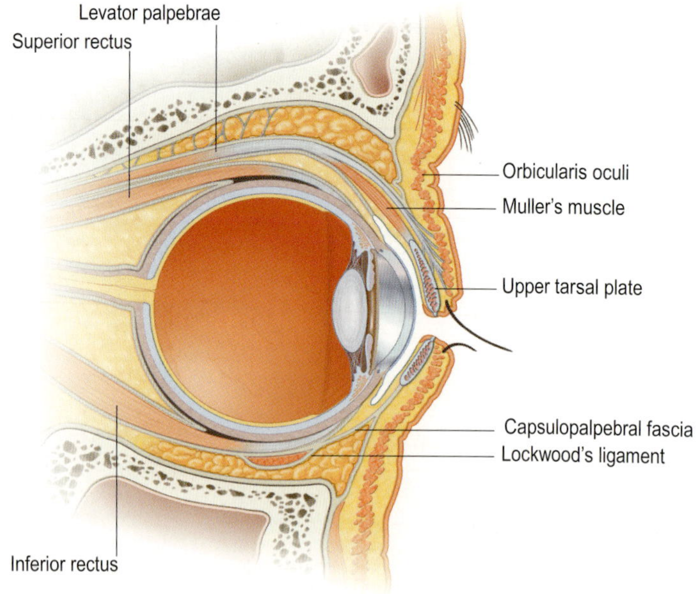

Figure 1.9 Eyelid anatomy. Each eyelid consists of an anterior lamella of skin and orbicularis muscle and a posterior lamella of tarsus and conjunctiva. The orbital septum forms the anterior border of the orbital fat.

Upper eyelid

- The orbital septum originates superiorly at the arcus and forms the anterior border of the orbit. It joins with the levator aponeurosis, just superior to the tarsus. The sling formed by the union of these two structures houses the orbital fat.
- The levator palpebrae superioris muscle originates above the annulus of Zinn. It extends anteriorly for 40 mm before becoming a tendinous aponeurosis below Whitnall's ligament. The aponeurosis fans out medially and laterally to attach to the orbital retinacula. The aponeurosis fuses with the orbital septum above the superior border of the tarsus and at the caudal extent of the sling, sending fibrous strands to the dermis to form the lid crease. Extensions of the aponeurosis finally insert into the anterior and inferior tarsus. As the levator aponeurosis undergoes senile attenuation, the lid crease rises into the superior orbit from its remaining dermal attachments while the lid margin drops.
- Müller's muscle, or the supratarsal muscle, originates on the deep surface of the levator near the point where the muscle becomes aponeurotic and inserts into the superior tarsus. Dehiscence of the attachment of the levator aponeurosis to the tarsus results in an acquired ptosis only after the Müller's muscle attenuates and loses its integrity.
- In the Asian eyelid, fusion of the levator and septum commonly occurs at a lower level, allowing the sling and fat to descend farther into the lid. This lower descent of fat creates the characteristic fullness of their upper eyelid. In addition, the aponeurotic fibers form a weaker attachment to the dermis, resulting in a less distinct lid fold ***(Fig. 1.10)***.

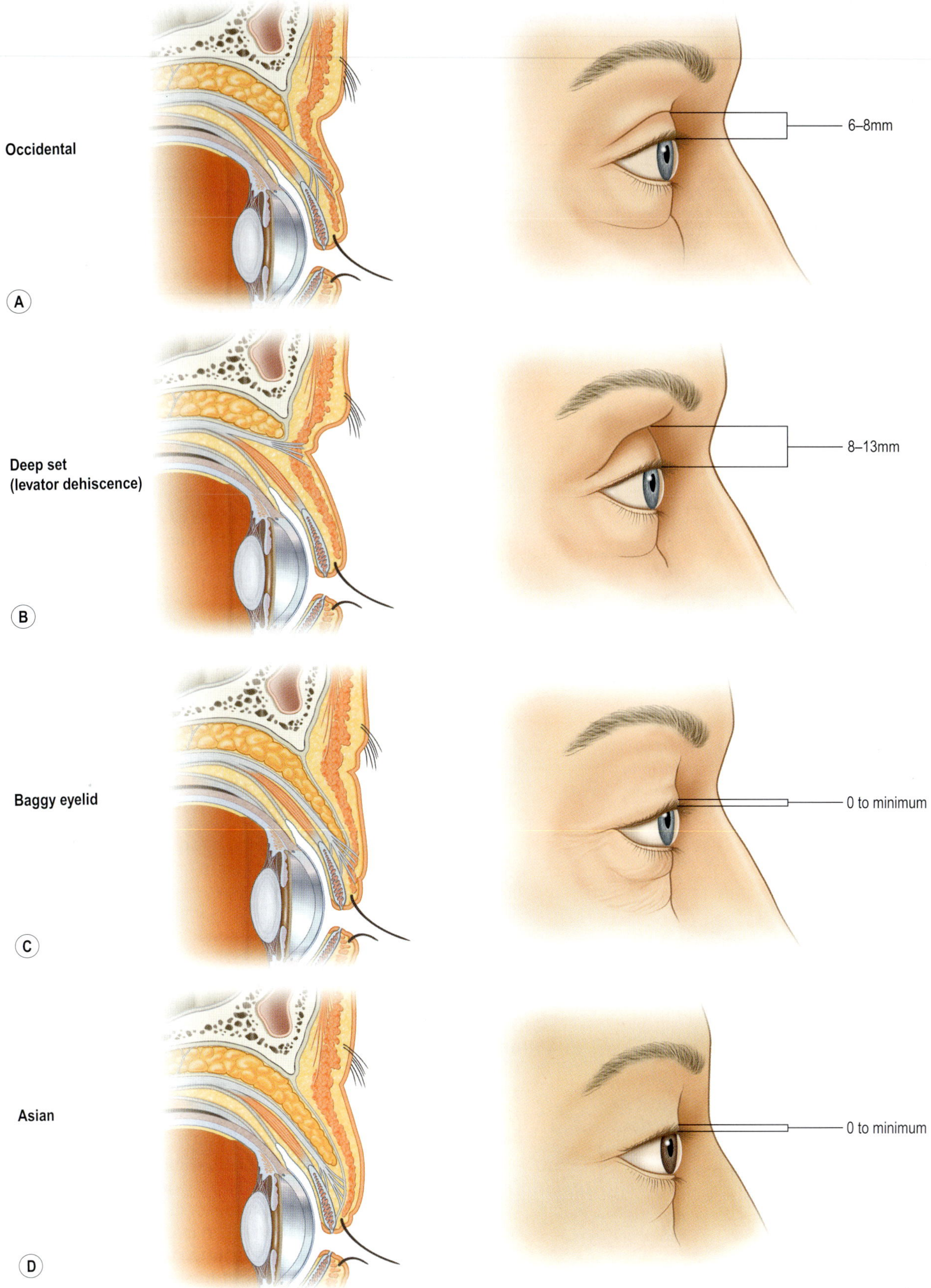

Figure 1.10 The anatomic variations in the upper eyelid displayed by different ethnic groups and the changes associated with senescence within each group allow for a convergence of anatomy. **(A)** The normal, youthful Asian upper eyelid has levator extensions inserting onto the skin surface to define a lid-fold that averages 6–8 mm above the lid margin. The position of the levator-skin linkage and the anteroposterior relationship of the preaponeurotic fat determine lid-fold height and degree of sulcus concavity or convexity (as shown on the right half of each anatomic depiction). **(B)** In the case of levator dehiscence from the tarsal plate, the upper lid crease is displaced superiorly. The orbital septum and preaponeurotic fat linked to the levator are displaced superiorly and posteriorly. These anatomic changes create a high lid crease, a deep superior sulcus, and eyelid ptosis. **(C)** In the aging eyelid, the septum becomes attenuated and stretches. The septal extension loosens, and this allows orbital fat to prolapse forward and slide over the levator into an anterior and inferior position. Clinically, this results in an inferior displacement of the levator skin attachments and a low and anterior position of the preaponeurotic fat pad. **(D)** The youthful Asian eyelid anatomically resembles the senescent upper lid with a low levator skin zone of adhesion and inferior and anteriorly located preaponeurotic fat. The characteristic, but variable, low eyelid crease and convex upper eyelid and sulcus are classic. (Adapted from Spinelli HM. *Atlas of Aesthetic Eyelid and Periocular Surgery.* Philadelphia: Saunders; 2004:59.).

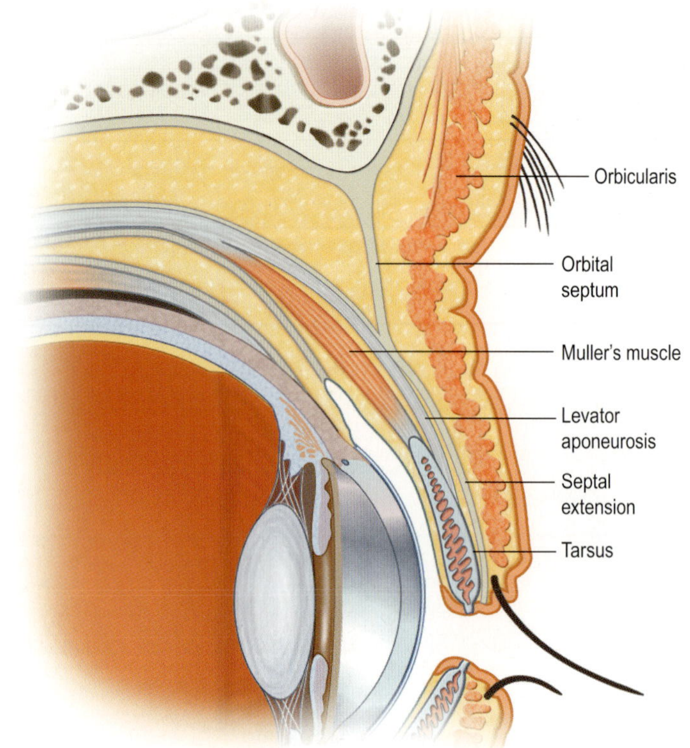

Figure 1.11 The orbital septum has an adhesion to the levator aponeurosis above the tarsus. The septal extension begins at the adhesion of the orbital septum to the levator and extends to the ciliary margin. It is superficial to the preaponeurotic fat found at the supratarsal crease. (Adapted from Reid RR, Said HK, Yu M, et al. Revisiting upper eyelid anatomy: introduction of the septal extension. *Plast Reconstr Surg*. 2006;117(1):65–70.)

Septal extension

- The orbital septum has an adhesion to the levator aponeurosis above the tarsus. The septum continues beyond this adhesion and extends to the ciliary margin. It is superficial to the preaponeurotic fat found at the supratarsal crease. The septal extension is a dynamic component to the motor apparatus, as traction on this fibrous sheet reproducibly alters ciliary margin position ***(Fig. 1.11)***. The septal extension serves as an adjunct to, and does not operate independent of, levator function, as mistaking the septal extension for levator apparatus and plicating this layer solely results in failed ptosis correction.

Lower eyelid

- The anatomy of the lower eyelid is somewhat analogous to that of the upper eyelid.
- The retractors of the lower lid, the capsulopalpebral fascia, correspond to the levator above.
- The capsulopalpebral head splits to surround and fuse with the sheath of the inferior oblique muscle. The two heads fuse to form the Lockwood suspensory ligament, which is analogous to Whitnall's ligament.
- It fuses with the orbital septum 5 mm below the tarsal border and then inserts into the anterior and inferior surface of the tarsus.
- The inferior tarsal muscle is analogous to Müller's muscle of the upper eyelid and also arises from the sheath of the inferior rectus muscle. It runs anteriorly above the inferior oblique muscle and also attaches to the inferior tarsal border.
- The combination of the orbital septum, orbicularis, and skin of the lower lid acts as the anterior barrier of the orbital fat. As these connective tissue properties relax, the orbital fat is allowed to herniate forward, forming an unpleasing, full lower eyelid. This relative loss of orbital volume leads to a commensurate, progressive hollowing of the upper lid as upper eyelid fat recesses.
- The capsulopalpebral fascia and its overlying conjunctiva form the posterior border of the lower orbital fat. Transection of the capsulopalpebral fascia during lower lid procedures, particularly transconjunctival blepharoplasty, releases the retractors of the lower eyelid, which can reduce downward traction and allow the position of the lower lid margin to rise.

Retaining ligaments

- A network of ligaments serves as a scaffold for the skin and subcutaneous tissue surrounding the orbit. The orbital retaining ligament directly attaches the orbicularis at the junction of its orbital and preseptal components to the periosteum of the orbital rim and, consequently, separates the prezygomatic space from the preseptal space. This ligament is continuous with the lateral orbital thickening, which inserts onto the lateral orbital rim and deep temporal fascia. It also has attachments to the superficial lateral canthal tendon (see Fig. 1.3, ***Figs 1.12, 1.13***). Attenuation of these ligaments permit descent of orbital fat onto the cheek. A midface lift must release these ligaments to achieve a supported, lasting lift.

Blood supply

- The internal and external carotid arteries supply blood to the orbit and eyelids ***(Fig. 1.14)***.
- The ophthalmic artery is the first intracranial branch of the internal carotid; its branches supply the globe, extraocular muscles, lacrimal gland, ethmoid, upper eyelids, and forehead.
- The external carotid artery branches into the superficial temporal and maxillary arteries. The infraorbital artery is a continuation of the maxillary artery and exits 8 mm below the inferomedial orbital rim to supply the lower eyelid.
- The arcade of the superior and inferior palpebral arteries gives a rich blood supply to the eyelids. The superior palpebral artery consists of a peripheral arcade located at the superior tarsal border – the area where surgical dissection occurs to correct lid ptosis and to define lid folds. Damage to a vessel within this network commonly results in a hematoma of Müller's muscle, causing lid

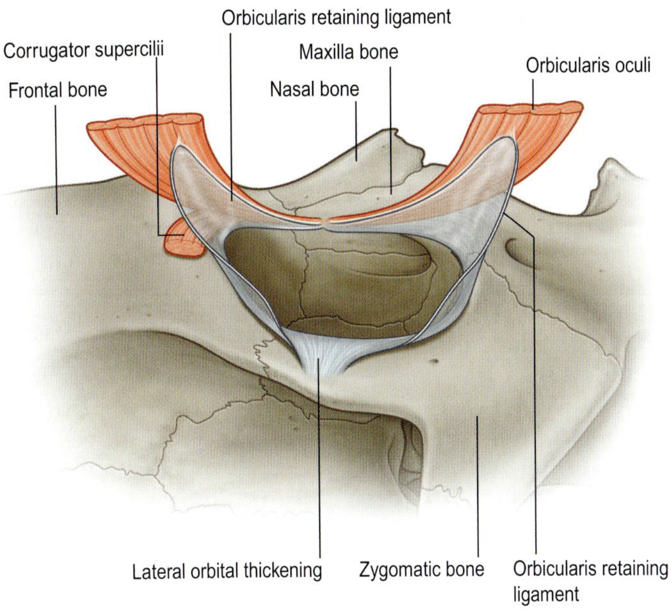

Figure 1.12 The orbicularis muscle fascia attaches to the skeleton along the orbital rim by the lateral orbital thickening (LOT) in continuity with the orbicularis retaining ligament (ORL). (Adapted from Ghavami A, Pessa JE, Janis J, et al. The orbicularis retaining ligament of the medial orbit: closing the circle. *Plast Reconstr Surg.* 2008;121(3):994–1001.).

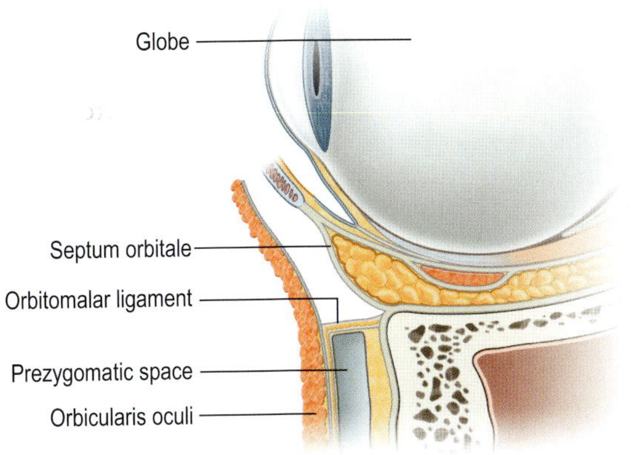

Figure 1.13 The orbital retaining ligament (ORL) directly attaches the orbicularis oris (OO) at the junction of its pars palpebrarum and pars orbitalis to the periosteum of the orbital rim and, consequently, separates the prezygomatic space from the preseptal space. (Adapted from Muzaffar AR, Mendelson BC, Adams Jr WP. Surgical anatomy of the ligamentous attachments of the lower lid and lateral canthus. *Plast Reconstr Surg.* 2002;110(3):873–884.)

ptosis for 2–8 weeks postoperatively. Likewise, on the lower lid, the inferior palpebral artery lies at the inferior border of the inferior tarsus.

- The supratrochlear, dorsal nasal, and medial palpebral arteries all traverse the orbit medially. Severing these arteries during fat removal, without adequately providing hemostasis, may lead to a retrobulbar hematoma, a vision-threatening complication of blepharoplasty.

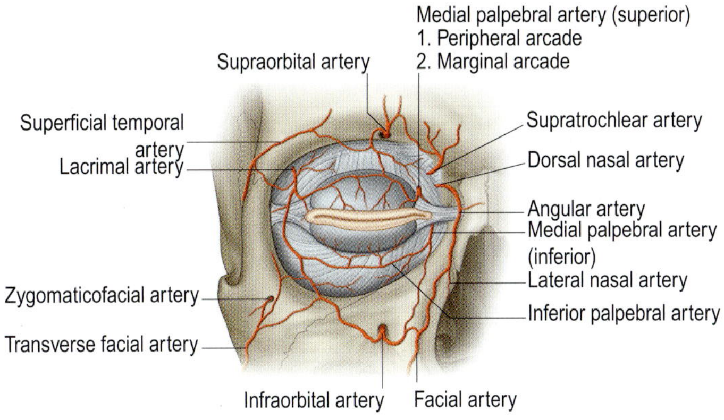

Figure 1.14 Arterial supply to the periorbital region.

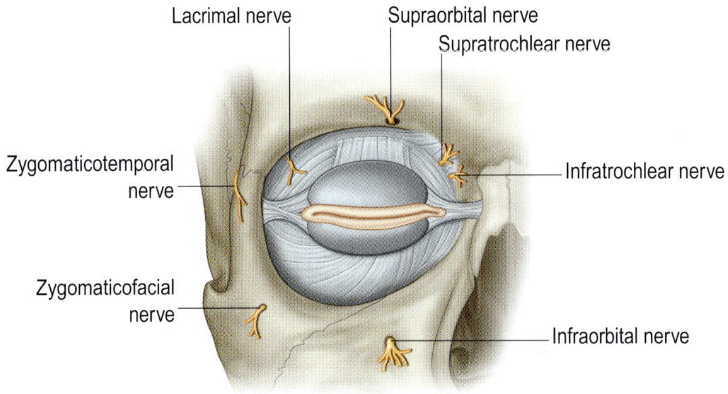

Figure 1.15 Sensory nerves of the eyelids.

Innervation: trigeminal nerve and facial nerve

- The trigeminal nerve along with its branches provides sensory innervations to the periorbital region ***(Fig. 1.15)***.
- A well-placed supraorbital block will anesthetize most of the upper lid and the central precoronal scalp.
- The maxillary division exits the orbit through one to three infraorbital foramina. It provides sensation to the skin of the nose, the lower eyelids, and the upper lid.
- The facial nerve supplies motor function to the lids ***(Fig. 1.16)***.
- Innervation of facial muscles occurs on their deep surfaces.
- Interruption of the branches to the orbicularis muscle from the periorbital surgery or facial surgery may result in atonicity due to partial denervation of the orbicularis with loss of lid tone or anomalous reinnervation and possibly undesirable eyelid twitching.
- The frontal branch of the facial nerve courses immediately above and is attached to the periosteum of the zygomatic bone. It then courses medially approximately 2 cm above the superior orbital rim to innervate the frontalis, corrugators, and procerus muscles from their deep surface.
- A separate branch travels along the inferior border of the zygoma to innervate the inferior component of orbicularis oculi.

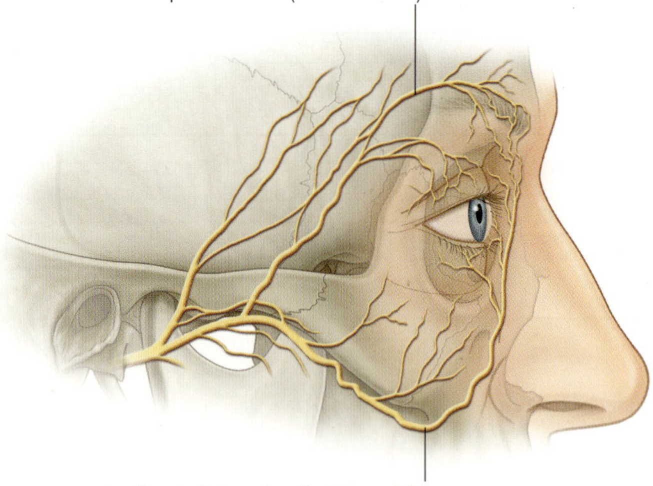

Figure 1.16 Anatomy of the brow and temporal region. The light green opaque area denotes the deep temporal fascia and the periosteum where sutures may be used to suspend soft tissue. Wide undermining, soft tissue suspension and canthopexy are safely performed here.

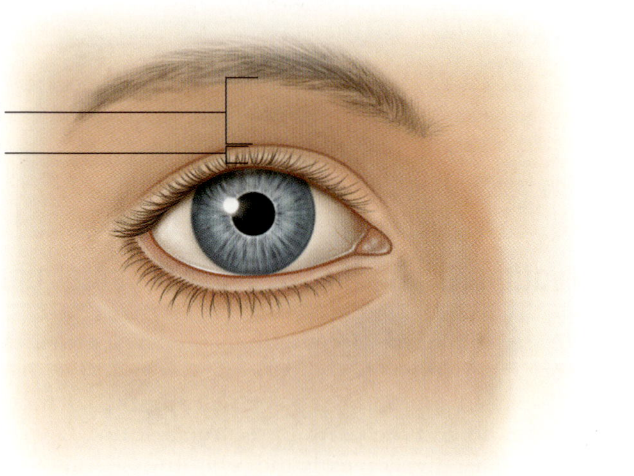

Figure 1.17 On relaxed forward gaze, the ideal upper lid should rest approximately 2 mm below the upper limbus. The lower lid ideally covers 0.5 mm of the lower limbus. The ratio of distance from the lower edge of the eyebrow to the open lid margin to the pretarsal skin ratio should be greater than 3.

Youthful, beautiful eyes

- The characteristics of youthful, beautiful eyes differ from one population to another but generalizations are possible and provide a needed reference to judge the success of various surgical maneuvers.
- Attractive, youthful eyes have globes framed in generously sized horizontal apertures (from medial and lateral), often accentuated by a slight upward tilt of the intercanthal axis ***(Fig. 1.17)***.
- The aperture length should span most of the distance between the orbital rims.
- In a relaxed forward gaze, the vertical height of the aperture should expose at least three-quarters of the cornea with the upper lid extending down at least 1.5 mm below the upper limbus (the upper margin of the cornea) but no more than 3 mm. The lower lid ideally covers 0.5 mm of the lower limbus but no more than 1.5 mm.
- In the upper lid, there should be a well-defined lid crease lying above the lid margin with lid skin under slight stretch, slightly wider laterally.
- Ideally, the actual pretarsal skin visualized on relaxed forward gaze ranges from 3 to 6 mm in European ethnicities.
- The Asian lid crease is generally 2–3 mm lower, with the distance from lid margin diminishing as the crease moves toward the inner canthus.
- Patients of Indo-European and African decent show 1 to 2 mm lower than European ethnicities.
- The ratio of distance from the lower edge of the eyebrow (at the center of the globe) to the open lid margin to the visualized pretarsal skin should never be less than 3–1 (see Fig. 1.1), preferably more.
- Scleral show is the appearance of white sclera below the lower border of the cornea and above the lower eyelid margin. In general, sclera show is contradictory to optimal aesthetics and may be perceived as a sign of aging, previous blepharoplasty, or orbital disease (e.g., thyroid disease).
- More than 0.5 mm of sclera show beneath the cornea on direct forward gaze begins to confer a sad or melancholy aura to one's appearance.
- The intercanthal axis is normally tilted slightly upward (from medial to lateral) in most populations.
- Exaggerated tilts are encountered in some Asian, Indo-European and African-American populations.

Preoperative considerations

- A thorough history and physical examination should be obtained – including an ophthalmic history (see Box 1.2).
- Physical exam should include evaluation for symmetry; globe shape, position and appearance; signs of aging; lid appearance; lid function and relative laxity.
- In the upper lid, excessive skin due to loss of elasticity and sun damage is one of the major causes of an aged appearance in the periorbital area.
- In addition to relaxed skin changes, excessive fat herniation can cause bulging, resulting in a heavy appearance to the upper lid area.
- Aging changes in the lower lid include relaxation of the tarsal margin with scleral show, rhytides of the lower lid, herniated fat pads resulting in bulging in one or all of the three fat pocket areas, and hollowing of the nasojugal groove and lateral orbital rim areas.
- Hollowing of the nasojugal groove area appears as dark circles under the eyes, mostly because of lighting and the shadowing that result from this defect.
- Contact lens wear poses particular risks when eyelid surgery is performed.

BOX 1.2 **Important information to obtain during history and physical examination**

- Medication use: particularly anticoagulants, anti-inflammatory and cardiovascular drugs, and vitamins (especially vitamin E).
- Herbal supplement use: herbs represent risks to anesthesia and surgery, particularly those affecting blood pressure, blood coagulation, the cardiovascular system, and healing.
- Allergies: medication and type.
- Past medical history: especially hypertension, diabetes, cardiovascular and cerebrovascular disease, hepatitis, liver disease, heart disease or arrhythmias, cancer, thyroid disease, and endocrine disease.
- Bleeding disorders or blood clots.
- Psychiatric disease.
- Alcohol and smoking history.
- Recreational drug use, which may interact with anesthesia.
- Exposure to human immunodeficiency virus and hepatitis virus.
- Any history of facial herpes zoster or simplex.

- Long-term contact lens wearing hastens the process of drying out the eyes.
- Traditional blepharoplasty techniques consistently produce vertical dystopia with increased scleral exposure, making the lens wear difficult if not dangerous.
- Ptosis and canthopexy surgery may alter the corneal curvature and require that contacts be refitted.
- The patient should discontinue contact lens wear in the perioperative period to allow healing without the need to manipulate the eyelids.
- Dry irritated eyes before surgery will lead to irritated eyes after surgery, and the surgeon may be blamed.
- Treatment options include artificial tears, ointment, anti-inflammatory drops, and punctal plugs or punctal closure.
- Exophthalmos, unilaterally or bilaterally, associated with a thyroid disorder should be completely stabilized for approximately 6 months before elective aesthetic surgery.
- Eyelid measurements are documented for use during ptosis surgery and, if necessary, for insurance purposes.
- In the typical person with the brow in an aesthetically pleasing position, 20 mm of upper lid skin must remain between the bottom of the central eyebrow and the upper lid margin to allow adequate lid closure during sleep, a well-defined lid crease, and an effective and complete blink.
- In the eyelid of the white individual, the aperture (distance between the upper and lower eyelids) average is 10–12 mm.
- The margin reflex distance (MRD), measured from the light reflex on the center of the cornea to the upper eyelid margin, ranges from 3 to 5 mm.
- True blepharoptosis is defined by the degree of upper lid infringement upon the iris and pupil.
- As the MRD decreases towards zero, the severity of blepharoptosis increases.
- Before method selection, the levator function must be determined by measuring the upper eyelid excursion from extreme downward gaze to extreme upward gaze; it generally ranges from 10 to 12 mm.

BOX 1.3 **Recommended photographic views**

- Full face, upright (at rest) frontal, oblique, and lateral views.
- Full face, upright, and smiling.
- Direct periorbital views in upward gaze and downward gaze and with eyes gently closed.
- A view with a finger slightly elevating the brows with the eyes open and another with the eyes closed.

- If ptosis exists, the type of repair depends upon the severity of the ptosis and the reliability of the levator to recreate smooth, upper lid elevation.
- Pseudoptosis occurs when excess upper lid skin covers the eyelid, depressing the eyelashes, forming hooding and simulating ptosis.
- Photographic evidence of this is often necessary for insurance purposes when a levator aponeurosis repair or an excisional blepharoplasty is planned.
- Brow ptosis is a common aspect of facial aging. It adds weight and volume to the upper eyelid to develop, or exacerbate, eyelid ptosis.
- The ability to differentiate the causes of droopy eyelids – brow ptosis (brow weight resting on the eyelids), dermatochalasis (excess skin), and blepharoptosis (levator attenuation or dehiscence) – will enable the surgeon to select the proper correction.
- There is a normal 10–12 mm projection of the globe seen in a lateral, as measured from the lateral orbital rim at the level of the canthal tendon to the pupil.
- Proptosis and enophthalmos are relative anterior and posterior displacement of the globe, respectively. Hertel exophthalmometry can be used to quantitate the degree of relative projection for documentation purposes.
- Assessment of tear production is a necessary but unreliable task.
- The Schirmer test:
  - Placing filter paper strips in the lateral third of the lower eyelid.
  - After 5 min, normal tear production should be greater than 15 mm; 5–10 mm indicates borderline tear secretion, and below 5 mm is hyposecretion.
- No other area of cosmetic surgery is more dependent on accurate photography than the periorbital region (Box 1.3).
- Before surgical planning, one must have a meaningful conceptualization of the desired result. Only then can the surgical maneuvers required be organized in a meaningful way (Box 1.4).

Operative techniques (Video 1.1)

Video 1.1

Simple skin blepharoplasty

- When skin-only excision is elected, it should occur above the supratarsal fold or crease, leaving that structure intact – this retains most of the definition of an existing lid fold.

BOX 1.4 **Preoperative periorbital plan**

The preoperative periorbital plan should include the following:

- The patient's specific concerns and desires for improvement.
- Brow position.
- Lower eyelid tonicity.
- Eyelid ptosis, retraction, or levator dehiscence.
- Exophthalmos or enophthalmos.
- Supraorbital rim prominence or hypoplasia.
- Suborbital malar and tear trough deformities.
- Excision of necessary skin, muscle, and fat – only if necessary.

- The supratarsal fold is located approximately 7–8 mm above the ciliary margin in women and 6–7 mm in men.
- The upper marking must be at least 10 mm from the lower edge of the brow and should not include any thick brow skin.
- The use of a pinch test for redraping the skin is helpful.
- The shape of the skin resection is lenticular in younger patients and more trapezoid-shaped laterally in older patients.
- The incision may need to be extended laterally with a larger extension, but extension lateral to the orbital rim should be avoided if possible, to prevent a prominent scar *(Fig. 1.18)*.

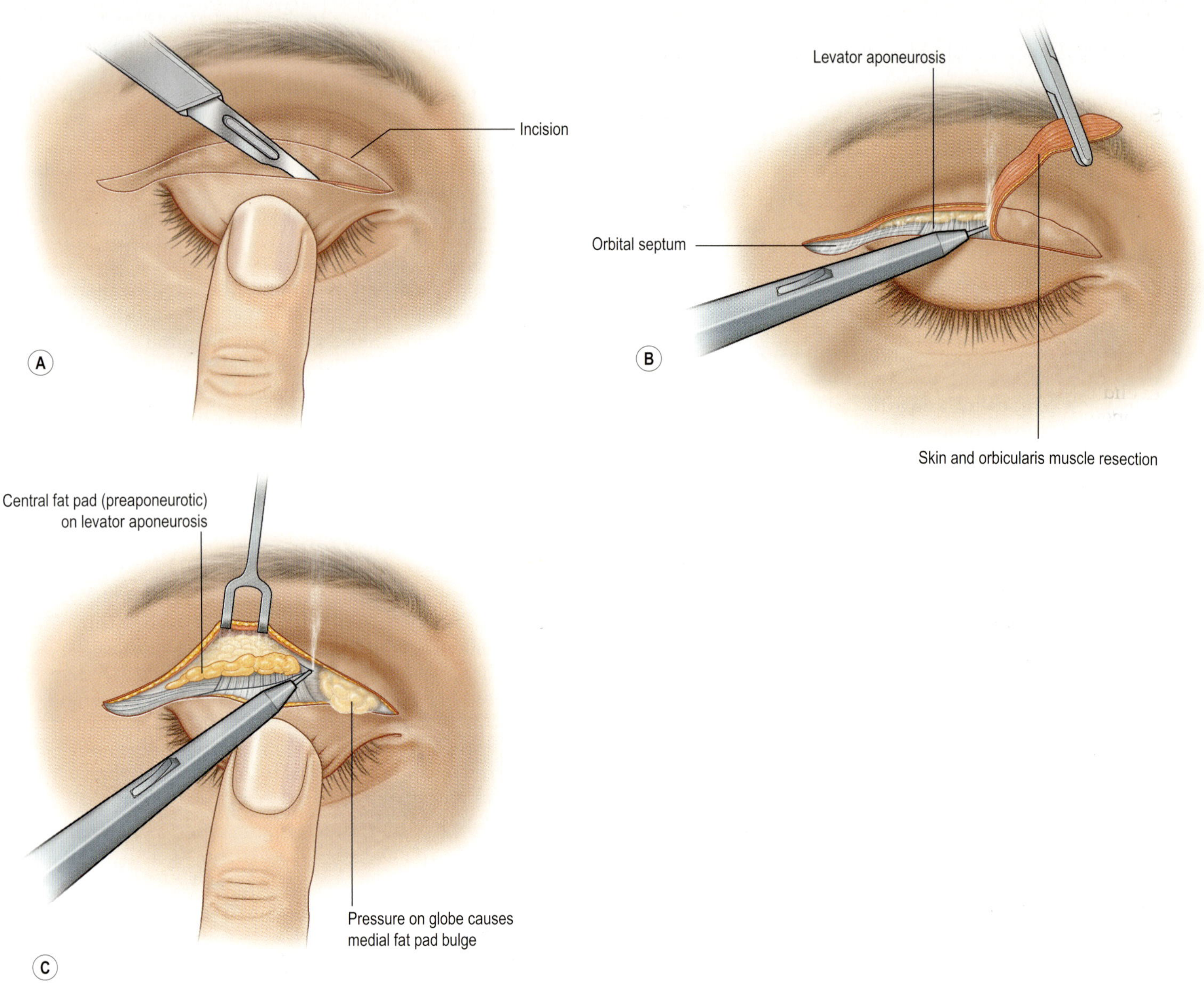

Figure 1.18 Simple skin excision blepharoplasty. **(A)** Digital traction and light pressure by the surgeon allow smooth quick incisions. **(B)** The skin may be elevated with the orbicularis muscle in one maneuver, proceeding from lateral to medial. **(C)** The orbital septum is then opened, exposing the preaponeurotic space. The underlying levator aponeurosis is protected by opening the septum as cephalad as possible. (Adapted from Spinelli HM. *Atlas of Aesthetic Eyelid and Periocular Surgery.* Philadelphia: Saunders; 2004:64.)

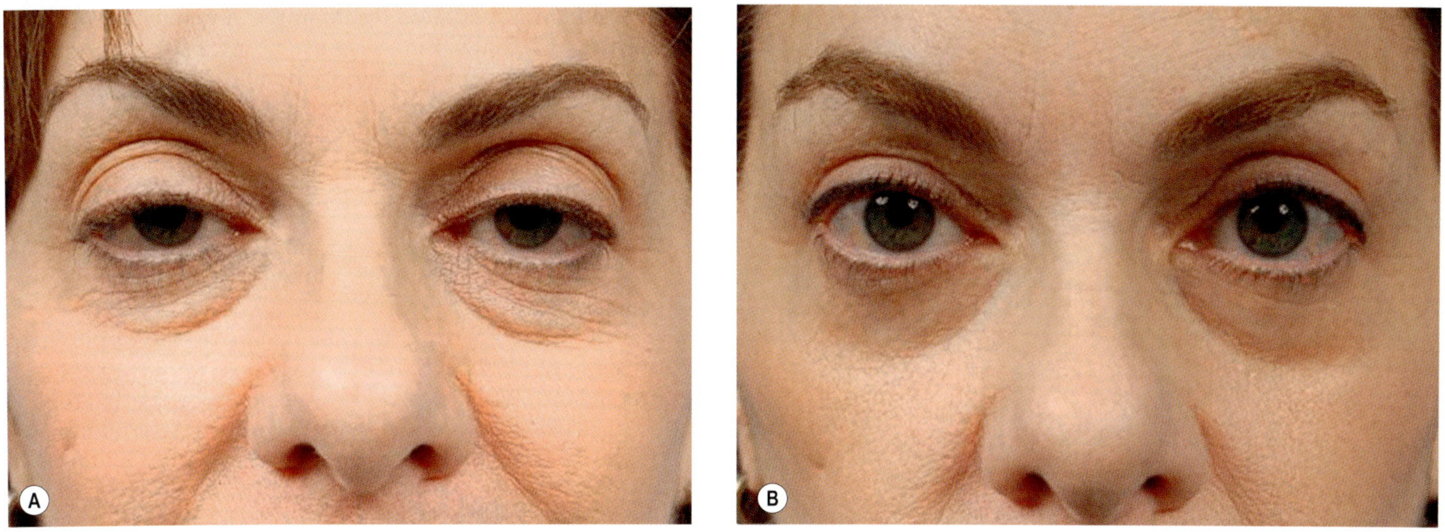

Figure 1.19 **(A)** Preoperative and **(B)** postoperative photograph depicting predictable results with simple skin excision blepharoplasty.

- Similarly, the medial markings should not be extended medial to the medial canthus because extensions onto the nasal side wall result in webbing.
- At the conclusion of the case, the patient should have approximately 1–2 mm of lagophthalmos bilaterally. *Figure 1.19* displays the predictable, restorative outcomes that can be achieved with skin excision alone.

Anchor (or invagination blepharoplasty)

- Anchor blepharoplasty involves the creation of an upper eyelid crease by attaching pretarsal skin to the underlying aponeurosis.
- Advantages of an anchor blepharoplasty are a crisp, precise, and well-defined eyelid crease that persists indefinitely.
- Disadvantages are that it is more time-consuming, requires greater surgical skills and expertise, and encourages greater frontalis relaxation as a result of more effective correction of the overhanging pseudoptotic skin.
- Key components of the anchor blepharoplasty include:
  - Minimal skin excision (2–3 mm) extending cephalad from the tarsus.
  - A 1–2 mm sliver of orbicularis must be removed in proportion to the amount of skin removed.
  - A small pretarsal skin and muscle flap are dissected from the aponeurosis and septum adhesion.
  - After sharply disinserting the aponeurosis from the tarsus, pretarsal fatty tissue can be removed to debulk the pretarsal skin.
  - Mattressed anchor sutures are placed connecting the tarsus to the aponeurosis and pretarsal skin *(Fig. 1.20)*.
  - Finally, a running suture approximates the preseptal skin incision.

Orbital fat excision

- A relative excess of retroseptal fat may be safely excised through an upper eyelid blepharoplasty incision.

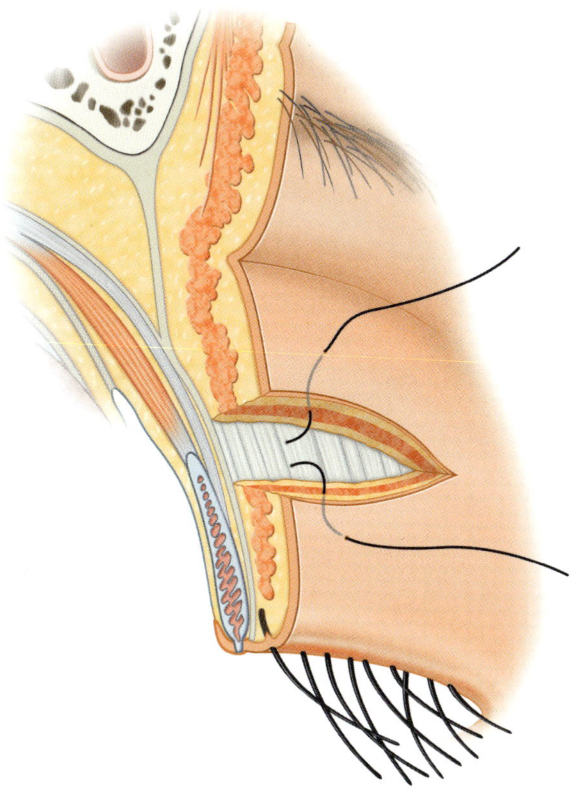

Figure 1.20 Anchor blepharoplasty technique. Attaching the dermis of the pretarsal skin flap to the superior aspect of the tarsus and to the free edge of the aponeurosis. (Adapted from Spinelli HM. *Atlas of Aesthetic Eyelid and Periocular Surgery.* Philadelphia: Saunders; 2004:69.)

- A small septotomy is made at the superior aspect of the skin excision into each fat compartment in which conservative resection of redundant fat has been planned.
- The fat is teased out bluntly and resected using pinpoint cautery.
- This fat usually includes the medial or nasal compartment, which contains white fat.

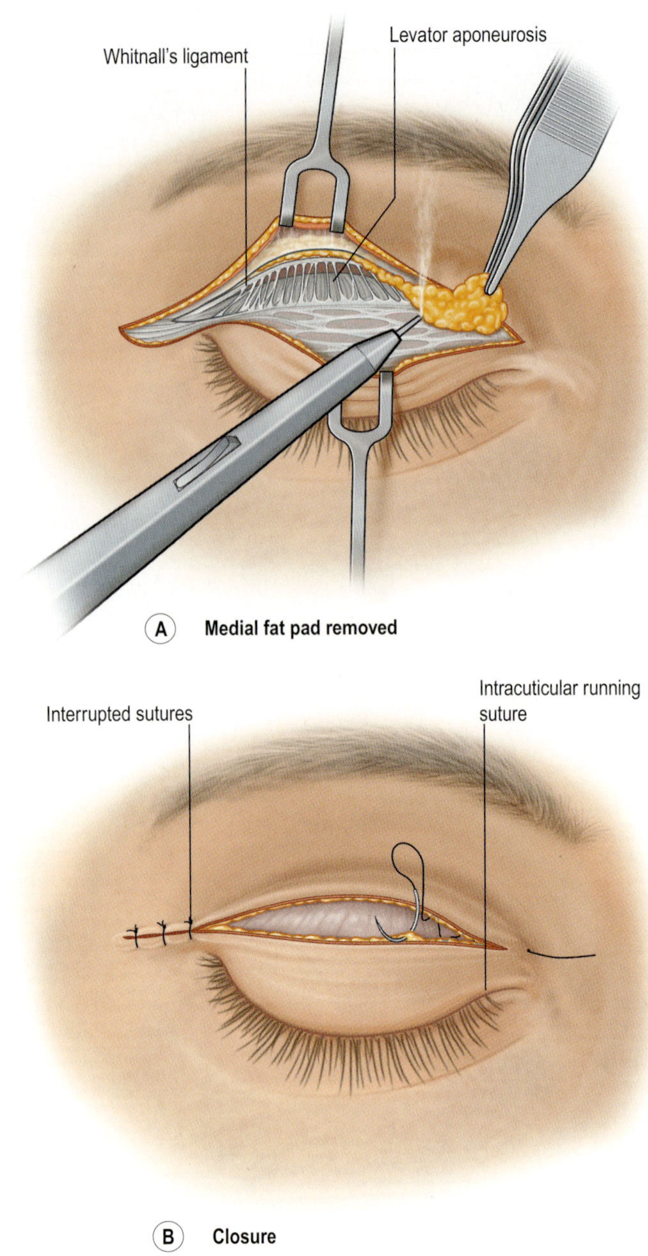

Figure 1.21 Simple skin excision blepharoplasty. **(A)** The medial fat pad may require digital pressure to expose and grasp; however, care should be taken not to overly resect fat when using digital pressure techniques. **(B)** Closure may then be performed with a combination of interrupted and running intracuticular sutures. (Adapted from Spinelli HM. *Atlas of Aesthetic Eyelid and Periocular Surgery.* Philadelphia: Saunders; 2004:65.)

- Yellow fat in the central compartment is usually more superficial and lateral.
- Gentle pressure on the patient's globe can reproduce the degree of excess while the patient lies recumbent on the operating room table ***(Fig. 1.21)***.
- Overall, undercorrection is preferred to prevent hollowing, which can be dramatic and recognized as an A-frame abnormality.
- The attenuated orbital septum may be addressed by using selective diathermy along the exposed caudal septum.
- Inflammation-mediated tightening can enhance septal integrity.
- Septal plication aid is unnecessary and may induce a brisk, restrictive inflammatory response.

Blepharoptosis

- During upper blepharoplasty, with the septum open and the aponeurosis and superior tarsus exposed, there is an ideal opportunity to adjust the level of the aperture.
- Inappropriate aperture opening can be due to upper lid ptosis or upper lid retraction.
- True ptosis repair involves reattachment of the levator aponeurosis to the tarsus, with or without shortening of applicable structures (e.g. aponeurosis, Müller's muscle, and tarsus).
- There are a variety of techniques to address blepharoptosis but they are outside the scope of this chapter. There is a significant learning curve to performing a ptosis repair, and even then, the ability to get perfect symmetry is elusive.
- In the setting of mild upper eyelid ptosis (approx. 1 mm), where the decision has been made to avoid a formal lid ptosis procedure, selective myectomy of the upper eyelid orbicularis can be performed to widen the lid aperture.
- The amount of muscle to be resected depends on a host of factors, including the severity of relative lid ptosis, brow position, and fold disparity ***(Fig. 1.22)*** and is titrated depending on the amount of effect desired.
- For 1 mm or less of relative upper lid ptosis, resection of at least 3–4 mm of orbicularis is required.
- No attempt is made to close orbicularis muscle in this resection, which could increase the risk of lagophthalmos.

The key components of formal lid ptosis correction include:

- Correct identification of the distal extensions of the aponeurosis and the orbital septal extension.
- The superior edge of the tarsus is freed from any dermal or tendinous extensions.
- Leaving a small cuff of filmy connective tissue (approx. 1 mm) on the tarsus will minimize bleeding from the richly vascularized area.
- Ensure that there is complete hemostasis by use of a fine forceps cautery, lifting all lid tissues away from the cornea and globe before cauterizing.
- Anchor the upper third of the tarsus to the remaining levator with 5–0 silk suture, placed as a horizontal mattress.
- The lid should be flipped to ensure that the suture is not exposed posteriorly on the tarsus, which could cause a troublesome corneal abrasion.
- If performed under sedation or local anesthetic, the level should be checked by having the patient open the eye.
- For cases under general anesthetic, one should attempt to create one to two times the amount of lagophthalmos relative to the preoperative ptosis.
- If there is any medial or lateral retraction or ptosis, the central suture should be repositioned medially or

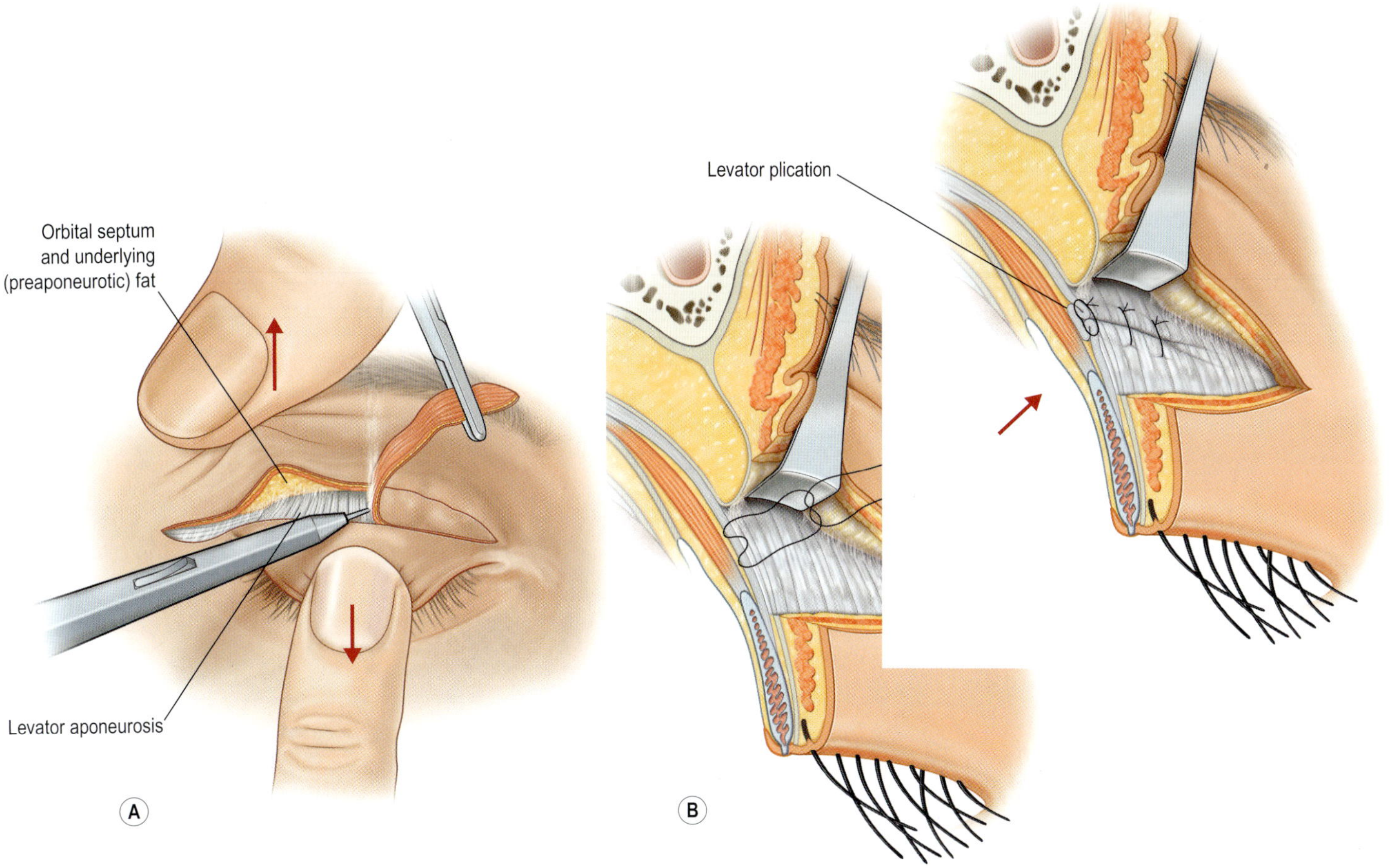

Figure 1.22 (A,B) Once the upper lid is incised, the levator may be modified (shortened/lengthened) in a number of ways, including simple plication. A suborbicularis skin flap can also be developed allowing access to preaponeurotic fat. (Adapted from Spinelli HM. *Atlas of Aesthetic Eyelid and Periocular Surgery.* Philadelphia: Saunders; 2004:69).

laterally as many times as needed, with adjustment to a pleasing lid height and contour.

- Both sides should be completed before the suture is permanently tied.

Lower lid blepharoplasty

- Lower blepharoplasty has evolved substantially. Although excellent aesthetic results can be achieved with transcutaneous lower blepharoplasty, lid retraction and ectropion are concerning complications. Conservative excisional techniques center on the concept of fat preservation. Transconjunctival lower blepharoplasty, although more conservative, does not eliminate the risk of lid malposition. An effective, lasting procedure should address the extrinsic and intrinsic support of the eye, which is weakened during the aging process.

Transconjunctival blepharoplasty

- Transconjunctival blepharoplasty is the preferred procedure for fat reduction in patients without excess skin and with good canthal position.
- It is less likely to lead to lower lid malposition than a transcutaneous approach.
- It minimizes but does not eliminate postoperative lower lid retraction.
- Transection of the lower lid retractors can cause a temporary rise in the lid margin, especially if they are suspended during the healing period.
- Previously suspected septal scarring through transconjunctival fat excision has not been shown to significantly alter lid posture or tonicity.
- The lower lid retractors (capsulopalpebral fascia and inferior tarsal muscle) and overlying conjunctiva lie directly posterior to the three fat pads of the lower lid.
- A broad and deep transconjunctival incision severs both conjunctiva and retractors but typically should not incise the orbital septum, orbicularis, or skin.
- The conjunctival incision is made with a monopolar cautery needle tip at least 4 mm below the inferior border of the tarsus – never through the tarsus ***(Fig. 1.23)***.
- A preseptal approach is obtained by entering the conjunctiva above the level of septal attachment to the capsulopalpebral fascia.
- A retroseptal approach involves a 1.5–2 cm incision lower down in the fornix, and is typically used to excise fat.
- It is preferable to leave the transconjunctival incision open.

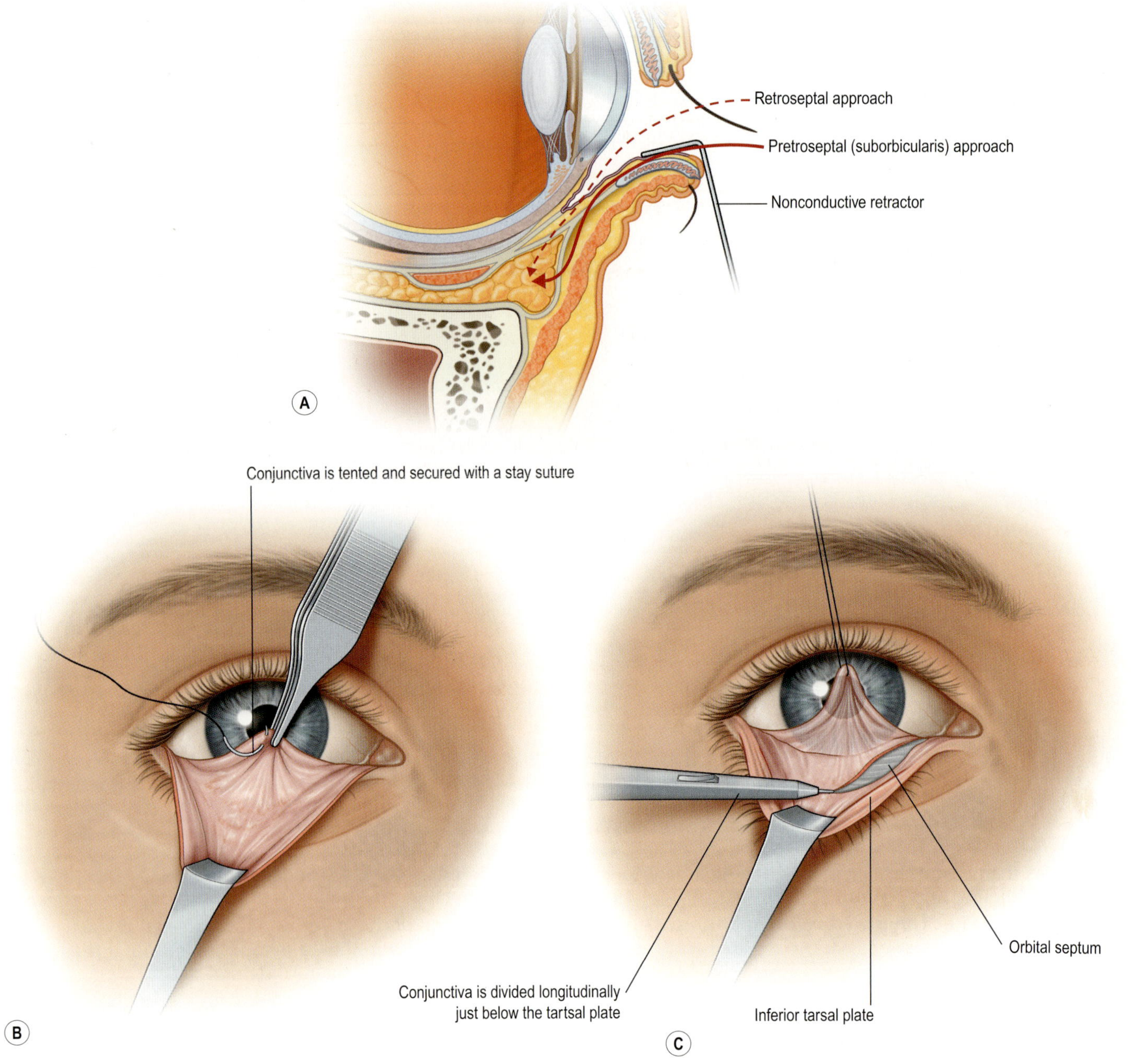

Figure 1.23 The transconjunctival approach to the retroseptal space may be in one of two ways: preseptal or retroseptal. The preseptal route requires entry into the suborbicularis preseptal space above the fusion of the lower lid retractors and the orbital septum. This will allow direct visualization of the septum, and each fat pad can be addressed separately in a controlled fashion. **(A)** A conjunctival stay suture is placed deep in the fornix and traction is applied superiorly while the lid margin is everted. This causes the inferior edge of the tarsal plate to rise toward the surgeon. **(B)** The conjunctiva and lower lid retractors are incised just below the tarsal plate entering the suborbicularis preseptal space. This plane is developed to the orbital rim with the assistance of the traction suture and a nonconductive instrument. **(C)** The conjunctiva and lower lid retractors are incised just below the tarsal plate entering the suborbicularis preseptal space. This plane is developed to the orbital rim with the assistance of the traction suture and a nonconductive instrument. (Adapted from Spinelli HM. *Atlas of Aesthetic Eyelid and Periocular Surgery.* Philadelphia: Saunders; 2004:86.)

- Suturing the wound may trap bacteria or cause corneal irritation.
- Conjunctival closure, when it is elected, is simplified by a monofilament pull-out suture that enters the eye externally, closes the conjunctiva, and exits through the skin and is taped.
- The incision through the conjunctiva and retractors gives excellent access to the orbital fat.
- A 6–0 silk traction suture passed through the inferior conjunctival wound and retracted over the globe gives wide access to the orbital fat, even helping to prolapse the fat into the wound. The thin film of synovium-appearing capsule encasing the orbital fat is opened, releasing the fat to bulge into the operative field ***(Fig. 1.24)***.
- Once fat is removed through a transconjunctival incision, excess skin can be removed through a subciliary position.
- Fat reduction may leave skin excess, leading to wrinkling.

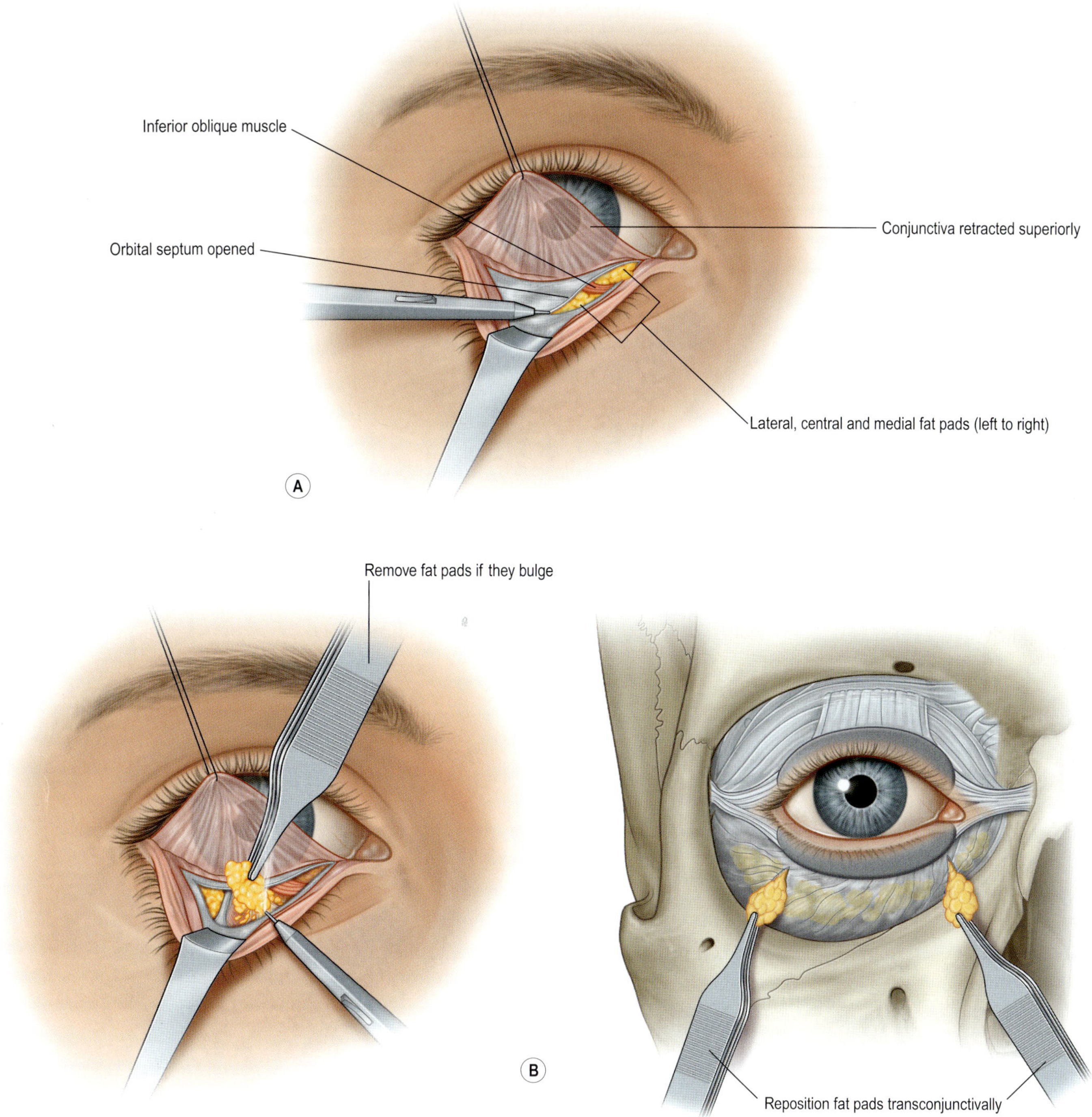

Figure 1.24 **(A)** The orbital septum may then be punctured and the inferior oblique muscle identified and preserved. **(B)** The fat pad may be addressed individually in-keeping with preoperative plans with either resection, repositioning, conservation or any combination of the these techniques. (Adapted from Spinelli HM. *Atlas of Aesthetic Eyelid and Periocular Surgery.* Philadelphia: Saunders; 2004:87.)

- A conservative "skin pinch" can be done to estimate skin removal, or alternatively, skin can be tightened by skin resurfacing with chemical or laser peels *(Fig. 1.25)*.
- One should be careful not to incise the orbital septum, which leads to increased postoperative retraction.
- This procedure works particularly well when there is an isolated fat pad, especially medially, accessed through a single stab incision through the conjunctiva.

Transcutaneous blepharoplasty

- A subciliary incision can be used to develop a skin flap or a skin-muscle flap.
- With either method, pretarsal orbicularis fibers should remain intact.
- For the skin-muscle flap, skin and preseptal orbicularis are elevated as one flap, while with a skin flap, the muscle and its innervation can be preserved.

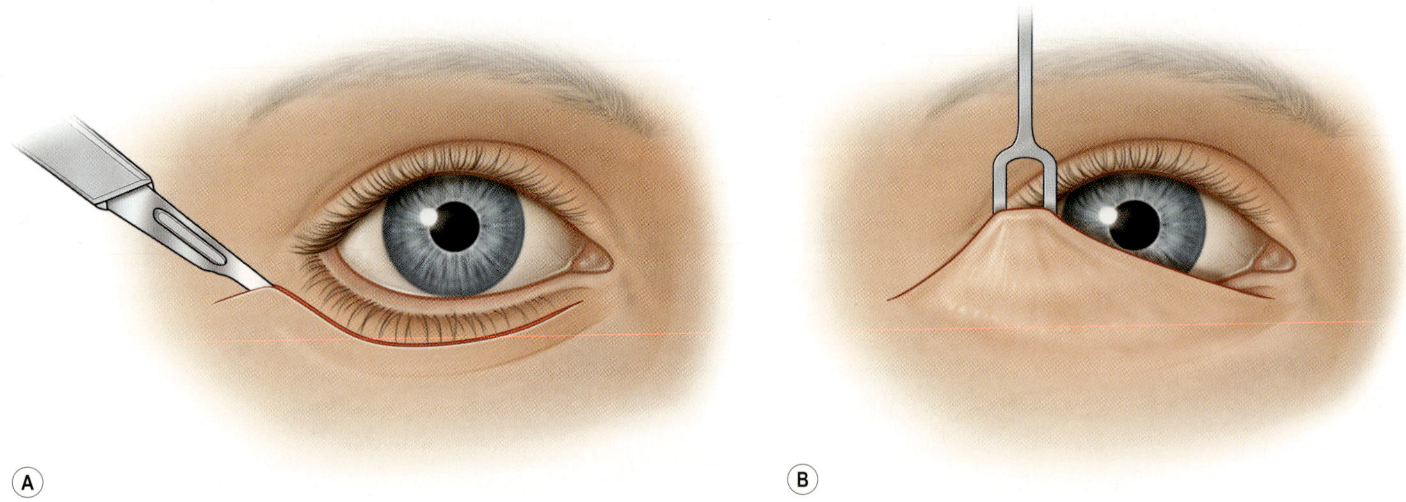

Figure 1.25 **(A)** Simple skin excision lower eyelid blepharoplasty. **(B)** Typical removal of redraped skin or skin-muscle from the lower lid, which can be the shape of an obtuse triangle, with the largest amount sacrificed laterally.

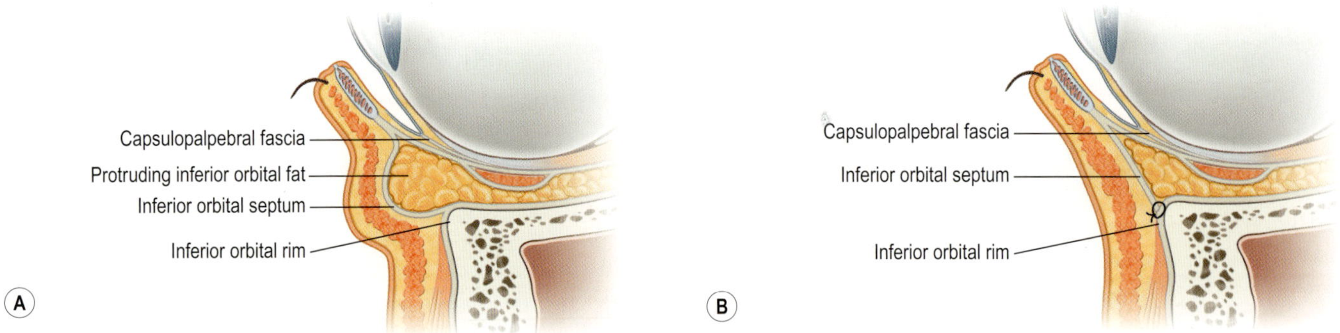

Figure 1.26 **(A,B)** Schematic representation of procedure for lower eyelid. Note that only the inferior orbital septum is plicated and sutured to the inferior orbital rim. (Adapted from Sensöz O, Unlu RE, Percin A, et al. Septoorbitoperiostoplasty for the treatment of palpebral bags: a 10-year experience. *Plast Reconstr Surg.* 1998; 101(6):1657–1663.)

- Periorbital fat, muscle, and skin can be addressed with either approach.
- Once the plane deep to the orbicularis is entered, dissection continues between the muscle and the orbital septum down to the level of the orbital rim.
- Periorbital fat can be excised through small incisions in the septum.
- The fat can also be retropositioned using capsulopalpebral fascia placation, or it can be transferred into the naso-jugular fold.

  Orbicularis muscle fibers and skin can be excised at closure.
- Care must be taken with muscle excision, which can lead to orbicularis denervation and lid malposition.

Orbital fat transposition

- An alternative to excising prominent orbital fat is to redrape the pedicled fat onto the arcus marginalis.
- Patients with tear trough deformities who have prominent medial fat pads are excellent candidates.
- Access to the medial and central fat pads is by the subciliary or transconjunctival incision.
- The minor degree of lateral fat pad prominence is generally insufficient to affect any change with repositioning.
- A supraperiosteal or a subperiosteal dissection of 8–10 mm caudal to the inferior orbital rim permits tension-free placement.
- The fat can be secured in place with interrupted absorbable sutures.
- Patients must be warned that various degrees of fat loss and hardening are possible. There is also a rare but described possibility of restrictive strabismus related to aggressive fat mobilization and fixation.

Orbital septum plication

- In this procedure, the herniated septum is plicated and repositioned to its normal anatomic site within the orbit.
- The fat is replaced in the retroseptal position to regain its original anatomic integrity ***(Fig. 1.26)***.

- Three to four 5–0 polyglycolic acid sutures are placed in a vertical fashion from medial to lateral.
- The protruding fat pads are invaginated and the integrity of the thin, flaccid septum is restored.
- Additional support may be gained with septo-orbitoperiostoplasty variation which plicates the flaccid septum and secures it to the periosteum of the inferior orbital rim.
- Because no disruption of the eyelid anatomy occurs, complications related to lid malposition such as lid retraction, scleral show, and ectropion are reduced.

Capsulopalpebral fascia plication

- The capsulopalpebral fascia can be plicated to the orbital rim either through a transcutaneous or a transconjunctival approach.
- In the transcutaneous method, dissection is carried out between the orbicularis and the septum down to the orbital rim; the capsulopalpebral fascia is then sutured to the orbital rim.
- In the transconjunctival method, the capsulopalpebral fascia is divided from the tarsus, and orbital fat is retroplaced, its position maintained by suturing the capsulopalpebral fascia to the periosteum of the orbital rim using a continuous running 6–0 nonabsorbable suture.
- The conjunctival gap of a few millimeters is allowed to reepithelialize ***(Fig. 1.27)***.
- One advantage of the transconjunctival approach is the division of lower eyelid depressors, which helps maintain the lower eyelid at an elevated level due to the unopposed action of the pretarsal orbicularis.

Orbicularis suspension

- Orbicularis repositioning can be used to eliminate hypotonic and herniated orbicularis muscle, soften palpebral depressions, and shorten the lower lid to cheek distance.
- The main steps include:
  - Elevation of a skin muscle flap.
  - Release of the orbicularis retaining ligament and resuspension of the orbicularis – frequently after lateral canthopexy.
  - Along the entire infraorbital rim, the orbicularis retaining ligament is divided.
  - Additional medial dissection is performed to release the levator labii when a tear trough deformity is present.
  - The skin muscle flap is draped in a superior lateral vector rather than a pure vertical vector.
  - Excision of skin and muscle are performed by removing a triangle of tissue lateral to the canthus, thereby minimizing the amount of tissue removed along the actual lid margin.
  - The lateral suspension of the orbicularis is to the orbital periosteum.
  - Lower lid support is gained by resuspension of the anterior (skin and muscle) and posterior lamellae (tarsus by canthopexy).

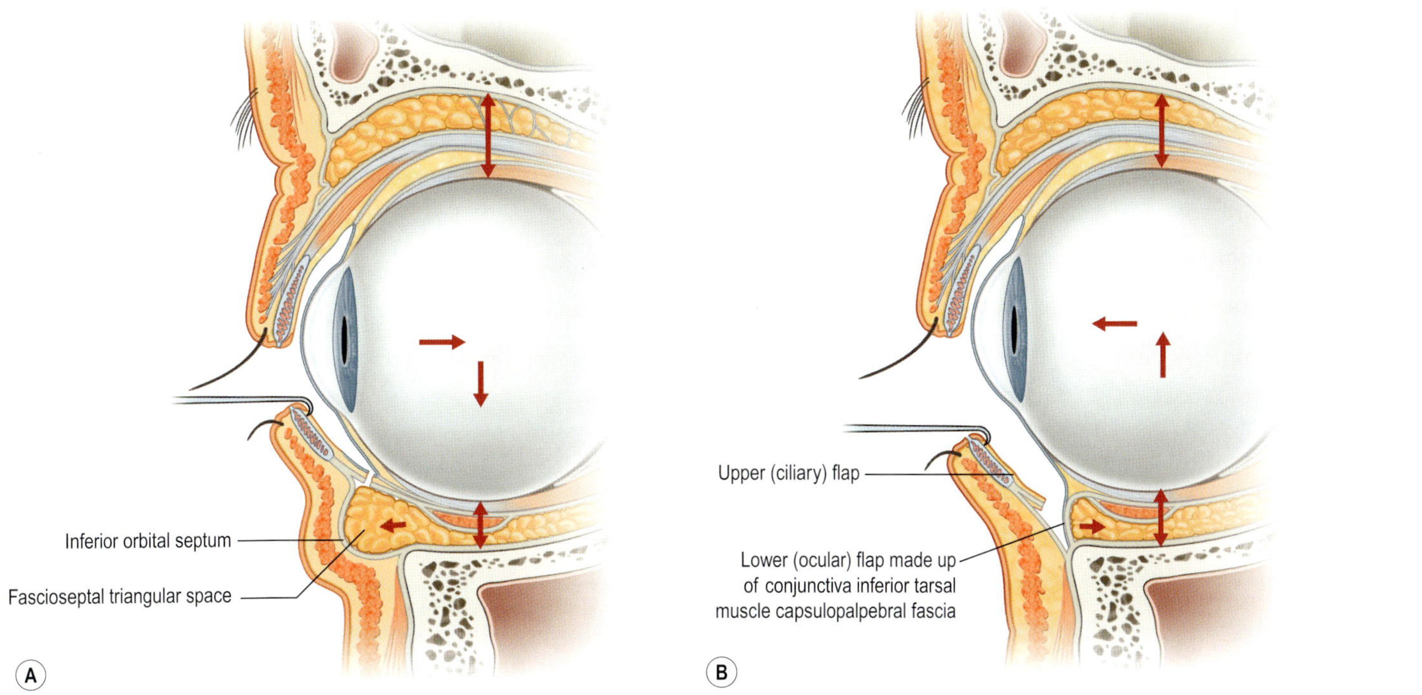

Figure 1.27 (A,B) Suturing the lower capsulopalpebral flap to the arcus marginalis to reduce and contain the herniated fat. (Adapted from Camirand A, Doucet J, Harris J. Anatomy, pathophysiology, and prevention of senile enophthalmia and associated herniated lower eyelid pads. *Plast Reconstr Surg*. 1997;100(3):1535–1538.)

- This technique is best suited for patients with scleral show, lid laxity, and a negative vector, which put them at risk for lid malposition in the postoperative period.
- Disadvantages are it inherently disrupts the orbicularis, which may lead to denervation, and mobilization of the levator labii muscles may put the buccal branch of the facial nerve at risk.

Canthopexy

- A lateral canthopexy can establish an aesthetically and functionally youthful eyelid *and* reduce the incidence of lower lid malposition and scleral show ***(Fig. 1.28)***.
- It has become an integral part of a lower lid blepharoplasty and midface lifting.
- A lateral canthopexy is recommended for moderate lid laxity, which is considered <6 mm of lid distraction away from the globe.
- This technique takes advantage of a bluntly dissected tunnel extending from the lateral upper lid blepharoplasty incision into the lateral aspect of a lower lid incision.

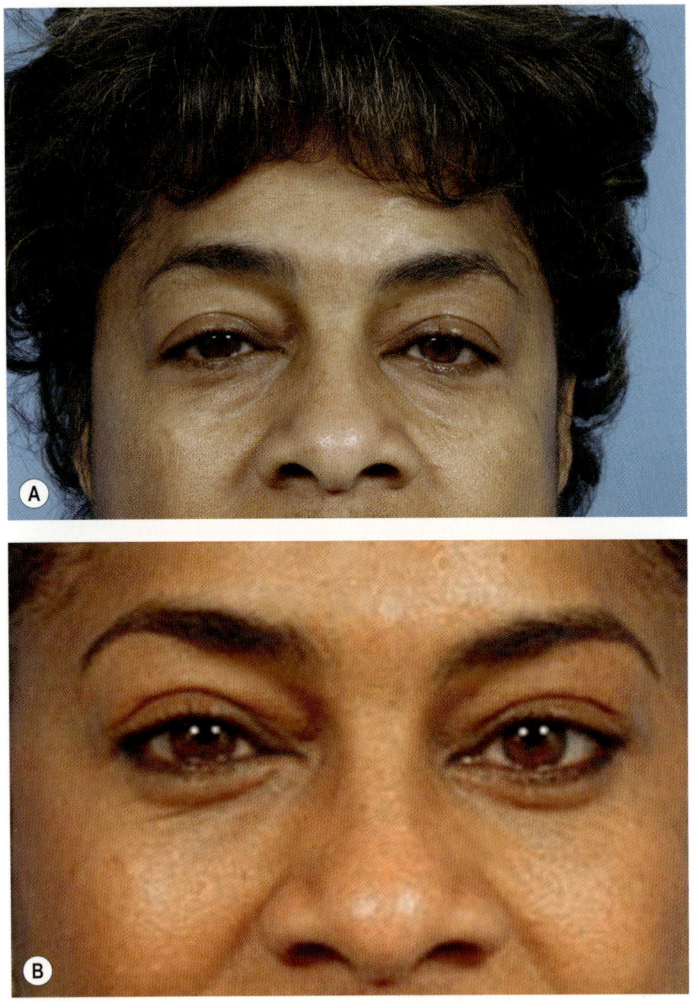

Figure 1.28 **(A)** Preoperative and **(B)** 5-year postoperative photograph of a patient with a lower lid blepharoplasty and canthopexy.

- Next, the lateral retinaculum and tarsal strap are bluntly dissected off the periosteum 5 mm in both directions (Figs 1.4, ***1.29***).
- A double-armed 4–0 Prolene or Mersilene is used to suture the tarsal plate and lateral retinaculum to the inner aspect of the lateral orbital rim periosteum above the Whitnall tubercle.
- Periosteum is thickest at the superior and lateral orbital rim, making it a secure suture site.
- The mattress suture is placed through the periosteum within the lateral orbital rim to maintain the posterior position of the lid margin against the globe.
- Bone canthopexy is technically possible through upper and lower lid incisions but is technically demanding.
- Wide exposure through a coronal brow lift provides the ideal environment and access.
- Bone fixation gives a profoundly longer lasting result than does periosteal fixation.
- Drill holes (1.5 mm drill bit) are placed 2–3 mm posterior to the lateral orbital rim.
- The inferior and superior holes are separated by 5–10 mm to allow suture separation and ligation ***(Fig. 1.30)***.
- The vertical position of the lateral canthal suture is dependent on eye prominence and preexisting canthal tilt. Patients with prominent eyes and negative vector morphology are at higher risk for lid malposition and require additional vertical support of the lateral canthus.
- While the standard position of the lateral canthopexy suture is most commonly at the lower level of the pupil, patients with prominent eyes or negative vectors require additional vertical positioning of the lateral canthal support suture at the superior aspect of the pupil.
- Lateral canthoplasty, which includes surgical division of the lateral canthus, is recommended for more significant lower lid laxity, defined by lid distraction >6 mm away from the globe.
- Lateral canthotomy, cantholysis of the inferior limb of the lateral canthal tendon, and release of the tarsal strap are performed.
- This dissection is followed by a 2–3 mm full-thickness lid margin resection, depending on the degree of tarsoligamentous laxity.
- The lateral commissure is carefully reconstructed by aligning the anatomical grey line with 6–0 plain gut.
- Final fixation to the lateral orbital periosteum can be as described above.

Midface lifting

- The middle third of the face, or midface, lies between the lateral canthal angle and the top of the nasolabial fold. It includes the lateral canthal tendon, the medial canthal tendon, the skin, fat, and orbicularis oculi muscle of the lower eyelids, the sub–orbicularis oculi fat pad, the malar fat pad, the orbitomalar ligament (orbicularis ligament), the orbital septum, and origins of the zygomaticus major and minor muscles and levator labii superioris.

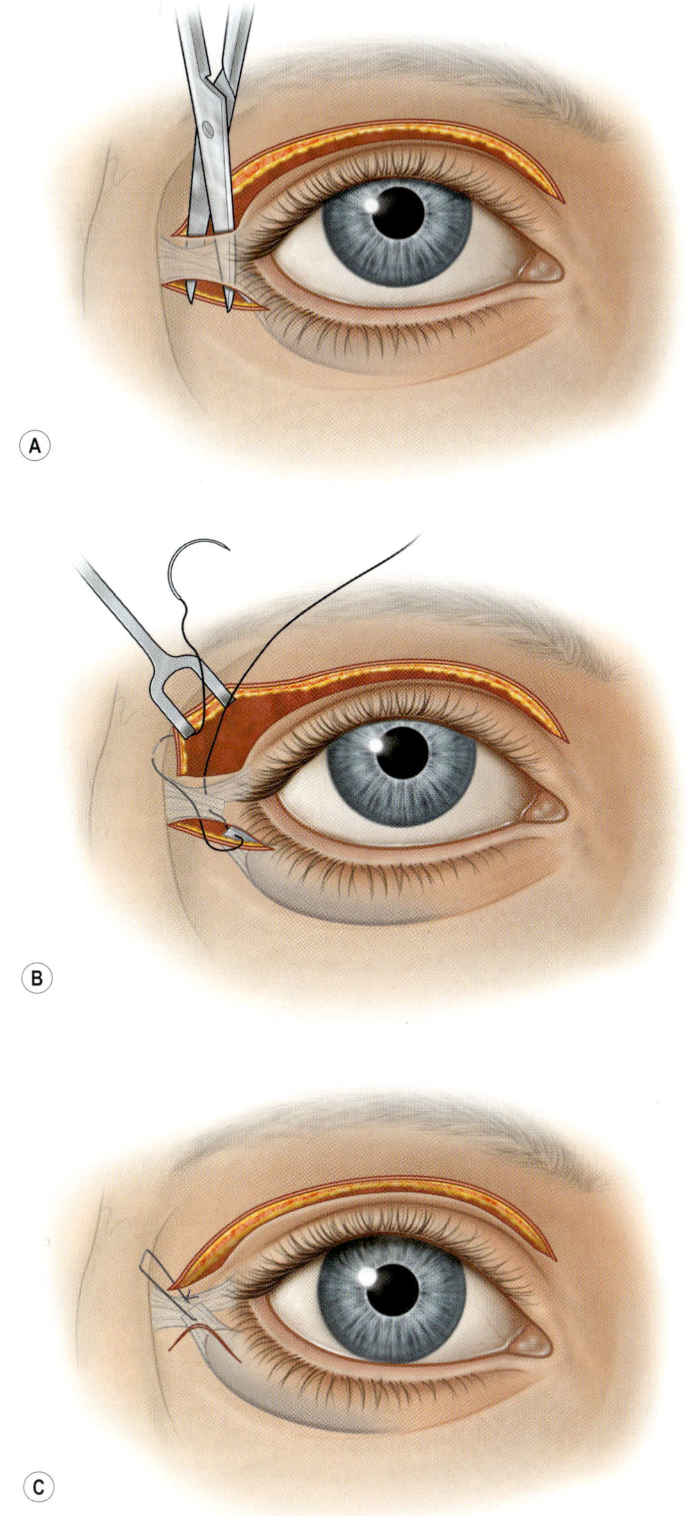

Figure 1.29 **(A–C)** Periosteal canthopexy. The inferior ramus of the lateral canthal tendon is secured and elevated to a raised position inside the orbital rim. Tension free suspension occurs with release of the tarsal strap and lateral orbital thickening.

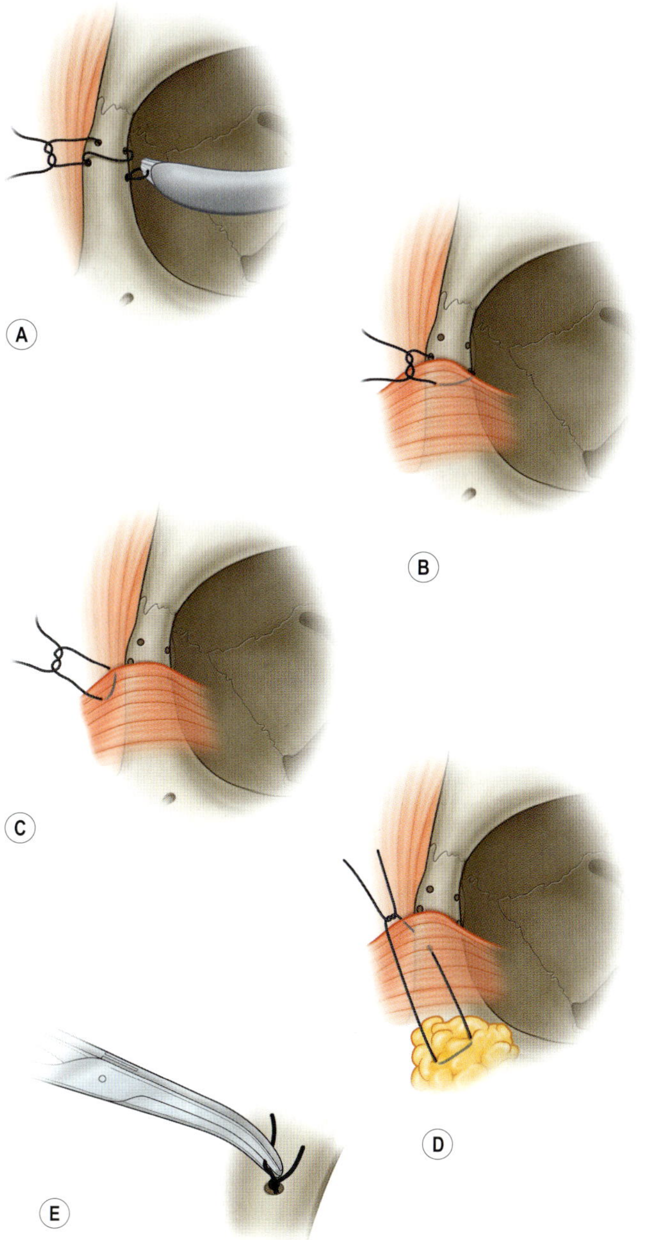

Figure 1.30 The canthopexy suture series for a two-layered canthopexy. **(A)** The canthopexy suture fixating the tarsal tail into the drilled hole. **(B)** The second-layer orbicularis suture. **(C)** Lateral sutures fix the lateral orbicularis to the deep temporal fascia. **(D)** If a midface lift is elected, an inferior drill hole can be made to fixate the midface tissues. **(E)** Bury the knot into the drill hole.

- When evaluating the midface for aesthetic surgery, all the structures listed above must be considered.
- The author's preferred technique includes approaching the midface through a transconjunctival incision.
- After repositioning or resection of orbital fat, the midface is elevated in a supraperiosteal plane.
- The attachment of the orbicularis oculi muscle to the orbital septum is preserved.
- Adequate release of the remaining, lax orbitomalar ligament then permits malar fat pad suspension in a

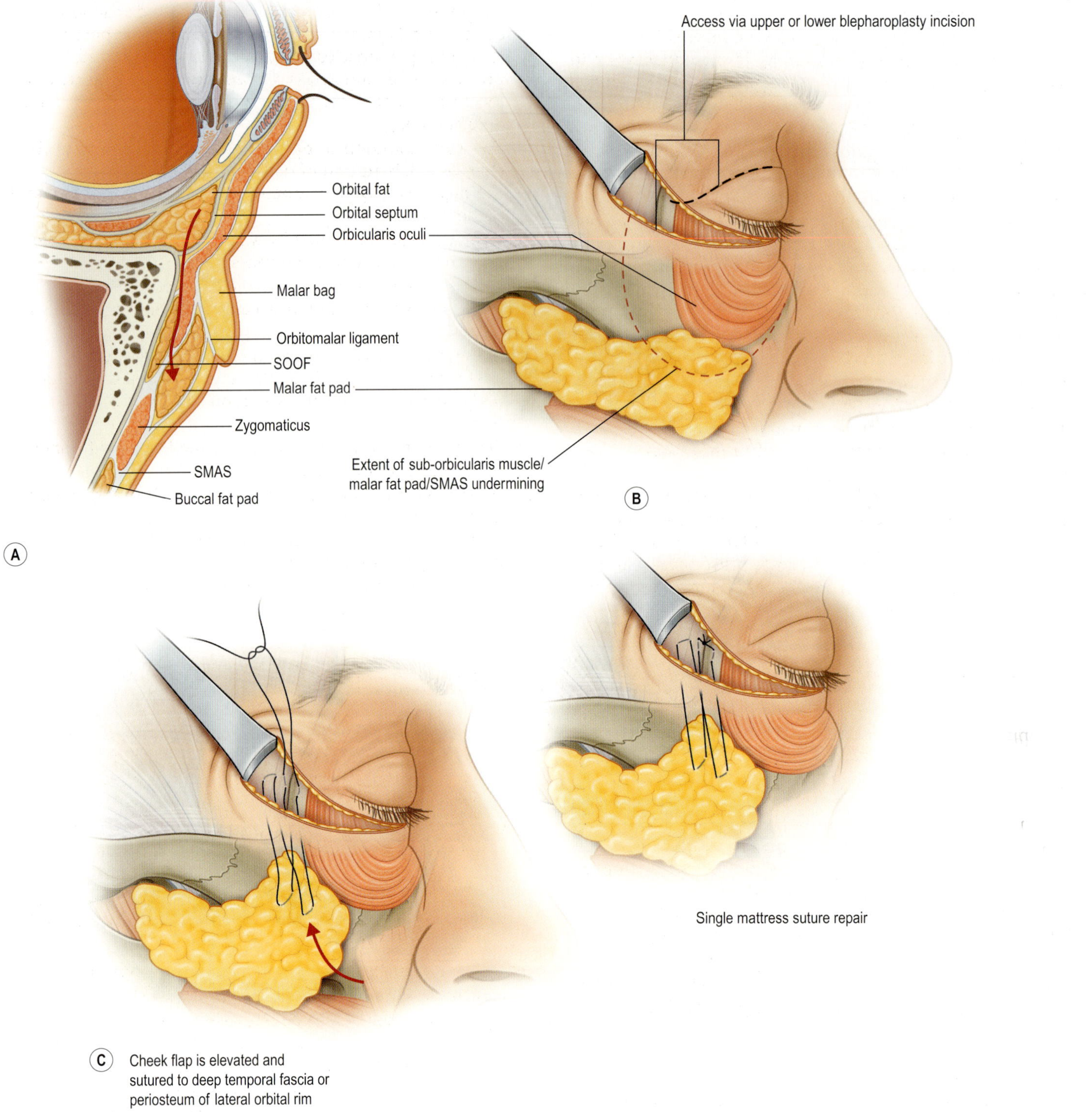

Figure 1.31 Midface lift. **(A)** The arrow in red depicts the plane of dissection to the midfacial structures in the cheek in a supraperiosteal approach. **(B)** Wide undermining of the periorbital ligamentous structures and lateral retinaculum may be transconjunctival or through the upper blepharoplasty incision. **(C)** Canthopexy and cheek suspension then proceed sequentially. (Adapted from Spinelli HM. *Atlas of Aesthetic Eyelid and Periocular Surgery.* Philadelphia: Saunders; 2004:129.)

superolateral vector to the lateral orbital rim and temporoparietal fascia *(Fig. 1.31)*.

- Canthopexy is then performed to redrape lower eyelid skin and recreate a youthful intercanthal angle. Finally, a skin only resection of the lower lid may be necessary to address any redundancy.

Postoperative considerations

- All patients are advised to expect swelling, bruising, some degree of ptosis, and tugging sensation on gazing upward. Although complete recovery takes months, patients generally look presentable approximately 2–3 weeks after surgery.

- Surgical literature has not advocated compression bandaging of the eyes after surgery. If one chooses not to use gently compressive bandages, postoperative edema can be reduced with cool compresses for up to 20 min intermittently during the initial 36 hours postoperatively.
- Patients are advised against using frozen compresses directly over their face in the setting of previous anesthetic use and pain medication.
- Additional recommendations include having the patient lie in a semi-recumbent position while resting and to avoid bedrest.
- Prescriptions for rewetting drops, Lacri-Lube® and antibiotic ophthalmic ointment can be given to reduce the incidence of exposure keratoconjunctivitis and dry eye symptoms in the immediate postoperative period.
- Patients are permitted to shower the next day and use antibiotic ointments as needed, for routine incisional care.
- It is also suggested that patients refrain from using contacts and to minimize the use of prescription eyeglasses.
- When no canthopexy is performed, half-inch Steri-Strips, retracted superiorly, are applied as a "cast" (with benzoin or Mastisol for security). This treatment tends to reduce lid retraction. Alternatively, a Frost suture placed in the lower lid margin and fixed to the brow suspends the lid during early healing.
- Visual changes, including diplopia, are generally temporary and can be attributed to wound reaction, edema and hematoma. Any damage to the superficial lying oblique muscles can be permanent and lead to postoperative strabismus. Conservative management is recommended; refractory cases should be referred to an ophthalmologist.
- The most common complication after blepharoplasty is chemosis. Disruption of ocular and eyelid lymphatic drainage leads to development of milky, conjunctival and corneal edema.
- Chemosis can be limited by atraumatic dissection, cold compresses, elevation and massage.
- It is usually self-limited and resolves spontaneously, though prolonged chemosis can be treated with topical steroids.
- Dry eye symptoms are also frequently cited in the postoperative phase. Patients may complain of foreign body sensation, burning, secretions and frequent blinking.
- Ocular protection can be achieved medically with liberal use of corneal lubricants.
- Additional complications such as lower lid malposition, lagophthalmos, undercorrection, asymmetry, and iatrogenic ptosis all require careful observation and photographic documentation.
- Reoperation should be performed no earlier than 3 months later.

Complications and outcomes

- Asymmetry is common postoperatively and can be caused by edema, bruising, and asymmetric sleep posture, but it also predictably follows undiagnosed preoperative asymmetry, including mild ptosis, made worse by the weight of postoperative edema.
- Patients should be advised that no reoperations are indicated before 8 weeks, and then only if the lids have stabilized and no edema or bruising is seen.
- The need for reoperations is infrequent, but when ptosis or exophthalmos is involved, incidence increases significantly to 10–30%.
- Retrobulbar hemorrhage is the most feared complication of eyelid surgery. Any complaint of severe orbital pain needs to be examined immediately, especially that of sudden onset.
- Acute management involves immediate evaluation, urgent ophthalmologic consultation and a return to the operation for evacuation of the hematoma.
- Medical treatments, in addition to operative exploration, include administration of high flow oxygen, topical and systemic corticosteroids and mannitol.
- Acute loss of vision mandates bedside suture removal and decompressive lateral canthotomy.
- Peribulbar hematoma, in contrast, does not threaten vision. It usually results from bleeding of an orbicularis muscle vessel. Small hematomas may resolve spontaneously, though larger hematomas can be evacuated in the office.

Further reading

Codner MA, Wolfi J, Anzarut A. Primary transcutaneous lower blepharoplasty with routine lateral canthal support: a comprehensive 10-year review. *Plast Reconstr Surg*. 2008;121(1):241–250.

Few JW. Rejuvenation of the African american periorbital area: dynamic considerations. *Semin Plast Surg*. 2009;23(1):198–206.

Few's survey-based study shows that one must prioritize a patient's ethnic identity and heritage when approaching the periorbital area in African-Americans.

Flowers RS. Canthopexy as a routine blepharoplasty component. *Clin Plast Surg*. 1993;20(2):351–365.

Flowers RS, Nassif JM, Rubin PA, et al. A key to canthopexy: the tarsal strap. A fresh cadaveric study. *Plast Reconstr Surg*. 2005;116(6):1752–1758.

Flowers and colleagues detail the anatomy of the lateral orbital retinaculum and highlight the importance of full dissection to achieve a tension-free canthopexy.

Hirmand H. Anatomy and nonsurgical correction of tear trough deformity. *Plast Reconstr Surg*. 2010;125(2): 699–708.

Mendelson BC. Fat preservation technique of lower-lid blepharoplasty. *Aesthet Surg J*. 2001;21(5):450–459.

Results shown in Mendelson's article demonstrate the safe, reproducible outcomes of a skin-only blepharoplasty and help swing the pendulum away from aggressive, fat excisional techniques.

Muzaffar AR, Mendelson BC, Adams Jr WP. Surgical anatomy of the ligamentous attachments of the lower lid and lateral canthus. *Plast Reconstr Surg.* 2002;110(3):873–884.

Reid RR, Said HK, Yu M, et al. Revisiting upper eyelid anatomy: introduction of the septal extension. *Plast Reconstr Surg.* 2006;117(1):65–70.

This cadaveric and histologic study identifies an extension of the orbital septum that must be identified and spared when performing a levator advancement for blepharoptosis.

Rohrich RJ, Coberly DM, Fagien S, et al. Current concepts in aesthetic upper blepharoplasty. *Plast Reconstr Surg.* 2004;3:32e–42e.

This continuing medical education article provides a concise description of upper eyelid aging and a step-by-step guide to popular rejuvenation techniques.

Spinelli HM. *Atlas of aesthetic eyelid and periocular surgery.* Philadelphia: Saunders; 2004.

Zide BM. *Surgical anatomy around the orbit: the system of zones.* 2nd ed. Philadelphia: Lippincott, Williams & Wilkins; 2006.

Chapter 2

Facelift

This chapter was created using content from Neligan & Warren, Plastic Surgery 3rd edition, Volume 2, Aesthetic, Chapter 11.1, Facelift: Principles, Richard J. Warren, Chapter 11.2, Facelift: Introduction to deep tissue techniques, Richard J. Warren, Chapter 11.3, Facelift: Platysma-SMAS plication, Dai M. Davies and Miles G. Berry, Chapter 11.4, Facelift: Facial rejuvenation with loop sutures, the MACS lift and its derivatives, Mark Laurence Jewell, Chapter 11.5, Facelift: Lateral SMASectomy, Daniel C. Baker, Chapter 11.7, Facelift: SMAS with skin attached –"the high SMAS" technique, Fritz E. Barton Jr., Chapter 11.8, Facelift: Subperiosteal facelift, Oscar M. Ramirez.

Brief introduction

- The classic stigmata of the aging face include:
  - Visible changes in skin, including folds, wrinkles, dyschromias, dryness, and thinning.
  - Folds in the skin and subcutaneous tissue created by chronic muscle contraction: glabellar frown lines, transverse forehead lines, and crow's feet over the lateral orbital rim.
  - Deepening folds between adjoining anatomic units: the nasojugular fold (tear trough), nasolabial folds, marionette lines, and submental crease.
  - Ptosis of soft tissue, particularly in the lower cheek, jowls and neck.
  - Loss of volume in the upper two-thirds of the face which creates hollowing of the temple, the lateral cheek, and the central cheek.
  - Expansion of volume in the neck and lateral jaw line which leads to the formation of jowls and fullness of the neck ***(Fig. 2.1)***.
- Aging of the face occurs in all its layers, from skin down to bone; no tissue is spared. The surgical significance of this concentric layer arrangement is:
  - Dissection can be done in the planes between the layers.
  - Anatomical changes in each of the layers can be addressed independently, as required to treat the presenting problem.
- Skin aging over time is both intrinsic and extrinsic. The net result is that facial skin loses its ability to recoil, a condition called elastosis.
- Intrinsic aging is the result of genetically determined apoptosis. The skin becomes thinner; there is a decrease in melanocytes, a reduced number of fibroblasts, and a loss of skin appendages. In the dermal matrix, there is fragmentation of the dermal collagen and impairment of fibroblast function.
- Extrinsic forces include sun exposure, cigarette smoke, extreme temperatures, and weight fluctuations.
- Important anatomic figures have been included: ***(Figs 2.2–2.8)***.

Preoperative considerations

- The quality of surgical result will be affected by many patient-related factors including the facial skeleton, the weight of facial soft tissue, the depth and location of folds, and the quality of the skin.
- Some issues can be reversed, others attenuated, and some may not be correctable at all.
- Incipient hypertension is common in the general population and can promote postoperative hematomas if it is not identified prior to surgery.

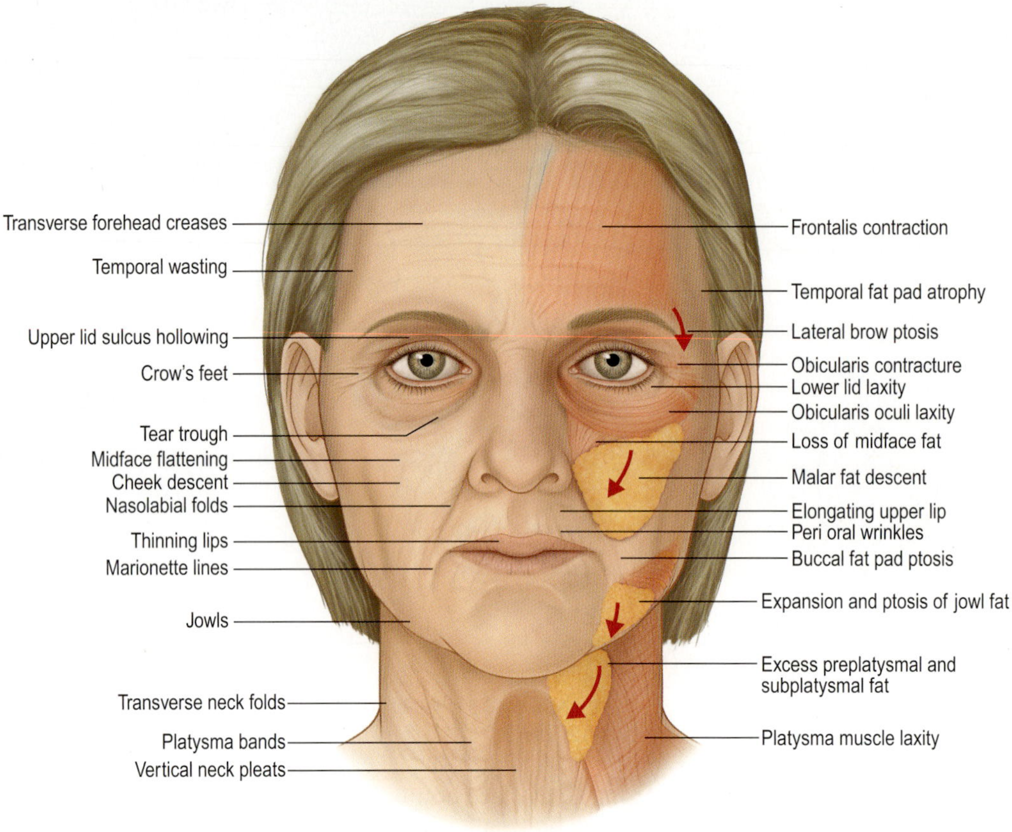

Figure 2.1 The aging face exhibits changes in the skin, superficial wrinkles, deeper folds, soft tissue ptosis, loss of volume in the upper third and middle third and increased volume in the lower third.

- Uncontrolled hypertension is a contraindication for surgery, while controlled hypertension is not a contraindication.
- Smokers have been shown to exhibit delayed wound healing due to microvasoconstriction and abnormal cell function.
- Nevertheless, there are significant short-term effects which can be reversed by abstaining from tobacco use for 2–3 weeks prior to surgery.
- Prior to surgery, the entire face should be properly assessed.
- The face should be assessed as a whole – looking for the equality of facial thirds, the degree of symmetry, and the overall shape (round, thin, wide).
- Surgeons should develop an organized way to examine all the zones of the face: forehead, eyelids, cheeks, the perioral area, and the neck.
- With the diversity of surgical techniques available, a surgeon should think like a sculptor – considering the face in three dimensions with a view to adding tissue in some areas, removing tissue in other areas, and repositioning tissue where indicated.
- The ear should be examined with a thought to the potential placement of incisions.
- Important factors: the size and orientation of the earlobe, the angle of attachment of the tragus, the difference in character of the cheek skin and tragal skin, and the size of the tragus, the density of the hair surrounding the ear, and the location of the hairline in the temple, the sideburn, and posterior to the ear.
- A careful assessment of the overlying skin is also important to determine if anything of a non-surgical nature is indicated before, during, or after facelift surgery.
- Excellent photographic documentation of the preoperative face is very important, and should include frontal, oblique, and profile views. Other optional views include the smile and close up views of the neck in repose and with platysma contracture.

Operative techniques

Subcutaneous facelift

- Classic procedure that tightens excess skin, and relies completely on skin tension to shift underlying facial soft tissue against the force of gravity.
- Advantages: relatively safe, relatively easy to do, and patient recovery is rapid.
- Effective for the thin patient with excess skin, and minimal ptosis of deep soft tissue.
- Disadvantage: skin placed under tension to support heavy underlying soft tissue will stretch, leading to a loss of surgical effect.

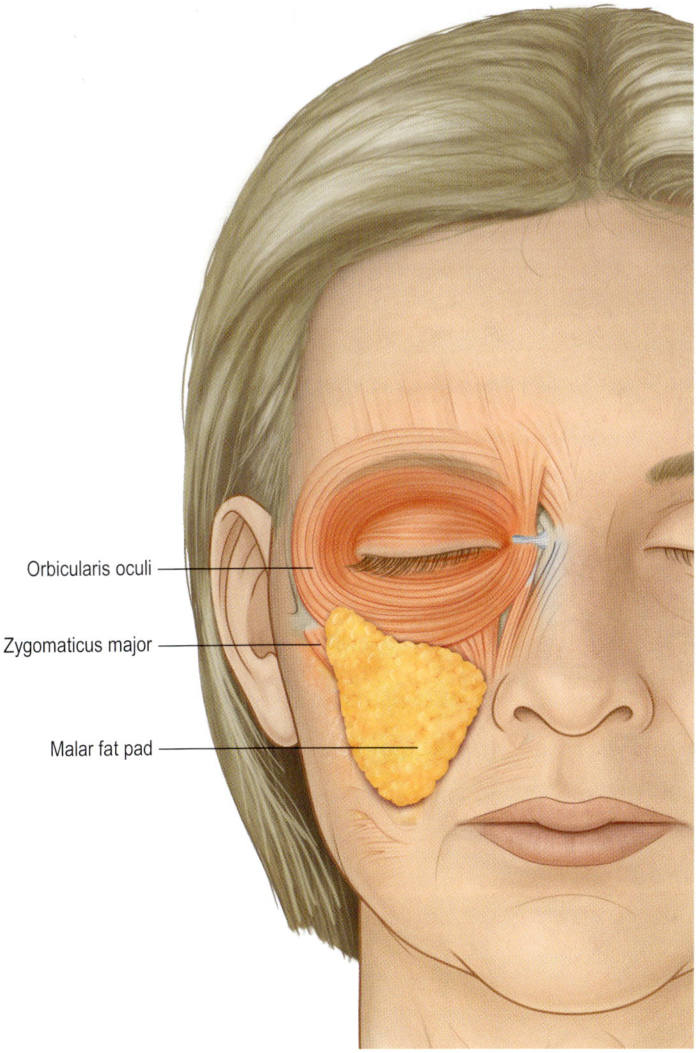

Figure 2.2 The malar fat pad is a triangular area of thickened superficial fat with its base along the nasolabial fold, and its apex over the superolateral malar prominence.

- Attempts to overcome this problem with excess skin tension may lead to distortion of facial shape, abnormal re-orientation of wrinkles, and local problems at the incision line including stretched scars and distorted earlobes.

Video 2.1

Facelift incisions (Video 2.1; Video 2.2)

Video 2.2

- In the temple area, the incision can be placed in the hair, at the anterior hairline, or a hybrid of the two, with an incision in the hair plus a transverse extension at the base of the sideburn *(Fig. 2.9A,B)*.
- The advantage of the incision in the hair is that it is hidden, but when the flap is drawn up, the anterior hairline and sideburn will shift; the degree of this depending on skin laxity.
- If the incision is placed at the anterior hairline, the scar is potentially more visible, but there will be no shift of the hairline.
- A transverse incision at the base of the sideburn is a compromise solution, which ameliorates much of the hairline shift, while preserving a largely hidden scar.
- Several factors should be assessed before committing to an incision within the temple hair.
- A preoperative estimate of skin redundancy will give the surgeon some sense of how far the skin flap will move.
- The distance between the lateral orbital rim and the temporal hairline should be assessed.
- In youth, this distance is generally <4–5 cm, while in older patients, the distance increases.
- If the distance is already excessive, or if the expected movement of the temporal hairline will create a distance over 5 cm, then an incision in the hair should be avoided (Fig. 2.9C).
- Anterior to the ear, the incision can be pretragal, or along the tragal edge (Fig. 2.9D,E).
- The advantage of the tragal edge incision is that it is hidden, but care must be taken to thin the flap covering the tragus in order to simulate a normal tragal appearance.
- Before committing to a tragal edge incision, the quality of tragal skin and that of facial skin must be compared; if the difference between the tragal skin and facial skin is too great, a tragal edge incision should be avoided.
- A pretragal incision is preferred in men as the hair-bearing portion of the cheek skin will not be drawn up onto the tragus.
- Around the earlobe, the incision can be placed either in the cleft of earlobe attachment or 1–2 mm distal to the cleft, leaving a cuff of skin along the earlobe. This cuff will ease the process of insetting the earlobe on skin closure.
- In the retroauricular sulcus, the incision can be placed directly in the conchal groove as it courses superiorly.
- The incision is often carried as high as the level of the external auditory canal, or slightly higher, at the level of the antihelix.
- An extension of the retroauricular sulcus incision toward the occipital hair-bearing region should be made when there is a need to remove excess redundant neck skin.
- A "short scar" facelift is one which avoids the occipital incision, and will suffice for many patients.
- The principle objectives for the occipital incision are to gain access to the neck in order to take up redundant neck skin, while making the incision as invisible as possible with little or no distortion of the occipital hairline *(Figs 2.10, 2.11)*.
- Either the temple dissection or the postauricular dissection can be done first, depending on surgeon preference.
- In the postauricular area, the flap is firmly attached to the deep cervical fascia of the sternocleidomastoid and the mastoid.
- This is the most common location to see skin flap necrosis, so the flap should be raised sharply under direct vision, keeping the dissection against the underlying deep fascia in order to maintain flap thickness.
- As the dissection continues inferior to the earlobe level, the surgeon must be cognizant of the great auricular nerve, where it is most at risk over the posterior border of the sternocleidomastoid.

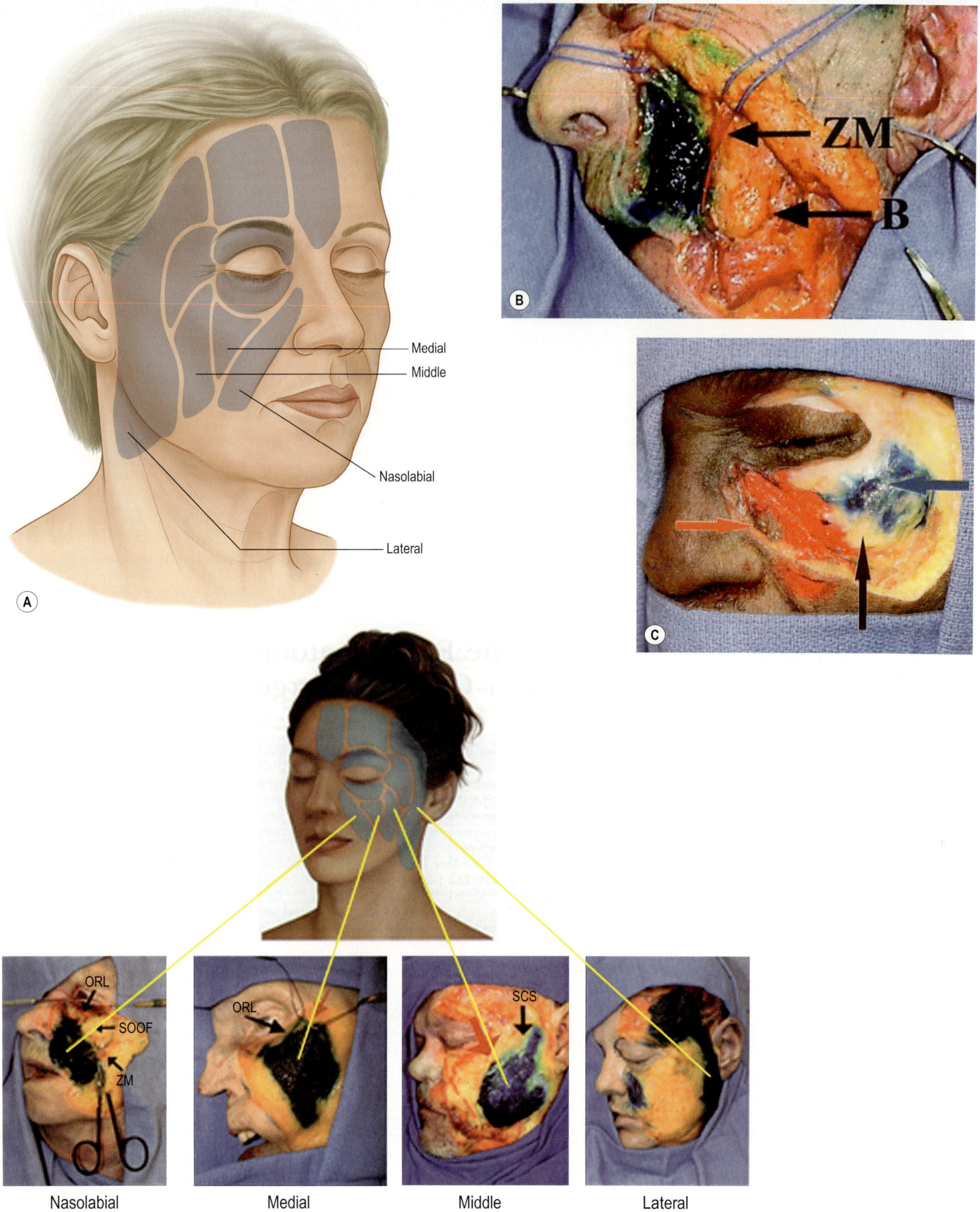

Figure 2.3 **(A)** Superficial facial fat is compartmentalized by vertically running septae. In the midcheek, from medial to lateral, these compartments are the nasolabial, medial, middle, and lateral compartments. The nasolabial and medial compartments make up the malar fat pad. **(B)** The deep facial fat is also compartmentalized by septae. The deep medial fat pad (here stained blue) is bounded above by the orbicularis retaining ligament, medially by the pyriform aperture, and laterally by the zygomaticus major (ZM) muscle and the buccal (labeled B) fat pad. **(C)** Over the body of the zygoma, the sub orbicularis oculi fat (SOOF) is deep fat. It is seen here with a medial portion (yellow) and a lateral portion (stained blue). It is bounded medially by deep medial fat pad (stained red). (**A** Courtesy of Rohrich RJ, Pessa JE. The fat compartments of the face: anatomy and clinical implications for cosmetic surgery. *Plast Reconstr Surg.* 2007;119:2219–2227; **B,C** Courtesy of Rohrich RJ, Pessa JE, Ristow B. The youthful cheek and the deep medial fat compartment. *Plast Reconstr Surg.* 2008;121(6):2107–2112).

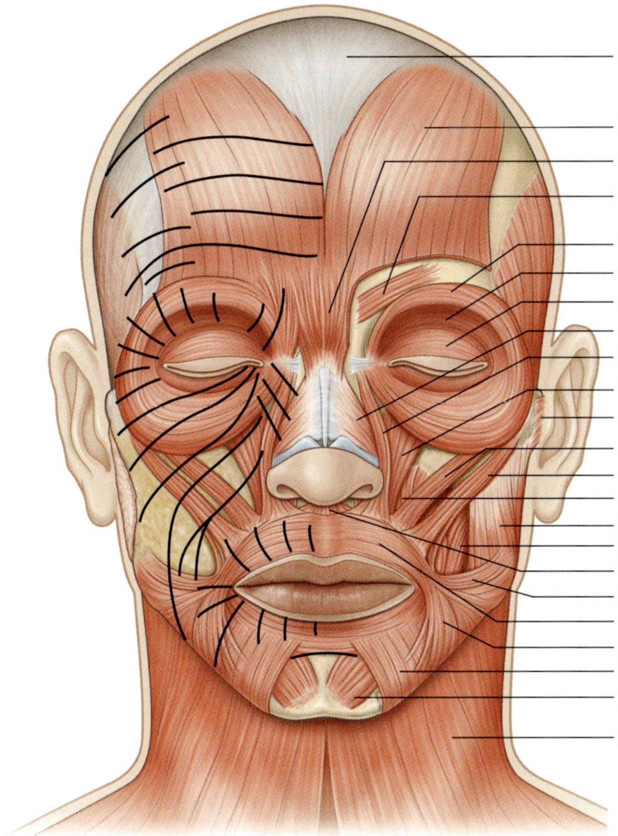

Figure 2.4 Muscles of facial expression. The solid lines demonstrate overlying skin creases caused by repeated contraction of the underlying muscles.

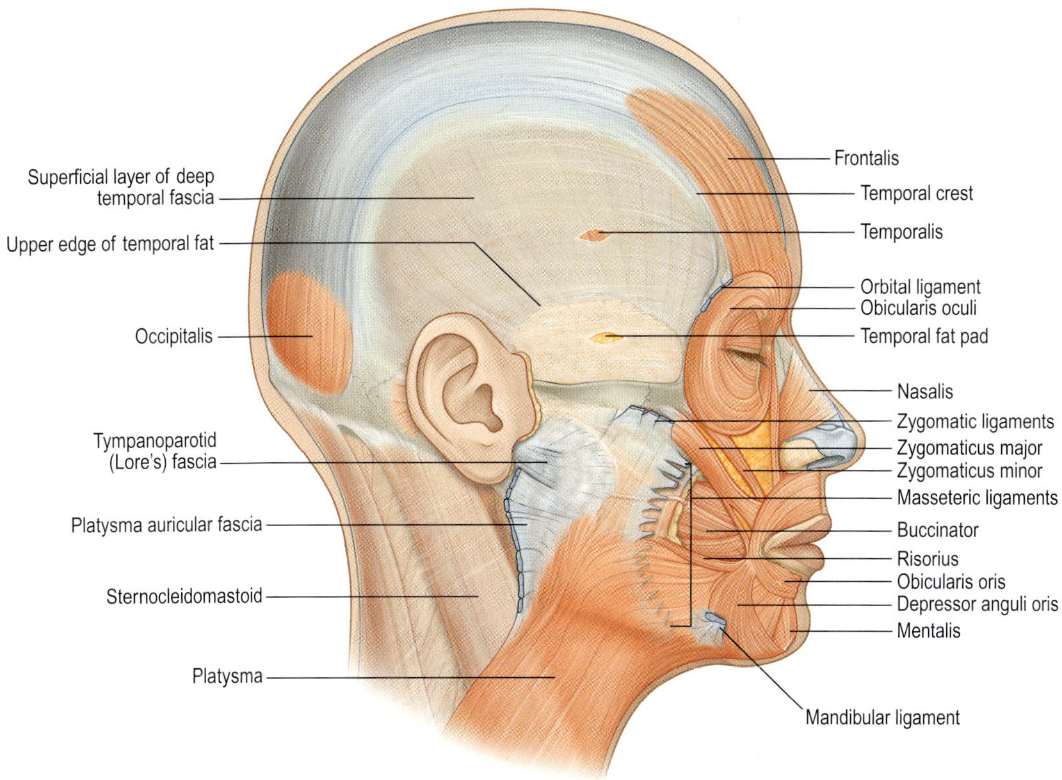

Figure 2.5 Facial soft tissue is tethered to underlying bone by the orbital, zygomatic and mandibular ligaments. Soft tissue is tethered to underlying deep fascia by the masseteric cutaneous ligaments and by an area of attachment anterior and inferior to the earlobe, known by a number of different terms: platysma auricular ligament (Furnas), platysma auricular ligament (Mendelson), parotid cutaneous ligament (Stuzin), and a distinct area anterior to the earlobe known as Lore's fascia.

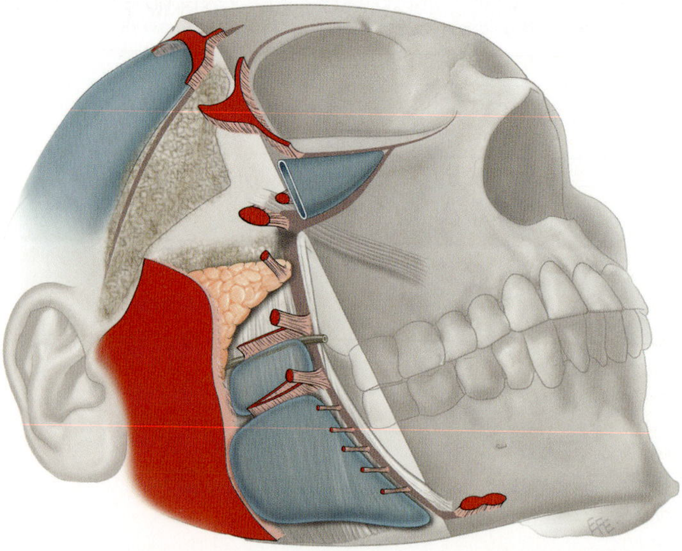

Figure 2.6 Mendelson's interpretation of soft tissue attachments. The fixed posterior soft tissue is held in place by the platysma auricular fascia (large red area). The anterior face is fixed by a vertical column of attachments: orbital ligament, lateral orbital thickening (superficial canthal tendon), zygomatic ligaments, masseteric ligaments, and mandibular ligament). The so-called "fixed SMAS" is that portion attached to the parotid and the posterior border of the platysma. Anterior to this, is the "mobile SMAS".

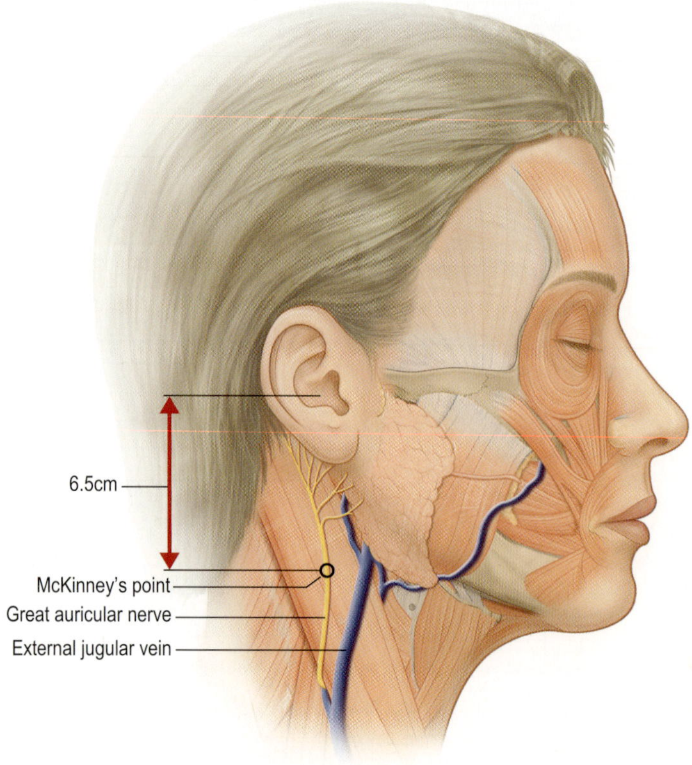

Figure 2.7 The great auricular nerve crosses the midportion of the sternocleidomastoid at McKinney's point, which is 6.5 cm inferior to the external auditory canal. It usually travels about 1 cm posterior to the external jugular vein. Anterior to McKinney's point, the nerve is covered by the superficial cervical fascia (SMAS), but at the posterior border of the sternocleidomastoid, the nerve is subcutaneous. The most common point of injury is at the posterior border of the sternocleidomastoid muscle.

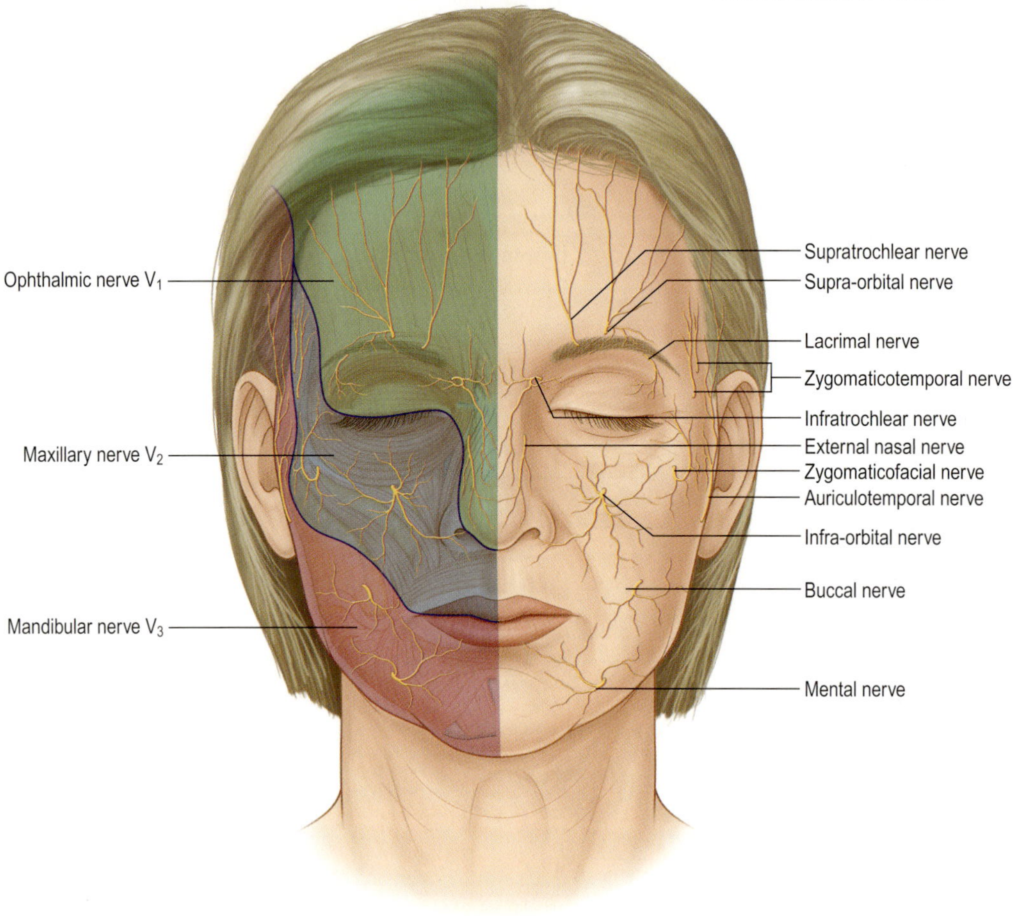

Figure 2.8 Major sensory nerves of the face.

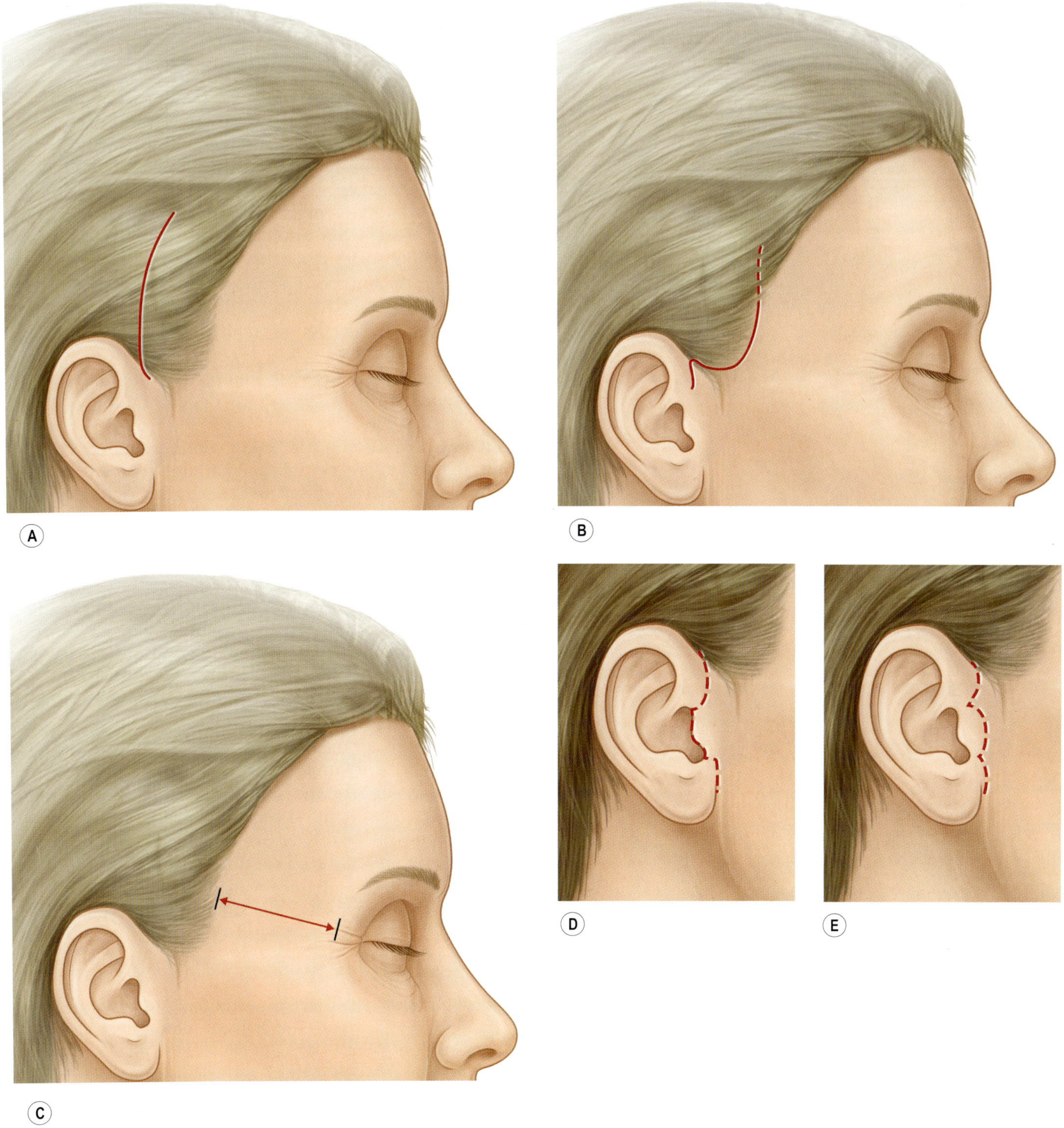

Figure 2.9 **(A)** The traditional hidden incision in the temple hair is appropriate when the temporal hairline will not be shifted adversely. **(B)** A temple incision along the hairline is used if a hidden incision will adversely shift the hairline. **(C)** The distance from the lateral orbital rim to the temporal hairline should not exceed 5 cm. **(D)** The retrotragal incision follows the edge of the tragus. **(E)** The pretragal incision is placed in the pretragal sulcus.

- By keeping the dissection in the subcutaneous plane, the great auricular nerve will be protected.
- In the temple, if the incision has been made along the anterior hairline, dissection is begun directly in the subcutaneous plane. If the incision has been made in the hair-bearing scalp of the temple, dissection can be carried out in one of two planes: superficial to the superficial temporal (temporoparietal fascia) which will continue directly into the subcutaneous facelift plane, or between the superficial temporal fascia and the deep temporal fascia.

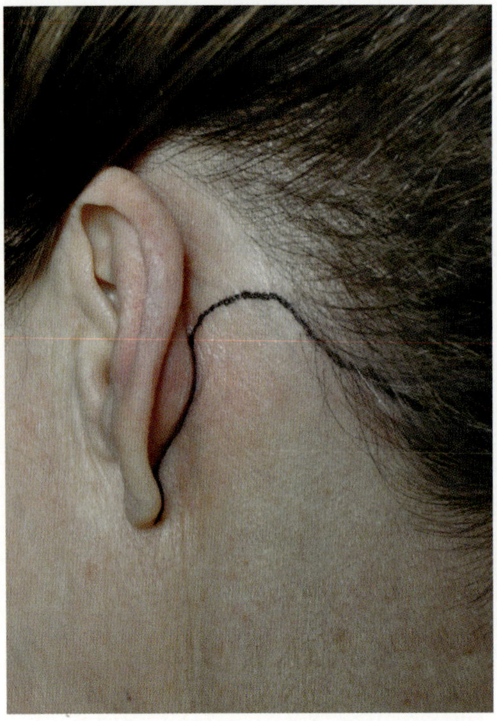

Figure 2.10 (A) When there is minimal to moderate skin shift expected, an appropriate incision will curve from the retroauricular incision directly into the occipital hair. **(B)** When a greater amount of skin is to be excised, a "Lazy S" incision, which partly follows the occipital hairline, is an appropriate choice.

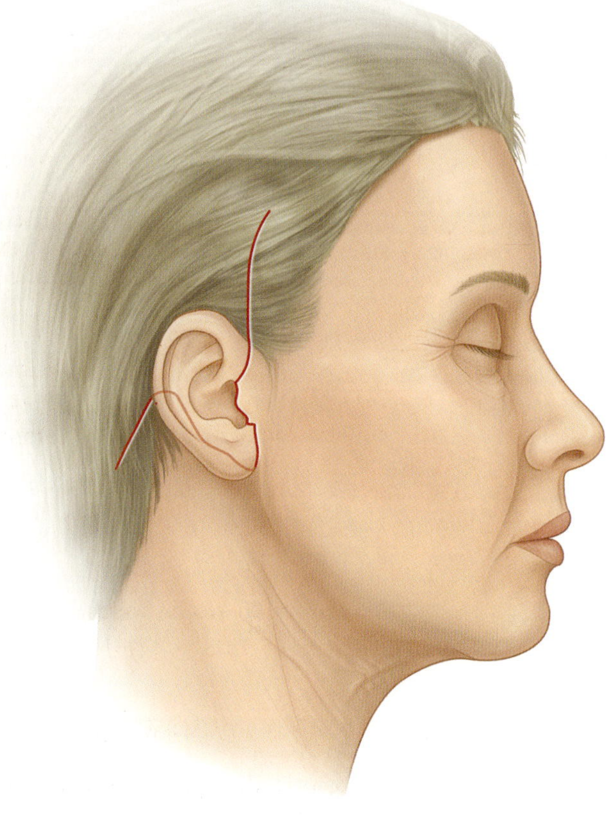

Figure 2.11 The traditional incision for a facelift flap curves vertically or slightly anteriorly in the temple, follows the contours of the ear, both anteriorly and posteriorly, and then angles into the posterior scalp.

- If the deeper approach is used, the dissection proceeds quickly against deep fascia, but at the anterior hairline, the dissection plane must transition into the subcutaneous facelift plane.
- This change of plane results in a narrow ribbon of superficial temporal fascia which will contain the superficial temporal artery and vein and branches of the auriculotemporal nerve which must be divided *(Fig. 2.12A)*.
- The superficial plane preserves the superficial temporal fascia and vessels, but can injure the hair follicles during the dissection unless care is taken (Fig. 2.12B).
- Anterior to the anterior hairline, the subcutaneous plane is then developed.
  - The level of dissection normally leaves 1–2 mm of fat on the dermis.
  - This results in a large random pattern skin flap the survival of which will entirely depend on the subdermal plexus.
- In the upper face, this dissection continues anteriorly until the orbicularis oculi is encountered where it encircles the lateral orbital rim. Depending on the type of deep plane surgery planned, the midcheek dissection may stop short of the malar fat pad, or alternatively, carry on over the fat pad, freeing it from the overlying skin in the temple and cheek.
- Lower in the cheek, immediately anterior to the ear and the earlobe, the skin is tethered to underlying structures by secure fascial attachments, but beyond this area, the subcutaneous dissection proceeds relatively easily.
- Once the skin flaps anterior and posterior to the ear have been raised, the two dissections are joined.
- The dissection can then be extended into the neck as far as the technique requires *(Figs 2.13, 2.14)*. (Video 2.3) Video 2.3
- After elevation of the subcutaneous tissues, management of the deep tissues can proceed, if needed.
- Once the deep tissues have been managed, skin flap mobilization and closure is performed:
  - Most techniques advance the skin flap along an oblique vector which is slightly more posterior than the vector for repositioning deep tissues.
  - In certain techniques, surgeons employ a nearly vertical vector to the skin flap.
  - One concept is to place the skin flap "where it lies", using the vector which facial skin naturally assumes when the patient is lying in the supine position.
  - Another guide is to advance the skin flap toward the temple along a vector which is perpendicular to the nasolabial fold.
- The anterior anchor point is immediately adjacent to the helix of the ear at the junction of the hair-bearing scalp.
- This will be the first of two anchor points; it can be held in place with a half buried mattress suture in order to minimize the chance of a visible suture mark *(Fig. 2.15)*.
- Posteriorly, the skin flap should be drawn along a vector which roughly parallels the body of the mandible.
- The second anchor point will be at the superior most extent of the postauricular sulcus at the point where the incision starts to transition posteriorly. Once again, a half buried mattress suture can be used.

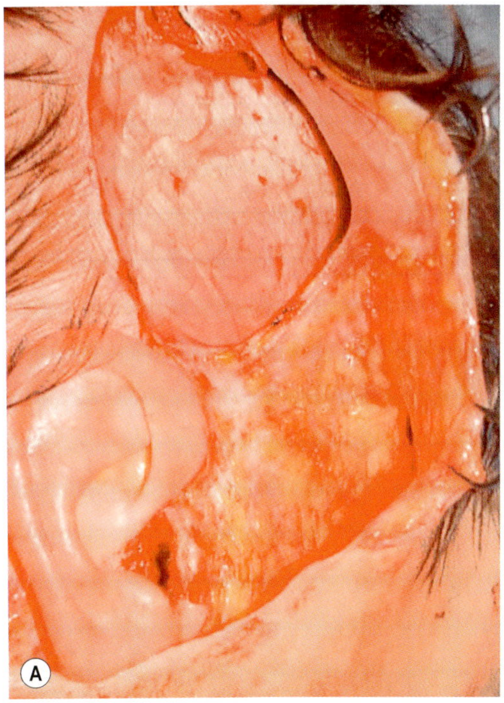

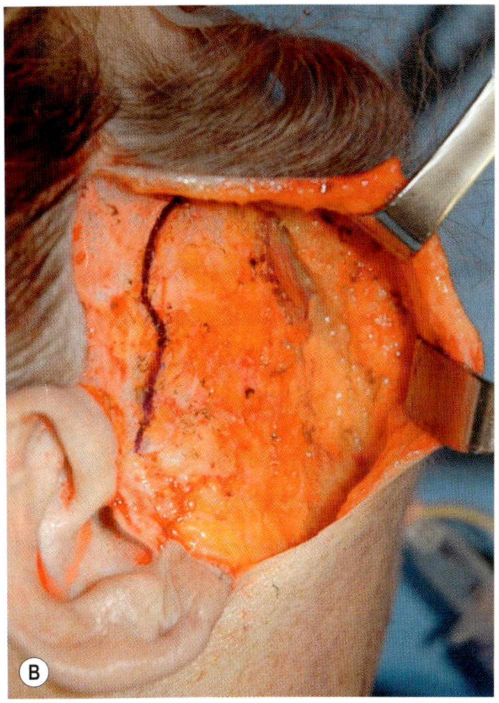

Figure 2.12 **(A)** Facelift flap has been raised in two different planes, initially deep to the superficial temporal fascia, against the deep temporal fascia (seen as an oval window), with a change of planes near the anterior temporal hairline into the subcutaneous plane. The "mesotemporalis" is a bridge of tissue which develops between these two planes. In order to unify the planes, it has been divided with ligation of the superficial temporal artery. **(B)** Facelift flap has been raised in a single subcutaneous plane, with dissection directly on the superficial temporal fascia and deep to the hair follicles of the scalp. The purple line outlines the course of the anterior branch of the superficial temporal artery.

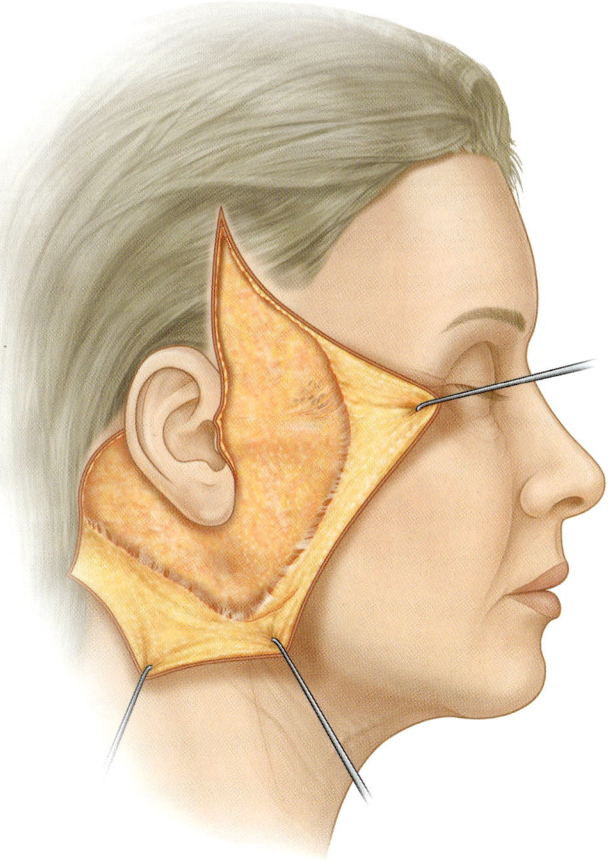

Figure 2.13 Subcutaneous facelift flap has been raised.

- At this point, trimming of the overlapping flap and suturing can be done in the temple and in the occipital region.
- The facelift flap is redraped in the desired direction with gentle tension.
- Attention is then turned to trimming excess skin around the ear, with absolutely no tension on the closure.
- If a tragal edge incision is used, the tragal flap is thinned and hair follicles are removed.
- In the retroauricular sulcus, there is normally little or no skin to be trimmed if the posterior flap has been correctly positioned.
- Earlobe inset is done last and is designed to angle 15° posterior to the long access of the ear *(Fig. 2.16)*.
- Skin trimming around the earlobe should be conservative.
- Tension on the earlobe can lead to distortions such as the pixy ear deformity and the malpositioned earlobe.

Midfacelift (blepharoplasty approach)

- In an attempt to lift the tissue immediately inferior to the infraorbital rim (the midface), an approach through the lower lid was developed which involves a subciliary or a transconjunctival blepharoplasty type incision followed by a dissection down over the face of the maxilla.

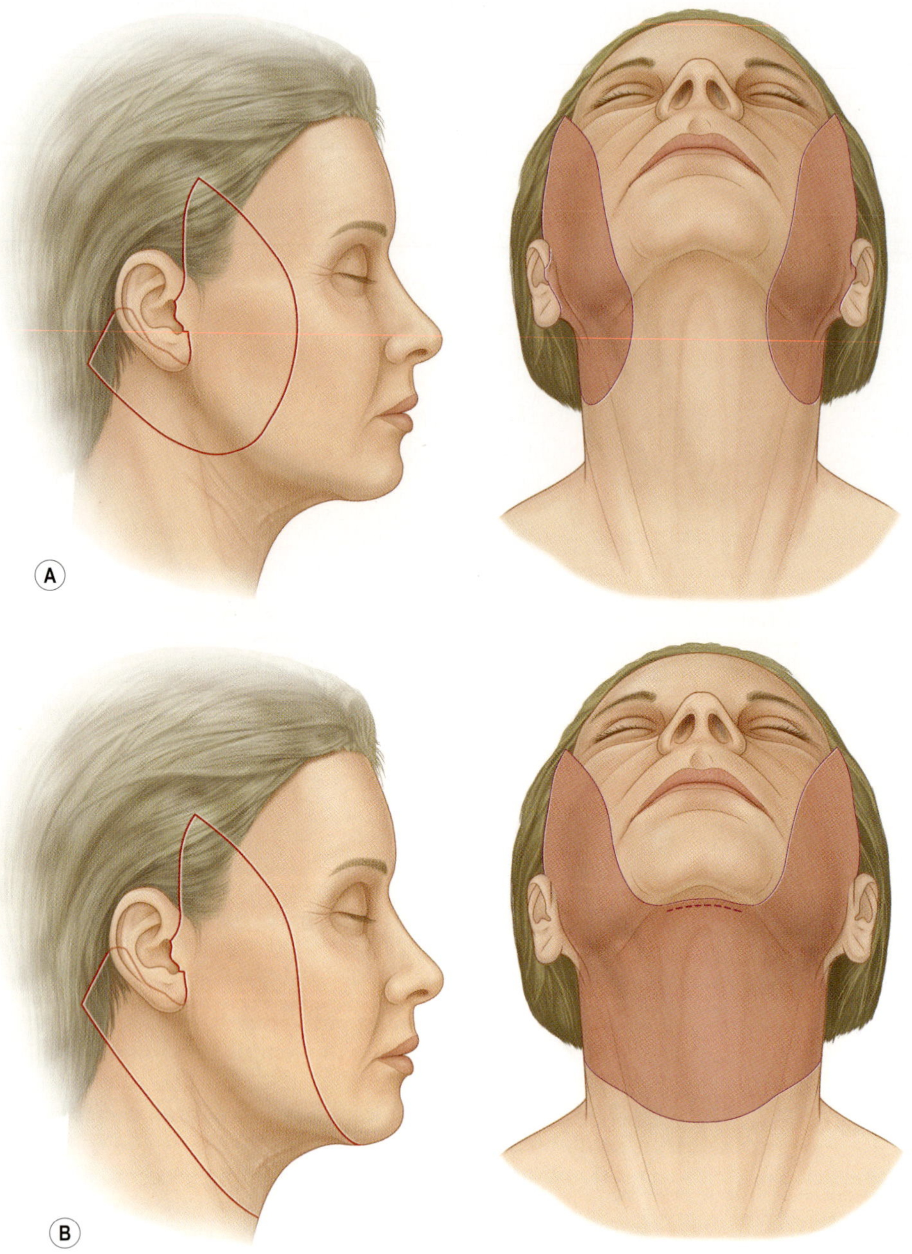

Figure 2.14 **(A)** Traditional subcutaneous flap dissection with no submental incision. **(B)** Traditional subcutaneous flap dissection with submental incision.

- Performed in either the subperiosteal plane, which requires an inferior periosteal release, or in a supraperiosteal plane.
- After mobilization of the cheek mass the soft tissue is fixated superiorly, either laterally along the lateral orbital rim, or more vertically with anchoring to the bone of the infraorbital rim.
- Disadvantages of the midfacelift: steep learning curve, and high incidence of revisions.

Video 2.4

SMAS plication (Video 2.4)

- Patients are prepared as for a standard facelift with tumescent infiltration (20 mL 0.5% bupivacaine and 1 mL 1:1000 adrenaline in 200 mL normal saline) into the subcutaneous plane.
- The incision extends vertically in the temporal scalp, along the anterior helical sulcus, then passes post-tragal, and on occasion into the postauricular sulcus *(Fig. 2.17)*.
- A postauricular extension is used where required and subcutaneous dissection tailored to each patient.
- The anterior SMAS is grasped in a postero-superior direction to provide a satisfactory effect on the jowl *(Fig. 2.18)*.
- The key suture, using 2-0 PDS (Johnson & Johnson Medical Ltd), is then inserted to attach this SMAS to the relatively immobile pre-auricular parotid-masseteric fascia.

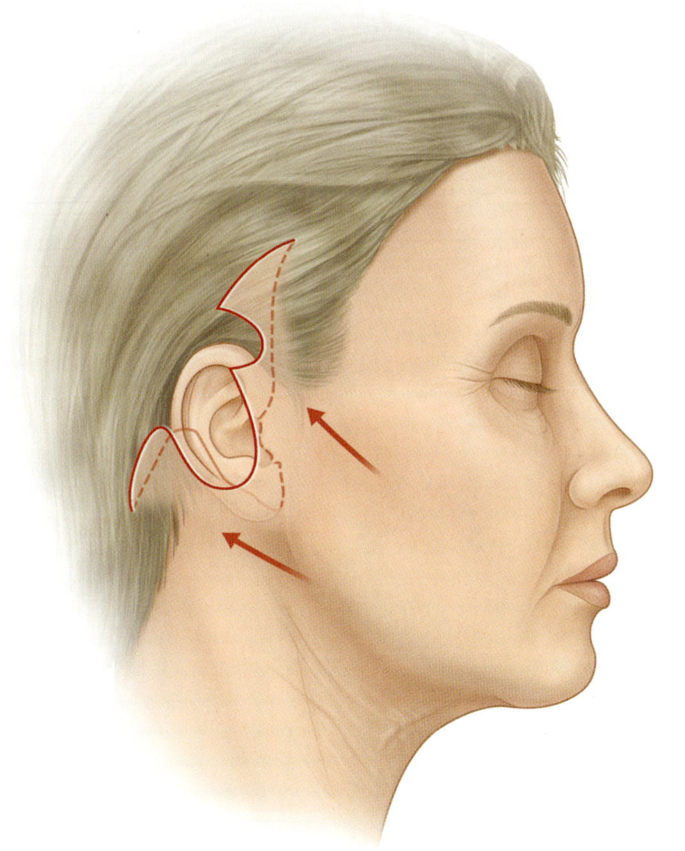

Figure 2.15 Diagram shows typical skin flap redraping along an oblique direction which is slightly less vertical than the vector along which deep tissues are moved. There is considerable variation in this; however, some techniques involve a more horizontal vector while other techniques utilize a nearly vertical vector.

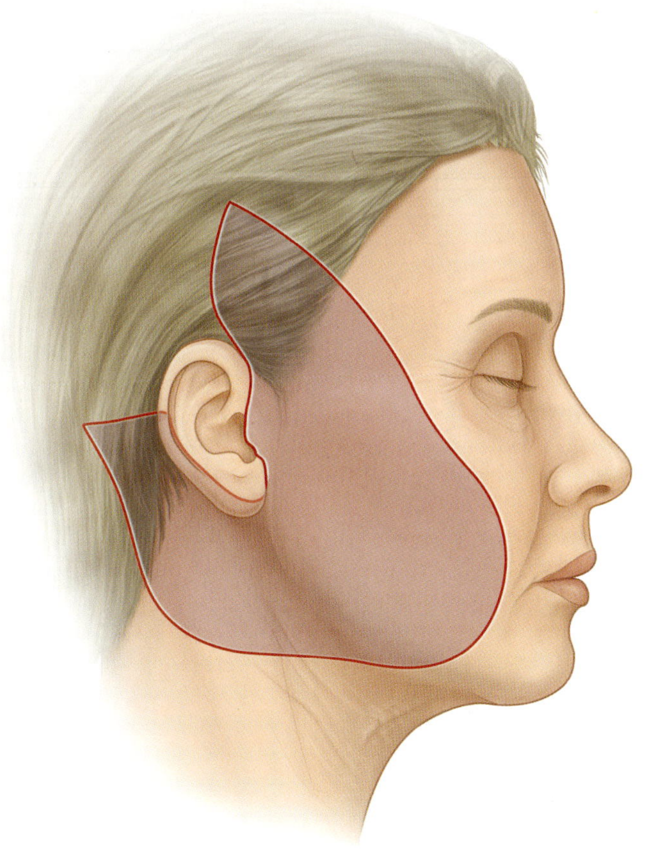

Figure 2.17 Incision and area of subcutaneous dissection employed with the PSP-lift. Note that the posterior extension is not always required, but is useful where excess skin remains in the neck after SMAS plication.

Proper insetting of the ear lobe

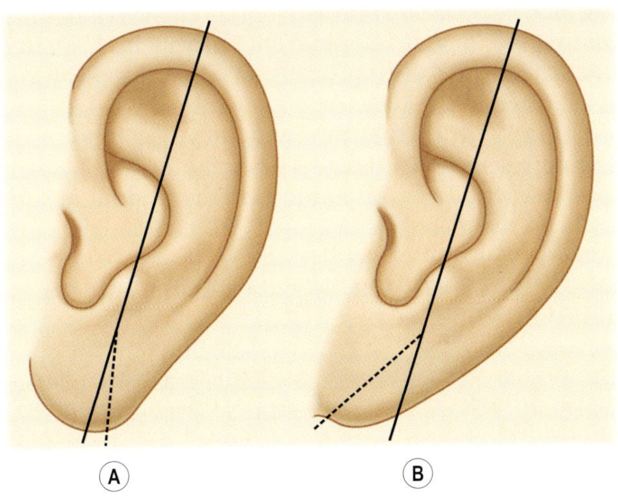

Figure 2.16 The earlobe should be inset with the long axis of the earlobe (dotted line) about 15° posterior to the long axis of the ear itself. If the earlobe is pulled forward, an unnatural appearance results.

- Further sutures complete plication of the cervical platysma, below the mandibular angle, to the mastoid fascia ***(Fig. 2.19)*** and any surface irregularities are addressed by suture imbrication with 3-0 Vicryl (Johnson & Johnson).
- Excess SMAS in the infra-lobular region is excised, following hydrodissection, and closed with 3-0 Vicryl.
- Following meticulous hemostasis, excess skin, with low tension traction only, is trimmed and the wound closed over a small suction drain with 4-0 and 6-0 nylon.
- A light, compressive facelift dressing remains overnight and is removed with the drain the following morning. These can be similarly removed immediately prior to discharge in day-case patients.
- Sutures are removed at 4–6 days.

Video 2.5

MACS-lift (Chapter 11.4) (Video 2.5)

- The patient is marked before the start of the procedure; key points are the planned incision, the degree of undermining, and the location of suture loops.
- The degree of skin flap undermining typically extends inferiorly just past the mandibular angle and anteriorly 5–6 cm in front of the ear.

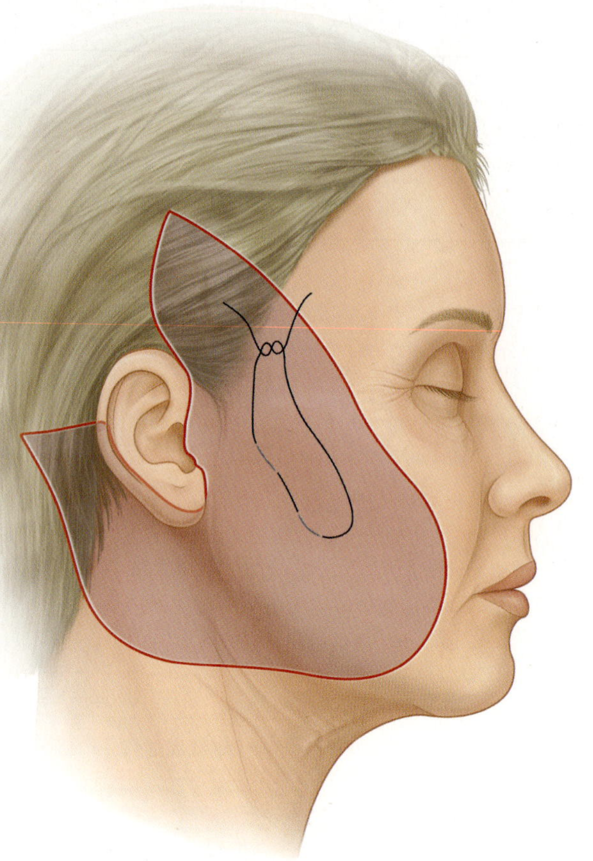

Figure 2.18 Placement of the first and key suture, which takes a generous bite of anterior SMAS and tractions it postero-superiorly onto the parotido-masseteric fascia. It can be trialed and its effect easily measured externally by observing reduction of the jowl and effacement of the nasolabial fold as the SMAS is tractioned and the suture tied.

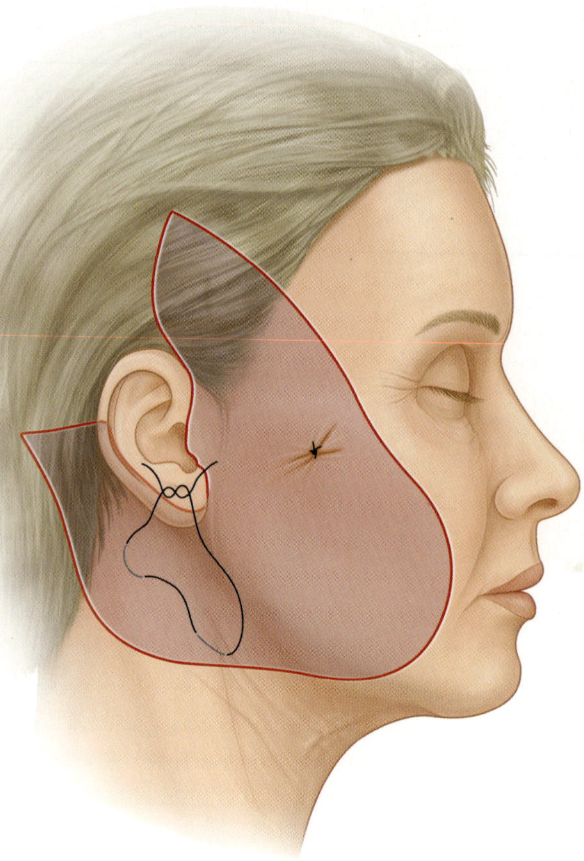

Figure 2.19 Tying the key suture produces a "dog-ear" of SMAS that produces a convenient malar autoaugmentation. A second suture passes between the posterior platysma and the mastoid fascia to complete the effect on the jowl and commence the necklift.

- If an extended MACS-lift is planned, undermining is marked over the malar prominence.
- If autologous fat grafting is considered, the fat is harvested, processed, and injected at the beginning, prior to the incisions for the MACS-lift.
- Local anesthetic containing epinephrine is injected along the incision line.
- The short scar incision extends from the earlobe below to the anterior hairline above.
- It follows the attachment of the earlobe from the retroauricular crease, around to the anterior attachment of the earlobe, following the tragal edge, the anterior helical attachment to the root of the helix, then across the lower portion of the sideburn and up the anterior hairline.
- Anteriorly, the incision is made in a zigzag pattern 1–2 mm within the hairline.
- In the standard MACS-lift, the incision is carried up to the level of the lateral canthus, while in the extended MACS-lift, the incision extends up to a point opposite the tail of the eyebrow.
- The deep temporal fascia anchor point is chosen to avoid the superficial temporal vessels and the temporal branch of the facial nerve.
- Small scissors are used to create a window in the subcutaneous tissue approximately 1 cm above the zygomatic arch and 1 cm in front of the helical rim in order to expose the deep temporal fascia ***(Fig. 2.20)***.
- When placing the suture into the temporalis fascia, the author sews away from the temporal vessel location.
- A single anchor point is used for both the neck loop and the cheek loop in order to diminish the amount of suture used and the palpability of knots. Absorbable monofilament sutures such as 0-polydiaxonone are preferred over non-absorbable polypropylene or braided polyester suture.
- The suture loop for the neck is placed first. Going inferiorly in the natural sulcus that is anterior to the tragus, firm bites between 1 cm and 1.5 cm long are taken into the SMAS.
- Progressing inferiorly past the angle of the mandible, two or three suture bites are taken into the platysma before the suturing is directed upward and back to the anchor point.
- A U-shaped loop about 1 cm wide is created and the knot is then tied at the anchor point under tension.
- Should additional reinforcement of the neck be desired, 2-0 polydioxanone sutures can be placed from the

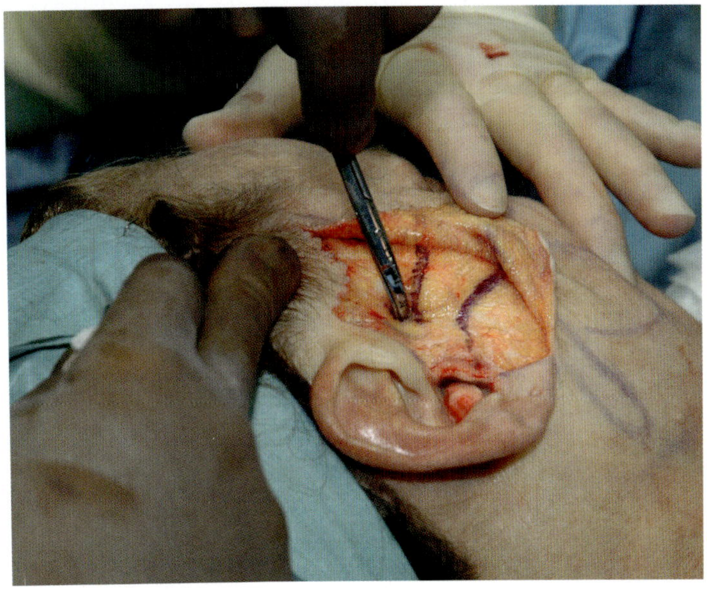

Figure 2.20 The short scar incision has been made, and the skin flap raised. The zygomatic arch is marked in purple. Note the marks on the skin designating the location of the suture loops. The scissors are dissecting a window down to the deep temporal fascia which will be used as the anchor point for the vertical and cheek suture loops.

platysma into the fascial zone of adherence just below the tragus (Lore's fascia) or from the platysma to the mastoid fascia.

- Suture knots in this area should be inverted to avoid knot palpability through the skin *(Fig. 2.21)*.
- The cheek loop is placed next. It originates at the same anchor point from the deep temporal fascia. Taking bites of the SMAS, suturing progresses inferiorly just anterior to the first loop and then curves more anteriorly, creating a wider loop above the jowl extending anteriorly as far as the skin flap has been raised.
- The overall angle of the cheek loop is approximately 30° across the cheek, as compared to the vertical neck loop.
- The suture is then tied under tension.
- Once the cheek loop is tied, it is possible to add a third loop for elevation of the malar fat; this constitutes the "extended MACS-lift" variant.
- A different anchor point is used anterior to the temporal branch of the facial nerve.
- This point can either be the deep temporal fascia just lateral to the lateral orbital rim, or the periosteum of the zygoma, approximately 1.5 cm lateral to the lateral canthal area.
- Access to either of these anchor points requires a small window in the orbicularis muscle where the fibers run vertically.
- This purse-string suture travels obliquely toward the malar fat pad where at a point 2 cm below the lateral canthus, the direction is reversed, creating a narrow U-shaped loop that is tight under tension.
- Tissue bunching is an integral problem with the MACS suture loops. It is resolved with imbrications with 4-0 polyglactin braided suture.

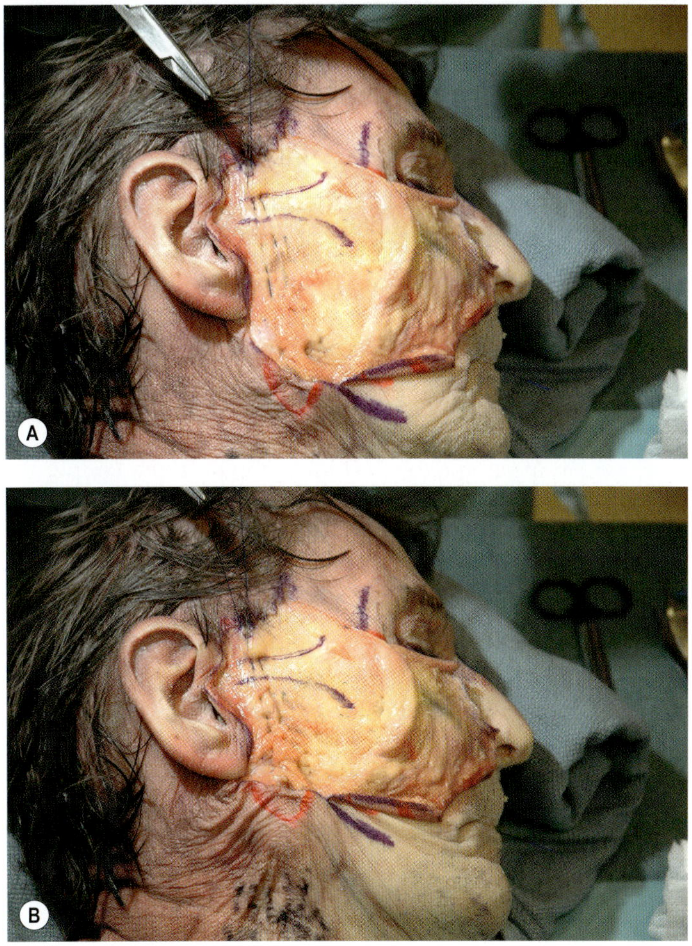

Figure 2.21 **(A,B)** Cadaveric example demonstrating placement and the effect of the vertical neck suture. The orientation is vertical, and neck traction depends on achieving excellent suture purchase of the platysma muscle below the angle of the mandible.

- Before leaving the deep tissue, it is necessary to place the skin flap over the tissue and observe for unresolved bunching and tissue tethering at the margins of the undermined area.
- Scissor removal of protruding fat may be needed in order to produce a smooth tissue surface inside the loops.
- Imbrication of tissue in the region just anterior to the tragus is important in order to preserve this normal sulcus.
- The skin flap is then redraped along a vertical axis and the excess skin is resected.
- The author's personal technique uses approximately 1 cc of fibrin glue (5 units/mL dilution) that is sprayed on the flaps and held for 3 min. This diminishes ecchymosis formation and eliminates the requirement for drains. Care must be given to not apply excessive fibrin glue as it can interfere with revascularization of the flaps.
- Wound closure is performed with absorbable 5-0 monofilament in the deeper layers and 5-0 and 6-0 polypropylene skin sutures placed as interrupted and continuous (horizontal mattress).

Lateral SMASectomy (Chapter 11.5)

- Virtually all of the author's procedural facelifts are performed with the patient under monitored intravenous propofol sedation. Patients are given oral clonidine, 0.1–0.2 mg, 30 min before surgery to control their blood pressure.
- The face and neck are infiltrated with local anesthesia, 0.5% lidocaine with 1:200000 epinephrine.
- Incisions are made in similar fashion as described above in the Subcutaneous facelift section.
- When the temporal hairline shift is assessed as minimal, the preferred incision is well within the temporal hair.
- When a larger skin shift is anticipated or the distance between the lateral canthus and temporal hairline is >5 cm, an incision a few millimeters within the temporal hairline is preferred.
- In short scar facelifting, efforts are made to end the incision at the base of the earlobe, but sometimes a short retroauricular incision is often necessary to correct a dog-ear after the facial flap rotation *(Fig. 2.22)*.
- Subcutaneous dissection is performed as outlined above.
- Dissection extends across the zygoma to release the zygomatic ligaments but stops several centimeters short of the nasolabial fold.
- In the cheek, dissection releases the masseteric-cutaneous ligaments and, if necessary, the mandibular ligaments.
- Subcutaneous dissection continues over the angle of the mandible and sternocleidomastoid for 5–6 cm into the neck, which exposes the posterior half of the platysma muscle.
- If a submental incision has been made, the facial and lateral neck dissection is connected through to the submental dissection.
- Some surgeons may employ closed suction assisted Lipoplasty in the neck and jowls.
- The outline of SMASectomy is marked on a tangent from the lateral malar eminence to the angle of the mandible, essentially in the region along the anterior edge of the parotid gland.
- In most patients, this involves a line of resection extending from the lateral aspect of the malar eminence toward the tail of the parotid gland.
- Usually, a 2–4 cm segment of superficial fascia is excised, depending on the degree of SMAS-platysma laxity *(Fig. 2.23)*.
- In SMAS resection, the author likes to pick up the superficial fascia region of the tail of the parotid, extending the resection from inferior to superior in a controlled fashion.
- When SMAS resection is being performed, it is important to keep the dissection superficial to the deep fascia and avoid dissection into the parotid parenchyma.
- The various vectors accomplish corrections of the anterior neck, the cervicomental angle, the jowls, and the nasolabial fold.
- The first key suture grasps the platysma at the angle of the mandible and advances it in a posterosuperior direction; it is secured with 2-0 Maxon (United States Surgical Corp., Norwalk, CT) to the fixed lateral SMAS overlying the parotid.
- This action lifts the cervical platysma and cervical skin.

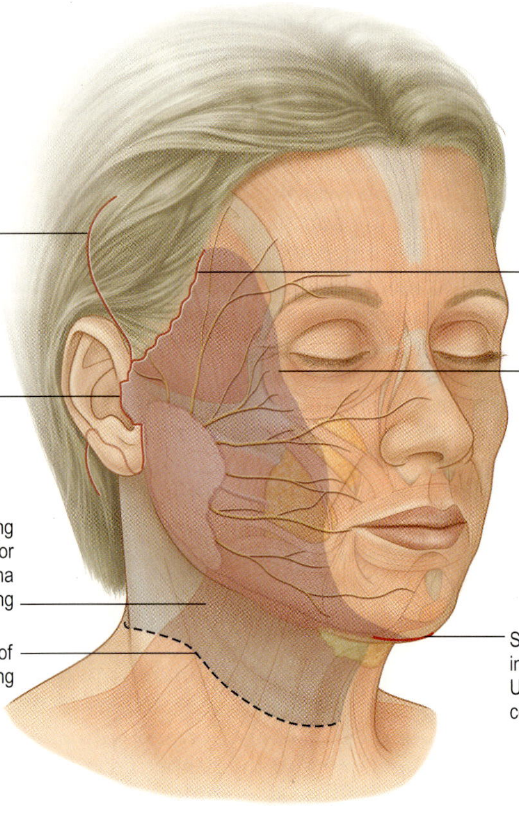

Figure 2.22 Incisions and extent of skin undermining.

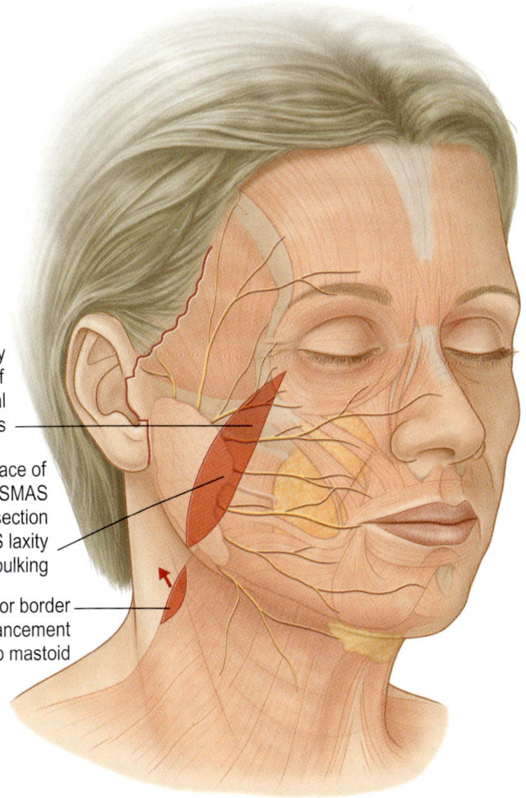

Figure 2.23 Lateral SMASectomy.

- After SMAS resection, interrupted 3-0 PDS buried sutures are used to close the SMASectomy, fixed lateral SMAS being evenly sutured to more mobile anterior superficial fascia.
- Vectors are usually perpendicular to the nasolabial fold.
- The last suture lifts the malar fat pad, securing it to the malar fascia.
- If firm monofilament sutures are used, such as PDA or Maxon, the sutures should be buried and sharp ends on the knot trimmed.
- Final contouring of any SMAS or fat irregularities along the suture line is completed with scissors.
- Skin redraping and closure completes the procedure *(Fig. 2.24)*.

Extended SMAS technique (Chapter 11.6)

(Figs 2.25-2.28)

SMAS with skin attached – the "high SMAS technique" (Chapter 11.7) (Video 2.6)

Video 2.6

- The initial incision location in the temporal area depends upon what is to be done with the forehead.
- If a bicoronal or hairline incision is to be utilized for the forehead, then that extension is used for the cheek dissection.
- If only an endoscopic approach or no forehead surgery is planned, then only a horizontal sideburn incision is done.

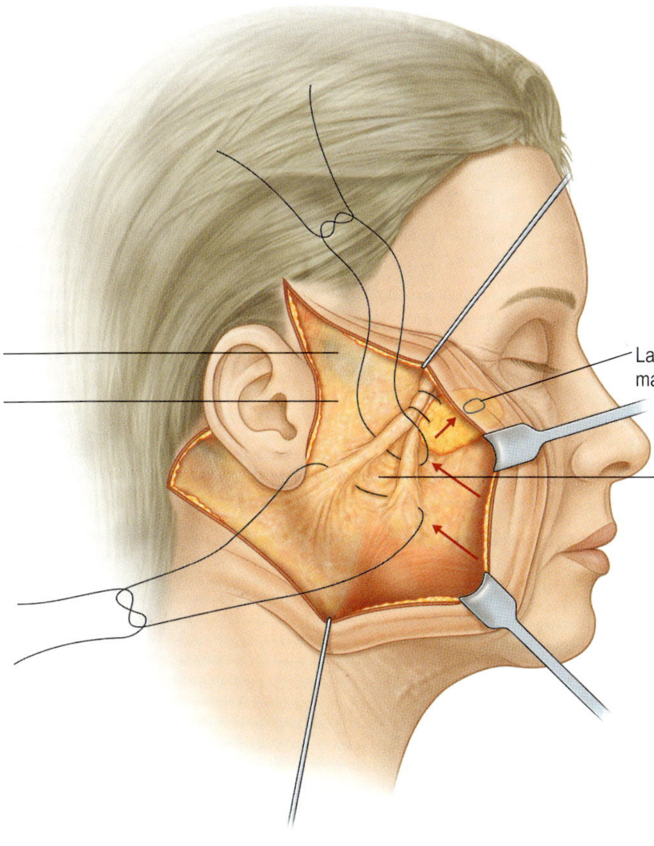

Figure 2.24 Optional plication of SMAS, for thin faces when debulking is not indicated.

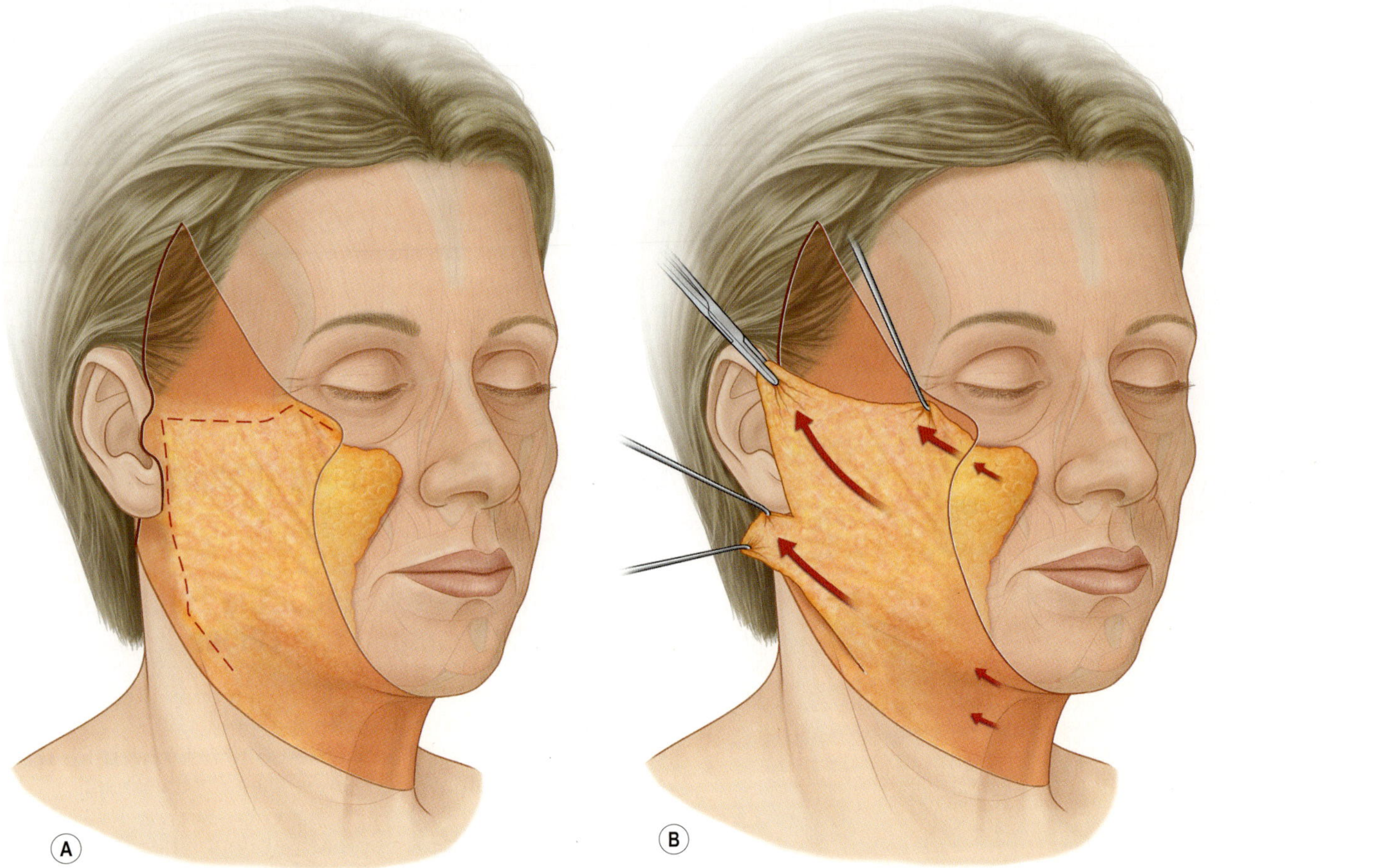

Figure 2.25 **(A)** If an extended SMAS dissection is to be performed, it is important not to widely undermine the skin all the way to the nasolabial fold, but rather to preserve some of the attachments that exist between the skin and the SMAS (the limit of subcutaneous undermining is the shaded area). If these attachments are left intact, this allows the surgeon to simultaneously re-suspend undissected anterior facial skin at the time of SMAS rotation and fixation. **(B)**It is important to understand which portion of the SMAS flap will affect facial contouring. In this diagram, the most superomedial aspect of the SMAS dissection affects contour along the nasolabial fold, whereas the more lateral portion of the SMAS dissection is used to re-elevate jowl fat upward into the cheek. A portion of the SMAS flap is rotated into the postauricular region with the vector of rotation of this portion of the SMAS dissection affecting submental and cervical contouring.

- A post-tragal auricular incision is used routinely in both males and females, except in dark skinned males with very dark, heavy beards.
- The cheek dissection is begun by elevating the skin in the pre-auricular area sharply.
- Above the level of the tragus, a subcutaneous tunnel is formed to the lateral border of the orbicularis oculi muscle.
- This tunnel will facilitate later horizontal division of the upper SMAS.
- From the tragus down, the skin flap is thinly dissected only to the extent of estimated skin excision *(Fig. 2.29)*.
- Care is taken not to overly separate the skin from the SMAS, especially at the upper corner where the previous tunnel was made.
- The lower extent of the subcutaneous cheek dissection extends below the mandibular border.
- If no previous neck skin dissection has been done, the submandibular skin dissection is carried approximately one-half way down the neck and one-half way to the midline.
- With the skin dissection complete, attention is turned to the SMAS. The safest place to penetrate the SMAS is between the top of the tragus and the bottom of the ear lobule where the SMAS is thickest.
- The proper dissection plane leaves a thin translucent fibrous layer over the visible parotid acini.
- As this dissection plane is extended anteriorly and inferiorly an areolar plane on the underside of identifiable platysma fibers can be visualized.
- Once in this areolar plane, dissection is carried to the anterior border of the parotid gland, and down the anterior border of the sternocleidomastoid muscle.
- At the anterior border of the parotid gland, the dissection method changes from sharp to blunt spreading in the anterior areolar plane.
- Over the parotid gland, the SMAS is fixed to the gland capsule – the so-called "fixed SMAS".
- Anterior to the parotid gland, in the buccal area, there is an areolar gliding plane which can be separated bluntly, to avoid any risk to the underlying facial nerve branches.
- It is imperative to maintain the filmy, near-transparent deep fascia over the masseter muscle, since the facial nerve branches lie just beneath.

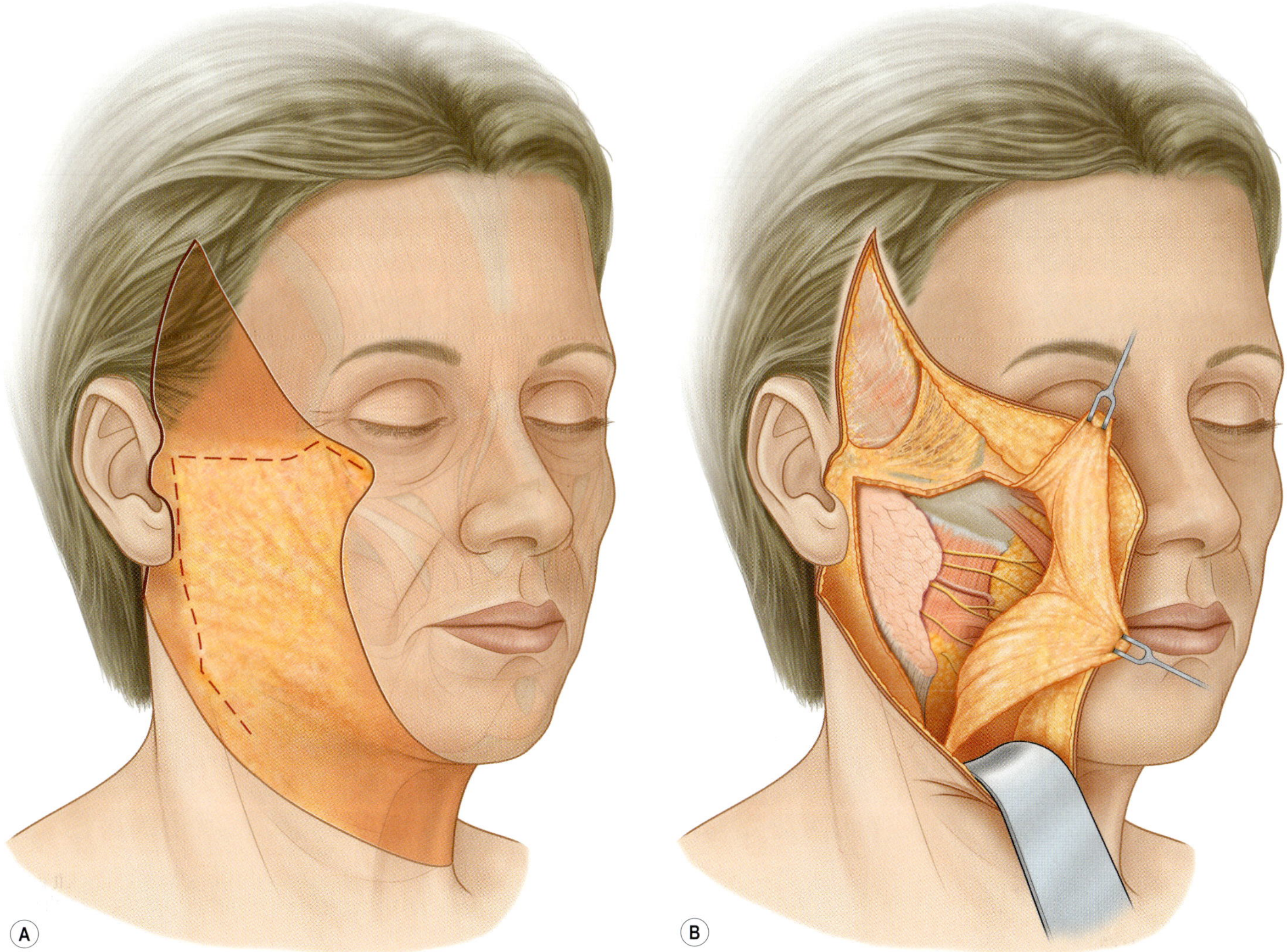

Figure 2.26 **(A)** In patients with malar deflation or malar pad descent, an extended SMAS dissection can be performed in which the SMAS dissection is extended into the malar region in an attempt to re-elevate ptotic malar fat back upward over the zygomatic prominence. The incisions begin at the junction where the zygomatic arch joins the body of the zygoma. From this point, the incision in the SMAS is angled superiorly toward the lateral canthus and along the lateral orbital rim. The incision in the SMAS is then carried medially and inferiorly toward the peripheral extent of skin flap undermining, angling toward the uppermost portion of the nasolabial fold (the amount of subcutaneous undermining is shaded in pink, whereas the amount of SMAS undermining is shaded in yellow.) **(B)** The malar-SMAS dissection is then performed in continuity with the cheek-SMAS dissection. Dissecting in the malar region carries the dissection directly along the superficial surface of the zygomaticus major and usually exposes the lateral aspects of the zygomaticus minor as well. To obtain adequate mobility in terms of SMAS dissection, it is necessary to elevate the malar portion of the dissection completely from the zygomatic eminence and free it from the zygomatic ligaments. To obtain mobility in terms of SMAS movement affecting the jowl contour, the uppermost portions of the masseteric cutaneous ligament commonly are divided, especially where they merge with the zygomatic ligaments of the malar area. If these fibers are not divided, they will restrict the upward redraping of jowl fat. On division of the upper portion of the masseteric cutaneous ligaments, the buccal fat pad becomes evident, and commonly the zygomatic nerve branches traversing toward the undersurface of the zygomaticus major muscle are visualized. This diagram illustrates the typical degree of mobilization performed in our extended SMAS dissection.

- Inferiorly, the dissection continues down the fascial fusion plane at the anterior border of the sternocleidomastoid muscle.
- Here a short 2–3 cm "back cut" in the investing fascia and platysma is made about 4 cm below the mandibular border.
- The "back cut" is made at this level to avoid any aberrant branches of the marginal mandibular facial nerve.
- The SMAS is divided horizontally above the zygomatic arch over to the lateral orbicularis.
- Using the visible edge of the orbicularis as a depth marker, the dissection is carried over the malar area to release the zygomatic retaining ligaments.
- With the inferior-lateral border of the orbicularis oculi muscle as a depth gauge, the dissection is carried over the lateral border of the zygomaticus major muscle into the subcutaneous plane.
- Dissection is then carried down the lateral border of the zygomaticus major muscle to the level of the modiolus ***(Fig. 2.30)***.
- In patients with minimal nasolabial fold depth, dissection stops short of the fold to preserve attachment of the fat to the cheek flap ***(Fig. 2.31)***.
- In patients with deep nasolabial folds, usually associated with a thin face, complete dissection across the nasolabial fold into the lip is done ***(Fig. 2.32)***.

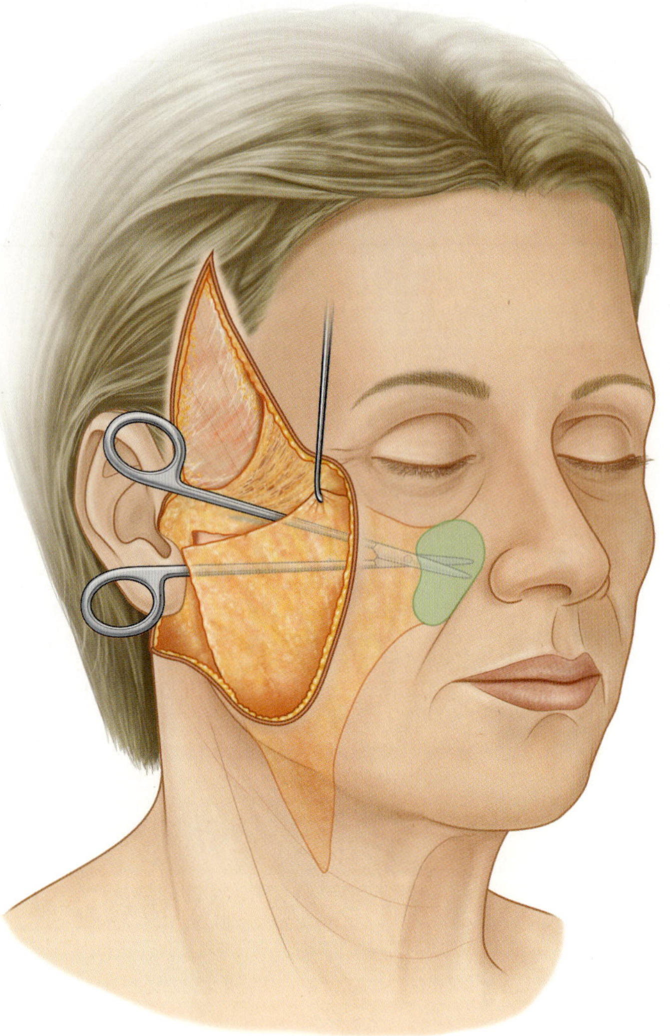

Figure 2.27 It is commonly necessary to extend the malar SMAS dissection more peripherally than the subcutaneous dissection to obtain adequate flap mobility of the soft tissues lateral to the nasolabial fold. This portion of the dissection is easily performed by simply inserting the scissors in the plane between the superficial surface of the elevators of the upper lip and the overlying subcutaneous fat. Once the scissors are inserted in the proper plane, the surgeon bluntly dissects in a series of passes past the nasolabial fold (area marked in green). As long as the scissors remain superficial to the elevators of the upper lip, motor nerve injury will be prevented. Usually three or four passes are required to obtain adequate flap mobility.

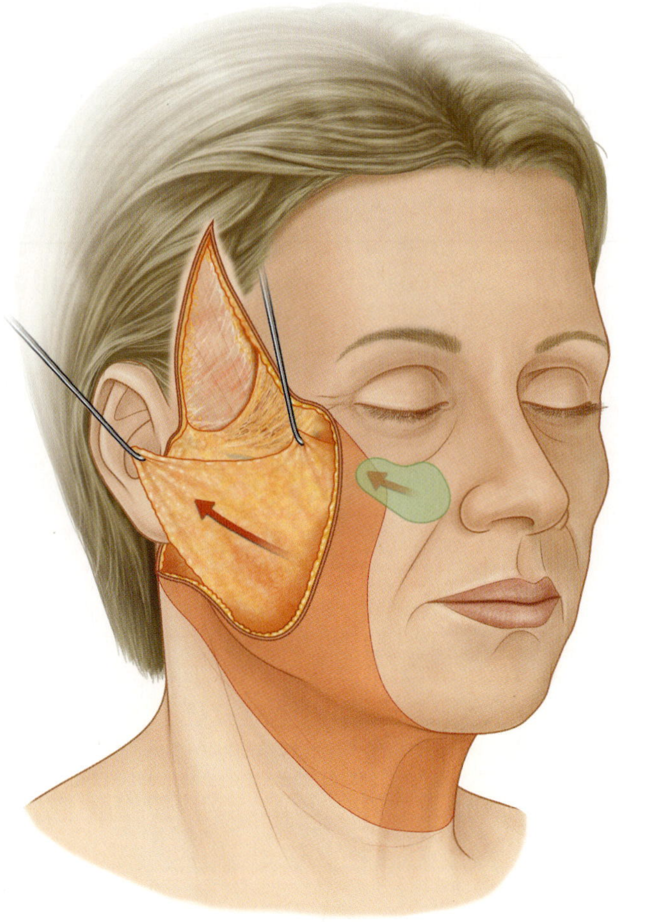

Figure 2.28 The vectors of redraping of the extended SMAS flap are determined according to the preoperative evaluation of the patient and are generally more cephalad than skin flap redraping.

- With completion of this release, the entire subcutaneous cheek mass, from mandible to orbit, will freely move superiorly.
  - It is paramount to mobilize the cheek in a pure vertical – not horizontal or oblique – direction. The primary vector is vertical along the lateral orbital rim *(Fig. 2.33)*.
- Key sutures are placed in the deep temporal fascia and in the mastoid fascia.
- The periauricular SMAS is then completely closed with a continuous suture to disperse the tension from the key sutures.
- Redundant skin is trimmed in place and closed in similar fashion as described above.

Subperiosteal midfacelift (Chapter 11.8) (Video 2.7)

Video 2.7

- In this author's particular technique, the subperiosteal midfacelift is often combined with a functional lower blepharoplasty in an effort to rejuvenate the lower eyelid while preserving its function.
- The midfacelift begins with Xylocaine 0.5% mixed with epinephrine at 1/200 000 dilution, which is infiltrated in the temporal and midface areas.
- The midface is approached from above through a temporal incision, and from below through an intraoral buccal mucosal incision.
- The length of the incision in the temporal area will depend on the technique used.
- In the open approach, the incision is either a coronal incision if the forehead lift is also done concomitantly or a limited temporal-frontal incision.
- Dissection in the temporal area separates the superficial temporal fascia from the temporal fascia proper in the upper temporal area, and the superficial temporal fascia from the intermediate temporal fascia in the lower temporal area.

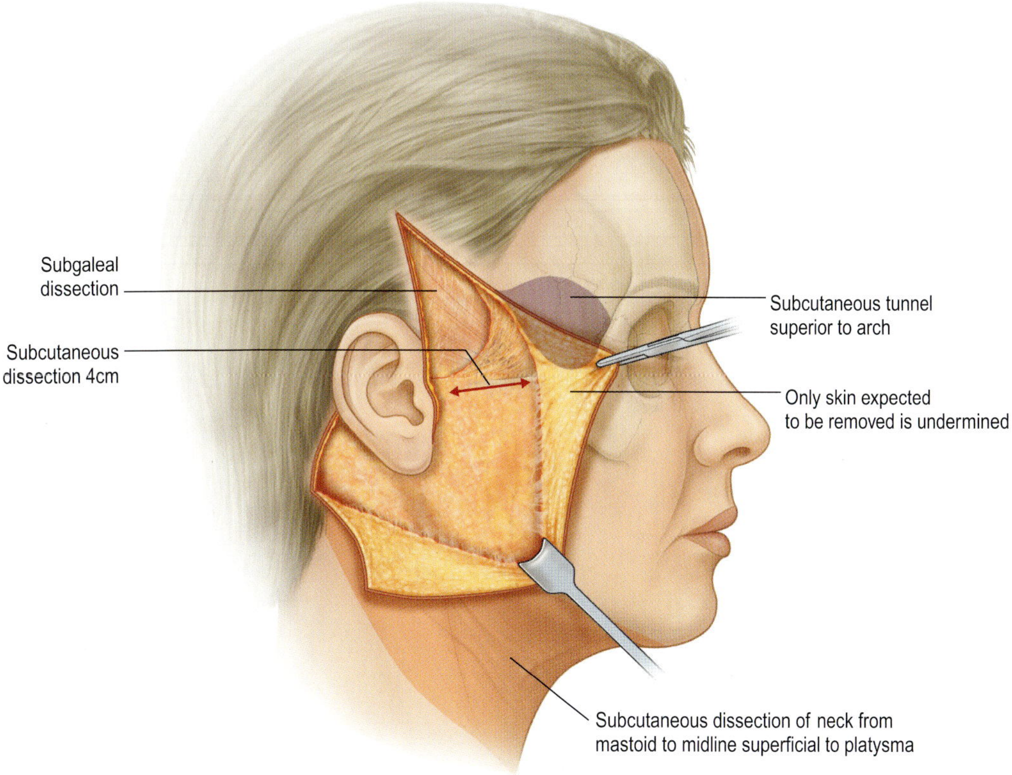

Figure 2.29 In the high SMAS technique, the skin flap is thinly dissected only to the extent of estimated skin excision.

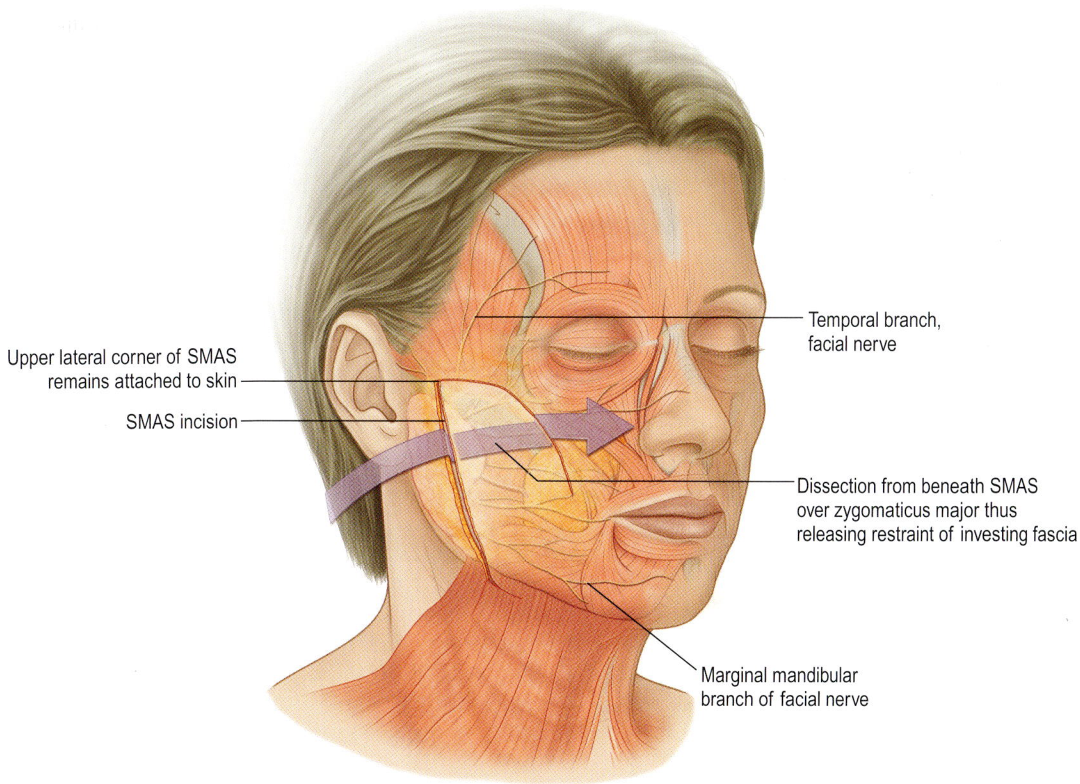

Figure 2.30 Complete release of the SMAS.

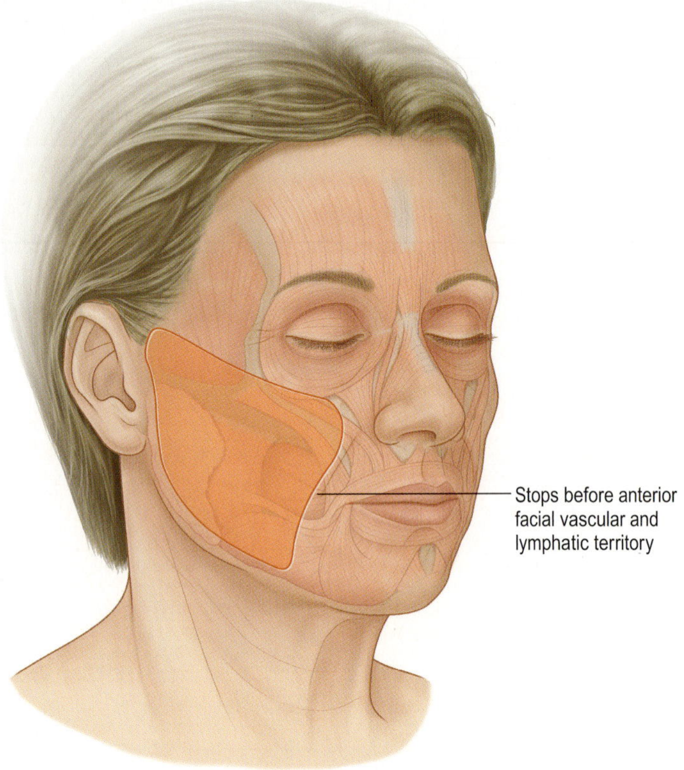

Figure 2.31 In patients with minimal nasolabial fold depth, dissection stops short of the fold to preserve attachment of the fat to the cheek flap

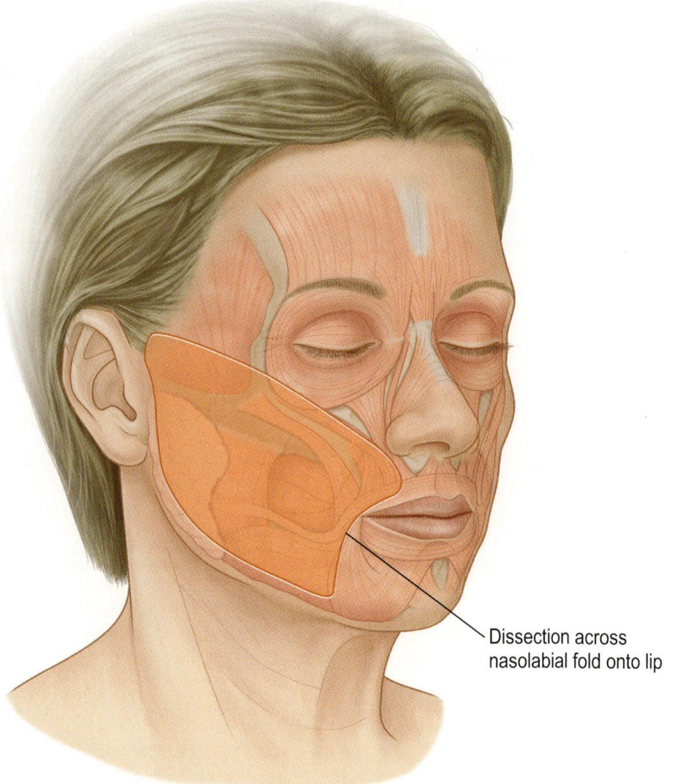

Figure 2.32 Cheek dissection across the nasolabial fold into the lip in patients with deep nasolabial folds.

- In the endoscopic technique, dissection continues in this plane until the superior border of the zygomaticus arch is reached.
- With upward traction of the temporal flap, the periosteum of the zygomaticus arch is elevated with a sharp periosteum elevator.
- In the open approach the intermediate temporal fascia with its attached intermediate fat pad is elevated 2–3 cm above the zygomaticus arch and the periosteum is dissected in continuity.
- This fascial flap will be used as an anchor suspension of the midface.
- Next, the intraoral buccal incision is made at the level of the first premolar and done either vertically or slightly obliquely.
- The initial incision is done through the mucosa only, then the buccinator muscle is spread with the periosteal elevator and a subperiosteal dissection is carried out on the maxilla and malar bones.
- Medially, this extends to the pyriformis area and laterally underneath the fascia of the masseter muscle.
- This lateral extension goes about 2.5 cm over the masseter tendon.
- Dissection superiorly is done to separate the orbicularis muscle attachments to the inferior orbital rim, thus releasing the arcus marginalis.
- The attachments around the infraorbital nerve are freed after the fixation points on the midface are applied and just before their fixation in the temporal fascia proper.
- Subperiosteal dissection of the midface is connected with the temporal optical cavity over the anterior two-thirds of the zygomatic arch ***(Fig. 2.34)***.
- Dissection includes elevation of the soft tissues from the external lateral orbital rim.
- The sutures applied to the midface have the following effects: suspension, volumetric remodeling, and lifting.
- The author routinely uses four sutures per side ***(Fig. 2.35)***:
- The first suture anchors the anterior central SOOF (suborbicularis oculi fat) to the most anterior portion of the temporal fascia proper near the lateral orbital rim using a 4-0 polydioxanone (PDS) suture.
- Prior to passing to the temporal area it can be anchored to the immediately superior arcus marginalis which will act as a pulley to direct the anterior SOOF towards the orbital rim area helping to efface the tear trough area.
- The second suture anchors the lateral SOOF to the compound periosteum/SOOF tissue 3 cm inferior and vertical to the lateral canthal tendon insertion using a 3-0 PDS suture.
- The third suture, the modiolus suspension, anchors the fibro-adipose tissue just inferior to the most anterior portion of the intraoral incision to the temporal region using a 4-0 PDS suture.
- The final suture is applied to the Bichat's or buccal fat pad.
- To place the suture, you must first open the anterior-medial wall of the fat pad, just medial to the masseter tendon using a blunt and long scissor.

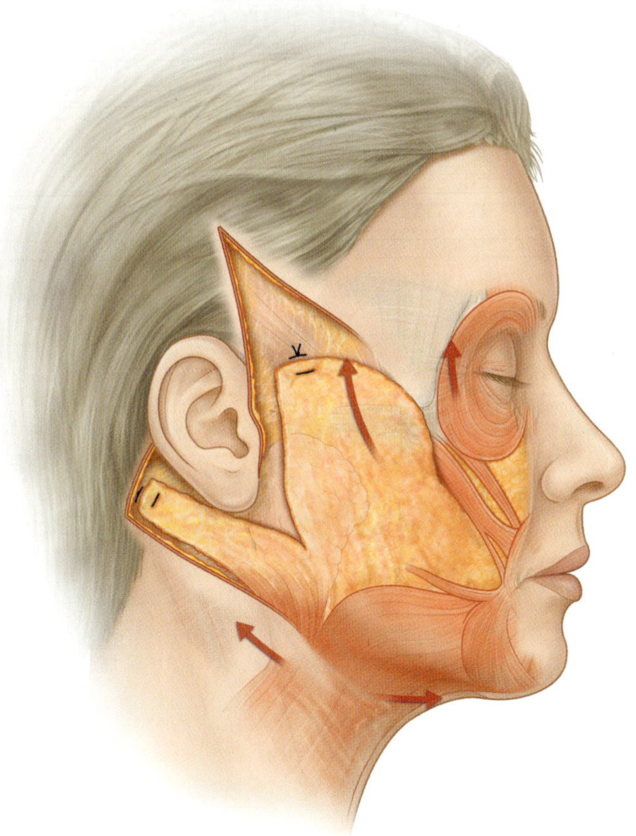

Figure 2.33 The cheek mass is suspended vertically (shown with key sutures), and the entire SMAS flap is closed with a continuous suture to disperse the tension from the key sutures. An orbicularis flap is then done to suspend the orbicularis.

- Once the blades of the scissors are opened, the fat pad will extrude from its encased buccal space.
- It is then gently pulled with two blunt scissors and delivered with external pressure on the cheek.
- Once the fat pad has been delivered, a 4-0 PDS suture with an RB1 needle is weaved into the fat pad utilizing two or three passes.
- This suture is then anchored to the loop of the SOOF suture applied beforehand, using a "piggy backing" technique.
- This limits the upward mobilization of the buccal fat pad and its potential avulsion.
- All the sutures anchored to the temporal area are done using the endoscopic sliding Peruvian fisherman's knot.
- A 2 mm "butterfly" drain is introduced via a mini stab incision.
- The last suspension suture is applied to the superficial temporal fascia at the inferior lip of the temporal entrance port and anchored to the temporal fascia proper above and anterior to it.
- The scalp is closed with staples.
- The midface cavity is irrigated with antibiotic solution and closure of the intraoral incision is done with interrupted 4-0 chromic catgut sutures.
- Once the midface lift is completed, the lower blepharoplasty can be performed.

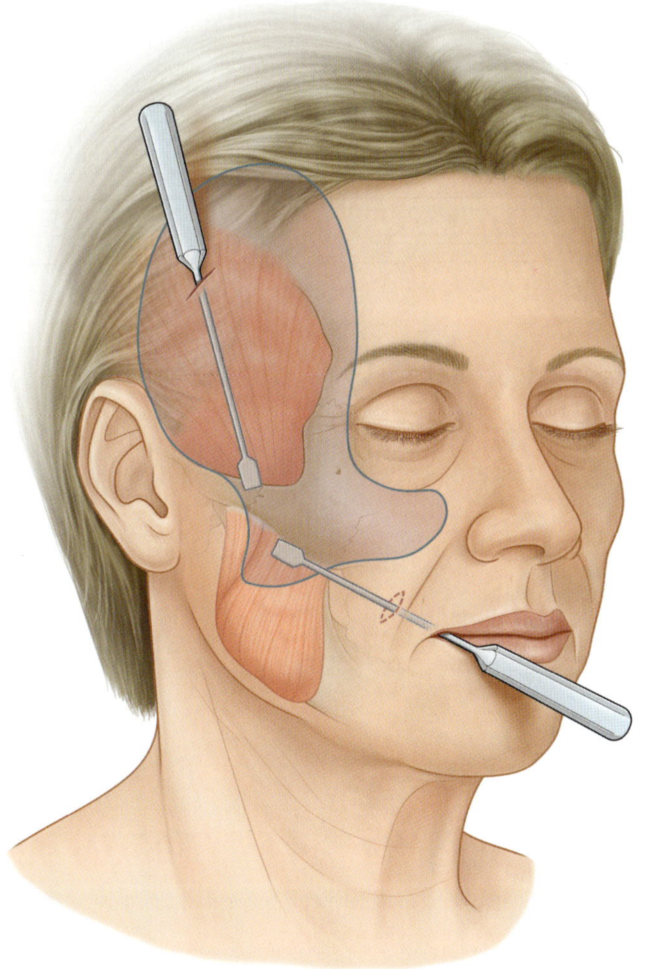

Fig. 2.34 The "endo-midface" is approached by a single temporal and an intraoral incision. For this reason, it is better called an endotemporo-midface procedure. The midface and temporal cavities are connected across the zygomatic arch. The subperiosteal dissection here is critical to avoid injuring the frontal branch of the facial nerve. The midface dissection extends under the masseteric fascia for 2–3 cm.

- For the lower blepharoplasty in this instance, this author makes a skin incision 2 mm below the ciliary border which is extended directly into the crow's foot area.
- The full thickness lower eyelid skin is "peeled" off the orbicularis muscle layer for an average of 1.5–2 cm inferiorly, creating a pure skin flap.
- The exposed lateral extension of the preseptal portion is anchored to the most anterior portion of the temporal fascia proper with a 5-0 or 6-0 Prolene suture.
- For this maneuver, a window in the lateral orbital portion of the orbicularis muscle is created with a blunt dissection.
- The lower eyelid incision can be closed as described in the blepharoplasty chapter.

Postoperative considerations

- Most surgeons use light dressings to protect the incisions and to act as an absorbent for wound drainage.

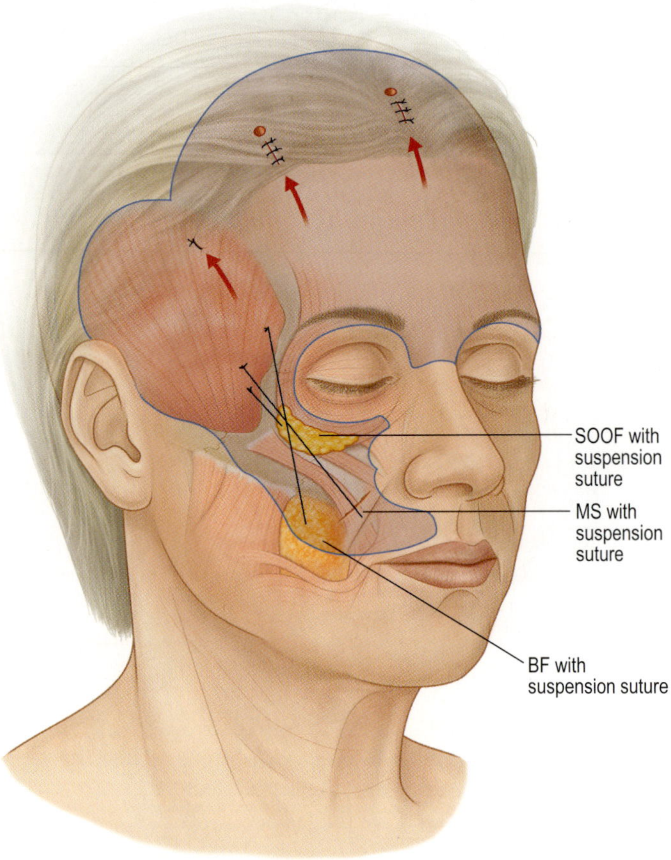

Fig. 2.35 An endoscopic browlift is shown in conjunction with an endoscopic midfacelift. For the midfacelift, four sutures are used to obtain the maximal remodeling and beneficial effect of the subperiosteal dissection. The anterior SOOF (suborbicularis oculi fat) effaces the infraorbital V deformity. The lateral SOOF lifts the midface. The MS (modiolus suspension) lifts the corner of the mouth. These three sutures also produce imbrication, thus increasing the anterior projection of the cheek. The last suture suspension is the buccal (Bichat's) fat pad (BF). This is the structure that helps more than any other to create the Ogee line of the midface.

- Dressings should not be tight or constrictive, but rather soft and comfortable and are typically removed on the first postoperative day.
- In the initial postoperative period, the patient is kept still and blood pressure is monitored closely.
- If an increase in blood pressure is endogenous, it should be treated pharmacologically.
- The patient should keep the head of the bed elevated, but avoiding flexion of the neck.
- Avoiding the use of a pillow for 10–14 days will help keep the patient's head in a neutral, non-flexed position.
- Cool packs to the face will increase comfort and help decrease swelling.
- Analgesics and antinauseants are used as necessary.
- Patients are usually permitted to have a shower and wash their hair when the incisions are sealed from the environment – usually 2–4 days postoperatively.
- Photographic documentation of the surgical result should be deferred for at least 6 months to allow for all postoperative swelling to settle completely.

Complications and outcomes

Hematoma

- Postoperative hematoma is the most common facelift complication.
- Incidence in women has been reported at 2–3%.
- Incidence in men has been reported between 4 and 8%.
- Hematomas typically develop in the first 12 h after surgery.
- If an expanding hematoma is identified it should be promptly drained.
- If skin flap compromise is suspected and there is a delay in returning to the operation, a temporary solution can be the removal of sutures in order to relieve pressure *(Fig. 2.33)*.

Sensory nerve injury

- A self-limiting paresthesia which usually recovers completely in 6–12 months can occur after facelift surgery.
- The great auricular nerve is the major sensory nerve at greatest risk of damage during facelift surgery.
- If knowingly transected during facelift surgery, either partial or complete, it should be repaired intraoperatively.

Motor nerve injury

- Damage to a facial nerve branch can easily go unnoticed by the surgeon until muscle paralysis is identified postoperatively. However, permanent paralysis is a rare event and has been reported to occur in less than 1% of cases.
- Persistent dysfunction may be due to surgical traction or the effect of cautery near a nerve branch; these issues can be expected to resolve spontaneously over days or weeks.
- If a facial nerve branch has been transected or wrapped in a suture, complete functional recovery may still be possible if the target muscle receives collateral innervation.
- The most commonly injured branches are thought to be the buccal branches, although long-term sequelae are rare due to multiple interconnections between nerve branches.
- Damaged temporal or marginal mandibular branches are less likely to recover because they are terminal branches with less collateral support.

Unsatisfactory scars

- Improper placement of incisions can lead to distortion of the ear and unnatural shifting of the hairline.
- Excessive tension can lead to loss of hair, depigmentation and widened scars, and/or hypertrophic scars.

Alopecia

- Loss of hair can occur along the incision line or within the hair-bearing scalp which has been raised as a flap.
- Permanent hair loss can be treated in some cases by mobilization of an adjacent flap of hair-bearing scalp.
- For significant alopecia, achieving adequate coverage with hair growth in the proper direction is best achieved with micro-hair-grafting.

Skin loss

- Factors which can contribute to the avascular loss of skin include excessive tension, an overly thin flap, hematoma, constrictive dressings, and perhaps the most damaging of all – smoking.
- Established skin necrosis should be dealt with conservatively; the majority of such cases will eventually heal spontaneously. Scar revision can be done at a later date.

Infection

- Infection is reported to be rare in facelift surgery, with various series indicating an incidence of less than 1%.

Further reading

Coleman SR. Facial recontouring with lipostructure. *Clin Plast Surg*. 1997;24(2):347.

A pioneer of facial fat grafting presents early experiences with lipoinjection of the face.

Coleman SR. *Structural fat grafting*. St Louis: Quality Medical; 2004.

This text is a comprehensive review of the history, basic science and technical details of fat harvest and fat injection.

Gosain AK, Amarante MTJ, Hyde JS, et al. A dynamic analysis of changes in the nasolabial fold using magnetic resonance imaging: Implications for facial rejuvenation and facial animation surgery. *Plast Reconstr Surg*. 1996;98:622.

A comparative MRI study demonstrates the changes in subcutaneous fat which develop with age. The authors conclude that superficial fat in the cheek becomes ptotic while the underlying elevators of the lip do not elongate with age.

Jones BM, Grover R. Avoiding hematoma in cervicofacial rhytidectomy: a personal 8-year quest. Reviewing 910 patients. *Plast Reconstr Surg*. 2004;113:381.

The authors review a large facelift series where the most common complication of facelift surgery, hematoma, is addressed. Variables thought to influence the formation of hematoma were reviewed, including the use of dressings, drains, soft tissue adhesives and epinephrine.

Marten TJ. Facelift planning and technique. *Clin Plast Surg*. 1997;24(2):269–308.

This review article covers the planning, surgical marking and technical details of two layer facelift surgery. Details regarding the skin incisions are emphasized.

Mitz V, Peyronie M. The superficial musculoaponeurotic system (SMAS) in the parotid and cheek area. *Plast Reconstr Surg*. 1976;58:80.

This paper is the first description of the superficial musculoaponeurotic system.

Rohrich RJ, Pessa JE. The fat compartments of the face: anatomy and clinical implications for cosmetic surgery. *Plast Reconstr Surg*. 2007;119:2219–2227.

Anatomic dissections are presented which demonstrate how the subcutaneous fat of the face is partitioned into multiple, independent anatomical compartments. In some locations, the septae dividing the fat compartments are aligned with retaining ligaments.

Rohrich RJ, Pessa JE, Ristow B. The youthful cheek and the deep medial fat compartment. *Plast Reconstr Surg*. 2008;121(6):2107–2112.

Anatomic dissections of deep facial fat are presented (fat which is deep to the muscles of facial expression). The deep fat is compartmentalized by septae, creating the deep medial fat pad, and the suborbicularis oculi fat.

Stuzin J. Restoring facial shape in facelifting: the role of skeletal support in facial analysis and midface soft-tissue repositioning (Baker Gordon Symposium Cosmetic Series). *Plast Reconstr Surg*. 2007;119:362.

This review discusses the changes in facial shape which occur with aging, the surgical means we have to correct these changes, and alterations which should be made with different degrees of underlying skeletal support.

Stuzin JM. Discussion: essays on the facial nerve: Part I. Microanatomy. *Plast Reconstr Surg*. 2010;125(3):890–892.

Stuzin JM, Baker TJ, Gordon HL. The relationship of the superficial and deep facial fascias: relevance to rhytidectomy and aging. *Plast Reconstr Surg*. 1992;89:441.

Anatomic dissections confirm the presence of retaining ligaments previously described by other authors as well as newly described masseteric ligaments. The authors discuss the support these structures supply between fixed bone and deep fascia and the superficial fascia.

Tzafetta K, Terzis J. Essays on the facial nerve: Part I. Microanatomy. *Plast Reconstr Surg*. 2010;125(3):879–889.

The authors review facial nerve anatomy and present anatomic findings which confirm extensive arborization between facial nerve branches. The discussion by Stuzin highlights clinically important issues.

3 Chapter

Rhinoplasty

This chapter was created using content from Neligan & Warren, Plastic Surgery 3rd edition, Volume 2, Aesthetic, Chapter 18, Open technique rhinoplasty, Rod J. Rohrich and Jamil Ahmad/ Chapter 19, Closed technique rhinoplasty, Mark B. Constantian.

SYNOPSIS (OPEN RHINO)

- Accurate preoperative analysis and clinical diagnosis set the foundation for successful primary open rhinoplasty.
- Open rhinoplasty allows anatomic exposure, identification, and correction of nasal deformities.
- Component dorsal hump reduction allows accurate and incremental reduction of the nasal dorsum while preventing problems with internal valve collapse or dorsal irregularities.
- Nasal tip suturing techniques allow control of definition without damaging the osseocartilaginous framework and compromising support.
- Knowledge of the normal course of recovery and potential complications is key to managing patient expectations in the postoperative period.

SYNOPSIS (CLOSED RHINO)

- Nature is predictable – therefore nasal phenomenology can be understood.
- Rhinoplasty has consistent "behavioral" rules, like all surgery – therefore the surgeon can control the result.
- Nasal deformities are not limitless or lawless but follow patterns – therefore their solutions follow patterns.
- Sequential intraoperative photography teaches nasal behavior and structural interactions.
- Follow the technical rules that apply to all other surgery: limit dissection, morbidity, and tension on closure.
- Reconstruct anatomically.
- Never forget function.
- Never forget the patient's own aesthetic.
- Remember that most problems are under the surgeon's control.
- Always follow your patients closely.

Brief introduction

- Regardless of your preferred technique, a thorough knowledge of nasal anatomy and understanding of nasal airflow and physiology are the foundations for successful aesthetic and functional rhinoplasty.
- Proponents of open rhinoplasty argue that closed rhinoplasty is difficult because the surgeon does not have good binocular vision through small incisions, the dissection is blind, the anatomy is complex, and the operation is technically difficult.
- Proponents of endonasal or closed rhinoplasty techniques point to two common considerations:
  - First, by separating columellar skin from the medial crura, the surgeon loses an important component of tip stability and projection, which therefore requires some method (suture fixation or columellar strut) to support the medial crura so that a new nasal tip can be made. The strut can impart rigidity to the columella and increases graft requirements.
  - In primary patients, this consideration may be unimportant, but in secondary patients, whose donor sites are already depleted, every bit of graft material counts.
  - Though incisions are limited, endonasal rhinoplasty is not a blind operation. Most procedures are performed under direct vision with greater access than endoscopic surgery permits.
  - The operative strategy, making skeletal changes through limited incisions and judging progress by feeling the surface, is precisely the same discipline required by suction-assisted lipectomy.
  - Limited pocket dissection minimizes the need for graft fixation and simplifies some procedures.
  - Solid or crushed grafts can be used in ways that would be tedious or impossible by the open approach, although some solutions have been described.

- In rhinoplasty, there are four common anatomic variants that predispose to unfavorable results:
- Low radix or low dorsum:
  - Low radix or low dorsum begins caudal to the level of the upper lash margin with the patient's eyes in primary gaze.
  - The low radix is one of several primary causes of nasal imbalance: an upper nose that seems too small for its lower nasal component.
  - When the radix begins lower than the upper lash margin, dorsal length is therefore shorter and so nasal base size appears larger.
  - If the surgeon reduces the nasal dorsum, the patient's preoperative skeletal and skin sleeve maldistribution will worsen and the lower nose will appear even larger.
  - The surgeon should instead either limit tip reduction or raise the dorsum segmentally or entirely to balance the nasal base.
- A narrow middle vault:
  - Arbitrarily defined as any upper cartilaginous vault that is at least 25% narrower than the upper or lower nasal third. This variant is a trait that places the patient at special risk for internal valvular obstruction, which can exist preoperatively or may be produced by dorsal resection.
  - Inadequate tip projection is defined as any tip that does not project to the level of the anterior septal angle.
  - Alar cartilages sufficiently strong to support the tip to the level of the septal angle are "adequately projecting"; alar cartilages too weak to do so are "inadequately projecting".
  - The practical value of this definition lies in its ability to define treatment: adequately projecting tips do not need increased support, whereas inadequately projecting tips do.
  - "Alar cartilage malposition" describes cephalically-rotated lateral crura whose long axes run on an axis toward the medial canthi instead of toward the lateral canthi, the position of orthotopic lateral crura.
  - This anatomic variation was first recognized by Sheen as an aesthetic deformity that produced a round or boxy tip lobule with characteristic "parentheses" on frontal view.
  - Malposition also has two additional ramifications that are not aesthetic:
  - First, the abnormal cephalic position of the lateral crura places them at special risk if an intercartilaginous incision is made at its normal intranasal location.
  - Second, most malpositioned lateral crura do not provide adequate external valvular support, and so malposition is not only associated with boxy or ball tips but also the leading cause of external valvular incompetence.
  - None of these four anatomical variants (low radix or low dorsum, narrow middle vault, inadequate tip projection, and alar cartilage malposition) always require treatment, but they do supply cautionary notes.
  - The most common grouping in both primary and secondary patients was the triad of low radix, narrow middle vault, and inadequate tip projection.
  - The second most common grouping was the association of all four anatomic traits.
- For many years, the following concepts provided the basis for analysis of the obstructed nose:
  - The bony and cartilaginous septal partition, deformed by congenital or traumatic causes, may obstruct the nasal airway.
  - Compensatory hypertrophy of the contralateral inferior turbinate frequently occurs, so that both airways eventually become obstructed.
- These concepts are more understandable if the reader considers airway size to be the product of at least four factors: (1) mucosal sensitivity to the environment or hereditary factors; (2) inferior turbinate hypertrophy from many causes; (3) septal deviation; and (4) position and stability of the lateral nasal wall during the dynamic process of ventilation.

Preoperative considerations

- Obtain information on the patient's medical and emotional suitability to undergo rhinoplasty.
- Feelings of inadequacy, immaturity, family conflicts, divorce, and other major life changes may be unhealthy motivating factors behind the patient seeking aesthetic surgery.
- Poor postoperative patient satisfaction is often based on emotional dissatisfaction as opposed to technical failure, and this can be avoided by the preoperative identification of these unhealthy motivating factors.
- Review past medical history and specifically note a history of allergic disorders, including hayfever and asthma, and other problems, including vasomotor rhinitis and sinusitis. These conditions should be controlled prior to rhinoplasty, however, patients should be informed that they may be exacerbated in the postoperative period and can persist for weeks to months.
- Nasal obstruction is usually found in patients with a long history of allergic rhinitis secondary to inferior turbinate hypertrophy. Engorgement of the inferior turbinates causes these symptoms to be worse at night. Patient's may also complain of headache because of the inadequacy of the inferior turbinate to warm inspired air.
- Prior nasal trauma and surgeries, including rhinoplasty, septal reconstruction/septoplasty and sinus surgery, should be noted.
- Smoking, alcohol consumption, and use of illicit drugs, in particular cocaine, can compromise outcomes. Medications including acetylsalicylic acid, nonsteroidal anti-inflammatory drugs, fish oil, and certain herbal supplements may cause increased risk of bleeding and postoperative ecchymosis.

Table 3.1 External nasal analysis

Frontal view	
Facial proportions	
Skin type/quality	Fitzpatrick type, thin or thick, sebaceous
Symmetry and nasal deviation	Midline, C-, reverse C-, S- or S-shaped deviation
Bony vault	Narrow or wide, asymmetrical, short or long nasal bones
Midvault	Narrow or wide, collapse, inverted-V deformity
Dorsal aesthetic lines	Straight, symmetrical or asymmetrical, well or ill defined, narrow or wide
Nasal tip	Ideal/bulbous/boxy/pinched, supratip, tip defining points, infratip lobule
Alar rims	Gull-shaped, facets, notching, retraction
Alar base	Width
Upper lip	Long or short, dynamic depressor septi muscles, upper-lip crease
Lateral view	
Nasofrontal angle	Acute or obtuse, high or low radix
Nasal length	Long or short
Dorsum	Smooth, hump, scooped out
Supratip	Break, fullness, polybeak
Tip projection	Over- or underprojected
Tip rotation	Over- or underrotated
Alar–columellar relationship	Hanging or retracted alae, hanging or retracted columella
Periapical hypoplasia	Maxillary or soft tissue deficiency
Lip–chin relationship	Normal, deficient
Basal view	
Nasal projection	Over- or underprojected, columellar–lobular ratio
Nostril	Symmetrical or asymmetrical, long or short
Columella	Septal tilt, flaring of medial crura
Alar base	Width
Alar flaring	

- Anatomic examination includes both external nasal analysis (Table 3.1) and internal nasal examination (Table 3.2). In addition, facial analysis plays a key role in achieving facial harmony after rhinoplasty.
- Standardized photography is obtained for every patient presenting for rhinoplasty and includes frontal, lateral, oblique, and basal views of the patient.
- It is useful to review photographs with the patient to identify areas of concern that can be addressed with

Table 3.2 Internal nasal exam

External valve	Collapse
Internal valve	Narrowing, collapse
Mucosa	Edema, irritation
Inferior turbinates	Hypertrophy
Septum	Deviation, tilt, spurs, perforation, cartilage
Masses	Polyps, tumors

surgery and deformities that may persist after surgery, including notches, grooves, and irregularities. Facial disproportions and asymmetries should be pointed out to the patient as these may require orthognathic surgery to address.
- Identifying the patient's expectations preoperatively is a key component to postoperative patient satisfaction and successful rhinoplasty.
- Common concerns include asymmetry, tip deformities, dorsum irregularities, and nasal airway obstruction.
- The patient should attempt to rank these concerns in order of importance.
- A patient who focuses on minor or uncorrectable problems or who has unrealistic expectations despite extensive discussion will likely be disappointed following surgery regardless of the aesthetic improvement; it is better to avoid operating on these patients.
- In general, the ideal candidate for surgery has legitimate concerns and realistic expectations, and is secure, well informed and understands the limitations of surgery.
- The acronym SYLVIA has been used to describe the ideal patient: secure, young, listens, verbal, intelligent, and attractive.
- The poor candidate for surgery has excessive concerns about minimal deformities and unrealistic expectations, and is insecure, poorly informed, and fails to recognize the limitations of surgery. These patients are likely to be unsatisfied following surgery regardless of the aesthetic improvement. They should be approached with caution and in most cases should not be operated on.
- The acronym SIMON has been used to describe this patient: single, immature, male, overly expectant, and narcissistic traits.
- Proper identification of causative factors of nasal airway obstruction is key to successful treatment. Nasal airway obstruction can have both medically and surgically correctable causes.
- Common surgically correctable causes include nasoseptal deviation, internal or external valve dysfunction, and inferior turbinate hypertrophy.
- Primary and secondary rhinoplasty patients differ in three characteristic ways.
  - First, the secondary patient's scarred, contracted soft tissues will not tolerate aggressive dissection, multiple incisions, or tight dressings.
  - Second, graft donor sites may have already been harvested, necessitating the use of more difficult

(distorted septum or concha), painful (costal), or frightening (calvarial) donor sources.
  - Third, the secondary rhinoplasty patient's morale is often more fragile. Having already invested money, time, discomfort, and emotion in one or more unsuccessful procedures, what secondary rhinoplasty patients' fear most and need least are additional disappointments.
- For secondary rhinoplasty patients, the surgeon should be careful to construct a plan that is based on a clear understanding of what is possible and founded on sound surgical and biologic principles that maximize the airway and respect the patient's aesthetic goals.
- Before agreeing to operate on a patient, the surgeon must be able to answer each of the following questions affirmatively:
  - *Can I see the deformity?* This question eliminates delusional patients or those with minimal defects that may not be surgically correctable.
  - *Can I personally fix it?* This criterion will vary from surgeon to surgeon and must be based on operative experience and ease in correcting specific problems.
  - *Can I manage the patient?* A patient who is unacceptably nervous, impossible to examine, or unwilling to comply with preoperative and postoperative instructions is a poor candidate, even if all other conditions are met.
  - *If there is a complication, will the patient remain controlled and cooperate with treatment?* No patient enjoys a complication, but there are those who, although disappointed, quietly understand and will await the proper time for revision. There are others who become hysterical, angry, disruptive, or accusatory and want an immediate correction.
  - *Does the patient accept the margin of error inherent in surgery?* This is the most important criterion. The patient's willingness to accept the imperfection that is inherent in surgery is a willingness to accept the imperfection that is inherent in being human.

Anatomical pearls

- It is helpful to conceptualize the nose as a system of two interrelated layers ***(Fig. 3.1)***.
- The outer layer, like a soft, elastic sleeve, slides over the inner semi-rigid layer and contains the entire investing nasal soft tissues plus the alar cartilages and their associated lining.
- The inner layer contains everything else (the bony and upper cartilaginous vaults, the nasal septum, and their associated linings.)
- This two-layer concept associates those structures that behave together anatomically and functionally, and provides an explanation for the "global" manifestations of some surgical changes (e.g., the effect of dorsal reduction or augmentation on nasal length).
- The internal nasal valve is formed by the articulation of the caudal and anterior (or dorsal) edges of the upper lateral cartilages with the anterior septal edge ***(Fig. 3.2)***.

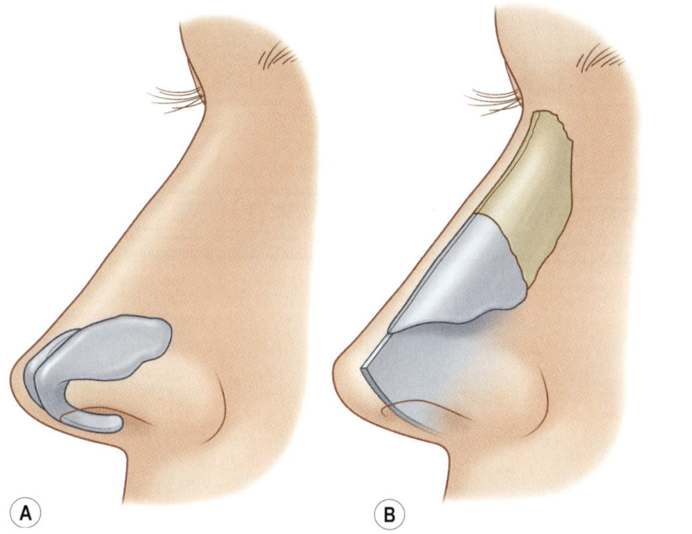

Figure 3.1 The structural layers of the nose, which separate those anatomical units that move together. The investing soft tissues and alar cartilages glide over the inner, fixed, semirigid layer, which contains the bony vault, the upper cartilaginous vault, and the nasal septum.

- The external nasal valve is composed of the cutaneous and skeletal support of the mobile alar wall (the alar cartilage lateral crura with their associated external and vestibular skin coverings).

Upper cartilaginous vaults

- The width and stability of the upper cartilaginous vault (formed by the upper lateral cartilages and the anterior septal edge), the critical area of the internal nasal valves, depend not only on the width of the bony vault but also on the height and width of the middle vault roof.
- Resection of the middle vault roof during hump reduction removes this most critical anterior stabilizing force on the upper lateral cartilages, which will fall medially and produce a characteristic "inverted V" deformity and consequent narrowing at the internal valves.
- Middle vault collapse virtually always occurs when the cartilaginous roof has been resected, whether or not osteotomy has been performed, but may not be visible if the overlying soft tissues are sufficiently thick.
- To avoid middle vault collapse and internal valvular incompetence, the surgeon should plan to reconstruct the normal distracting forces by a substantial dorsal graft or by spreader grafts, which provide the same degree of functional mean nasal airflow improvement (see below).

Middle and lower cartilaginous vaults

- The upper lateral cartilages are supported caudally by their relationship to the cephalic margins of the lateral crura in the region of the so-called "scroll".
- Radical alar cartilage resection can compromise middle vault support and may leave an external deformity typified by deepening and lengthening of the alar creases.

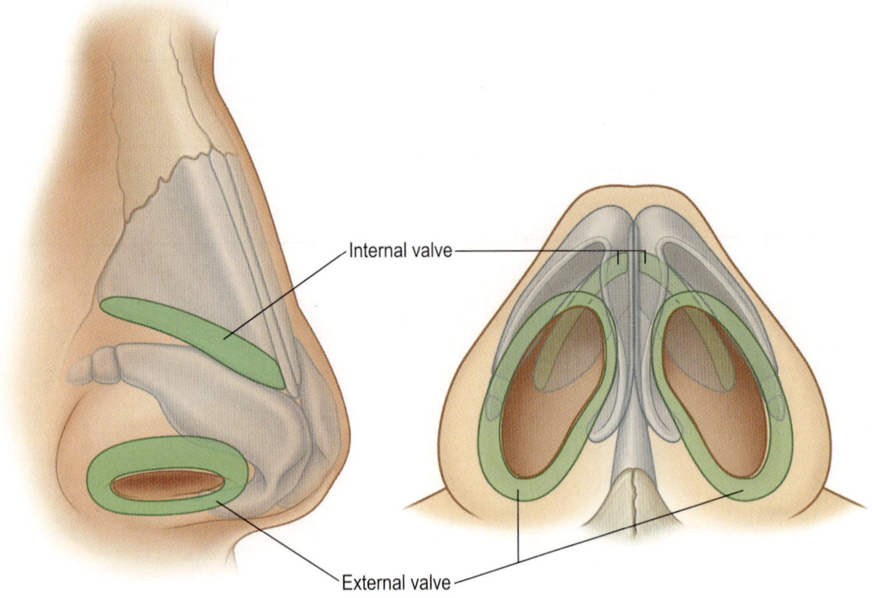

Figure 3.2 The nasal valves. The internal valves are formed by the articulation of the upper lateral cartilages with the anterior (dorsal) septal edge; the external valves are formed by the alar cartilage lateral crura and their associated investing soft tissue cover.

- Resect the upper lateral cartilages submucosally only when failure to do so would allow them to prolapse into the airway or when necessary to shorten the nose.
- The point of intersection of the upper and lower lateral cartilages creates the "watershed" area between the internal and external nasal valves, and aggressive surgery in this area also affects external valvular competence, particularly in patients whose alar cartilage lateral crura are cephalically rotated.

Dorsum and tip

- Tip projection, that is, the intrinsic ability of the alar cartilages to support the tip lobule independent of dorsal height, depends on alar cartilage middle crural size, shape, and substance.
- Septal deviation can involve deviation of the septal cartilage, perpendicular plate of the ethmoid bone, or vomer away from the midline and can cause obstruction of one or both of the nasal airways, along with external deviation of the nose.
- Nasal deviations can generally be classified into three basic types: (1) caudal septal deviations; (2) concave dorsal deformities; and (3) concave/convex dorsal deformities (Table 3.3).
- Septal tilt is the most common type where the quadrangular cartilage and perpendicular plate of the ethmoid are straight but the quadrangular cartilage is tilted to one side internally and to the opposite side externally. Hypertrophy of the inferior turbinate contralateral to the side of internal deviation is usually present.
- The turbinates exist as three or four bilateral extensions from the lateral nasal cavity.
- The inferior turbinate consists of highly vascular mucoperiosteum covering a thin semicircular conchal bone and is involved in regulation of filtration and humidification of inspired air.

Table 3.3 **Classification of nasal deviations**

I. Caudal septal deviation
a. Straight septal tilt
b. Concave deformity (C-shaped)
c. S-shaped deformity
II. Concave dorsal deformity
a. C-shaped dorsal deformity
b. Reverse C-shaped dorsal deformity
III. Concave/convex dorsal deformity (S-shaped)

- In combination with the internal nasal valve, the anterior extent of the inferior turbinate can be responsible for up to two-thirds of the upper-airway resistance.
- Inferior turbinoplasty is performed in patients with nasal airway obstruction secondary to inferior turbinate hypertrophy refractory to medical management.
- Overly aggressive surgical management may be complicated by bleeding, mucosal crusting and desiccation, ciliary dysfunction, chronic infection, malodorous nasal drainage, or atrophic rhinitis.
- In most cases, inferior turbinoplasty with outfracture of the inferior turbinate or submucous resection is adequate to achieve significant improvement ***(Fig. 3.3)***.
- In cases of severe inferior turbinate hypertrophy, submucous resection of the inferior turbinate is indicated.
- Autologous grafts are preferential to homografts and alloplastic implants because of their high biocompatibility and low risk of infection and extrusion.
- Disadvantages include donor site morbidity, graft resorption, and unavailability of sufficient quantities of graft material.
- Grafts are most commonly obtained from septal, ear, and costal cartilage. Other sites include calvarial, nasal bone, and the olecranon process of the ulna.

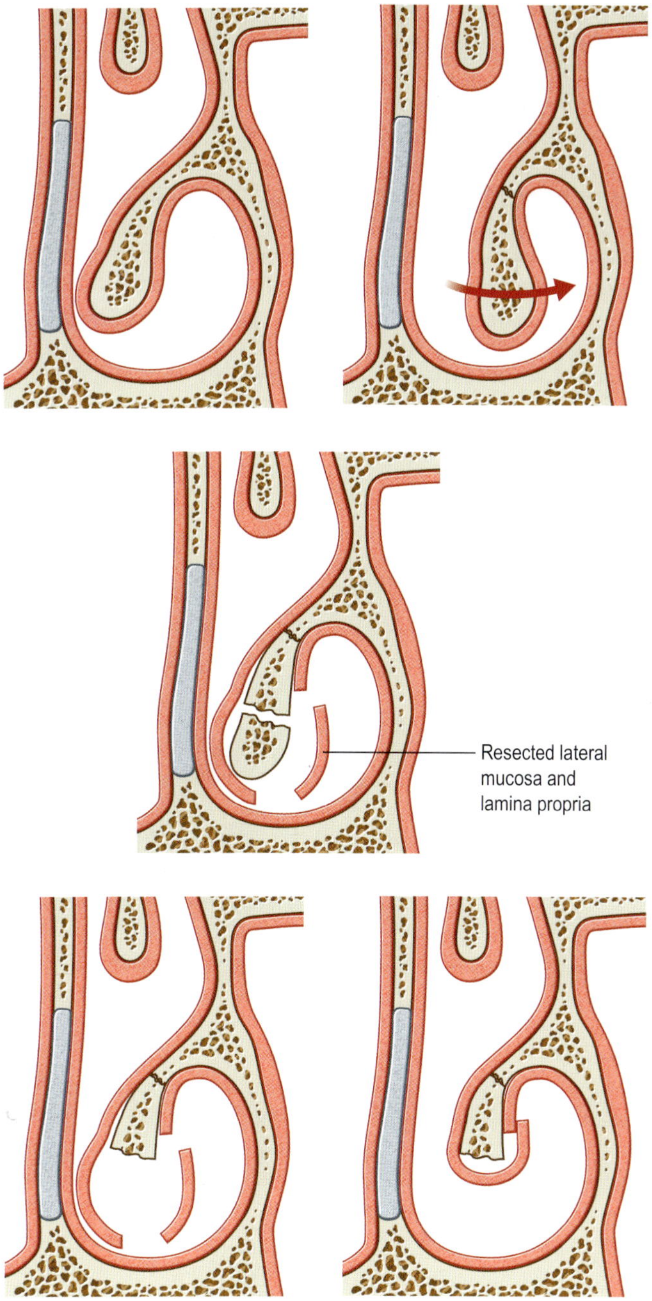

Figure 3.3 Inferior turbinate outfracture and submucous resection.

- Concerns regarding donor site morbidity, graft availability, and graft resorption will necessitate the use of homologous or alloplastic implants.
- Septal cartilage is the primary choice for autogenous grafts in rhinoplasty. It can be used in all areas including tip grafts, dorsal onlay grafts, columellar strut grafts, and nasal spreader grafts. It is easily harvested, leaves minimal donor site morbidity, and is available in the operative field.
- The ear can provide a significant amount of cartilage for rhinoplasty when septal cartilage has been depleted. It can be used for tip grafts, dorsal onlay grafts, alar contour grafts, and reconstruction of the lower lateral cartilages. However, its flaccidity does not allow it to be used where structural support is necessary. Donor site morbidity and scarring are minimal.
- Costal cartilage provides abundant autogenous graft material. It can be used for tip grafts, columellar strut grafts, nasal spreader grafts, alar cartilage grafts, and dorsal onlay grafts. Given the size, amount, and intrinsic qualities, costal cartilage lends itself well to use as a dorsal onlay graft and where structural support is required.
- It can be carved into any shape. However, allowing at least 30 min to pass prior to carving allows initial warping to occur, minimizing late deformity.
- The straightest, smoothest cartilage graft is used for the nasal dorsum to reconstruct this dominant area covered by thin soft tissues.
- If septum is available, it is used. Failing that, use rib cartilage for the dorsum.
- Bone that may be unsuitable elsewhere can be used instead for spreader grafts, lateral wall grafts, or alar wall grafts. And primarily in closed techniques, solid or lightly crushed cartilage scraps can fill regional depressions.
- The key principle in all augmentation is to match the graft material to the patient's soft tissue characteristics and to his or her aesthetic goals.
- Unmodified rib cartilage is stiff, ear cartilage is rubbery, and septal cartilage is the most "plastic".
- Thicker skin needs more augmentation to provide a given result but will hide more underlying flaws.
- Thinner skin requires softer, well contoured grafts that will not show excessively.
- A graduated approach to nasal tip surgery requires a combination of techniques including the cephalic trim, the use of a columellar strut graft, nasal tip suturing, and nasal tip grafting.
- Compared with the closed approach, the open approach may cause mild loss of tip projection due to disruption of ligamentous support and increased skin undermining. As such, columellar strut graft and nasal tip suturing techniques are often employed to maintain nasal tip support during open rhinoplasty.
- Nasal tip grafts are used in primary rhinoplasty only if adequate tip projection, definition, or symmetry cannot be obtained by the use of the previously discussed techniques. Visible nasal tip grafts are used infrequently in primary rhinoplasty because of the potential for long-term resorption leading to asymmetries or sharp angulations requiring revision.
- Tip suturing techniques (Table 3.4) are used to refine the tip by controlling the subtle contours of the lower lateral cartilages.
- When nasal tip grafts are used, it is important that they have smooth, tapered edges. Nasal tip grafts of all shapes and sizes have been described ***(Fig. 3.4)***.
- The presence of deformities of the alar rims such as alar notching or retraction, facets of the soft tissue triangles, malposition of the lateral crura, or functional problems including external valve collapse may require the use of lateral crural horizontal mattress sutures, lower lateral crural turnover flaps, alar contour or lateral crural strut grafts to correct.

- Nasal osteotomies are a key component to shape the bony vault in rhinoplasty. They are used to narrow a wide bony vault, close an open-roof deformity, or straighten deviated nasal bones.
- The goals of nasal osteotomies are maintenance or creation of smooth dorsal aesthetic lines and obtaining a desirable width of the bony vault.

Table 3.4 **Tip suturing techniques**

Medial crural suture
Interdomal suture
Transdomal suture
Joined transdomal suture
Intercrural septal suture
Lateral crural mattress suture

- Osteotomies can be classified by approach (external or internal), type (lateral, medial, transverse, or a combination), and level (low-to-high, low-to-low, or double-level) ***(Fig. 3.5)***.
- A transition zone of decreased bony thickness exists along the frontal processes of the maxilla near its junction with the nasal bone, from the pyriform aperture to the radix.
- This area of relatively thin bone allows for consistent osteotomies and predictable fracture patterns.
- Relative contraindications to the use of osteotomies during rhinoplasty include patients with short nasal bones, elderly patients with excessively thin nasal bones, those with relatively thick nasal skin, and some noncaucasian patients with extremely low and broad noses.

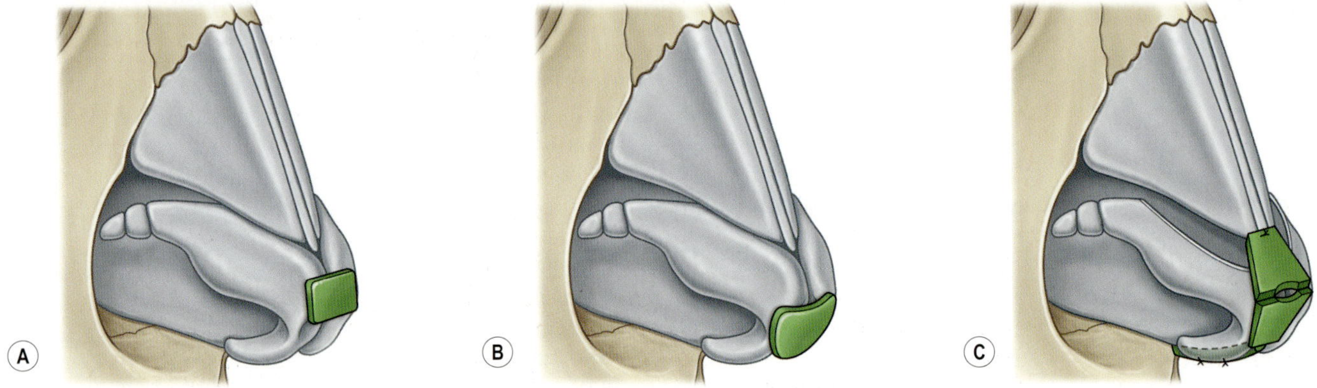

Figure 3.4 Nasal tip cartilage grafts. **(A)** Supratip; **(B)** infratip; **(C)** anatomic.

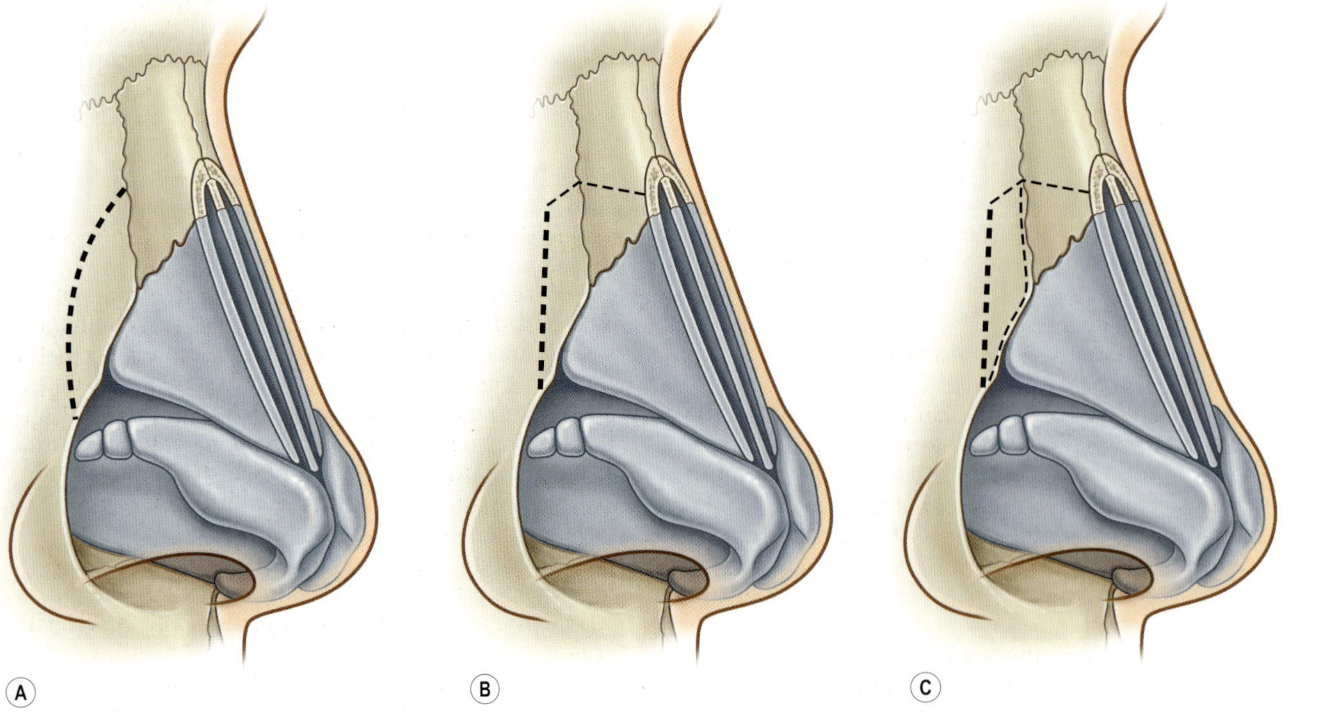

Figure 3.5 Percutaneous discontinuous lateral nasal osteotomies. **(A)** Low-to-high; **(B)** low-to-low; **(C)** double-level (right).

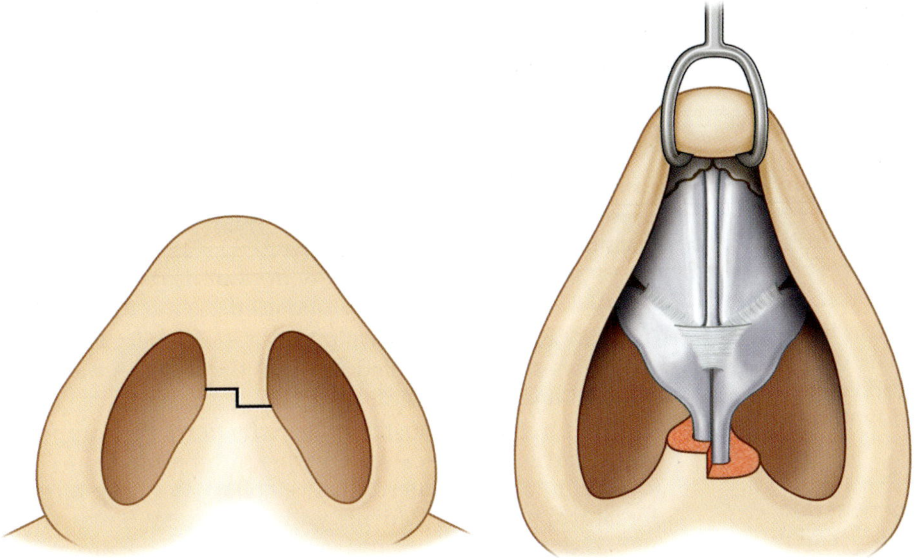

Figure 3.6 Transcolumellar stair-step incision.

Operative techniques

Video 3.1

Open rhinoplasty (Video 3.1)

- It is our preference to perform primary open rhinoplasty under general endotracheal anesthesia.
- Prior to sterile prep, the nose and septum are infiltrated with a total of 10 mL 1% lidocaine with 1:100 000 epinephrine.
- Oxymetazoline-soaked cottonoid pledgets are inserted into the nasal cavities. One drop of methylene blue is instilled in the oxymetazoline to differentiate this from the local anesthesia and prevent inadvertent injection.
- Comparable hemostasis can be obtained using lidocaine with oxymetazoline while avoiding the use of a controlled substance with potential cardiac effects, as seen with cocaine.
- Adequate exposure during primary open rhinoplasty is best obtained using a transcolumellar incision with infracartilaginous extensions.
- Several transcolumellar incisions are commonly used, including stair-step, inverted-V, and transverse.
- Blood supply to the nasal tip is preserved with the transcolumellar incision provided that extensive defatting of the nasal tip or extensive alar base resections above the alar grooves are not performed.
- We prefer to use a stair-step incision made at the narrowest part of the columella (usually its midportion, *Fig. 3.6*), which camouflages the scar, provides landmarks for accurate closure, and prevents linear scar contracture.
- The incision is carried into the nasal vestibule and then continued along the caudal border of the medial crus towards the middle crus of the lower lateral cartilage.

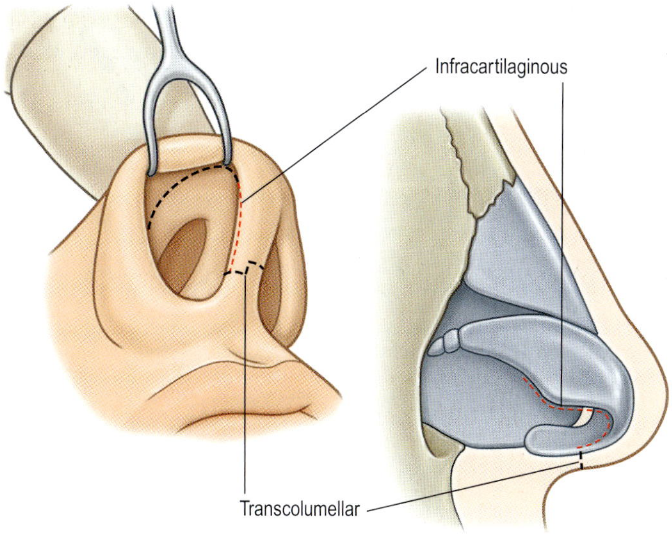

Figure 3.7 Transcolumellar stair-step incision with infracartilaginous extensions.

- After everting the ala using external digital pressure against a double hook placed within the alar rim, a separate incision is started at the caudal border of the lateral crura and connected with the medial incision, caudal to the middle crus ***(Fig. 3.7)***.
- Fine dissecting scissors are used to elevate the nasal skin in a supraperichondrial plane starting from the columellar incision in a superior direction to the nasal tip.
- Next, dissection is started over the lateral crus and continued in a medial direction connecting the supraperichondrial dissection planes over the middle crus.
- Dissection to elevate the nasal skin in the supraperichondrial plane is carried superiorly to 2 mm above the keystone area.

- A Joseph elevator is then used to elevate nasal skin in a subperiosteal plane off nasal bones to radix.
- This dissection over the nasal bones is only performed in the central area to allow for bony dorsal hump reduction, while the lateral periosteal attachments of the bony side wall should not be disrupted as they provide necessary stability to the bony vault after percutaneous osteotomies have been performed.

Component dorsal hump reduction

- Dorsal hump reduction without careful attention to the anatomic and physiologic functions of the nasal dorsum and internal nasal valve can lead to irregularities of the nasal dorsum, excessive narrowing of the midvault, the inverted-V deformity, and underresection or overresection of the osseocartilaginous hump.
- We prefer a graduated approach using component dorsal hump reduction (Table 3.5) over earlier techniques of composite dorsal hump reduction ***(Fig. 3.8)***.
- Preservation of the upper lateral cartilages during dorsal reduction of the cartilaginous septum is important in achieving smooth dorsal aesthetic lines.
- Equal resection of the septum and upper lateral cartilages results in rounding of the dorsum and excessive resection of the upper lateral cartilages results in the inverted-V deformity.

Table 3.5 **Component dorsal hump reduction**

Separation of the upper lateral cartilage from the septum
Incremental reduction of the septum proper
Incremental dorsal bony reduction (using a rasp)
Verification by palpation
Final modifications, if indicated (spreader grafts, suturing techniques, osteotomies)

- For dorsal reduction of the bony hump less than 3 mm, a down-biting diamond rasp is used to reduce the bony dorsum incrementally.
- Rasping should proceed along left and right dorsal aesthetic lines and then centrally, employing short excursions of the rasp for maximal control.
- Care is taken to avoid avulsing the attachments of the upper lateral cartilages from the undersurface of the nasal bones.
- If a larger reduction of the bony dorsum is required, a guarded 8 mm osteotome can be used.
- The osteotomy should start at the caudal aspect of the nasal bones and is directed towards the radix. A rasp is used for final adjustments.
- Only in limited circumstances is reduction of the upper lateral cartilages indicated. Overresection must be avoided to prevent internal valve collapse or long-term dorsal irregularities. Patients with short nasal bones and high and narrow osseocartilaginous framework are at higher risk for these problems.
- Spreader grafts may be added, and are indicated in primary rhinoplasty to recreate the dorsal aesthetic lines, widen the midvault, or correct the deviated nose ***(Fig. 3.9)***.
- They may be fashioned from harvested septal cartilage and are typically 5–6 mm in height and 30–32 mm in length and can be placed either unilaterally or bilaterally.
- If indicated for improvement of the dorsal aesthetic lines they can be visible, placed above the plane of the dorsal septum, and if indicated to improve function of the internal nasal valve they can be invisible, placed below the plane of the dorsal septum.
- Spreader grafts are secured to the septum using 5-0 PDS horizontal mattress sutures.
- Following re-establishment of the cartilaginous midvault, percutaneous osteotomies are performed to correct widened or asymmetrical nasal bones, or close the open-roof deformity if present after dorsal reduction.

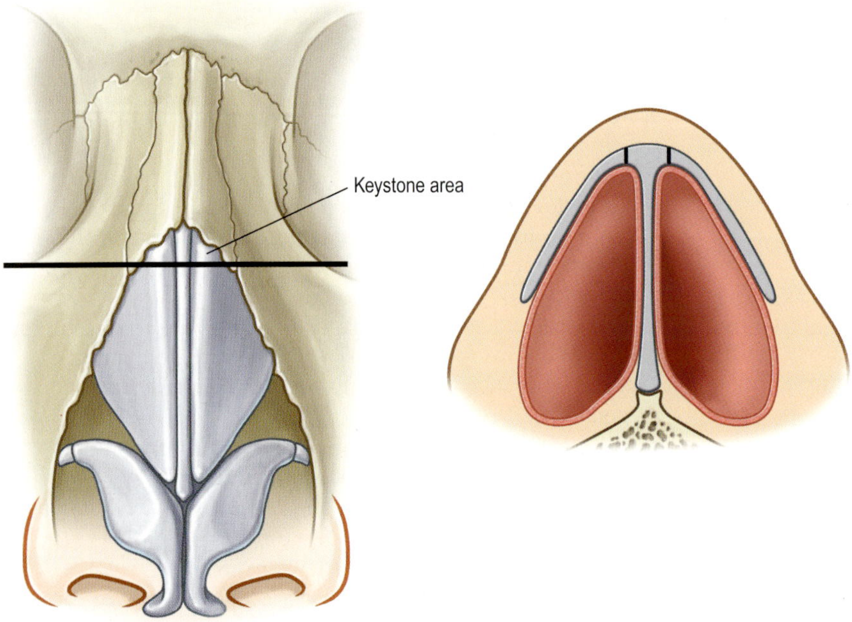

Figure 3.8 Nasal dorsum.

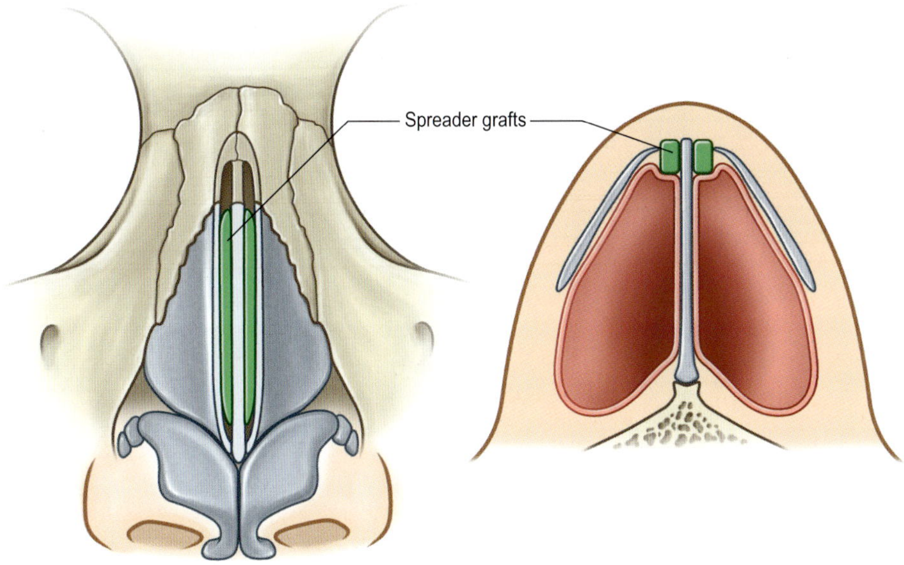

Figure 3.9 Dorsal spreader grafts.

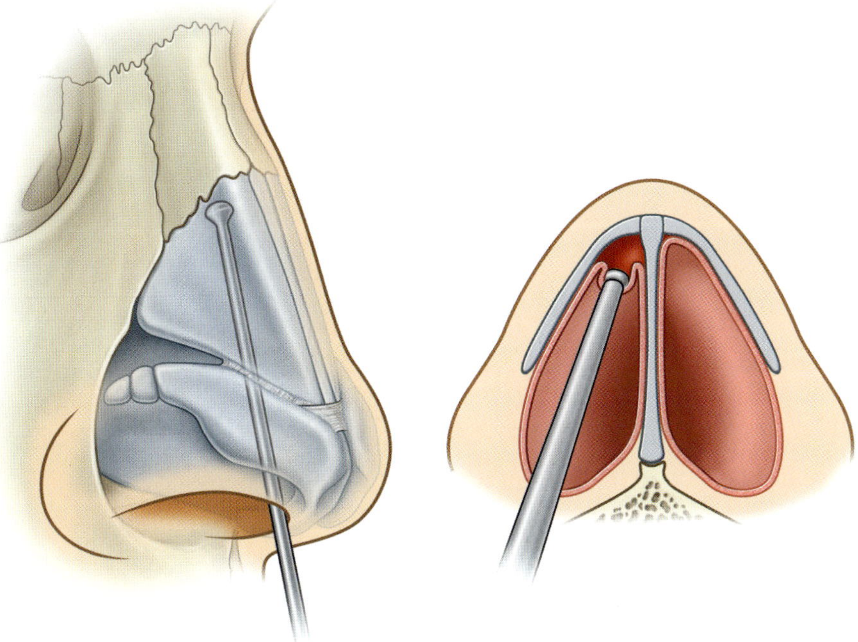

Figure 3.10 Submucoperichondrial dissection.

Septal reconstruction

- Exposure of all deviated structures through the open approach.
- Release of all mucoperichondrial attachments to the septum, especially the deviated part.
- Straightening of the septum, and if necessary septal reconstruction, while maintaining an 8–10 mm caudal and dorsal L-strut.
- Restoration of long-term support with buttressing caudal septal batten or dorsal nasal spreader grafts.
- If necessary, submucous resection of hypertrophied inferior turbinates.
- Precisely planned and executed external percutaneous osteotomies.

Septal graft harvest

- A 15-blade scalpel is used to score the mucoperichondrium of the septal angle
- A Cottle elevator is used to develop the submucoperichondrial pocket on one side of the septum ***(Fig. 3.10)***.
- Dissection should be continued to the maxillary crest and posteriorly to the vomer ***(Fig. 3.11)***.

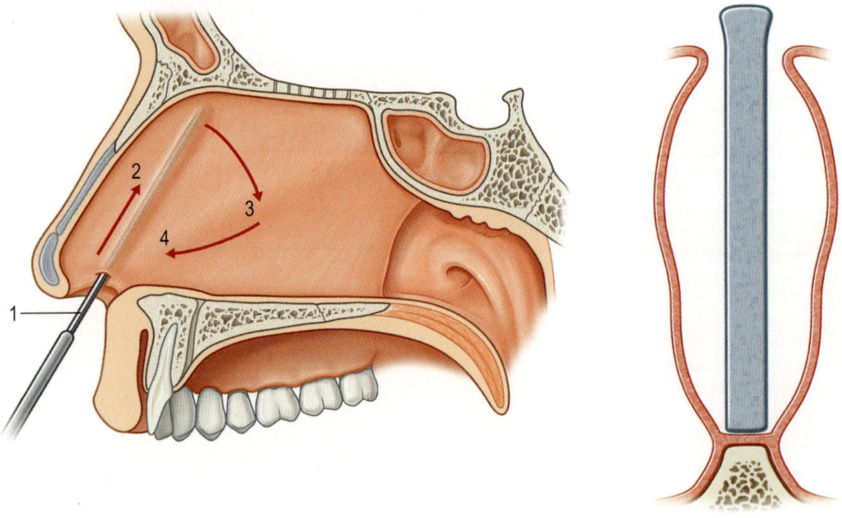

Figure 3.11 Submucoperichondrial flaps.

- The contralateral mucoperichondrium may be left attached to the septum and only the portion of the septal cartilage to be harvested is released. This method leaves contralateral mucoperichondrium attached to the L-strut for more support and decreases the amount of dissection and dead space with the potential for hematoma formation.
- Alternatively, development of these submucoperichondrial pockets can be performed bilaterally, allowing for improved visualization.
- Care is taken to avoid perforations of the mucosa. Anterior perforations should be repaired with 5-0 chromic gut sutures while posterior perforations can be left as they allow for drainage of any blood.
- An 8–10 mm wide dorsal and caudal L-strut is created using a 15-blade scalpel to incise the septal cartilage parallel to the dorsal edge of the septum from the perpendicular plate of the ethmoid to a point 8–10 mm from the caudal edge of the septum ***(Fig. 3.12)***. This incision is then continued posteriorly and parallel to the caudal edge of the septum until the crest of the maxilla.
- During septal cartilage harvest, pressure on the L-strut must be avoided to prevent its fracture. If this occurs, it should be repaired to restore nasal support.
- After cartilage grafts have been fashioned, any excess material should be replaced between the mucoperichondrial flaps in case it is required in subsequent procedures.
- The mucoperichondrial flaps can be sutured together using a 5-0 chromic gut quilting suture and are bolstered by placement of Doyle splints to support the mucoperichondrial flaps and minimize dead space.

Ear cartilage

- An anterior approach is used if autogenous graft material is required for tip grafts or lower lateral cartilage reconstruction ***(Fig. 3.13)***.
- A posterior approach is used if a longer, more malleable piece of cartilage is required.

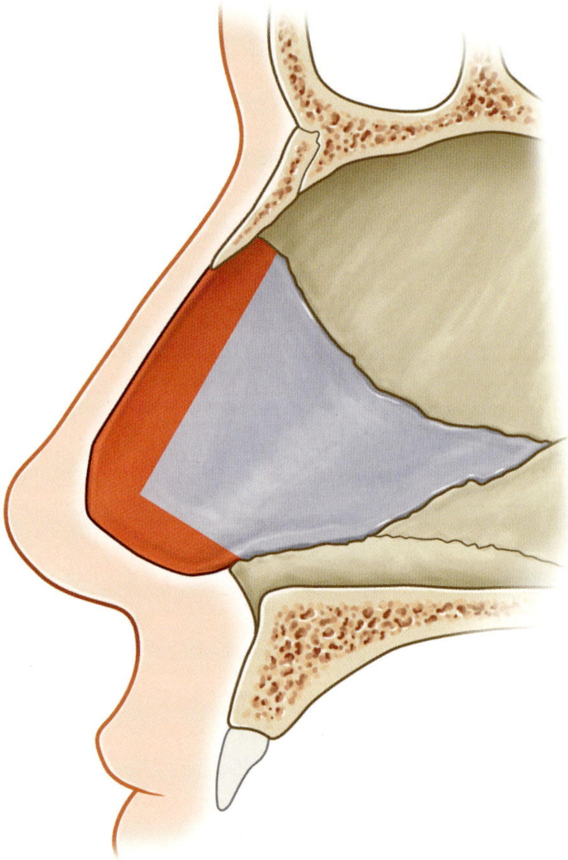

Figure 3.12 Septal L-strut.

- Hemostasis is obtained and the incision is closed with a 5-0 plain gut running suture.
- A tie-over Xeroform-cotton bolster held in place with a 3-0 nylon suture through the anterior and posterior auricular skin is used to obliterate dead space and prevent hematoma formation.
- This is removed on postoperative day 3.

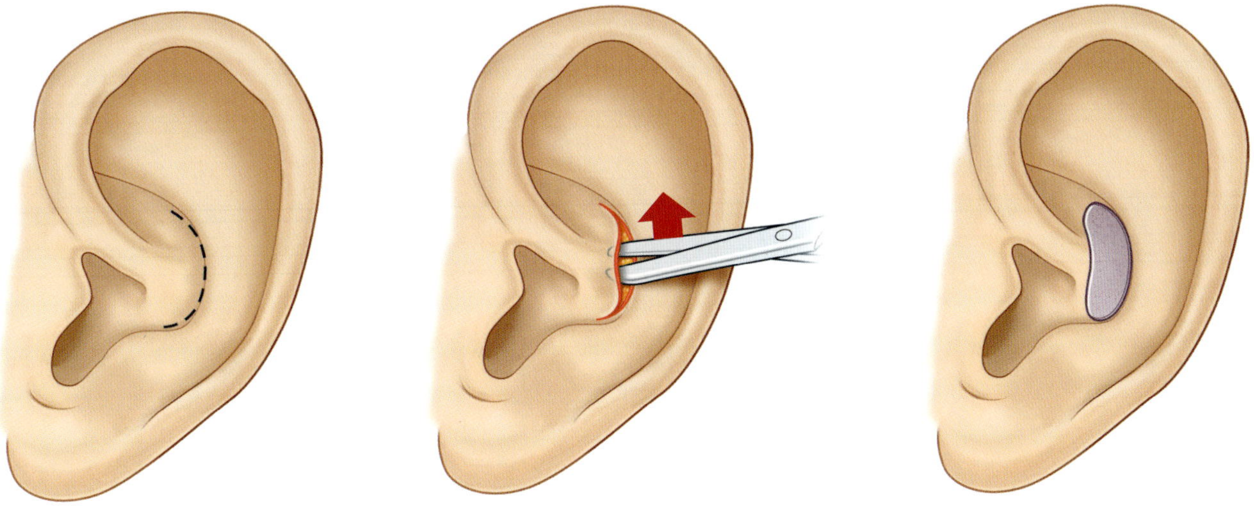

Figure 3.13 Harvesting ear cartilage.

Costal cartilage

- Various authors have described harvesting costal cartilage from different ribs but it is the author's preference to harvest the ninth rib because it is straight medially and provides 4–5 cm of autogenous graft material ***(Fig. 3.14)***.
- If there is concern about pneumothorax during costal cartilage harvest, the wound is filled with saline and positive-pressure ventilation can be performed by the anesthesia provider to ensure that there are no gas bubbles escaping from the chest cavity.
- If the parietal pleura has been violated, the tip of a red rubber catheter is inserted into the defect and a 3-0 Vicryl pursestring suture is performed around the catheter. The anesthesia provider performs a Valsalva maneuver while suction is applied to the red rubber catheter. As the catheter is withdrawn, the pursestring suture is tied to seal the parietal pleural defect followed by wound closure.
- An upright chest X-ray should be performed postoperatively to confirm resolution of the pneumothorax.

The nasal tip

- Cephalic trim should be performed with the bulbous or boxy tip ***(Fig. 3.15)***.
- Paradomal fullness is secondary to prominence of the cephalic border of the middle and lateral crura of the lower lateral cartilages.
- Cephalic trim of this area reduces paradomal fullness and helps to define the tip and narrow the distance between the tip defining points.
- A rim strip of at least 5 mm is preserved for adequate support of the external valve.
- Calipers should be used to measure the rim strip accurately.

Columellar strut graft

- An intercrural columellar strut graft is used to maintain or increase nasal tip projection, and aids in unifying the nasal tip. It can be either floating or fixed ***(Fig. 3.16)***.
- A floating columellar strut graft is used more commonly to maintain tip projection and is positioned between the medial crura and rests in the soft tissues 2–3 mm anterior to the nasal spine.
- A fixed columellar strut graft is used to increase tip projection and is positioned between the medial crura and rests on the nasal spine.
- The columellar strut graft is typically fashioned from septal cartilage, to measure 3 × 2 mm.
- The columellar strut graft is placed in a pre-dissected pocket and with the tip defining points held at the same level, a 25 G needle is placed through the medial crura and columellar strut graft to stabilize the complex for suturing.
- A 5-0 PDS suture is used to stabilize the medial crura to the columellar strut graft, followed by two additional 5-0 PDS sutures to unify the nasal tip complex.
- The columellar strut graft is then trimmed to alter or refine the infratip lobule.

Nasal tip suturing techniques **(Fig. 3.17)**

- Medial crural sutures: used to correct medial crural asymmetries, to reduce flaring, to control the overall width of the columella, and stabilize a columellar strut.
- Interdomal sutures: used to increase infratip columellar projection and definition, further increase tip projection, or narrow the interdomal distance.
- Transdomal sutures: used to control dome asymmetry ***(Fig. 3.18)***.
- Intercrural septal sutures: used to alter tip rotation ***(Fig. 3.19)*** (usally a 5-0 clear nylon is used for permanency).
- Lateral crural mattress sutures: used to reduce the convexity and straighten the lateral crus ***(Fig. 3.20)***.

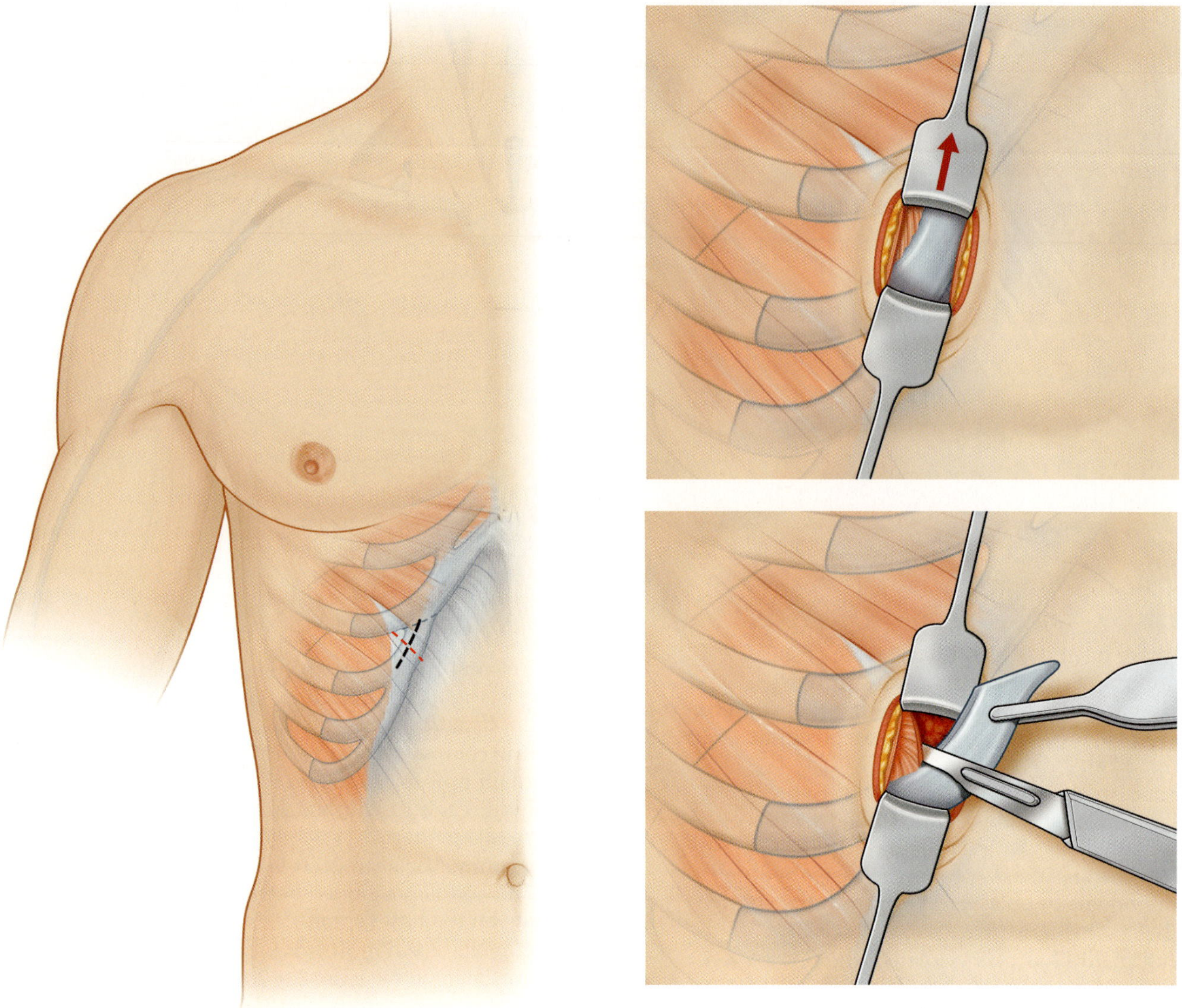

Figure 3.14 Harvesting costal cartilage.

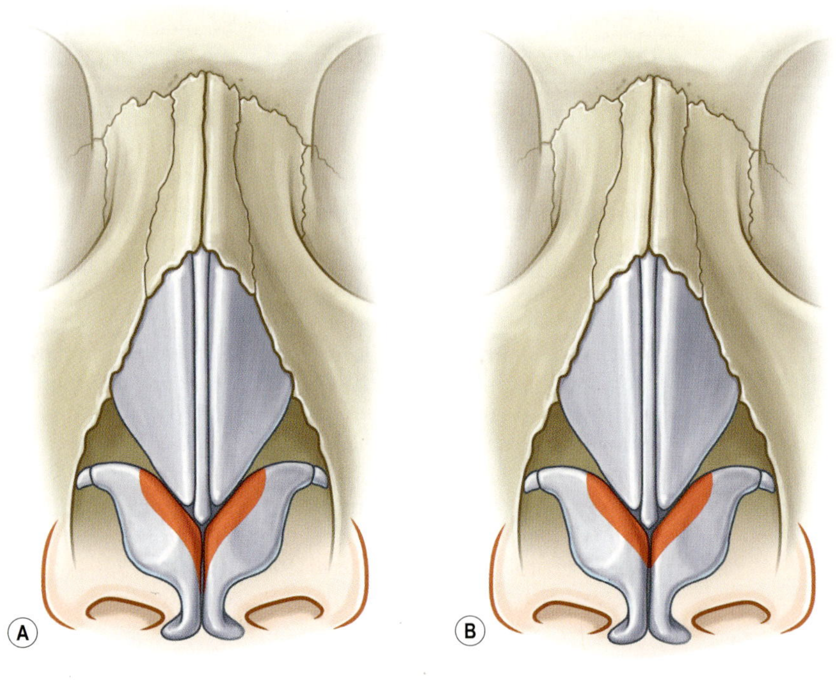

Figure 3.15 Cephalic trim. **(A)** Lateral and middle crura; **(B)** lateral crus (right).

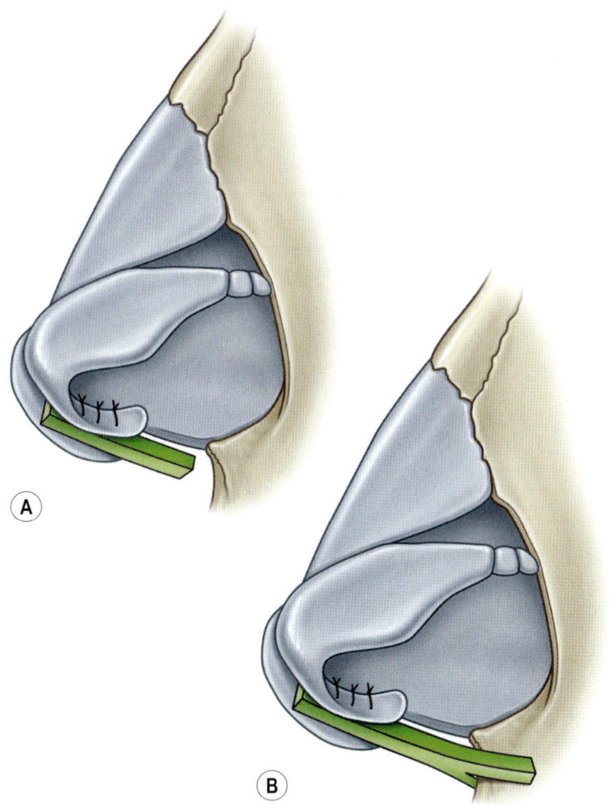

Figure 3.16 **(A)** Floating and **(B)** fixed columellar strut grafts.

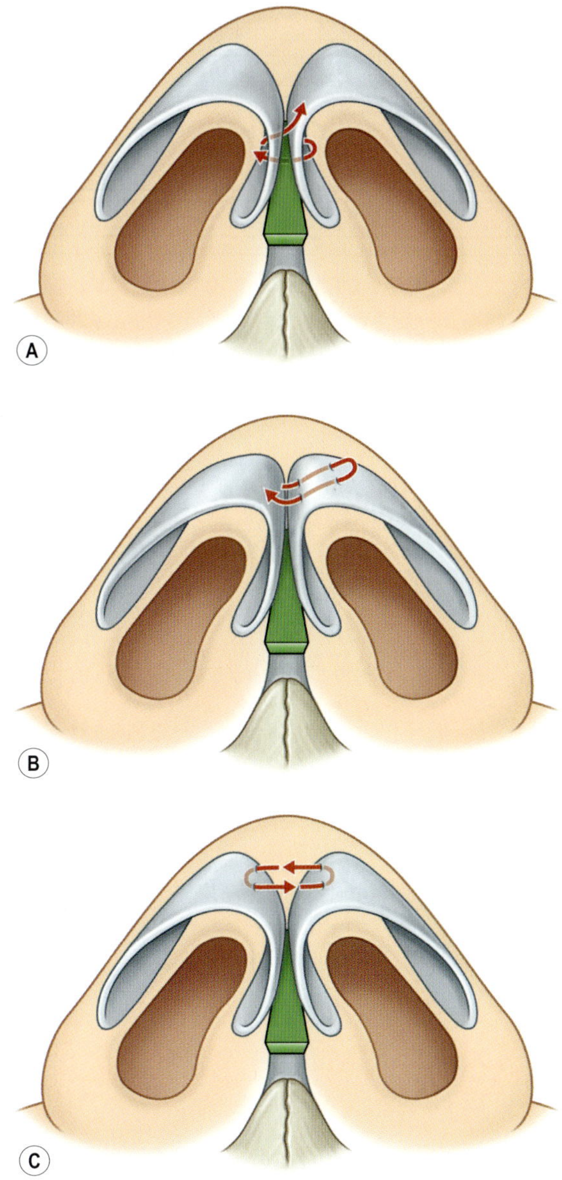

Figure 3.17 Nasal tip suturing techniques. **(A)** Medial crural; **(B)** transdomal; **(C)** interdomal.

Nasal tip grafting techniques

- A shield graft: used to increase tip projection, and improve definition of the tip and the infratip lobule.
- Placed adjacent to the caudal edges of the anterior middle crura and extends into the tip. It is placed so that it extends 2–3 mm past the tip defining points and should be sutured with at least two 5-0 PDS sutures to the caudal margins of the dome and medial crura.
- Approximately 8 mm wide and 10–12 mm long. The width of the base of the graft is the same as the distance between the caudal margins of the medial crura.
- An onlay graft: placed horizontally over the alar domes and is used to camouflage tip irregularities and can provide increased tip projection.
- Cartilage removed from the lower lateral cartilages after cephalic trim is usually sufficient for use as an onlay graft.
- An anatomic tip graft: in primary rhinoplasty, the anatomic tip graft is reserved for the patient with inadequate tip projection or thick skin.
- A combination of the shield and onlay grafts and reflects the surface anatomy of the ideal tip.

Alar contour grafts

- Used as a simple and effective method to correct and prevent alar notching or retraction, and facets of the soft tissue triangles, after correcting the tip deformity ***(Fig. 3.21)***.

Lateral crural strut grafts

- Used to support weak lateral crura, prevent collapse of the external nasal valve, address malposition of the lateral crura, or increase tip projection ***(Fig. 3.22)***.
- A 4 × 25 mm lateral crural strut graft rests on the pyriform aperture posteriorly. The anterior aspect of the graft is placed deep to the lateral crus and secured with two or three 5-0 PDS simple interrupted sutures.

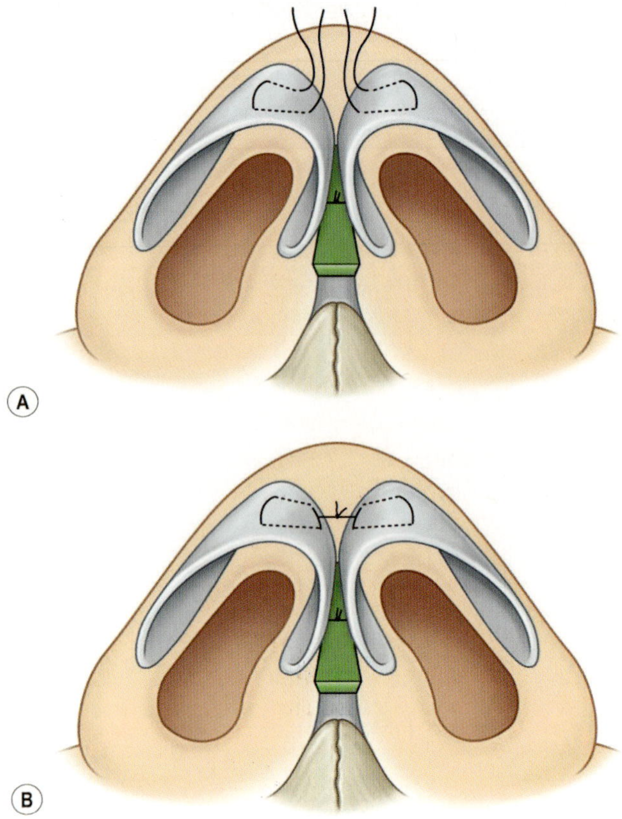

Figure 3.18 **(A, B)** Joined transdomal sutures.

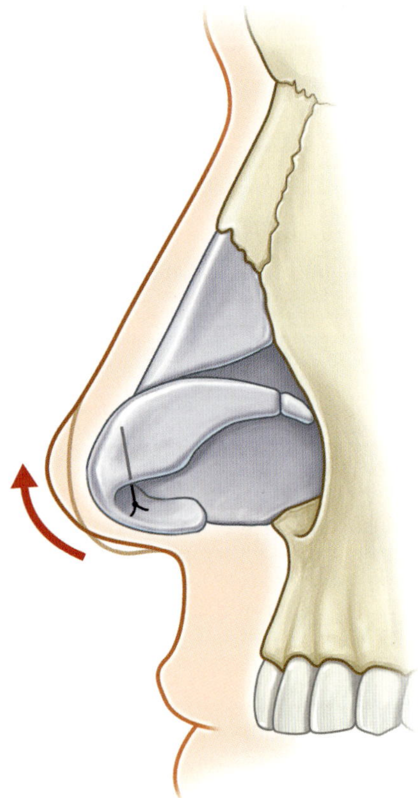

Figure 3.19 Intercrural septal suture.

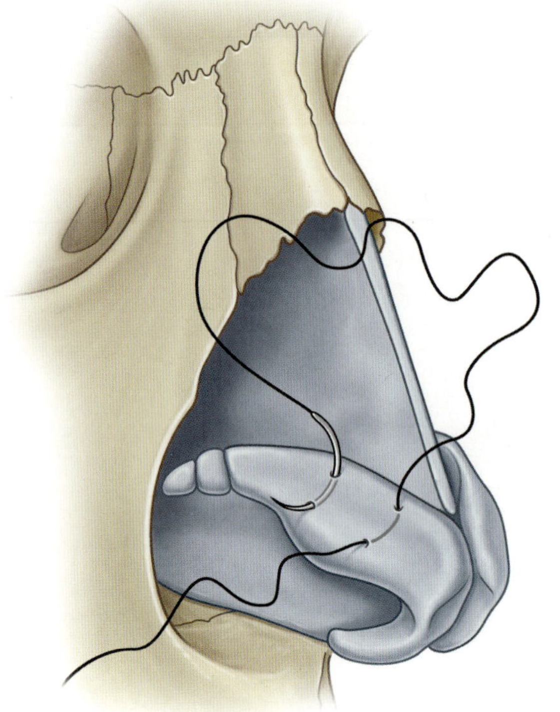

Figure 3.20 Lateral crural mattress suture.

The alar–columellar relationship

- The alar–columellar relationship demonstrated on the lateral view is dictated by the relative positions of the alar rim and the columella to a line drawn through the long axis of the nostril ***(Fig. 3.23)***. The ideal distance from the long axis to both the alar rim superiorly and the columella inferiorly is 1–2 mm.
- Six classes of alar–columellar relationship have been described:
- Class I (Hanging columella): the distance from the long axis to the columella is greater than 2 mm while the distance from the long axis to the alar rim is 1–2 mm.
  - Correction involves resection and reapproximation of the membranous septum to reposition the columella superiorly. It may also be necessary to resect part of the caudal septum or medial crura if they contribute to the hanging columella.
- Class II (secondary to alar retraction): the distance from the long axis to the columella is 1–2 mm while the distance from the long axis to the alar rim is greater than 2 mm.
  - Correction may involve caudal repositioning of the lateral crus, the use of alar contour or lateral crural strut grafts, or composite grafts from the septum or concha.
- Class III: A combination of both classes I and II and requires the use of techniques described for both classes.
- Class IV (hanging ala): the distance from the long axis to the columella is 1–2 mm while the distance from the long axis to the alar rim is less than 1 mm.

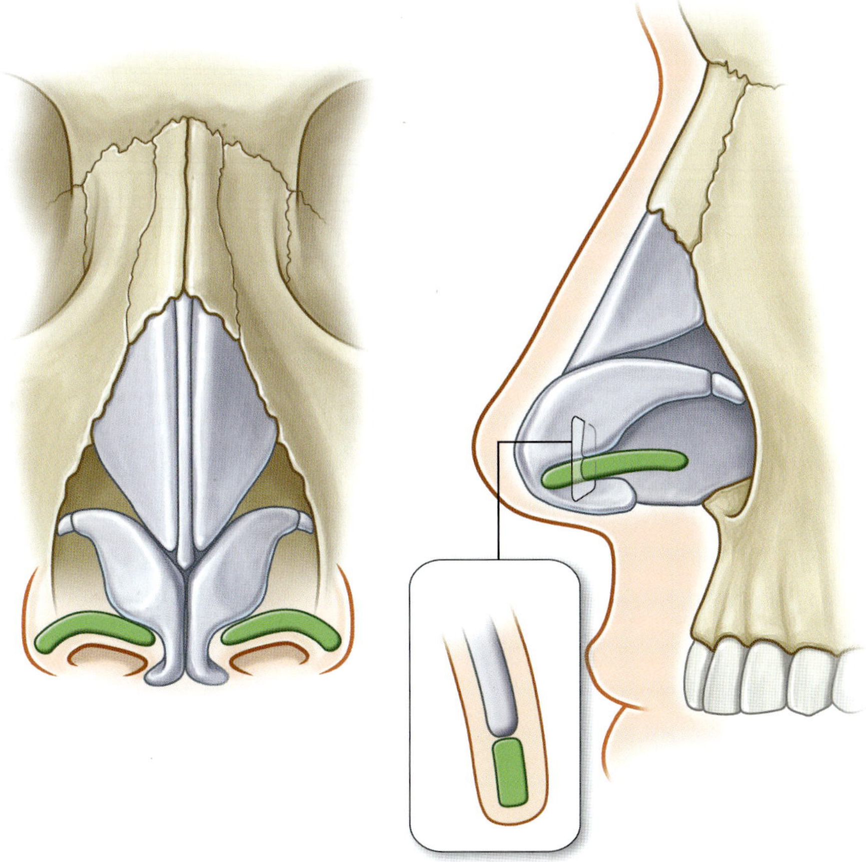

Figure 3.21 Alar contour grafts.

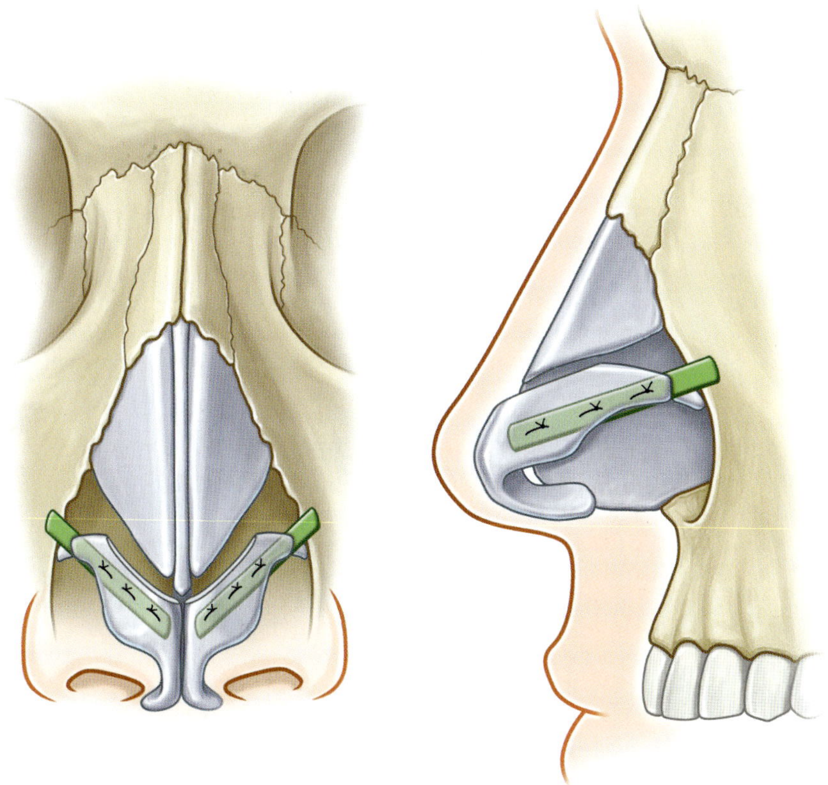

Figure 3.22 Lateral crural strut grafts.

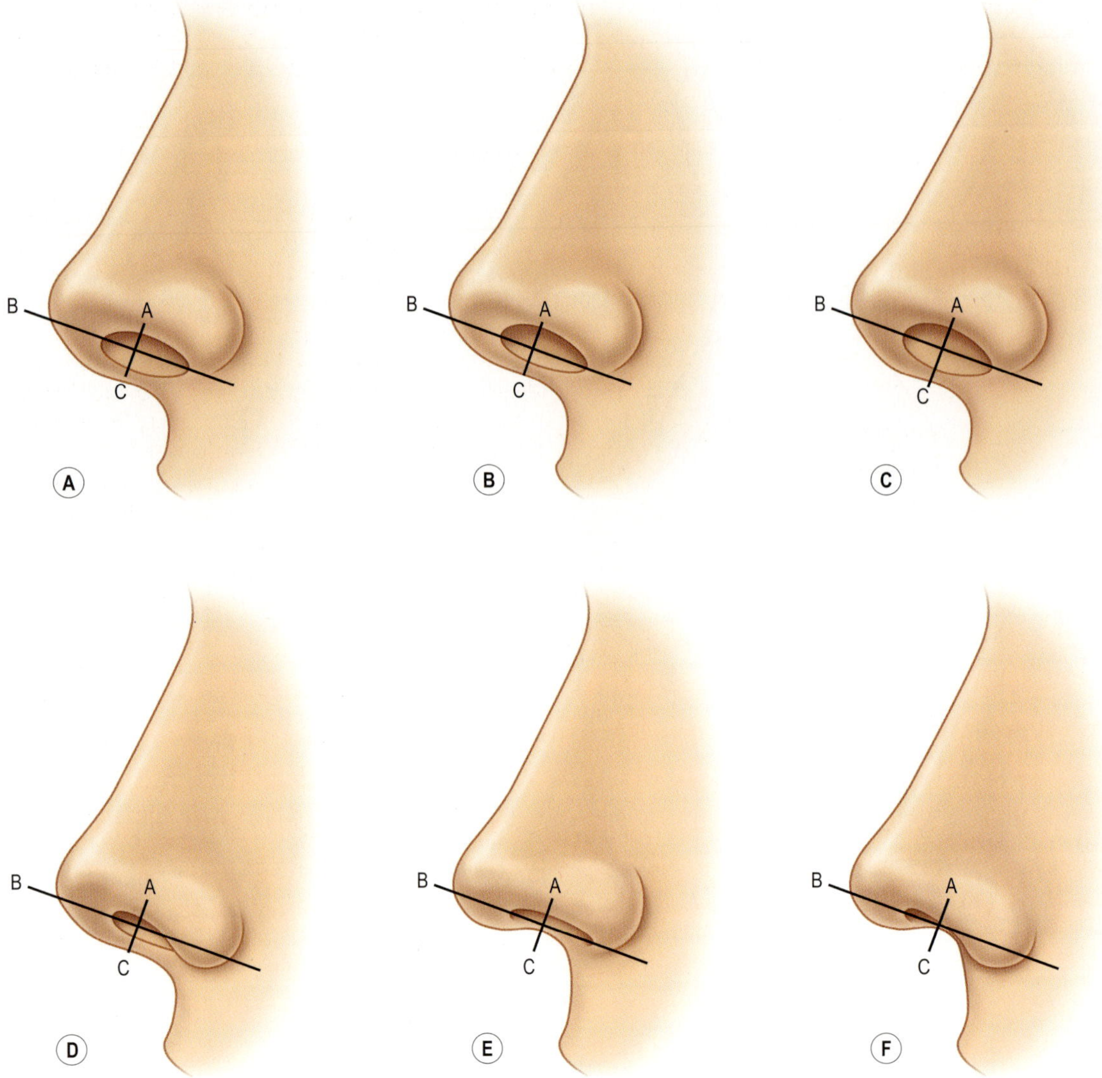

Figure 3.23 Alar–columellar relationships. **(A)** Class I; **(B)** class II; **(C)** class III; **(D)** class IV; **(E)** class V; **(F)** class VI.

  - Correction involves resection of a horizontal ellipse of vestibular skin no more than 3 mm in width to raise the hanging ala.
- Class V (secondary to columellar retraction): the distance from the long axis to the columella is less than 1 mm while the distance from the long axis to the alar rim is 1–2 mm.
  - Correction involves placing a contoured columellar strut graft between the medial crura to push the columellar skin inferiorly.
- Class VI: a combination of both classes IV and V and requires the use of techniques described for both classes.

Percutaneous lateral nasal osteotomies

- Various authors have described their experience using different approaches, including intranasal, intraoral, and percutaneous techniques. We prefer percutaneous lateral discontinuous osteotomies because this technique results in a more controlled fracture with less intranasal trauma while minimizing morbidity, including bleeding, ecchymosis, and edema ***(Fig. 3.24)***.
- A 2 mm incision is made in the nasofacial groove at the level of the inferior orbital rim and a sharp 2 mm straight osteotome is inserted through the incision and parallel to the surface of the maxilla, down through the periosteum.
- A lateral subperiosteal sweep to the bony nasofacial groove is performed to displace the angular artery laterally and prevent its injury.
- The discontinuous osteotomy is performed from inferiorly, preserving the caudal aspect of the frontal process of the maxilla at the pyriform aperture to prevent collapse of the internal nasal valve, to the level of the medial canthus superiorly and then continued into a superior oblique osteotomy medially.
- The osteotomy should not be continued superior to the medial canthus to avoid injury to the lacrimal system.
- After the osteotomies have been completed, the thumb and index finger are used to exert gentle pressure to perform a greenstick fracture of the nasal bones to

reposition them in the desired location. If more than gentle pressure is required, the osteotome should be reinserted to ensure that there are no significant areas of nonosteotomized bone between the discontinuous perforations.

Closure

- Closure of the incisions is begun by lining up the transcolumellar stair-step incision in the midline and at the junction of the columellar skin and nasal vestibule bilaterally.
- This closure must be meticulously performed to prevent notching leading to a noticeable columellar scar.
- The bilateral infracartilaginous incisions are closed next with simple interrupted sutures using 5-0 chromic gut.

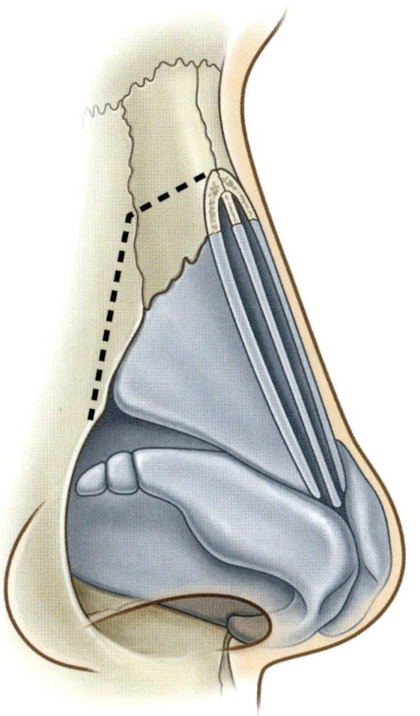

Figure 3.24 Percutaneous discontinuous lateral nasal osteotomies.

- The mucosa should be exactly reapproximated, particularly around the middle crura, to prevent distortion of the soft triangle or webbing at the nasal vestibule.

Alar base surgery

- Alar base surgery is indicated for abnormalities including alar flaring, nostril asymmetry, excessively large nostrils, elongated alar side walls, widened alar base, large alae, and alar asymmetry ***(Fig. 3.25)***.
- Alar flaring is the most common problem requiring modification of the alar base. The relationship between the alar and basal planes, alar base width, and the nostril shape and size should be taken into consideration when choosing the appropriate surgical technique.
- Alar flaring in the presence of normal nostril shape and symmetry is corrected by limiting excision to the alar lobule; the incision is not continued into the vestibule. The incision is not made directly in the alar-cheek groove but within 1 mm of the groove, allowing for an everted closure with improved scarring. In addition, 1–2 mm of the alar base is preserved, preventing alar base notching.
- Alar flaring with nostril asymmetry or excessively large nostrils requires a wedge excision of the alar lobule and vestibule. The alar lobule incision is continued into the vestibule 2 mm above the alar groove. The medial incision is made using an 11-blade scalpel angled 30° laterally, resulting in a small medially based flap. Straight-line closure is avoided to prevent distortion of the nostril or notching of the nostril sill.

Closed Rhinoplasty

Access

- The operation is routinely performed under general anesthesia.
- The patient is placed supine with the arms and legs padded and the knees slightly flexed; the operating table is in 10–15° reverse Trendelenburg position to minimize bleeding.
- After induction of general anesthesia, the nose is blocked with a freshly prepared solution of 1% lidocaine with

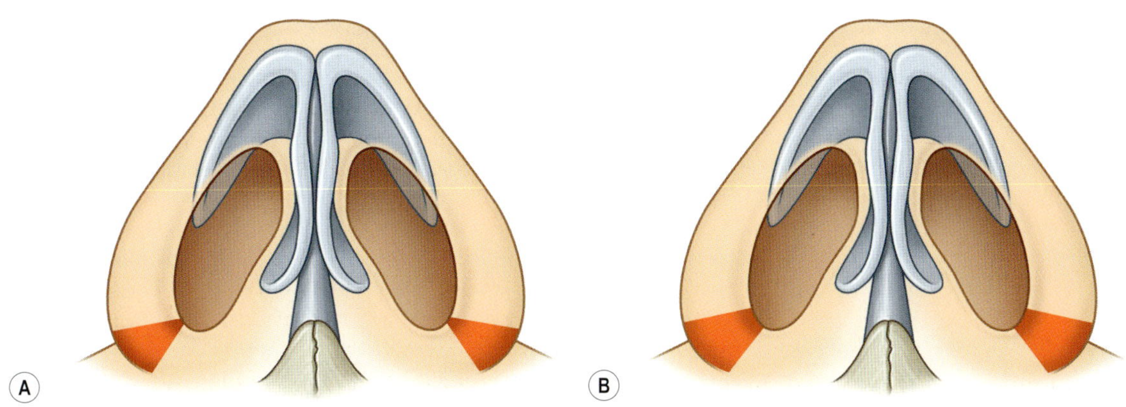

Figure 3.25 Alar base surgery. **(A)** Alar flaring; **(B)** alar flaring with modification of nostril shape.

epinephrine 1:100000 (20 mL of 1% lidocaine plus 0.2 mL of epinephrine 1:1000).

- Infiltration begins at the nasal root, along each lateral nasal wall, into the columella, across the maxillary arch, and into the alar lobules to vasoconstrict the branches of the primary supplying vessels (angular, anterior ethmoidal, superior labial) and the relevant nerves (anterior ethmoidal, infraorbital, infratrochlear).
- This infiltration usually consumes about 7 mL of the anesthetic solution, the rest of which is saved for the septal surgery.
- Nasal vibrissae are shaved with a No. 15 blade, and the nose is thoroughly cleansed internally with a povidone–iodine solution.
- Internal preparation of the nose should be even more fastidious than skin preparation, not the reverse, remembering that the nasal lining is the real operative surface.
- For hemostasis and anesthesia of the nasopalatine nerve, the internal nasal and posterior nasal branches of the anterior ethmoidal nerve, the internal nasal branch of the nasociliary nerve, and the nasal branch of the anterior superior alveolar nerve, two cotton packs soaked in 4% cocaine solution and squeezed dry with sterile gauze are placed in each airway. Only 4 mL of 4% tinted cocaine solution is made available for each patient (160 mg), safely below the maximum allowable dosage (200 mg).
- The patient's face is prepared and draped.
- The author ordinarily skeletonizes the nose through unilateral or bilateral intracartilaginous incisions ***(Fig. 3.26)***, depending on whether alar cartilage modification will be necessary.
- The incision runs from the lateral end of the caudal reflection of the upper lateral cartilage around the septal angle.

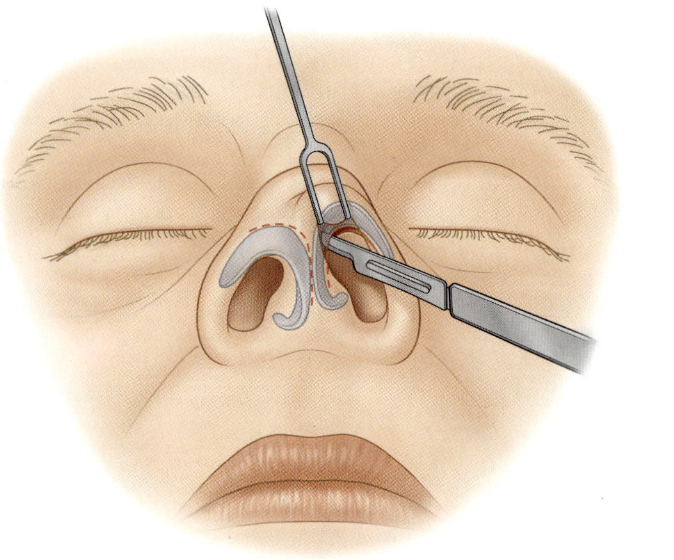

Figure 3.26 The intercartilaginous incision, which can be lengthened into a transfixing incision if necessary, gives access to the dorsum, upper and lower lateral cartilages, and the septal angle. Dorsal modification; upper and lower lateral cartilage resection; spreader, radix, dorsal, and lateral wall grafts can all be performed through this excellent access point under direct vision.

- With Joseph scissors ***(Fig. 3.27)*** and then a broad Cottle periosteal elevator, the soft tissues are elevated over the bony and upper cartilaginous vaults only as necessary for access.
- It is important for the surgeon to obtain smooth elevation of all soft tissues to ensure good cover and avoid dermal injury.
- If no transfixing incision is necessary, the intercartilaginous incision stops at the junction of the anterior and middle thirds of the membranous septum.
- If the caudal septum requires shortening, the incision can be carried toward the anterior nasal spine.

Dorsal resection

- Producing a straight dorsum from a convex one is not a simple matter.
- The surgical plan must consider: (1) radix position; (2) dorsal height, and (3) the adequacy of tip support.
- The author performs the dorsal resection under direct vision using a sharp Fomon rasp.
- Resection of the dorsal border of the septum is accomplished with a No. 11 blade from which the tip has been broken to avoid lacerating the contralateral dorsal skin.
- The dorsum should feel and appear perfectly smooth through the skin surface after dorsal resection.

Nasal spine–caudal septum

- Caudal septal resection may change the relationship of the columella to nostril rim, nasal length, subnasale contour, and upper lip carriage.
- If the nasolabial angle and upper lip relationships are satisfactory, no transfixing incision and no caudal septal or nasal spine modifications are necessary.
- If columellar position is satisfactory but the subnasale is full, a short incision can be made in the posterior membranous septum and septal floor, the nasal spine exposed and resected with a small rongeur.

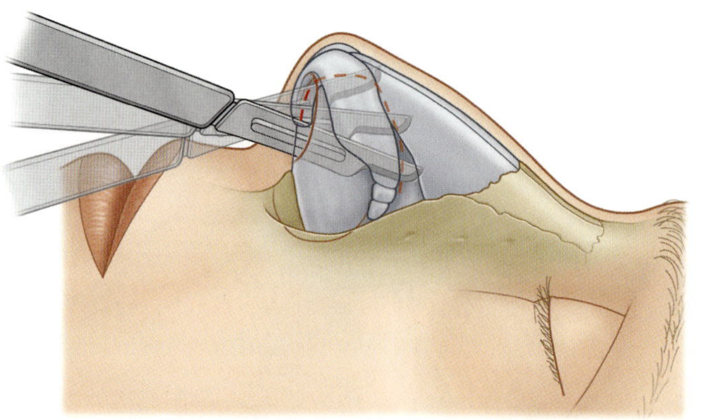

Figure 3.27 The intercartilaginous skeletonizing incision begins at the apex and proceeds laterally only as far as necessary. Dorsal access and visualization are easiest for a right-handed surgeon through a left-sided incision, and vice versa. If the surgeon does not need to shorten the upper or lower lateral cartilages, only a single intercartilaginous incision is needed.

- If the columella is low but the nasolabial angle is satisfactory, the caudal or membranous septum is resected, paralleling the nostril rims and without shortening the nose. Finally, if the columella is low or the nasolabial angle is acute, more caudal septum and membranous septum is resected anteriorly than posteriorly.
- Be cautious about over-resection; 1 or 2 mm makes the difference between normal columellar position and retraction.

Alar cartilage resection

- In the majority of primary rhinoplasties in which only conservative reductions of the cephalic lateral crura edges are necessary, the cartilages are modified retrograde through the intercartilaginous incisions.
- If the cartilages are distorted, they can be delivered as bipedicle flaps by intercartilaginous and infracartilaginous incisions.
- If only the arch needs interruption (e.g., to narrow the tip or to resect a "knuckle" at the lateral genu), only that portion of the alar cartilage should be exposed.
- If the lateral crus or dome areas are so distorted that a simple reduction or tip grafting will not provide the intended result, the distorting structures can be dissected free from the vestibular and overlying skin and (1) resected and replaced after modification; (2) resected and replaced by septal cartilage grafts, or (3) delivered as a medially based flap, and replaced along the alar rims.
- Radical freeing of the lateral crura, dome resection, or division of the alar cartilage arch reduces tip projection and so tip grafts are necessary to reconstruct the lobule. Lining should never be resected to avoid vestibular stenoses and iatrogenic airway obstruction.

Upper lateral cartilages: shortening the nose

- A variety of interventions shorten the nose. In descending order of their effect, they are dorsal resection, caudal septal resection, resection of the cephalic edges of the alar cartilage lateral crura, and resection of the anterocaudal ends of the upper lateral cartilages.
- The posterior edges of the upper lateral cartilages should be left to abut the lateral crura; mucosa should never be resected.
- The caudal edge of the upper lateral cartilage can be drawn downwards by a single hook in its lining, exposing the caudal edge for submucosal resection with Joseph scissors.

Septoplasty, spreader graft tunnels

- Septoplasty is performed to relieve an airway obstruction from septal deflection and to provide graft material for the reconstruction itself.
- The surgeon should leave 15–20 mm intact, undissected cartilage along the nasal dorsum and 15 mm caudally in performing any submucous resection to preserve stability and to make spreader graft placement simpler.
- Recent trauma (within 3 months) is an indication to postpone the rhinoplasty until any fractures have healed and until postoperative edema allows accurate judgment of the aesthetic contours.
- If they are needed, spreader graft tunnels are performed before septoplasty.
- Spreader graft tunnels are facilitated by prior infiltration beneath the mucoperichondrium with local anesthetic.
- By identifying the septal angle, the surgeon can incise to cartilage beneath each mucoperichondrial flap and develop the tunnels themselves with the sharp end of a Cottle perichondrial elevator.
- Each tunnel must follow the dorsal septal edge and should extend beneath the caudal edge of the bony arch on each side, leaving a narrow mucoperichondrial attachment along the top edge.
- For septoplasty access, the initial mucoperichondrial incision is made 15 mm above (cephalad to) the caudal septal edge.
- Using first the sharp and later the blunt end of a Freer elevator in one hand and a Frazier suction in the other, dissection proceeds under the mucoperichondrial flap onto the perpendicular plate of the ethmoid and over any posterior bony obstructions.
- Once the first flap has been developed, the sharp end of the elevator can cut the septal cartilage at the site of the opening incision and dissection then proceeds on the second side.
- Elevation of the perichondrium at the junction of septal cartilage and vomer is particularly difficult because the periosteal and perichondrial fibers are interlaced.
- Because the periosteal fibers are stronger, the mucosal flaps are less likely to tear if the surgeon begins dissection beneath the maxillary and vomerine mucoperiosteum and works cephalad.
- The first septal cut is made 15–20 mm below the dorsal septal edge with angled Knight septal scissors, which cut through septal cartilage and ethmoid.
- Make sure that both blades are within the mucoperichondrial flaps before making the cut.
- A parallel cut is performed 10 mm inferiorly, and using Killian septal forceps, the first graft, now free on three sides, can be twisted so that the ethmoid fractures and is removed in one piece.
- This maneuver often provides an initial graft of 25–30 mm long containing the flattest, thickest, longest piece of septal cartilage, ideal for a dorsal graft.
- Dissection continues posteriorly and caudally with the sharp end of a Cottle perichondrial elevator.
- The septal cartilage in the vomerine groove can often be dislodged by a bit of judicious wiggling with a narrow osteotome.
- With an osteotome and septal forceps, additional pieces of vomer or perpendicular plate of the ethmoid can be removed if obstructing or if additional graft material is needed, always working under direct vision.

- In areas of severe deflection, tears in the mucoperichondrial flaps may be unavoidable, but the surgeon should nevertheless proceed cautiously and repair any tears.
- Close the septal pocket with 4-0 chromic mattress sutures.

Turbinectomy

- Partial inferior turbinectomy, defined as a trim of the anterior edge sufficient to obtain 3 mm clearance to the septum or nasal floor, is valuable adjunctive airway treatment if indicated.
- Turbinate crushing and outfracture may suffice in patients whose turbinates contain significant cystic bone and in whom adequate airway size can be achieved without resection.
- When resection is necessary, biopsy forceps allow smaller, more incremental changes than angled scissors.
- The raw surfaces left will contract and epithelize, further reducing the size of the remaining turbinate.

Graft placement and wound closure

- Close some of the wounds with 5-0 plain catgut sutures before placing grafts so that their position will be easier to maintain.
- This sequence keeps grafts from slipping out of one incision as the surgeon closes another.

Osteotomy

- Before performing any osteotomy, the surgeon should be sure that one is necessary.
- If the lower nasal third is already appropriately wider than the bony vault, narrowing the upper nose further may be counterproductive by making the nasal base appear larger.
- If there is a high septal deviation, bilateral osteotomies may create a newly asymmetric nose because one nasal bone will move medially farther than the other.
- In the elderly patient (in whom comminution of the nasal bones may occur), the patient who wears heavy eyeglasses, or the patient with nasal bones extending less than one-third the distance to the septal angle (in whom middle vault width depends partially on bony vault width), the surgeon may wish to omit osteotomy.
- Finally, osteotomy may lengthen a long nose further by reducing support beneath a large skin sleeve.
- A single lateral osteotomy that begins intranasally, low at the pyriform aperture, and ends higher toward the nasal root (at the attachment of the nasal pyramid to the maxilla) is effective and seems the most anatomically correct.
- Gentle digital pressure causes a greenstick fracture at the remaining cephalic attachment and will re-form the bony pyramid.
- Use a guarded osteotome facing the button laterally to constantly assure correct orientation.

Alar wedge resection

- In considering the degree of resection, the surgeon should assess the proportion of tip lobular size to nostril length, remembering that tip grafting (if part of the preoperative plan) will increase tip lobular size and may eliminate the need for nostril reduction.
- Because the alar rim has both external and vestibular skin surfaces, the requirements of each must be assessed and treated individually.
- If nostril size is excessive, however, it is important to preserve a medial flap at the sill to lessen the possibility of alar notching.
- Even with the medial flap, excess resection of even 1 mm can notch the nasal floor.
- Be conservative.
- An external incision made slightly outside the alar crease is preferable in order not to destroy this important landmark, a unique structure that simple skin repair does not reduplicate.
- Accurate closure with 6-0 nylon suffices and this suture should be removed by 5 days; 5-0 plain catgut is used for the nasal floor.

Spreader grafts

- Although septal cartilage provides the ideal spreader graft, strips of costal or conchal cartilage, ethmoid, or vomer may be used instead ***(Fig. 3.28)***.
- After spreader grafts are placed, caudal slippage can be avoided by a single 4-0 plain catgut transfixing suture placed at the septal angle.

Lateral wall and columellar grafts

- Cartilage provides the ideal lateral wall graft, split tangentially or crushed to fit the defect.
- Augment the columella through a short lateral incision in the membranous septum, limiting cephalic dissection so that the grafts provide adequate augmentation but do not disappear between the medial crura.

Tip grafting

- The surgeon who uses tip grafts commonly finds that they not only increase tip projection but also alter tip lobular and nostril contour; increase lobular volume (reducing relative nostril size); impart a different ethnic character; and enlarge the nasal base, therefore changing the balance between dorsal height and tip projection.
- Tip grafts are placed through an infracartilaginous incision on the side from which the surgeon operates.
- It is important to dissect the recipient pocket adequately, but not so liberally that the grafts cannot create the required support and projection.
- Complete access incision closure is mandatory to minimize infection.
- The grafts should be manipulated as little as possible and rinsed in saline in an antibiotic solution before insertion.

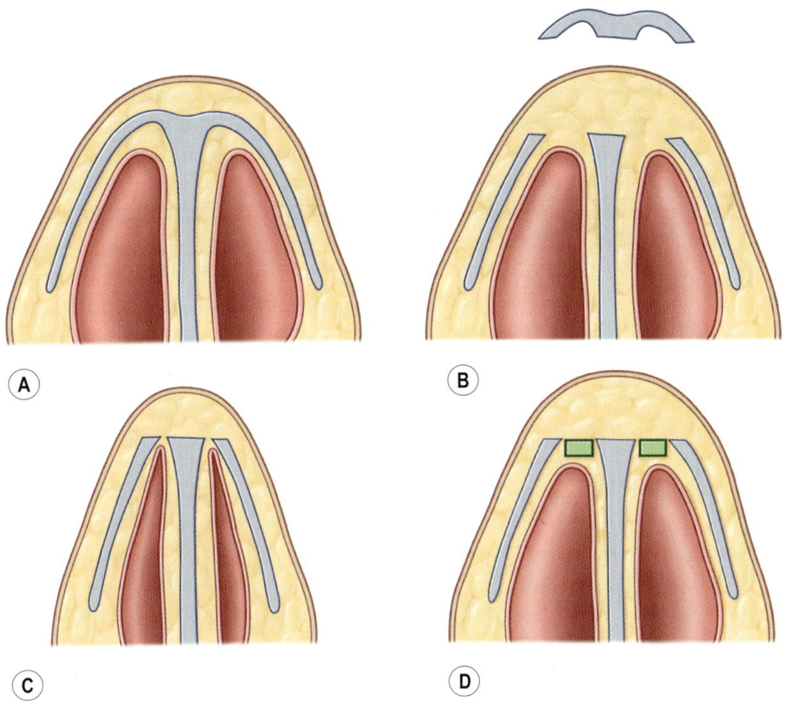

Figure 3.28 **(A)** Septal cartilage is not uniform in thickness, but broadens along its anterior edge, where it becomes confluent with the upper lateral cartilages and forms the middle vault roof. **(B)** Any dorsal resection thicker than 2 mm interrupts this cartilaginous arch and removes the widened septal area, regardless of whether the mucosa is intact. **(C)** The surgeon has now created a disequilibrium in which the upper lateral cartilages are no longer held apart by the spreading action of the intact roof. Even if the internal valves were not incompetent preoperatively, they are now. **(D)** Spreader grafts recreate the former intact septal width and reconstitute competent internal valves. Thus spreader grafts are indicated whenever the internal valves are incompetent preoperatively or when the surgeon resects an intact cartilaginous roof, unless the nasal contour independently suggests a substantial dorsal graft (which duplicates the functional effect of spreader grafts).

- The author now places tip grafts in almost every patient, except for those whose preoperative tip aesthetics are excellent.

Postoperative considerations

- Postoperative care begins preoperatively with a thorough review of the plan of care and expected postoperative recovery.
- SteriStrips are often applied starting at the supratip break, carefully contouring the soft tissue to the underlying osseocartilaginous skeleton and then continuing superiorly along the dorsum with SteriStrips of progressively shorter length.
- A Denver dorsal splint (Shippert Medical Technologies, Centennial, CO) is shaped over a cylindrical object with a diameter similar to the width of the osseous base of the nose. This splint is applied over the superior two-thirds of the dorsum and the edges are compressed medially to support the osteotomized nasal bones. The inferior edge of this splint should be superior to the supratip area.
- If septal reconstruction and/or inferior turbinoplasty was performed, Doyle septal splints (Micromedics, St Paul, MN) are applied to avoid hematoma formation deep to the mucoperichondrial flaps, support and stabilize the structures, protect the septal mucosa, and prevent synechiae formation between adjacent mucosal surfaces.
- These splints are covered with antistaphylococcal antibiotic ointment, inserted into each of the nasal cavities and secured using a 3-0 nylon horizontal mattress suture through the membranous septum, loosely tied to prevent ischemia of this delicate tissue.
- Both Denver and Doyle splints are removed, typically on postoperative day 7, along with any columellar sutures. If the patient has undergone extensive septal reconstruction, the splints are left in place for approximately 10 days. Alar base sutures are also removed on postoperative day 10.
- A nasal drip pad is fashioned using 2×2 gauze and held in place under the nose with paper tape secured to tape on the cheeks.
- Despite better symmetry, a straighter bridge, or increased tip contour, many patients are disappointed 1 week after surgery and need repeated assurance that the nose is still swollen.
- Generally, most of the nasal swelling and ecchymosis will resolve within 3–4 weeks of following surgery; however soft tissue edema, both external and internal, may take 6–12 months to resolve and external subtle nasal definition and internal nasal airflow will continue to improve over this period.
- First- or second-generation cephalosporins are generally used for antibiotic prophylaxis.
- Some surgeons will prescribe a short course of high-dose corticosteroids which is started intraoperatively and continued in the early postoperative period to minimize edema and ecchymosis.
- Intraoperatively, 8 mg intravenous dexamethasone can be given and continued postoperatively in the form of oral methylprednisolone (Medrol Dose Pack) for 6 days. Although the efficacy of high-dose corticosteroids remains debatable, newer data suggest their utility in open rhinoplasty.
- Postoperative pain and discomfort are highly variable. In general, oral narcotic analgesia is used for several days, after which nonsteroidal anti-inflammatory drugs are adequate.

- During the initial 48 hours following rhinoplasty, the patient should keep his/her head elevated greater than 30° degrees and gently apply cold compresses to help decrease postoperative edema and ecchymosis.
- Head elevation should be continued until there is no longer edema in the morning. This is typically 7–10 days.
- The patient should avoid any straining, including strenuous activity or heavy lifting, for 3 weeks. Trauma and pressure on the nose, including wearing glasses, should be avoided for 6 weeks.
- The following sequence generally occurs in most patients during the first postoperative year:
  - The nose becomes longer and "deskeletonizes" as upper lip edema abates, so that the nasolabial angle decreases and the nostrils become less visible.
  - The nasal base rotates caudally, depending on skin elasticity and the degree of skeletal support; the long preoperative nose has the greatest tendency to elongate postoperatively.
  - The profile assumes its final postoperative shape sooner than the frontal view; the nose narrows on frontal view for at least 12–18 months, particularly in the middle third. During this time, the unsupported middle vault narrows and demarcates from the caudal edges of the bony vault. The nasal skin tries to assume its preoperative shape, a characteristic that has particular implications for tip grafting: the flatter, more contracted preoperative tip will compress tip grafts and alter postoperative contour more than the larger tip with a more pliable soft tissue cover.
  - Skeletal irregularities or asymmetries may appear (and sometimes disappear).
  - Areas of underlying skeletal change or grafts may become visible and suggest the need for revision; conversely, early postoperative improvement may become obscured by soft tissue contraction and thickening.

Complications and outcomes

- Following rhinoplasty, most patient dissatisfaction is seen in the lower third of the nose, including the nasal tip, followed by the middle and upper thirds.
- Poor results in the lower third typically arise from nasal tip asymmetries, notching of the alae, and inadequate tip rotation.
- Common problems in the middle third include supratip fullness or a pinched supratip.
- Complaints in the upper third include excessive reduction of the dorsum, asymmetrical or ill-defined dorsal aesthetic lines, and other dorsal irregularities.
- The reported incidence of significant complications following rhinoplasty ranges from 1.7 to 18%.
- Common complications following rhinoplasty include bleeding, infection, prolonged edema, deformities and deviation, and nasal airway obstruction (Table 3.6).
- Epistaxis is one of the most common complications following rhinoplasty. Most patients, particularly those who have undergone septal or turbinate surgery, have moderate bleeding for the first 48–72 h postoperatively, after which drainage subsides.

Table 3.6 **Complications following rhinoplasty**

Anosmia
Arteriovenous fistula
Bleeding (ecchymosis, epistaxis, hematoma)
Deformities and deviation
Epiphora
Infection (cellulitis, abscess, granulomas, toxic shock syndrome)
Intracranial injury
Nasal airway obstruction (external valve collapse, internal valve collapse, septal deviation, synechiae, vestibular stenosis)
Nasal cyst formation
Nasolacrimal apparatus injury
Prolonged edema
Scarring
Septal perforation

- A total of 3% of patients, however, classically re-bleed between postoperative days 5 and 10.
- Head elevation greater than 60°, oxymetazoline nasal spray into the affected nostril, and gentle pressure for 15 minutes are usually enough to stop any mild epistaxis.
- If epistaxis persists, removal of Doyle splints and silver nitrate cautery, followed by anterior nasal packing can be attempted.
- If bleeding remains refractory, posterior nasal packing should be considered along with hospital admission for observation.
- In less than 1% of patients, major epistaxis occurs and should be addressed in the operating room with exploration and cauterization. Inferior turbinate resection is usually the source.
- If all of the above measures fail, consultation for angiographic embolization should be obtained.
- Regardless of the location, all hematomas should be drained.
- Hematomas deep to the skin will cause fibrosis leading to scarring and contour deformities affecting the final nasal appearance.
- Septal hematomas (ecchymotic septal mass that resembles a "blackberry") can create septal perforations or necrosis of septal cartilage leading to a saddle-nose deformitiy.
- Hematomas can usually be drained in the office with appropriate lighting. Following drainage, the area should be packed to prevent recurrence for 24 hours and then reinspected.
- Although infections are rare following rhinoplasty, diligent physical examination to identify early signs of infection allows early initiation of treatment to prevent serious complications such as tissue necrosis, toxic shock syndrome, and cavernous sinus thrombosis. In the event of an infection, internal nasal splints or packing may need to be removed.
- In cases of severe cellulitis, the patient may need to be admitted for intravenous antibiotics. Abscesses are usually found at the nasal dorsum, nasal tip, and the septum. Any abscess identified should be drained and

irrigated, and purulent material should be cultured to guide antibiotic therapy.

- Toxic shock syndrome has been described after rhinoplasty with the use of both nasal packing and internal nasal splints.
- It is an acute, multisystem disease caused by release of exotoxins from *Staphylococcus aureus* or *Streptococcus pyogenes* causing excessive activation of inflammatory cells and release of inflammatory cytokines, often resulting in tissue damage and organ dysfunction.
- Patients can present with fever, a diffuse macular erythroderma rash, desquamation, nausea, vomiting, diarrhea, tachycardia, and hypotension.
- Removal of nasal packing or internal nasal splints, administration of intravenous antibiotics, supportive care, and intensive care unit monitoring are indicated in this rare event.
- Soft tissue edema in the early postoperative period is largely prevented by preoperative patient education about postoperative care and recovery, perioperative corticosteroid use, head elevation, taping, and application of cold compresses. Most edema will resolve within 4 weeks.
- Septal perforations occasionally occur after difficult septoplasties but can be minimized by cautious dissection over the vomer, by repairing tears in the mucoperichondrial flaps, and by placing 1 mm silicone splints on each side of the septal partition before the nose is packed.
- Even with these precautions, the occasional septal perforation may be unavoidable and is usually asymptomatic.
- Small perforations may cause a curious whistling.
- Larger perforations cause crusting, epistaxis, and rhinitis as the turbulent airflow spins through the perforated mucosa.
- Temporary rhinitis may occur for several weeks postoperatively, particularly when an obstructed airway has been improved.
- Late soft tissue edema persists several months to more than a year postoperatively and represents scar remodeling. It can be seen in situations such as secondary rhinoplasty or patients with thick skin.
- Patients should be reassured that it will resolve on its own.
- In certain circumstances where excessive scarring threatens to cause loss of definition, such as in the supratip area or radix, corticosteroid injection may be indicated to decrease the production of scar tissue.
- Triamcinolone acetate 3–5 mg (10 mg/mL) mixed with 2% lidocaine in a 1:1 ratio is injected into the supratip area with a 27 G needle.
- Depending on the clinical scenario, injections may be administered as early as 1 week postoperatively and repeated at 4- and 8-week intervals.
- Deformities may be identified in the postoperative period. Mild deformities should be observed. If they persist beyond 1 year, surgical treatment is required. Significant deformities should be corrected as soon as they are identified to avoid patient dissatisfaction.
- Deviations are managed similarly to deformities. Mild deviation may be corrected using nasal molding techniques. The patient is instructed to apply controlled pressure using his/her thumb along the nasal side wall 3–4 times per day for 4–6 weeks postoperatively. If the deviation is significant or persistent beyond 1 year, surgical treatment is required.
- Following rhinoplasty, most patients experience transient nasal airway obstruction secondary to edema. This typically resolves over 2–3 weeks as edema subsides.
- When nasal airway obstruction persists after 3 weeks, internal nasal examination using a topical vasoconstrictor should be performed to identify the cause.
- If it is secondary to edema, nasal decongestants can be used but topical vasoconstrictors should not be used for more than 7 days because of rebound congestion following cessation of these medications.
- If an anatomical cause of obstruction is identified, such as internal nasal valve collapse or synechiae, surgical treatment will be required but should be delayed for at least 1 year to allow for complete resolution of edema and maturation of scar tissue.
- The "post-rhinoplasty red nose" is a cutaneous manifestation of postoperative circulatory readjustment and is displayed varyingly in patients; many never develop this condition, whereas others develop it after the first rhinoplasty.
- Most improve spontaneously during the first postoperative year. When the condition persists, laser treatment is simple and effective.
- Lacrimal duct injury, cerebrospinal fluid rhinorrhea, cavernous sinus thrombosis, meningitis, permanent anosmia, recurrent intradermal cysts and blindness after corticosteroid injection for supratip deformity have been reported but are fortunately uncommon.
- Although it is difficult to determine an exact revision rate following primary open rhinoplasty, a recent survey revealed that 58% of those surveyed cited their revision rate less than 5% while another 33% reported their revision rate between 6 and 10%.

Further reading

Constantian MB. *Rhinoplasty: craft and magic*. St Louis: Quality Medical; 2009.

The author's complete text. Covers nasal phenomenology, so that preoperative and postoperative deformities can be seen to form patterns; therefore the solutions are not limitless but also form patterns. The rhinomanometric improvement in airflow is given for each case where the information was available, and analysis and exposition of intraoperative changes are emphasized. Chapters cover not only rhinoplasty analysis and technique but anatomic variants, function, right brain training for rhinoplasty, body dysmorphic disorder, and the author's own complications.

Edwards B. *A new drawing on the right side of the brain*. New York: Penguin Putnam; 1999.

A delightful and instructive adventure into art. Most of us lose the ability to "see" what is really in front of us as the left brain begins to dominate at about age 10, which is why most adults draw at that level of sophistication. Yet plastic surgery, not only rhinoplasty but breast reduction, TRAM flap shaping, forehead flaps, and many other procedures benefit from the ability to call upon right-brain skills at will. This book teaches how, in an entertaining way.

Fomon S, Gilbert JG, Caron AL, et al. Collapsed ala: pathologic physiology and management. *Arch Otolaryngol*. 1950;51:465.

A classic paper on what we now call external valvular collapse by a pioneer who intuitively understood what the next generation of surgeons forgot: that each airway has two sides.

Ghavami A, Janis JE, Acikel C, et al. Tip shaping in primary rhinoplasty: an algorithmic approach. *Plast Reconstr Surg*. 2008;122:1229–1241.

Underprojection and lack of tip definition often coexist. Techniques that improve both nasal tip refinement and projection are closely interrelated. The authors present a simplified algorithmic approach to creating aesthetic nasal tip shape and projection in primary rhinoplasty to aid the rhinoplasty surgeon in reducing the inherent unpredictability of combined techniques and improving long-term aesthetic outcomes.

Gunter JP, Rohrich RJ. Management of the deviated nose: the importance of septal reconstruction. *Clin Plast Surg*. 1988;15:43–55.

Gunter JP, Landecker A, Cochran CS. Frequently used grafts in rhinoplasty: nomenclature and analysis. *Plast Reconstr Surg*. 2006;118:14e–29e.

Howard BK, Rohrich RJ. Understanding the nasal airway: principles and practice. *Plast Reconstr Surg*. 2002;109:1128–1146.

Phillips KA. *The broken mirror: understanding and treating body dysmorphic disorder*. New York: Oxford University Press; 2005.

A text written by a noted authority on body dysmorphic disorder, intended for the lay public but so well referenced that it can be an introduction and reference work for the interested physician as well.

Rohrich RJ, Krueger JK, Adams Jr WP, et al. Achieving consistency in the lateral nasal osteotomy during rhinoplasty: an external perforated technique. *Plast Reconstr Surg*. 2001;108:2122–2130.

The lateral nasal osteotomy is an integral element in rhinoplasty. The authors present a reproducible and predictable technique for the lateral nasal osteotomy and discuss the role of the external perforated osteotomy technique in reproducing consistent results in rhinoplasty with minimal postoperative complications.

Rohrich RJ, Raniere Jr J, Ha RY. The alar contour graft: correction and prevention of alar rim deformities in rhinoplasty. *Plast Reconstr Surg*. 2002;109: 2495–2505.

Deformity of the alar rim is a common problem after primary and secondary rhinoplasty. It is caused by congenital malposition, hypoplasia, or surgical weakening of the lateral crura, with the potential for both functional and aesthetic consequences. The authors describe the use of the alar contour graft to provide the foundation for the re-establishment of a normally functioning external nasal valve and an aesthetically pleasing alar contour.

Rohrich RJ, Gunter JP, Deuber MA, et al. The deviated nose: optimizing results using a simplified classification and algorithmic approach. *Plast Reconstr Surg*. 2002;110:1509–1523.

The deviated nose frequently causes both functional and aesthetic problems. The authors present a classification and approach to the deviated nose that relies on accurate preoperative planning and precise intraoperative execution of corrective measures to return the nasal dorsum to midline, restore dorsal aesthetic lines, and maintain airway patency. An operative algorithm is described that emphasizes simplicity and reproducibility.

Rohrich RJ, Janis JE, Kenkel JM. Male rhinoplasty. *Plast Reconstr Surg*. 2003;112:1071–1085.

Rohrich RJ, Muzaffar AR. Rhinoplasty in the African-American patient. *Plast Reconstr Surg*. 2003;111:1322–1339.

Rohrich RJ, Muzaffar AR, Janis JE. Component dorsal hump reduction: the importance of maintaining dorsal aesthetic lines in rhinoplasty. *Plast Reconstr Surg*. 2004;114:1298–1308.

Dorsal hump reduction may result in dorsal irregularities caused by uneven resection, overresection or underresection of the osseocartilaginous hump, the inverted-V deformity, excessive narrowing of the midvault, and collapse of the internal valve. The authors present a technique for component dorsal hump reduction that allows a graduated approach to the correction of the nasal dorsum by emphasizing the integrity of the upper lateral cartilages when performing dorsal reduction.

Rohrich RJ, Ahmad J. Rhinoplasty. *Plast Reconstr Surg*. 2011;128:49e–73e.

Sheen JH, Sheen AP. *Aesthetic rhinoplasty*. 2nd ed. St Louis: Mosby;1987:988–1011.

This two volume text is the 2nd edition of the book that started the revolution in rhinoplasty of the 1980s and beyond. Our entire rhinoplasty lexicon derives from it. Virtually all of the text is still current and any surgeon seriously interested in learning rhinoplasty and its modern roots should own and study a copy.

Chapter 4

Otoplasty

This chapter was created using content from Neligan & Warren, Plastic Surgery 3rd edition, Volume 2, Aesthetic, Chapter 22, Otoplasty, Charles H. Thorne.

SYNOPSIS

- Analysis. Analyze the problem in thirds.
- Endpoint. Know what normal looks like, so you know your surgical endpoint.
- Do not be destructive. Do not do anything to the ear that cannot be reversed.
- Skin is precious but weak. Preserve skin in the sulcus and do not rely on skin tension to maintain ear position.
- Lobule. Consider lobule setback in every case.
- Asymmetry. In asymmetric cases, operate on both ears most of the time.
- Facelifts are otoplasties. Do not deform the tragus, lobule or sulcus.

Brief introduction

- "Otoplasty" refers to surgical changes in the shape or position of the ear.
- The most common indication is the patient with prominent, but normally shaped, ears.
- The single most important exercise for the surgeon, before performing any procedure in the otoplasty spectrum, is to have the characteristics of a normal ear firmly in his/her mind. With proper choice of technique, the surgeon can usually avoid the uncorrectable problems of over-correction and unnatural contours ***(Figs 4.1, 4.2)***.
- It has also never been shown that an otoplasty retards auricular growth.

Preoperative considerations

- Otoplasty is unique in that it is perhaps the only cosmetic procedure that can be performed in childhood, and both parents and grandparents may be involved in surgical decision making for the patient who cannot yet express himself or herself.
- The overall size and shape of the ear is evaluated to determine if the ear is prominent with an otherwise normal size and configuration, or if there are abnormalities in addition to the prominence.
- The upper third of the ear is evaluated to determine if it is prominent, if the antihelix/superior crus of the triangular fossa is well formed and if the helical rim is well defined.
- The middle third of the ear is evaluated to determine if the concha is overly deep or protruding.
- The relationship between the antihelix and the helix is examined to determine if any underdevelopment of the antihelix/superior crus in the upper third extends into the middle third or if it is confined to the upper third.
- The lobule is evaluated to determine if it is prominent.
- Even if the lobule is not particularly prominent on initial examination, it may become prominent once the upper two-thirds of the ear have been corrected
- Asymmetry is noted, mostly because patients and families will always comment on it.
- In asymmetric cases it is usually preferable to operate on both ears rather than attempt to set back only the prominent ear to match its less prominent counterpart (see Fig. 4.1).
- The degree of prominence/deformity and the age at presentation will determine when a surgical recommendation is made.

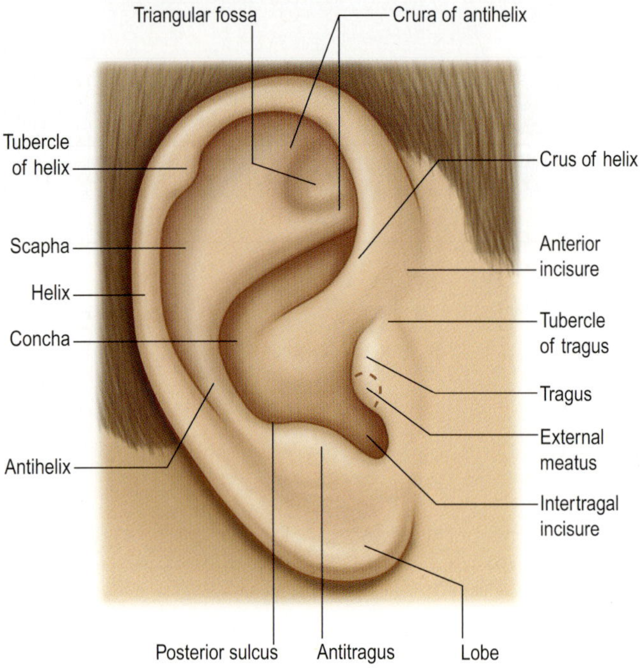

Figure 4.1 Anatomical structures of the ear. The tubercle of the helix is synonymous with Darwinian's tubercle. (Reprinted with permission from Janis JE, Rohrich RJ, Gutowski KA. Otoplasty. *Plast Reconstr Surg.* 2005;115(4):60e–72e.)

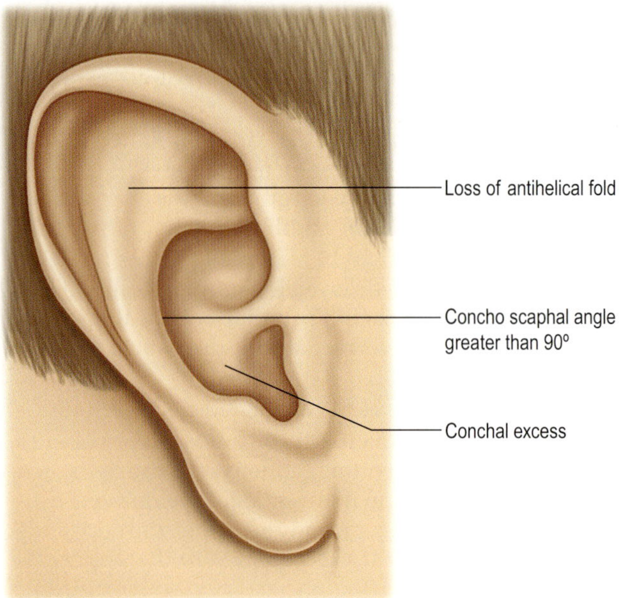

Figure 4.2 Main components of the prominent ear. (Reprinted with permission from Janis JE, Rohrich RJ, Gutowski KA. Otoplasty. *Plast Reconstr Surg.* 2005;115(4):60e–72e.)

- For young children with very prominent ears and whose parents desire early correction, otoplasty is recommended as early as age 4 years.
- Four years of age can be viewed as a minimum for most otoplasty procedures.
- When the entire ear requires reconstruction, as in microtia, this author prefers to wait until approximately 10 years of age.
- In some cases, the parents may want the child to participate in the decision process and that will necessitate later intervention.
- It is common to have patients present at approximately 18 years of age, when they are legally independent, or later when they have earned the money for the procedure.
- It is not unusual for adults at almost any age to request correction, either because they have wanted it all their lives or because their desire to have other procedures (e.g., a facelift), has led to the realization that their ears are also prominent.

Anatomic/technical pearls

- While the delicate, complex contours of the ear may be difficult to create *de novo* (i.e., microtia), anatomic considerations are minimal in standard otoplasty.
- There is abundant blood supply, making almost any combination of incisions acceptable without the risk of necrosis.
- There are no motor nerves in the neighborhood. The terminal branches of the great auricular nerve will always be injured but normal sensory function usually returns.
- The one anatomic structure that can be compromised in otoplasty is the external auditory canal (conchal setback narrows the meatus). Otherwise, the anatomic considerations of otoplasty are those of preservation:
  - Preservation of the sulcus.
  - Preservation of the natural softness of the auricular contours.
  - Preservation of the normal landmarks such as the posterior wall of the concha (i.e., the middle third of the antihelix).
- Otoplasty surgery is all about the endpoint. The right endpoint can be achieved with a thorough knowledge of a normal ear. If the surgeon remembers the following regarding how the ear should look from various vantage points it will aid tremendously in the intraoperative decision-making:
  - From the front, the helical rim should be visible, poking out from behind the antihelix.
  - From the side, the contours of the ear should be round and soft, never sharp.
  - From behind (and this is the most helpful to the surgeon who is sitting behind the patient intraoperatively), the contour of the helical rim should be a straight line, not a "C", or a "hockey stick", or any other shape. If the helical contour is a straight line, it almost ensures that a harmonious correction will be achieved.
  - Regardless, if the ultimate correction is slightly under- or slightly over-corrected, a harmonious correction will read as "normal" to the outside world and almost all patients will be happy. This is perhaps the single most important lesson from this chapter.

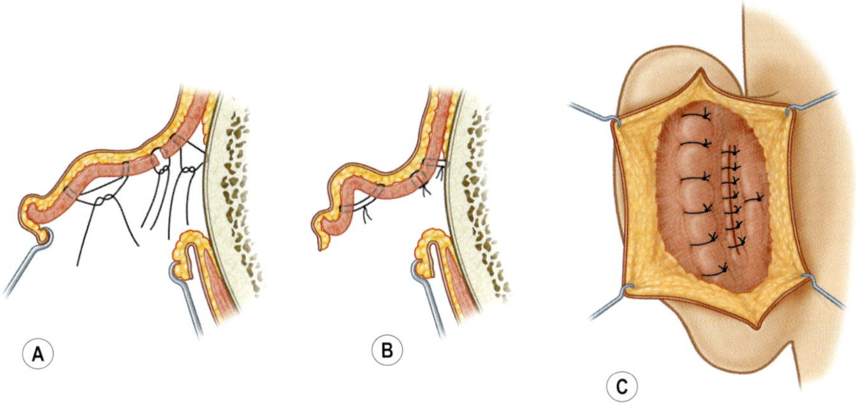

Figure 4.3 Technique for the standard otoplasty. The combination of Mustarde sutures, conchal resection/closure and concha-mastoid sutures is shown. **(A)** Suture placement. **(B)** Suture tightened and ties appropriately. **(C)** Position of sutures as shown from the surgeon's vantage point.

- The last judgment is how close to the head the ear should be placed. The final position of the ear should be over-corrected minimally to allow for some relapse, but not enough to create an unsatisfactory result if no relapse should occur.

Operative techniques

Standard otoplasty for prominent ears of normal size

- The incision is made in the retroauricular sulcus.
- In the upper third of the ear, it can be extended up to the back of the ear to provide adequate exposure to place Mustarde sutures between the triangular fossa and scapha.
- No skin is excised, except a small triangle from the medial surface of the lobule (not the retrolobular skin), taking care to preserve enough tissue for a normal earlobe and retrolobular sulcus.
- This skin excision on the lobule is frequently necessary for repositioning of the lobule at the end of the procedure.
- The cartilage is exposed on the posterior (medial) surface of the ear and soft tissue is excised from deep to the concha.
- In the region of the earlobe, deep dissection is performed under the concha in preparation for lobule repositioning. Branches of the great auricular nerve will be seen and divided.
- Mustarde concha–scapha and triangular fossa–scapha sutures are placed using 4-0 clear nylon sutures on an FS-2 needle *(Fig. 4.3)*.
- The number of sutures depends on the how far into the middle third of the ear the antihelical deficiency extends.
- These sutures are placed in order to create a soft curvature to the antihelix and no attempt is made to correct the prominence of the ear at this point.
- The Mustarde sutures are not parallel to each other but, instead, are arranged like spokes on a wheel, all pointing toward the top of the tragus (center of the wheel).
- Care is taken to create a superior crus that curves anteriorly such that it terminates almost parallel to the inferior crus.
- If the superior crus is created such that it is a direct, cephalad extension of the antihelix (straight line), the result will appear unnatural and amateurish.
- A small crescent of cartilage (≤3 mm at its widest point) is excised from the posterior wall of the concha, at its junction with the conchal floor.
- The defect in the concha is closed primarily using numerous 4-0 nylon sutures.
- It is important that the conchal resection be placed precisely as lack of attention to the placement of the conchal resection is a common cause of complications.
- If the resection is too large or if it is too far up the posterior conchal wall, then it will irrevocably deform the antihelix.
- If the resection is too far anterior, in the floor of the concha, it will not decrease the height of the posterior conchal wall and the closure may be visible.
- A conchal setback suture (Furnas suture) is then placed between the reduced concha and the mastoid fascia using a single 3-0 nylon or 3-0 PDS suture.
- This combination of a small conchal resection and a small conchal setback avoids the distortion of a large conchal resection and the unreliability of a large conchal setback.
- This author avoids conchal setback alone in all but the mildest cases as it can narrow the external auditory meatus to the point of significant stenosis *(Fig. 4.4)*.
- The earlobe is repositioned by closing the triangular defect on the medial surface of the lobule created by the skin excision *(Fig. 4.5)*.
- The 5-0 PDS sutures do not just approximate the skin; rather, they approximate the skin AND take a bite of the concha deep in the sulcus (similar to Gosain and Recinos).
- Ideally, the endpoint of earlobe repositioning should be slight over-correction because the skin will stretch over time.
- The skin is approximated using 5-0 plain gut sutures *(Figs 4.6, 4.7)*.

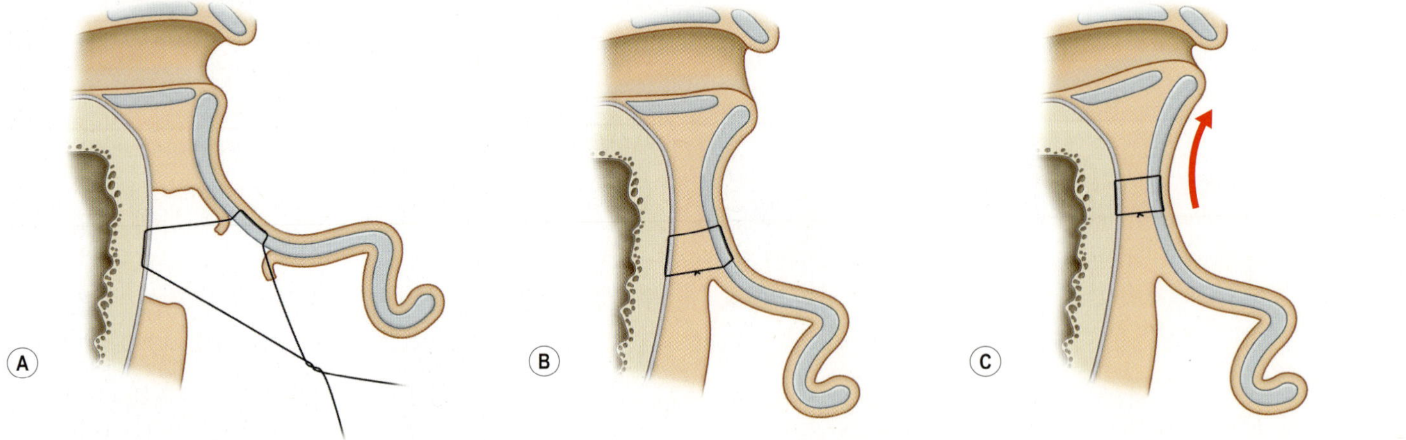

Figure 4.4 Placement of Furnas concha-mastoid sutures. Note that suture placement too close to the external auditory canal can constrict the canal (far right). (Reprinted with permission from Janis JE, Rohrich RJ, Gutowski KA. Otoplasty. *Plast Reconstr Surg.* 2005;115(4):60e–72e.)

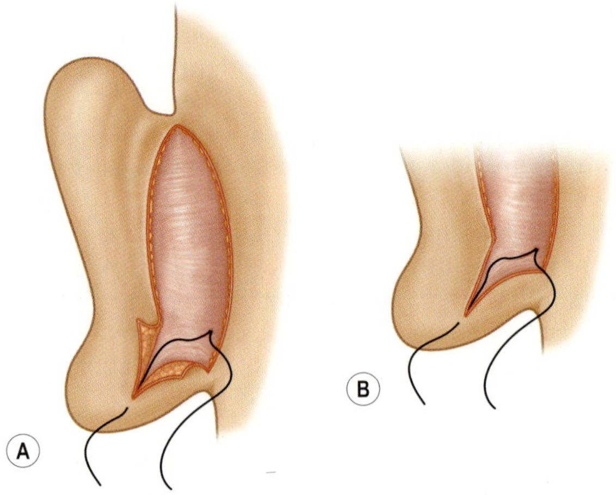

Figure 4.5 Lobule repositioning. The technique for lobule repositioning is shown. A triangle of skin is excised on the earlobe, never compromising the appearance of the lobe or the ability for the patient to wear earrings. Sutures are placed close to the skin defect while catching a bite of the concha deep in the closure.

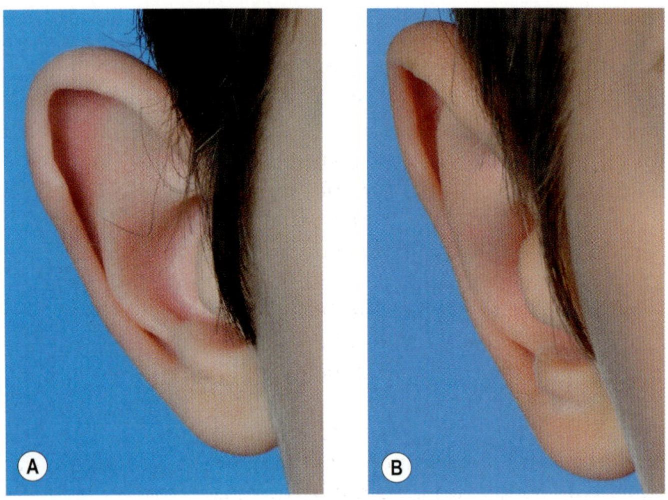

Figure 4.6 Otoplasty. The patient is shown before **(A)** and after **(B)** standard otoplasty. The upper, middle and lower thirds of the ear have been set back in a harmonious fashion. The contours are soft and natural.

Otoplasty for large ears or ears with inadequate helical rim definition

Incision

- An incision is made on the lateral (visible) surface of the ear, just inside the helical rim (or where the helical rim would be if it is underdeveloped).
- In addition, an incision in the retroauricular sulcus may also be required depending on what additional maneuvers are required.
- The lateral incision is extended through the cartilage. The posterior surface of the cartilage is dissected, just as if a standard posterior incision had been made.
- In the case of excessively large ears, the scaphal cartilage (and perhaps some scaphal skin) are trimmed to the desired size and shape.
- Care is taken to excise more cartilage than skin.
- At this point the helical rim will be too long for the new scapha and will require shortening at the end of the procedure.
- Mustarde sutures are placed if necessary through this anterior access.
- Conchal resection/setback and earlobe repositioning are performed through a separate incision in the sulcus if necessary ***(Fig. 4.8)***.
- A wedge is then removed from the helical rim so that it will fit the scapha, which is now of lesser circumference.
- The desired resection will leave the helix the correct length for the new scapha and allow closure without excess tension.
- The helix is reapproximated carefully using horizontal mattress sutures of 5-0 nylon sutures attempting to evert the skin edges to avoid notching.
- The lateral incision is closed with a combination of a few interrupted 5-0 plain sutures and a running 6-0 plain suture.

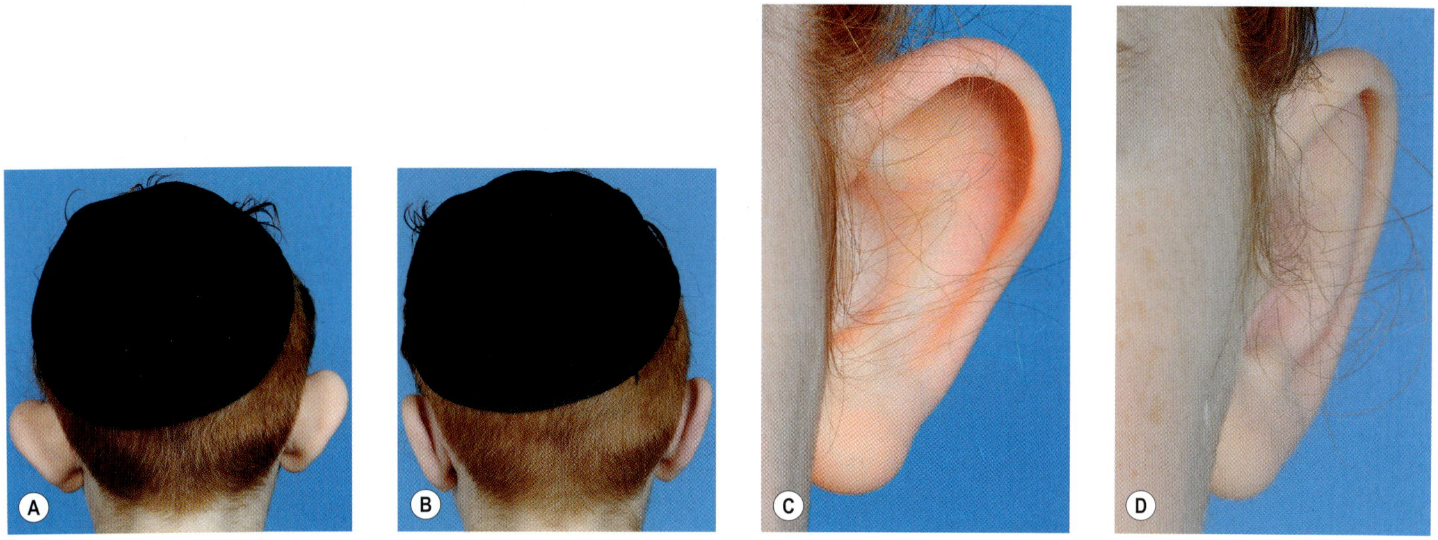

Figure 4.7 Otoplasty. **(A,B)** Posterior view before and after otoplasty. The helical rim contour is straight and the scars are hidden within the sulcus. **(C,D)** Frontal view showing harmonious correction and soft natural contours.

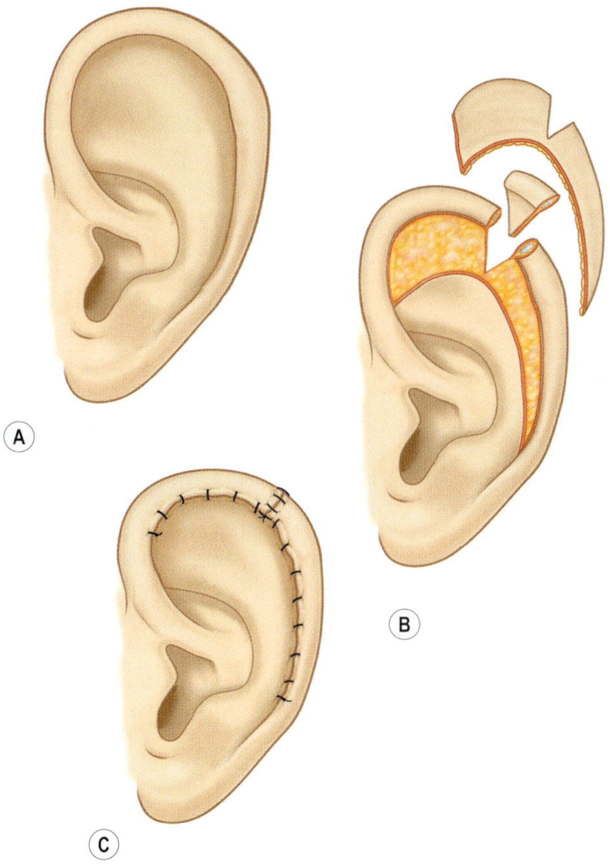

Figure 4.8 Ear reduction. The technique of ear reduction is shown. (Redrawn from Argamaso RV. Ear reduction. *Plast Reconstr Surg.* 1990;85(2):316.)

Otoplasty for constricted ears

- Constricted ears are tremendously variable and no single technique is applicable to all. Tanzer divided constricted ear deformities into three types: type 1 – involving only the helix, type II – involving the helix and scapha, type III – extreme cupping of the ear.
- The simplest constricted ear deformity is the "lop ear", in which the upper pole of the ear is turned over. There is always deficiency of tissue in this region.
- In some cases, it is adequate to excise directly the leading edge of the overhanging skin and cartilage to create a less hooded appearance.
- In more significant deformities (Tanzer type II), it is necessary to expand the overhanging cartilage with radial cuts and reinforce the area with a conchal graft.
- Other constricted ears may appear prominent because the helical circumference is inadequate as if the helix has been tightened excessively like a drawstring, forcing the ear forward. Thus the ear cannot lie flat because the excessively short helical rim draws the auricle into a cup.
- Any attempt to set back a constricted ear must be accompanied by elongation of the helix.
- The most common technique for elongating the helix is by a variation of the incision described above for large ears.
- The incision is made inside the helical rim and extended anteriorly around the crus of the helix into the preauricular region to the junction of the ear and the temporal scalp.
- The crus of the helix is then mobilized and when standard otoplasty maneuvers are performed, the crus of the helix is recruited into the helical rim.
- The donor site in the concha is closed primarily as if the crus of the helix had been taken for a composite graft to the nose.

- Any excess or unusable crus of the helix is discarded.
- In the case of more severely constricted ears (Tanzer type III), it is preferable to discard the cartilage and construct a framework as if the patient had classic microtia.

Otoplasty for cryptotia

- Cryptotia is the rare condition where the upper portion of the ear is buried beneath the temporal scalp. The ear can often be pulled out of the scalp to examine it.
- Correction is performed by pulling the ear out of its bed in the scalp, incising around it in order to release it fully, and resurfacing the defect behind the upper pole of ear with a skin graft or a local flap.
- In some cases, the auricular cartilage is normal in contour and only requires the soft tissue rearrangement described above for correction.
- In other cases, the cartilage is misshapen, as in a lop ear, and requires cartilage grafting to augment the deficient native cartilage framework in addition to the soft tissue considerations.

Otoplasty for Stahl's ears

- Stahl's ear is defined by an abnormal crus extending superolaterally and the deformity is variable.
- In the mildest cases, the extra crus is barely noticeable and can be ignored and the otoplasty performed as if it were a standard case of prominent ears.
- More severe deformities include excess scapha in the region of the abnormal crus and termination of the abnormal crus in a point ("Mr Spock" ears).
- In the most severe cases, there is also complete absence of the normal superior crus.
- Correction of the deformity mandates resection of the abnormal crus.
- The author makes an incision inside the helical rim as described above but *not* through the cartilage.
- The skin is carefully dissected off the lateral surface of the cartilage *(Fig. 4.9)*.
- The abnormal crus is resected and placed as an onlay graft to reconstruct the absent superior crus.
- The cartilaginous defect left by the resected crus is closed primarily and the skin is then reapproximated.

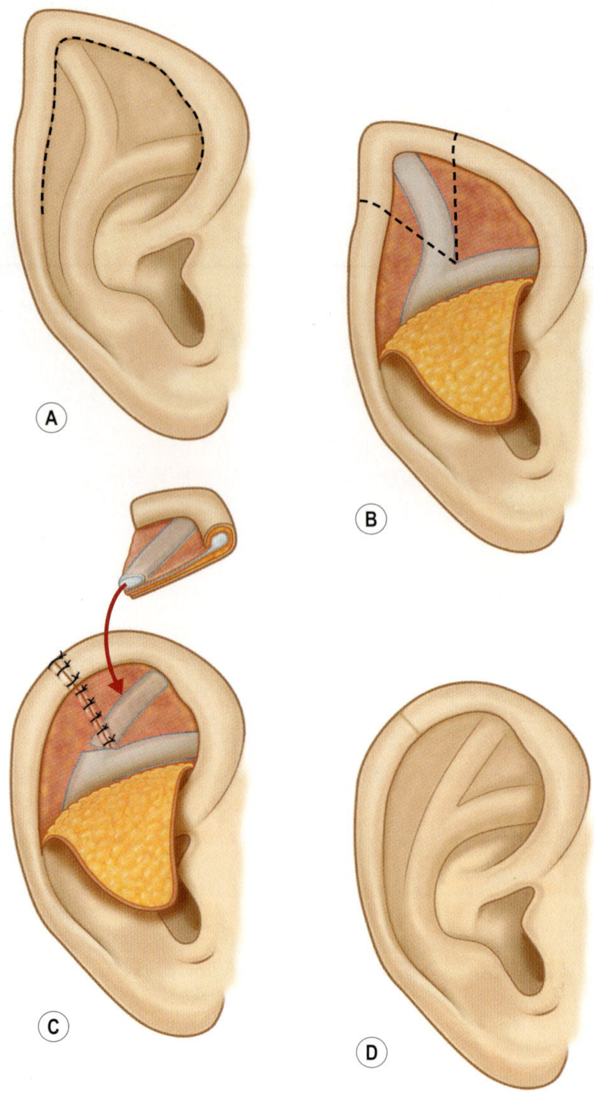

Figure 4.9 Correction of Stahl's ear. The lateral skin is reflected, the abnormal crus is excised, the cartilage defect is closed primarily and the cartilage from the excised crus is used as an onlay graft to recreate the normal superior crus. **(A)** The skin incision is shown inside the helical rim. **(B)** The abnormal crus is excised. **(C)** The cartilage defect is reapproximated and the excised cartilage is placed as an onlay graft to reconstruct the superior crus. **(D)** The final result. (Redrawn from Kaplan HM, Hudson DA. A novel surgical method of repair for Stahl's ear; a case report and review of current treatment modalities. *Plast Reconstr Surg.* 1999;103:566–569.)

Correction of aging, elongated ear lobes

- A number of techniques have been described and the anatomy of the individual patient dictates the design.
- The most common procedure in the author's hands, however, is amputation of the caudal border of the lobule with scar placement on the back side of the earlobe where it is not visible.
- The ideal contour is drawn on the lobule. The excision is designed asymmetrically so that the incision is made caudal to this line on the lateral surface and cephalic to it on the medial surface.
- This asymmetry leads to greater resection from the medial side of the ear lobe and creates a longer skin flap on the lateral surface.
- The lateral flap is thinned so it is more mobile than its medial counterpart.
- The combination of the asymmetric design, the thinner lateral flap and the fact that the ends of the defect are not located precisely on the margin of the lobule but rather slightly medial to it, result in the ultimate scar being hidden on the medial surface of the lobule. Numerous sutures, meticulous tapering and some patience are required for the best outcome.

Correction of earring-related complications

- While a number of procedures have been described for correction of elongated piercings, the author has found that simple excision and closure is most effective.

- This technique applies to both elongated earring holes and those that have torn completely through the lobule margin.
- In the case of a complete traumatic cleft lobule, a Z-plasty can be added in an effort to avoid a notch.
- In reality, an everted closure using horizontal mattress sutures seems to yield equivalent results at the lobule margin.
- The medial and lateral skin is closed with nylon sutures, and no deep, absorbable sutures are used.
- Avoiding absorbable sutures in the subcutaneous tissue of the lobe seems to minimize the inflammation and shorten the recovery and the waiting period before re-piercing.
- The earlobes can be re-pierced in 6 weeks, depending on how stiff and fibrotic they are after the repair.

Correction of facelift deformities around the ear

- Facelift deformities of the ear are frequently unfixable, leading to lesson number one in facelifting: AVOID THEM. Problems fall into the following categories:
  - Deformities of the lobule (pixie ear): the result of excessive anterior and inferior traction on the lobule due to inexpert trimming of the facelift flap. Such deformities are completely avoidable but difficult to correct.
  - The facial skin should be trimmed so that the ear can barely be pulled out from under it.
  - Deformities of the tragus: consist of either anterior traction on the tragus, amputation of some of the tragal cartilage or excess facial skin at the bottom of the tragus that serves as an across-the-room surgical signature.
  - There is little that can be done for the first two conditions, since too much tissue has been removed.
  - A lack of definition of the caudal tragus can be corrected by removing a triangle of skin from the caudal aspect of the tragus to recreate the natural, right-angle contour.
  - Deformities of the retroauricular sulcus: placing facelift incisions high up on the back of the ear repeatedly may result in thinning of the skin and a pulled back appearance.
  - Once the deformity is created, there is no solution except release of the ear and placement of a full thickness skin graft.
  - Unsightly scarring: can frequently be improved by excision and additional facelifting maneuvers as long as no tension is placed on the closure.
  - The facelift flap should be redraped and trimmed so the edges are touching. While a few sutures are placed, no sutures should really be necessary in the preauricular region or the postauricular sulcus.
  - Hypertrophic scars are more problematic. Therefore, revision of scars should be approached with trepidation.
  - Kenalog injection is helpful and eliminates the need for revision in many cases.
  - If recurrent hypertrophic scars or real keloids develop, the author recommends scar revision with postoperative radiation beginning immediately on the day of the scar revision.

Postoperative considerations

- A piece of Xeroform and a soft bulky dressing are placed on the skin. The purpose of the dressing is to protect the repair, keep the skin of the ear moist, and to absorb drainage.
- No attempt is made to put pressure on the ear and often a doughnut of gauze is placed around each ear specifically to avoid pressure.
- The dressing is left in place 3–5 days depending on when the most convenient day for an office visit occurs.
- The patient or family is instructed to wear a loose headband at night only. The goal is to have no pressure on the ear during the day and only enough at night to prevent inadvertent pulling forward of the repaired auricle.
- The nocturnal headband is continued for 4–6 weeks, although most patients confess to discarding it much sooner than that. Remember, the headband should only be tight enough so that it does not fall off.

Complications and outcomes

- Most patients who undergo otoplasty are satisfied with the results, making the procedure gratifying for the surgeon as well.
- Suture complications are relatively common:
  - The Nylon Mustarde sutures may eventually protrude through the posterior skin. This may occur within the first few weeks or not for years.
  - In some cases, the sutures are associated with inflammation or a granuloma.
  - Suture removal immediately cures any apparent infection and does not seem to lead to recurrence of the prominent ear.
- The second most common complication is under-correction or recurrence:
  - While this is not ideal, it is far better in this author's opinion than over-correction or distortion.
- Infection and hematoma may also occur.
- Unfortunately, patients requesting secondary procedures are not uncommon. The most common complaints of these patients are:
- Over-correction. This can usually be improved by removing sutures, undermining skin and occasionally placing a skin graft.
- Visible cartilage irregularities or unnatural contours. Firmin has the best and most impressive series of patients in this category in whom she has removed the damaged cartilage and placed expertly carved pieces of rib cartilage.

- Unpleasing shape of the ear (e.g. telephone ear, protruding lobules).
- Unpleasing shapes of the ear such as telephone ear (where the middle third of the ear is over-corrected relative to the upper and lower poles) can usually be improved significantly simply by restoring the natural contour harmony.
- Under-correction, usually of the upper pole of the ear. Often easily corrected by revision otoplasty.

Further reading

Argamaso RV. Ear reduction with or without setback otoplasty. *Plast Reconstr Surg*. 1989;83(6):967–975.

Converse JM, Wood-Smith D. Technical details in the surgical correction of the lop ear deformity. *Plast Reconstr Surg*. 1963;31:118–128.

Firmin F. Ear reconstruction in cases of typical microtia. Personal experience based on 352 microtic ear corrections. *Scand J Plast Reconstr Surg Hand Surg*. 1998;32(1):35–47.

Furnas DW. Correction of prominent ears by concha mastoid sutures. *Plast Reconstr Surg*. 1968;42: 189–193.

Gosain AK, Recinos RF. A novel approach to correction of the prominent lobule during otoplasty. *Plast Reconstr Surg*. 2003;112(2):575–583.

Kajikawa A, Ueda K, Asai E, et al. A new surgical correction of cryptotia: A new flap design and switched double banner flap. *Plast Reconstr Surg*. 2009;123(3):897–901.

Kaplan HM, Hudson DA. A novel surgical method of repair for Stahl's ear: a case report and review of current treatment modalities. *Plast Reconstr Surg*. 1999;103(2):566–569.

Luckett WH. A new operation for prominent ears based on the anatomy of the deformity. *Surg Gynecol Obstet*. 1910;10:635.

McDowell AJ. Goals in otoplasty for protruding ears. *Plast Reconstr Surg*. 1968;41:17–27.

Matsuo K, Hirose T, Tomono T, et al. Nonsurgical correction of congenital auricular deformities in the early neonate. A preliminary report. *Plast Reconstr Surg*. 1984;73:38–51.

This is the first report showing the enormous potential for neonatal molding of congenital ear deformities.

Mustarde JC. The correction of prominent ears using simple mattress sutures. *Br J Plast Surg*. 1963;16: 170–178.

Spira M. Otoplasty: what I do now – a 30-year perspective. *Plast Reconstr Surg*. 1999;104(3):834–840.

Stenstroem SJ. A "natural" technique for correction of congenitally prominent ears. *Plast Reconstr Surg*. 1963;32:509–518.

The technique of otoabrasion is described. The technique was fully embraced by a large number of surgeons.

Tanzer RC. The constricted (cup and lop) ear. *Plast Reconstr Surg*. 1975;55:406–415.

Thorne CH. Otoplasty. *Plast Reconstr Surg*. 2008;122(1): 291–292.

The author of this chapter demonstrates his preferred otoplasty technique in a video and emphasizes the role of endpoint visualization when performing the procedure.

Webster GV. The tail of the helix as a key to otoplasty. *Plast Reconstr Surg*. 1969;44(5):455–461.

This paper describes a technique for repositioning the lobule that is a classic but with which the author of this chapter has not had success.

Chapter 5

Abdominoplasty

This chapter was created using content from Neligan & Warren, Plastic Surgery 3rd edition, Volume 2, Aesthetic, Chapter 25, Abdominoplasty procedures, Dirk F. Richter and Alexander Stoff.

SYNOPSIS

- Assessment of the abdominal region includes a detailed medical and physical history, including pregnancies, prior surgeries especially in the lower truncal area, and weight changes. Preoperative identification of any existing ventral hernia including diastasis recti is imperative.
- Essential abdominal exam findings include the existence and localization of vertical and horizontal tissue excess, the relationship between fatty excess and skin excess, and examination of the umbilical stalk with exclusion of umbilical hernia.
- Further perioperative adjuncts include preoperative bowel evacuation for reduction of intraabdominal pressure, careful intraoperative tissue handling, maintainance of an adequate body temperature, sufficient medical thromboembolism prophylaxis, precise intraoperative preparation with respect to anatomical key points, postoperative compression treatment and early management of postoperative complications such as seromas.
- The fleur-de-lis abdominoplasty allows an improvement of the entire abdominal area with simultaneous tightening of the waist circumference. Hereby it is essential to initially assess and temporarily close the vertical line prior to resection of the lower abdominal redundant tissue. Care should be taken to avoid extending the vertical incision line cranially between the breasts.
- In patients after massive weight loss, aesthetic outcome will improve by high-lateral-tension and fleur-de-lis abdominoplasty. However, in most cases circumferential truncal procedures are necessary for superior results.
- The preservation of the loose areolar epifascial tissue allows preservation of subfascial lymphatic vessels which reduces the incidence of seroma formation.
- It is mandatory to analyze any suspected skin tumor in the area of excised tissue.

Brief introduction

- Abdominoplasty is one of the most commonly performed aesthetic procedures which encompasses not only aesthetic features but also structural reconstruction of the abdominal wall.
- Due to the number of variations and modifications of abdominoplasty procedures, it is critical to select the appropriate technique based upon patient characteristics in order to minimize morbidity and postoperative disability while providing a desirable and predictable result.
- Pregnancy is the most common cause of abdominal wall aesthetic deformities because the skin and musculoaponeurotic structures are stretched beyond their biomechanical capability to retract.
- Massive weight loss after dieting or bariatric surgery results in excess, inelastic skin and subcutaneous tissue and a laxity of the abdominal wall musculature.
- Fat accumulation occurs in a distribution pattern that varies according to the gender. Normal anatomic abdominal proportions can be found in ***Figure 5.1***.
  - Women tend to add local adiposity in the lower trunk and hip region as well as posterior thigh region which can result in cellulite, or fibrous septa within the subcutaneous tissue.
  - Men tend to add intraabdominal adipose tissue resulting in an increase in abdominal girth.

Preoperative considerations

- In addition to standard documentation of other medical co-morbidities and medications, the medical history should also include documentation of the following: a detailed weight history including current BMI, history of

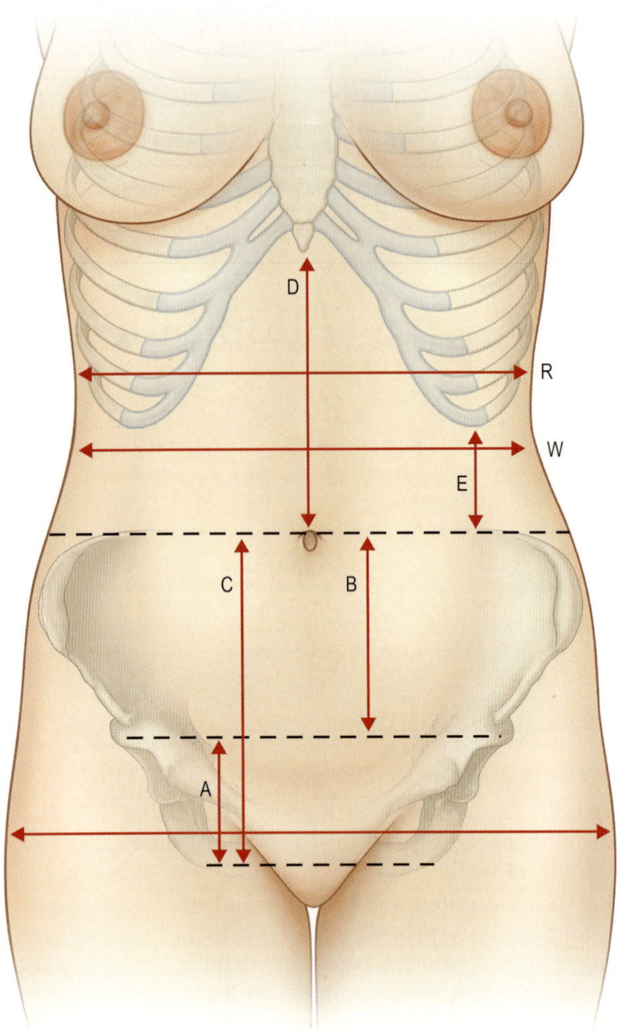

Figure 5.1 Anatomical landmarks. Normal abdominal anatomic proportions. The approximate measurements for an average female abdomen are listed. These vary according to individual height and bone structure. The umbilicus is located in line with the most superior point of the iliac crest in 99% of patients. **A,** Distance between top of mons and anterior vilvar commissure. Average height is 5–7 cm. **B,** Distance between umbilicus and top of mons. Average height is 11–13 cm. **C** (=A + B) Distance between umbilicus and top of anterior and vulvar commissure (C=D). **E,** distance between the costal margina and the iliac crest. The proportion of this distance to the width of the base of the rib cage (R) determines whether the patient is long waisted or short waisted. The normal proportion (E : R) is roughly 1 : 3 (long waisted approaches 1 : 2, short waisted approaches 1 : 3).The rib cage tapers inferiorly. A more narrow lower rib cage relative to the width under the armpits helps to emphasize the waist by creating a subtle V. **H,** hip width. A wider pelvis than rib cage emphasizes the waist; the waist is more defined when R<H. **W,** Natural waist – the narrowest point of the torso. (Note that the umbiculus usually sits below the natural waist by about 1–4 cm). Relative to the hips, this waist-to-hip (W : H) ratio in healthy women is roughly 0.72 : 1; in healthy men, it is roughly 0.83 : 1. Note that the natural contour of the healthy abdomen reveals a subtle epigastric sagittal depression transitioning to a mild infraumbilical convexity. A subtle vertical sulcus at the lateral rectus border, which is more distinct in a muscular person, may also be seen.

weight fluctuations, and/or history of prior bariatric procedures; a detailed pregnancy history including number of pregnancies/children and history of cesarean section; history of other abdominal surgeries, including suction assisted lipectomy, and abdominal hernias.

- Physical examination should be performed in the seated and upright positions, and should focus on the following findings and measurements:
  - Quality of skin.
  - Thickness of adipose tissue by pinching.
  - Number and location of folds.
  - Location of abdominal wall defects.
  - Patient's favored clothings.
  - Preexisting scars.
  - Status of abdominal musculature.
  - Distance from umbilicus to top of mons, from umbilicus to sternal notch, and from anterior vulva commissure to top of mons.
  - Waist and hip measurement, waist-to-hip ratio.
- In cases of diagnostic uncertainly, a computed tomography or magnetic resonance imaging test can be helpful in determining the presence of hernia.
- Patient weight should be stable for at least 12 months preoperatively; with any desired weight loss achieved prior to the surgery.
- Cessation of smoking should occur ideally 6 weeks prior to the surgery and after, but at the least 2 weeks prior and for at least 2 weeks postoperative to minimize the risk for postoperative wound complications.
- Patients should take antiseptic showers in the evening and morning prior to the surgery, the abdominal folds and the umbilicus should be cleaned thoroughly with cotton sticks and antiseptic solutions.
- Anticoagulant drugs must be avoided prior to surgery. The patient should also avoid perioperative use of various homeopathic drugs and nutritional supplements, which can induce bleeding.

Anatomic pearls

- The abdominal wall is embryonically derived in a segmental manner, reflected in blood supply and innervation.
- The umbilicus:
  - Situated in the midline, approximately 9–12 cm above the mons pubis.
  - The periumbical area is characterized by a round or eliptoid shape with a slight depression of 4–6 cm in diameter.
  - The fascia surrounding the umbilicus can be unstable with an increased incidence for hernias, resulting in a risk of bowel injury during umbilical dissection.
  - The blood supply to the periumbilical area is supplied by branches from the subdermal plexus, from both deep inferior epigastric arteries as well as the median umbilical ligament.
- The skin of the abdomen has areas of increased adherence to the underlying fascia ("zones of adherence"), such as the anterior superior iliac crest and the linea alba.
- The abdominal subcutaneous tissue is divided by two layers of fascia, the superficial Camper's fascia and the deep Scarpa's fascia, a strong fibrous layer of connective

tissue which is continuous with the fascia lata of the thigh.

- The superficial fat layer has a more compact character with smaller lobules and a rich vascularization, while the deeper fat layer contains larger lobules with a more scattered pattern.
- The abdominal musculature includes four paired muscles, which are the rectus abdominis, connected in the median linea alba, the external oblique and internal oblique and the transversus abdominis muscle, which incorporate into the anterior and posterior rectus sheath at the linea semilunaris *(Fig. 5.2)*.
- The abdominal lymphatic system is divided into a supraumbical system which drains into the ipsilateral axillary lymph node basin and an infraumbilical drainage system which drains into the ipsilateral superficial inguinal lymph node basin.
- The lymph vessels in the infraumbical area pass through the subscarpal plane, explaining the importance of Scarpa's fascia preservation in abdominal wall surgery.
- Huger described different zones of the abdominal blood supply which should guide the surgeon in planning and performing a safe operation *(Fig. 5.3)*:
  - Zone 1: the midline supplied by the vertically oriented deep epigastric arcade.
  - Zone II: the lower abdominal circulation supplied by the superficial epigastric, superficial external pudendal, and superficial circumflex iliac systems.
  - Zone III: the lateral aspect of the abdominal wall (flanks) supplied by the 6 lateral intercostal and 4 lumbar arteries.
- In standard abdominoplasty procedures, the cutaneous blood supply to zone I and a main part of zone II is disrupted, resulting in an abdominal flap perfusion mainly supplied by zone III. Therefore it is crucial to study any preoperative existing scar, such as subcostal cholecystectomy incisions. In certain circumstances, even a vertical midline incision can jeopardize flap perfusion.
- Cutaneous sensation of the abdominal wall is derived from the anterior and lateral cutaneous branches of the intercostal nerves 8 to 12.
- The anterior branches pass between the internal oblique and transversus abdominis muscles, enter the rectus abdominis muscle and reach the overlying fascia and skin.
- The lateral cutaneous branches penetrate the intercostal muscles in the midaxillary line, ending in the subcutaneous layer.
- Both branches are responsible for the overlapping of the sensory dermatomes T5 to L1.
- The ilioinguinal and iliohypogastric nerves, not involved in innervation of the abdominal wall, can be disrupted and injured in lateral transverse lower abdominal incisions, resulting in consistent sensory loss in the area of the groin and medioventral thigh *(Fig. 5.4)*.
- Patients with significant health risks, with unrealistic surgical goals and body dysmorphic disorder are primary contraindications for an elective abdominoplasty procedure.
- Relative contraindications to abdominoplasty include right, left, or bilateral upper quadrant scars, further severe co-morbid conditions (e.g., heart disease, diabetes, morbid obesity, cigarette smoking), eventual future plans for pregnancy, a history of thromboembolic disease, and morbid obesity (BMI >40).
- Patients with disposition to keloids or hypertrophic scars have to be informed, and must accept the postoperative scarring associated with these conditions.

Operative technique (Video 5.1, Video 5.2, Video 5.3)

Video 5.1
Video 5.2
Video 5.3

Marking and positioning

- The patient should be marked preoperative in the upright position. Borders of underwear, where possible, should be marked in an attempt to place the scar in a hidden position *(Fig. 5.5)*.
- The expected resection should be estimated by the pinch test *(Fig. 5.6)*.
- The lower incision line will run parallel to the scar line and is normally below the abdominal fold, and 6–7 cm superior to the vulvar commissure.
- The upper incision line is an estimate and should be tailored intraoperatively depending on tension.
- Local fat depots are marked for guidance with adjunctive liposuction.
- Perioperative thromboprophylaxis with sequential compression devices should be implemented in all patients having abdominal wall surgery. In many cases, the intraoperative and postoperative use of heparin may also be indicated.
- While antibiotic prophylaxis is not universally required, it may be indicated as a single preoperative dose, especially if a hernia is present.
- Patient positioning on the operating room table should include adequate padding of feet, knees, buttocks, back (especially for hyperlodosis cases), shoulders, and head. In addition, the patient's hips should be placed at the level of the break in the table for adequate flexion during the wound closure portion of the case.

Mini abdominoplasty

- Characterized by a transverse incision that is shorter than the incision used in full abdominoplasty procedures.
- Indicated in patients with a mild to moderate skin laxity and tissue excess of the lower (infraumbilical) abdomen, together with a sufficient distance between the symphysis and the umbilicus.
- Common for young women with a pre-existing Pfannenstiel incision to benefit from this technique.
- A distance of at least 9 cm between the upper resection line and the umbilicus should be strictly respected to avoid an unaesthetic appearance. If, after skin resection, the distance is expected to be less than 9 cm, umbilical transposition should be preferred *(Fig. 5.7)*.

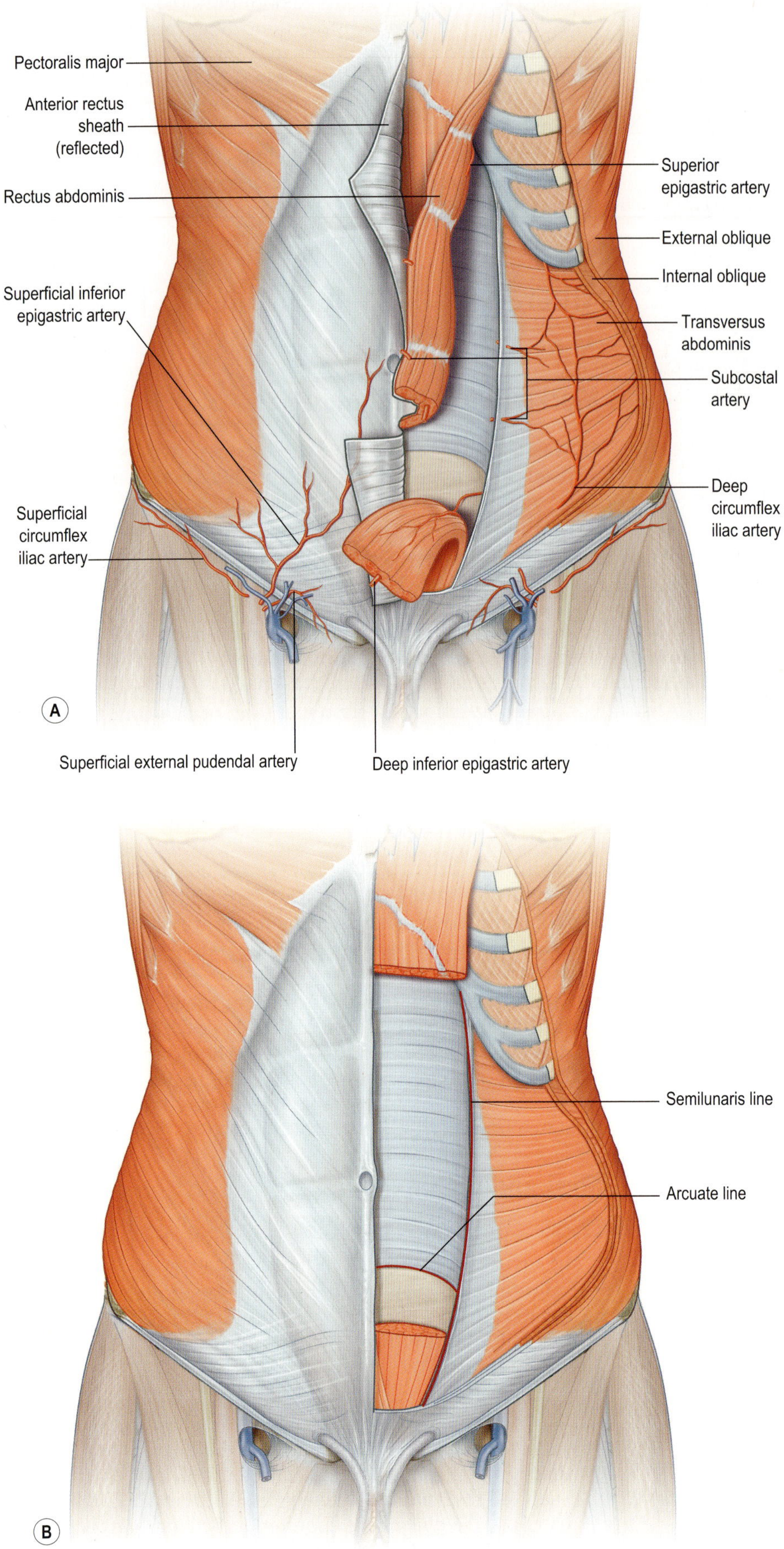

Figure 5.2 **(A)** Anatomy of the musculature of the abdominal wall with arterial supply. **(B)** Arcuate line and linea semilunaris.

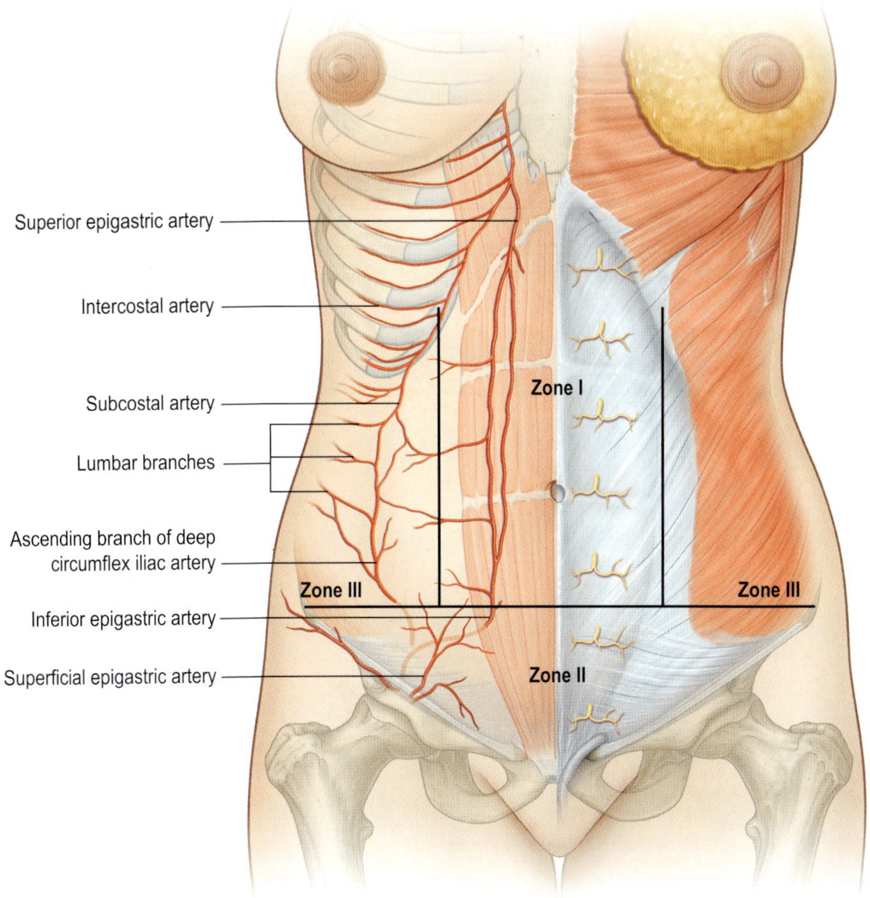

Figure 5.3 Zones of blood supply (Huger WE, 1978).

Table 5.1 Indication for different techniques

	Mini	Modern	Short-T	Standard	HLT	Anchor	Circular	Reverse
Lower abdomen	+	++	++	+++	+++	+++	+++	0
Periumbilical	(+)	+	+	++	++	+++	++	(+)
Upper abdomen	0	(+)	+	++	++	+++	++	+++
Diastasis/hernia	(+)	+	++	++	++	+++	++	(+)
Flanks/hips/thighs	0	0	0	(+)	+	++	+++	0

- The primary limitation of this procedure is the presence of upper abdominal skin folds and rolls; these patients will require one of the more extensive procedures described subsequently in this chapter.

Abdominoplasty with umbilical transection *(Fig. 5.8)*

- Abdominoplasty with a prefascial release and transposition of the umbilicus without circumferential release from the abdominal flap thereby avoiding a perumbilical scar.
- Therefore, this technique represents a good alternative between mini abdominoplasty and standard abdominoplasty procedures.

Standard abdominoplasty *(Fig. 5.9)*

- Indicated in patients presenting with skin and soft tissue excess of the upper and lower abdomen who will accept a periumbilical scar.
- The inferior incision is made first and carried down through scarpa fascia to the rectus fascia.
- The abdominal flap elevated in a suprafascial plan.
- Through a circumferential, peri-areolar incision, the umbilicus is freed from the abdominal flap.

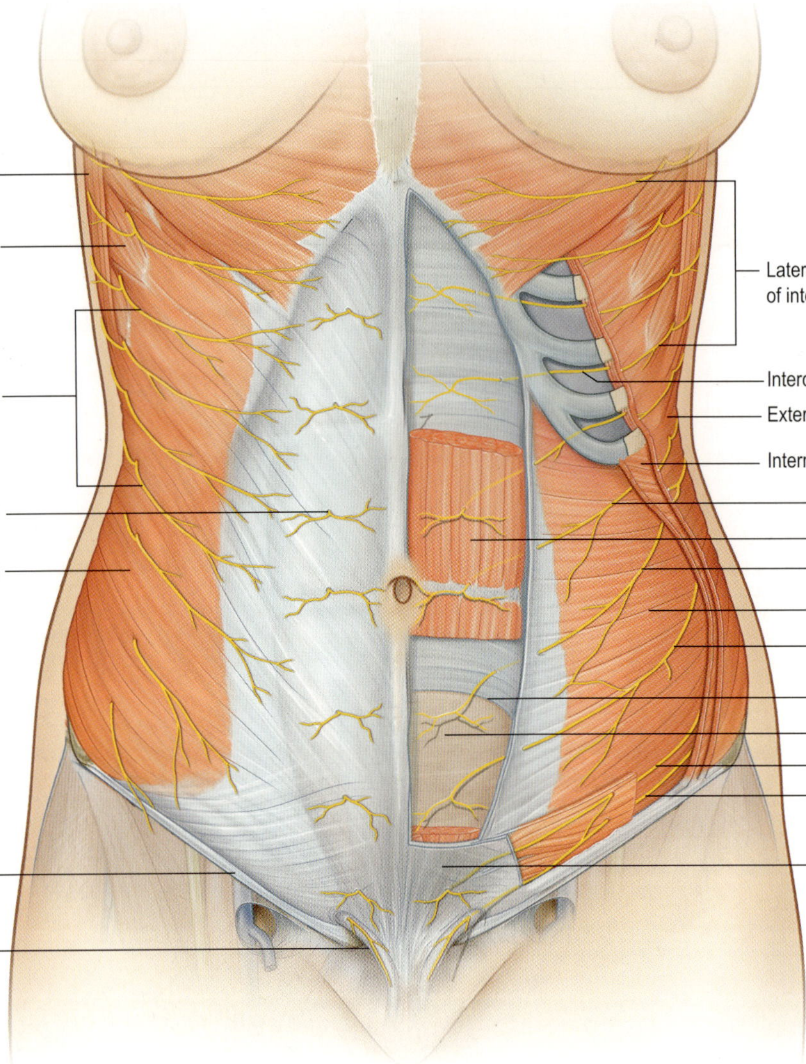

Figure 5.4 Abdominal nerves.

- Supraumbilically, the abdominal flap is undermined primarily in the midline to the level of the xiphoid.
- In cases of rectus diastasis, plication of the anterior rectus sheath from the xiphoid to the symphysis is accomplished using non-absorbable suture material.
- Paramedian plication of the anterior rectus sheath may facilitate a correction of an asymmetrically located umbilical stalk or for accentuation of an hourglass figure with further waist tightening.
- The patient is flexed at the hip approximately 30° and the abdominal flap is pulled infero-medially to determine the appropriate position of the superior skin incision.
- Once the superior skin incision is made, the medial portion of the wound is temporarily closed to allow marking of the new location for the umbilicus.
- Wound closure is performed in layers, and if significant dead space exists, progressive tension sutures may be used.
- The umbilicoplasty can be performed in many ways including skin incisions involving an elliptoid, chevron, or shield shape.
- The umbilicus is best secured using absorbable deep-dermal sutures and a running skin closure.
- Two subcutaneous drains are often inserted to assist with postoperative fluid drainage.

High-lateral-tension (HLT) abdominoplasty

- Extended modification of the traditional abdominoplasty procedure that also treats the hips and the lateral thigh.
- A modified skin incision/resection is utilized to lead to more conservative resection centrally with wider excision of the lateral skin ***(Fig. 5.10)***.
- Suitable for patients that want their hips and lateral thighs addressed, patients after massive weight loss, and

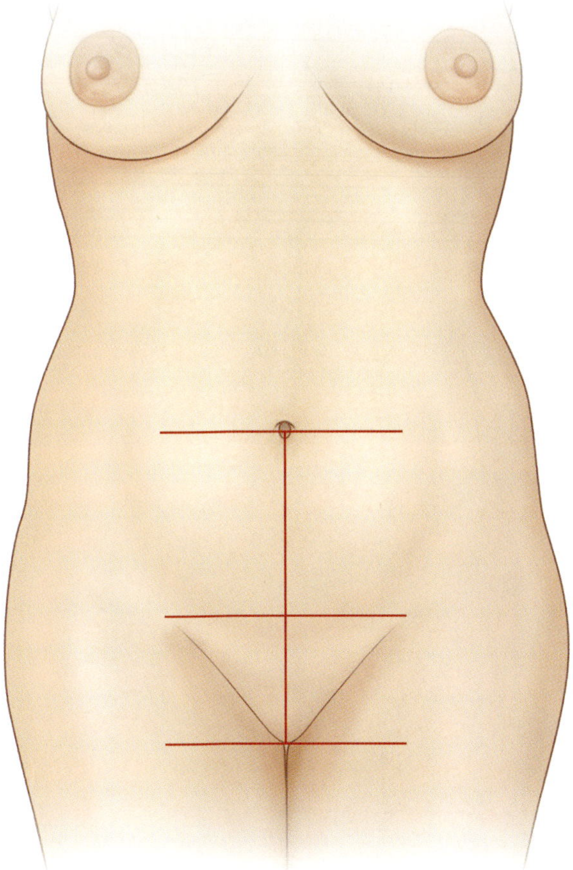

Figure 5.5 Markings are to be performed with respect to the anterior vulva commissure and the umbilicus.

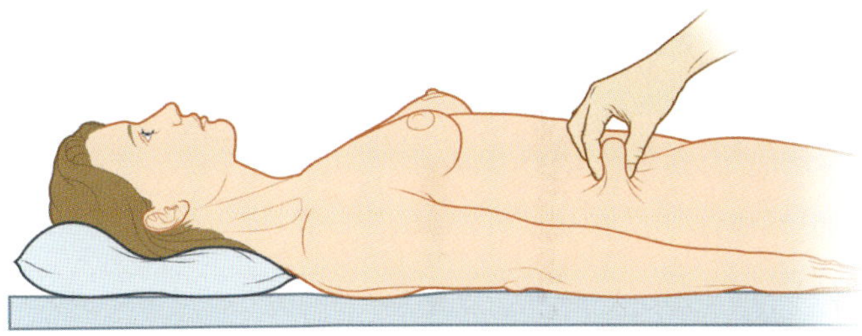

Figure 5.6 Pinching of the abdominal tissue in upright and supine position.

in patients for whom an abdominoplasty is deficient and a lower body-lift is beyond their needs ***(Fig. 5.11)***.

Fleur-de-lis abdominoplasty

- Includes a vertical midline scar that allows elimination of horizontal and vertical skin/subcutaneous tissue redundancy.
- Suitable for patients suffering from a tissue excess of the lower and particularly of the upper abdomen in the horizontal direction. This often includes patients after massive weight loss and in those who have preexisting midline abdominal scars.

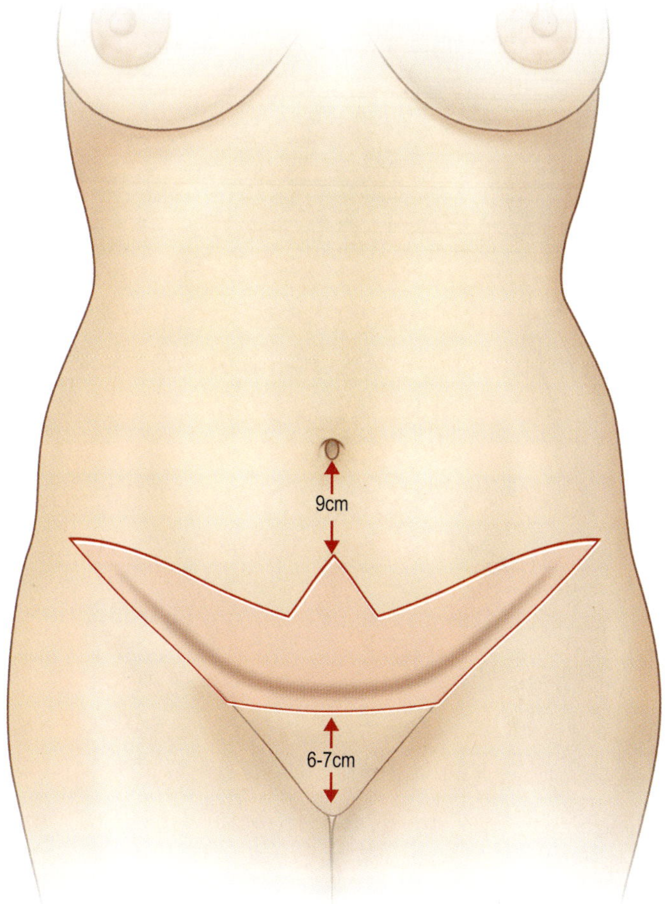

Figure 5.7 Preoperative markings for a short scar abdominoplasty. The red line demonstrates the resulting scar line. It is essential to respect the umbilico-pubic distance. The distance from the upper resection line to the umbilicus should be at least 9 cm.

- The key in planning this procedure is to independently assess the horizontal and vertical excess of skin and fat tissue ***(Fig. 5.12)***.
- In this technique, the umbilicus must be integrated into the vertical scar.
- In general, the vertical resection should be performed first and prior to horizontal resection to reduce the risk of over-resection ***(Fig. 5.13)***.

Reverse abdominoplasty

- Performed in patients who require tightening of skin in the upper abdomen alone.
- The most common indication is the massive weight loss patient who has undergone a conventioanal abdominoplasty and still suffers from persistent skin and soft tissue excess of the upper abdomen.
- The marking is performed with the patient in upright position. The patient is asked to slightly bend forward for demonstration of tissue excess. This enables an optimal assessment of the vertical

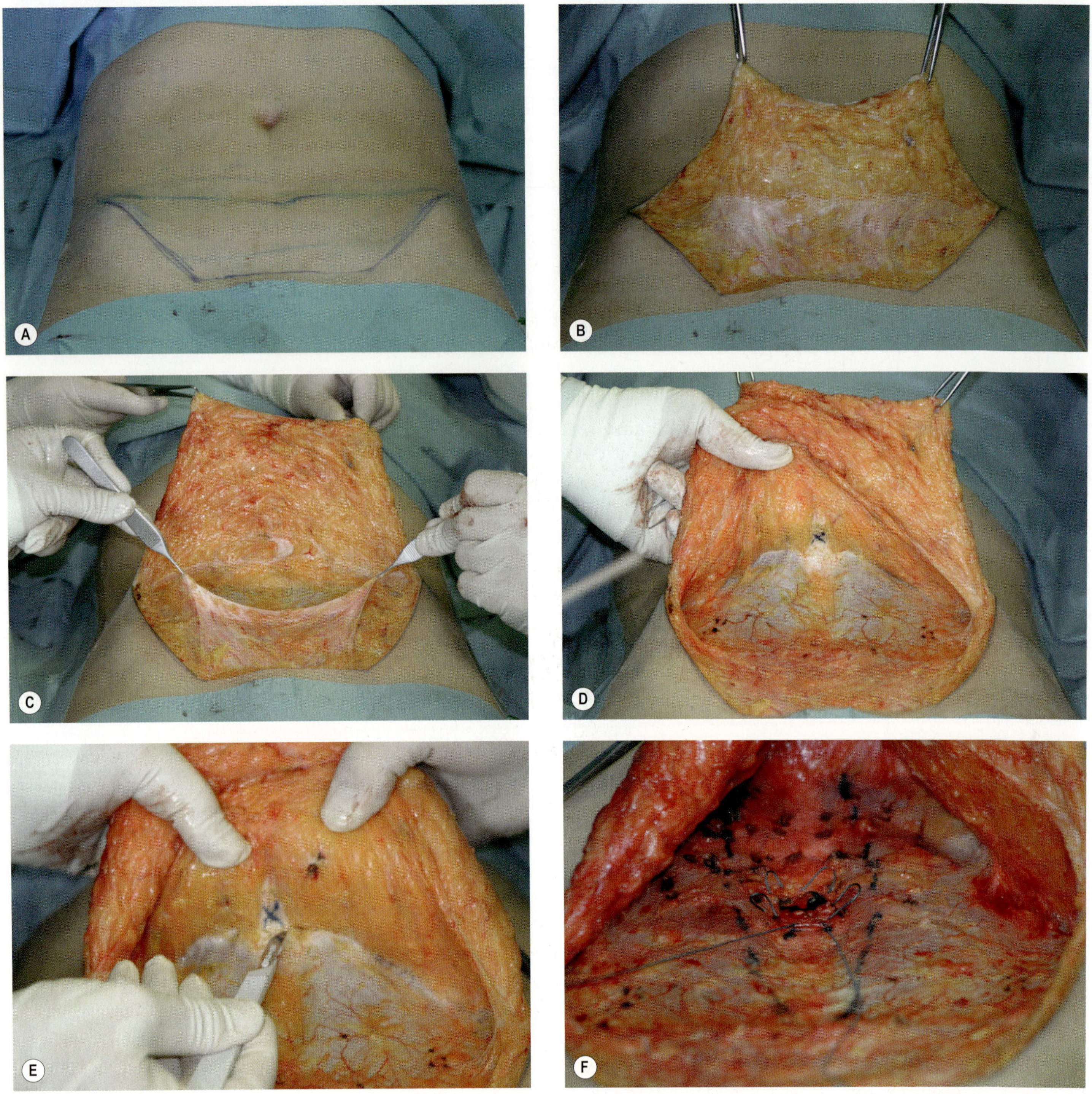

Figure 5.8 Intraoperative view of abdominoplasty with umbilical transection. **(A)** Markings in the supine position; **(B,C)** preservation of scarpa fascia; **(D,E)** preparation of the umbilical stalk; **(F)** closure of the umbilical base with non-resorbable suture material;

and horizontal tissue excess. The inframammary fold is then marked extending laterally to the anterior axillary line. The width of resection is generally less then 15 cm *(Fig. 5.14)*.

- In selective cases, the excess tissue may be utilized deepithelialized and rotated cranially for autologous augmentation of the breast as part of a mastopexy procedures.

Vertical abdominoplasty

- The vertical abdominoplasty refers to a purely vertical incision with lateral mobilization of abdominal soft tissue.
- Indicated in patients with a preexisting scar in the abdominal midline who seek improvement of abdominal contour without additional transverse scars.

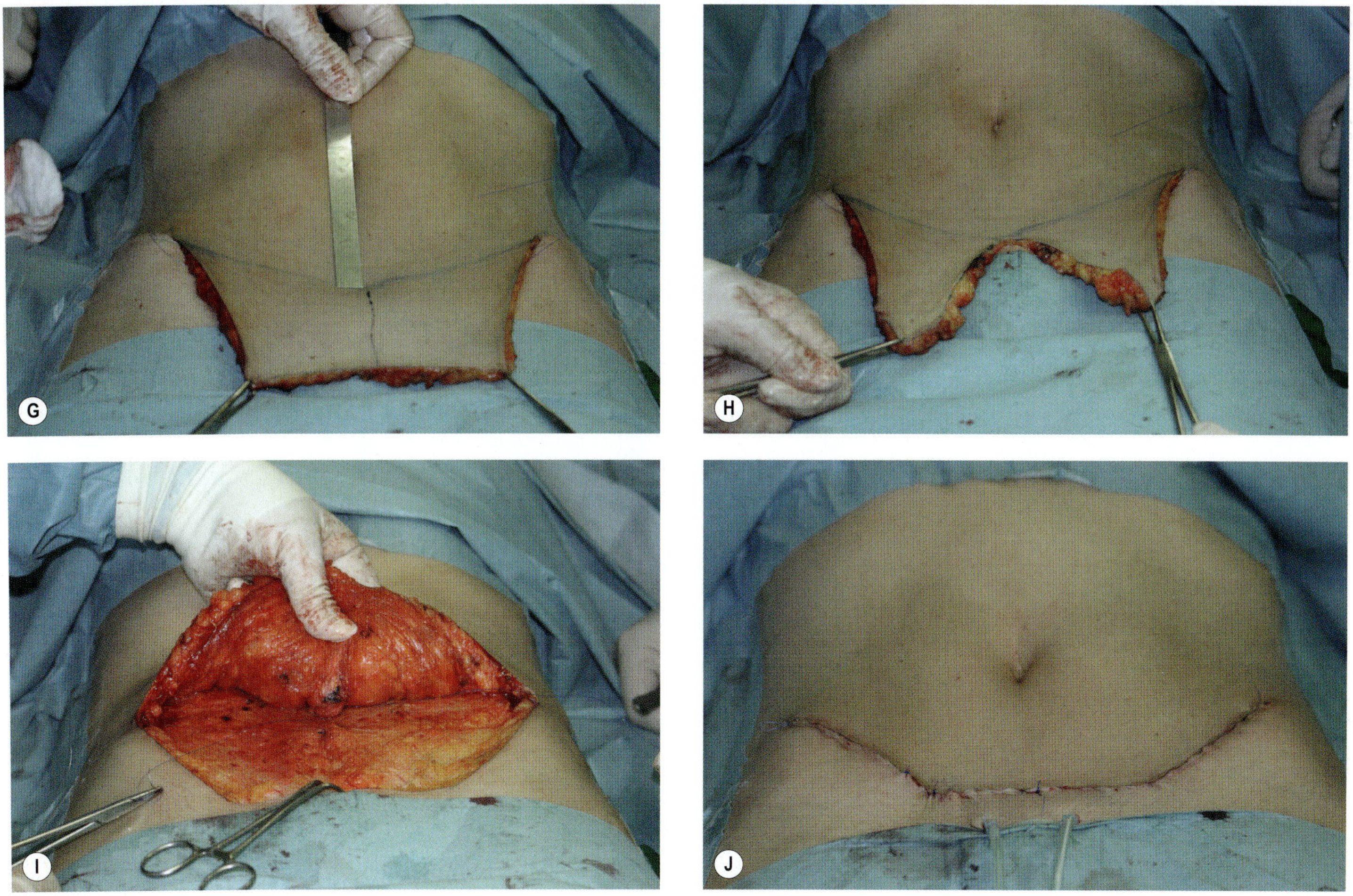

Figure 5.8, cont'd **(G,H)** assessment of the distance between upper resection line and the umbilicus with resection of the redundant tissue; **(I)** refixation of the umbilical stalk to the anterior rectus sheath and **(J)** the intraoperative result.

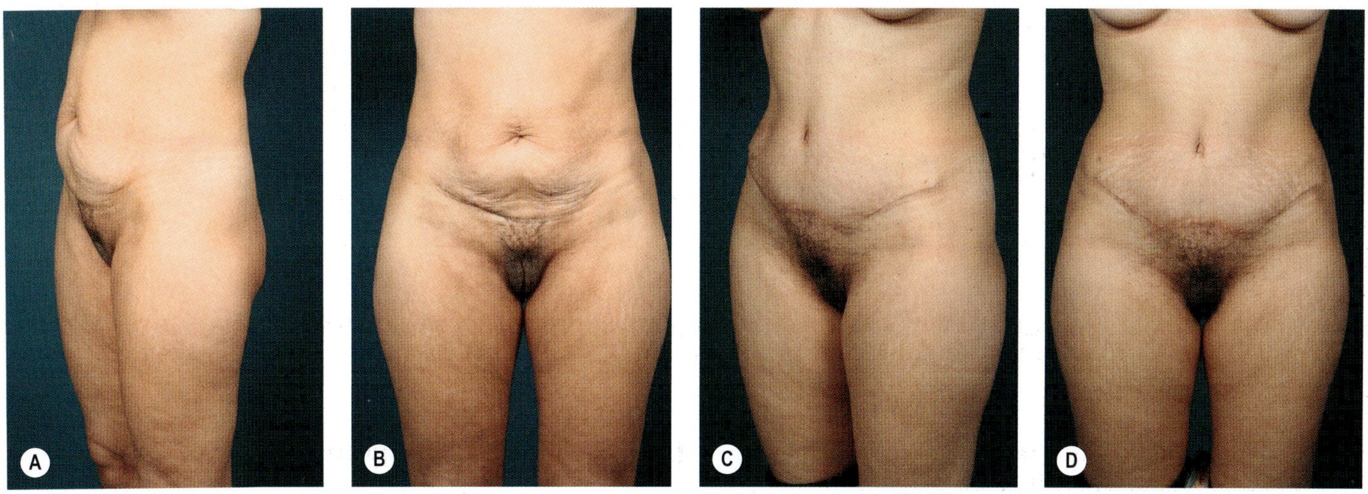

Figure 5.9 A 42-year-old woman with remarkable amount of striae distensae in the periumbilical region after a single pregnancy. Pre- and postoperative oblique and front images of a standard abdominoplasty procedure with incomplete elimination of striae.

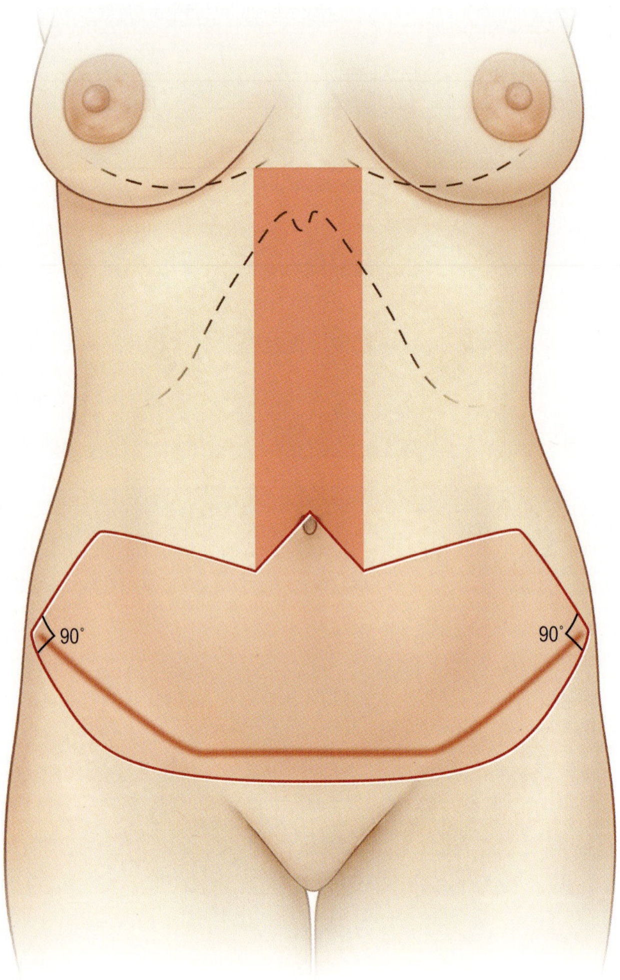

Figure 5.10 HLT abdominoplasty pattern.

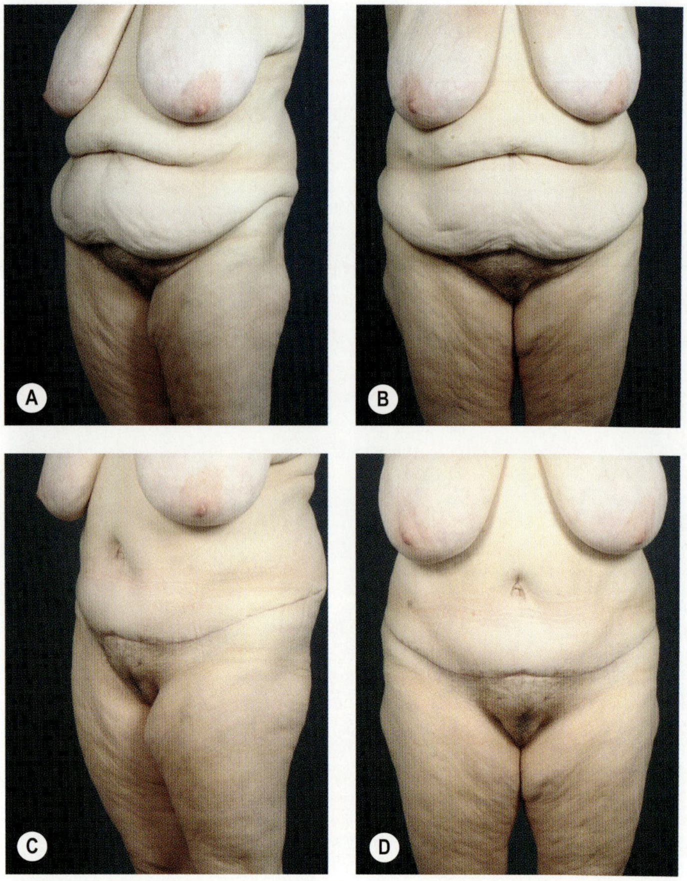

Figure 5.11 A 54-year-old patient with a massive skin and soft tissue redundancy at the abdominal and flank region. Pre- and 3 months postoperative oblique and front images of an HLT abdominoplasty procedure with fascial tightening without any additional liposuction.

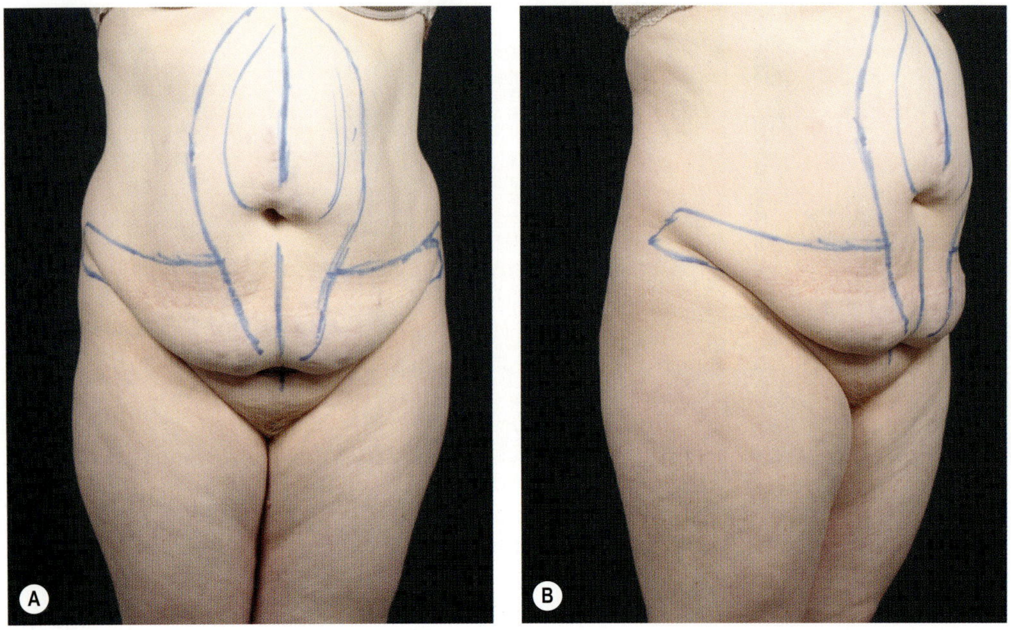

Figure 5.12 Fleur de lis markings.

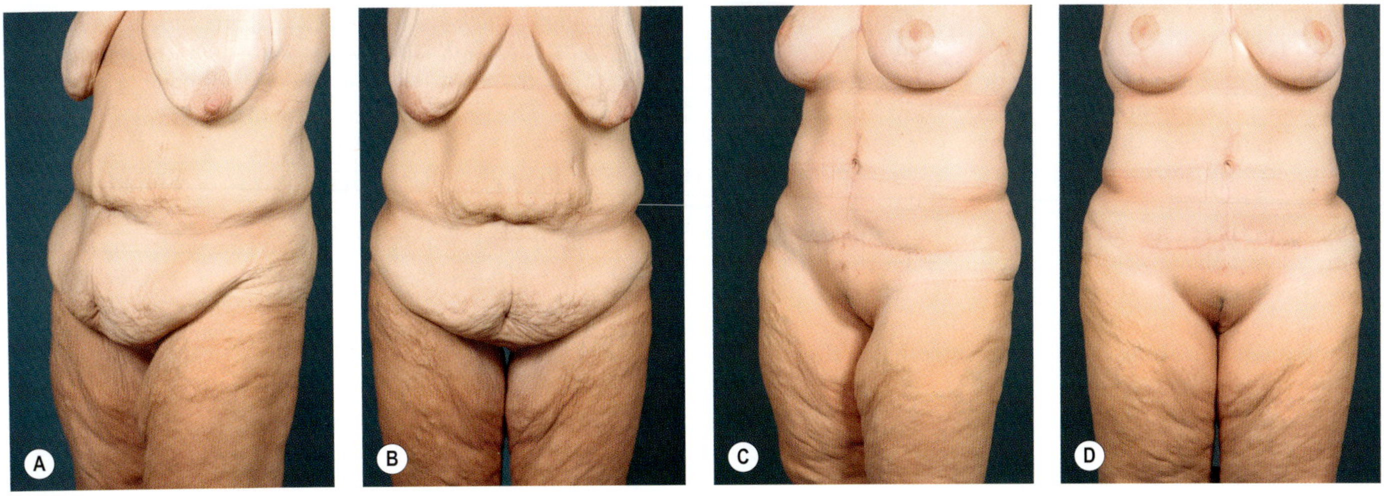

Figure 5.13 A 49-year-old patient with weight reduction of 50 kg with circumferential skin excess in the abdominal, flank, lateral/medial thigh and gluteal region. After rejecting a lower bodylift, the patient underwent a fleur-de-lis abdominoplasty. Pre- and 3 months postoperative oblique and front images of a fleur-de-lis abdominoplasty procedure with fascial tightening.

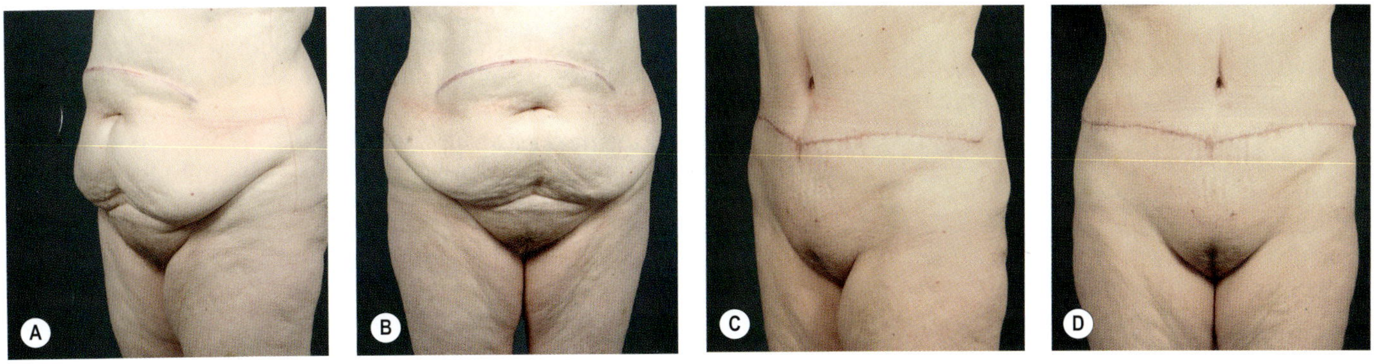

Figure 5.14 A 52-year-old patient after an open laparotomy procedure with a transverse scar. Pre- and postoperative front view following a reverse abdominoplasty procedure.

Postoperative considerations

- The operation can be performed as outpatient or inpatient surgery.
- Drains are left in place until discharge is less then 30 ml in 24 h.
- The patient should rest in a relaxed position with a flexion of approximately 30° at the hip joint.
- This position should be retained for 2–3 weeks postoperatively in order to assure a tension free healing of the scar.
- Sporting activities should be omitted for 6 weeks postoperatively, and in cases of fascial reconstruction for 8 weeks.
- Patient should be advised to avoid saunas and tanning beds.
- A compression garment should be worn for the same period of time.

Complications and outcomes

- Patients can expect postoperative pain or soreness, numbness of the abdominal flap, bruising, general fatigue and discomfort due to increased abdominal tension for many weeks.
- Local complications include hematoma, seroma, wound infection, fat necrosis, wound dehiscence, parasthesias, and persisting numbness.
- Seromas are the most common problem and are usually handled with serial punctures and drainage.
- Persistent seromas may require an indwelling drain, or in the case of a late encapsulated seroma, a secondary surgical procedure.
- Minor wound dehiscence is common and is normally a self-limiting problem.
- Many local problems of a cosmetic nature can result from abdominoplasty including lateral dog ears, widened or

hypertrophic scars, malpositioned scars, and numerous cosmetic problems directly related to the umbilicus.
- Most of these problems can be avoided with proper preoperative planning and attention to surgical detail.
- If liposuction has been done simultaneously, issues pertaining to that procedure include contour irregularities and dermal tethering.
- Systemic complications include deep vein thrombosis, pulmonary embolism, respiratory compromise due to increased intraabdominal pressure, and systemic infections including toxic shock syndrome.
- All of these complications are potentially lethal and must be dealt with expeditiously.
- Abdominoplasty, especially when combined with other procedures such as liposuction, has a higher systemic complication rate than any other type of routine cosmetic surgical procedure.

Further reading

Aly AS. *Body Contouring after Massive Weight Loss*. St Louis: Quality Medical; 2006.

This work is published by a currently "leading postbariatric surgeon." Aly has composed a unique work on all reliable techniques for body contouring of patients after massive weight loss.

Bozola AR. Abdominoplasty: same classification and a new treatment concept 20 years later. *Aesthet Plast Surg*. 2010;34(2):181–192.

Costa-Ferreira A, Rebelo M, Vásconez LO, et al. Scarpa fascia preservation during abdominoplasty: a prospective study. *Plast Reconstr Surg*. 2010;125(4):1232–1239.

Dellon AL. Fleur-de-lis abdominoplasty. *Aesthet Plast Surg*. 1985;9:27.

Dellon first published, in 1985, his approach to a vertical and horizontal restoration of the abdominal wall through a combined resection, the "fleur-de-lis" technique.

Huger Jr WE. The anatomic rationale for abdominal lipectomy. *Am Surg*. 1979;45(9):612–617.

Hunstad JP, Repta R. *Atlas of Abdominoplasty*. Philadelphia: Saunders Elsevier; 2009.

This major work on all current abdominoplasty procedures is written by a leading authority on this subject, covering all topics from patient selection, incision placement, ancillary procedures up to all possible complications by highlighting key considerations for a safe and successful performance.

Lockwood T. High lateral-tension abdominoplasty with superficial fascial system suspension. *Plast Reconstr Surg*. 1995;96:603–608.

This article describes the principles and details of this new approach to abdominoplasty. It offers an alternative technique, especially in patients after massive weight loss with limited treatment of the flanks.

Pitanguy I. Abdominolipectomy. An approach to it through an analysis of 300 consecutive cases. *Plast Reconstr Surg*. 1967;40:384.

Saldanha OR, Pinto EB, Matos WN Jr, et al. Lipoabdominoplasty without undermining. *Aesthet Surg J*. 2001;21(6):518–526.

Song AY, Jean RD, Hurwitz DJ, et al. A classification of contour deformities after bariatric weight loss: the Pittsburgh Rating Scale. *Plast Reconstr Surg*. 2005;116(5):1535–1546.

Rubin, as a currently "leading postbariatric surgeon" has published an interesting work on the different deformities in patients after bariatric weight loss, which may serve as a guideline for plastic surgeons during preoperative planning and for evaluation of their postoperative outcomes.

Chapter 6

Facial injuries

This chapter was created using content from Neligan & Rodriguez, Plastic Surgery 3rd edition, Volume 3, Craniofacial, Head and Neck Surgery, Chapter 3, Facial fractures, Eduardo D. Rodriguez, Amir H. Dorafshar and Paul N. Manson.

SYNOPSIS

- The teachings of John Converse, Nicholas Georgiade and Reed Dingman provided the benchmark for an entire generation of surgeons in facial injury repair.
- The treatment concepts discussed in this chapter were developed at the University of Maryland Shock Trauma Unit and ultimately employed at the International Center for Facial Injury Reconstruction at Johns Hopkins.
- The proportion of severe injuries seen at these centers is high.
- The treatment concepts, however, may be modified for common fractures and less significant injuries.
- Greater emphasis has been placed on minimizing operative techniques and limited exposures, whereas the decade of the eighties witnessed craniofacial principles of broad exposure and fixation at all buttresses for a particular fracture across all degrees of severity.
- Presently, the treatment of injuries is organized both by severity and anatomic area to permit the smallest exposure possible to achieve a good result. (CT based facial fracture treatment).

Brief introduction

- Bone and soft tissue injuries in the facial area should be managed as soon as the patient's general condition permits.
- Classically, facial soft tissue and bone injuries are not acute surgical emergencies, but both the ease of obtaining a good result and the quality of the result are better with early or immediate management.
- Less soft tissue stripping is required, bones are often easily replaced into their anatomic position and easier fracture repairs are performed.
- The definitive radiographic evaluation is the craniofacial CT scan with axial, coronal and sagittal sections of bone and soft tissue windows. However, the clinical examination remains the most sensitive detection of the character and functional implications of the facial injury.
- Access to the craniofacial skeleton can be achieved through strategic incision placement ***(Fig. 6.1)***.

Preoperative considerations

- Management begins with an initial physical examination and is followed by a radiologic evaluation accomplished with computerized tomographic (CT) scanning (Table 6.1).
- Bone injuries are suggested by soft tissue symptoms such as contusions, abrasions, ecchymosis, edema, and distortion of the facial proportions.

Frontal bone and sinus injury patterns

Brief introduction

- The frontal sinuses are paired structures that begin to be detected at 3 years of age. Significant pneumatic expansion does not begin to occur until approximately 7 years, with full sinus development complete by the age of 18 to 20.
- The frontal sinuses are lined with respiratory epithelium, which consists of a ciliated membrane with mucus

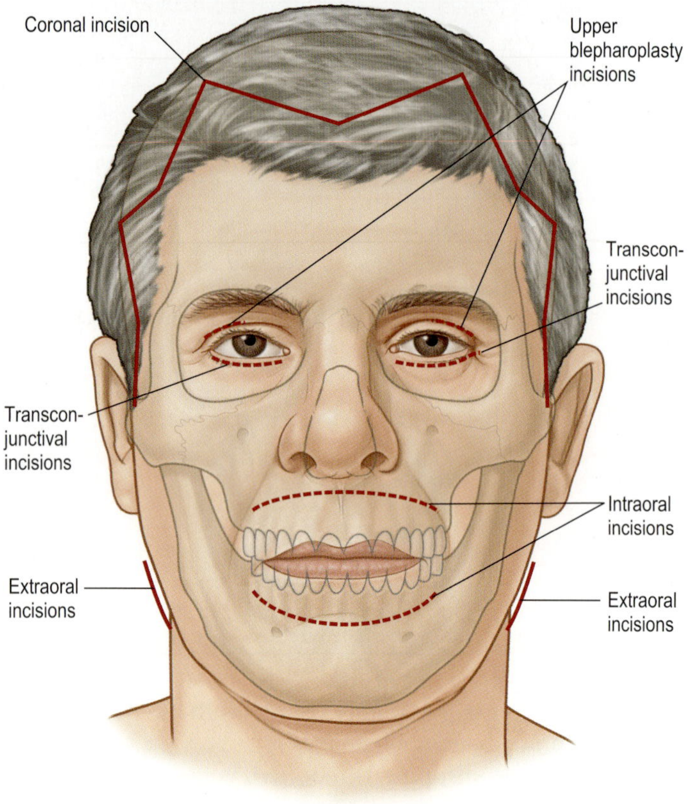

Figure 6.1 Cutaneous incisions (solid line) available for open reduction and internal fixation of facial fractures. The conjunctival approach (dotted line) also gives access to the orbital floor and anterior aspect of the maxilla, and exposure may be extended by a lateral canthotomy. Intraoral incisions (dotted line) are also indicated for the Le Fort 1 level of the maxilla and the anterior mandible. The lateral limb of an upper blepharoplasty incision is preferred for isolated zygomaticofrontal suture exposure if a coronal incision is not used. A horizontal incision directly across the nasal radix is the one case in which a local incision can be tolerated over the nose. In many instances, a coronal incision is preferable unless the hair is short or the patient is balding.

secreting glands. A blanket of mucin is essential for normal function and the cilia beat this mucin in the direction of the nasofrontal ducts.

- When injured, they serve as a focus for infection, especially if duct function is impaired.
- One-third of fractures involve the anterior table alone, and 60% involve the anterior table and posterior table and/or ducts.
- Forty percent of frontal sinus fractures have an accompanying dural laceration.

Preoperative considerations

- Lacerations, bruises, hematomas, and contusions constitute the most frequent signs of frontal bone or sinus fractures.
- Occasionally, the first presentation of a frontal sinus fracture may be an infection or symptom of frontal sinus obstruction, such as mucocele, or abscess formation. Infection in the frontal sinus may produce serious complications because of its location.

Table 6.1 **Key components of initial evaluation**

I. ABCs

II. History
1. Mechanism of injury (was the patient restrained, mobile, stationary)?
2. Time of injury (i.e., how much time has elapsed since injury)?
3. Penetrating vs. blunt injury?
4. What type of object involved (e.g., fist, bat, windshield, etc.)?
5. Does the patient complain of any symptoms to particular facial area (e.g., numbness, pain)?
6. How does it feel when the patient bites down – pain? Do teeth feel "normal"? Does bite "feel normal"?
7. Does the patient complain of visual problems, nasal problems, hearing problems, or abnormal/painful bite?
8. Any significant PMH, meds, allergies, social history (e.g., diabetes, aspirin, coumadin, steroid use, ETOH, etc.)?

III. Exam
1. Inspect face/head for asymmetry, lacerations, abraisions, hematomas, ecchymoses (especially periorbital), epistaxis
2. Document any bony irregularities, enophthalmos, proptosis, telectanthus
3. Document visual acuity (e.g., Can you read my ID badge from 12 inches away?)
4. Check pupils and ocular muscles
   a. Is there a hyphema (blood in the anterior chamber)
   b. Are extra-ocular movements intact or is there a restriction in gaze
   c. Are pupils reactive and equal
5. Inspect oral cavity – pay particular attention to dentition, occlusion, lacerations
6. Palpate the facial bones and soft-tissue: document bony step-offs, crepitance, mobile segments, significant pain, and numbness
   a. Palpate orbital rims
   b. Palpate radix and nasal bridge for instability, crepitance
   c. Check for integrity/mobility of medial canthus
   d. Palpate zygoma/zygomatic arch
   e. Palpate frontal bone, maxilla/maxillary sinus, cranium
   f. Palpate TMJ at rest and through mandible ROM
   g. Palpate mandible along its length
   h. Using gloved hand, palpate teeth for instability, fractures, etc.
   i. Using gloved hand, grab maxilla/alveolus and check for midface instability/pain
   j. Inspect nasal passages and external auditory canal to rule out septal hematoma, CSF rhinorrhea, otorrhea
7. Perform sensory exam of all branches of trigeminal nerve (supraorbital, infraorbital, marginal mandibular)
8. Perform motor exam of facial nerve – raise eyebrows, smile, grit teeth, close eyes tightly

IV. Imaging
1. CT face/orbits (1.5–3 mm cuts along facial bones with coronal/sagittal/axial reconstructions)
2. CT Cspine (overall, 2–4% incidence of Cspine injury with facial fractures)
3. Sometimes a Panorex is warranted. (Often study of choice for mandible fracture, can miss symphyseal fractures – requires normal Cspine)

V. Adjuncts
1. Ophthalmology consult – if any sign/concern for ocular injury/visual disturbance

- Frontal sinus fractures should be characterized by describing both the anatomic location of the fracture, including involvement of the anterior table, posterior table, or both, and their degree of displacement.
- Indications for operative management include:
- Depression of the anterior table.
- Radiographic demonstration of involvement of the nasofrontal duct with presumed future non-function.
- Obstruction of the nasofrontal duct with persistent air fluid levels.
- Mucocele formation.
- Fractures of the posterior table that are displaced and presumably have lacerated the dura resulting in a cerebrospinal fluid leak.
- While some authors recommend exploration of any posterior table fracture or any fracture in which an air fluid level is visible, most explore posterior wall fractures only if their displacement exceeds the width of the posterior table.

Anatomical pearls

- The nasofrontal duct passes through the anterior ethmoidal air cells to exit adjacent to the ethmoidal infundibulum beneath the middle meatus.
- Blockage prevents adequate drainage of normal mucous secretions and predisposes to the development of mucoceles.
- The reported average interval between the primary injury and development of frontal sinus mucocele is 7½ years.

Key technical considerations

- The best technique of exposure is the coronal incision. Occasionally, a laceration may be used.
- Any depressed frontal sinus fracture of the anterior wall potentially requires exploration and wall replacement in an anatomical position to prevent contour deformity.
- If the nasofrontal duct is compromised, obliteration of the sinus is required and commonly involves stripping of the mucosa, burring of the bone, and occlusion with well-designed "formed-to-fit" calvarial bone plugs or soft tissue ***(Fig. 6.2A–C)***.
- If most of the posterior bony wall is intact, the entire frontal sinus cavity may be filled either with fat or cancellous bone.
- If the posterior table is missing, or significantly displaced, the sinus should be "cranialized". In cranialization, the posterior wall of the frontal sinus is removed, effectively making the frontal sinus a part of the intracranial cavity.

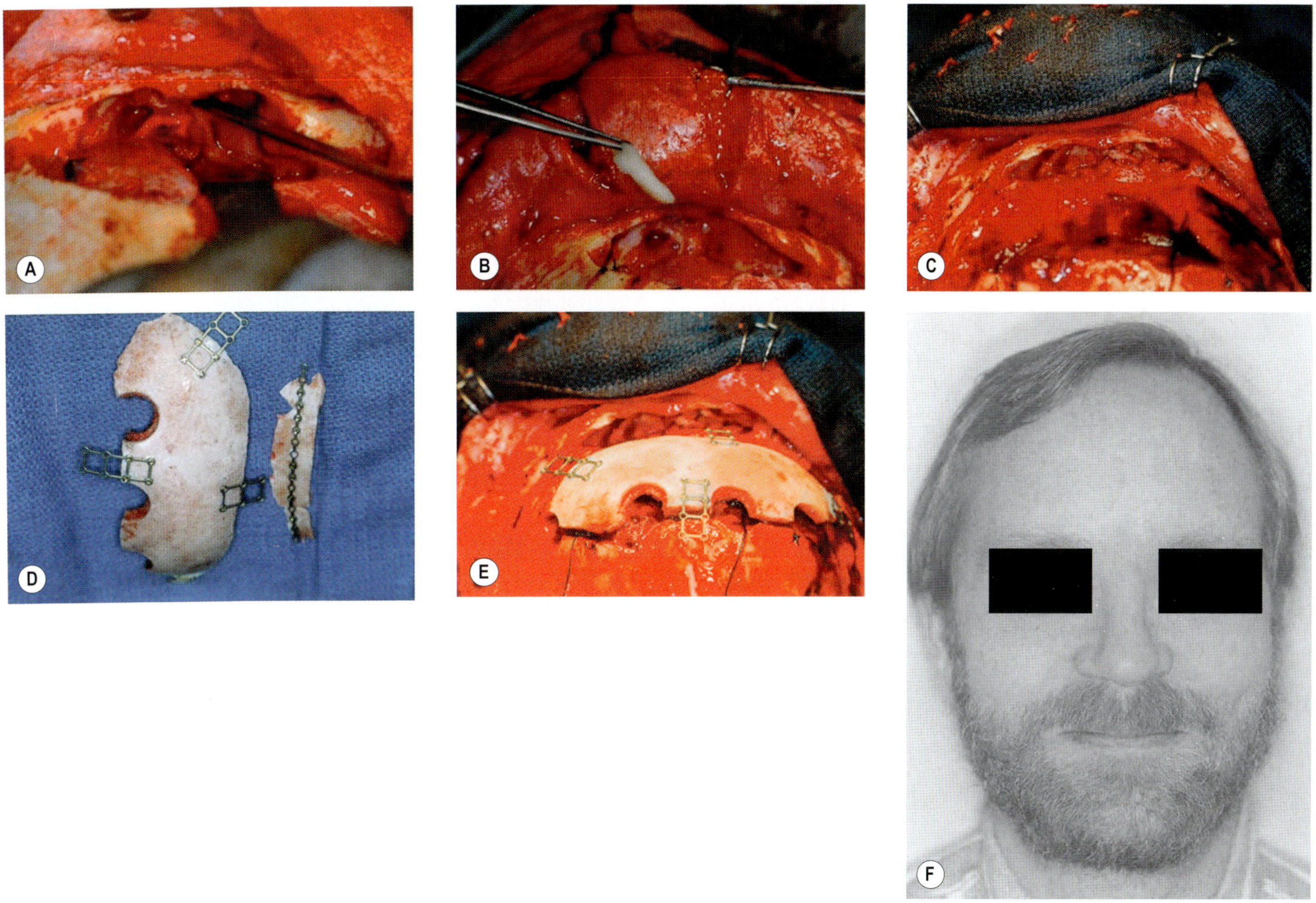

Figure 6.2 **(A)** Nasofrontal duct. **(B)** Bone plug for nasofrontal duct and galeal flap. **(C)** Bone obliteration of frontal sinus. **(D)** "Back table" surgery for bone replacement. **(E)** Bone reconstruction and cranialization of the frontal sinus; intracranial neurosurgery. **(F)** Postoperative result.

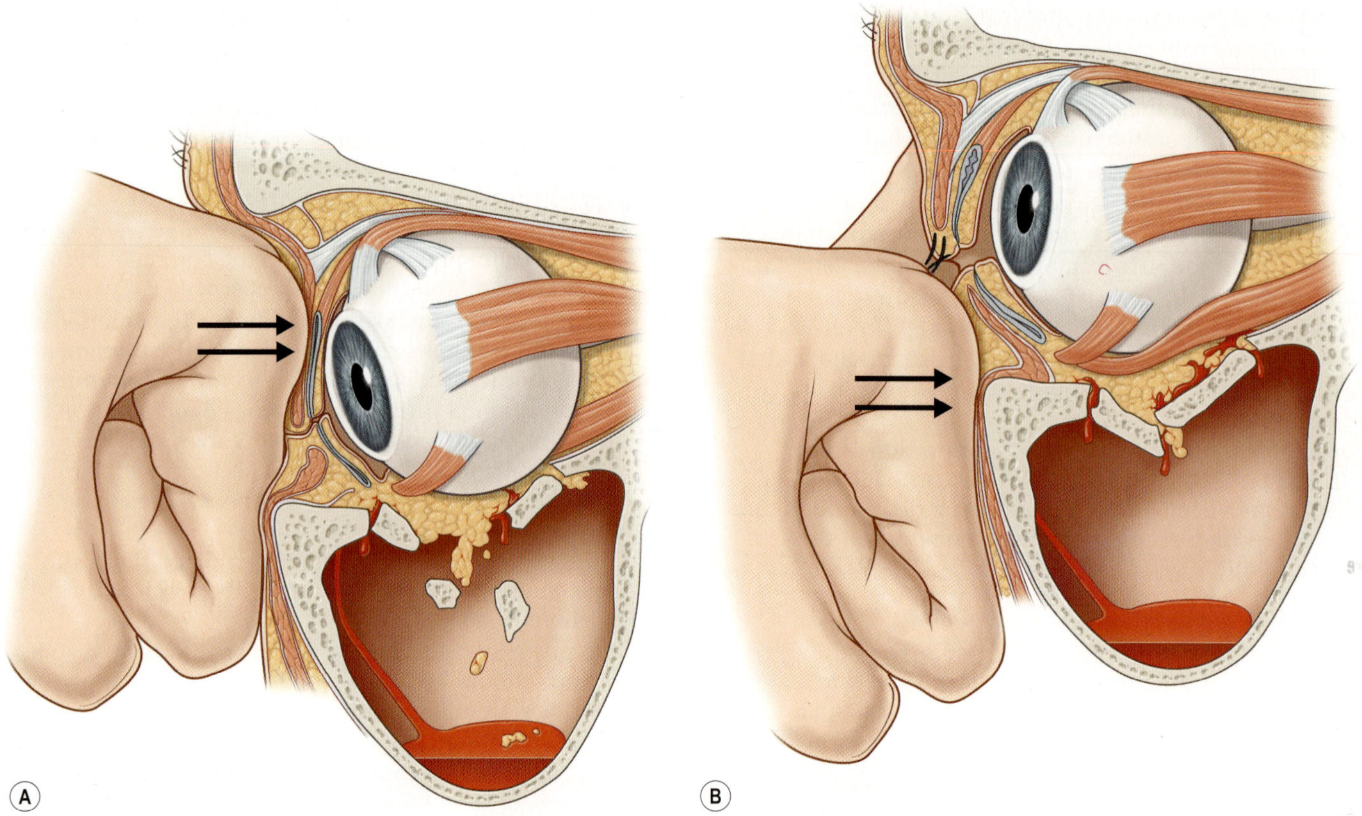

Figure 6.3 **(A)** Mechanism of blow-out fracture from displacement of the globe itself into the orbital walls. The globe is displaced posteriorly, striking the orbital walls and forcing them outward, causing a "punched out" fracture the size of the globe. **(B)** "Force transmission" fracture of orbital floor.

The "dead space" may be filled with cancellous bone or left open. Any communication with the nose by the nasofrontal duct or with the ethmoid sinuses should be sealed.

- A galeal flap with a pedicle of the superficial temporal artery can be a useful method for vascularized soft tissue obliteration of frontal bone problems.

Outcomes and complications

- Complications of frontal bone and sinus fractures include:
  - CSF fluid rhinorrhea.
  - Pneumocephalus and orbital emphysema.
  - Absence of orbital roof and pulsating exophthalmos.
  - Carotid-cavernous sinus fistula.

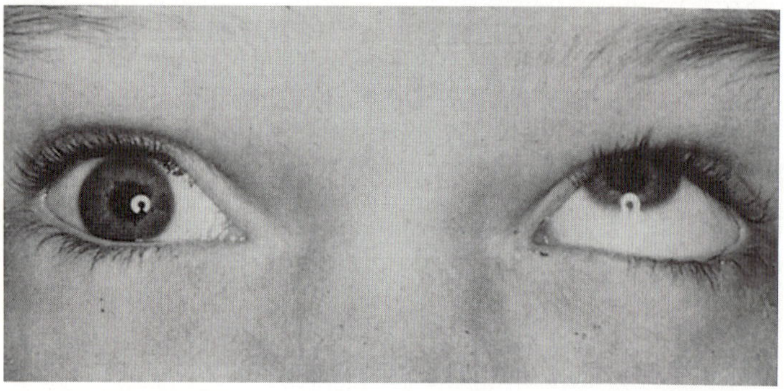

Figure 6.4 Blow-out fracture in a child produced by a snowball. Note the nearly complete immobility of the ocular globe and the enophthalmos. Such severe loss of motion implies actual muscle incarceration, an injury that is more frequent in children than in adults. This fracture deserves *immediate* operation with release of the incarcerated extraocular muscle system. It is often accompanied by pain on attempted rotation of the globe and sometimes nausea and vomiting. These symptoms are unusual in orbital floor fractures without true muscle incarceration.

Orbital fractures

Brief introduction

- Orbital fractures may occur as isolated fractures of the internal orbit or may involve both the internal orbit and the orbital rim.
- An orbital blow-out fracture is caused by the application of a traumatic force to the rim, globe or soft tissues of the orbit accompanied by sudden increase in intraorbital pressure and subsequent fracture through the orbital floor ***(Fig. 6.3)***.
- In children, the mechanism is more frequently like that of a trapdoor, rather than the "blow-out" fracture seen in adults ***(Fig. 6.4)***.
- As opposed to incarceration of fat adjacent to the inferior rectus muscle, children more frequently "scissor" or capture the muscle directly in the fracture site.

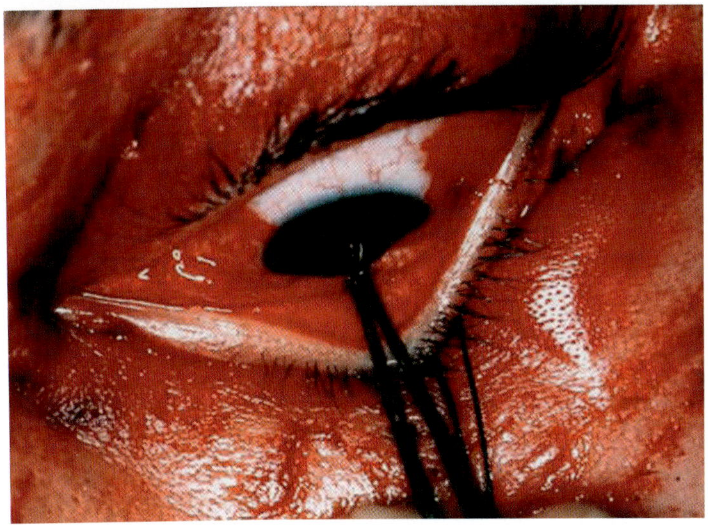

Figure 6.5 The forced duction test. Clinical photograph. A drop of local anesthetic instilled into the conjunctival sac precedes the procedure.

- Muscle incarceration is an urgent situation that demands immediate release of the incarcerated muscle.
- The patient with true muscle entrapment may experience pain on attempted eye motion as well as nausea, vomiting, and an oculocardiac reflex (nausea, bradycardia, and hypotension).
- The purpose of orbital floor reconstruction/replacement in this scenario, whether a bone graft or an inorganic implant, is to re-establish the size and the shape of the orbital cavity. This replaces the orbital soft tissue contents and allows scar tissue to form in an anatomic position.
- A forced duction test is performed by grasping the orbital conjunctiva with forceps and testing the range of motion of the globe *(Fig. 6.5)*.
- Limitation of forced rotation or motion is a positive test for entrapment of extraocular muscles.
  - This test should be performed:
  - Before dissection.
  - After dissection
  - After the insertion of each material used to reconstruct the orbital wall.
  - Just prior to closure of the incisions.

Preoperative considerations

- Indications for surgical treatment of orbital fractures:
- Diplopia caused by incarceration of muscle or the fine ligament system, documented by forced duction examination and suggested by CT scans.
- Radiographic evidence of extensive fracture, such that enophthalmos would occur.
- Enophthalmos or exophthalmos produced by an orbital volume change.
- Visual acuity deficit, increasing and not responsive to medical dose steroids, implying that optic canal decompression would be indicated.
- "Blow-in" orbital fractures that involve the medial or lateral walls of the orbit, and severely constrict orbital volume, creating increased intraorbital pressure.
- Goals of surgical management:
- Disengage entrapped structures and restore ocular rotatory function.
- Replace orbital contents into the usual confines of the normal bony orbital cavity, including restoration of both orbital volume and shape.
- Restore orbital cavity walls which, in effect, replaces the tissues into their proper position and dictates the shape into which the soft tissue can scar.

Anatomical pearls

- The orbits are conceptualized in thirds progressing from anterior to posterior.
- Anteriorly, the orbital rims consist of thick bone.
- The middle third of the orbit consists of thin bone, while the bone structure thickens again in the posterior third.
- The orbital bone structure is thus analogous to a "shock-absorbing" device in which the middle portion of the orbit breaks first, followed by the rim.
- The optic foramen is situated at the junction of the lateral and medial walls of the orbit posteriorly and is well above the horizontal plane of the orbital floor. The foramen is located 40–45 mm behind the inferior orbital rim.

Key technical considerations

- Exposure considerations:
  - Endoscopic approaches through the maxillary sinus permit direct visualization and repair of the orbital floor and manipulation of the soft tissues without an eyelid incision *(Fig. 6.6)*.
  - Lower eyelid incisions have the least incidence of ectropion of any lid incision location but tend to be the most noticeable.
  - Subciliary incisions near the upper margin of the lid leave the least conspicuous cutaneous scar, although they have the highest incidence of lid retraction.
  - Transconjunctival incisions can be performed in the preseptal or retroseptal plane and avoid external scars. Occasionally, a lateral canthotomy or caruncular extension is necessary to widen exposure to the lateral and medial orbit, respectively.

Complications and outcomes

- Diplopia: usually the result of muscle contusion, but can be the result of incarceration of muscle, soft tissue adjacent to the muscles, or nerve damage to cranial nerve III, IV, and VI.
- Enophthalmos: second major complication of blow-out fractures usually due to enlargement of the orbital volume.

- Retrobulbular hematoma: signaled by globe proptosis, congestion and prolapse of the edematous conjunctiva. Diagnosis is confirmed by a CT scan imaged with soft tissue windows. It is usually not possible to drain retrobulbar hematomas.
- Ocular (globe) injuries and blindness.
- Implant migration, late hemorrhage around implants and implant fixation.
- Ptosis of the upper lid: true ptosis of the upper lid should be differentiated from "pseudoptosis" resulting from the downward displacement of the eyeball in enophthalmos.

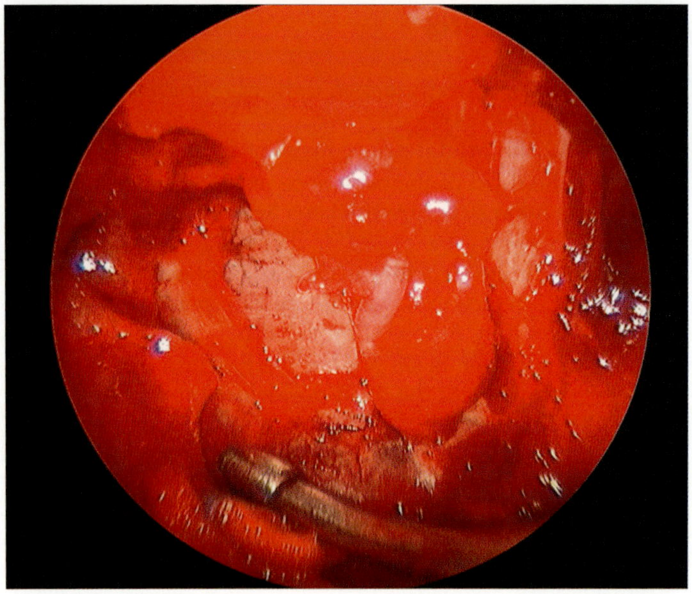

Figure 6.6 Endoscopic approach through the maxillary sinus permits direct visualization of the orbital floor and manipulation of the soft tissue and floor repair.

- Scleral show, ectropion and entropion – vertical shortening of the lower eyelid.
- Infraorbital nerve anesthesia.
- The "superior orbital fissure" syndrome: when a roof fracture extends posteriorly to involve the superior orbital fissure and its contents (CN III, IV, V, VI). Signaled by: restricted gaze and numbness of the forehead, brow, medial portion of upper lid, and medial upper nose.
- The "orbital apex" syndrome: when a roof fracture extends posteriorly to involve the superior orbital fissure and optic foramen and their contents (CN II, III, IV, V, VI). Signaled by: all symptoms of the superior orbital fissure syndrome with visual acuity change or blindness.

Nasal fractures

Brief introduction

- Most nasal fractures are initially reduced by closed reduction *(Fig. 6.7)*.
- In practice, closed reduction is frequently deferred until the edema has partially subsided and the accuracy of the reduction may be confirmed by visual inspection and palpation.
- In more severe frontal impacts where loss of nasal height and length occurs, or in nasoethmoidal orbital fractures, the use of open reduction and primary bone or cartilage grafting is beneficial to restore the support of the nose to its original volume *(Fig. 6.8)*.
- Naso-orbital ethmoid (NOE) fractures are severe fractures of the central one-third of the upper midfacial skeleton. They comminute the nose, the medial orbital rims and

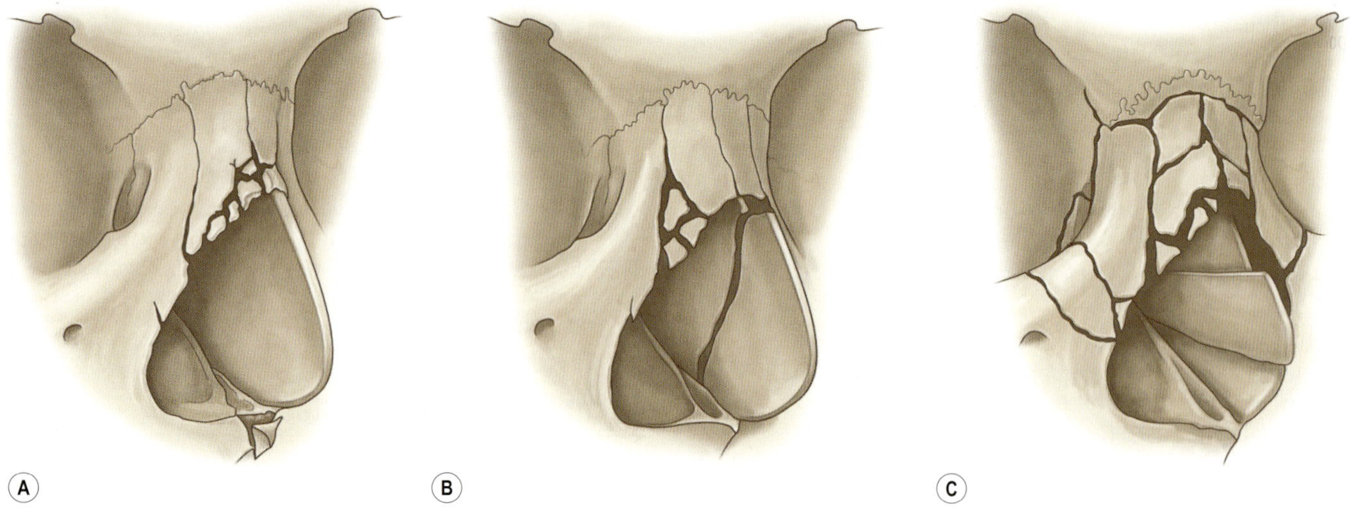

Figure 6.7 Frontal impact nasal fractures are classified by degrees of displacement, as are lateral fractures. **(A)** Plane I frontal impact nasal fracture. Only the distal ends of the nasal bones and the septum are injured. **(B)** Plane II frontal impact nasal fracture. The injury is more extensive, involving the entire distal portion of the nasal bones and the frontal process of the maxilla at the piriform aperture. The septum is comminuted and begins to lose height. **(C)** Plane III frontal impact nasal fractures involve one or both frontal processes of the maxilla, and the fracture extends to the frontal bone. These fractures are in reality nasoethmoidal-orbital fractures because they involve the lower two-thirds of the medial orbital rim (central fragment of the nasoethmoidal-orbital fracture) as well as the bones of the nose.

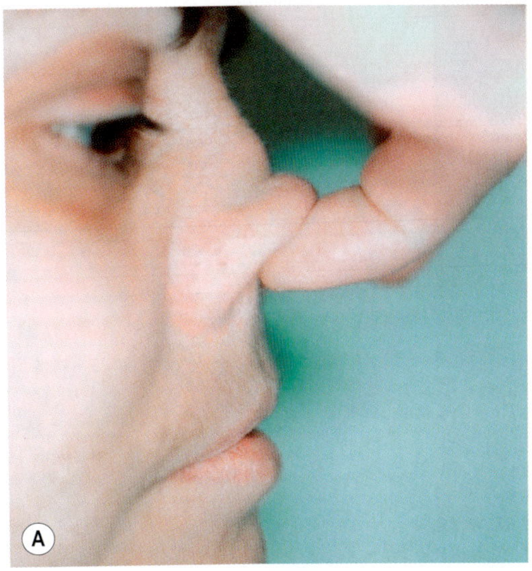

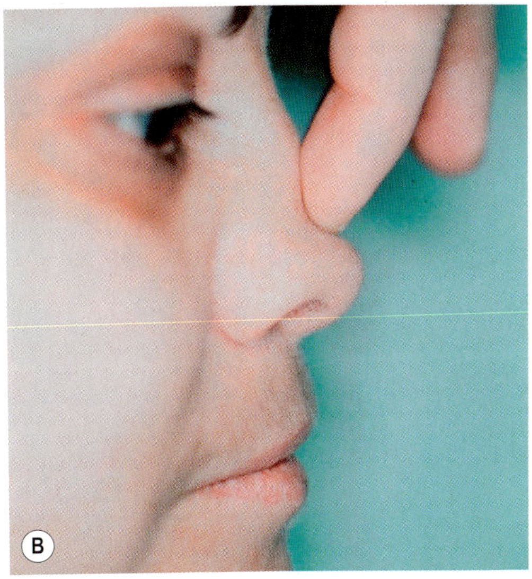

Figure 6.8 Palpation of the columella **(A)** and dorsum **(B)** detects superior rotation of the septum and lack of dorsal support. There is an absence of columellar support and dorsal septal support.

the piriform aperture. NOE fractures are isolated in one-third of cases and in two-thirds of cases extend to involve the frontal bone, zygoma or maxilla. One-third is unilateral and two-thirds are bilateral injuries. The central feature is the displacement of the section of the medial orbital rim carrying the attachment of the medial canthal ligament.

Preoperative considerations

- The appearance of NOE fractures is typical:
  - The nose is flattened.
  - There is a loss of dorsal nasal prominence.
  - An obtuse angle is noted between the lip and columella.
  - The medial canthal areas are swollen and distorted with palpebral and subconjunctival hematoma.
  - Directly over the medial canthal ligaments, crepitus or movement may be palpated with external pressure.
  - Traumatic telecanthus (increase in distance between medial canthal ligaments) and/or traumatic orbital hypertelorism (increase in distance between the orbits and globe) is present.

Anatomical pearls

- The diagnosis of an NOE fracture requires at a minimum four fractures that isolate the frontal process of the maxilla from adjacent bones:
  - Fracture of the nose.
  - Fracture of the junction of the frontal process of the maxilla with the frontal bone.
  - Fracture of the medial orbit (ethmoidal area).
  - Fracture of the inferior orbital rim extending to involve the piriform aperture and orbital floor.
- NOE fractures can be classified into one of three types:
  - Type I: an incomplete fracture which is displaced only inferiorly at the infraorbital rim and piriform margin ***(Fig. 6.9)***.
  - Type II: comminuted fracture with the fracture remaining outside the canthal ligament insertion ***(Fig. 6.10)***.
  - Type III: either avulsion of the canthal ligament (uncommon) or extension of the fracture underneath the canthal ligament insertion ***(Fig. 6.11)***.

Technical considerations

- Exposure: typically requires three incisions: (1) a coronal (or an appropriate laceration or local incision); (2) a lower eyelid incision; and (3) a gingival buccal sulcus incision.
- In all cases of NOE fractures, one must identify and classify what is happening to the bone of the medial orbital rim which bears the medial canthal attachment.
- Displacement of the medial canthal bone fragment is the "sine qua non" of the NOE injury.
- The most essential feature of NOE reduction is the transnasal reduction of the medial orbital rims by a wire placed posterior and superior to the canthal ligament insertion. It should be emphasized that the transnasal reduction wires must be passed posterior and superior to the lachrymal fossa in order to provide the proper direction of force to recreate the preinjury bony position of the central fragments.

Complications and outcomes

- Untreated hematomas of the nasal septum may result in subperichondrial fibrosis and thickening with partial nasal airway obstruction.
- Senechia formation usually occurs between the septum and the turbinates.
- Nasal obstruction may occur as a result of fracture malunion of the piriform margin, especially if displaced medially.

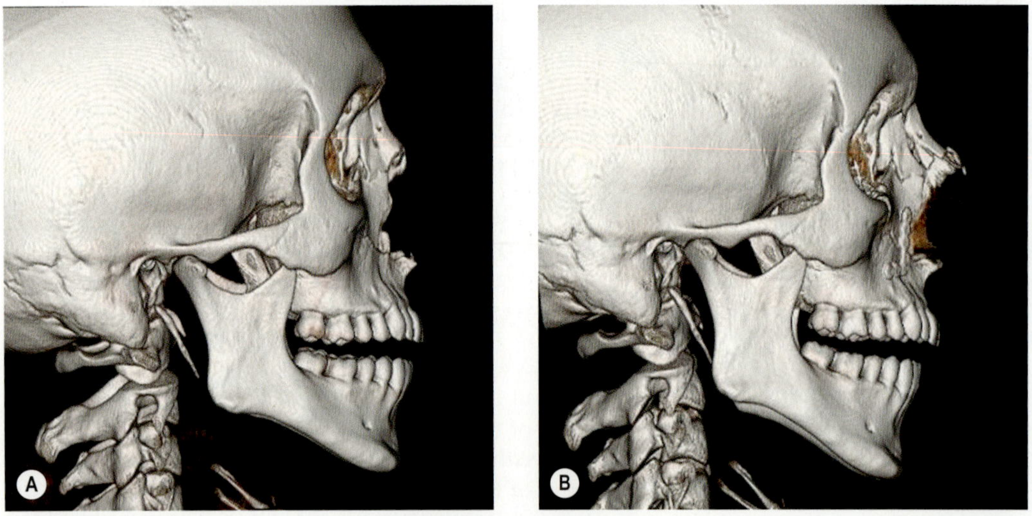

Figure 6.9 (A,B) Lateral image of 3D craniofacial computer tomography scan of a Type 1 naso-orbital ethmoidal fracture injury pattern pre and post open reduction and internal fixation of midface fractures using the inferior alone approach.

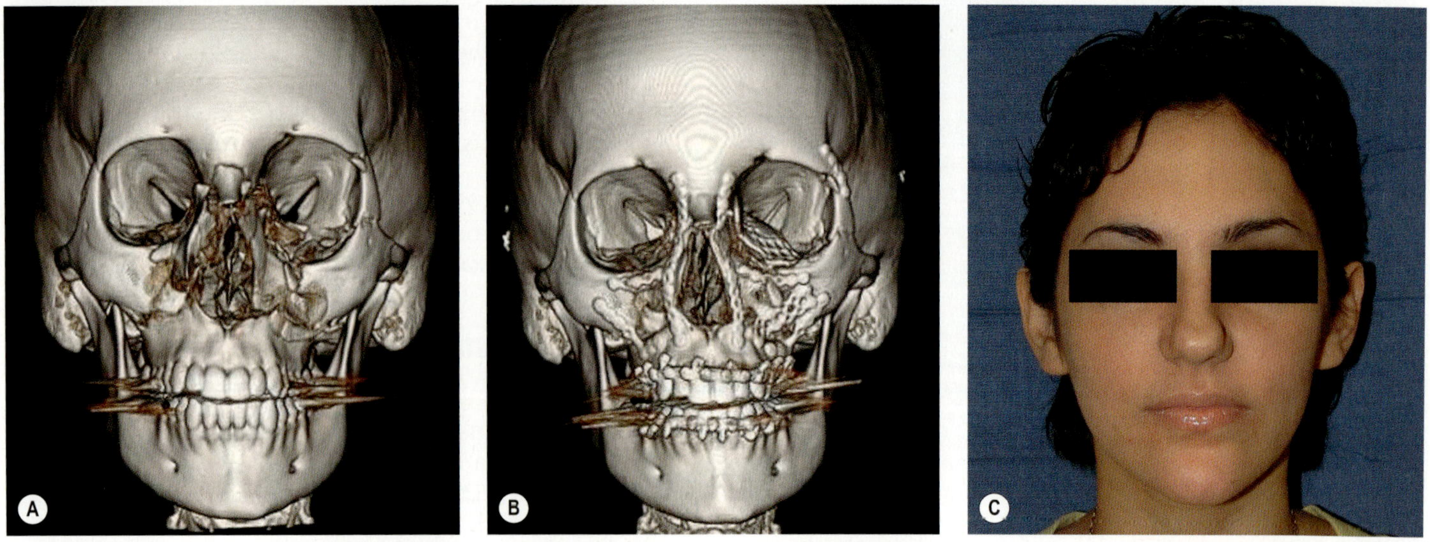

Figure 6.10 (A,B) Frontal 3D craniofacial computer tomography scan of a Type II naso-orbital ethmoidal fracture injury pattern in a 23-year-old female who sustained craniofacial injuries following being struck by a motor vehicle as a pedestrian, pre and post open reduction and internal fixation of midface fractures. **(C)** Postoperative frontal photograph view of patient approximately 12 months from surgery.

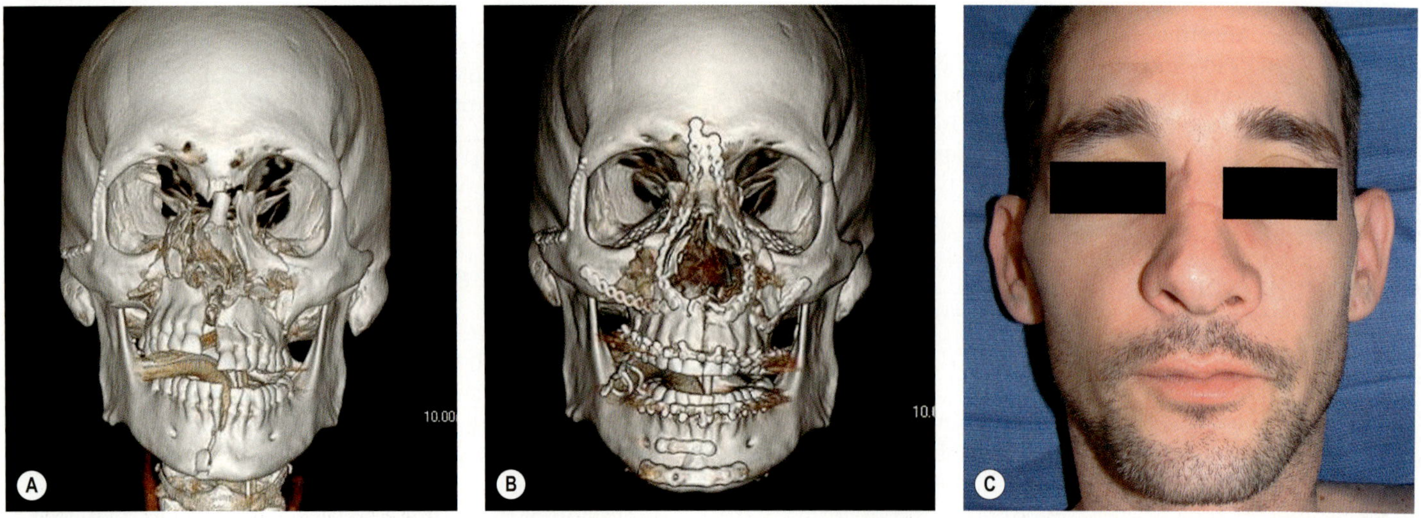

Figure 6.11 (A,B) Frontal 3D craniofacial computer tomography scan of Type III naso-orbital ethmoidal and a Le Fort II type injury pattern in a 33-year-old who sustained craniofacial injuries following being thrown off a motorcycle without a helmet, pre and post open reduction and internal fixation of midface and mandibular fractures. **(C)** Postoperative frontal photograph view of patient 6 months from surgery.

- Malunion.
- Special considerations for NOE fractures:
  - Frontal sinus obstruction.
  - Nasal functional impairment.
  - Nasal deformity.
  - Enophthalmos.

Zygoma fractures

Brief introduction

- The zygoma, a major buttress of the midfacial skeleton, forms the malar eminence and the lateral and inferior portions of the orbit *(Fig. 6.12)*.

Preoperative considerations

- When disrupted, the zygoma is usually displaced in a downward, medial, and posterior direction *(Fig. 6.13)*.
- The direction of displacement, however, varies with the direction of the injuring force and with the pull of the attached muscles.
- About half of fracture dislocations of the zygoma result in separation at the zygomaticofrontal (ZF) suture, which is palpable through the skin over the upper lateral margin of the orbit.
- The lateral canthal attachment is directed towards Whitnall's tubercle located approximately 10 mm below the zygomaticofrontal suture.
- When the zygoma is displaced inferiorly, the lateral attachment of the eyelids is also displaced inferiorly giving rise to an antimongoloid slant of the palpebral fissure.

Anatomical pearls

- The zygomatic bone has a quadrilateral shape with several processes that extend to reach the frontal bone, the maxilla, the temporal bone (zygomatic arch), and orbital processes of the sphenoid and maxilla.

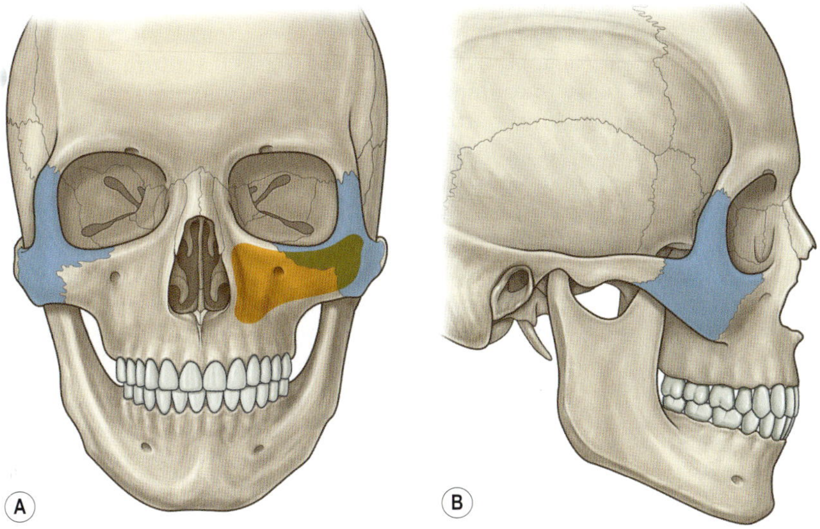

Figure 6.12 The zygoma and its articulating bones. **(A)** The zygoma articulates with the frontal, sphenoid, and temporal bones and the maxilla. The orange-shaded area shows the portion of the zygoma and maxilla occupied by the maxillary sinus. **(B)** Lateral view of the zygoma. (From Kazanjian VH, Converse J. *Surgical Treatment of Facial Injuries*, 3rd ed. Baltimore, Williams & Wilkins, 1974.)

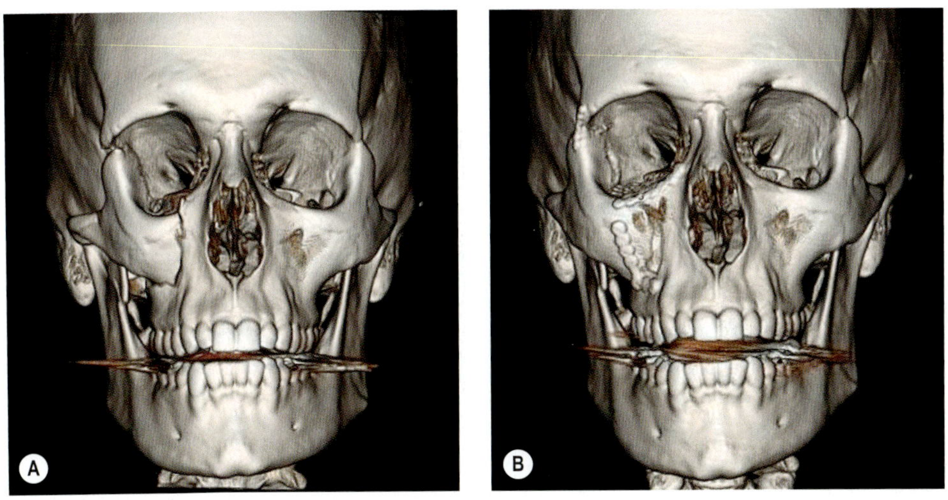

Figure 6.13 (A,B) Frontal 3D craniofacial computer tomography scan of a right zygomaticomaxillary fracture in a 22-year-old male who sustained craniofacial injuries following a sports related injury, pre and post open reduction and internal fixation of the right zygomaticomaxillary complex and orbital floor fractures.

- The bone furnishes attachments for the masseter, temporalis, zygomaticus major and minor, and the zygomatic head of the quadratus labii superiorus muscles.
- The zygomaticotemporal and zygomaticofacial nerves pass through this region to innervate the soft tissues over the region of the zygomaticofrontal junction and malar eminence.

Technical considerations

- If the ZF suture demonstrates significant diastasis then it must be stabilized. Exposure of the ZF suture is most easily accomplished through the lateral portion of an upper blepharoplasty incision which is made directly over the ZF suture 8–10 mm above the lateral canthus. Alternately, it may be approached through a brow laceration, coronal incision, or by superior dissection from a subciliary or transconjunctival lower lid incision with lateral canthotomy.
- Fractures with extreme posterior displacement, and those with lateral displacement of the zygomatic arch benefit from the addition of a coronal incision which allows exposure of the entire zygomatic arch and roof of the glenoid fossa as well as the ZF suture and the lateral orbital wall.
- Medially displaced arch fractures, whether isolated or part of a more extensive zygomatic fracture, may be managed through a temporal/Gillies approach.
- Fractures amenable to closed reduction include medial displaced isolated arch fractures, and simple large segment or single piece zygoma fractures without comminution at the buttresses or complete fracture at the ZF suture.

Complications and outcomes

- Bleeding.
- Maxillary sinusitis.
- Nonunion.
- Malunion.
- Infraorbital nerve injury.
- Orbital complications:
  - Diplopia.
  - Visual loss.
  - Globe injury.
  - Enophthalmos or exophthalmos.
  - Lid position abnormalities.
- Ankylosis of the temporomandibular joint from impacted arch fractures abutting the coronoid process.
- Oral–antral fistula.
- Miniplate complications.

Midface fractures

Brief introduction

- The midface is a system of sinus cavities interspersed between skeletal buttresses which provide vertical and horizontal structural support. If fractured or malpositioned, the buttresses must be anatomically reconstructed or reduced to re-establish pre-injury facial bone architecture ***(Fig. 6.14)***.
- Vertical buttresses include the nasal septum, and the paired nasomaxillary, zygomaticomaxillary, and pterygoid buttresses ***(Fig. 6.15)***.
- Horizontal buttresses include the inferior orbital rims and associated orbital floor, the paired zygomatic arches, and the palate at the level of the maxillary alveolus.
- Le Fort fractures represent the common patterns of severe midface fractures as characterized by Rene LeFort in 1901. The typical Le Fort fracture consists of combinations of these patterns, rather than pure bilateral Le Fort I, Le Fort II, or Le Fort III fractures ***(Fig. 6.16)***.
- Le Fort I fractures are those which traverse the maxilla horizontally above the level of the apices of the maxillary teeth. These fractures separate the entire alveolar process of the maxilla, vault of the palate and the inferior ends of

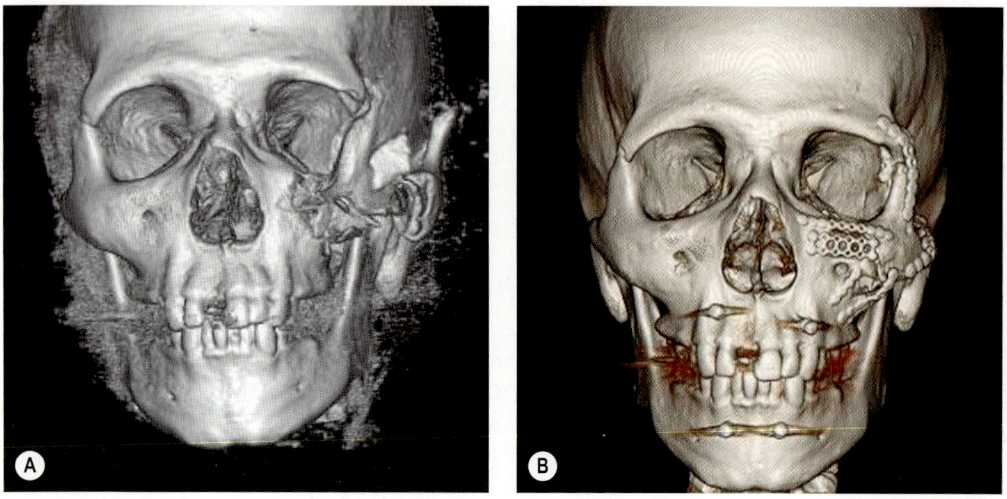

Figure 6.14 Frontal 3D craniofacial computer tomography scan of a Le Fort II type injury in a 33 year old who sustained craniofacial injuries following a high speed motor vehicle collision, pre and post open reduction and internal fixation of the left orbital and zygomaticomaxillary complex.

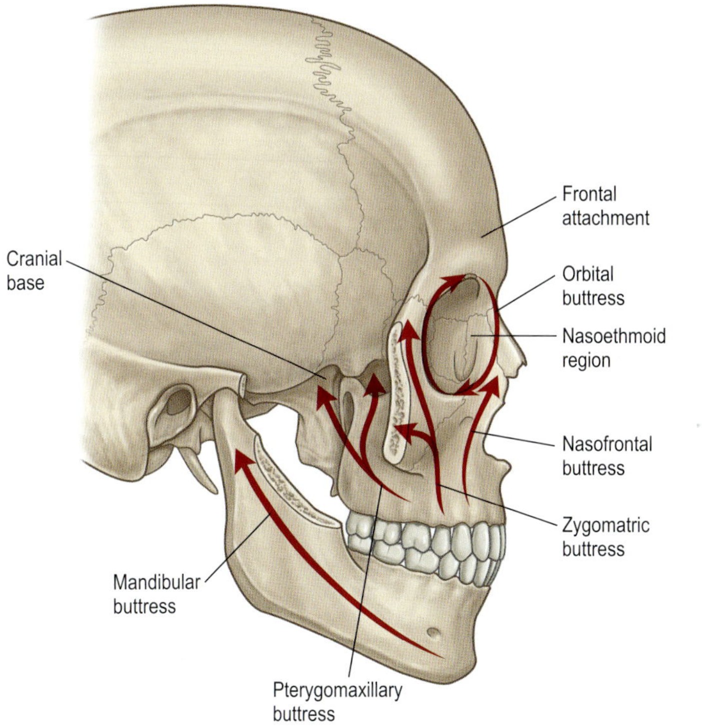

Figure 6.15 The vertical buttresses of the midfacial skeleton. Anteriorly, the nasofacial buttress skirts the piriform aperture inferiorly and composes the bone of the medial orbital rim superiorly to reach the frontal bone at its internal angular process. Laterally, the zygomaticomaxillary buttress extends from the zygomatic process of the frontal bone through the lateral aspect of the zygoma to reach the maxillary alveolus. A component of the zygomaticomaxillary buttress extends laterally through the zygomatic arch to reach the temporal bone. Posteriorly, the pterygomaxillary buttress is seen. It extends from the posterior portion of the maxilla and the pterygoid fossa to reach the cranial base structures. The mandibular buttress forms a strong structural support for the lower midface in fracture treatment. This support for maxillary fracture reduction must conceptually be achieved by placement of both jaws in intermaxillary fixation. The other "transverse" maxillary buttresses include the palate, the inferior orbital rims, and the superior orbital rims. The superior orbital rims and lower sections of the frontal sinus are also known in the supraorbital regions as the frontal bar and are technically frontal bone and not part of the maxilla. (From Manson PN. Hoopes JE, Su CT. Structural pillars of the facial skeleton: an approach to the management of Le Fort fractures. *Plast Reconstr Surg.* 1980;66:54.)

the pterygoid processes in a single block from the upper craniofacial skeleton ***(Fig. 6.17)***.
- Le Fort II fractures are those which result in a pyramidally shaped central maxillary segment. This fracture begins above the level of the apices of the maxillary teeth laterally and posteriorly in the zygomaticomaxillary buttress and extends through the pterygoid plates in the same fashion as the Le Fort I fracture. The fracture lines travel medially and superiorly to pass through the medial portion of the inferior orbital rim and extend across the nose ***(Fig. 6.18)***.
- Le Fort III fractures, or craniofacial dysjunction, may occur when the fracture extends through the zygomatico-frontal suture and the nasal frontal suture and across the floor of the orbits to effectively separate all midfacial structures from the cranium ***(Fig. 6.19)***.

Technical considerations

- Treatment of maxillary fractures is initially oriented toward the establishment of an airway, control of hemorrhage, closure of soft tissue lacerations and placement of intermaxillary fixation (IMF). IMF reduces the fracture, reduces movement and bleeding, and is the single most important treatment of a maxillary fracture.
- Simple fractures of the maxillary alveolar process can usually be digitally repositioned and held in reduction with arch bars. Fixation of the alveolar segment should be maintained for at least 4–12 weeks or until clinical immobility has been achieved.
- The goals of Le Fort fracture treatment are:
  - Restoration of midfacial height and projection through buttress reduction and fixation.
  - Provide proper occlusion.
  - Restore the integrity of the nose and orbit.
- Management of LeFort I fractures may only require IMF. Although in most cases the alveolus should be opened through a gingival buccal sulcus incision with plate and screw fixation at the nasomaxillary and zygomaticomaxillary buttresses.
- Le Fort II fractures are managed with IMF placement, exposure through a gingival buccal sulcus incision and lower lid incision for reduction and fixation at the zygomaticomaxillary and nasomaxillary buttresses and at the inferior orbital rims. The need for opening fractures crossing the nose must be assessed by the CT scan and the displacement at the nasofrontal junction.
- Open reduction of Le Fort III fractures generally involves combining procedures at the Le Fort I, Le Fort II and zygomatic levels in a single operation.

Postoperative considerations

- Cleansing and aspiration of the nose and mouth is very important.
- The presence of a fever in patients with facial fractures should always prompt a sinus evaluation by radiographs if the fever cannot be explained by other sources.
- Any foul odor to the breath necessitates inspection, cleaning and/or a return to the operating room for irrigation and a thorough examination.

Complications and outcomes

- Complications of maxillary/midface fractures include:
  - Airway compromise.
  - In severe cases, bleeding may require anterior–posterior nasopharyngeal packing, manual reduction of the displaced maxilla and intermaxillary fixation, or in extreme circumstances angiographic embolization or external carotid and superficial temporal artery ligation.
  - Infection.
  - CSF rhinorrhea.
  - Blindness.

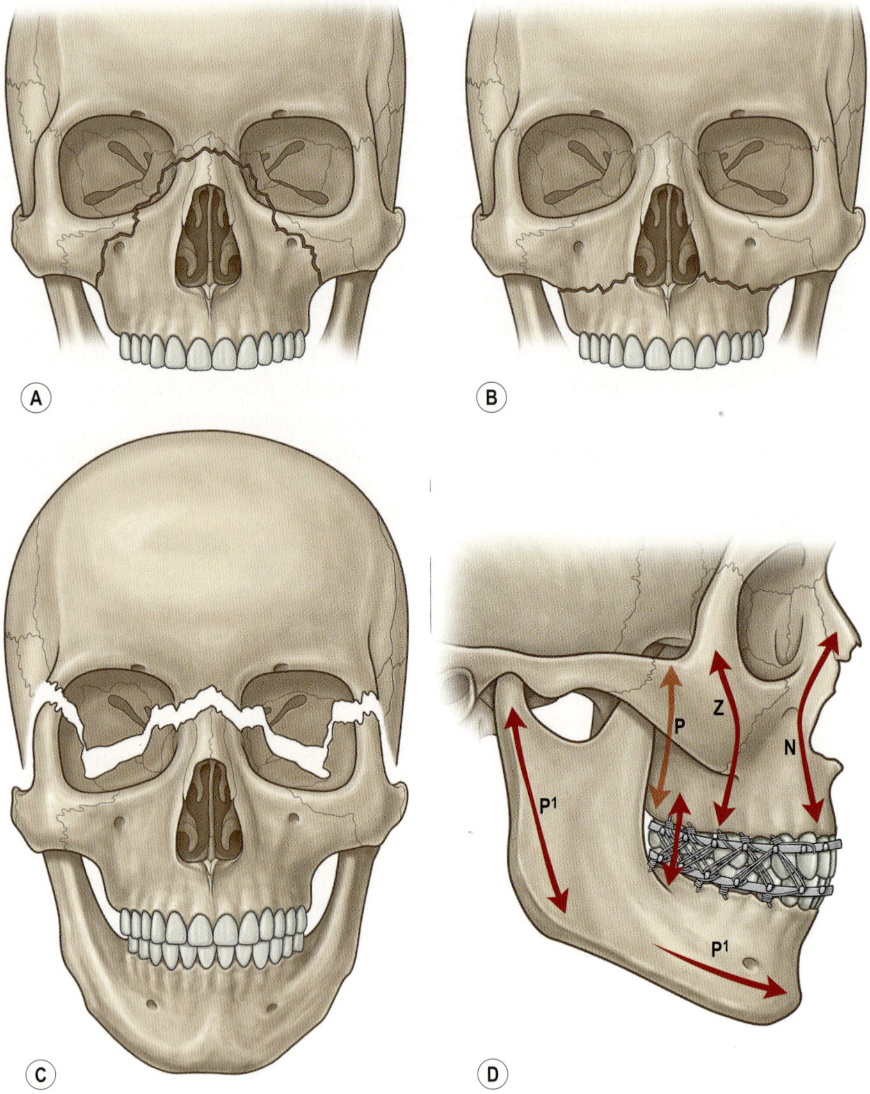

Figure 6.16 The Le Fort classification of midfacial fractures. **(A)** The Le Fort I (horizontal or transverse) fracture of the maxilla, also known as Guérin fracture. **(B)** The Le Fort II (or pyramidal) fracture of the maxilla. In this fracture, the central maxilla is separated from the zygomatic areas. The fracture line may cross the nose through its cartilages or through the middle nasal bone area, or it may separate the nasal bones from the frontal bone through the junction of the nose and frontal sinus. **(C)** The Le Fort III fracture (or craniofacial disjunction). In this fracture, the entire facial bone mass is separated from the frontal bone by fracture lines traversing the zygoma nasoethmoid, and nasofrontal bone junctions. **(D)** Buttresses of the midface. N: nasofrontal buttress; Z: zygomatic buttress; P: pterygomaxillary buttress; P^1: posterior height and anteroposterior projection must be maintained in complicated fractures. This is especially true in Le Fort fractures accompanied by bilateral subcondylar fractures. (**A–C** from Kazanjian VH, Converse J. *Surgical Treatment of Facial Injuries,* 3rd ed. Baltimore, Williams &Wilkins, 1974.)

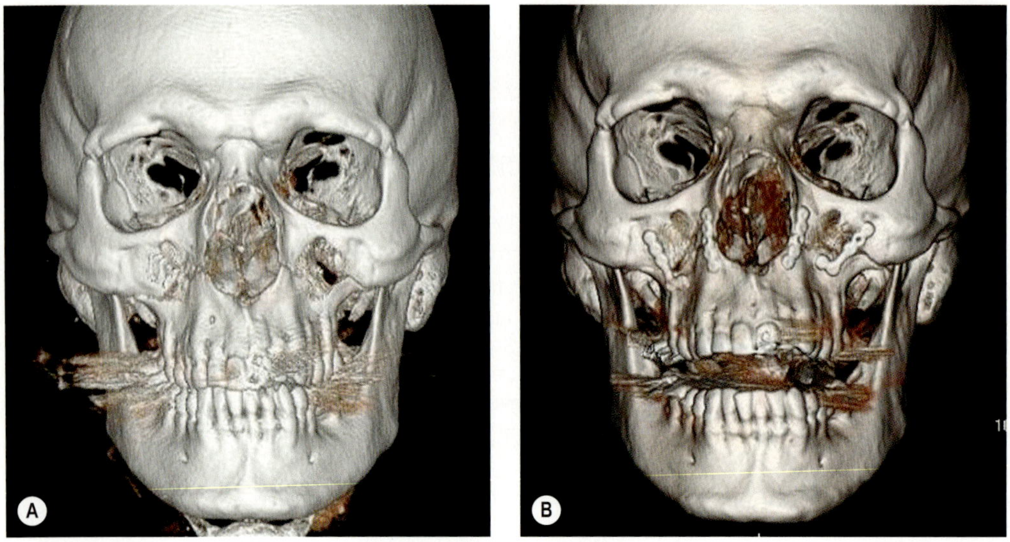

Figure 6.17 Frontal 3D craniofacial computer tomography scan of a Le Fort I type injury pre and post open reduction and internal fixation.

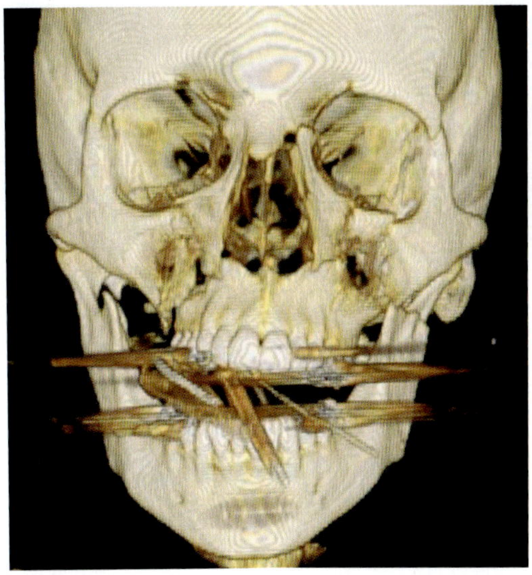

Figure 6.18 Frontal 3D craniofacial computer tomography scan of a Le Fort II type injury pre and post open reduction and internal fixation.

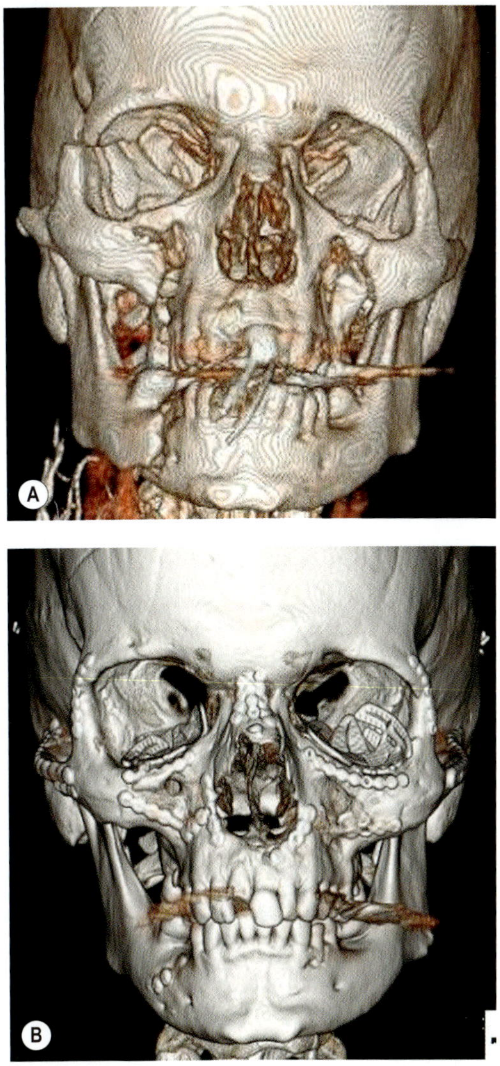

Figure 6.19 Frontal 3D craniofacial computer tomography scan of a Le Fort III type injury pre and post open reduction and internal fixation.

- Late complications:
  - Nonunion and bone grafting.
  - Malunion.
  - Malocclusion.
  - Nasolacrimal duct injury.

Mandible fractures

Brief introduction

- Craniofacial fractures frequently involve the jaws, which will invariably produce malocclusion.
- The mandible is a strong bone, but has several weak areas that are prone to fracture including:
  - The subcondylar area.
  - Angle.
  - Distal body.
  - The mental foramen.
- Timely loss of teeth results in atrophic changes of the alveolar bone and alters the structural characteristics of the mandible.
- Fractures often occur through the edentulous areas rather than through the areas better supported by adequate tooth and alveolar bone structures.
- In general, a tooth in the fractured segment may be extremely important, and should be retained, as the tooth acts as an occlusal stop and provides some stability for fracture alignment.
- Class I mandible fractures: fractures with teeth on either side of the fracture site (symphysis, parasymphysis, body) ***(Fig. 6.20)***.
- Class II fractures: fractures where teeth are present only on one side of the fracture site (posterior body, angle).
- Class III fractures: fractures which have no teeth on either side of the fracture site (ramus, condyle).

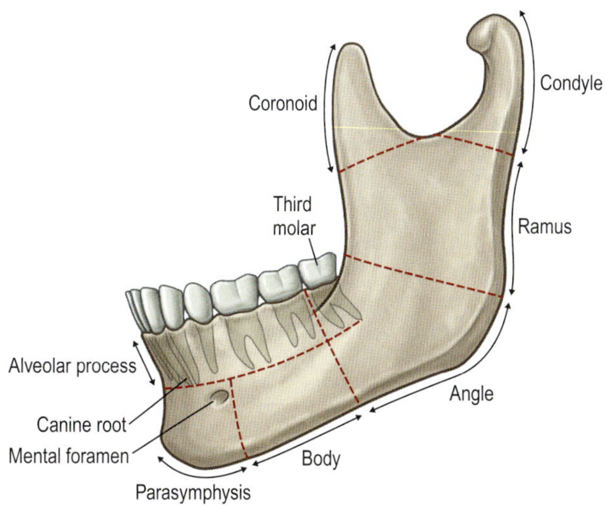

Figure 6.20 Classification of mandibular fractures.

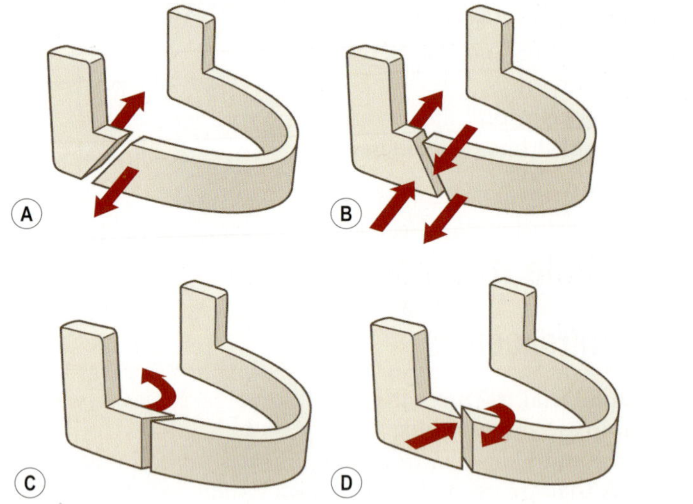

Figure 6.21 In **(A)** and **(C)**, the direction and bevel of the fracture line did not resist displacement due to muscle action. The arrows indicate the direction of muscle pull. In **(B)** and **(D)**, the bevel and direction of the fracture line resist displacement and oppose muscle action. The direction of the muscle pull in fractures beveled in this direction would tend to impact the fractured bone ends. (After Fry WK, Shepherd PR, McLeod AC, Parfitt GJ. *The Dental Treatment of Maxillofacial Injuries,* Oxford, Blackwell Scientific, 1942.)

Preoperative considerations

- Key diagnostic signs of mandible fractures:
  - Mobility or distraction at the fracture site with manual manipulation.
  - Crepitation with motion.
  - Malocclusion.
  - Inability to move the jaw.
  - Pain and/or tenderness with speech or motion.
- Indications for ORIF of mandible fractures:
  - Favorable or unfavorable Class I fractures where stability is desired ***(Fig. 6.21)***.
  - Class II and Class III fractures.
  - Comminuted fractures ***(Fig. 6.22)***.
  - Displaced fractures and those subject to rotation.
  - Edentulous fractures.
  - The desire to avoid IMF in the postoperative period.
  - Combined fractures of the upper and lower jaws.
  - Uncooperative (head injured) patients.
- Extraction of an impacted 3rd molar is recommended if it is preventing alignment of the fracture fragments, partially erupted and/or inflamed, or if the tooth root is exposed.
  - It is important to note that extraction of impacted 3rd molars may result in greater bone instability and conversion to comminution.
- Most condylar or subcondylar fractures are generally treated with closed reduction, with or without IMF ***(Fig. 6.23)***.
  - In children, growth considerations create a capacity for both regeneration and remodeling which is not present in adults.
  - Some shortening of the ramus height is almost inevitable with a closed approach and is first heralded by a premature contact in the molar dentition on the fractured side, which produces a subtle open bite in the contralateral occlusion.
- Absolute indications for open treatment of condylar/ subcondylar fractures are ***(Fig. 6.24)***:
  - Dislocation into the middle cranial fossa or external auditory canal.
  - Lateral extracapsular displacement.
  - Inability to obtain adequate occlusion.
  - Open joint wound with foreign body or gross contamination.
- Relative indications for open treatment of condylar/ subcondylar fractures include:
  - Angulation between the fractured fragments in excess of 30°.
  - Fracture gap between the bone ends exceeding 4–5 mm.
  - Significant lateral override and lack of contact of the ends of the fractured fragments.

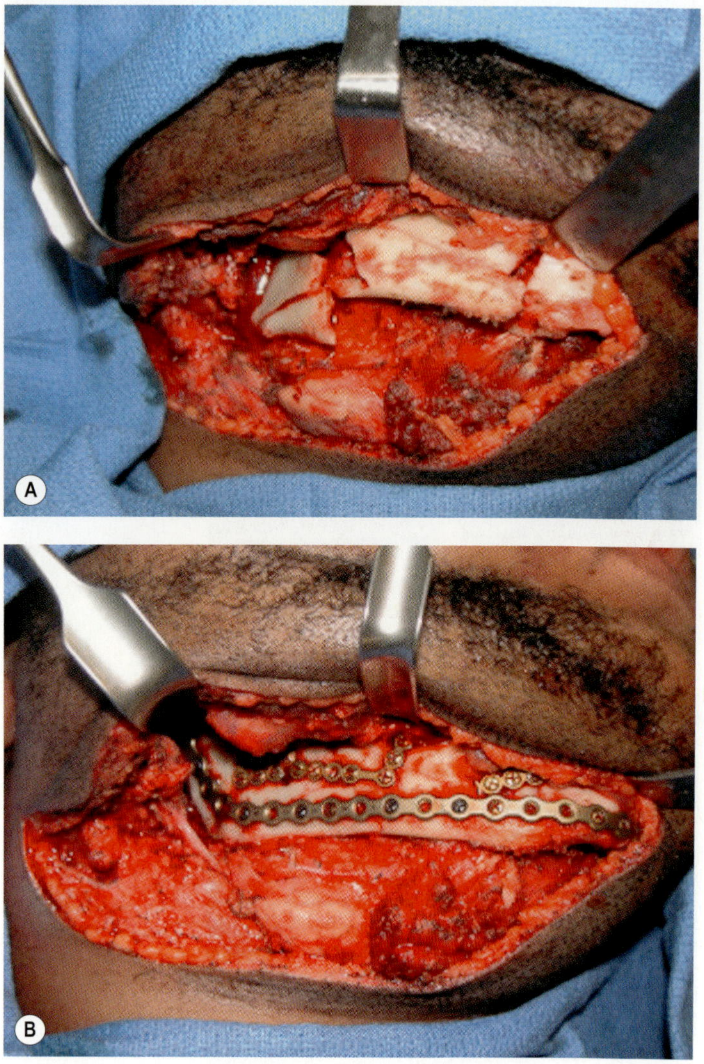

Figure 6.22 **(A,B)** Intraoperative photograph of comminuted mandibular fracture in a 23-year-old male following attempted homicidal gunshot wound to the face pre and post open reduction and internal fixation via the extra-oral approach using multiple miniplates.

  - Bilateral subcondylar fractures in a patient who has no dentition and where a splint is unavailable or when splinting is impossible because of alveolar ridge atrophy.
  - Bilateral or unilateral subcondylar fractures when splinting is not recommended for medical reasons or where adequate physiotherapy is impossible.
  - Bilateral condylar fractures associated with comminuted midfacial fractures.
  - Bilateral subcondylar fractures with associated gnathologic problems, such as (1) retrognathia or prognathism, (2) open bite with periodontal problems or lack of posterior support, (3) loss of multiple teeth and later need for elaborate reconstruction, (4) bilateral condylar fractures with unstable occlusion due to orthodontics, and (5) unilateral condylar fracture with unstable fracture base.
- Edentulous mandibular fractures represent less than 5% of the mandibular fractures and commonly occur through the most atrophic portions where the bone is thin and weak (typically the body) ***(Fig. 6.25)***.
- Many fractures are bilateral or multiple, and displacement of a bilateral edentulous body fracture is often severe and a challenging condition to treat.
- Closed fractures demonstrating minimal displacement may be treated with a soft diet and avoidance of dentures; however, in these cases observation is critical to be sure that healing occurs within several weeks without further displacement.
- Most fractures are better treated with fixation using large reconstruction "locking" plates.

Anatomical pearls

- Unique to mandibular fractures, mandibular movements are determined by the action of reciprocally placed muscles attached to the bone.
  - When fractures occur, displacement of the segments is influenced by the pull of the muscles attaching to the segments.
- The direction of the fracture line may oppose forces created by these muscles.
- Mandibular fractures can be classified as "favorable" or "unfavorable" according to their direction and bevel of displacement. In some fractures, the muscular force would pull the fragments into a position favorable for healing, whereas in other fractures, the muscular pull is unfavorable resulting in separation at the fracture site ***(Fig. 6.26)***.

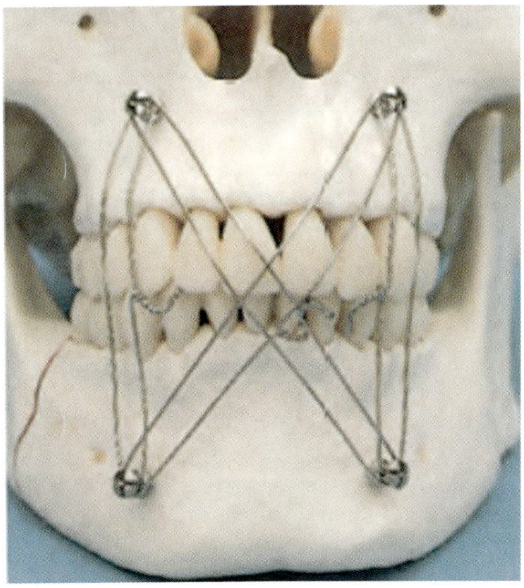

Figure 6.23 The use of intermaxillary fixation screws for intermaxillary fixation. These devices do not provide the stability or flexibility obtained from arch bars and full intermaxillary fixation. Numbers of patients have been thought to be in good occlusion with this technique when actually they were in an open bite, were malreduced, and required osteotomy or fracture revision. Crossed wires may also be used to buttress the screw support obtained. (Courtesy of Synthes Maxillofacial, Paoli, Pa.)

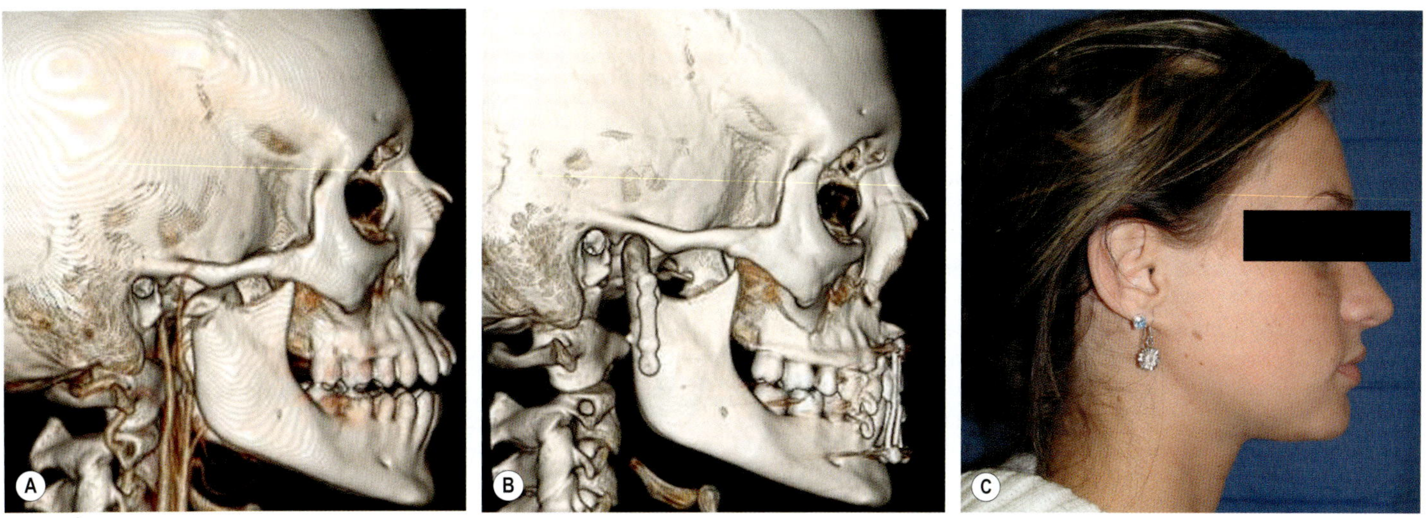

Figure 6.24 (A,B) Lateral view of 3D craniofacial computer tomography on a 20-year-old female involved in a motor vehicle collision who sustained craniofacial injuries, pre and post open reduction and internal fixation of a right mandibular subcondylar fracture via a retromandibular extra-oral approach. Note that the patient also had a Le Fort II type fracture that was treated with closed reduction and interdental fixation. **(C)** Lateral profile view photograph of patient one year postoperatively.

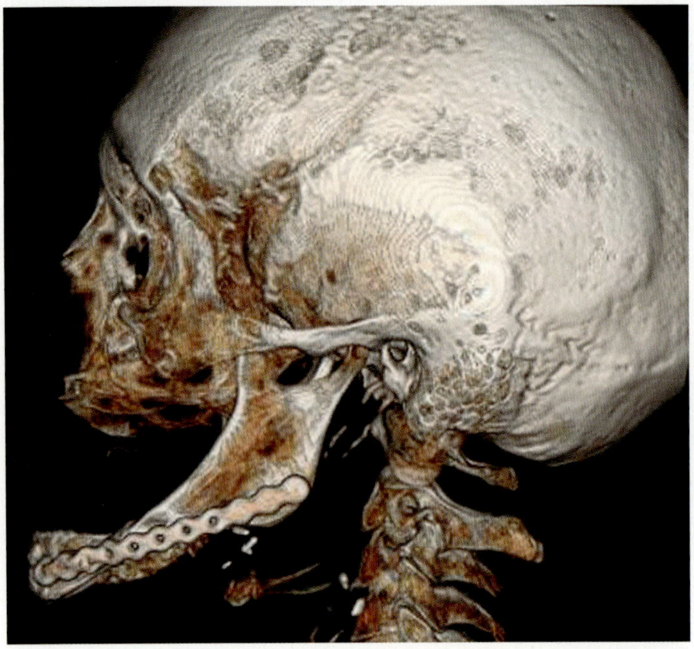

Figure 6.25 Lateral view of 3D craniofacial computer tomography on a 64-year-old edentulous female with a history of oseogenesis imperfecta; who was referred for treatment of a malunion of a left mandibular fracture postoperative open reduction and internal fixation using a load bearing mandibular plate and iliac bone grafting via an extra-oral approach.

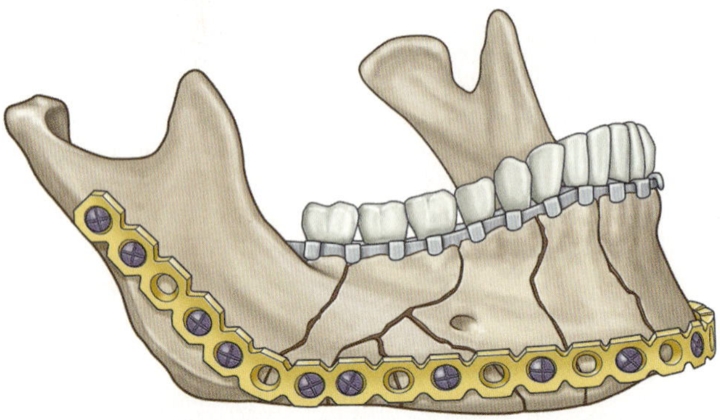

Figure 6.26 Large reconstruction plate spans fractures of the entire body. (Courtesy of Synthes Maxillofacial, Paoli, Pa.)

- Horizontally favorable: mandibular fractures that are directed from lingual to buccal cortex in a forward direction. In this fracture pattern, the pull of the muscles of mastication holds the fragments together at the fracture site.
- Horizontally unfavorable: fractures directed from lingual to buccal cortex in a posterior direction. In this pattern, the muscle groups displace the fracture fragments.
- Vertically unfavorable: fractures directed from superior to inferior in a posterior direction.
- Vertically favorable: fractures directed from superior to inferior in a forward direction.
- In general, class I fractures are broadly exposed with an intraoral degloving technique to allow adequate exposure for plate and screw fixation.
- In symphysis and parasymphysis fractures, both a muscular and mucosal closure of intraoral incisions is preferred.
- Class II fractures require open reduction and fixation.
- The type and strength of plate needed to control the non-toothbearing fragment and displacement of the fracture will vary according to the direction and bevel of the fracture and the position of the teeth and surrounding muscles.
- Generally, a larger inferior border plate with a smaller superior border plate is preferred.
- In non-displaced or favorable angle fractures, the Champy technique may be used.
- Class III fractures that are non-displaced and immobile may be treated by a soft diet with close follow up, although the majority should be managed with rigid fixation using superior and inferior border plates.

Technical considerations

- In select cases (non-displaced or favorable fractures) management by IMF alone is possible.
- In unfavorable fractures, panfacial fractures, or those in which early function is desired, internal fixation is preferred.
- Dental wiring and fixation techniques include arch bars and IMF screws.
- Arch bars are ligated to the external surface of the dental arch by passing 24 or 26 G steel wires around the arch-bar, and around the necks of the teeth.
- The wires are twisted tightly to individual teeth to hold the arch bars in the form of the dental arch.
- If segments of teeth are missing, or if anterior support of the arch bar is needed to balance the forces generated by elastic traction anteriorly, the arch bar may be stabilized by additional wires passed to the skeleton (skeletal wires).
- IMF screws are a rapid method of immobilizing the teeth in occlusion, given good dentition and uncomplicated fracture types (see Fig. 6.23).
- The number and position of the IMF screws is based on the fracture type, fracture location and surgeon preference.
- Screws must be positioned superior to the maxillary tooth roots and inferior to the mandibular tooth roots.

Operative techniques

- The general approaches to mandible fractures are:
  - Establish proper occlusion.
  - Anatomically reduce the fractured bones into their normal position.
  - Utilize fixation techniques that hold the fractured bone segments in occlusion and normal position until healing has occurred. Open reduction internal fixation (ORIF) can often permit limited function while healing is occurring.
  - Control infection.

- General principles of reduction and fixation:
  - Superior and inferior border stabilization is the general rule.
  - The use of the "locking plate" minimizes the requirement for precise plate bending.
  - Comminuted fractures require larger fixation plates, and are conceptually fractures with "bone loss", where the plate itself bears the entire load of fixation (see Fig. 6.26).
- Champy and miniplate fixation:
  - Speeds exposure and is more tolerant for mandibular shape and occlusion versus more rigid plates.
  - The malleable plates minimize malreductions from "plate bending errors" common to stiff larger plates.
  - Does not result in the maximum rigidity achieved with the large plates, but is generally sufficient for good immobilization at fracture sites with minimal movement, such as a favorable and minimally displaced angle fracture.
- Lag screw technique *(Fig. 6.27)*:
  - Indicated in non-comminuted parasymphysis or symphysis fractures where a long length of screw can be tolerated.
  - In this technique, the first cortex in the bone is over-drilled to the major diameter of the screw while the second segment of the screw path is drilled to the minor diameter of the screw. This allows the screw head to engage only the bone in the first section and as the screw is tightened into the second section of the fracture, the screw head impacts the cortex toward the fracture site as it is tightened.
  - Generally, two lag screws are recommended for each fracture to be stable, for if one becomes loose, the fracture would be unstable by virtue of the rotation.
- Extraoral approach to mandible fractures:
  - The position of an external mandibular incision should always respect the location of the marginal mandibular branch of the facial nerve.
  - Subperiosteal dissection should be performed.
  - The fragments at the inferior border of the fracture are aligned with clamps and occlusal reduction should be checked.
  - A superior border plate is secured first at the upper border of the mandible and fixed with unicortical screws and the occlusion is again checked.
  - The lower border plate and screws are then applied. A larger plate may be utilized and bicortical screw placement is preferred.
- Intraoral approach:
  - Any fracture in the horizontal or vertical mandible is usually amenable to an intraoral approach and is the preferred exposure for symphysis, parasymphysis, and noncomminuted angle fractures. The body region is also able to be reduced but may require use of a percutaneous Trocar approach for drilling and screw placement.

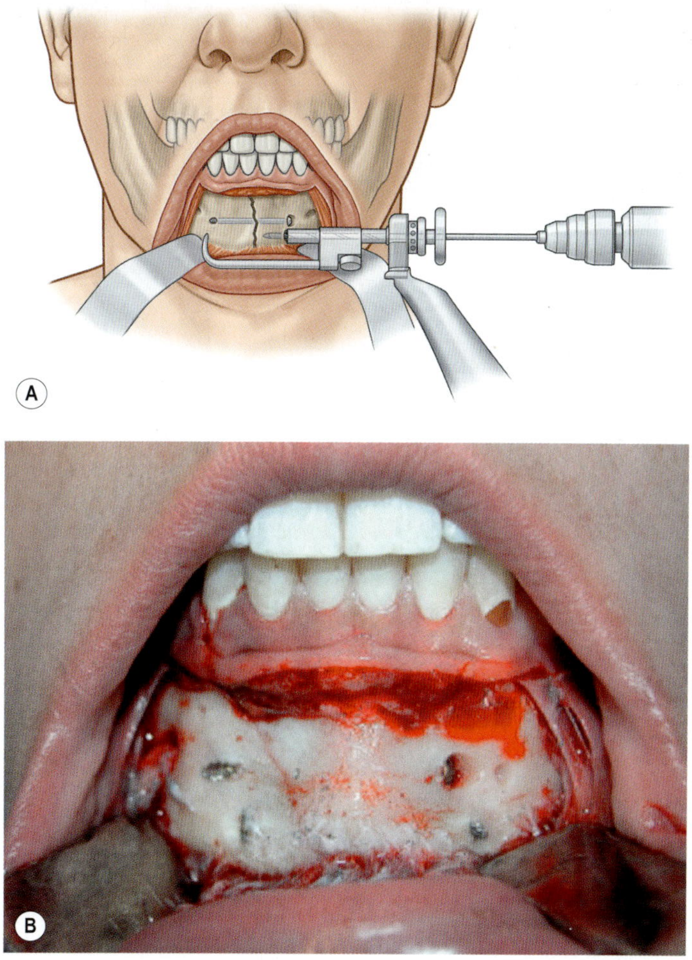

Figure 6.27 **(A)** Placement of two horizontal lag screws to reduce and stabilize a parasymphysis fracture using a trocar device. (Courtesy of Synthes Maxillofacial, Paoli, Pa.) **(B)** Intraoperative photograph of open reduction and internal fixation of mandibular symphseal fracture using lag screws.

Complications and outcomes

- Malocclusion.
- Hardware infection and migration.
- Increased facial width and rotation of the mandible.
- Non-union.
- Osteomyelitis.

The panfacial injury

Brief introduction

- Conceptually, panfacial fractures involve all three areas of the face: frontal bone, midface, and mandible.

Preoperative considerations

- Various sequences have been suggested such as "top to bottom", "bottom to top", "outside to inside", or "inside to outside". In reality, it does not make any difference

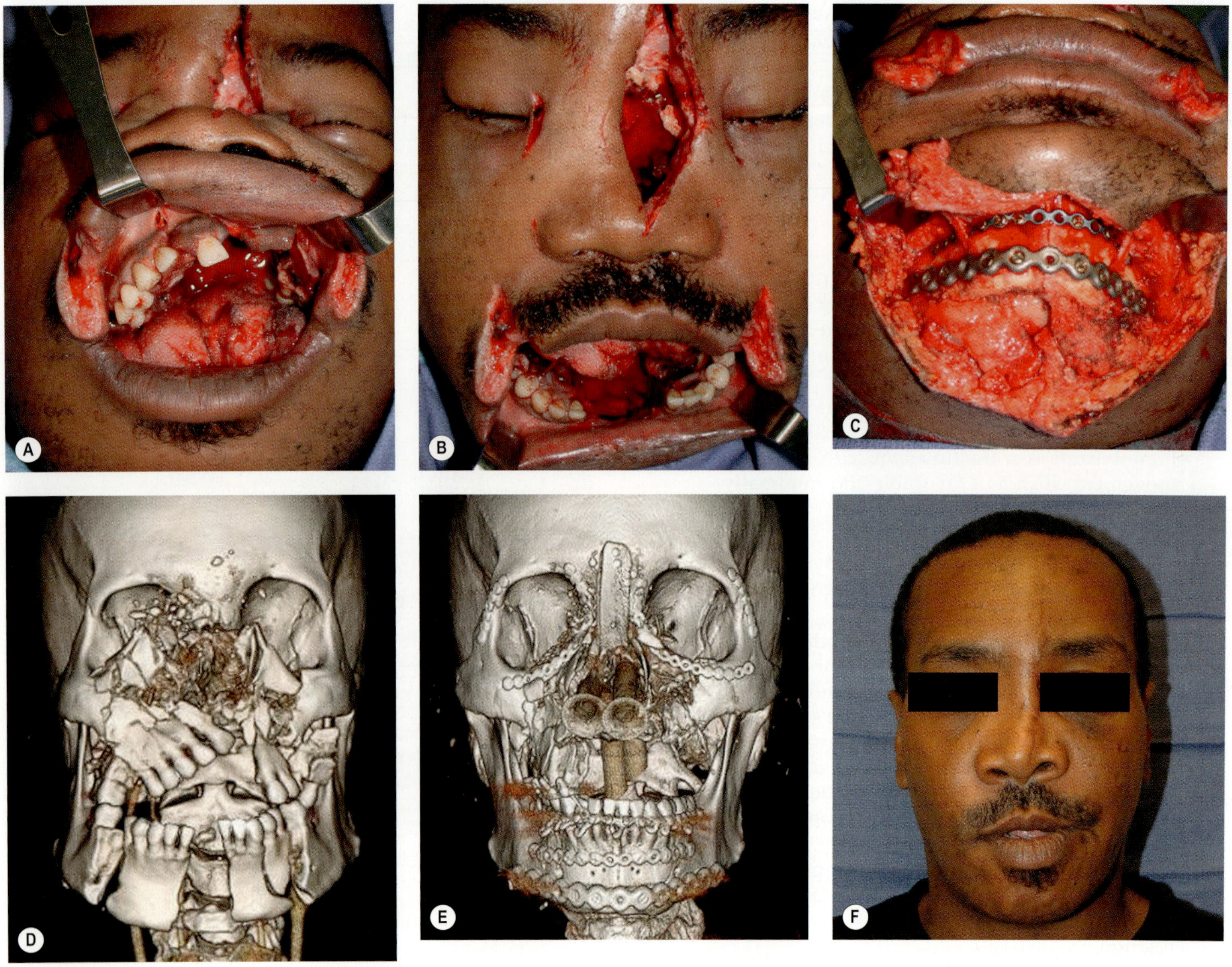

Figure 6.28 **(A,B)** Frontal photographs of a 34-year-old male following a self-inflicted gunshot wound injury to the face demonstrating severe midfacial and mandibular fractures. **(C)** Intraoperative photographs following open reduction and internal fixation of mandibular fractures using a load bearing mandibular plate and a monocortical miniplate fixation via an extra-oral approach. **(D,E)** Frontal 3D craniofacial computer tomography scan of the patient pre and post open reduction and internal fixation of midfacial and mandibular fractures. **(F)** Postoperative photograph 1 year following surgery.

what the order is as long as the order makes sense and leads to a reproducible, anatomically accurate bone reconstruction.

- In our experience, it is more predictable to stabilize the occlusion by relating the maxilla to the mandible than by relating the inferior maxilla to the superior maxilla.

Technical considerations

- Presently, a one-stage restoration of the architecture of the craniofacial skeleton is the preferred method of treatment using open reduction of all fracture sites with plate and screw fixation.
- Regional incisions such as the coronal, transconjunctival, upper and lower gingival buccal sulcus and the retromandibular incisions provide the complete exposure.
- In each subunit of the face, the important dimension to be considered first is facial width.

Complications and outcomes

- Lack of facial projection.
- Enophthalmos.
- Malocclusion.
- Increased facial width.
- Positional deformities seen in the frontal region:
  - Posterior and inferior positioning of the superior orbital rims.
  - Flattened frontal contour.
- Soft tissue deformities, including descent, diastasis, fat atrophy, and ectropion, thickening and rigidity.
- Temporal wasting: usually caused by lack of periosteal closure over the zygomaticofrontal suture.

Ballistics injuries to the face

Brief introduction

- Recently, immediate reconstruction and immediate soft tissue closure with "serial-second-look" procedures has become the standard of care.
- Ballistic injuries are classified into low, medium, and high-energy deposit injuries.
- In formulating a treatment plan for ballistic injuries, it is helpful to identify the entrance and exit wounds, the presumed path of the bullet, and to appreciate the mass and velocity of the projectile, so that the extent of internal areas of tissue injury can be predicted.
- Conceptually, soft tissue injury and bone injury, and soft tissue loss and bone loss must all be individually assessed.

Technical considerations

- Low velocity gunshot wounds involve little soft tissue and bone loss and have limited associated soft tissue injury outside the exact path of the bullet.
- Appropriate for immediate definitive bony stabilization and primary soft tissue closure with limited debridement necessary.
- Intermediate and high velocity ballistic injuries to the face are characterized by extensive soft tissue and bone destruction ***(Fig. 6.28)***.
- These injuries must be managed with a specific treatment plan that involves stabilization of existing bone and soft tissue in anatomic position, maintenance of this stabilization throughout the period of soft tissue contracture, and eventual bone and soft tissue reconstruction.
- "Second look" procedures, which generally occur at 48-hour intervals, are important with these injuries to re-open the soft tissue and define additional areas of soft tissue necrosis, drain hematomas and/or developing fluid collections, and assure bone integrity.
- In some cases, it may be possible to plan a more complex reconstruction of bone and soft tissue simultaneously by loco-regional flaps and/or composite free tissue transfer.

Further reading

Champy M, Lodde JP, Schmidt R, et al. Mandibular osteosynthesis by miniature screwed plates via a buccal approach. *J Maxillofac Surg*. 1978;6:14.

Clark N, Birely B, Manson PN, et al. High-energy ballistic and avulsive facial injuries: Classification, patterns, and an algorithm for primary reconstruction. *Plast Reconstr Surg*. 1996;98:583–601.

Dingman RO, Grabb WC. Surgical anatomy of the mandibular ramus of the facial nerve based on the dissection of 100 facial halves. *Plast Reconstr Surg*.1962;29:2166.

Ellis 3rd E. Treatment methods for fractures of the mandibular angle. *Int J Oral Maxillofac Surg*. 1999;28(4):243–252.

Gruss JS, MacKinnon SE, Kassel EE, et al. The role of primary bone grafting in complex craniomaxillofacial trauma. *Plast Reconstr Surg*. 1985;75:17.

Le Fort R. Etude experimentale sur les fractures de la machoire superieur. *Rev Chir Paris*. 1901;23:208,360,479.

Original article describing the various fracture patterns associated with traumatic craniofacial injury. We associate the author's name to the different types of fracture patterns recognized.

Manson PN, Su CT, Hoopes JE. Structural pillars of the facial skeleton. *Plast Reconstr Surg*. 1980;66:54.

Significant article describing the anatomical buttresses of the craniofacial skeleton that are required for reconstruction to maintain facial width and height.

Markowitz B, Manson P, Sargent, et al. Management of the medial canthal tendon in nasoethmoid orbital fractures: The importance of the central fragment in treatment and classification. *Plast Reconstr Surg*. 1991;87:843–853 .

Landmark article on the classification types of nasoethmoidorbital region. Knowledge of this fracture pattern classification assists with the treatment of this complex surgical condition.

Rodriguez ED, Stanwix MG, Nam AJ, et al. Twenty-six-year experience treating frontal sinus fractures: a novel algorithm based on anatomical fracture pattern and failure of conventional techniques. *Plast Reconstr Surg*. 2008;122(6):1850–1866.

Landmark article describing the longest experience with treating frontal sinus fractures and provides an algorithm for its treatment based on their outcomes, to minimize long-term complications.

Tessier P, Guiot G, Rougerie J, et al. Osteotomies cranio-naso-orbital-facials. *Hypertelorism Ann Chir Plast*. 1967;12:103.

An article by the father of craniofacial surgery describing the possibilities of an intracranial approach for orbital reconstructive surgery.

7 Chapter

Local flaps for facial coverage

This chapter was created using content from Neligan & Rodriguez, Plastic Surgery 3rd edition, Volume 3, Craniofacial, Head and Neck Surgery, Chapter 10, Cheek and lip reconstruction, Peter C. Neligan, Chapter 18, Local flaps for facial coverage, Ian T. Jackson.

SYNOPSIS

- Always consider the defect when planning a flap.
- Assess availability and laxity of local tissue.
- Rob Peter to pay Paul but only if Peter can afford it.
- Match the flap to the defect, not the defect to the flap.
- Keep your reconstruction as simple as possible.
- Good cosmesis is vital but function trumps cosmesis.
- Do not burn bridges.
- If unsure of how to proceed, for whatever reason, use a temporizing approach.

Cheek reconstruction
- Local tissue should be used whenever possible.
- Local and regional flaps work well.
- Color match is important.
- For composite defects of lips and cheeks, each component defect can be reconstructed as a separate unit.

Lip reconstruction
- Accurate three layered closure of lip defects is imperative to preserve function.
- Local tissue should be used whenever possible.
- Small defects can be closed by direct repair:
  - Defects up to 25% the width of the upper lip can be closed.
  - Defects up to 30% the width of the lower lip can be closed.
- Intermediate defects are best reconstructed with local flaps.
- Total or sub-total lip defects are best reconstructed with free tissue.

Brief introduction

- Flaps on the face have many designs and these are related to the area to be reconstructed and the size of the defect. It must not be forgotten, however, that there are only certain basic well-defined tissue manipulations; these are based on the concepts of advancement, transposition, and rotation (Video 7.1; Video 7.2).
- When a wound is closed tightly or a flap which seems too small is used and yet the defect is closed, the biomechanical properties of creep and stress relaxation have been harnessed, and the skin elongates over time (Table 7.1).
- For simplicity, key concepts for facial coverage will be grouped according to anatomic area.

Video 7.1

Video 7.2

Forehead and scalp

- The characteristics of the forehead vary considerably with age and nationality.
- All foreheads have a limited amount of spare skin and, as a result, wide undermining and freeing are necessary to deal with many skin defects.
- The forehead is surrounded by a frame with distinct outlines, mainly of hair that should not be disturbed, where possible.

Technical pearls

- In the forehead, vertical donor sites are preferred to horizontal sites, which may cause an upward shift of the eyebrows or downward repositioning the forehead hairline ***(Fig. 7.1)***.

- In larger defects, a triple rhomboid may be used; this necessitates an excision of a hexagonal design ***(Fig. 7.2)***.
- Careful planning and assessment of the availability of loose skin in all three areas of flap harvest is essential.

Table 7.1 **Viscoelastic properties of the skin**

Creep	When a sudden load is applied and kept constant, skin will stretch
Stress relaxation	A constant load on the skin will cause lengthening. With time, the load required to maintain the lengthening decreases. This explains why white flaps will frequently become pink with time

- In the temporal area, 3.5 cm flaps can be used, but this requires great care in order to prevent too great a shift of the hairline. This applies to reconstruction of any area on the non-hair-bearing scalp in proximity to the hairline edge ***(Fig. 7.3)***.
- Direct advancement flaps are possible but can only close smaller defects.
- Island flaps are used only occasionally; they are frequently based on subcutaneous tissue rather than on definite blood vessels. This necessitates taking great care to maintain every subcutaneous strand possible and tension must be minimized.
- Bilobed flaps can be used, but they tend to trapdoor or pincushion and are therefore obvious in any form of indirect lighting.
- Large forehead reconstruction is treated by tissue expansion; this allows reconstruction by simple

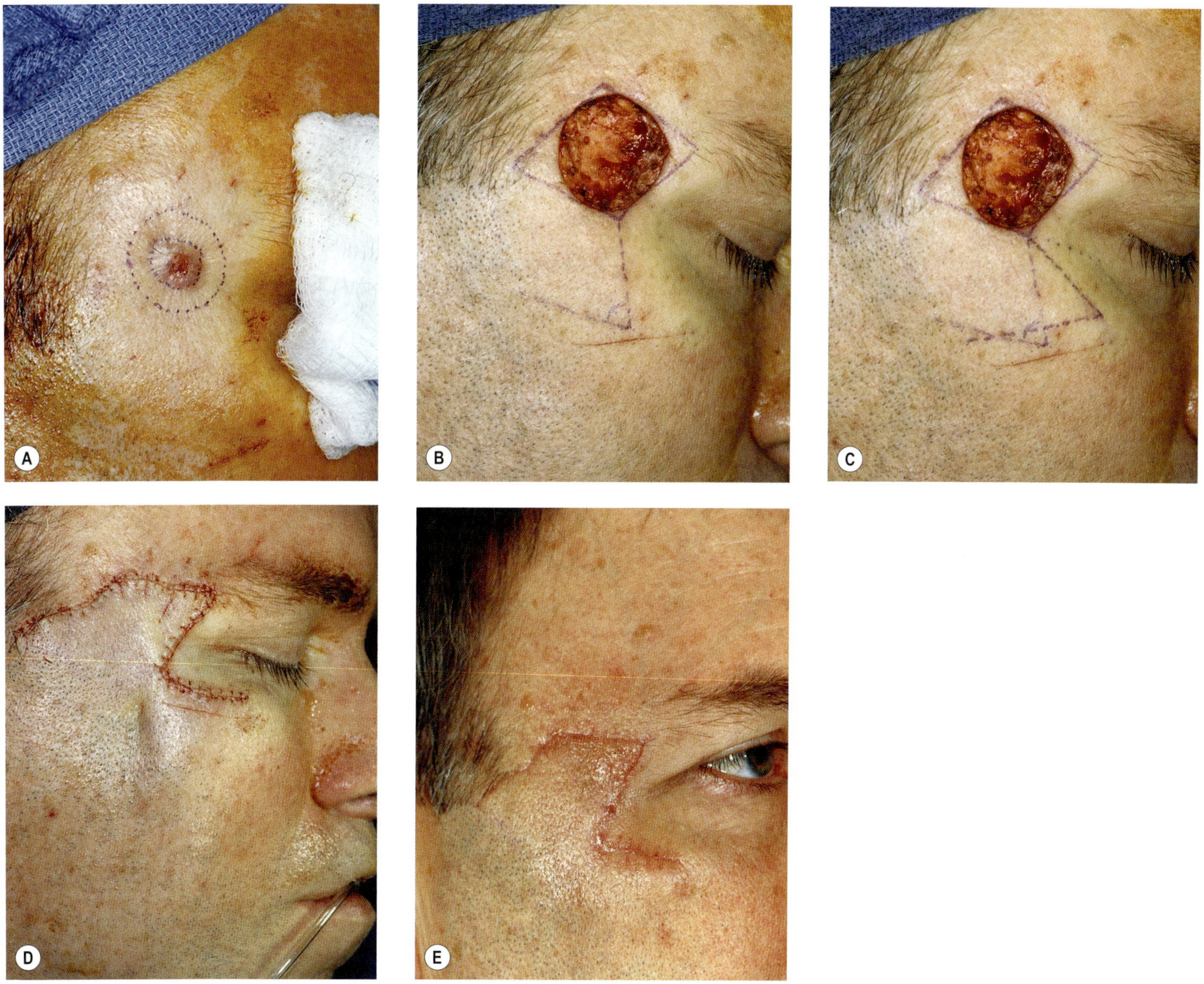

Figure 7.1 Rhomboid flap. **(A)** Melanoma *in situ* right temple. **(B,C)** Lesion excised. Limberg flap designed for repair of 2×2 cm defect. **(D,E)** Dufourmentel flap designed and transferred to defect.

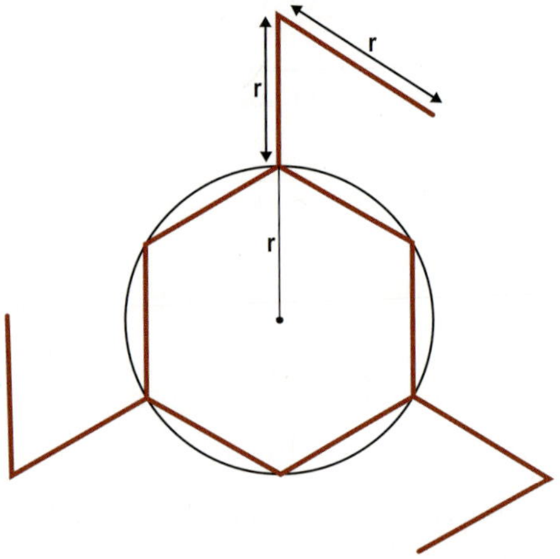

Figure 7.2 Triple rhomboid flap. Circular cutaneous defect conceptualized as hexagon. Sides of hexagon are equal to radius **(r)** of circle. First side of flap created by direct extension equal in length to radius at alternative corners to prevent sharing of common sides. Second side of flap designed parallel to adjacent side of hexagon. (From Bray DA. Rhombic flaps. In: Baker SR, Swanson NA, eds. *Local Flaps in Facial Reconstruction.* St Louis: Mosby; 1995:155, Fig 6, with permission.)

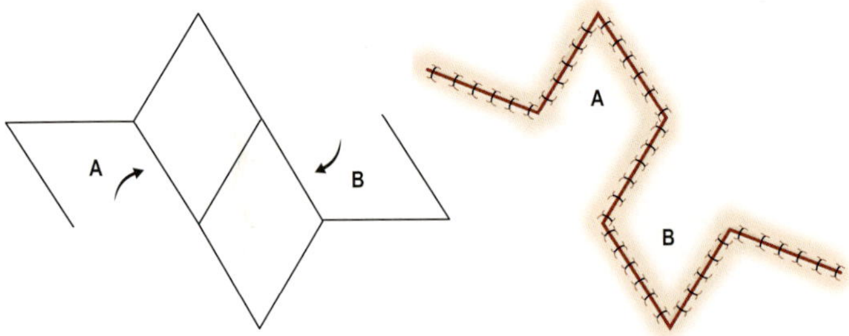

Figure 7.3 Bilateral rhombic flaps designed for repair of large defect. Defect divided into two adjacent rhombuses **(A,B)** to assist with designing rhombic flaps.

advancement or one of the expanded flaps described previously *(Fig. 7.4)*.

- Post-expansion size increases will decrease when the expander is removed and this must be taken into consideration when planning the reconstruction. Thus, a degree of over-expansion is strongly advised.

Eyebrow reconstruction

- The eyebrow is complex and reconstruction is difficult, this is because hair grows in a fixed pattern that is not uniform and is difficult to reproduce exactly.

Technical pearls

- A scalp island flap based on the temporal blood supply can be used, but the hair must be trimmed.
- The hair is often too dense and does not grow in the correct manner; however, the reconstructed eyebrow can be much appreciated by the patient, especially in the burned patient in whom both eyebrows are frequently involved.
- An alternative technique is micro-hair transplants with frequent trimming. These, unfortunately, rarely produce the unique anatomy and the density of the eyebrow hair. *(Fig. 7.5)*.

Nasal reconstruction

- Many different flaps for nasal reconstruction have been described.

Technical pearls

- In the bridgeline region, the glabella is the preferred donor site, and the variety of flaps can be the direct advancement type *(Fig. 7.6)*, transposition *(Fig. 7.7)*, bilobed *(Fig. 7.8)*, rhomboid (see Fig. 7.1), or island *(Fig. 7.9)*.
- On the lateral aspect of the nose, bilobed (see Fig. 7.8), rotation *(Fig. 7.10)*, or transposition flaps *(Fig. 7.11)* – all can provide excellent results. Fortunately, there is often more skin available in this area than expected.
- To provide an acceptable nasal tip reconstruction, the bilobed flap is ideal, though, as already mentioned, it does have a tendency to trapdoor.
- The long advancement flap of Rintala, which looks unreliable, usually works well but can cause some apprehension on the part of the surgeon and the patient due to skin color changes (see Fig. 7.11).
- Laterally, a nostril is made by dissecting a skin pocket and lining it with a skin graft and cartilage, which will provide the required support if necessary.
- Approximately 2–3 weeks after the initial reconstruction, this composite is brought down to reconstruct the rim and the alar region (see Fig. 7.11).
- A composite graft from the ear is an excellent choice when the nostril is to be reconstructed.
- The maximal dimensions of a composite graft are approximately 1 cm^2; for defects greater than this, a composite flap of helical root is an excellent solution.
- When a more complex reconstruction is required (e.g., bilateral alar rims and columella), the total central forehead should be used.
- The key to complete survival of the flap is the position of its base; this should be at the medial canthal level or below. In this way, the vascular anastomosis on the side of the nose between the cheek and forehead vessels is used to give length to the flap.
- The reason for poor results and failures is usually due to elevating the flap pedicle based on the brow area.
- The forehead is closed directly, but if there is tension in the area just anterior to the hairline, it should be left to close secondarily. The scar resulting from this rarely, if ever, requires any reconstruction
- The pedicle is divided at 2–3 weeks, depending on the inset, and the nasal tip is fashioned. Apart from thinning, it is unusual to require further adjustments *(Fig. 7.12)*.

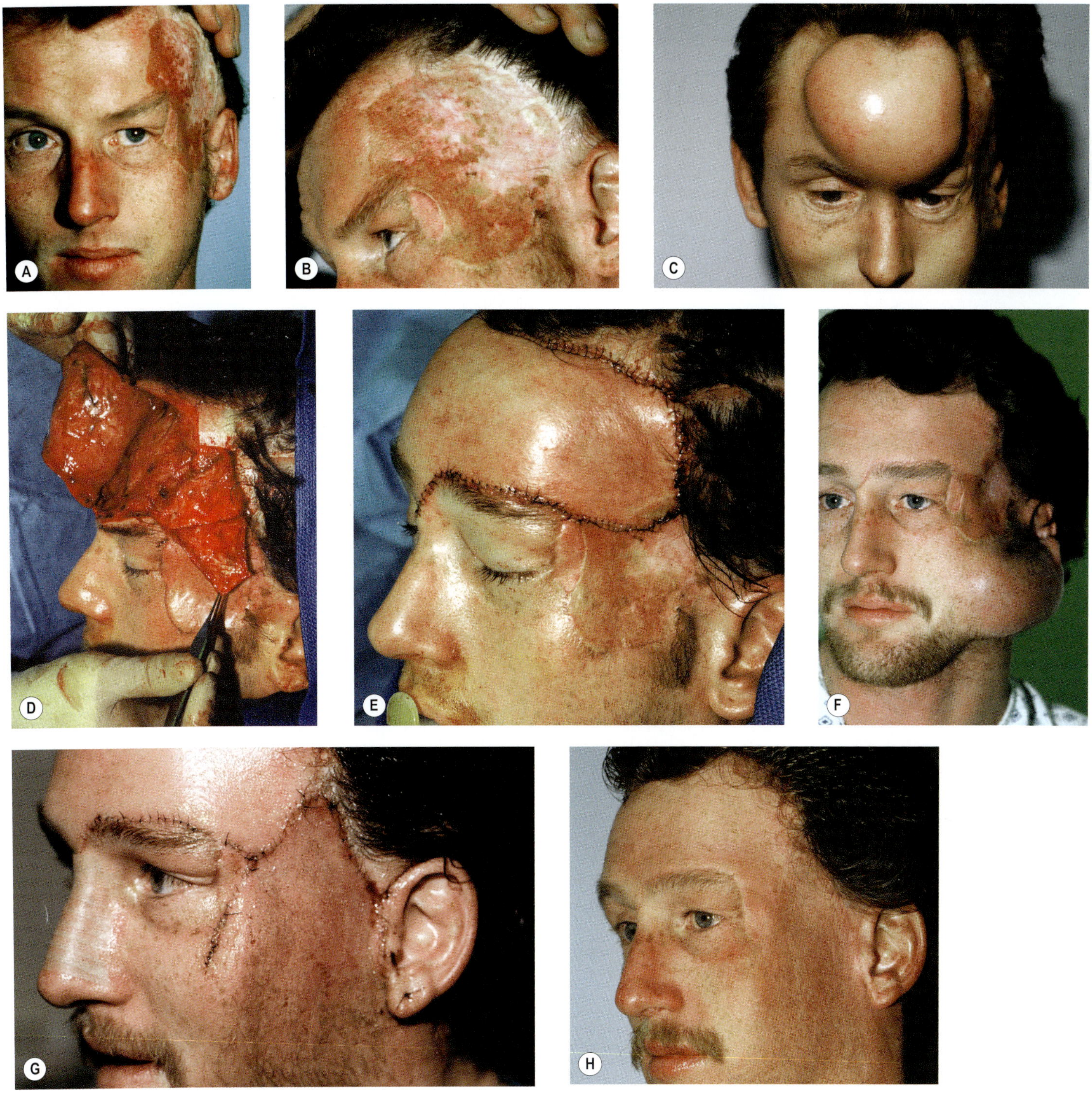

Figure 7.4 Tissue expansion to achieve defect closure. **(A,B)** Skin graft covering temple, anterior parietal scalp, and lateral cheek. **(C)** Expanded forehead skin. **(D)** Following tissue expansion, expanded forehead skin used to cover defect created by partial resection of skin graft. **(E)** Expansion provided sufficient skin to cover temple. **(F)** Tissue expander beneath lateral cheek skin. **(G)** 6 days following removal of skin graft from cheek and reconstruction with expanded cheek advancement flap. **(H)** 6 months' postoperative.

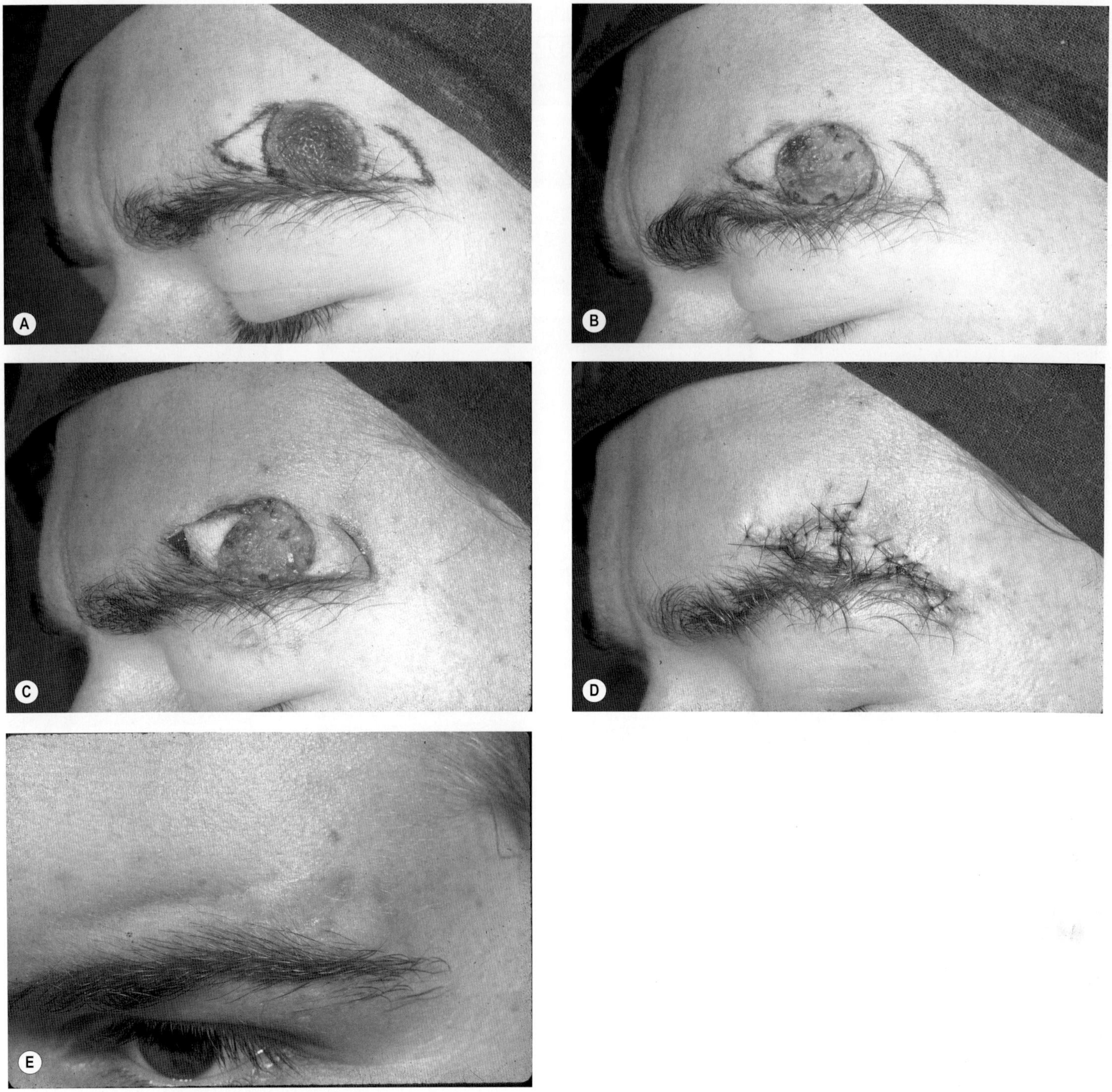

Figure 7.5 Nevus of left supraorbital area involving eyebrow – hatchet flap reconstruction. **(A)** The planned excision has been drawn out together with bilateral hatchet flaps. **(B)** Nevus has been excised. It can be seen that the flap pedicles are superior for the lateral flap and inferior for the medial flap. **(C)** The flaps are elevated. **(D)** The flaps are transposed, and the secondary defect is closed. **(E)** Satisfactory end result with the eyebrow in a good position.

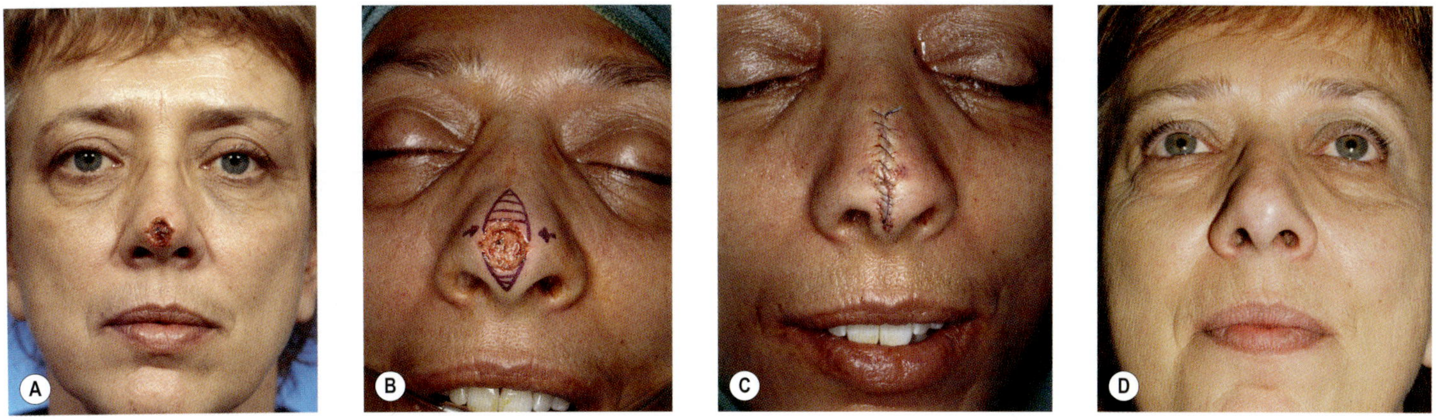

Figure 7.6 Reconstruction of nasal defect with lateral advancement flaps. **(A)** 0.5×0.5 cm skin defect of nasal tip. **(B)** Primary wound closure planned. Anticipated standing cutaneous deformities (marked by horizontal lines). **(C)** Deformities excised and wound closed. **(D)** 1.5 years' postoperatively.

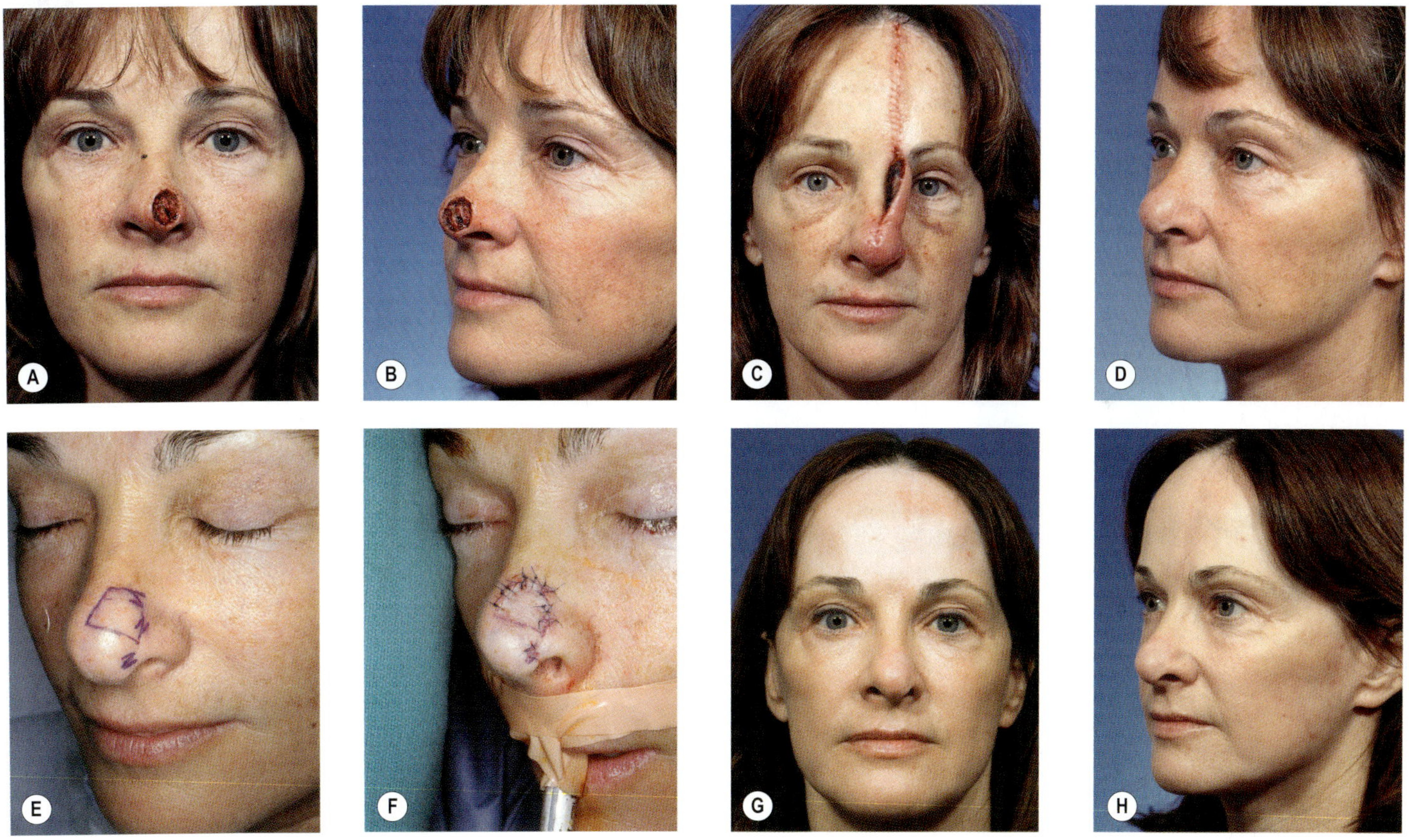

Figure 7.7 Reconstruction of lateral nasal defect with forehead flap. **(A,B)** 1.5×1.5 cm skin defect of nasal tip. **(C)** Interpolated paramedian forehead flap used to repair defect. **(D)** 9 months' postoperative. Depressed scar surrounds lateral aspect of flap and mild trap-door deformity is present. **(E)** Nose marked for planned contouring procedure. Three Z-plasties positioned along depressed scar. **(F)** Flap thinned and Z-plasties performed. **(G,H)** 4 months following Z-plasties and full face carbon dioxide laser peel.

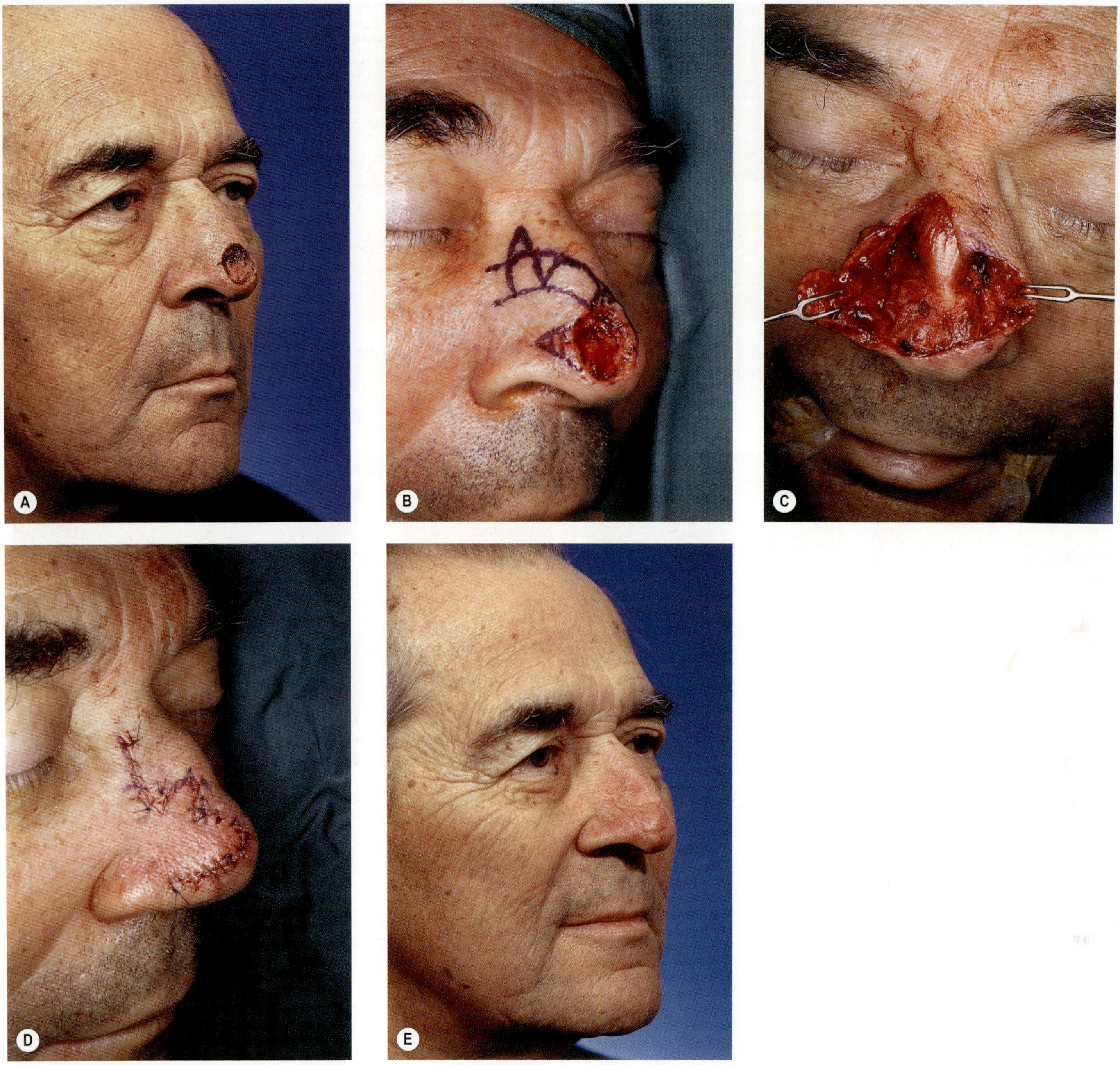

Figure 7.8 Closure of nasal defect with bilobed flap. **(A)** 1×1 cm skin defect of tip. **(B)** Bilobed flap designed for repair. Anticipated standing cutaneous deformity marked for excision in alar groove. Linear axis of each lobe designed 45° from each other with primary lobe axis positioned 45° from axis of defect. **(C)** Transfer of flap requires complete undermining of entire nasal skin. **(D)** Flap in place. **(E)** 1 year postoperative. No revision surgery performed.

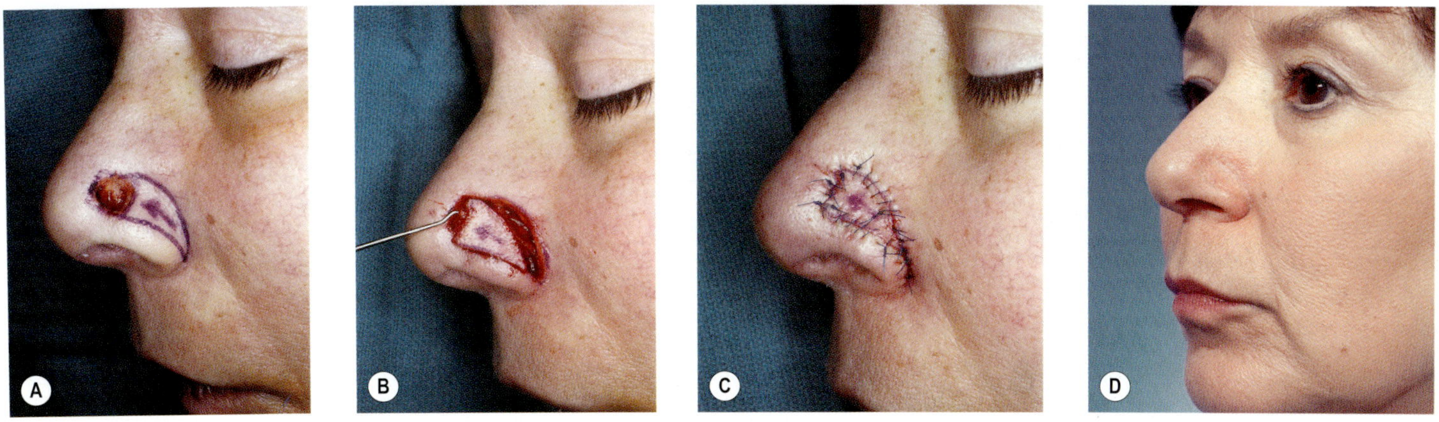

Figure 7.9 **(A)** 0.8×0.7 cm skin defect of alar groove. V–Y island subcutaneous tissue pedicle advancement flap designed for repair. **(B)** Flap incised and advanced on nasalis muscle. **(C)** Flap in place. **(D)** 4 months' postoperative.

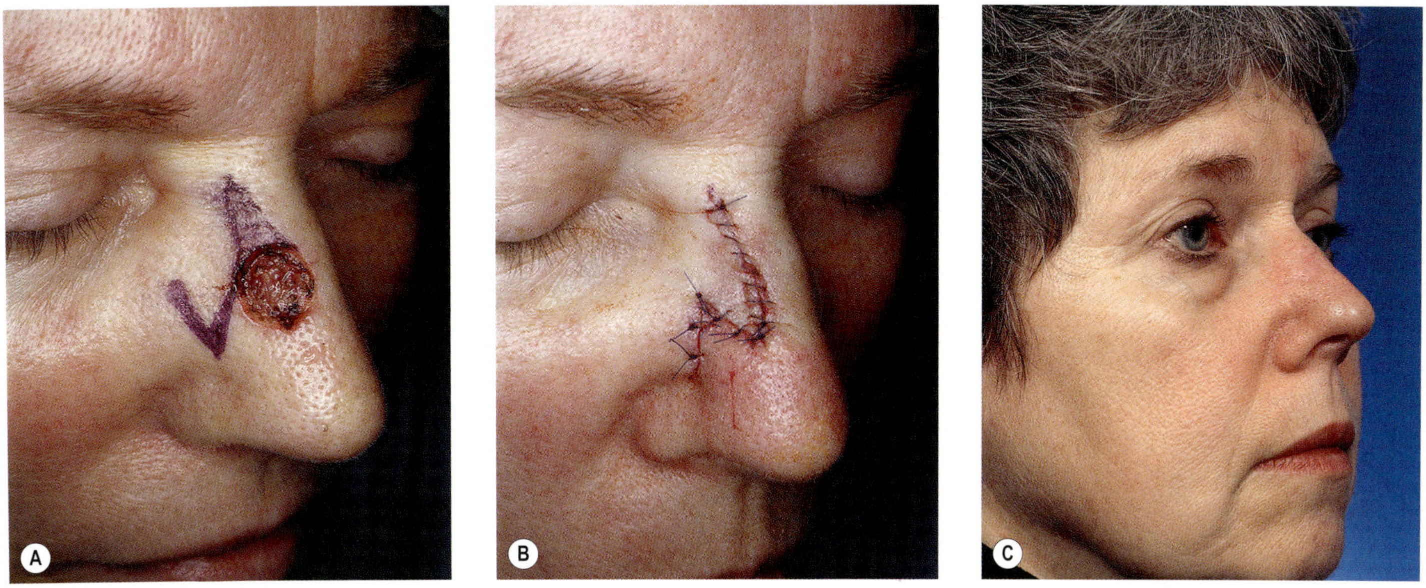

Figure 7.10 **(A)** 1×0.8 cm skin defect of the dorsum. Transoperative flap designed for repair. Anticipated standing cutaneous deformity marked by horizontal lines. **(B)** Flap transposed. **(C)** 6 months postoperative. No revision surgery performed.

- If there is any concern about vascularity, the flap base is delayed.
- If a total nasal reconstruction is required, a larger amount of forehead skin is harvested in the transverse dimension, but again, the base should be positioned at or below the medial canthal ligament.
- The septal mucosa is used for lining.
- If nasal support is needed, a cranial bone graft from the outer table of the skull can be used.
- For closure of the midline forehead defect, the skin can frequently be mobilized extensively and advanced. If there is concern, a tissue expander can be inserted to expand the whole forehead. This gives a large amount of skin with a good blood supply.
- Noses may be prefabricated elsewhere (e.g., on the forearm using a radial flap) and subsequently transferred by microvascular techniques.

Eyelids

Technical pearls

Partial lower lid defects

- Lesions are frequently resected in a V fashion and the resulting defect can be carefully closed in layers.

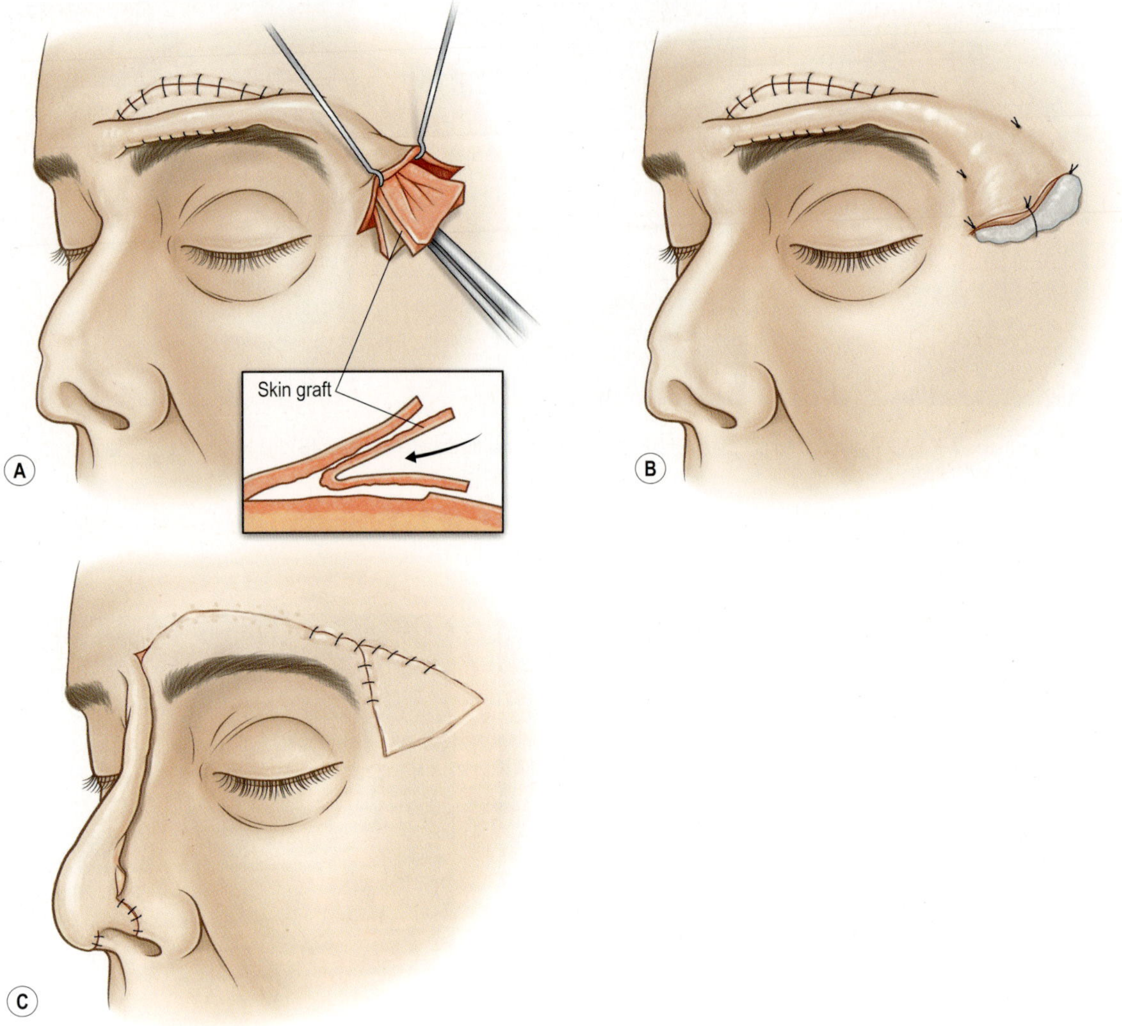

Figure 7.11 Transverse forehead flap for composite nasal tip defect. **(A)** At initial elevation of the flap, a septal mucosa graft is prelaminated within the distal flap to provide eventual nasal lining. **(B)** A bolster dressing is applied to the septal mucosa graft. **(C)** At a second stage the flap is rotated and inset.

- If this is not possible, the lower portion of the lateral canthal ligament is divided through a small lateral canthal incision. This allows the lid to move medially, and closure can be obtained without tension.
- If there is too much tension, the incision and dissection are taken further laterally on the cheek. Closure is then obtained without difficulty. The lateral incision is closed with a Z-plasty in order to reduce any skin tension.
- An extensive defect requires that a portion of nasal septum, with mucosa attached on one side, be inserted with the mucosa toward the globe in order to form an internal lamella.
- A portion of ear cartilage, with perichondrium in place of the mucosa, can also be used for support.
- A cheek rotation flap of the required size then provides external cover.
- If the cheek skin is insufficient, prior expansion of the lateral cheek skin should be performed, or a narrow midline forehead flap can be used.

Partial upper lid defects

- Reconstruction of the upper lid is a more difficult problem because the lid is vital for protection of the eye.
- It is best for the surgeon to sit at the head of the operating table and think of the upper lid as the lower lid and use the same techniques described for the lower lid modified to the required shape and size of the upper lid.
- Any failure of reconstruction, particularly in the vertical dimension, may cause conjunctivitis and/or impair vision. Without an adequate upper lid, the eye will be at risk for exposure, scarring, and loss of vision. Experience in eyelid surgery is essential.

Advancement flap

- For a triangular defect in the upper lid (e.g., after tumor resection), an incision is made horizontally from the lateral canthus, followed by division of the superior limb

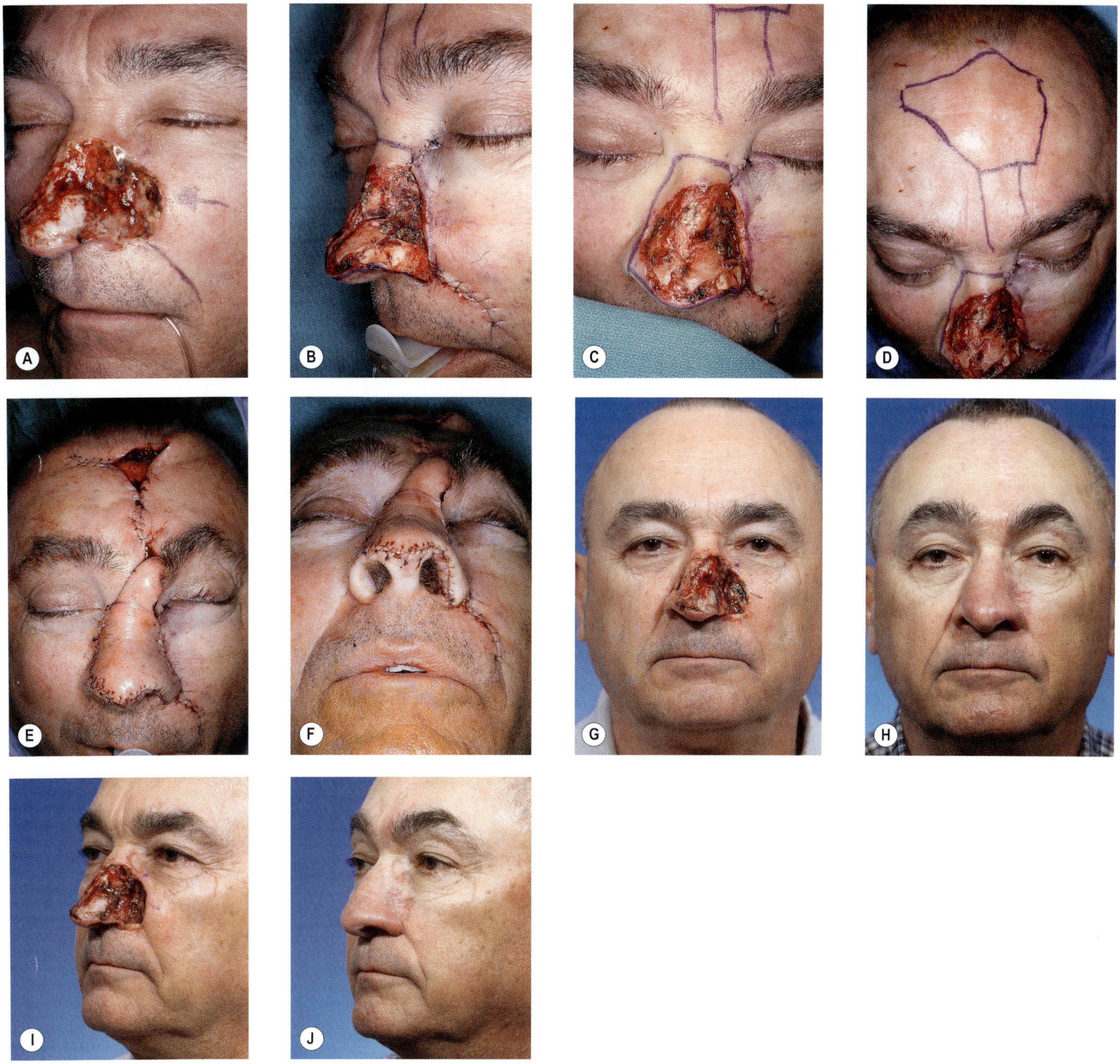

Figure 7.12 Reconstruction of nasal tip and dorsum with forehead flap after resection of basal cell carcinoma. **(A)** 4 × 6 cm skin defect of dorsum, nasal tip, sidewall, and ala extending into cheek. Cheek advancement flap designed to repair cheek component of defect. **(B)** Cheek flap advanced to nasal facial sulcus. Auricular cartilage graft positioned for ala framework. **(C)** Remaining skin of dorsum and sidewall aesthetic units marked for excision. **(D)** Interpolated paramedian forehead flap design as covering flap. **(E,F)** Forehead flap transferred to nose. Portion of donor site left to heal by secondary incision. **(G–J)** Preoperative and 1 year, 4 months' postoperative. Contouring procedure performed.

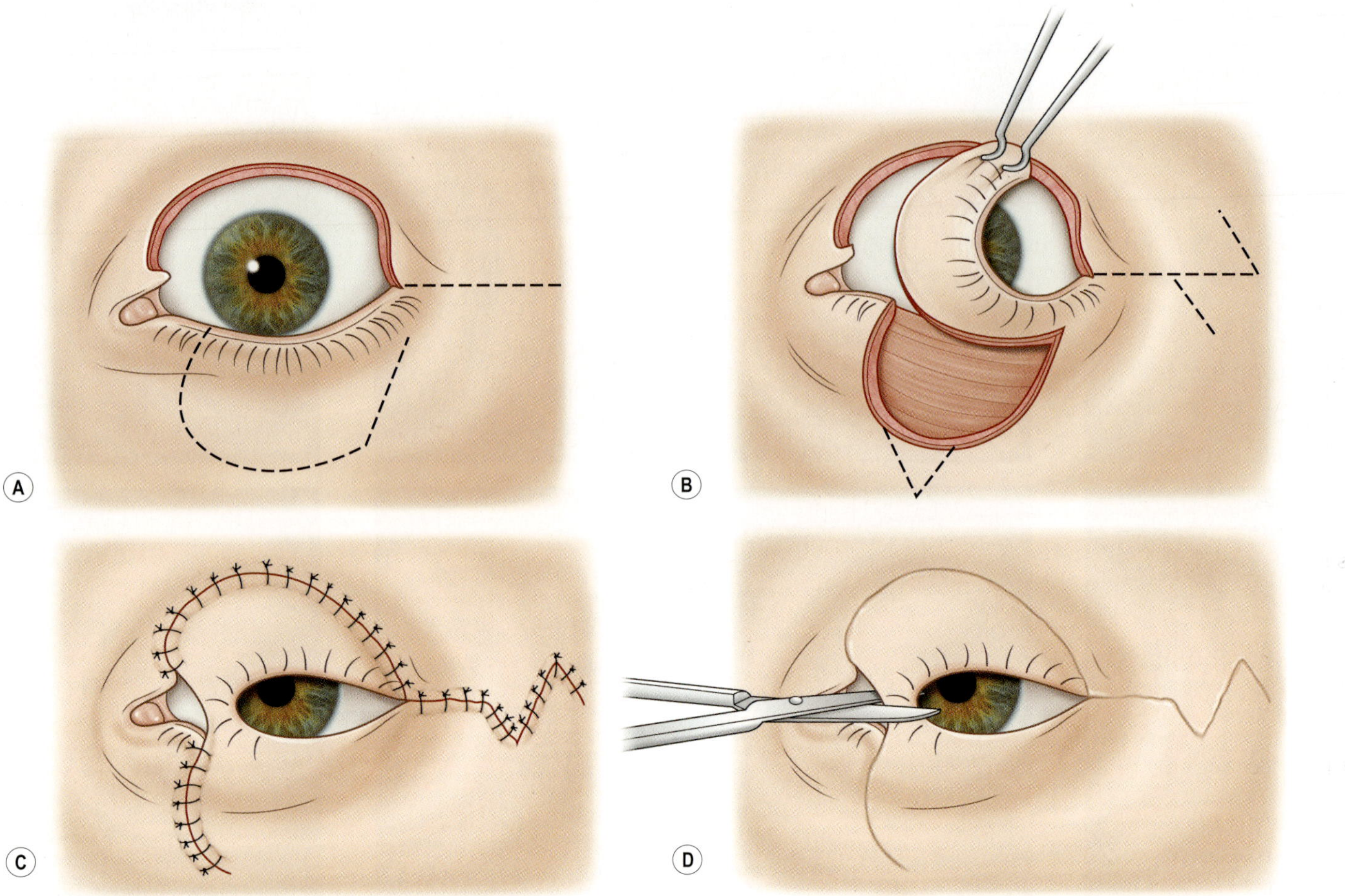

Figure 7.13 Reconstruction of total upper eyelid defect with lower lid transposition. **(A–D)** Illustration of planned reconstruction of an upper eyelid defect with lower lid transposition.

of the lateral canthal ligament. An incision is also made in the conjunctiva of the superior fornix. This alone will allow small defects to be closed.

- As in the lower lid, accurate suturing and repositioning of the gray line, the lash line, and the rim conjunctival junction is essential.

Lid-switch flap (Abbé flap) *(Fig. 7.13)*

- By using the same principles as the Abbé flap on the lip, a similar reconstruction can be used for defects of the upper lid.
- There are marginal vessels in the lid, and a full-thickness V flap (the defect of which should close easily) can be taken from the lower lid, swung up, and sutured into the upper lid in layers.
- The lower lid defect closure requires the edges to come together directly without tension.
- If this does not occur, a small lateral canthal incision is made, and the inferior limb of the lateral canthal tendon is divided.
- If this is not sufficient, a long transverse incision from the canthus out to the temporal skin (incorporating a Z-plasty if necessary) will suffice to obtain tensionless closure.

Free grafts

- For larger defects, free, full-thickness lid replacements (composite grafts) have been employed.
- A full-thickness lid replacement is used as a composite graft if a portion of conjunctiva and subconjunctival tissue can be preserved as described in the last segment.
- A full-thickness graft can be taken from the lower lid, and the conjunctiva is excised from the graft, leaving just enough for the full-thickness defect. The full-thickness skin portion remaining will be enough to allow the graft to survive; however, meticulous reconstructive technique is imperative. The lower lid defect is closed as described previously.

Large and total upper lid defects

- For larger defects, the lower lid is used and the significant lower lid defect is reconstructed.

- A large full-thickness portion of lower lid is moved up on its marginal vascular pedicle.
- As the portion of lower lid is turned up, the full thickness of the cheek is advanced medially and grafted with nasal septum on its inner surface, as required.
- These pedicled lid reconstructions are left attached for 2–3 weeks, depending on the vascularity of the upturned flaps.
- Once the upper lid reconstruction is in position, small adjustments are often necessary. Rearrangements are usually required for the lateral canthus and occasionally to the edge of the lower lid or to provide adjustment of lower lid height.
- When a healthy eye is present, a lid can be prefabricated on the forehead. A pocket the size of the lid is designed and a mucosal graft is inserted. When this reconstruction is complete, it is brought down on a vascular pedicle to replace the lid. The pedicle is divided at 3 weeks. This protects the eye, but movement is minimal, unless there is some remaining orbicularis which can be used immediately or at a later date.

Total lower lid defects

- These result from tumor resection, from trauma, or when the lower lid is used to reconstruct the upper lid (see Fig. 7.13). Reconstruction of the total lower lid is primarily performed for cosmesis.
- The lower lid can be reconstructed with a cheek rotation flap which is lined with oral mucosa or more satisfactorily using nasal septal cartilage with its perichondrium intact. In other instances, a forehead flap may be necessary.

Medial canthal defects

- Generally, forehead flaps provide a reliable and reasonably good method of reconstruction. These flaps must be lined with mucosa; however, additional support is not required because of the inherent flap rigidity. It is very important to place a flap of sufficient size into the medial canthal area. Failure to do this results in troublesome epiphora.

Cheek

- Skin tumors are common in this area. The whole range of flaps can be used – rotation, advancement, transposition, and island type – with many variations required and usually available for each type of reconstruction. Occasionally, for extremely large defects, a free flap may be required.
- The most important feature to consider when planning cheek reconstruction is skin color.
- Although we think of the cheek as a separate esthetic unit, reconstruction of the cheek will frequently impact on nearby units.
- Whenever possible, local tissue is the first choice in reconstructing the cheek as it provides tissue of like texture, similar color, and with identical characteristics such as dermal appendages and hair growth.
- When there is insufficient local tissue and time is available for staged reconstruction, tissue expansion may be an option.
- The only indication to use distant tissue in cheek reconstruction is in the situation where there is insufficient local tissue.
- Older patients generally have greater skin laxity which will often allow smaller cheek wounds to frequently be converted to an ellipse and closed directly.
- It is important to be cognizant of the relaxed skin tension lines and to keep all scars parallel to these lines if possible.

Cheek rotation flap

- Because the cheek area is relatively large, rotation flaps may be designed in many sizes, depending on the position, shape and size of the defect to be reconstructed ***(Figs 7.14, 7.15)***.
- Cheek flaps can be based anteriorly or posteriorly:
  - Basing the flap posteriorly allows mobilization of the jowls so that this excess can be moved up onto the face.
  - Basing the flap anteriorly allows for mobilization of neck skin up onto the face.
- Extending the incision down onto the chest significantly increases the arc of the rotation of the flap. This incorporates a back-cut which allows for better flap mobility of the flap as well as facilitating closure of the secondary defect.
- The possibility of ectropion as a complication of a cheek rotation advancement flap is a very real one.
- To avoid ectropion and pull on the lower lid, the cheek flap should be suspended from the underlying bony skeleton either using peri-osteal sutures or with an anchoring device such as a Mitek anchor.
- Particular care must be exercised in female patients to avoid advancing hair-bearing skin from the sideburn area onto the cheek. This can be avoided by placing the incision around the sideburn in these cases (Fig. 7.14).

Advancement flaps

- Advancement flaps can be used at any location on the cheek. As with the rotation flap, the advancement flap can be of any size. It is best to use natural lines, even if they diverge away from the defect, because this will still give a better and more natural cosmetic end result ***(Fig. 7.16)***.
- When an advancement flap is used to close a square defect, there are areas of excess skin related to the Burow's triangles, these are resected.
- Composite cheek and nose defects require composite reconstructions. The nose is resurfaced with a full-thickness skin graft, and an advancement flap again with excision of Burow's triangles is used to reconstruct the cheek ***(Fig. 7.17)***.

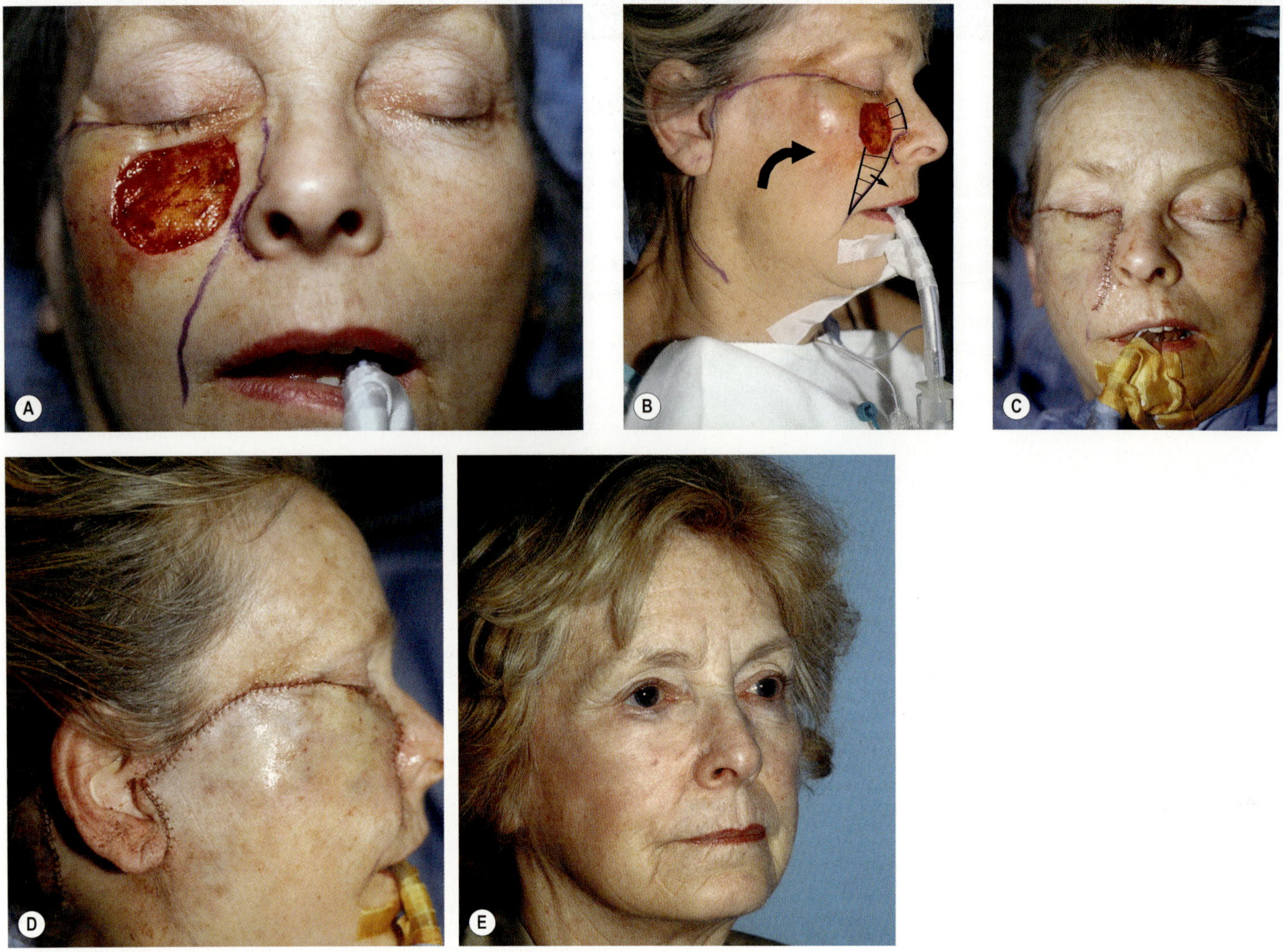

Figure 7.14 Rotation cheek flap. **(A)** 4×3 cm medial cheek defect. Flap designed for repair. Incision for flap placed in subciliary line. Nasofacial sulcus and melolabial creases marked. Skin between defect and nasofacial sulcus and melolabial crease removed to position advancing border of flap in aesthetic boundary. **(B)** Incision for flap extended to preauricular crease and posterior auricular sulcus. Anticipated standing cutaneous deformity marked with horizontal lines on melolabial fold. **(C,D)** Flap in position. Note incision lines at level of lateral canthus. Medial border of flap positioned in nasofacial sulcus and melolabial crease. **(E)** Postoperative result with normal eyelid position and well-camouflaged scars.

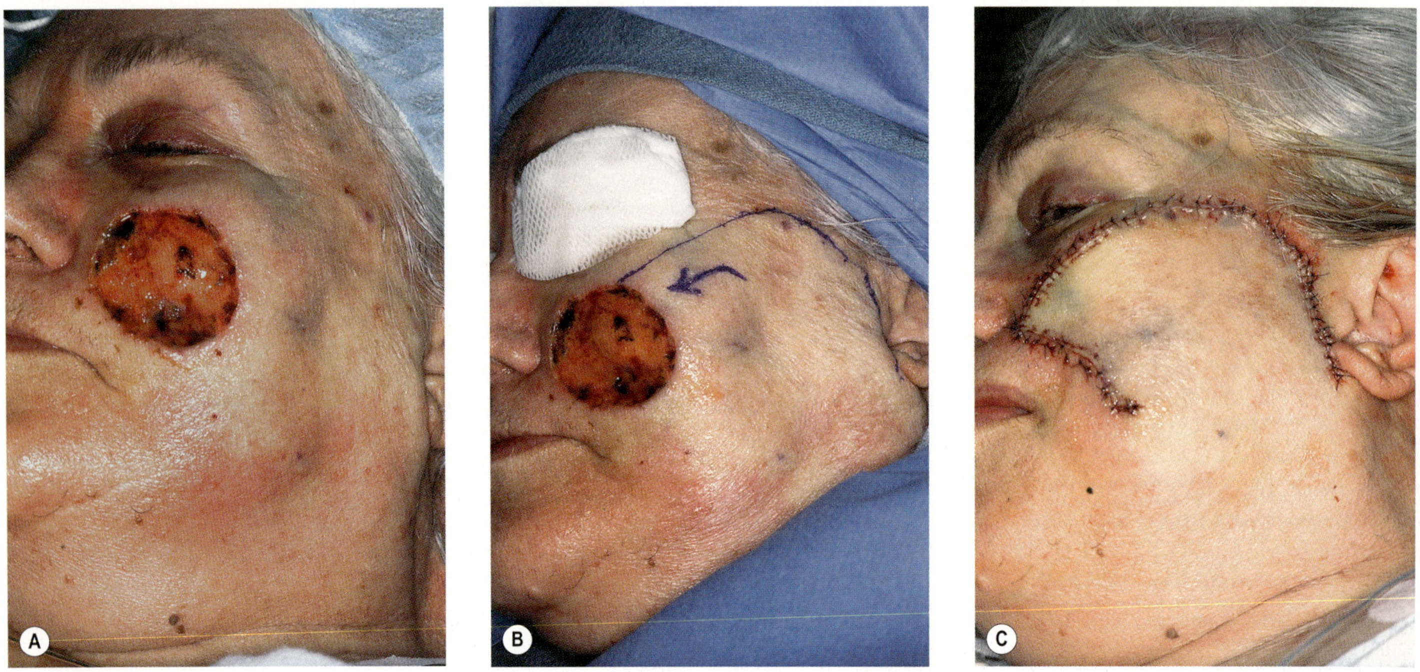

Figure 7.15 Cheek rotation flap to close cheek defect. **(A)** 3 × 3 cm skin defect of medial cheek. **(B)** Rotation flap designed for repair. **(C)** Flap in place. Standing cutaneous deformity excised parallel to melolabial crease. (Courtesy of Shaun R. Baker MD.)

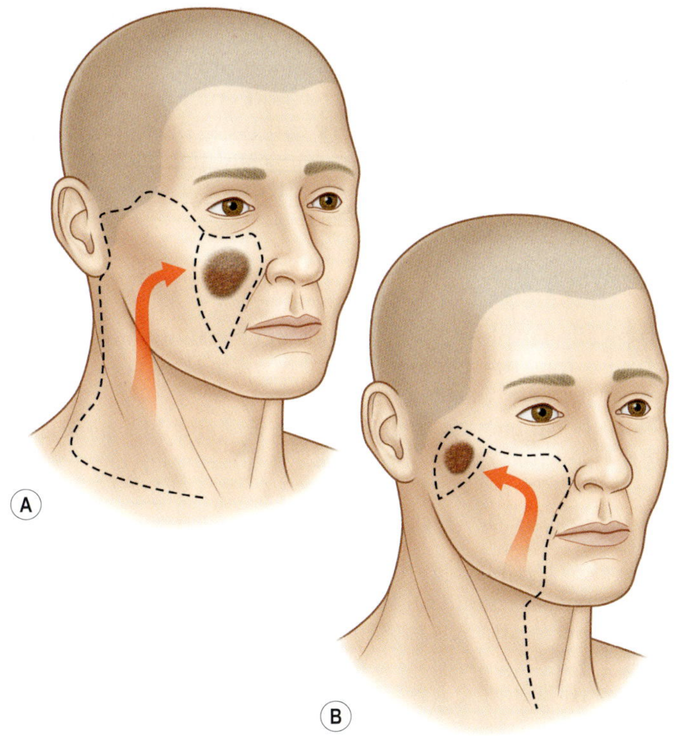

Figure 7.16 **(A)** A medially-based cheek rotation flap. **(B)** A laterally-based cheek rotation flap.

Transposition flaps

- A transposition flap is elevated from a nearby area and moved to close a defect while the base of the flap remains intact. Geometric flap planning is required.
- The rhomboid flap is an ideal example.
- The lesion is resected in a rhomboid design.
- Before this reconstruction, it is necessary to determine the location of excess skin by pinching the area between the thumb and index finger and determining the location of a 120° angle opposite this.
- The flap can then be taken from the area with the most available skin.
- As the flap is fitted into the defect, the donor site becomes significantly reduced and is closed directly (see Fig. 7.1).

Finger flap

- The finger flap is similar to the rhomboid flap with removal of the corners, although it is usually longer and narrower. Because the cosmetic result is not optimal, it is not advisable to use this flap for facial reconstruction.

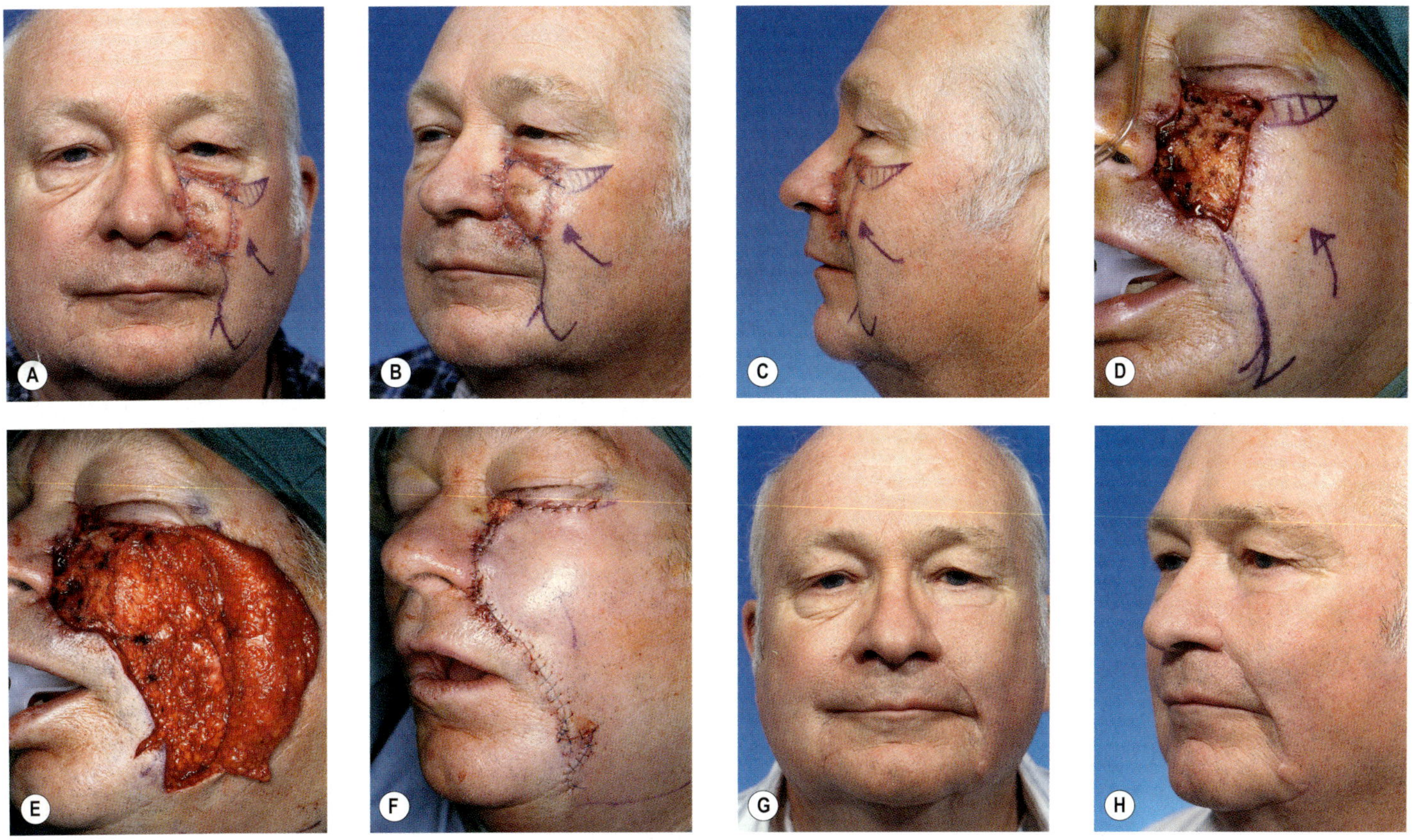

Figure 7.17 **(A–C)** Melanoma *in situ* of medial cheek; 5×3 cm area marked for excision using square technique to ensure tumor-free margins. **(D–F)** Pivotal advancement flap designed for repair of defect following resection of lesion. Anticipated standing cutaneous deformity marked with vertical lines. Z-plasty designed at base of flap to eliminate need for equalizing Burow's triangle. **(G,H)** Melanoma excised, flap dissected. (Courtesy of Shaun R. Baker MD.)

Island flap

- This technique can be used for advancement or transposition, but it must be employed with care because of the tendency to pincushion.
- The island flaps tend to be round or triangular.
- The triangular flap is less likely to pincushion. It is better to keep the dermis intact, but unfortunately, this is not always possible.
- The advantage of this variety of flap is that it is a one-stage procedure, and it is probably more flexible than the conventional flap.
- If care is not taken, these flaps can be devascularized more easily than standard pedicled flaps. This can occur by traction on or twisting of the pedicle or because of a tunnel that is too narrow and constricts the pedicle, compromising flap survival (see Fig. 7.9).

The submental artery flap **(Fig 7.18)**

- Advantages of the submental flap include similar skin color and texture, and a conveniently hidden scar under the chin.
- Based on the submental branch of the facial artery, this flap can easily be tunneled up into the cheek.
- In males it is important to remember that this flap resides in the hair-bearing portion of the chin.
- This flap is an excellent choice for small to moderate sized defects.
- An increasing arc of rotation can be achieved in two ways:
  - Division of the facial artery cephalad to the submental branch allows dissection of the facial artery to its origin off the external carotid, supplying a few extra centimeters of pedicle length and antegrade flow.
  - Division of the facial artery caudal to the submental branch allows pedicle elevation and flap perfusion in a retrograde fashion which is adequate to sustain the flap.

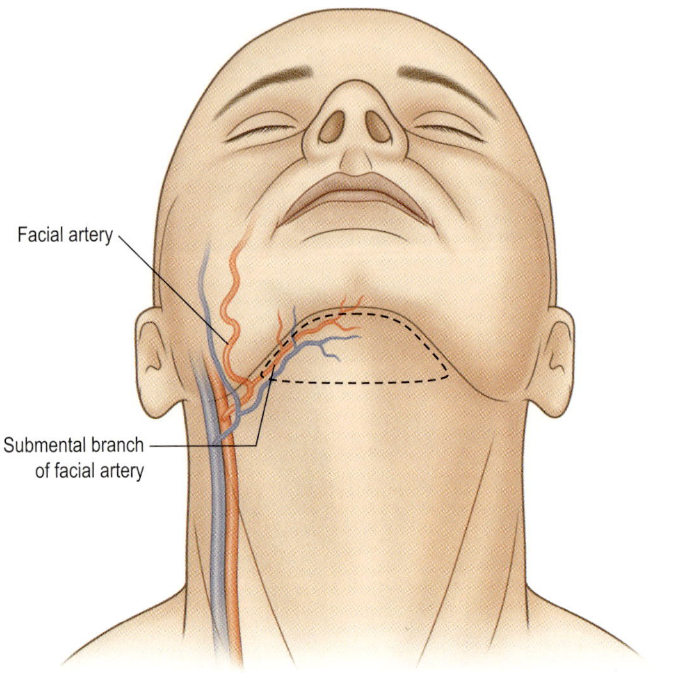

Figure 7.18 Schematic diagram of the vascular supply of the submental flap. Note the separate vein draining the flap.

Free tissue transfer

- Typically employed for large defects without sufficient local tissue, or in instances where more than soft tissue reconstruction is required.
- Flap choice is often dependent on defect characteristics and need for composite tissue.

Scapular and parascapular flaps

- The skin territory of the scapular and parascapular flap is sufficiently large to allow for closure of the largest cheek defect while at the same time closing the donor defect directly.
- Depending on the size of defect, the flap can be folded on itself in the case of through and through defects, to provide lining and cover or alternatively, scapular and parascapular flaps can be harvested on the transverse and descending branches of the circumflex scapular artery respectively, to provide lining and cover.
- The scapula can also be taken with bone and this can be used effectively to reconstruct the bony contour of the cheek.

Anterolateral thigh flap

- The anterolateral thigh flap is an alternative to the scapular/parascapular flap.
- Color match is not as good in lighter skinned patients.
- The flap can be harvested with or without fascia depending on need for thin or bulky flaps.

Other flap options

- The radial forearm flap.
- The rectus abdominis myocutaneous flap.

Lips

- The upper lip and lower lip must be considered individually because the methods used for reconstruction are not always applicable to both locations ***(Fig. 7.19)***.
- Goals of lip reconstruction:
  - Preservation of function.
  - Reconstitution of orbicularis oris.
  - Three layered closure.
  - Accurate alignment of vermillion.
  - Maintenance of relationship between upper and lower lips.
  - Optimization of cosmesis ***(Fig. 7.20)***.

- Given their critical importance functionally and aesthetically, a thorough knowledge of the lip anatomy is imperative (*Fig. 7.21,* Table 7.2).

Technical pearls

- Local tissue should be used whenever possible.
- Small defects can be closed by direct repair.
- Intermediate defects are best reconstructed with local flaps.
- Total or subtotal lip defects are best reconstructed with free tissue *(Fig. 7.22).*

Operative techniques

*Wedge resection **(Figs** 7.22, **7.23)***

- Up to 25% of the upper lip can be resected and repaired directly.
- Up to 30% of the lower lip can be resected and repaired directly.
- Careful approximation of the muscle layer ensures a functional repair.
- Consider a W resection for larger wedges in order to keep the scar above the mental crease.

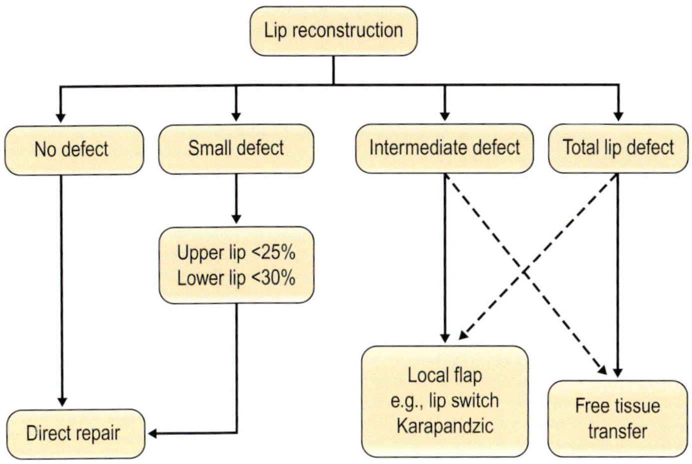

Figure 7.19 An algorithmic approach to lip reconstruction.

*Lip switch flaps: Abbé **(Fig. 7.24)** and Estlander flaps **(Fig. 7.25)***

- Width of the flap should be half the width of the defect.
- Height of the flap should be the same as height of the defect.
- Pedicle of Abbé flap should be placed at the midpoint of the defect.
- Pedicle division at 14–21 days.

Table 7.2 **Critical anatomy of the lips**

Arterial supply of the upper and lower lips	Sup. and Inf. labial a. (from the facial a.)
Sensory innervation	Maxillary and mandibular divisions of the trigeminal n. (CN V)
Important muscular anatomy	
Orbicularis oris	Function to protrude the lips away from the facial plane, and also approximates the lips to the alveolar arch
Zygomaticus major	Major lip elevator; innervated by buccal branch of facial n. (CN VII)
Levator anguli oris	Major lip elevator; innervated by buccal branch of facial n. (CN VII)
Depressor anguli oris	Major lip depressor; innervated by mandibular branch of facial n. (CN VII)
Platysma	Major lip depressor; innervated by mandibular branch of facial n. (CN VII)
Modiolus	A 1 cm thick fibrovascular region where the levator and depressor muscle fibers intersect and attach firmly to the dermis. It is located approximately 1.5 cm lateral to the oral commissures. The modiolus significantly affects the appearance of the oral commissures with movement. Disruption can lead to abnormal appearance of the mouth at rest or during function.

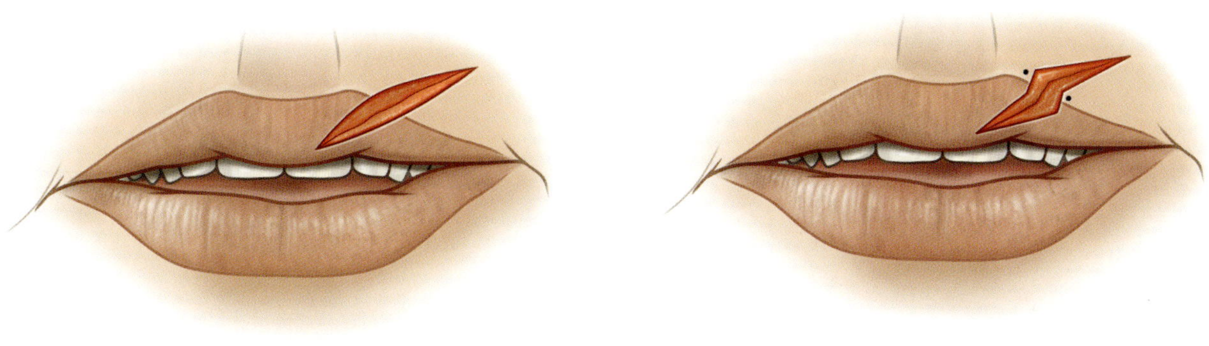

Figure 7.20 Breaking up the linear scar by introducing a vertical element to an excision will allow for more precise closure as the vermillion borders can be accurately approximated (marked with dots). Furthermore, the resulting scar will not be linear and will therefore be less likely to contract.

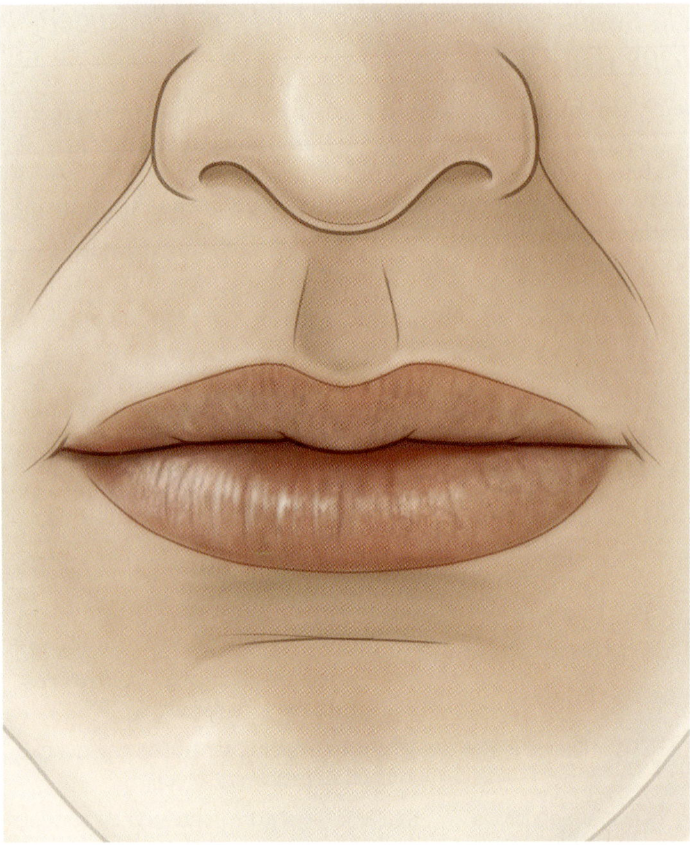

Figure 7.21 The aesthetic landmarks of the lips are seen. The curve of the upper lip resembles a bow, known as Cupid's bow. The central concavity of the upper lip is the philtrum, bounded on either side by the conves philtral columns. The lateral elements of the upper lip are bounded by the philtral ridge medially, the nasal vestibule and alar base superiorly and the nasolabial fold laterally. The mental crease separates the lower lip from the aesthetic unit of the chin.

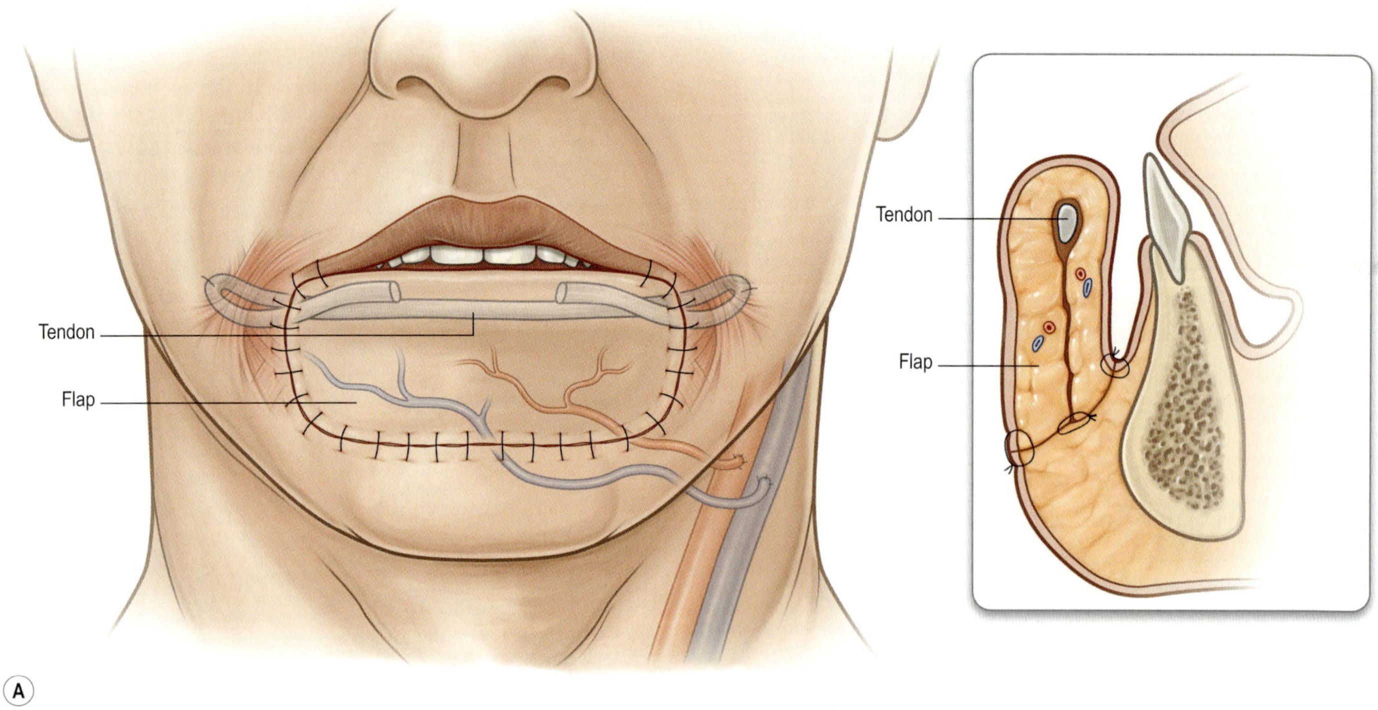

Figure 7.22 **(A)** Schematic of palmaris/radial forearm flap reconstruction of the lower lip showing the Palmaris tendon woven through the remaining orbicularis muscle.

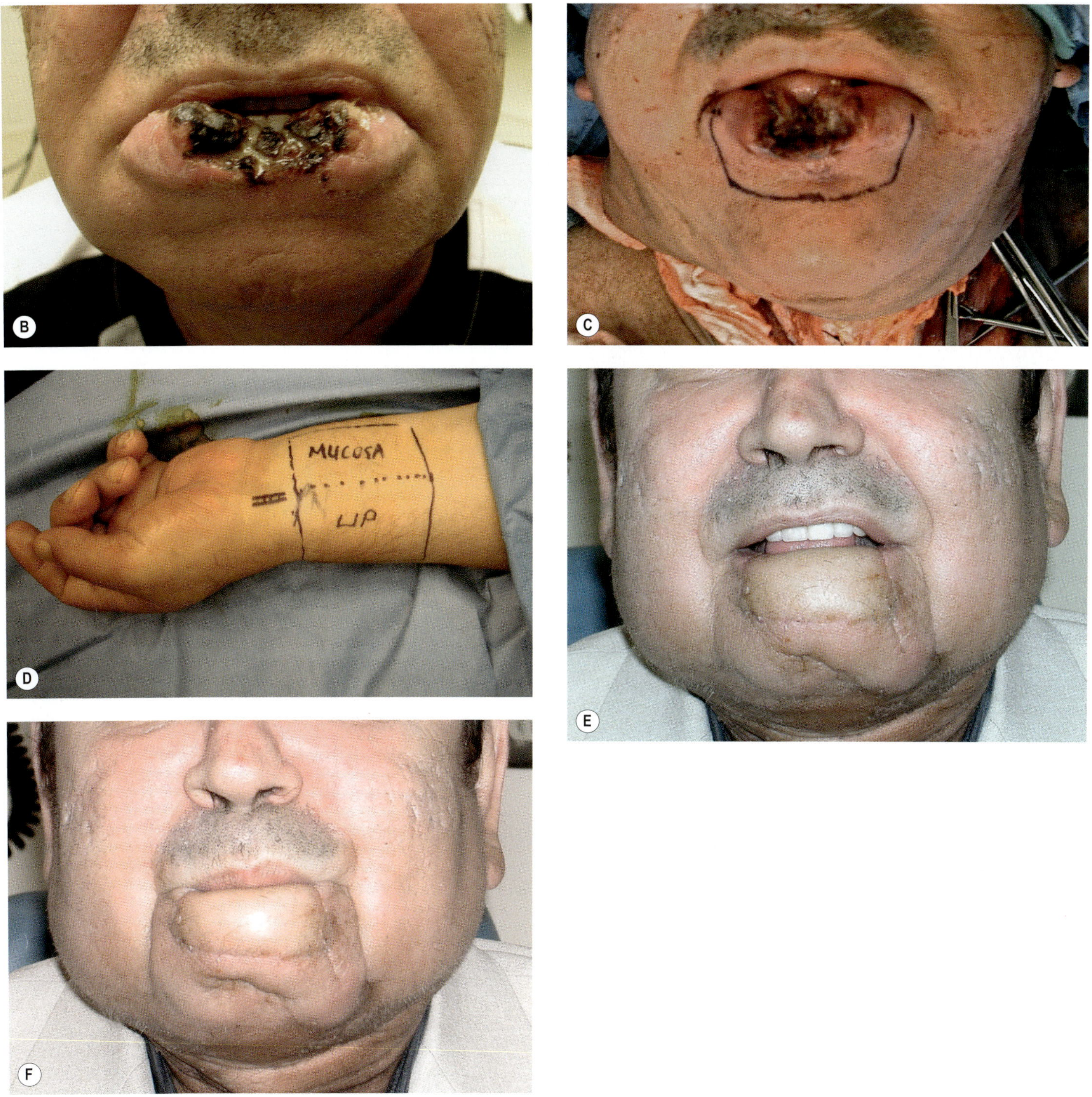

Fig. 7.22, cont'd **(B)** Patient shown with a large squamous cell carcinoma of the lower lip. **(C)** Resection of the lower lip planned. **(D)** The planned radial forearm flap. Note the different dimensions of the skin and mucosal segments of the flap. **(E)** Postoperative appearance. **(F)** Note that the patient can purse his lips and has good oral competence.

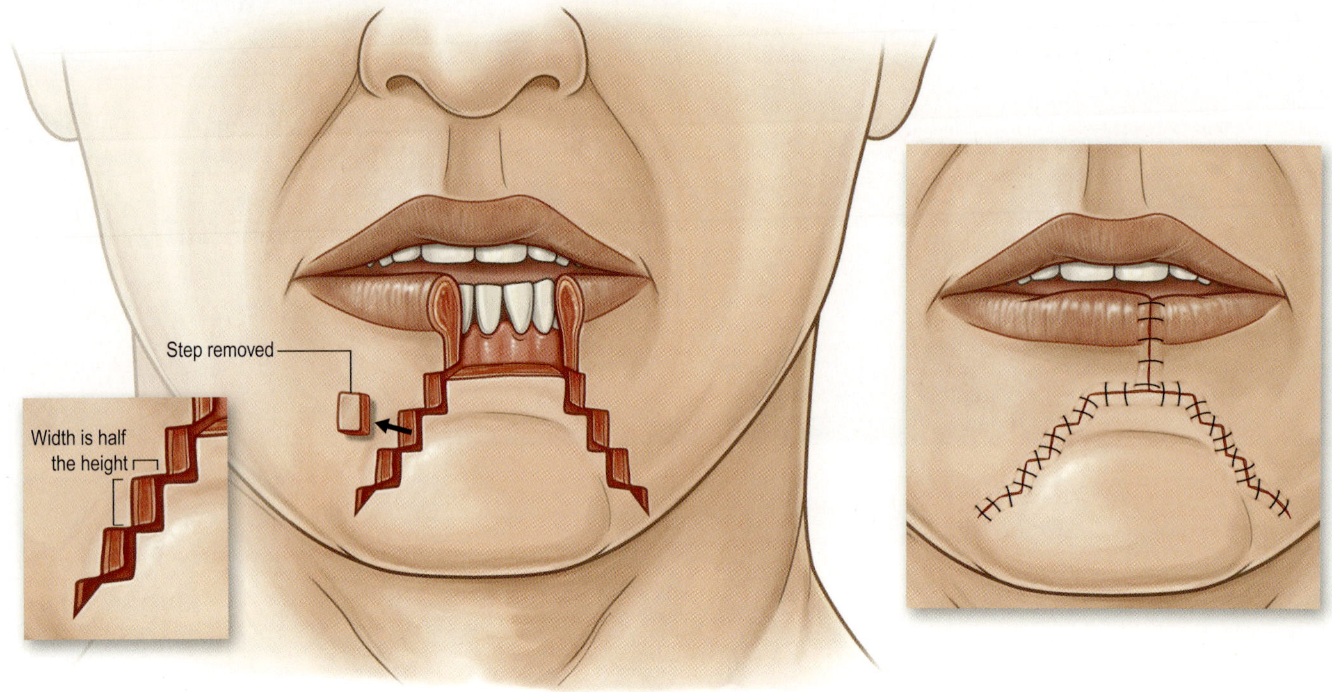

Figure 7.23 Schematic of a step flap reconstruction. Note that the steps are excised to allow the flaps to advance. Note also that the scar remains above the mental crease.

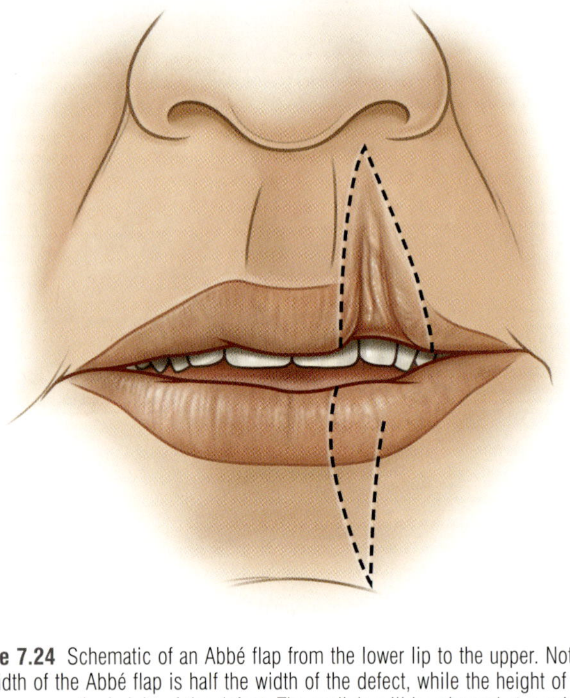

Figure 7.24 Schematic of an Abbé flap from the lower lip to the upper. Note that the width of the Abbé flap is half the width of the defect, while the height of the flap is the same as the height of the defect. The pedicle will be planned at a point opposite the mid-portion of the defect and will end up at the medial end of the defect following rotation of the flap.

Large, composite or total lip defects

- Typically require large local flaps, such as the Karapandzic, Gillies *(Fig. 7.26)*, or Fukimori Gate Flap *(Fig. 7.27)* or free tissue transfer.

Ear

- The areas of the ear most often requiring excision and reconstruction are the rim and the conchal area.

Rim defects

- It is frequently possible to excise a rim lesion and advance the rim by incising full thickness down to the lobule. There is no residual defect with this method *(Fig. 7.28)*.
- If there is concern about the viability of the tip of this flap or if the defect is larger, the posterior skin is dissected up and may be included into the rim.
- A larger flap with a large base has a better blood supply and is more likely to survive. It does not result in any ear deformity.
- In some instances, superior and inferior rim flaps will be used in conjunction with one another.
- Larger defects are better reconstructed by postauricular flaps *(Fig. 7.29)*.
- The flap is elevated and sutured to the anterior edge of the defect.
- After 3 weeks, a large flap is incised in the postauricular area, dissected up to provide laxity, and brought to the ear rim to provide more tissue.
- It is trimmed as necessary and sutured in place. Deep sutures can help in forming the shape as required.

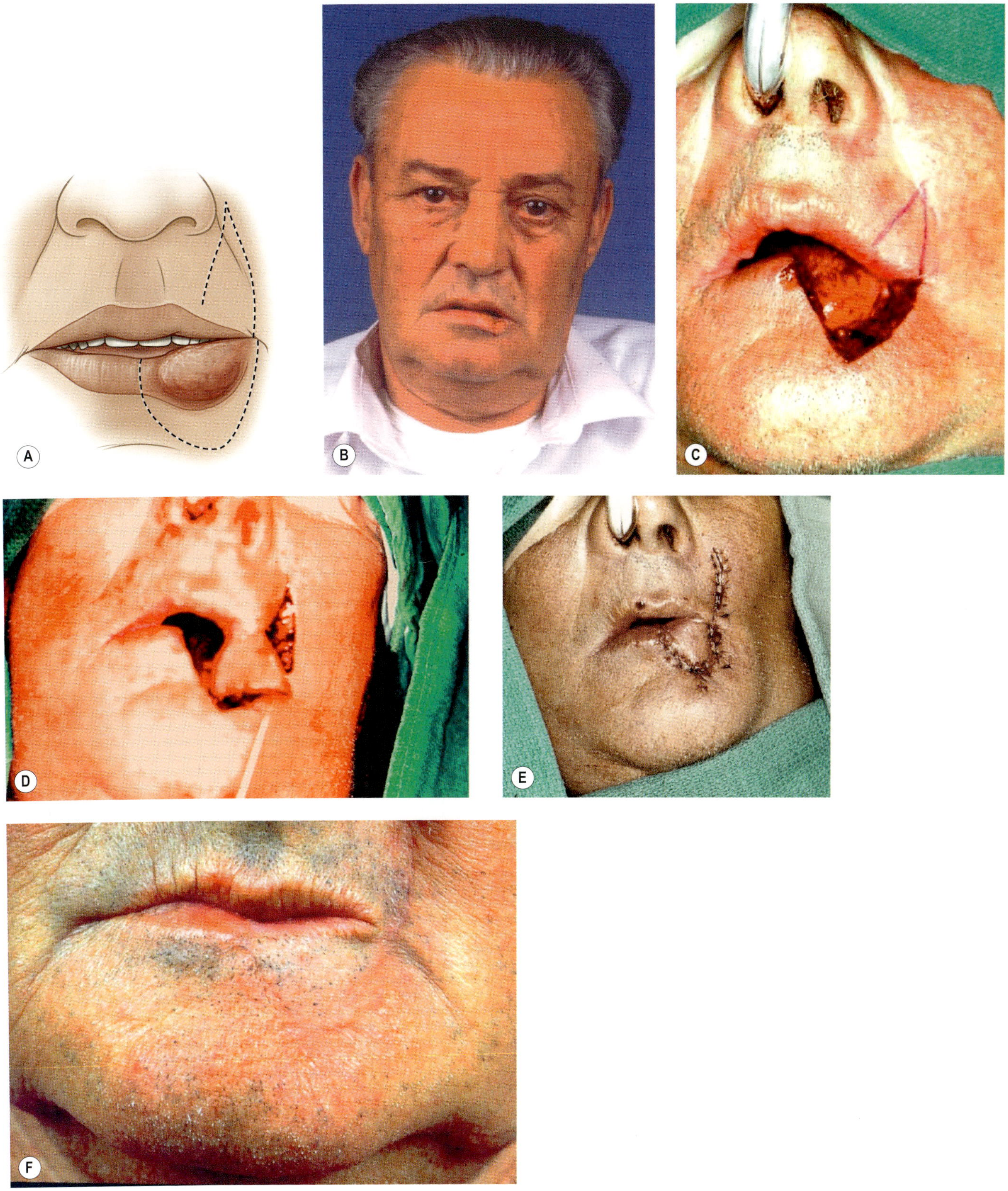

Figure 7.25 **(A)** Schematic of Estlander flap designed to reconstruct a defect of the lower lip. **(B)** Patient with squamous cell carcinoma of the lower lip. **(C)** The lesion has been excised and the flap designed. Note the dimensions of the flap. The width is half that of the defect but the height is the same as the height of the defect. **(D)** The flap is being rotated into the defect. **(E)** Final inset of the flap and closure of the donor defect. **(F)** Final appearance. Note the slight blunting of the commisure.

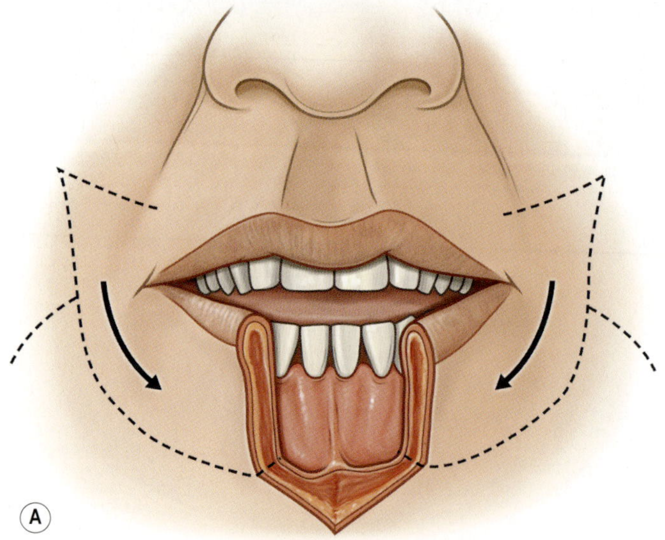

Figure 7.26 A schematic of the Gillies fan flap is shown. Note the releasing incisions on the upper lip that allow the flaps to rotate and advance.

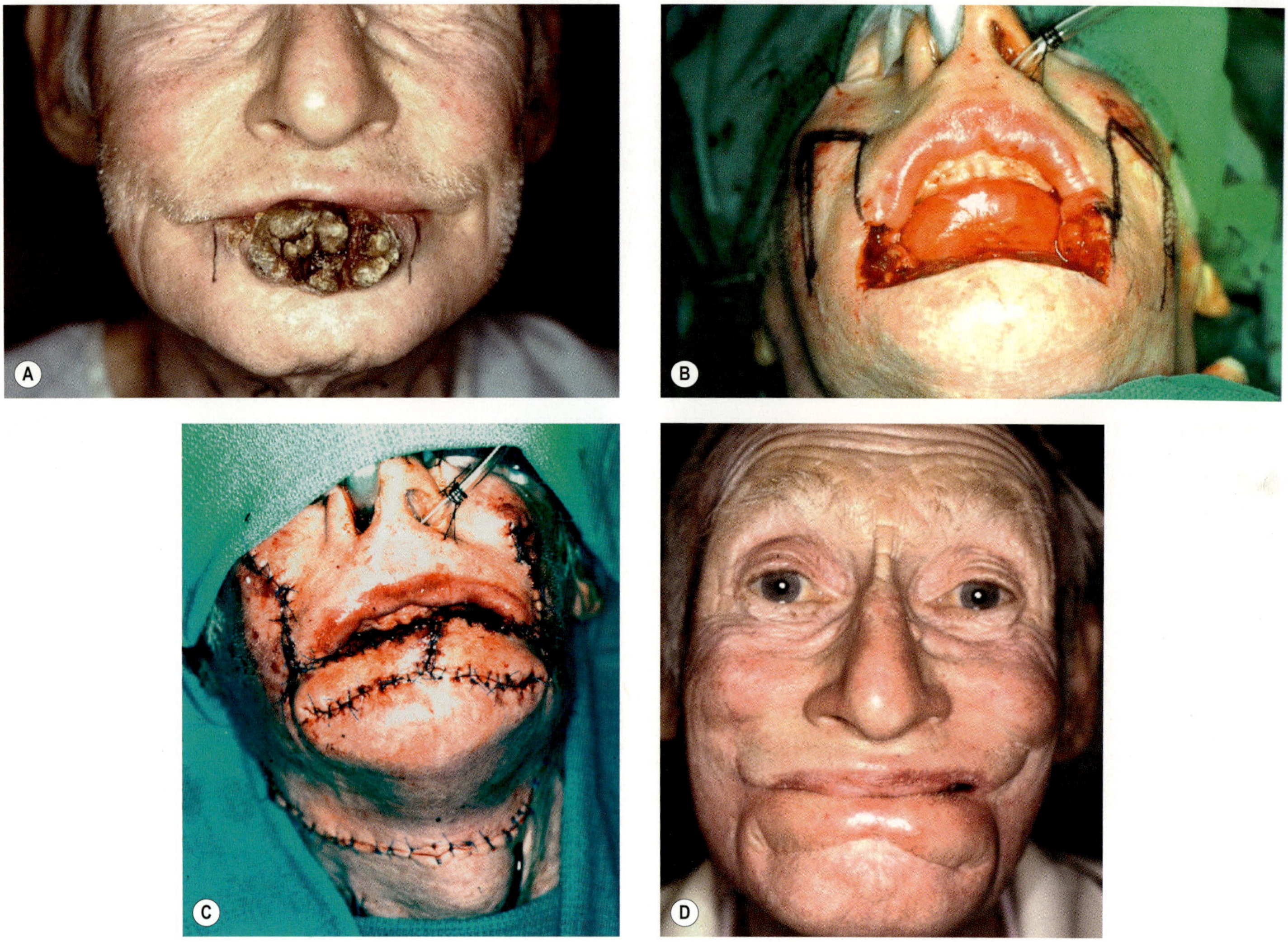

Figure 7.27 **(A)** Patient with a large squamous cell carcinoma of the lower lip requiring total resection. **(B)** The resection is complete and bilateral Fukimori gate flaps have been designed. **(C)** The flaps are rotated into the defect and the secondary defects closed. **(D)** Postoperative appearance showing significant deformity of the lower face.

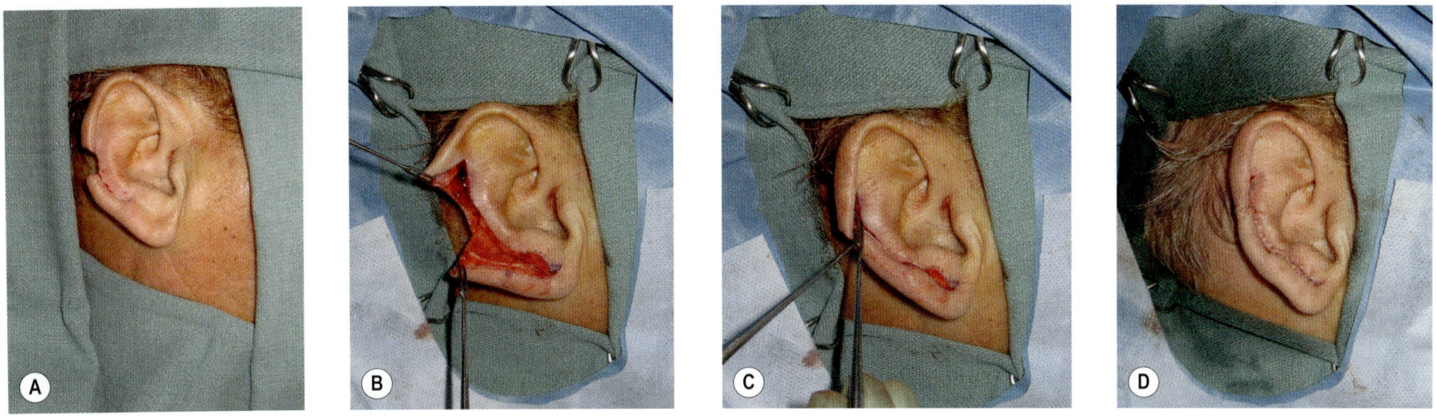

Figure 7.28 **(A)** Helical defect following resection of a basal cell carcinoma. **(B)** Helical flaps are raised based on the posterior skin. **(C)** Flaps are dissected until advancement and closure without tension is possible. **(D)** Final appearance following closure. (Courtesy of Dr David Mathes.)

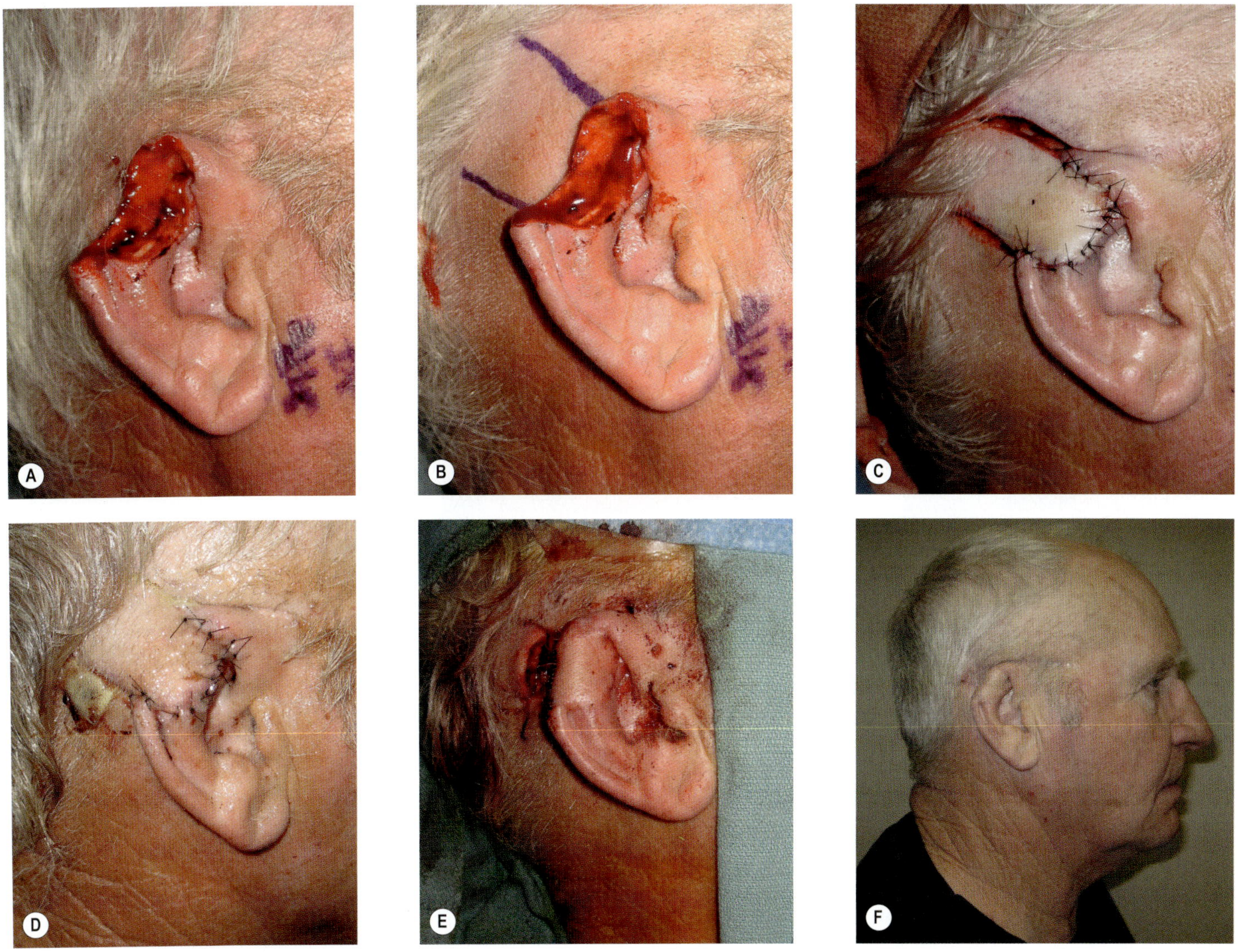

Figure 7.29 **(A)** Defect of upper ear after resection of squamous cell carcinoma. **(B)** Postauricular flap is designed, **(C)** raised and inset into defect. **(D)** Appearance prior to pedicle division and **(E)** following pedicle division. The intervening defect is skin grafted most easily with a post-auricular graft harvested more inferiorly than the defect and closed directly. **(F)** Late appearance. (Courtesy of Dr David Mathes.)

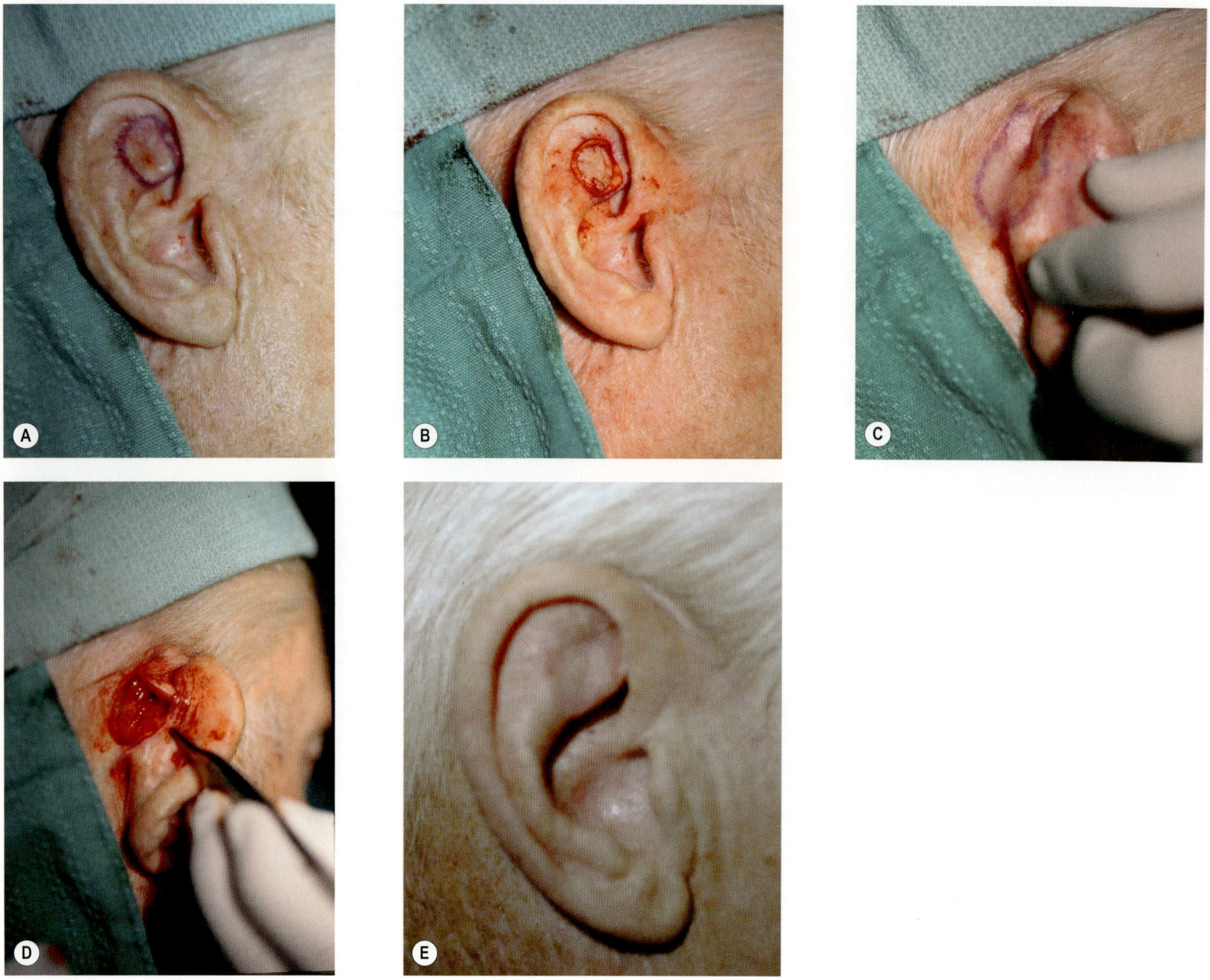

Figure 7.30 **(A)** A 72-year-old man with a basal cell in the upper ear, marked for excision. **(B)** Defect includes anterior skin and underlying cartilage. **(C)** Postauricular, superiorly based flap outlined. **(D)** Flap raised and tunneled into anterior defect. Small segment of flap is de-epithelialized and secondary defect is closed directly. **(E)** Final appearance of healed flap. (Courtesy of Dr Peter Neligan.)

Anterior concha

- If a lesion of significant size occurs in the anterior concha, resurfacing will be required.
- To achieve this, the lesion is resected together with the underlying conchal cartilage. The ear is then distracted forward, and a flap is designed with a central vertical pedicle based on the ear mastoid groove.
- The skin anterior and posterior to the groove is elevated, with some division of the subcutaneous hinge superiorly and inferiorly, it can be rotated into the ear defect.
- The posterior edge of the postauricular island is sutured to the posterior edge of the defect, and the anterior edge of the island is sutured to the anterior edge of the defect. The posterior defect is closed directly ***(Fig. 7.30)***.
- In a large degloving of the ear, a temporal fascial flap is used to cover the defect. The flap is then covered with a full-thickness skin graft.
- This is a rare injury, but this technique can also be used in reconstruction of the congenitally absent ear.

Further reading

Abbé R. A new plastic operation for the relief of deformity due to double harelip. *Plast Reconstr Surg*. 1968;42(5):481–483.

Cordeiro PG, Santamaria E. Primary reconstruction of complex midfacial defects with combined lip-switch procedures and free flaps. *Plast Reconstr Surg*. 1999;103(7):1850–1856.

Free flaps are generally the preferred method for reconstructing large defects of the midface, orbit, and maxilla that include the lip and oral commissure; commissuroplasty is traditionally performed at a second stage. Functional results of the oral sphincter using this reconstructive approach are, however, limited. This article presents a new approach to the reconstruction of massive defects of the lip and midface using a free flap in combination with a lip-switch flap. This was used in 10 patients. One-third to one-half of the upper lip was excised in seven patients, one-third of the lower lip was excised in one patient, and both the upper and lower lips were excised (one-third each) in two patients. All patients had maxillectomies, with or without mandibulectomies, in addition to full-thickness resections of the cheek. A switch flap from the opposite lip was used for reconstruction of the oral commissure and oral sphincter, and a rectus abdominis myocutaneous flap with two or three skin islands was used for reconstruction of the through-and-through defect in the midface. Free flap survival was 100%. All patients had good-to-excellent oral competence, and they were discharged without feeding tubes.

Curran AJ, Neligan P, Gullane PJ. Submental artery island flap. *Laryngoscope*. 1997;107(11):1545–1549.

This paper describes the anatomy of the submental artery perforator flap. The artery is a branch of the facial artery. The perforators run alongside the anterior belly of digastric, which is harvested with the flap. Two cases are presented of lower face reconstruction using the submental flap.

Hofer SO, Posch NA, Smit X. The facial artery perforator flap for reconstruction of perioral defects. *Plast Reconstr Surg*. 2005;115(4):996–1003.

The concept of the facial artery perforator flap is discussed in a study of five clinical cases. The article concludes that this is a versatile flap due to a large arc of rotation and an aesthetically pleasing donor site. It is an ideal flap for one-stage reconstruction without secondary revisions.

Jackson IT. Use of tongue flaps to resurface lip defects and close palatal fistulae in children. *Plast Reconstr Surg*. 1972;49:537–541.

This paper describes the technique of using an anterior tongue flap to reconstruct the vermillion, as well as more extensive lip defects. It also describes the use of the tongue flap for repair of palatal fistulae. In dentate patients, it is particularly important to ensure that precautions are taken to prevent the patient from biting the flap.

Jackson IT. *Local Flaps in Head and Neck Reconstruction*. 2nd ed. St Louis: Quality Medical; 2007.

Jeng SF, Kuo YR, Wei FC, et al . Total lower lip reconstruction with a composite radial forearm palmaris longus tendon flap: a clinical series. *Plast Reconstr Surg*. 2004;113(1):19–23.

Large, full-thickness lip defects after head and neck surgery continue to be a challenge for reconstructive surgeons. The reconstructive aims are to restore the oral lining, the external cheek, oral competence, and function (i.e., articulation, speech, and mastication). These authors' refinement of the composite radial forearm-palmaris longus free flap technique meets these criteria and allows a functional reconstruction of extensive lip and cheek defects in one stage. A composite radial forearm flap including the palmaris longus tendon was designed. The skin flap for the reconstruction of the intraoral lining and the skin defect was folded over the palmaris longus tendon. Both ends of the vascularized tendon were laid through the bilateral modiolus and anchored with adequate tension to the intact orbicularis muscle of the upper lip. This procedure was used in 12 patients.

Karapandzic M. Reconstruction of lip defects by local arterial flaps. *Br J Plast Surg*. 1974;27:93–97.

In this classic paper, Dr Karapandzic describes the procedure which allows for preservation of the neurovascular bundles of the orbicularis oris in order to reconstruct defects of the lips. This classic description focuses on reconstruction of lower lip defects.

Keskin M, Kelly CP, Yavuzer R, et al. External filling ports in tissue expansion: confirming their safety and convenience. *Plast Reconstr Surg*. 2006;117(5):1543–1551.

Kroll SS. Staged sequential flap reconstruction for large lower lip defects. *Plast Reconstr Surg*. 1991;88(4):620–627.

Langstein H, Robb G. Lip and perioral reconstruction. *Clin Plast Surg*. 2005;32:431–445.

Limberg AA. The planning of local plastic operations on the body surface: theory and practice. In: Wolfe SA, ed. trans. *Planirovanie Mestnoplasticheskikh Operatsiina Poverkhnosti Tela, 1906*. Lexington MA: Collamore Press; 1984.

McGregor IA. Eyelid reconstruction following subtotal resection of the upper or lower lid. *Br J Plast Surg*. 1973;26:346–354.

McGregor JC, Soutar DS. A critical assessment of the bilobed flap. *Br J Plast Surg*. 1981;34:197–205.

Mustardé JC. Eyelid repairs with costochondral grafts. *Plast Reconstr Surg*. 1962;30:267–272.

Neligan PC. Strategies in lip reconstruction. *Clin Plast Surg*. 2009;36(3):477–485.

Injury or surgical trauma can result in significant alterations of normal lip appearance and function that can profoundly impact the patient' s self-image and quality of life. Neuromuscular injury can lead to asymmetry at rest and during facial animation, and distressing functional disabilities are common. Loss of labial competence may interfere with the ability to articulate, whistle, suck, kiss, and contain salivary secretions. For smaller defects, reconstruction can be very effective. Reconstructing an aesthetically pleasing and functional lip is more difficult with larger defects.

Shestak KC, Roth AG, Jones NF, et al . The cervicopectoral rotation flap – a valuable technique for facial reconstruction. *Br J Plast Surg*.1993;46(5):375–377.

Webster J. Crescentic peri-alar cheek excision for upper lip flap advancement with a short history of upper lip repair. *Plast Reconstr Surg*. 1955;16:434–464.

8 Chapter

Cleft lip repair

This chapter was created using content from Neligan & Losee, Plastic Surgery 3rd edition, Volume 3, Pediatric Plastic Surgery, Chapter 23 Repair of unilateral cleft lip, Philip Kuo-Ting Chen, M. Samuel Noordhoff and Alex Kane, Chapter 24, Repair of bilateral cleft lip, John B. Mulliken.

SYNOPSIS (UNILATERAL LIP REPAIR)

Principles of unilateral cleft lip repair

- Presurgical nasoalveolar molding.
- Modification of surgical techniques.
  - Mohler's rotation incision.
  - Mucosal flaps for nasal floor reconstruction, correction of mucosal deficiency in piriform area.
  - Eliminate the perialar incision on advancement flap, limiting scars around the ala base and nostril floor.
  - Mobilization of alar base.
  - Nasal floor reconstruction with complete mucosal closure.
  - Muscle release and reconstruction to simulate the philtral column.
  - Anchoring of advancement flap to nasal septum for centralizing the Cupid's bow.
  - Correction of central vermillion deficiency with triangular vermillion flap from lateral lip.
  - Semi-open rhinoplasty with a reverse U incision on the cleft side and rim incision on the non-cleft side.
  - Atraumatic dissection to release the fibrofatty tissue from lower lateral cartilages.
  - Advancement and fixation of the cleft side lower lateral cartilage to the non-cleft side lower lateral cartilage and to the skin in an over-corrected position.
  - Definition of the ala-facial groove with alar transfixion sutures.
- Postoperative maintenance of over-correction with silicone nasal conformer.

SYNOPSIS (BILATERAL LIP REPAIR)

- A child born with bilateral cleft lip should not have to suffer because of an ill-conceived and poorly executed primary repair. The operative principles for synchronous nasolabial repair are established:
  - Maintain symmetry.
  - Secure primary muscular continuity.
  - Design proper philtral size and shape.
  - Construct the median tubercle from lateral labial elements.
  - Position/secure the lower lateral cartilages and sculpt the nasal tip and columella.
- The techniques based on these principles are within the repertoire of a well-trained surgeon whose practice is focused on children with cleft lip. Only the philtral columns and dimple seem just beyond the surgeon's craft.
- Preoperative dentofacial orthopedic manipulation of the premaxilla is necessary to permit synchronous closure of the primary palate. The surgeon must repair the bilateral cleft lip and correct the nasal deformity in three-dimensions based on knowledge of anticipated changes in the fourth-dimension. Modifications of the techniques used in repair of the most common complete form are needed for the less common bilateral variants, such as, binderoid, complete with intact secondary palate, symmetrical incomplete, and asymmetrical complete/incomplete.
- Outcomes can be assessed using preoperative and serial photography and documentation of revision-rates. Direct anthropometry is the "gold-standard" for quantification of the changing nasolabial features; however, it requires training and experience. Intraoperative anthropometry is used to record baseline dimensions and is repeated as the child grows. Two-dimensional photogrammetry is applicable for certain linear and angular measurements if properly scaled. Computerized three-dimensional photogrammetry is a new methodology for quantifying nasolabial appearance. It is both accurate and reliable, and someday could be employed in intra- and inter-institutional comparative studies.

Brief introduction

- The multidisciplinary approach is essential to the satisfactory treatment of the cleft patient including: surgeons, orthodontists, speech pathologists, pedodontists, prosthodontists, otolaryngologists, social workers, psychologists, as well as a photographer.
- The techniques presented for the unilateral cleft lip repair are based on the experience of the members of the Chang Gung Craniofacial Center over a period of 30 years in a Chinese population. They have also been tested in other racially diverse centers. The improved outcomes result from an integrated approach with presurgical management, surgical refinements and postsurgical maintenance.
- It is generally believed that isolated cleft palate is a genetic entity distinct from unilateral cleft lip with or without cleft palate.
- This conclusion arises from both epidemiologic studies and the fact that embryologic events leading to cleft lip/palate and cleft palate occur at somewhat different times (3–7 weeks versus 5–12 weeks).
- It has long been assumed that both genetic and epigenetic factors play important roles in the etiology of clefts, and this is supported by the varying incidence of clefting with ethnicity, geographic location, and socioeconomic conditions.
- The incidence of cleft lip/palate in white newborns is approximately 1 in 1000 (Table 8.1); isolated cleft palate occurs in about 0.5 in 1000.
- While there are more than 250 syndromes associated with orofacial clefting, most cases occur as an isolated abnormality; so-called non-syndromic cleft lip/palate.
- In a large review of their center's experience, Rollnick and Pruzansky identified other malformations in 35% of cleft lip/palate patients and 54% of cleft palate patients.
- Cleft lip/palate has an unequal gender distribution, favoring boys over girls, whereas this relationship is reversed in cleft palate only.
- Cleft lip/palate affects the left side more often.
- A common question from parents pertains to their risk of having another child with a cleft lip/palate:
  - Unaffected (i.e., non-cleft) parents who have one child with cleft lip/palate have an estimated recurrence risk of 4%, increasing to 9% if two children are affected.
  - If one parent is affected, the risk of having a child with cleft lip/palate is also 4%, increasing to 17% if there is already both an affected parent and an affected child.
  - As the degree of familial relationship increases, recurrence risk decreases: first-, second-, and third-degree relatives have 4%, 0.7%, and 0.3% risk, respectively.
  - Recurrence risk increases with the severity of the cleft.

Table 8.1 Incidence of cleft lip/palate in differing ethnic groups

Ethnicity	Incidence per 1000 births
American Indian	3.6
Japanese	2.1
Chinese	1.7
White	1.0
African-American	0.3

Data from Wyszynski DF, Beaty TH, Maestri NE. Genetics of nonsyndromic oral clefts revisited. *Cleft Palate Craniofac J.* 1996;33:406–417. Vieira AR, Orioli IM. Candidate genes for nonsyndromic cleft lip and palate. *ASDC J Dent Child.* 2001;68:229, 272–279.

Preoperative considerations

- With the assistance of ultrasound, prenatal diagnosis of cleft lip is usually made after 16–20 weeks' gestation.
- Three-dimensional ultrasonography has improved the accuracy of cleft lip diagnosis and is helpful for prenatal counseling because parents can visualize the face of the fetus clearly.
- A genetic diagnosis and evaluation for other systemic conditions should be done at the time when a prenatal diagnosis of the cleft is made.
- The newborn cleft baby should have a pediatric evaluation and parents are counseled about feeding and given information for subsequent care and treatment.
- Depending on surgical preference, presurgical nasoalveolar molding may be started at 2 weeks or even earlier.
- If utilized, it usually takes 3–4 months before the completion of the nasoalveolar molding.
- There are several different treatment plans for surgical correction of the cleft lip deformity ***(Fig. 8.1, Fig. 8.2)***; however, generally timing is as follows:
  - Alveolar/nasoalveolar molding:
  - If utilized, typically begins by 2 weeks of age.
- Lip repair typically occurs around 3 months of age:
  - With presurgical nasoalveolar molding, a definitive cheiloplasty is done at the age of 3–5 months, when the alveolar gap is narrowed and nasal deformity is improved.
  - When presurgical orthopedics is not available or if the child is older than 3 months, a definitive cheiloplasty with nasal correction is performed.
  - If there is a wide cleft (>12–15 mm) and an associated tissue deficiency, a nasolabial adhesion cheiloplasty is done at 3 months, followed by a definitive cheiloplasty at about 9 months.
- If the child has an associated cleft palate, a palatoplasty is typically performed at 9–12 months.
- Timing of alveolar bone grafting relates to the eruption of the central incisor and canine and is frequently determined by the orthodontist usually at the age of 7–11 years.
- Early intervention for velopharyngeal insufficiency is done as soon as possible on the basis of speech evaluation and nasopharyngoscopy.

- Secondary correction of nasal deformities and orthognathic surgery, when indicated, are delayed until facial growth is complete.
- Bilateral cleft lip presents in three major anatomic forms *(Fig. 8.3)*:
  - bilateral symmetrical complete (50%).
  - bilateral symmetrical incomplete (25%).
  - bilateral asymmetrical (complete/incomplete) (25%).
- The extent of the palatal cleft usually corresponds to the severity of the labial clefts.
- *Minor-form* cleft lip extends 3–5 mm above the normal Cupid's bow peak, i.e., 50% or less of the normal cutaneous labial height.
- Other features are: deficient vermillion on medial side of the cleft; cutaneous groove and muscular depression; hypoplastic median tubercle; and minor nasal deformity.

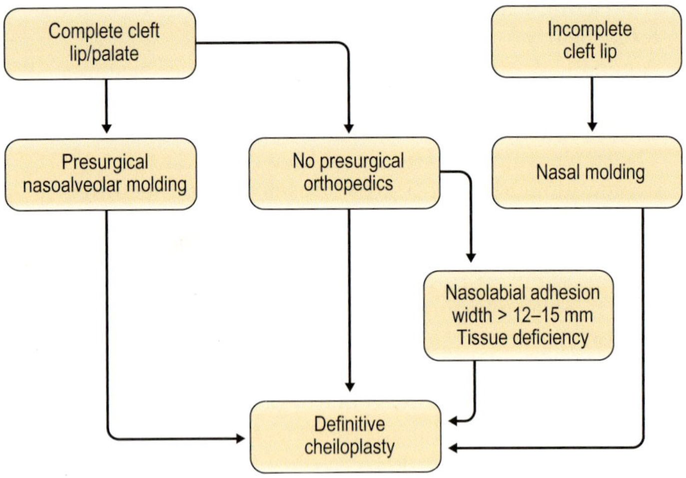

Figure 8.1 Overall cleft treatment plan in the Chang Gung Craniofacial Center.

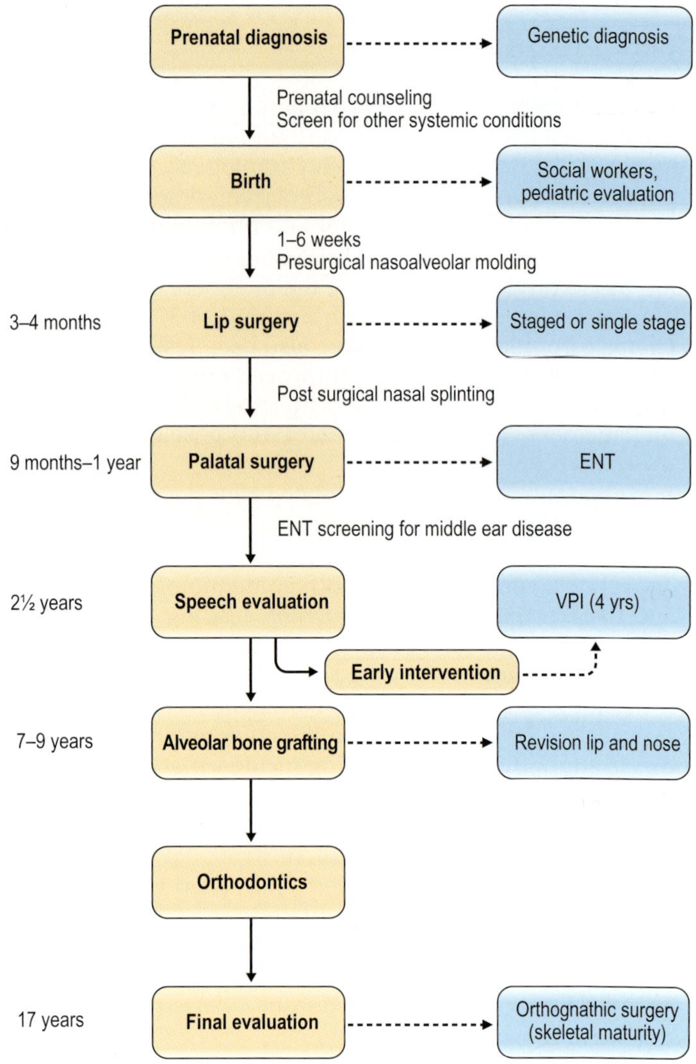

Figure 8.2 Surgical algorithm for unilateral cleft lip repair in the Chang Gung Craniofacial Center.

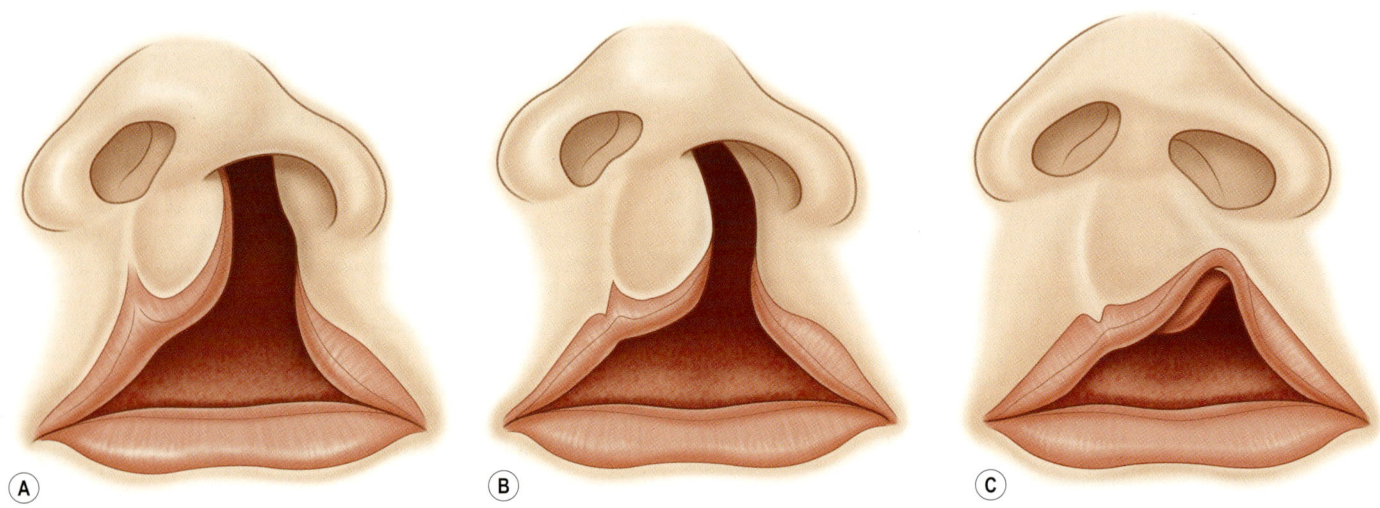

Figure 8.3 Examples of asymmetrical bilateral cleft lip. **(A)** Left complete and right minor-form; **(B)** left complete and right microform; **(C)** left incomplete and right mini-microform.

- *Microform* cleft lip is characterized by a notched vermillion–cutaneous junction in which the Cupid's bow peak is elevated less than 3 mm above normal.
- Other features are the same as in a minor-form, but they are less obvious.
- Nasal deformities include small depression of the sill, slightly slumped alar genu and 1–2 mm lateral displacement (and often under-rotation) of the alar base.
- *Mini-microform* cleft lip is distinguished by a disruption of the white roll (vermillion–cutaneous junction) without elevation of the Cupid's bow peak.
- Usually there is a notch of the free mucosal margin. Muscular depression (particularly noticeable below the nostril sill) is variable as is the cleft nasal deformity.
- This detailed subcategorization of the contralateral side in an asymmetrical bilateral cleft lip is important because the extent of vermillion–cutaneous disjunction determines the operative strategy.
- Synchronous bilateral nasolabial repair is indicated for a contralateral incomplete cleft lip, including a minor-form.
- Correction of a contralateral microform or mini-microform is usually deferred until closure on the greater side.
- Alignment of the three maxillary elements sets the skeletal stage for synchronous bilateral nasolabial repair and minimizes the nasolabial distortions that occur during rapid growth of early childhood.
- After retrusion and centralization of the premaxilla, the philtral flap can be designed in proper proportions, the nasal tip cartilages can be anatomically positioned, and the alveolar clefts can be closed, which stabilizes the maxillary arch and usually eliminates oronasal fistulas.
- There are two dentofacial orthopedic strategies: passive and active.
- Passive strategies include nasoalveolar molding (NAM) devices.
- Active strategies include the Latham appliance *(Fig. 8.4)*.

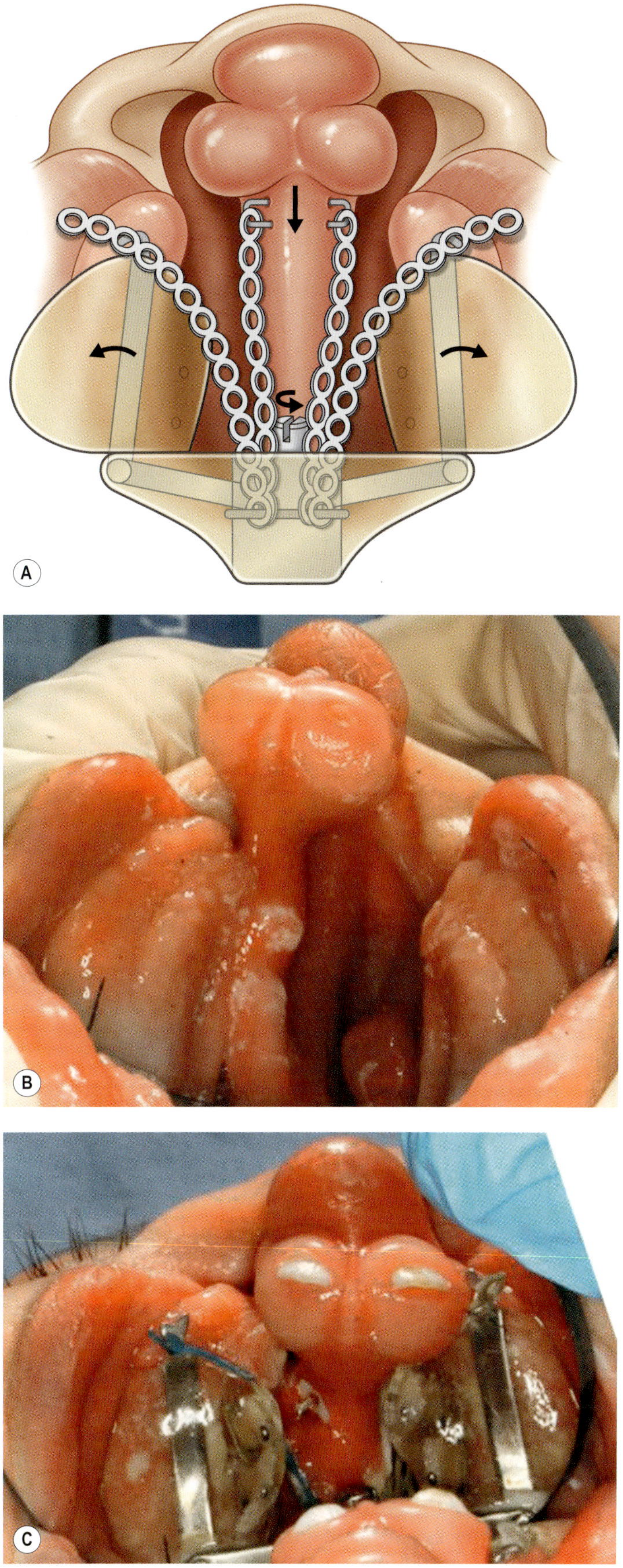

Figure 8.4 **(A)** Latham appliance; **(B)** prior to insertion of device; **(C)** 6 weeks following dentofacial orthopedic manipulation.

Anatomical/technical pearls

- Areas of vital concern to the surgeon: the amount of tissue medial to the base of the ala, the vertical height of the lateral lip, the horizontal length of the lateral lip, and the epidermal extension from the columella onto the premaxilla.
- The discrepancy between the height from the central point of the base of columella to the two peaks of the Cupid's bow is critical for leveling of the Cupid's bow.
- Vertical length of the lip is more important aesthetically compared with the horizontal length.
- Therefore, vertical length is seldom sacrificed for horizontal length columella and nasal floor skin.

The vermillion beneath the cleft-side Cupid's bow is always deficient compared with the counterpart vermillion width on the non-cleft side *(Fig. 8.5)*.

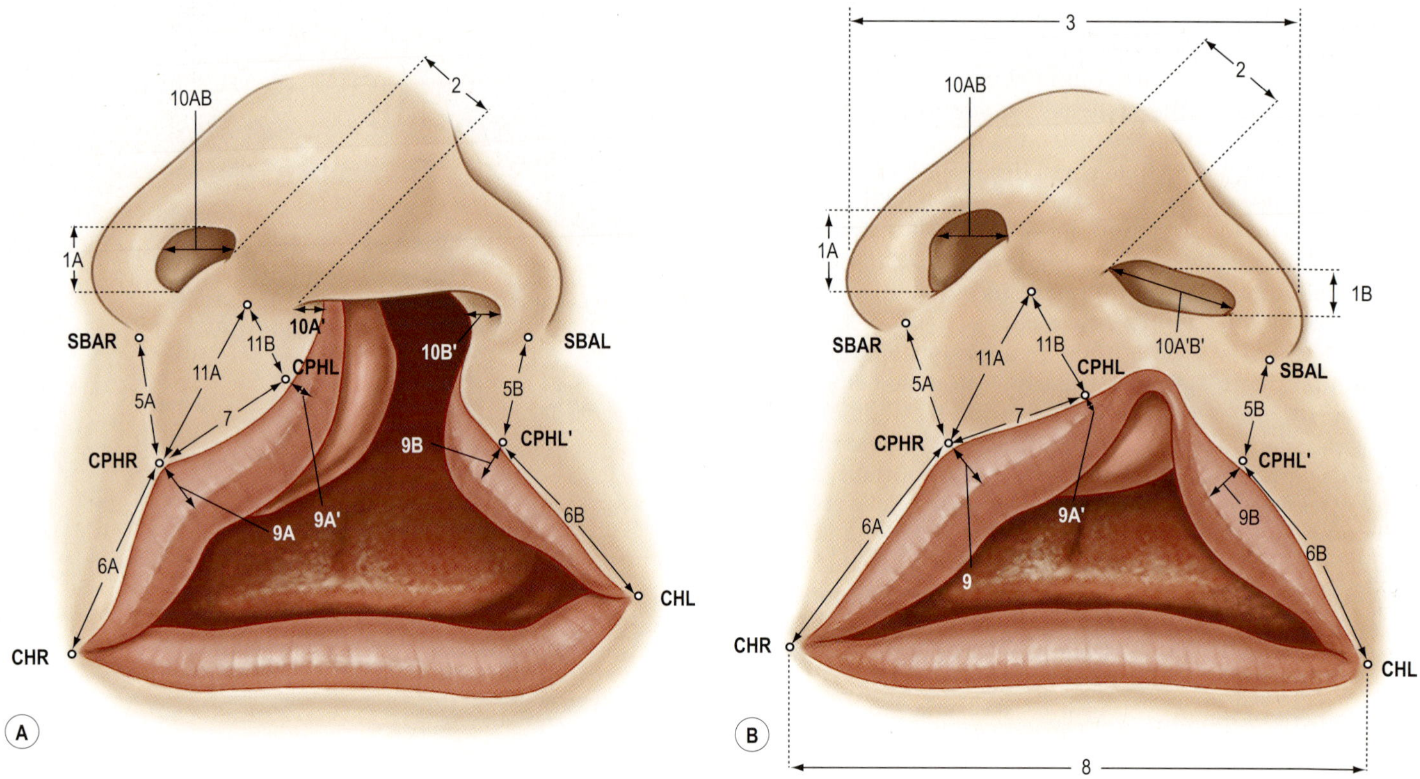

Figure 8.5 (A) Unilateral complete cleft with anthropometric markings for measurements: CHR, CHL, commissure; right and left horizontal length; right and left vertical length; CPHR, non-cleft-side philtral column; CPHL, cleft side Cupid's bow; central Cupid's bow; CPHL', cleft-side philtral column; SBAR, SBAL, right and left base of ala. **(B)** Similar markings for the incomplete cleft lip. (From Noordhoff MS, Chen YR, Chen KT, et al. The surgical technique for the complete unilateral cleft lip-nasal deformity. *Plast Reconstr Surg.* 1995;2:167–174.)

- Inadequate reconstruction of this deficient vermillion will result in free border deformities as seen in a straight-line vermillion closure.
- The vermillion medial to the base of the philtral column fits into the deficient vermillion beneath the Cupid's bow.
- The key concepts of the rotation-advancement surgical technique in the unilateral cheiloplasty are as follows:
  - Mohler's rotation incision.
  - Mucosal flaps for nasal floor reconstruction, correction of mucosal deficiency in piriform area.
  - Eliminate the perialar incision on advancement flap, limiting scars around the ala base and nostril floor.
  - Mobilization of alar base.
  - Nasal floor reconstruction with complete mucosal closure.
  - Muscle release and reconstruction to simulate the philtral column.
  - Anchoring of advancement flap to nasal septum for centralizing the Cupid's bow.
  - Correction of central vermillion deficiency with triangular vermillion flap from lateral lip.
  - Sem-iopen rhinoplasty with a reverse U incision on the cleft side and rim incision on the non-cleft side.
  - Atraumatic dissection to release the fibrofatty tissue from lower lateral cartilages (LLCs).
  - Advancement and fixation of the cleft side LLC to the non-cleft side LLC and to the skin in an over-corrected position.
  - Definition of the alar-facial groove with alar transfixion sutures.
- The following principles for repair of bilateral cleft lip were induced based on study of the literature and observations of residual deformities:
  - *Maintain nasolabial symmetry*. Even the slightest differences between the two sides of the lip and nose will become more obvious with growth. Symmetry is the one advantage a bilateral cleft lip has over its unilateral counterpart. It must be maintained.
  - *Secure muscular continuity*. Construction of a complete oral ring permits normal labial function, eliminates the lateral bulges, and minimizes later distortion of the philtrum and interalar widening.
  - *Design the philtral flap of proper size and shape*. The philtrum rapidly elongates and widens, particularly at the columellar–labial junction.
  - *Construct the median tubercle using lateral vermillion-mucosal elements*. There is no white roll in the prolabium. Retained vermillion lacks normal coloration and fails to grow to full height.

5. *Position the slumped/splayed lower lateral cartilages and sculpt excess soft tissue in nasal tip and columella*. These maneuvers are necessary to establish normal nasal tip projection and columellar length/width.

Video 8.1

Operative techniques

Video 8.2

Unilateral cleft lip (Video 8.1; Video 8.2)

Alveolar molding: external taping

- The external taping (non-surgical lip adhesion) is the simplest technique for both presurgical molding of the maxillary halves and approximation of the alveolus.
- A strip of Micropore tape is placed across the cleft to approximate the upper lips. The objective of the tape is to simulate effects of an adhesion cheiloplasty and reposition the maxillary segments into proper alignment.

Nasoalveolar molding

- Liou's method utilizes a molding bulb attached to a dental plate as an outrigger to mold the nose along with external taping of the lip.
- The device is held to the palate with dental adhesives.
- The force from taping and counterforce from the molding bulb provide the combined force necessary to bring the alveolus into proper position.
- The nasal molding and alveolar molding are done at the same time, taking approximately 3 months.
- Newer devices contain an internal spring.
- Grayson's method utilizes nasal molding *after* alveolar approximation to avoid overstretching the nasal cartilage.
- The appliance consists of an acrylic or resin plate which fits over the maxillary dental arch (alveolar ridges), an acrylic retention arm or button, and a nasal stent.
- This technique should be started within the first 2 weeks after birth; careful monitoring is required every 1–2 weeks for a period of 3–6 months to complete it.

Rotation advancement cheiloplasty for complete clefts

- The following points and measurements are made, with a caliper, at the time of surgery:
  - The points of the Cupid's bow on the epidermis–vermillion junction line (the white skin roll).
  - The vermillion–mucosa junction line (the red line).
  - This clearly defines the intervening vermillion and also helps identify the deficient vermillion beneath the cleft-side Cupid's bow.
  - The base of the ala and the commissure (see Fig. 8.5).
  - The base of the cleft-side philtral column is difficult to identify.
  - It is located where the white skin roll changes direction and where the vermillion first becomes widest, usually 3–4 mm lateral to the converging point of red line and white skin roll.

Medial incisions

- After the above markings are made, a Mohler's rotation incision line is marked as a curving line from CPHL going upward into the base of columella then turning back to the nasolabial junction of the non-cleft side philtral column ***(Fig. 8.6)***.
- The height of this rotation incision should be the same as the height of the non-cleft side philtral column.
- The angle of the backcut is dependent on the width of columella.
- If the columella is wide, a wider angle can be made.
- The incision across the free border of the lip at CPHL should be at right angles to the axis of the white skin roll to facilitate subsequent lip closure.
- After the incision is made, the muscle is freed from the skin in the subdermal plane for a distance of 2–3 mm (***Fig. 8.7,*** inset).
- The muscle dissection on the non-cleft side should reach the nasal floor of the non-cleft side for adequate releasing of the abnormal muscle insertion to the columellar base.
- Traction on the free border of the lip will determine if the rotation is adequate, that is, both sides of the Cupid's bow at the same level ***(Fig. 8.8)***.
- Even if the rotation is inadequate, extending the incision across the non-cleft-side philtral column should be avoided, as it will result in a vertically long lip. If the rotation fails to level the Cupid's bow, nothing further is done until after muscle repositioning.
- The C-flap incisions are made on a line that extends from point CPHL along the junction of skin and mucosa to the most lateral point of the skin overlying the premaxilla ***(Fig. 8.9)***.
- The incision on the premaxilla then turns superiorly at the junction of the columellar skin and septal mucosa for a distance of 5 mm or even longer ***(Fig. 8.10)***.
- Blunt-tip tenotomy scissors are used to separate the medial crura of the cleft side lower lateral cartilage (see Fig. 8.10).

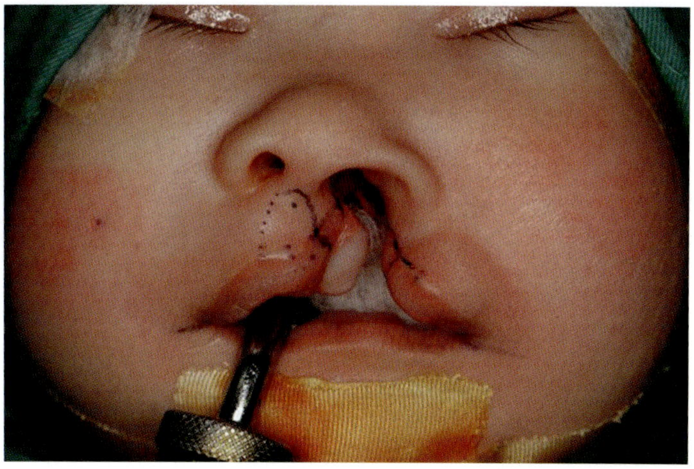

Figure 8.6 Preoperative marking: CPHR, IS, CPHL, CPHL′ and CHL as described in Figure 8.5. The C-flap (C) and C-flap mucosa (CM) are marked. The dotted line on the lip is the red line, which is the junction between vermillion and mucosa. Incision lines are shown on the lip extending from point CPHL lateral to the columella on the skin edge overlying the premaxilla extending superiorly along the junction line of columella skin and septal cartilage mucosa. The cleft-side base of the philtral column is also marked (CPHL′). The proposed incision lines are marked with the rotation incision in a Mohler's fashion. A small triangular white skin roll flap is designed above the CPHL′.

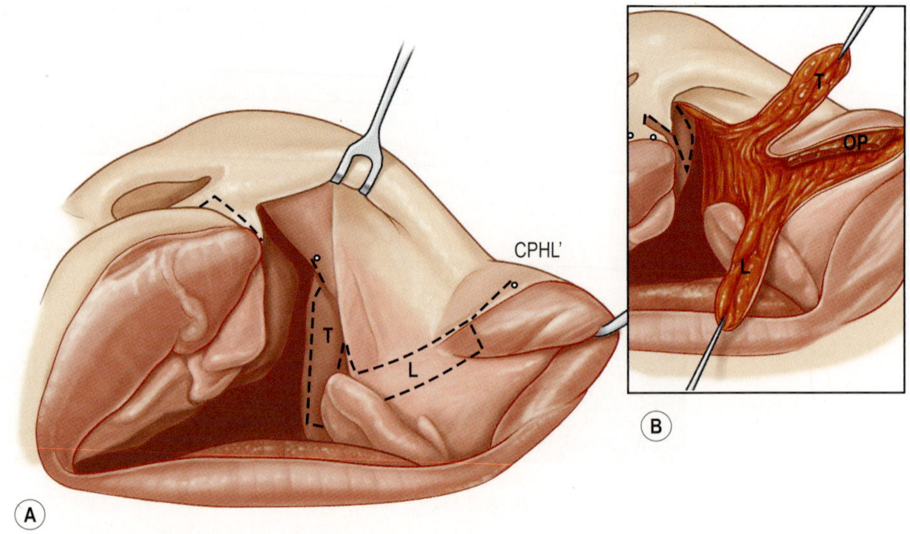

Figure 8.7 The orbicularis peripheralis muscle (OP) is released in a subdermal plane. The abnormally inserted fibers of the nasalis, depressor septi, and levator muscles are released from the base of the ala. Inset **(B)**: the muscle is freed from the skin in the subdermal plane for a distance of 2–3 mm.

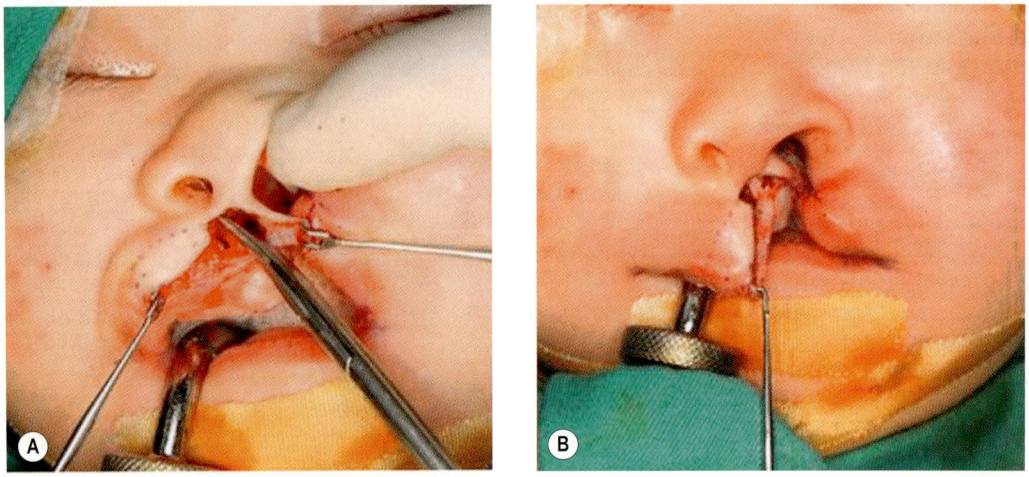

Figure 8.8 **(A)** Traction on the free border of the lip helps to determine if the rotation is adequate. **(B)** The muscle dissection on the rotation flap should reach the nasal floor on non-cleft side.

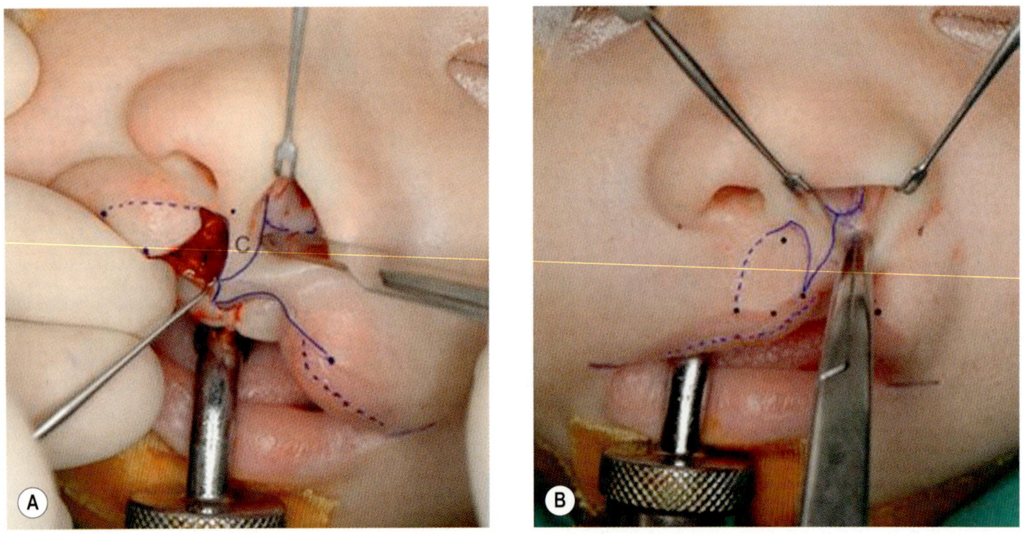

Figure 8.9 The incision lines for C-flap and nasal floor: a transverse incision is made inside the nasal floor at the junction of skin and mucosa leaving ample tissue on piriform area and premaxilla.

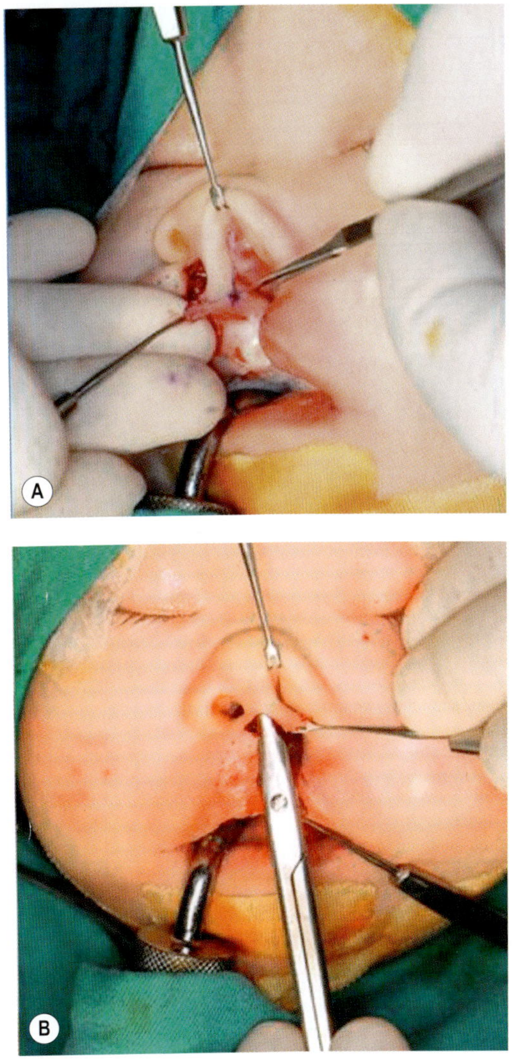

Figure 8.10 **(A)** The incision line of the C-flap. **(B)** A blunt-tip scissors is used to release the foot plate of the medial crura of the cleft side lower lateral cartilage.

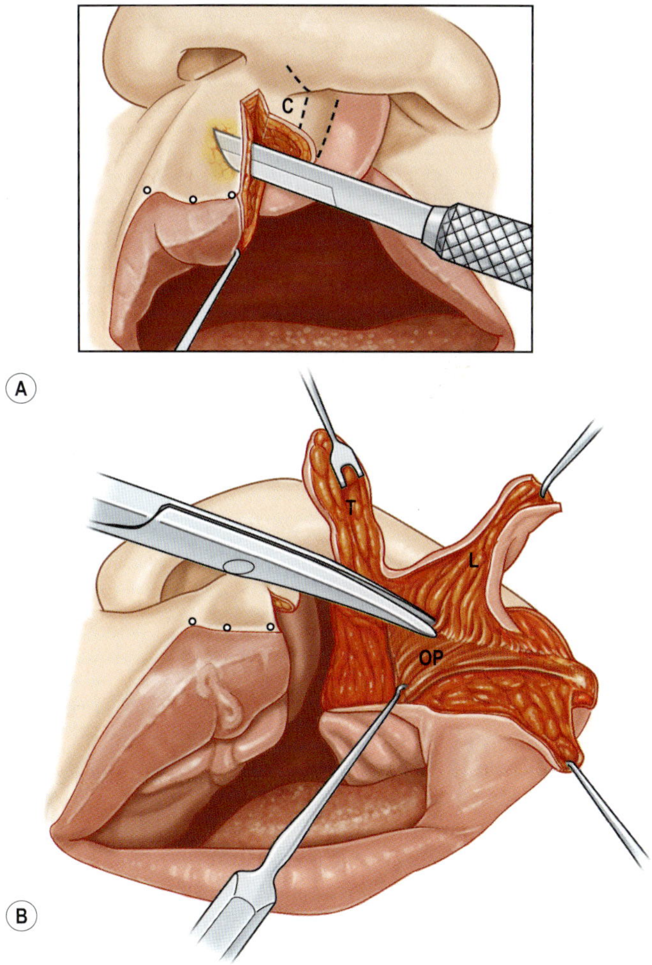

Figure 8.11 **(A)** The tip of the C-flap adjacent to CPHL is rotated medially to fill the defect on columellar base after a Mohler's incision. **(B)** The completed dissection with an elevated turbinate **(T)** and mucosal flap **(L)** based on the maxilla. Markings for the mucosal flap L, based on maxilla and inferior turbinate flap T. The L-flap based on the maxilla extends to the converging red line and white skin roll, leaving the vermillion between this point and CPHL' available for reconstruction of the deficient vermillion beneath the cleft side of the Cupid's bow.

- This allows mobilization of the C-flap and repositioning of the downward displaced footplate of the medial crura of the cleft side lower lateral cartilage.
- The tip of the C-flap (point at CPHL) is rotated medially to fill in the defect on the columellar base after the Mohler's incision ***(Fig. 8.11)***.
- An L-flap is marked based on the maxilla, extending on the free border of the lip to the point where the red line and white skin roll converge, preserving the vermillion on the lateral lip.
- The skin incision line on the free border of the lip starts from point CPHL' and a triangular shaped small WSR flap is designed (see Fig. 8.6).
- The width of the WSR flap is exactly the same as the width of WSR above the point CPHL'.
- The length of the WSR flap is only 1–2 mm.
- The incision line is then continued along the skin–mucosal junction on the piriform up to the inferior edge of the inferior turbinate then turning inward to include an inferior turbinate flap (see Fig. 8.11).
- The incision line on the inferior turbinate extends from the piriform rim inward on the upper and lower edges of the inferior turbinate for a distance of 1.5 cm, where a transverse cut is made.
- The inferior turbinate flap (T) is elevated in a retrograde fashion based on the vestibular skin.
- After elevation of the L and T flaps, the attachments of the LLC to the maxilla and ULC are released, allowing easy mobilization of the LLC and the lateral lip.
- Even in wide clefts, mobilization of the lip and cartilage is easily accomplished without an extensive dissection over the maxilla (see Fig. 8.11).
- The lateral lip mucosa is incised and dissected free for only 2 mm as excessive dissection contributes to scarring and should be avoided.
- The orbicularis peripheralis muscle is bunched up as a disorganized mass of fibers with numerous dermal

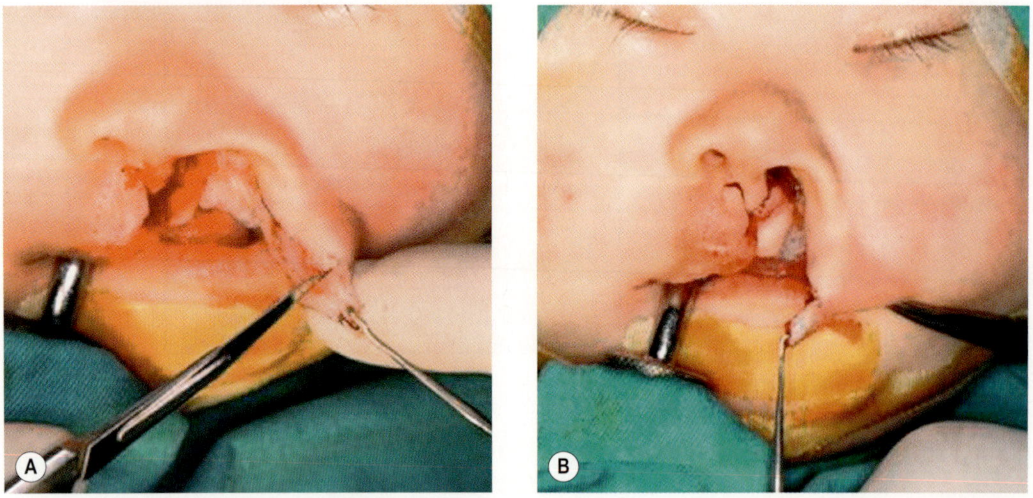

Figure 8.12 (A,B) The incision along the skin edge from CPHL′ to the base of the inferior turbinate and elevation of the OM flap on the lateral lip. The OM flap is elevated to its base beneath the philtral column (CPHL′) in such a way that the volume of muscle at its base CPHL′ is similar to the volume of muscle at the opposite point CPHR on the non-cleft side of the lip.

insertions, by use of a blunt-nosed tenotomy scissors, the orbicularis peripheralis muscle is dissected along the edge of the dermis to a line extending from the base of the ala to the base of the philtral column CPHL′.

- The dissection is continued on a subdermal plane superiorly under and around the base of the ala.
- This releases the abnormal insertions of the paranasal muscles including the transverse portion of the nasalis muscle, the depressor septi, and the levator muscles of the upper lip and ala.
- The angular artery is used as a landmark for the muscle dissection around the alar base.
- The extent of dissection should be lateral to the vessel to assure most of the abnormal muscle insertions to the alar base are released.
- Release of the muscle from the overlying skin and ala allows the tethered, bunched-up muscle to be stretched, effectively elongating the lateral lip.
- The skin will also stretch in a similar manner, gaining increased vertical height (see Fig. 8.7).
- The orbicularis marginalis (OM) flap is incised along the free border of the lip to include the orbicularis marginalis muscle, the vermillion medial to point CPHL′, and the corresponding mucosa posteriorly.
- The OM flap is elevated to its base beneath the philtral column (CPHL′) in such a way that the volume of muscle at its base CPHL′ is similar to the volume of muscle at the opposite point CPHR on the non-cleft side of the lip.
- The OM flap is cut squarely and not beveled *(Fig. 8.12)*.
- The LLC is repositioned superiorly and fixed to the ULC with interrupted polyglactin sutures *(Fig. 8.13)*.
- The T-flap based on vestibular skin is rotated 90° to fill in the defect on piriform rim.
- Its superior edge is sutured to the piriform edge.
- The T-flap corrects mucosal deficiency and allows repositioning of the LLC and ala without restriction.

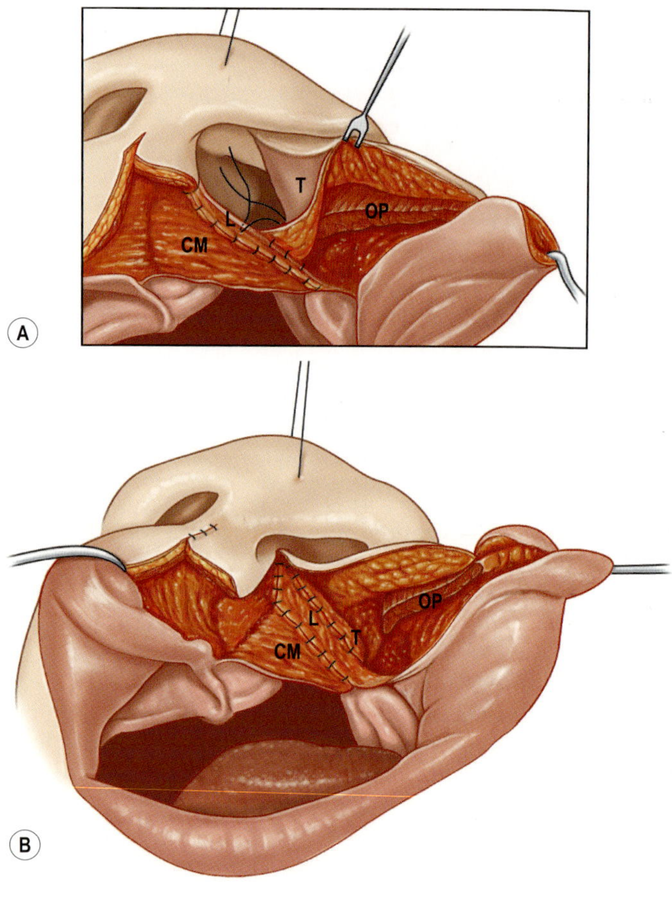

Figure 8.13 (A) The LLC is freed from its fibrous attachments to the maxilla and ULC. There is no dissection over the maxilla. The LLC is elevated with a traction suture and fixed to the ULC in an elevated position. The turbinate flap **(T)** is rotated into the piriform area. The nostril floor is reconstructed with the L-flap behind the columella, and the CM flap mucosa is sutured lateral to the maxilla. **(B)** Completion of nostril floor reconstruction with advancement of the vestibular skin rotating the alar base inward. There is good mucosal closure with no open areas for secondary healing and scar contracture. OP, orbicularis peripheralis muscle.

- The L-flap is rotated medially behind the columella and attached to the perichondrium of the previous incision behind the columella.
- The inferior edge of the T-flap is sutured to the superior edge of the L-flap with interrupted 5–0 polyglactin sutures.
- The C-flap mucosa is rotated laterally and placed below the L-flap.
- It is attached to the maxilla and sutured to the inferior edge of the L-flap.
- This gives good mucosal coverage of the nostril floor and lateral nostril wall without any raw surface or tension.
- The vestibular skin with attached ala is advanced over the mucosal bridge to the uppermost point of the previous incision behind the columella.
- The upper free edge of the vestibular skin flap and bridging T and L flaps are closed with interrupted 5–0 polyglactin sutures.
- This gives a good two-layer closure of the nostril floor and effectively corrects the tissue deficiency in this area.
- The vestibular skin is advanced as far as necessary to achieve a slightly over-corrected nostril width.
- This also advances and rotates the ala inward into a position slightly over-corrected to the opposite side.
- Final positioning and closure of the nostril floor are done after muscle reconstruction (see Fig. 8.13).
- The muscle is approximated with a 5–0 polydioxanone.
- A key suture is placed in the center of the muscle, opposite points CPHL and CPHL′ and pulled downward to level the Cupid's bow.
- This is to assure the correct placement of each muscle suture.
- The first stitch is passed through the caudal edge of the nasal septum, catching the tip of the muscle (which is originally inserted above and lateral to the cleft side alar base) in the advancement flap in a mattress fashion and anchored to the septum.
- This anchoring suture helps to pull the lateral lip medially and centralize the Cupid's bow.
- The muscle sutures are placed in such a way that the lateral muscle is overlapping above the medial muscle to increase the muscle thickness and simulate a philtral column.
- The muscle in OM flap is also sutured in a mattress fashion to avoid any depression in this area after operation ***(Fig. 8.14)***.
- The vermillion flap is marked and incised on the OM flap, while the OM flap is held under tension.
- A No. 11 blade is laid on the incision line, drawing the knife across to ensure an accurate cut.
- After the vermillion flap is incised, an incision is made along or above the red line of the lip beneath the Cupid's bow opposite point CPHL, thus opening the lip for eventual insertion of the vermillion flap after muscle approximation.
- The width of the vermillion flap should correct the vermillion deficiency under the Cupid's bow.
- The tip of the vermillion flap should not cross the natural lip tubercle ***(Fig. 8.15)***.

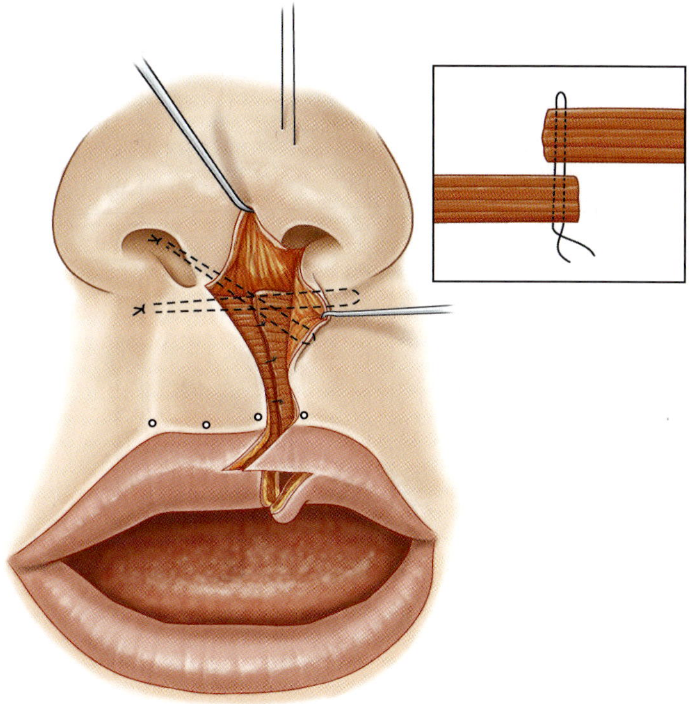

Figure 8.14 Orbicularis peripheralis muscle closure (with septal anchoring suture). Inset: Overlapping the lateral muscle on the medial muscle for philtral column reconstruction.

Closure

- Points CPHL and CPHL′ are approximated with a fine 7–0 absorbable polyglactin suture.
- The excess mucosa opposite points CPHL and CPHL′ on the free border of the lip is trimmed.
- The vermillion triangular flap should fit into the medial opening beneath the Cupid's bow ***(Fig. 8.16)***.
- Incisions on the vermillion are closed with continuous 7–0 polyglactin suture.
- The lateral lip buccal mucosa is trimmed and closed with interrupted fine absorbable sutures.
- The upper edge of the buccal mucosa is sutured to the C-flap mucosa that bridges the alveolar gap.
- This gives a complete mucosal closure without tension.
- The other tip of the C-flap (the most lateral point of skin overlying the premaxilla) is brought laterally. No lateral horizontal skin incision for the lateral advancement flap is made initially, as now the surgeon can better visualize how to make appropriate incisions that will eliminate incisions around the ala.
- If the alar base and the peak of the Cupid's bow on the cleft side are still high, an incision is made inside the cleft side nasal floor.
- If the alar base is already leveled after muscle reconstruction, a nasal floor incision is made.
- The tip of the advancement flap is sutured to the most lateral point on the junction of the C-flap and the rotation flap.
- The suture line on the lateral part of the rotation flap thus mimics the philtral ridge.

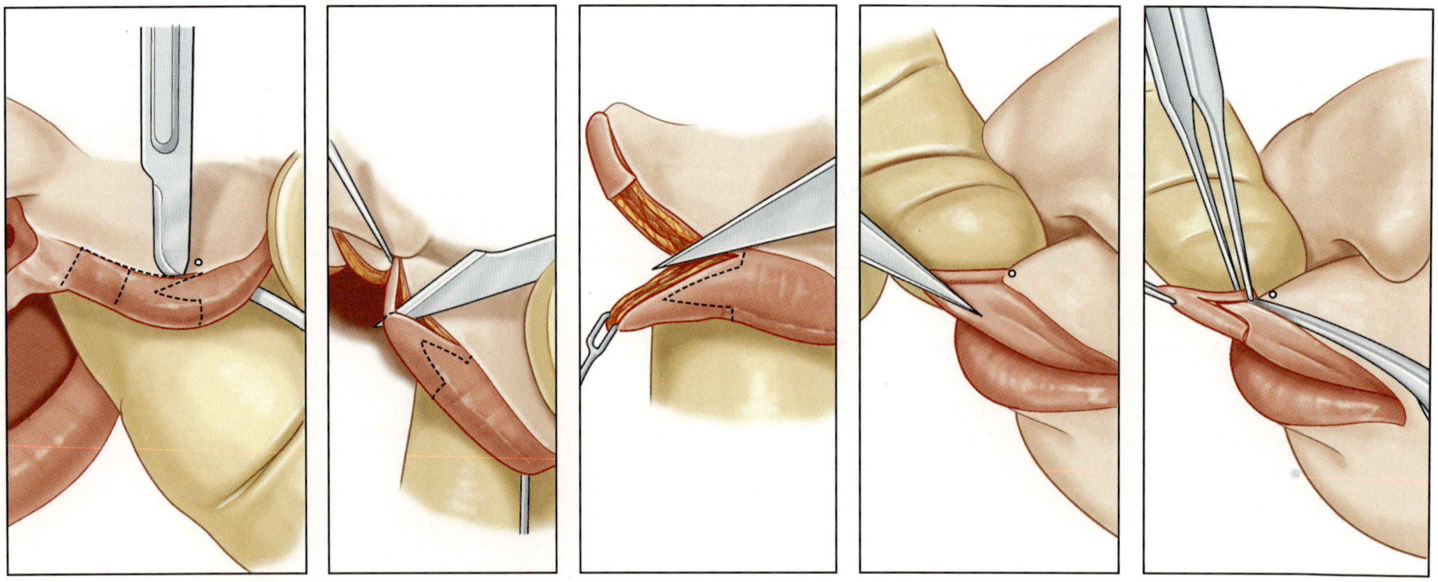

Figure 8.15 The vermillion flap is marked and incised on the OM flap while the OM flap is held under tension. The width of the vermillion flap should correct the vermillion deficiency under the Cupid's bow. The tip of the vermillion flap should not cross the natural lip tubercle.

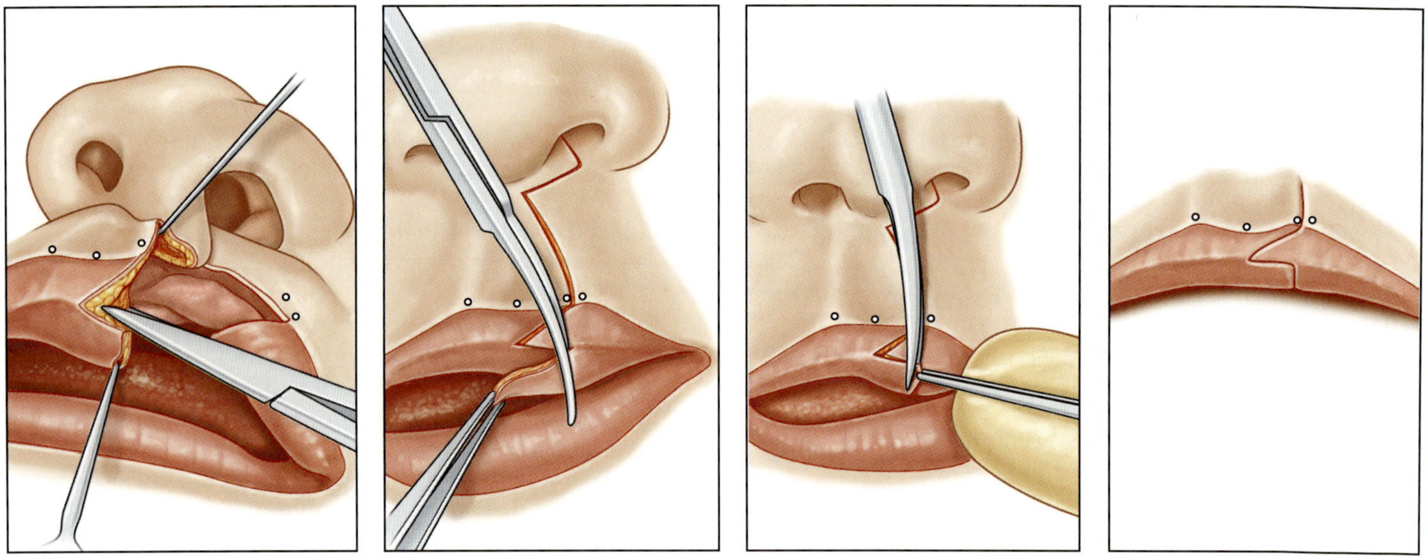

Figure 8.16 Medially, the lip is opened on the red line beneath the Cupid's bow for insertion of the vermillion flap. The excessive tissue on both medial and lateral lips is carefully trimmed.

- Excess skin on the nostril floor is excised as necessary with careful preservation of the nasal sill.
- The nasal floor is closed with 5–0 polyglactin sutures and lip skin is closed with 7–0 polyglactin sutures ***(Fig. 8.17)***.
- The small triangular WSR flap on the lateral lip is directly approximated to the medial lip to reconstruct the bulging of the WSR.
- If the WSR on the medial lip is less prominent, a small horizontal incision can be made slightly above the point; CPHL and the WSR flap from lateral lip can be inserted into medial lip for augmentation of the WSR above the CPHL.
- It is important to make any necessary minor adjustments before finishing the operation. The cleft side Cupid's bow must be adequately rotated.
- If it is slightly elevated, a small hook is used to place the Cupid's bow under tension and a short transverse incision is made above the white skin roll to release the Cupid's bow into its proper position.
- An appropriately sized small triangular skin flap, 1–2 mm in width, is incised from the lateral lip and filled into the defect above the white skin roll and secured with fine 7–0 polyglactin sutures ***(Fig. 8.18)***.
- This small triangular skin flap is also helpful to improve the lip pout as it tightens the skin above the white skin roll.

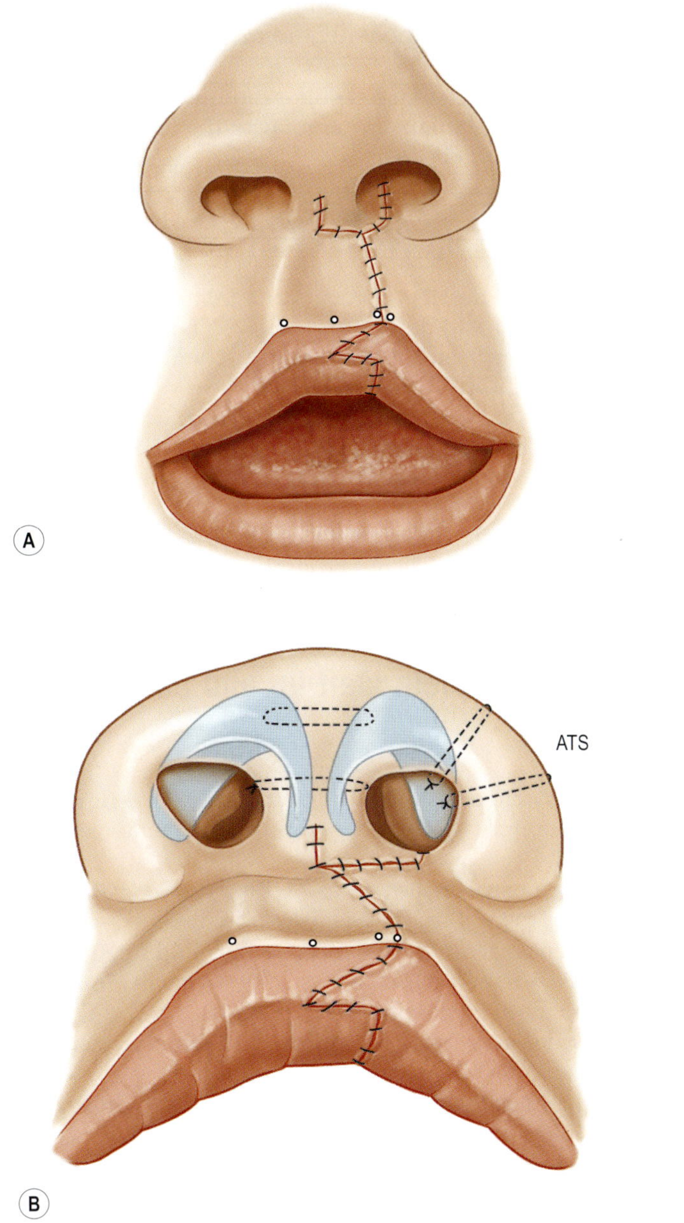

Figure 8.17 **(A)** Complete wound closure with columella elongation with the Mohler's rotation incision; note the laterally positioned philtral column. **(B)** Alar transfixion sutures (ATS) of 5–0 absorbable monofilament are placed with traction on the LLC. One suture is placed in the vestibular skin. The remaining sutures catch the leading edge of the LLC, pass through the alar-facial groove and back near the rim of the ala, and are tied on the inner side. Notching of the skin disappears within 1–2 weeks.

Addressing the cleft nasal deformity

- Most surgeons address the cleft nasal deformity at this stage by releasing the fibrofatty tissue over the nasal tip and LLC, and repositioning the LLCs through a "semi-open" approach.
- To release the fibrofatty tissue on the nasal tip and LLC, dissection is carried out over the LLCs using sharp scissors.
- The extent of dissection on the cleft side should be lateral to the groove on the caudal edge of the LLC to correct this groove.

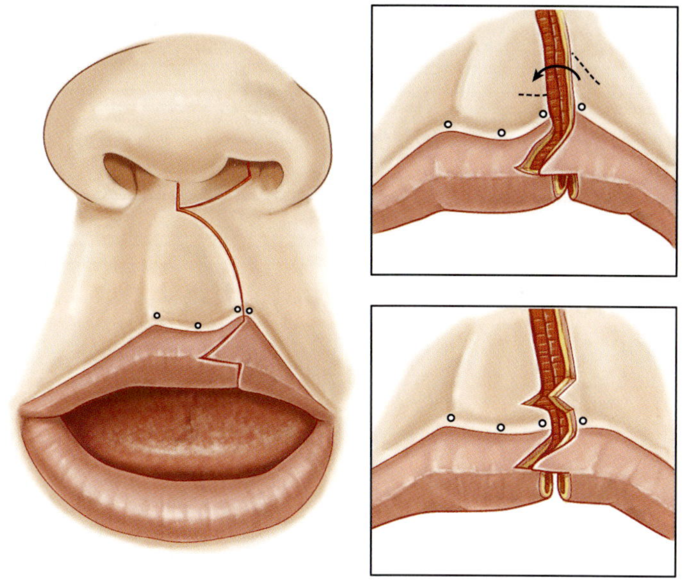

Figure 8.18 The skin closure is depicted to show inadequate rotation and peaking of the Cupid's bow. A horizontal incision is made above CPHL on the cleft side of the Cupid's bow to rotate it down. An appropriately sized triangular flap from the lateral lip skin is inserted into this defect to correct the deformity.

- The LLCs are approximated with 5–0 polydioxanone mattress sutures for medial rotation of the cleft side LLC.
- The stitches are placed more laterally on the cleft side LLC for over-correction. Through-and-through sutures placed on the medial crura for further support to the LLCs.
- The most important factor in achieving alar symmetry is releasing the abnormally attached paranasal muscles.
- In reconstructing the nostril floor, the alar base is advanced farther to its proper width compared with the normal side.
- The alar-facial groove is further accentuated by the approximation of the lip musculature.
- Mobilization of the alar base on cleft side will accentuate the vestibular webbing inside the cleft side nostril and alar transfixion sutures can help reduce this.
- Two sutures are usually required:
  - The lower suture is used to close the dead space and tack the vestibular webbing.
  - The upper suture catches the leading edge of the LLC and helps to support the LLC.
  - Skin dimpling from the sutures disappears 2 weeks after surgery (see Fig. 8.17).

Adjustments at cheiloplasty

- Making the necessary minor adjustments to achieve a satisfactory result is the enjoyment and challenge of cleft surgery. Every cleft is different and always needs minor adjustments.

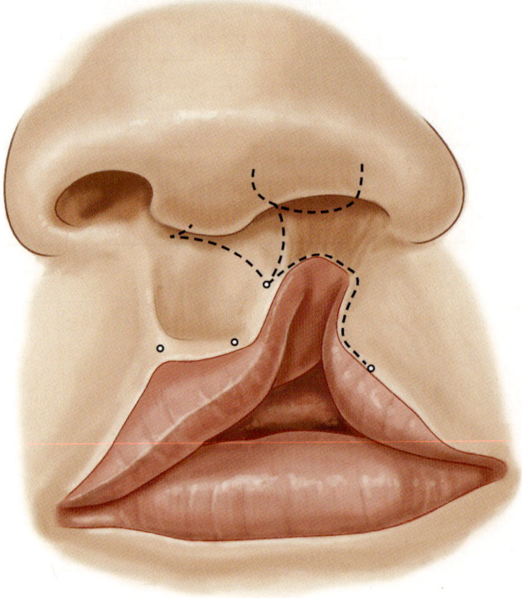

Figure 8.19 Markings for incision lines in incomplete clefts with incision made along the free edge of the skin.

Rotation advancement cheiloplasty for incomplete clefts

- The incomplete cleft lip is sometimes surprisingly difficult to reconstruct.
- The rotation incision and muscle dissection is made similar to complete clefts in a Mohler's fashion. The C-flap is raised similar to complete clefts. The incision on the advancement flap is made along the cleft edge. The WSR flap is also designed ***(Fig. 8.19)***.
- The technique and extent of muscle dissection is similar to complete clefts. Less muscle dissection tends to leave the abnormal muscle insertions to the alar base, which will cause the lateral and downward displacement of the alar base in secondary deformities. The OM flap is raised as in complete clefts.
- The local tissue on the nasal septum and piriform area is turned over and sutured to each other, matching the height of the nasal floor on non-cleft side nostril.
- Muscle reconstruction is performed as in complete clefts, using an anchoring suture to the septum for centralizing Cupid's bow. Overlapping mattress muscle sutures are used to reconstruct the philtral column.
- Nasal correction is performed as in complete clefts with a rim incision on non-cleft side nostril and reversed U incision (semi-open) on cleft side. The cartilage dissection, cartilage repositioning, alar transfixion sutures are the same.

Microform cleft lip

- Surgical correction of microform cleft lip has received less attention in the literature because of its minor deformity.
- Efforts have been made to eliminate the external scar as with traditional rotation-advancement or straight-line closures.
- The authors' preference is still a modified rotation advancement cheiloplasty similar to the technique used in incomplete cleft lips.

Bilateral cleft lip (Video 8.3)

Video 8.3

- The technical details for repair of a bilateral complete cleft lip and nasal deformity are given below, followed by modifications used for the major anatomic variants of bilateral cleft lip.
- The steps are portrayed as they proceed, which often requires turning attention from the lip to the nose, then back to the lip again, and ending with the final touches to the nose.
- Some leeway in the sequence of the procedure is possible but, in general, this is not advisable, until considerable experience is gained in these procedures.

Bilateral, complete cleft lip and palate

Markings

- The anatomic points are designated using the standard anthropometric initialisms, as in the unilateral cleft patient.
- With the nostrils held upward with a double-ball retractor, the philtral flap is drawn first.
- Its dimensions are determined by the child's age at repair (usually 5–6 months), and less so by ethnicity.
    - The length of the philtral flap (sn-ls) is set at 6–7 mm (normal male 11.4±1.3 mm at 6–12 months); usually it is the same as the cutaneous prolabium.
    - If the prolabial element is overly long, the philtral flap should be shortened appropriately.
    - The width of the philtral flap is set at 2 mm at the columellar–labial junction (cphs-cphs) and 3.5–4 mm between the proposed Cupid's bow peaks (cphi-cphi) (normal male 6.7±1.0 mm at 6–12 months).
    - The sides of the philtral flap should be drawn slightly concave in anticipation of slight bowing with growth.
- Flanking flaps are drawn which will be de-epithelialized and will come to lie beneath the lateral labial flaps in an effort to simulate elevation of philtral columns.
- The proposed Cupid's bow peaks are carefully noted on the lateral labial elements, and marked just atop the white roll above the vermillion-cutaneous junction.
- Curvilinear lines are drawn at the juncture of the alar bases and lateral labial elements. ***(Fig. 8.20)***.

Labial dissection

- First, all labial lines are lightly scored, the philtral flanking flaps are de-epithelialized, the extra prolabial skin is discarded, and the philtral flap is elevated (including subcutaneous tissue) up to the anterior nasal spine.

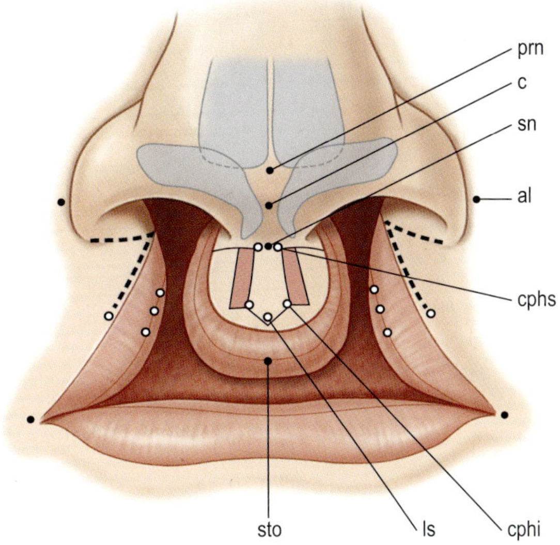

Figure 8.20 Markings for synchronous repair of bilateral cleft lip and nasal deformity. Open circles denote tattooed dots. Anthropometric points: nasion; pronasale (prn); highest point of columella nasi (c); subnasale (sn); ala nasi (al); crista philtri superior (cphs); crista philtri inferior (cphi); labiale superius (ls); stomion (sto).

- The lateral white-roll-vermillion-mucosal flaps are incised; however, stop these incisions about 2–3 mm short of the tattooed lateral Cupid's bow peak-points.
- The lateral labial elements are disjoined from the alar bases, and the basilar flaps are freed from the piriform attachments by incision along the lower section of the cutaneo-mucosal junction.
- The mucosal incisions are extended distal along the gingivolabial sulcus to the premolar region.
- With a double-hook on the muscular layer, the lateral labial elements are widely dissected off the maxillae in the supraperiosteal plane.
- The non-dominant ring finger is held on the infraorbital rim (to protect the globe) as the dissection is further extended over the malar eminence ***(Fig. 8.21)***.
- Extensive release of the lateral labial segments is a critical maneuver so as to minimize tension at the muscular and cutaneous closure.
- The orbicularis oris bundles are dissected in the subdermal and submucosal plane for 1 cm, or a little further if necessary ***(Fig. 8.22)***.

Alveolar closure

The lateral nasal mucosal flaps are released from beneath the inferior turbinates, the medial nasal mucosal flaps are elevated from the premaxilla, and the nasal floors are closed.

The premaxillary mucosal incisions are continued on each side and vertical incisions are made in the facing gingiva of the lesser segments.

The alar base flaps are advanced medially and the inner edge is sutured to the anterior edge of the constructed nasal floors.

The thin strip of vermillion is trimmed off the premaxillary mucosa and the remaining mucosal flange is secured high to the premaxillary periosteum to construct the posterior side of the central gingivolabial sulcus ***(Fig. 8.23)***.

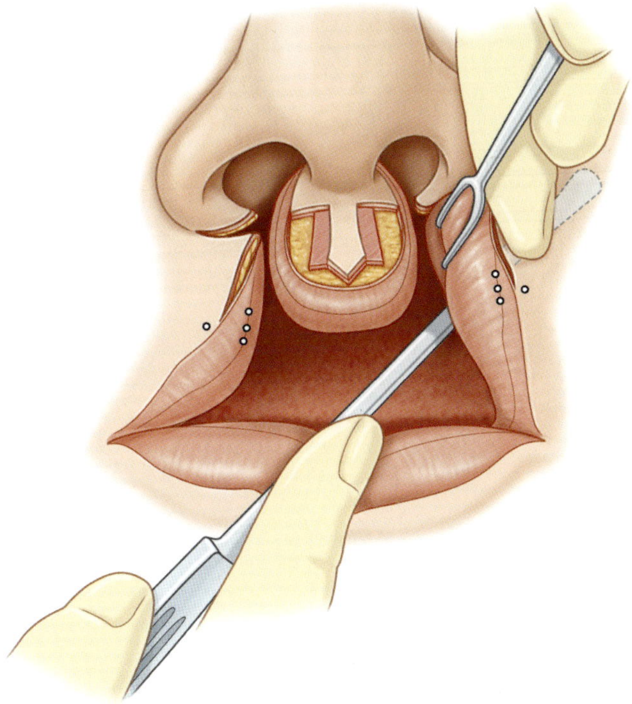

Figure 8.21 Lateral labial elements dissected off maxilla in supra-periosteal plane, extending over the malar eminences.

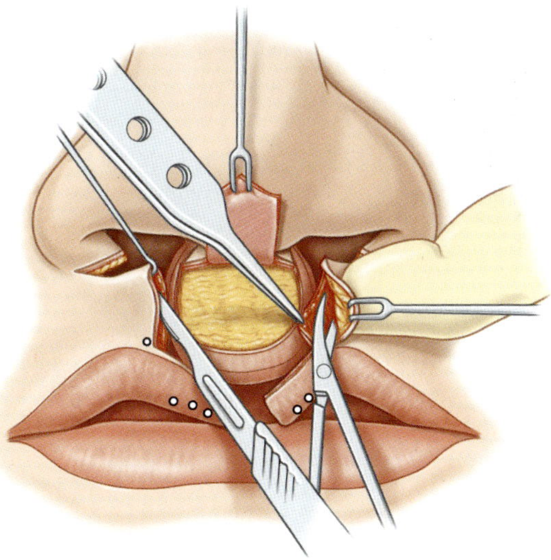

Figure 8.22 Dissection of orbicularis oris muscle bundles in subdermal and submucosal planes.

Labial closure

- Advancement of the lateral labial elements during closure of the sulci is critical.
- A back-cut is made at the distal end of the sulcal incision, and each sulcus is closed while the labial flap is being pulled mesially with a double hook.

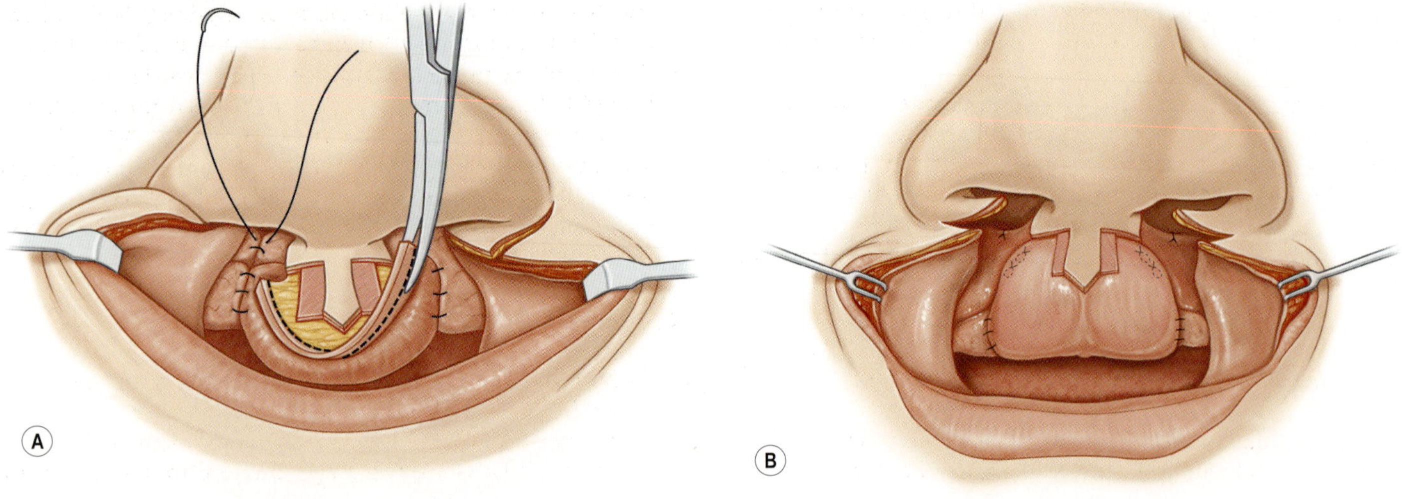

Figure 8.23 **(A)** After completion of gingivoperiosteoplasty, redundant premaxillary vermillion trimmed. **(B)** Remaining premaxillary mucosal flange sutured to periosteum forming posterior wall of anterior gingivolabial sulcus.

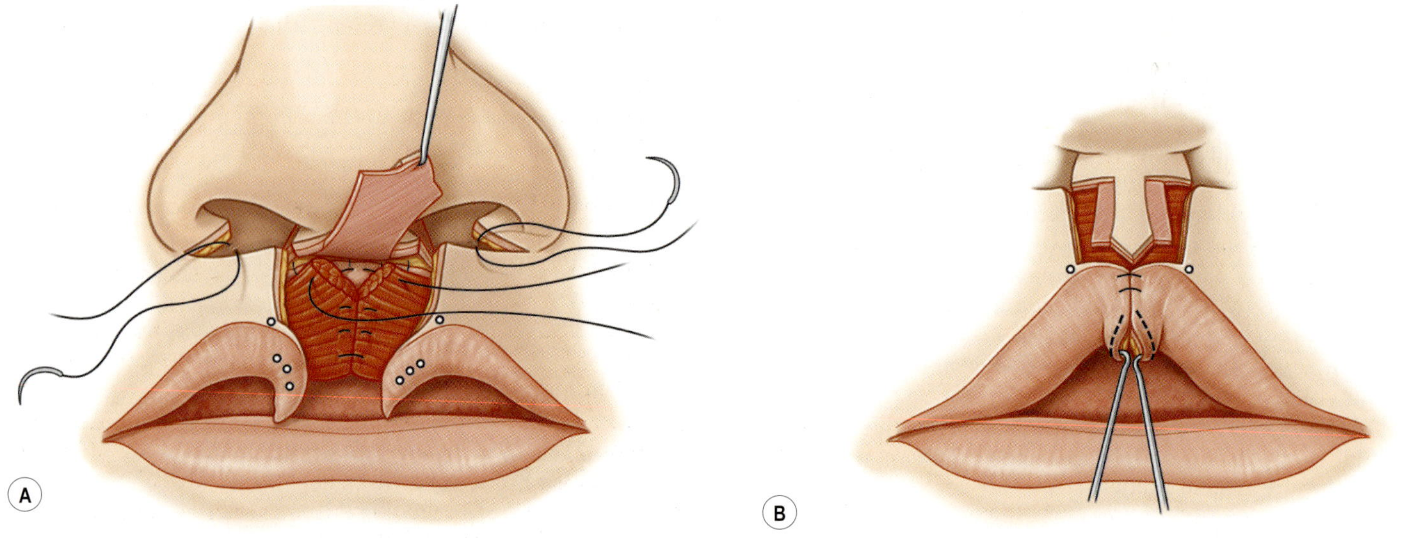

Figure 8.24 **(A)** Apposition of orbicularis oris from inferior-to-superior; uppermost suture placed through periosteum of anterior nasal spine. **(B)** Lateral white-roll-vermillion-mucosal flaps trimmed to construct median tubercle and Cupid's bow.

- The advanced lateral labial mucosa forms the anterior wall of the central gingivolabial sulcus.
- The orbicular bundles are apposed (end-to-end), inferiorly-to-superiorly, using simple polydioxanone sutures.
- Prior to completion of the muscular closure, a polydioxanone suture is placed on each side through the maxillary periosteum in the region of the origin of the depressor alae nasi and left untied.
- A polypropylene suture suspends the uppermost muscular elements to the periosteum of the anterior nasal spine ***(Fig. 8.24A)***.
- Construction of the median tubercle begins with placement of a fine chromic suture, about 3 mm medial to the tattooed lateral Cupid's bow peak-point, joining the white-roll-vermillion-mucosal flaps in the midline (Fig. 8.24B).
- The excess vermillion-mucosa is successively trimmed from each flap, and the flaps are accurately aligned to form the median raphe.
- Nasal dissection and positioning the lower lateral cartilages
- The slumped/splayed lower lateral cartilages are visualized through bilateral rim incisions ("semi-open" approach).
- Fibrofatty tissue is dissected off the anterior surface of and in between the cartilages:
- This is aided by elevation with a cotton-tipped applicator on the mucosal underside.
- Dissection is continued across the dorsal septum to expose the upper lateral cartilages ***(Fig. 8.25)***.
- With direct visualization, a horizontal mattress suture of 5–0 polydioxanone (1/2 circle cutting needle) is placed between the genua and left untied.

- Another mattress suture is inserted through each upper lateral cartilage and then through the ipsilateral lateral crus.
- Often it is possible to place a second suture to suspend the lateral crus to the upper lateral cartilage.
- Holding an intranasal cotton-tipped applicator, beneath the genu and tenting the nostril roof, facilitates the insertion and tying of these sutures ***(Fig. 8.26)***.
- The C-flap on each side of the columellar base is trimmed to 3–5 mm in length ***(Fig 8.27A)***.
- The alar bases are advanced medially, rotated endonasally, and sutured side-to-end to the C-flaps.
- Next, the tips of the alar base flaps are trimmed to complete closure of the sills.
- A "cinch suture" of polypropylene is placed through the dermis of each alar base, passing under the philtral flap, and tied to narrow the inter-alar dimension (al-al) to less than 25 mm (normal male 26±1.4 mm at 6–12 months).
- The maxillary periosteal sutures, placed earlier, are brought above the muscular layer, inserted through the alar bases (superficial to the "cinch suture") and tied.
- This suture simulates the depressor alae nasi and also: (1) forms the cymal shape of the sills; (2) prevents alar elevation with smiling; (3) minimizes postoperative nasal widening (see Fig. 8.27B).

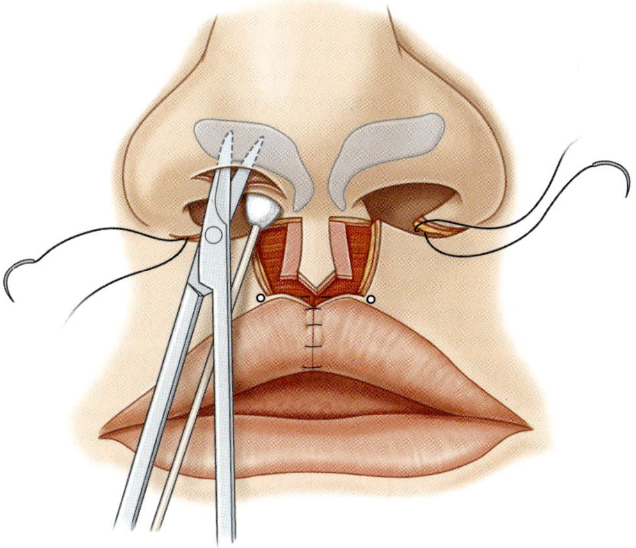

Figure 8.25 Lower lateral cartilages exposed through rim incisions. Cotton-tipped applicator elevates nostril and helps display genua.

Final touches

- Fashioning a philtral dimple seems just beyond the surgeon's skill, nevertheless, it is worth trying.
- One way to simulate this depression is to suture the dermis in the lower one-third of the philtral flap down to the orbicularis layer.
- The tip of the philtral flap is inset into the handle of the Cupid's bow.
- The leading edge of the lateral labial flaps should not be trimmed before apposition to the philtral flap.
- A little extra lateral labial tissue helps to simulate the columns.
- There should be no tension at the philtral closure, which is done with fine, interrupted dermal and percutaneous sutures.
- The cephalic margin of the labial flaps must be trimmed, corresponding to the position and cymal configuration of the sills ***(Fig. 8.28)***.
- Closure of the labial flaps to the sills proceeds laterally-to-medially.
- After anatomic positioning of the lower lateral cartilages, it is obvious that there is redundant domal skin in the soft triangles and in the upper columella.
- This extra skin is excised in a crescentic fashion from the leading edge of the rim incisions and extending inferiorly along each side of the columella (see Fig. 8.28).
- This resection narrows the nasal tip, defines and tapers the midcolumella, and elongates the nostrils.

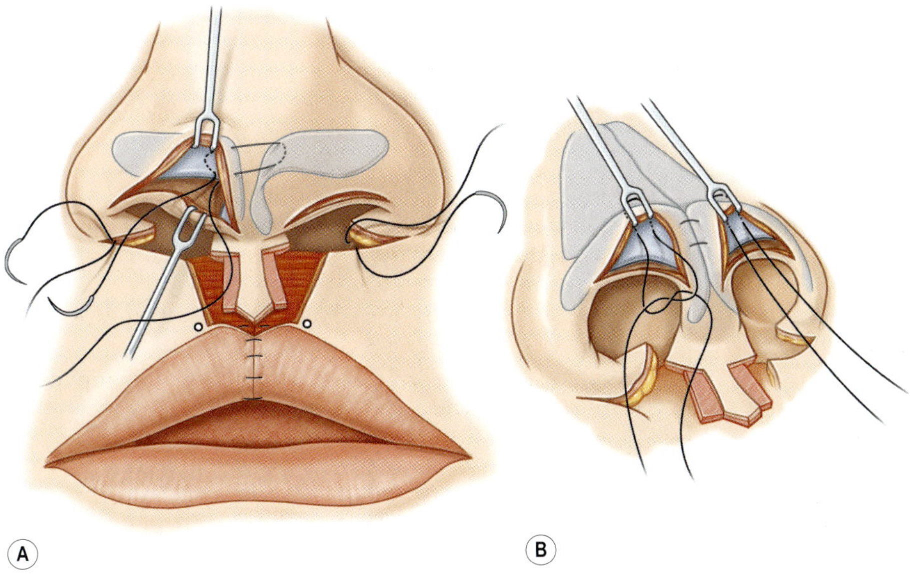

Figure 8.26 Positioning dislocated and splayed lower lateral cartilages: **(A)** Apposition of genua with interdomal mattress suture; **(B)** suspension over ipsilateral upper lateral cartilage with inter-cartilaginous mattress suture.

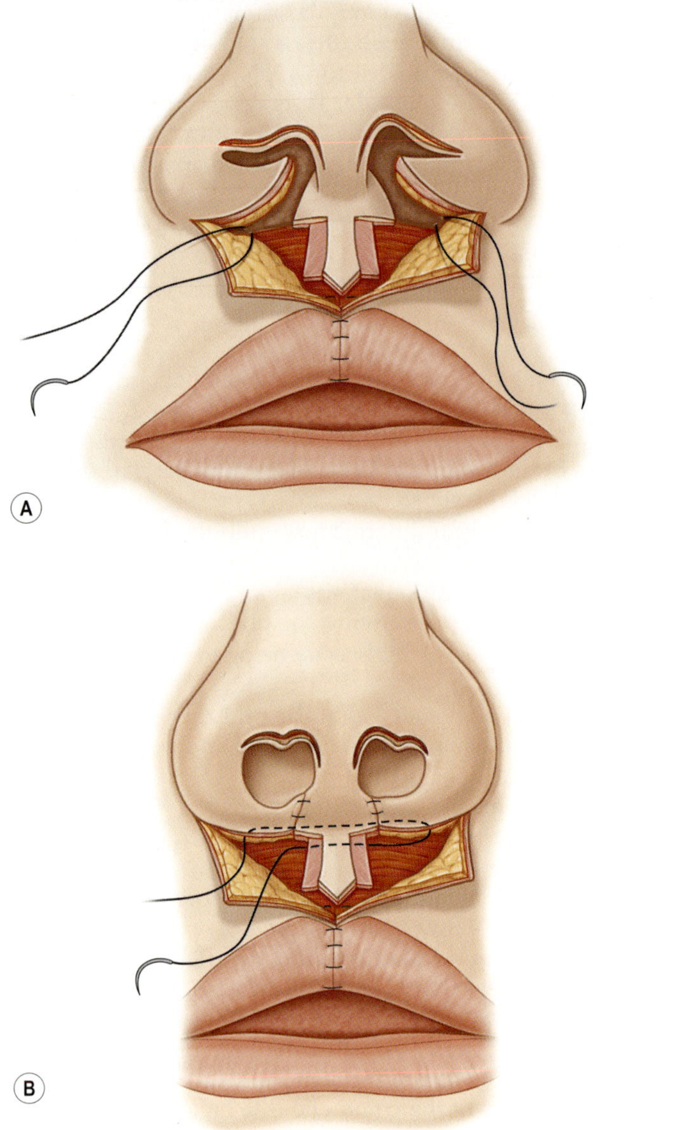

Figure 8.27 **(A)** Columellar flaps shortened and alar bases trimmed. Note bilateral sutures in maxillary periosteum below alar bases – these sutures were inserted prior to completion of muscular closure. **(B)** Alar base flaps rotated endonasally and secured (side-to-end) to C-flaps. Interalar distance narrowed with cinch suture. Right maxillary periosteal suture to alar base has been tied – note cymal configuration (depression) of lateral sill.

- Apposition of the genua also accentuates the extra lining (oblique webbing) in the lateral vestibules.
- Lenticular excision on the cutaneous side of the intercartilaginous junction flattens this lateral ridge (see Fig. 8.28, inset).
- Immediately postoperative nasolabial anthropometry is documented and placed in the child's record *(Fig. 8.29)*.
- The constructed columella (sn-c) is usually 5–6 mm, (normal male 4.7±0.8 mm at 5 months).
- After the measurements, a strip of ¼ inch Xeroform® gauze is wrapped around a 19 G silicone tubing and a 1 cm segment is inserted into each nostril.
- These vented "stents" are removed after 48 h.
- Prolonged nostril splinting is difficult to maintain, likely to damage the sills, and unnecessary.

Late presentation of bilateral complete cleft lip/palate

- Rather than attempt labial closure over a protrusive premaxilla, consider ostectomy and set-back. There are two alternatives: (1) premaxillary set-back and nasolabial repair or (2) premaxillary set-back and palatoplasty.
- The second alternative, premaxillary set-back, gingivoperiosteoplasties, and palatoplasty, is the safer procedure.
- It is recommended if the child is nearing age 1 year or older when speech is the first priority.
- Bilateral nasolabial repair on a solid maxillary foundation is scheduled later.

Bilateral incomplete cleft lip

- One-quarter of all double labial clefts are incomplete cleft lip; most are symmetrical.
- Of all the bilateral variants, this is the most easily repaired.
- The design and execution are the same as for the bilateral complete form, including adjustments based on expected nasolabial changes with growth.
- There are two technical considerations that need to be underscored.
- Construction of the median tubercle:
- Usually formed using the lateral white-roll-vermillion-mucosal flaps, in the rare instance of a bilateral lesser-form (<50% of cutaneous labial height) and a prominent central white roll, the prolabial vermillion-mucosa may be utilized as the central segment.
- Columellar length:
- If columellar length is normal for the infant's age and the lower lateral cartilages are in nearly normal position, it may be unnecessary to position the cartilages and sculpt the tip. (*Fig. 8.30,* Table 8.2).

Table 8.2 Intraoperative anthropometry. Fast-growing features made smaller and slow-growing dimensions made larger than normal age/sex-matched values

Intraoperative	Patient (6 months)	Normal (6–12 months)
n-sn	20.0[a]	27.0±1.7
al-al	24.5[a]	26.5±1.4
sn-prn	12.3[a]	9.1±1.2
sn-c	6.0[a]	4.3±0.9
cphs-cphs	2.0	NA
cphi-cphi	5.0[a]	6.7±1.0
sn-ls	7.0[a]	11.4±1.3
sn-sto	14.5	15.8±1.5
ls-sto	7.0[a]	4.4±1.0

Normal values expressed as norm±SD. [a]Values outside SD. NA, not available.

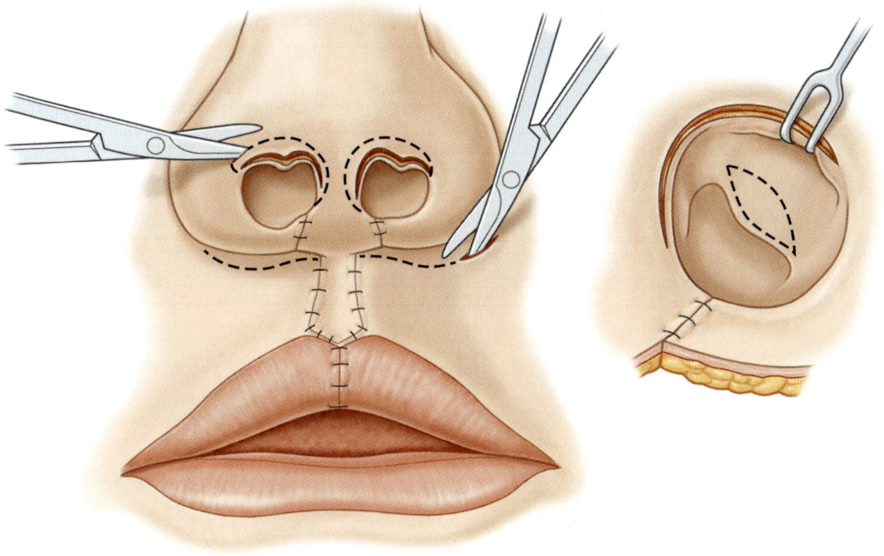

Figure 8.28 Crescentic excision of expanded domal skin and lining extended into upper columella. Cyma-shaped resection of superior margin of lateral labial elements to fit curve of the alar base and sill. Lenticular excision of lateral vestibular web (inset).

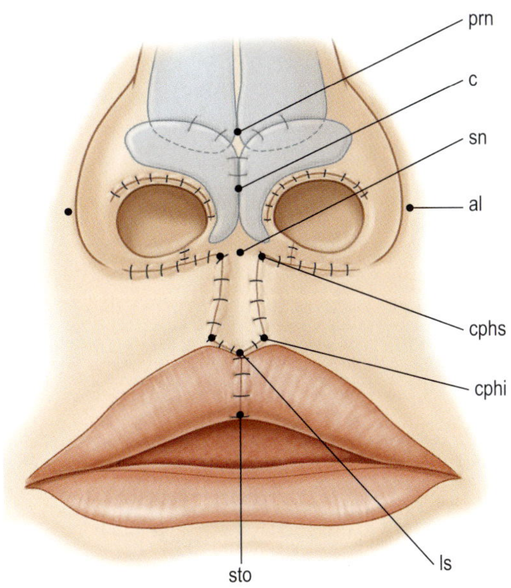

Figure 8.29 Completed bilateral complete cleft lip/nasal repair. Pronasale (prn); highest point of columella nasi (c); subnasale (sn); ala nasi (al); crista philtri superior (cphs); crista philtri inferior (cphi); labiale superius (ls); stomion (sto).

Asymmetrical bilateral (complete/incomplete) cleft lip

- Symmetry, the first principle of bilateral labial repair, should be foremost in mind when planning and executing closure of an asymmetrical variant.
- An algorithm for timing and techniques for repair of asymmetrical bilateral cleft lip is shown in ***Figure 8.31***.

Postoperative considerations

- A soft nipple with good flow is used with bottle-feeding.
- Feeding is started as soon as the baby desires.
- Parents are instructed in suture-line care and how to keep the nostrils clean.
- Antibiotic ointment is often placed on the suture line after it is cleaned, keeping it from drying out or crusting.
- Postsurgical molding with silicone nasal conformers has been used in many centers to support the lower lateral cartilages during the healing phase and to prevent contracture and nasal stenosis.
- If used, the parents are instructed to use the conformers full-time for 6 months to 1 year if possible.
- Success in nasal conformer use depends more upon the cooperation of the parents rather than the compliance of the patients.
- After bilateral lip repair, Dr Mulliken utilizes a Logan bow, which is taped to the cheeks to protect the labial repair and to hold an iced-saline sponge over the wound for 24 h postoperatively.
- Percutaneous sutures are removed 5–6 days postoperatively under general anesthesia using mask induction and insufflation.
- After suture removal, a ½ inch transverse Steri-Strip® (3M Health Care, St Paul, Minnesota) can be trimmed and placed over the labial scars to aid healing.
- If placed, the tape is typically changed as needed for 6 weeks.
- After adequate healing has occurred, the parents are instructed how to perform digital massage to hasten scar maturity and counseled about the importance of application of sun-block ointment (***Fig. 8.32***, Table 8.3).

Complications and outcomes

- A symmetrical balanced lip is the goal of cleft lip repair. Patient and parental satisfaction is largely dependent upon psychosocial adaptation.
- Complications can include lip asymmetry, infection, dehiscence, and hypertrophic scarring.

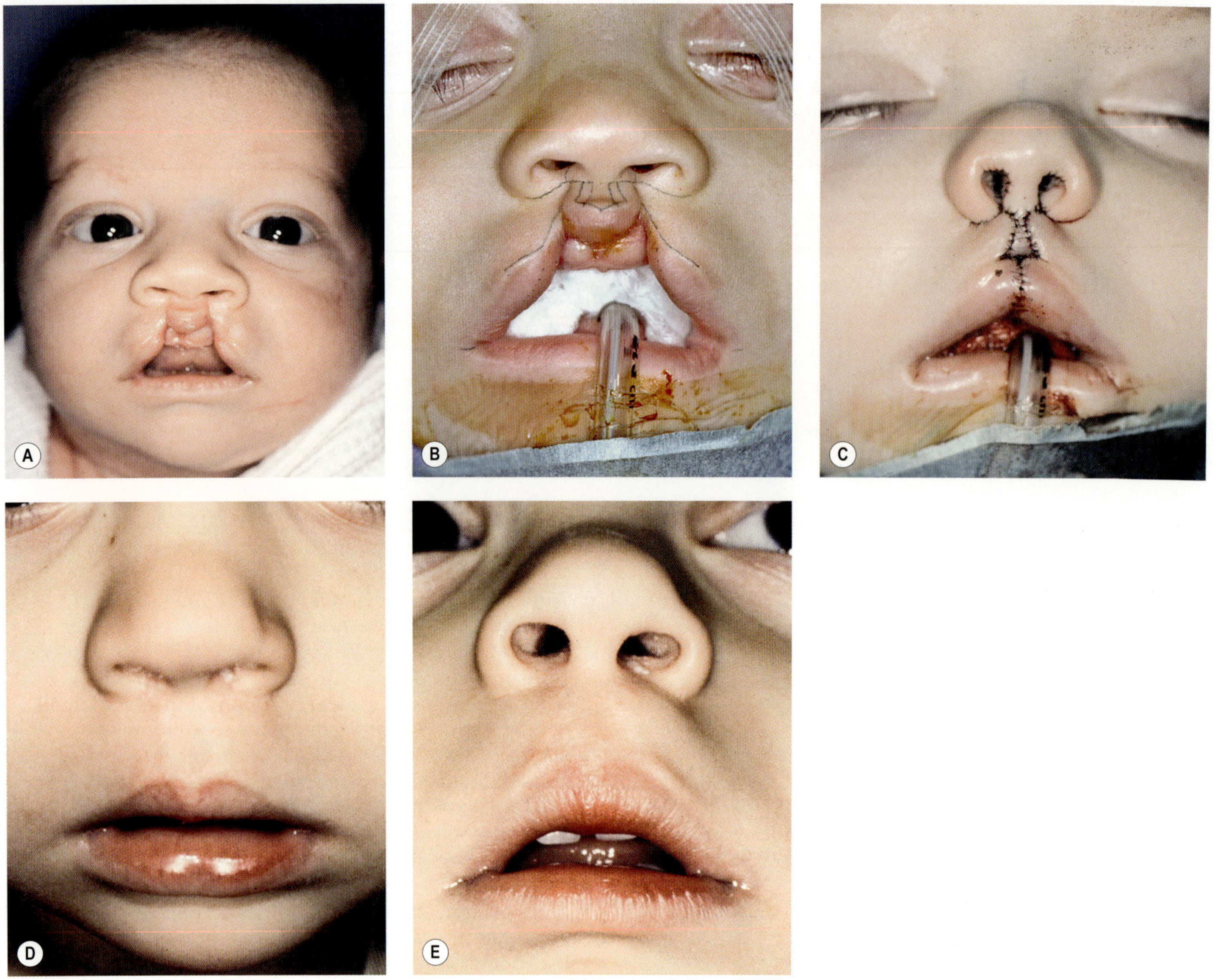

Figure 8.30 **(A)** Bilateral symmetrical incomplete cleft lip. **(B)** Markings for synchronous closure at age 6 months. **(C)** Following nasolabial repair. **(D,E)** Appearance at age 1.5 years.

- It is not uncommon to have notching at the height of Cupid's bow on the cleft side as well as vermillion irregularities.
- Symmetry is the one major advantage of a bilateral complete cleft lip as compared to a unilateral complete cleft lip.
- Any nasolabial asymmetry following closure and further distortions with growth will become increasingly obvious before the child attends school.
- In a study of 50 consecutive non-syndromic children (median age 5.4 years), the revision rate was 33% for those with bilateral complete cleft lip/palate as compared to 12% for those with bilateral complete cleft lip/alveolus and intact secondary palate
- The most common labial revision was resuspension of prolapsed anterior gingivolabial mucosa. This problem has since been minimized by trimming prolabial vermillion and securing the remaining mucosa to the premaxillary periosteum.

Table 8.3 **Immediate postoperative anthropometry documents under-corrected fast-growing features and over-corrected slow-growing features compared with normal values**

Intraoperative	Patient (7 months)	Normal (6–12 months)
n-sn	20.0[a]	26.9±1.6
al-al	24.5	25.4±1.5
sn-prn	10.5	9.7±0.8
sn-c	6.0[a]	4.7±0.8
cphs-cphs	1.5	NA
cphi-cphi	4.5[a]	6.5±1.1
sn-ls	5.5[a]	10.7±1.1
sn-sto	11.2[a]	16.0±0.8
ls-sto	6.2	5.3±1.4

Normal values expressed as norm±SD. [a]Values outside SD. NA, not available.

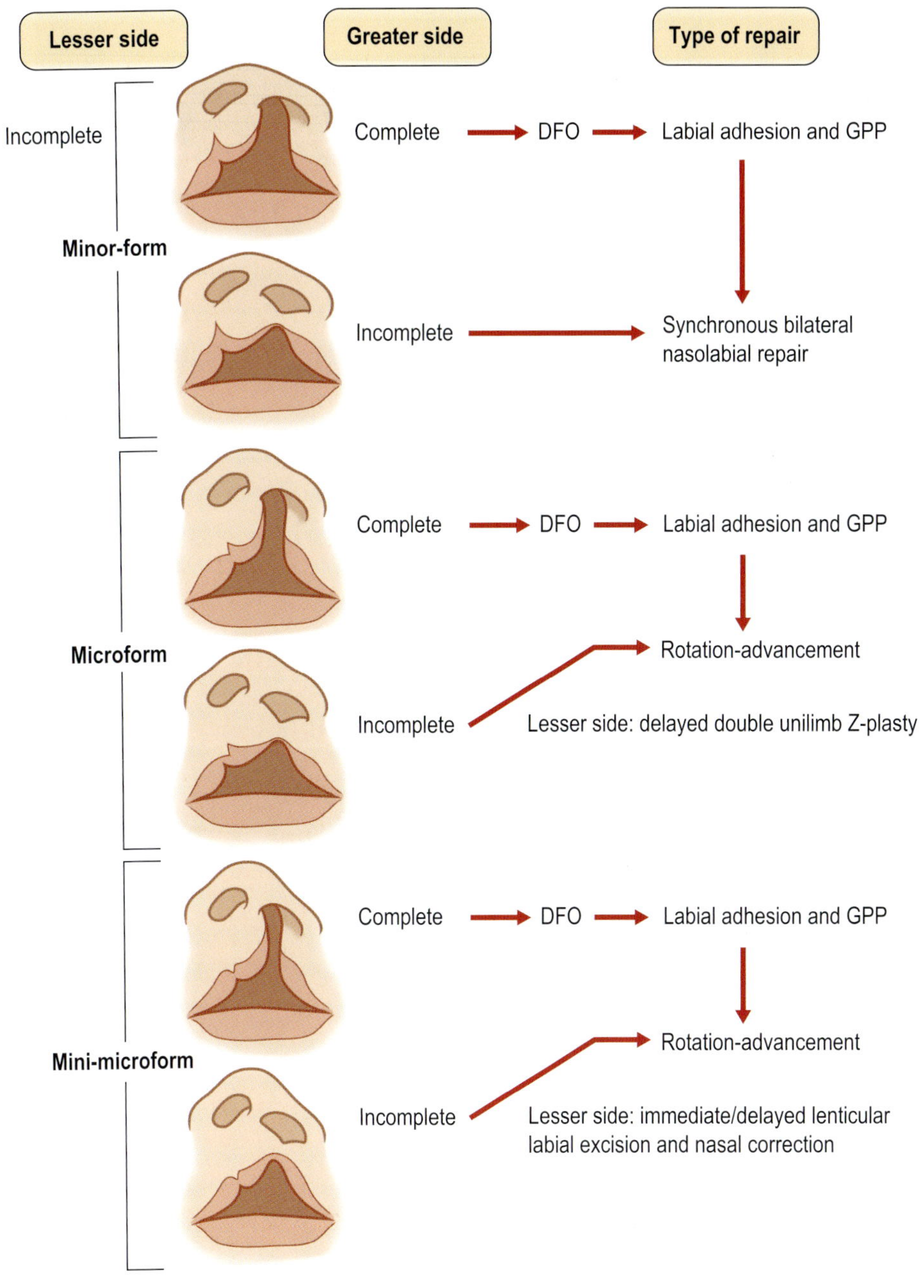

Figure 8.31 Algorithm for correction of asymmetrical bilateral cleft lip (complete/incomplete) and contralateral incomplete or lesser-form cleft. DFO, dentofacial orthopedics; GPP, gingivoperiosteoplasty. (Modified from Yuzuriha et al. 2008.)

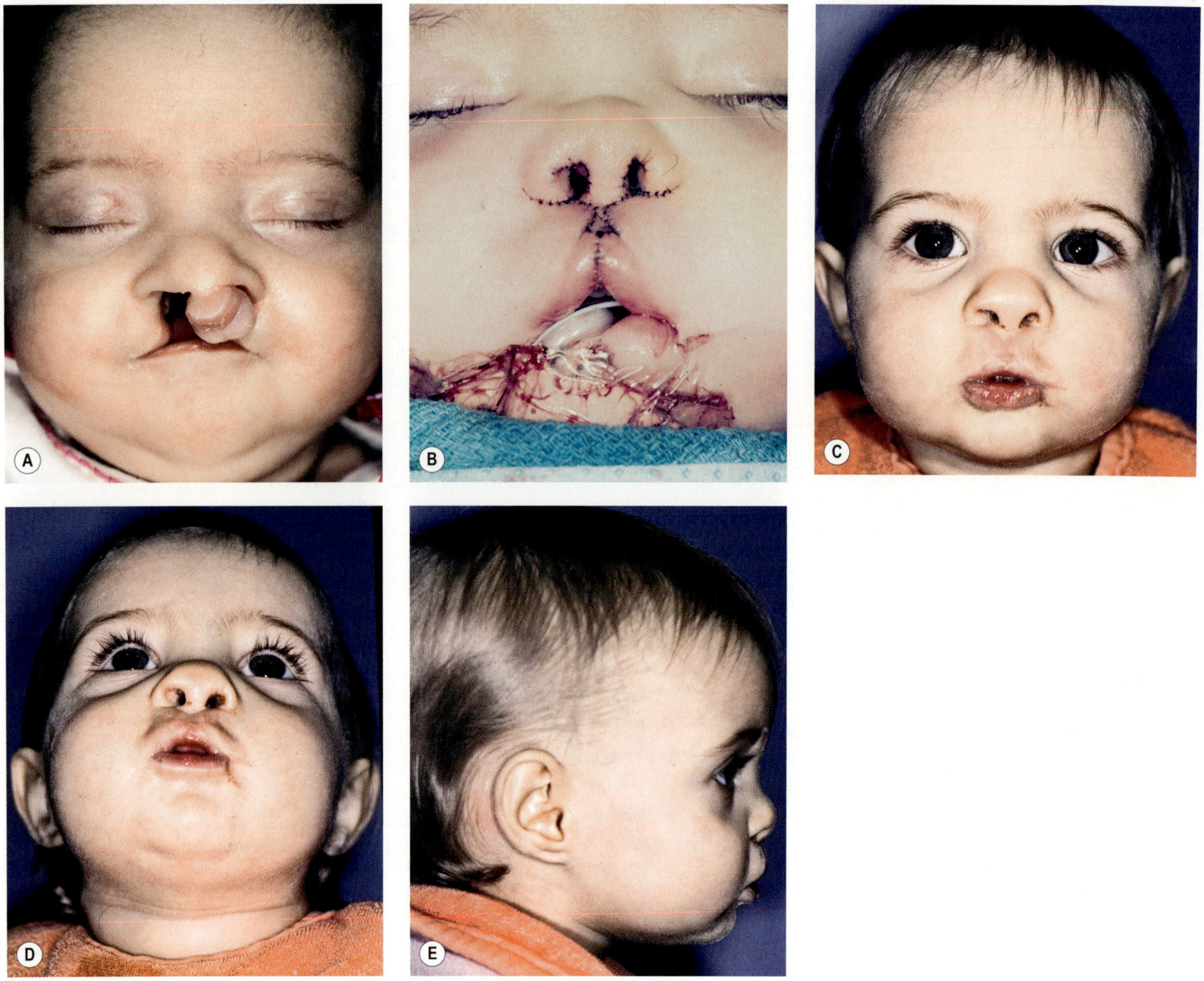

Figure 8.32 (A) Bilateral complete cleft lip/palate. **(B)** Following synchronous nasolabial repair at 6 months. **(C,D,E)** At 4 months postoperative. Note columella/tip projection, hint of a philtral dimple, and normal columellar-labial angle.

Further reading

Barillas I, Dec W, Warren SM, et al. Nasoalveolar molding improves long-term nasal symmetry in complete unilateral cleft lip-cleft palate patients. *Plast Reconstr Surg*. 2009;123(3):1002–1006.

This paper demonstrated that the lower lateral and septal cartilages are more symmetric in patients with nasoalveolar molding compared with the surgery-alone patients. Furthermore, the improved symmetry can be maintained at 9 years of age.

Cutting CB, Grayson BH, Brecht L, et al. Presurgical columellar elongation and primary retrograde nasal reconstruction in one-stage bilateral cleft lip and nose repair. *Plast Reconstr Surg*. 1998;101:630–639.

The article describes the prototype of a nasoalveolar molding appliance in preparation for synchronous nasolabial repair by Cutting's technique. The authors underscore that expansion of nasal lining is as important as stretching columellar skin. The principle of primary positioning the lower lateral cartilages is applied as described in this chapter; however, the technique differs.

Farkas LG, ed. *Anthropometry of the Head and Face*. 2nd ed. New York: Raven Press; 1994.

Grayson BH, Garfinkle JS. Nasoalveolar molding and columellar elongation in preparation for primary repair of unilateral and bilateral cleft lip and palate. In: Losee JE, ed. *Comprehensive Cleft Care*. New York: McGraw Hill; 2009:701–720.

Lee CT, Garfinkle JS, Warren SM, et al. Nasoalveolar molding improves appearance of children with bilateral cleft lip-cleft palate. *Plast Reconstr Surg.* 2008;122:1131–1137.

This study provides further proof of the principle of primary nasal correction. Photogrammetry was used to document columellar length in patients with bilateral cleft lip/palate who had nasal repair by the two-stage forked flap method versus primary nasal correction after nasoalveolar molding; both groups were compared to age-matched controls. Measurements to age 3 years showed nearly normal columellar length in the primary repair group without need for further nasal procedures, whereas secondary operations were recommended for all children who had forked flap columellar lengthening.

Liou EJ, Subramanian M, Chen PKT, et al. The progressive changes of nasal symmetry and growth after nasoalveolar molding: a three-year follow-up study. *Plast Reconstr Surg.* 2004;114(4):858–864.

This paper revealed that in patients with unilateral complete cleft lips, the nasal asymmetry was significantly improved after nasoalveolar molding and was further improved after primary cheiloplasty. However, after surgery, the nasal asymmetry significantly relapsed in the first year postoperatively and then remained stable and well afterward. The authors recommend (1) narrowing down the alveolar cleft as well as possible by nasoalveolar molding; (2) overcorrecting the nasal vertical dimension surgically; and (3) maintaining the surgical results using a nasal conformer.

Lo L-J, Wong F-H, Mardini S, et al. Assessment of bilateral cleft lip nose deformity: A comparison of results as judged by cleft surgeons and laypersons. *Plast Reconstr Surg.* 2002;110:733–741.

Millard Jr DR, ed. *The unilateral deformity. Cleft Craft: The Evolution of Its Surgery.* Vol I. Boston: Little, Brown; 1976.

Millard Jr DR. *Cleft Craft: The Evolution of Its Surgery.* Vol II. Boston: Little, Brown; 1977.

One definition of a "classic" is a great book that is often cited, but seldom read. In his conversational style of writing, Millard recounts the history of bilateral cleft lip repair as if he was an observer. The novice may find the organization of the book a little difficult to follow. Nevertheless, reading Millard's text is analogous to watching a master-surgeon in the operating room. The more experienced the visitor, the more gained by the experience.

Mohler L. Unilateral cleft lip repair. *Plast Reconstr Surg.* 1995;2:193–199.

This paper introduced a modification of the original rotation-advancement technique by changing the direction of the rotation incision to the "mirror-image of the noncleft side philtral column" that resulted in a more natural looking lip.

Morris HL, ed. *Multidisciplinary Management of Cleft Lip and Palate.* Philadelphia: WB Saunders; 1990:18–26.

Mulliken JB, Martinez-Perez D. The principle of rotation advancement for repair of unilateral complete cleft lip and nasal deformity: technical variations and analysis of results. *Plast Reconstr Surg.* 1999;104:1247–1260.

Mulliken JB, Burvin R, Farkas LG. Repair of bilateral complete cleft lip: Intraoperative nasolabial anthropometry. *Plast Reconstr Surg.* 2001;107:307–314.

Mulliken JB, Wu JK, Padwa BL. Repair of bilateral cleft lip: Review, revisions, and reflections. *J Craniofac Surg.* 2003;14:609–620.

Mulliken JB, Burvin R, Padwa BL. Binderoid complete cleft lip/palate. *Plast Reconstr Surg.* 2003;111:1000–1010.

The authors define a rare subset of patients who have complete cleft lip/palate, nasolabiomaxillary underdevelopment, and orbital hypertelorism. One-half of the patients have a bilateral complete deformity, characterized by a diminutive single-toothed premaxilla. Necessary modifications in primary repair and in secondary correction of the hypoplastic soft tissue and skeletal elements are described.

Noordhoff MS, Huang CS, Wu J. Multidisciplinary management of cleft lip and palate in Taiwan. In: Bardach J, Noordhoff MS, Chen PK. *Unilateral cheiloplasty.* In: Mathes ST, ed. Plastic Surgery. Vol 4. Philadelphia: WB Saunders; 2006.

Salyer KE, Genecov E, Genecov D. Unilateral cleft lip-nose repair: A 33-year experience. *J Craniofac Surg.* 2003;14(4):549–558.

A 33-year experience in over 750 patients with a proven method of repair for primary unilateral cleft lip-nose is presented in this paper. Approximately 35% of them needed a minor revision in preschool age and most of them received an aesthetic rhinoplasty after growth was completed. This long-term experience showed that with primary nasal reconstruction, self-esteem was enhanced in cleft patients.

Wong JY, Oh AK, Ohta E, et al. Validity and reliability of craniofacial anthropometric measurements of 3D digital photogrammetric images. *Cleft Palate Craniofac J.* 2008;45:232–239.

Yeow VK, Chen PKT, Chen YR, et al. The use of nasal splints in the primary management of unilateral cleft nasal deformity. *Plast Reconstr Surg.* 1999;103(5):1347–1354.

This paper shows that postoperative nasal splinting in the primary management of the unilateral cleft nasal deformity serves to preserve and maintain the corrected position of the nose after primary lip and nasal correction, resulting in a significantly improved aesthetic result. The authors recommend that all patients undergoing primary correction of complete unilateral cleft deformity use the nasal retainer postoperatively for a period of at least 6 months.

Yuzuriha S, Oh AK, Mulliken JB. Asymmetrical bilateral cleft lip: Complete or incomplete and contralateral lesser defect (minor-form, microform, or mini-microform). *Plast Reconstr Surg.* 2008;122:1494–1504.

This paper focuses on a subgroup of asymmetrical bilateral clefts that present with a lesser-form variant that is contralateral to a complete or incomplete cleft lip. The lesser forms are defined based on extent of disruption at the vermilion–cutaneous junction: minor-form, microform, and mini-microform. These designations determine the methods of repair and correlate with frequency and types of revisions that are usually necessary.

9 Chapter

Cleft palate

This chapter was created using content from Neligan & Losee, Plastic Surgery 3rd edition, Volume 3, Pediatric Plastic Surgery, Chapter 25, Cleft Palate, William Y. Hoffman.

SYNOPSIS

- Normal speech is the primary goal of cleft palate repair; minimizing effects of maxillary growth is also important but ultimately secondary.
- Cleft palate repair prior to 1 year of age (ideally 9–10 months) results in better speech outcomes than later repairs.
- The levator veli palatini muscle is longitudinally oriented in the cleft palate patient. Realignment of the muscle to a transverse and posterior position in the soft palate is the key to a successful functional result.
- Eustachian tube function is abnormal in cleft patients due to abnormal position of the tensor veli palatini muscle; this must be addressed in every cleft palate patient, usually with ventilating tubes.

Brief introduction

- The failure of fusion of the frontonasal and maxillary processes gives rise to the cleft of the primary palate, which includes the lip, alveolar process, and the hard palate anterior to the incisive foramen.
- This results in a cleft in the typical location between the premaxilla and the lateral maxilla, on either one or both sides.
- The lateral palatal shelves fuse later than the primary palate, around 7–8 weeks' gestation, as they rotate from vertical to horizontal orientation.
- This fusion proceeds from anterior to posterior, which helps to understand the spectrum of clefts of the secondary palate.
- The levator palatini and other pharyngeal muscles are derived from the fourth branchial arch and are innervated by cranial nerve X (vagus). The sole exception to this is the tensor palatini muscle, which arises from the first branchial arch and is innervated by cranial nerve V (trigeminal).
- The incidence of otitis media effusion has been found to be 96–100% in cleft palate patients.
- It is estimated that there is a 20–30% incidence of pure tone hearing loss in cleft palate patients by audiography.
- It has long been suggested that closure of the palate reduces risk of permanent hearing loss

Preoperative considerations

Sub-mucous cleft palate

- Sub-mucous cleft palate occurs when the palate has mucosal continuity but the underlying levator palatini muscle is discontinuous across the midline and longitudinally oriented, similar to the muscle anatomy in overt clefts of the palate ***(Fig. 9.1)***.
- Calnan's classic triad is diagnostic of this condition:
  - A midline clear zone (zona pellucida).
  - A bifid uvula.
  - A palpable notch in the posterior hard palate.
  - With contraction of velar musculature, a distinct midline muscle diastasis may be seen (see Fig. 9.1).
- The significance of a sub-mucous cleft may be difficult to assess clinically; the child with sub-mucous cleft palate is often undiagnosed in infancy.
- It has been reported that 45–55% of patients with isolated sub-mucous cleft palate are symptomatic

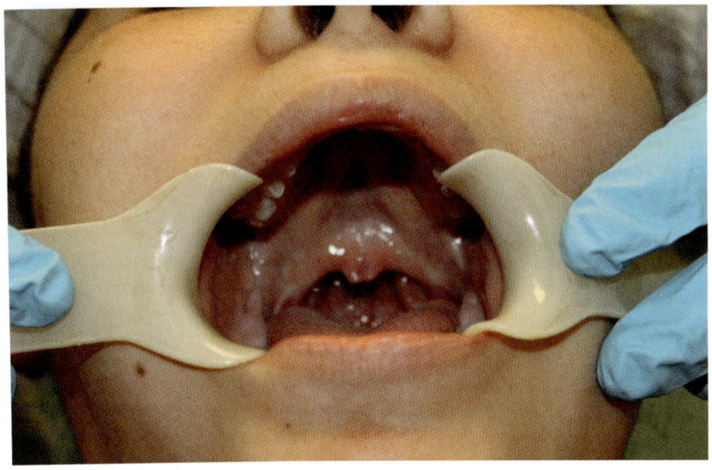

Figure 9.1 Sub-mucous cleft palate – note bifid uvula and thinning of central palate. On palpation there is a notch in the posterior hard palate rather than a posterior nasal spine.

with regard to speech, serous otitis media, or hearing loss.

- However, an infant identified with sub-mucous cleft palate need not routinely undergo repair because a significant number of individuals with sub-mucous cleft palate will not develop velopharyngeal insufficiency.
- Rather, these patients should be closely monitored with serial speech evaluations and audiometric surveillance.
- Patients who present with velopharyngeal insufficiency and sub-mucous cleft palate on examination require full evaluation, including speech evaluation and endoscopy.
- Even in the absence of obvious findings on clinical examination, anatomic abnormalities are found in most patients (>90%) at the time of surgery.
- Corrective surgical technique for sub-mucous cleft palate is focused on anatomic correction of the velar muscle diastasis.
- Although pharyngeal flaps and sphincter pharyngoplasty have been proposed as primary means of treatment, most surgeons focus on repair of the abnormal levator muscle position.
- The Furlow double opposing Z-plasty (see below) is an ideal procedure for these patients because there is no width discrepancy to overcome.

Pierre Robin sequence

- Pierre Robin described the triad of micrognathia, glossoptosis, and respiratory distress.
- 60–90% of patients diagnosed with Pierre Robin sequence have cleft palate.
- Infants with Pierre Robin sequence also have increased incidence of associated anomalies, particularly cardiac and renal problems.
- Newborns with Pierre Robin sequence may have severe respiratory and feeding difficulty because of the posterior displacement of the tongue.
- Initial treatment consists of placing the child prone and use of gastric lavage feeding tubes to push the tongue forward.
- Nasal airways have been used for the same purpose with reported success rates of 80–90%.
- If these conservative measures fail, surgical management of the airway may be required.
- A tongue–lip adhesion has been used as an alternative to tracheostomy and is generally effective.
- More recently, mandibular distraction osteogenesis has been used in neonates with success in averting tracheostomy.
- Palatoplasty in children with Pierre Robin sequence must be carefully timed with growth of the child, particularly the mandible, as closure of the palate narrows the effective area for respiration and can lead to respiratory distress.
  - If the mandible attains reasonable size in the first year of life, palate repair can still be performed safely before 1 year of age.
  - In the rare patient who has previously undergone tracheostomy, the palate should be repaired before decannulation.
  - The risk of airway compromise after palatoplasty reaches 25%, with an emergent tracheostomy or reintubation rate of 11% at one institution.

Syndromes

- Cleft palate without associated cleft lip has been reported to be associated with a syndrome in as many as 50% of cases, while cleft lip and palate together have an incidence of syndromes of about 30%.
- Van der Woude syndrome is associated with a mutation in the interferon regulatory factor 6 (IRF6) gene; this is an autosomal dominant syndrome associated with lower lip sinus tracts ("lip pits"), and has variable penetrance including the full range of cleft lips as well as palates.
- Velocardiofacial syndrome is associated with a 22q chromosomal deletion, detected by fluorescent immunohybridization (FISH). These children have a characteristic "bird-like" facial appearance, soft palate dysfunction, developmental delay, and various cardiac conditions.
- The same deletion gives rise to DiGeorge syndrome with associated B-cell and immune dysfunction.
- Infants with profound developmental delay and severely shortened life span projection should have surgical intervention delayed or should undergo palatoplasty under special circumstances only.
- Palate repair in severely disabled children can lead to altered airway status and obstructed upper airway in those with neuromuscular delay.

Growth

- At birth the average weight is the same for cleft and unaffected newborns. However, cleft infants have been shown to exhibit poor weight gain in early infancy.
- After repair of the palate, average growth returns to normal compared with unaffected children by the age of 4 years.

- Children with orofacial clefting stabilize and continue normal growth to at least 6 years of age, with no statistically significant differences in height and weight when compared to unaffected children.
- In later childhood, however, the average weight and height of children with cleft palate appears to diminish compared with those of control subjects.

Feeding and swallowing

- Oral intake is divided into two separate activities: generation of suction force (negative intraoral pressure) and swallowing.
- For negative intraoral pressure to be produced, the velum seals off the pharynx posteriorly; the lips close anteriorly, and negative pressure is produced by moving the tongue away from the palate and by opening the mandible which effectively increases the intraoral volume within a closed system.
- If the individual is unable to close the nasopharynx or to generate a seal of the lips, or if the palate is not intact at the point of contact with the tongue, negative pressure cannot be produced.
- In the cleft palate infant, the communication between the oropharynx and nasopharynx prevents a seal of the tongue against the palate, and negative pressure cannot be generated. Suckling is therefore not productive, and breast-feeding is ineffective.
- Swallowing involves a coordinated, complex interaction of the tongue and pharynx and is dependent on neuromuscular control and rhythmic coordinated contraction of the tongue and pharynx.
- Children with clefts generally do *not* have difficulty with swallowing and aspiration unless intrinsic neuromuscular abnormality of the tongue or pharynx is present.
- When the palate has an open cleft, food may reflux into the nasal passage.
- Nasal reflux is irritating to the nasal mucosa and can predispose to sinusitis and ulceration.
- In the older child, a persistent communication through a fistula in the palate may result in regurgitation of food through the nose, which is socially unacceptable.
- Most infants with clefts are unable to breast-feed. Infants who are unable to breast-feed because of cleft palate have a number of options for feeding including nipples, crosscutting of standard nipples, long soft nipples that place the liquid at the posterior tongue, and special flow bottles.
- All of these techniques are effective, and selection is generally by personal preference and the baby's acceptance of the method.
- Other key considerations are elevated head positioning during feeding and careful observation of feeding time and volume ingested.
- Weight gain and skeletal growth confirm success of the feeding regimen. Once the palate is successfully closed surgically, special feeding methods are generally unnecessary.

Speech

- The primary goal of palatoplasty is normal speech.
- Patients can grow and even thrive, despite feeding difficulties, but speech cannot be normalized if the palate is not repaired.
- The ability to partition the oropharynx and nasopharynx is crucial for normal speech production.
- The palate elevates during production of any sounds requiring positive pressure in the oropharynx; the levator palatini is primarily responsible for this movement ***(Fig. 9.2)***.
- Speech is a complex issue, and many factors may influence speech development in a child with a cleft palate.
- In addition to the importance of the palate itself, speech development may be influenced by motor or neurologic developmental delay (often seen in syndromes), by hearing, and by environmental stimuli.
- If palate function is not corrected, velopharyngeal insufficiency results, with speech that is hypernasal, often with hoarse quality due to difficulty in directing airflow through the mouth.
- When complete closure cannot be anatomically or functionally obtained, compensatory mechanisms for sound production are learned.
- These are maladaptive patterns that interfere with global intelligibility and include glottal stops and pharyngeal fricatives.
- Two crucial aspects of palatoplasty are important in optimal speech outcome: (1) surgical technique and (2) timing of palate repair.
- Most would agree that the best speech results are correlated with closure of the palate near the time of the infant beginning language acquisition, which for the normal-developing child is before 12 months of age.
- Despite the absence of hard evidence supporting earlier palate repairs, a growing body of opinion seems to support palate repair around 9–10 months of age for children with apparently normal development.
- Very early repair of the palate (6 months or younger) has been proposed by some surgeons, primarily as a means of improving feeding; however, long-term results are lacking for any large cohort of these patients.

Maxillary growth

- Palatoplasty has been shown to detrimentally affect maxillary growth.
- Many children with repaired cleft palate display typical findings of transverse maxillary deficiency requiring orthodontic widening of the maxilla once permanent teeth have erupted.
- There may be a sagittal growth deficiency as well; whereas 35–40% of children will develop an anterior crossbite, as many as 15–20% of children with cleft palate go on to require a Le Fort I maxillary advancement in some series.
- Although it might seem preferable to wait until a more advanced age for palate repair, given the growth effects

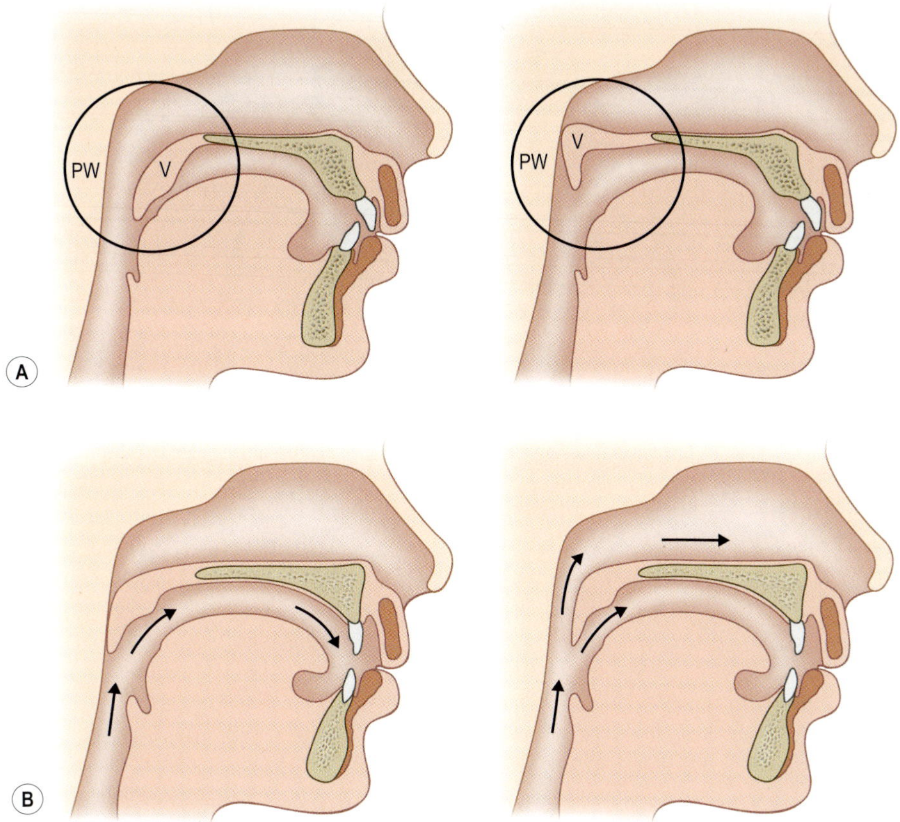

Figure 9.2 **(A)** In the lateral cephalogram, the soft palate or velum ("V") is shown at rest (above left) and during speech, making contact with the posterior pharyngeal wall ("PW") (above right). **(B)** This line drawing shows the air flow during normal speech (left), with the velum making contact with the posterior pharynx to direct air out the mouth. If the velum is too short or movement is inadequate (right), air can escape through the nose during speech, creating velopharyngeal insufficiency (VPI).

on the maxilla, it is far more difficult to establish normal speech in older children after cleft repair than to correct occlusion with a combination of orthodontic treatment and orthognathic surgery.

Anatomical considerations

- It is critical to understand the normal anatomy of the levator palatini muscle and the derangement of this anatomy that occurs in all clefts of the palate, including sub-mucous cleft palate *(Fig. 9.3)*.
- Normally, the levator muscle forms a transverse sling across the posterior half of the soft palate, and contraction causes the soft palate to move superiorly and posteriorly, contacting the posterior pharyngeal wall for velar closure, usually at the level of the adenoid pad.
- In addition to being discontinuous across the cleft, the levator muscle runs more or less longitudinally along the cleft margin before it inserts aberrantly into the posterior border of the hard palate.
- This results in ineffective contraction and inability to close the palate against the posterior pharyngeal wall.
- Air escape through the nose during speech produces a characteristic hypernasal quality.
- In addition, there is abnormal fusion with the tendon of the tensor veli palatini muscle, which impairs its function and contributes to cleft otopathology.
- Although the primary palate and the secondary palate form at different stages of embryonic development, cleft palate is most commonly seen in combination with cleft lip.
- The alveolar portion of the cleft lies between the maxillary lateral incisor and canine tooth roots resulting in malposition of the maxillary lateral incisor and cuspid in both the deciduous and permanent dentition.
- The maxillary lateral incisor on the cleft side is absent in 80–90% of cleft patients.
- Unilateral complete cleft palate is characterized by direct communication between the entire length of the nasal passage and oropharynx.
- The nasal septum is deviated and buckled toward the cleft side.
- Absence of a portion of the inferior piriform aperture and hypoplasia of the lateral nasal bony platform at the maxillary wall contribute to the cleft nasal deformity:
- The nasal base is depressed, the ala collapses, and the floor widens.
- The unilateral complete cleft is a full-thickness palatal defect of nasal mucosa, bony palate, velar musculature, and oral mucosa and all of these deficiencies must be addressed during the cleft palate repair or later at the time of alveolar cleft bone grafting.
- In the bilateral complete cleft lip and palate, the premaxillary segment containing the central and lateral incisor tooth roots is discontinuous from the alveolar arch.

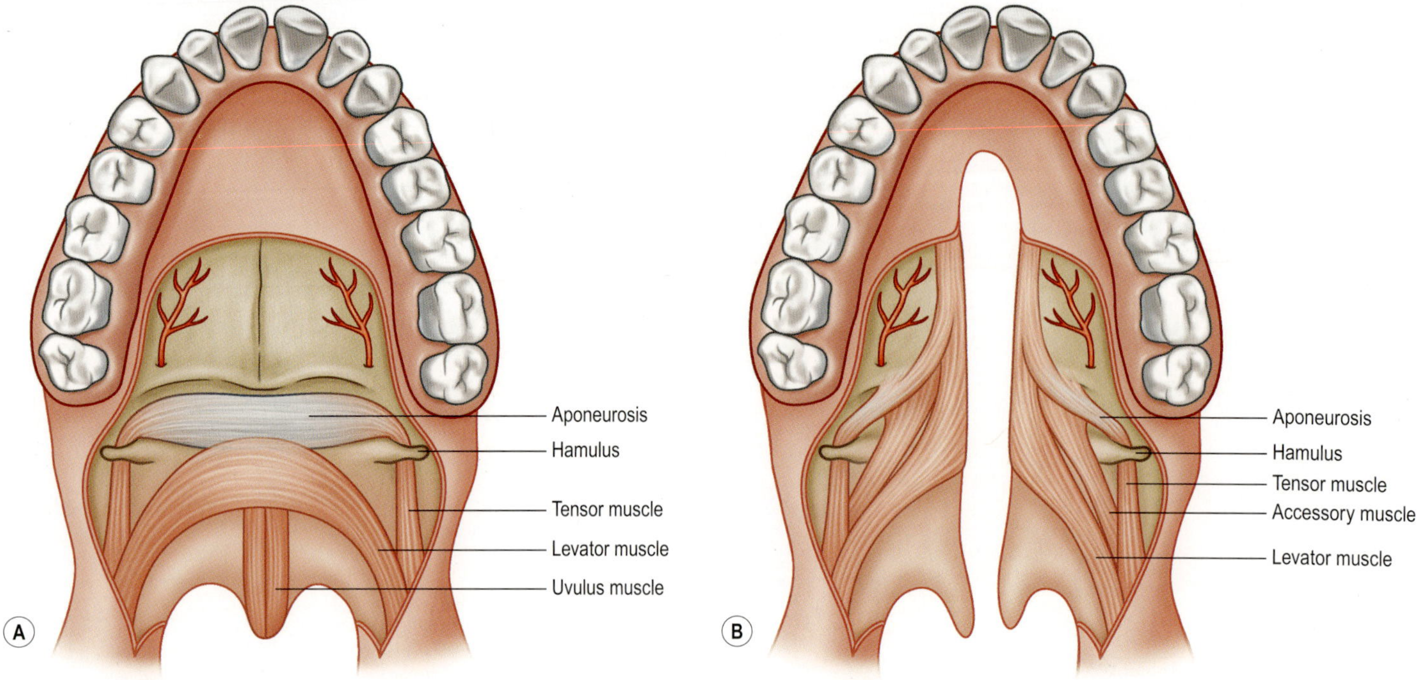

Figure 9.3 **(A)** Normal anatomy: the levator veli palatini muscle can be seen forming a sling across the soft palate; the tensor veli palatini is shown coming around the hamulus to fuse with the levator. **(B)** Cleft palate: the muscles are seen running more or less parallel with the cleft margin.

- The lateral segments often collapse inward and lingually, resulting in "locking out" of the premaxilla.
- Preoperative management with presurgical infant orthopedics (PSIO) may help prevent or treat lateral segment collapse and correct the anterior position of the premaxilla.
- Kernahan proposed a standardized reporting form to distinguish the variable presentations of cleft lip and palate, shown in *Figure 9.4*.
- The greater palatine neurovascular bundle emerges through the greater palatine foramen through the lateral posterior hard palate.
- Circumferential freeing of the palatal attachments around the pedicle and gentle stretching of the pedicle out of the foramen are essential to obtain a tension-free closure of the oral flap.
- In general, the goal is to obtain complete nasal and oral closure from front to back.
- In wide clefts, this may not be possible, particularly on the nasal surface.
- The most difficult area for closure, around the junction of the hard and soft palate, is the most common location for fistulas.

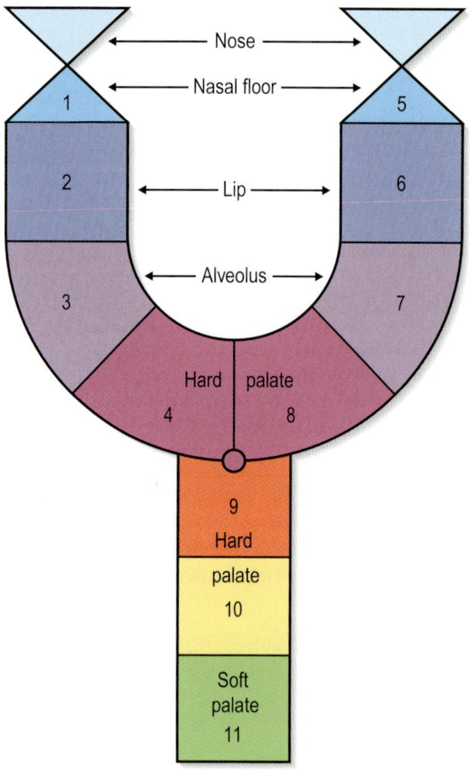

Figure 9.4 Kernohan's classification of clefts allows for standardized reporting of the severity of both cleft lip and palate.

Operative techniques

General technical considerations

- The use of a RAE endotracheal tube facilitates placement of the Dingman gag without kinking the tube.

- The Dingman gag, the most commonly used instrument for exposure, compresses the tongue and causes ischemia:
  - If it is used for longer than 2 h, significant postoperative tongue swelling can occur.
- Lidocaine 0.5% and epinephrine 1:200 000 are infiltrated into the palate 7–10 min before incision.
- A rolled towel under the shoulders will extend the neck; it is important to ensure that the child does not have any syndromes that predispose to cervical spine anomalies.
- The use of curved needle holders facilitates suture placement without obstruction of vision.

von Langenbeck

- Bernhard von Langenbeck introduced the use of mucoperiosteal flaps to close clefts of the secondary palate in the late 1800s.
- The initial description of the technique involved a simple approximation of the cleft margins with a relaxing incision that began posterior to the maxillary tuberosity and followed the posterior portion of the alveolar ridge.
- Intravelar veloplasty, or repair of the levator palatini muscle, as described below, is added today to reproduce the normal muscle sling ***(Fig. 9.5)***.

V-Y pushback (Veau–Wardill–Kilner)

- The essence of the pushback repair is the central V incision on the hard palate that is then closed in a straight line, creating length on the oral side of the closure ***(Fig. 9.6)***. This involves:
  - Circumferential dissection with release of the periosteum behind the greater palatine vessels.
  - The nasal tissue is released and left open: some authors have proposed providing nasal lining either with septal flaps, or with buccal mucosa ***(Fig. 9.7)***.
  - The soft palate is addressed with repair of the cleft margins and transverse closure of the levator muscle.
- Advantage:
  - Providing increased length for the palate and places the levator muscle in a more favorable position.
- Disadvantages:
  - Large open areas are left anteriorly and on the nasal surface; as these close by contraction, a good deal of the length gain is lost.
  - The contraction of the oral mucosal defects results in loss of maxillary width anteriorly.
  - Flattening of the arch.
  - Closure anteriorly is a single layer of nasal mucosa only, which gives rise to a higher fistula rate than in other techniques.

Two-flap palatoplasty

- Bardach and Salyer originally described a technique of freeing mucoperiosteal flaps from the cleft margins only, arguing that the arch of the cleft would provide the length needed for central closure.
- The more extensive two-flap palatoplasty is a modification of the Langenbeck technique, extending the relaxing incisions along the alveolar margins to the edge of the cleft.

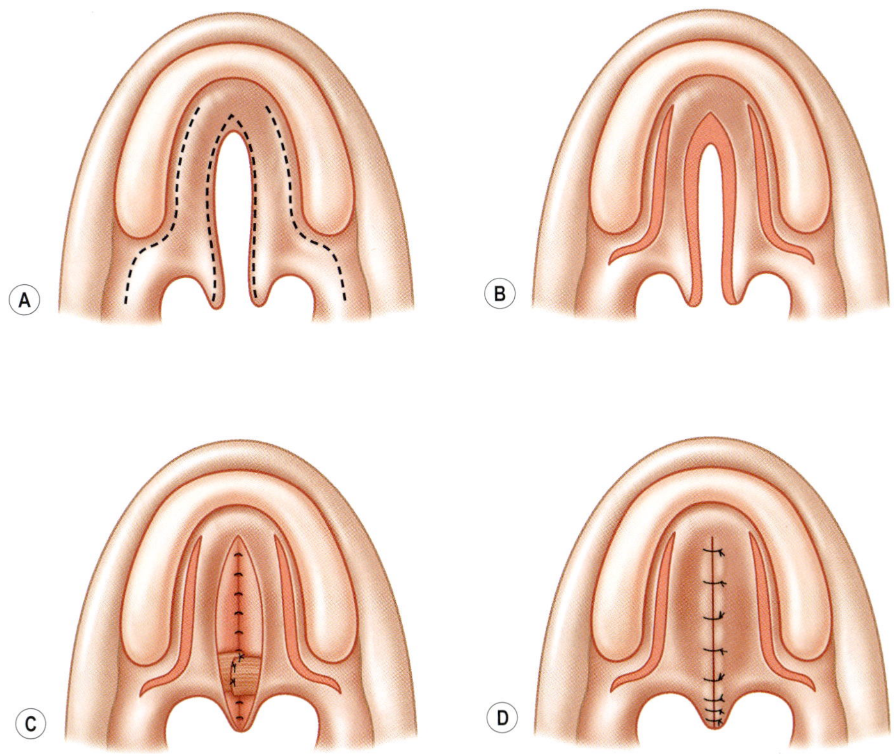

Figure 9.5 von Langenbeck repair. **(A)** Relaxing incisions are made behind the alveolar ridge, creating bilateral bipedicle flaps for midline closure. The greater palatine vessels must be preserved. **(B)** The cleft margins are incised in a manner to leave adequate nasal mucosa for complete closure. **(C)** Closure of the nasal mucosa and muscle repair. **(D)** Final appearance.

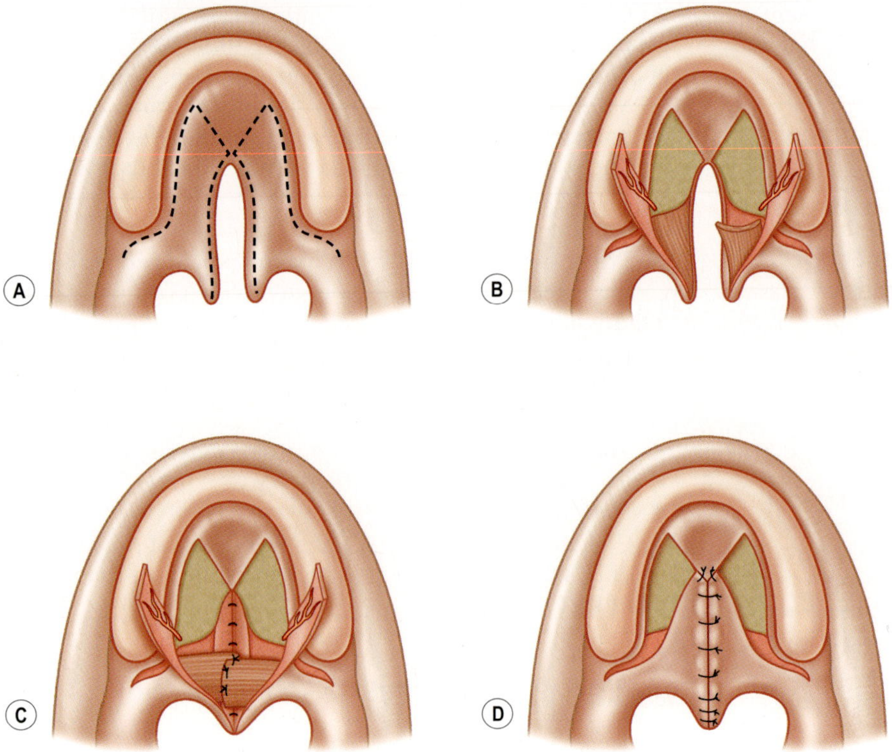

Figure 9.6 Pushback repair. **(A)** Design of anterior "W" incision. **(B)** Elevation of bilateral mucoperiosteal flaps based on palatine vessels. The levator veli palatini muscles are freed from the posterior border of the hard palate. **(C)** The muscles are repaired across the midline of the soft palate. **(D)** The "Y" closure creates additional length but also leaves large raw areas bilaterally.

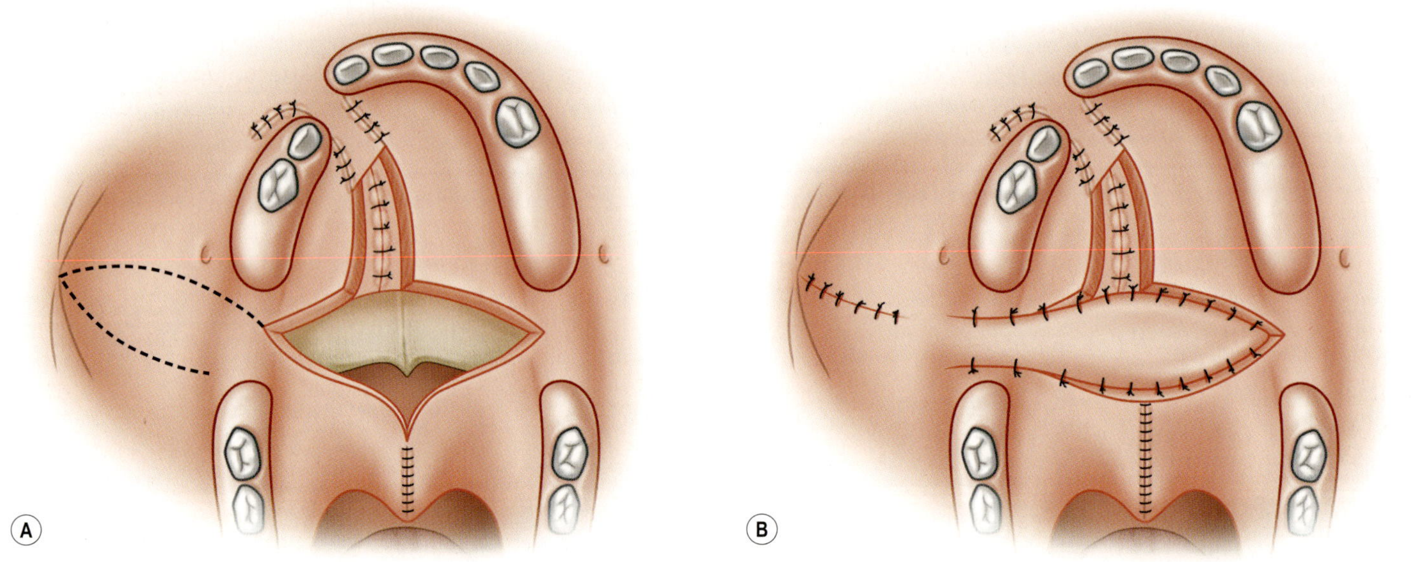

Figure 9.7 **(A)** Buccal mucosal flap. Kaplan advocated use of this flap to elongate the nasal mucosa. **(B)** Flap transposed into the nasal surface. In some situations, bilateral flaps can be used with the second flap lining the oral surface.

- The flaps are designed entirely dependent on the circulation from the palatine vessels
- In a complete unilateral cleft, the flap from the greater (medial) segment can be shifted across the cleft and closed directly behind the alveolar margin.
- This virtually eliminates fistulas in the anterior hard palate.
- The soft palate closure is accomplished with a straight-line closure in the typical two-flap technique.
- Intravelar veloplasty is an essential part of this closure *(Fig. 9.8)*.

Vomer flaps

- There is confusion about the terminology applied to anterior closure of the nasal mucosa in complete cleft lip and palate.

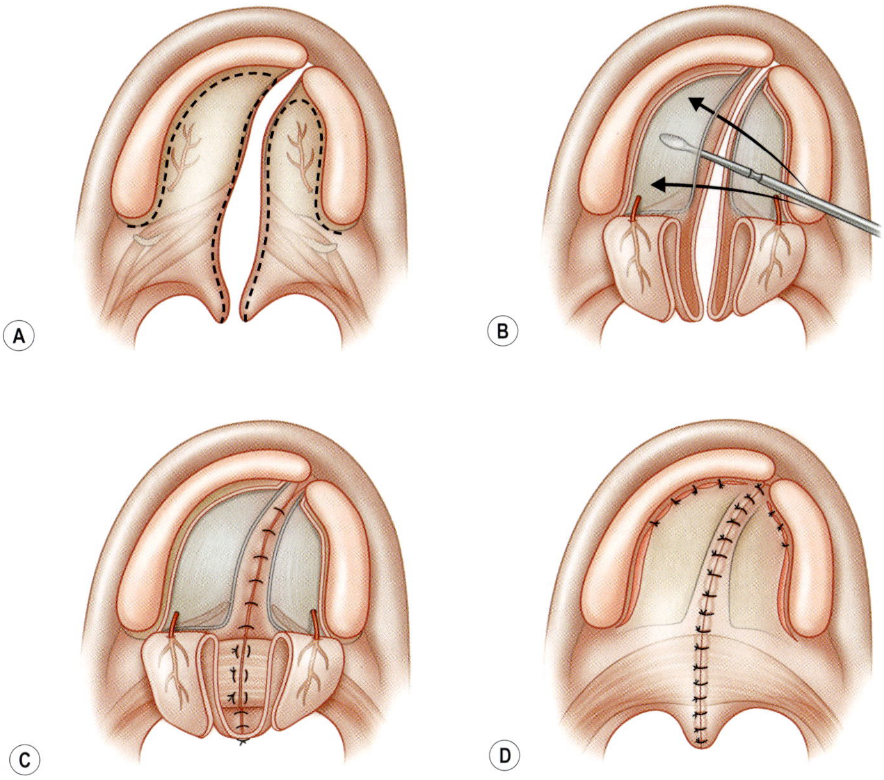

Figure 9.8 Two flap palatoplasty. **(A)** The incisions are similar to the Langenbeck repair but meet the cleft margin just behind the alveolar ridge. **(B)** Mucoperiosteal flaps are developed on both sides with preservation of the greater palatine vessels. **(C)** The levator veli palatini muscle is freed from the posterior border of the hard palate and sutured across the midline. **(D)** Final closure. It is often possible to close much of the lateral incision and minimize raw areas.

- The original vomer flap is described as inferiorly based; an incision is made high on the septum, and the flap is reflected downward to provide a single-layer closure on the oral side.
- A high number of patients with maxillary retrusion, presumably from injury to the vomer-premaxillary suture, as well as a high fistula rate and changed to a two-layer anterior closure.
- Similar problems have not been found with superiorly based vomer flaps.
- It involves:
  - Reflecting the mucosa from the septum near the cleft margin.
  - Dissecting only enough to close the nasal mucosa of the opposite side.
  - In bilateral cleft palate, this requires a midline incision along the septum, and two flaps are reflected in each direction.
  - Results in a two-layer closure of the hard palate mucosa, with low fistula rates and less effect on maxillary growth.

Double opposing Z-plasty (Furlow)

- Furlow first described his technique for palate closure in the 1980s, adapting the Z-plasty principle to palatal closure.
- A Z-plasty is developed on both the oral and nasal surfaces of the soft palate but in opposite directions.
- For both of the Z-plasties, the central limb is the cleft margin, and the posteriorly based flap is designed to include the levator muscle.
- Furlow recommended that the posteriorly based oral flap be on the left side for a right-handed surgeon because the elevation of the muscle from the nasal mucosa is the most difficult part of the dissection *(Fig. 9.9)*.
- This technique addresses closure of the soft palate in a manner that provides complete nasal and oral closure as it re-establishes the levator sling (intravelar veloplasty).
- The chief problem may arise in very wide clefts, in which the distance to be traversed by the Z-plasty may be excessive.
- Alternatively, relaxing incisions have been described to allow the flaps to advance.
- Another alternative is to extend the relaxing incision along the lateral border of the soft palate to allow oral closure and to use acellular dermal matrix for any nasal defects.
- A third alternative is to employ a straight line for closure in wide cases, reserving the Z-plasty as a secondary procedure if needed for speech.

Two-stage palate repair

- The problem of maxillary growth after cleft palate repair has led some surgeons to advocate a two-stage approach to palatoplasty, with earlier repair of the soft palate only and later repair of the hard palate.
- The general protocol:

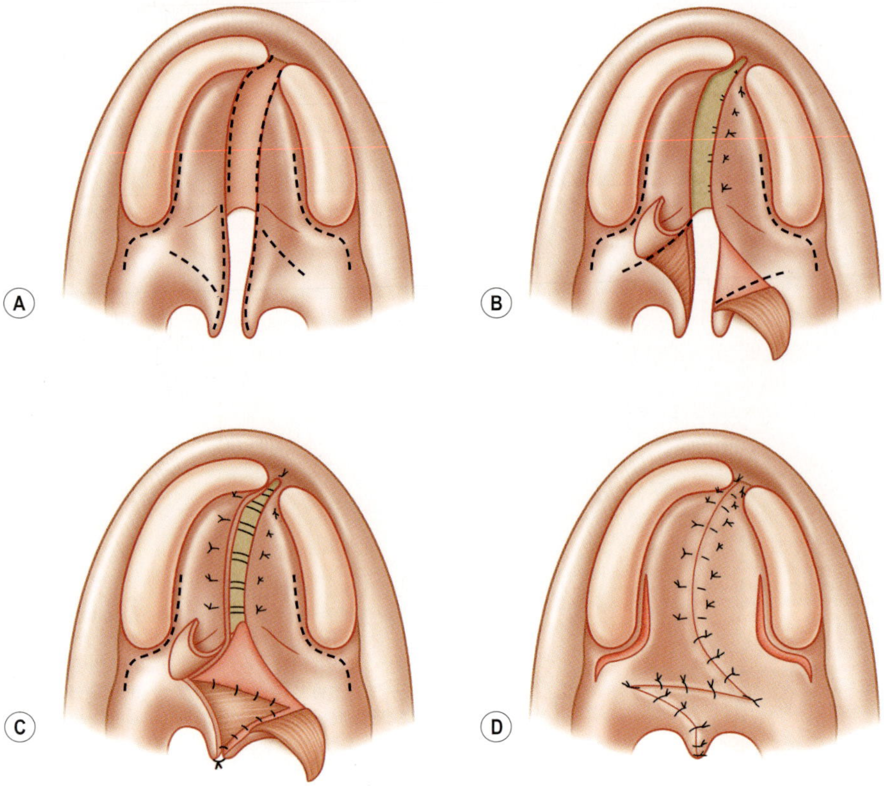

Figure 9.9 Furlow double opposing Z-plasty. **(A)** The oral flap design is shown with the posteriorly based flap on the left side. If necessary the relaxing incisions can be continued up to the cleft margin behind the alveolus, similar to the two flap palatoplasty (Fig. 9.7) for the hard palate closure. **(B)** The left sided oral flap is raised with the levator muscle, the right sided flap above the muscle. The reverse pattern is planned for the oral side. A vomer flap is shown closing the nasal mucosa anteriorly. **(C)** The nasal flaps are transposed and the anterior oral mucosa closed. **(D)** The final appearance after transposition of the oral flaps.

  - Repair of the soft palate at the same time as the cleft lip repair, around 4–6 months.
- The hard palate is obturated and repaired at about 4–5 years of age.
- Earlier ages have subsequently been proposed for hard palate repair, usually around 18–24 months.
- The rationale for this approach has been that the hard palate cleft narrows during the time between procedures, requiring less dissection and thus resulting in less maxillary growth disturbance.

Postoperative considerations

- Postoperative hypoxemia is not uncommon, but generally resolves after 24–48 h.
- The use of a traction suture in the tongue during the immediate period after extubation may avoid the need for utilizing any oral devices for maintaining the airway.
- Some centers use nasal trumpets routinely to improve ventilation.
- Monitoring with continuous pulse oximetry and minimizing narcotic use will help to avoid catastrophic problems.
- Acetaminophen 15 mg/kg alternating with ibuprofen 10 mg/kg will usually give adequate pain relief.
- Any patient who has had prolonged surgery (over 2 h) with the mouth gag in place should be observed for at least 48 h for tongue edema.
- Children with Pierre Robin sequence and any other children with syndromes that may affect breathing must be observed closely, even in an ICU setting.
- There are inevitably raw surfaces which may ooze for 12–24 h.
- Bleeding can be reduced by surgery that takes less than 90–120 min because the epinephrine will still have some effect during emergence from anesthesia.
- Light pressure on the hard palate repair at the conclusion of the procedure will often control bleeding as well.
- The author has found that application of ice packs to the posterior neck is almost always effective in stopping postoperative bleeding in recovery or on the ward.
- Postoperative feeding is generally limited to liquids for 10–14 days, to prevent particulate matter lodging in the areas that are left open at the end of the procedure.
- The parents must learn to time feeding for 30 min or so after analgesic administration.
- Arm splints may be used as well to prevent children from putting their fingers, or more likely foreign objects, in their mouth.

Complications and outcomes

- Fistula formation is a source of nasal regurgitation of fluids and may be a source of persistent nasal air loss even in the face of a functioning soft palate.
- Use of the Furlow repair was shown to markedly reduce fistulas relative to the V-Y pushback or von Langenbeck

technique; however, the width of the cleft is an important factor to consider.

- Normal speech is the primary goal of cleft palate repair.
  - In the majority of studies in which some form of muscle repair is utilized, good speech results are obtained about 85–90% of the time.
  - Syndromic patients will always have poorer results for a variety of reasons, but their good outcomes may be in the 50–60% range.
- Normal maxillary growth is the secondary goal of palate repair.
  - Avoidance of large raw surfaces on the hard palate will improve maxillary growth long term, and minimizing scar tissue will have a salutary effect as well.
  - Fistula formation requiring additional procedures will increase scar tissue and often decrease maxillary growth.
  - The need for maxillary advancement is highly variable, from 10–40% in non-syndromic cleft patients.
  - Syndromic patients have a higher rate of maxillary hypoplasia, which may well be genetically determined.

Further reading

Bardach J. The influence of cleft lip repair on facial growth. *Cleft Palate J*. 1990;27:76–78.

Chen PK-T, Wu J, Hung KF, et al. Surgical correction of sub-mucous cleft palate with Furlow palatoplasty. *Plast Reconstr Surg*. 1996;97:1136–1146.

Sleep apnea is a recognized adverse outcome of pharyngeal flaps performed for velopharyngeal insufficiency (VPI). This report demonstrates that Furlow palatoplasty is a reliable alternative to pharyngeal flaps for the correction of VPI in the context of submucous cleft palate.

Cutting C, Rosenbaum J, Rovati L. The technique of muscle repair in the soft palate. *Operative Techniques Plast Surg*. 1995;2:215–222.

Denny AD, Talisman R, Hanson PR, et al. Mandibular distraction osteogenesis in very young patients to correct airway obstruction. *Plast Reconstr Surg*. 2001;108:302–311.

This clinical series correlates airway measurements before and after distraction with functional outcomes. The authors conclude that distraction improves tongue base position such that airway space is effectively increased.

Emory Jr RE, Clay RP, Bite U, et al. Fistula formation and repair after palatal closure: an institutional perspective. *Plast Reconstr Surg*. 1997;99:1535–1538.

The authors report an 11.5% post-palatoplasty fistula rate. Local flaps are advocated to repair these lesions.

Furlow Jr LT. Cleft palate repair by double opposing Z-plasty. *Plast Reconstr Surg*.1986;78:724.

Furlow describes his palatoplasty in the context of a 22-patient case series. Optimistic speech outcomes are reported.

Huang MH, Lee ST, Rajendran K. A fresh cadaveric study of the paratubal muscles: implications for eustachian tube function in cleft palate. *Plast Reconstr Surg*. 1997;100:833–842.

Cadaveric dissections were performed to clarify possible ramifications of palatal clefting on eustachian tube function. Functional hypotheses are drawn from morphological findings.

Kaplan EN. The occult submucous cleft palate. *Cleft Palate J*. 1975;12:356–368.

Robin P. Glossoptosis due to atresia and hypotrophy of the mandible. *Am J Dis Child*. 1934;48:541–547.

Rohrich RJ, Byrd HS. Optimal timing of cleft palate closure. Speech, facial growth, and hearing considerations. *Clin Plast Surg*. 1990;17:27–36.

10 Chapter

Lower extremity reconstruction

This chapter was created using content from Neligan & Song, Plastic Surgery 3rd edition, Volume 4, Lower Extremity, Trunk and Burns, Chapter 5, Reconstructive surgery: lower extremity coverage, Joon Pio Hong.

SYNOPSIS

- The reconstructive surgery for the lower extremity has evolved from a staged approach to proving best solutions for functional and cosmetic outcome.
- This chapter covers the classical approach with a gradual change of principle that advocates a one-stage elevator approach.
- Special considerations should be given to overcome the complexity of lower extremity reconstruction, such as diabetes and chronic infection.
- Finally, introduction of perforator flaps, the use of multiple flaps by combination, and supermicrosurgery will help you design and widen the reconstructive choice for the lower extremity.

Brief introduction

- Lower extremity reconstruction following severe trauma, cancer ablation and chronic infections remains challenging, as multiple structures including bone, muscle, vessels, nerves and skin may be involved.
- In the recent years, the management of lower extremity has evolved with numerous new techniques and innovations leading to greater salvage opportunities.
- If the extremity cannot be salvaged, the next goal is to maintain maximal functional length with good soft tissue coverage on the stump to bear the prosthesis for functional gait.
- Extremity salvage is a long and complex process, thus patient education, motivation, and compliance along with family support will be critical during physical and psychological recovery.
- Although early amputation and prosthetic treatment was thought to offer the potential of faster recovery and lower cost, recent reports have provided different views.
- The Lower Extremity Assessment Project, or LEAP study showed no significant difference in outcome at 2 years.

Preoperative considerations

- The primary goal of surgical reconstruction of the lower extremity wound is to restore or maintain function.
- Although evaluations such as Mangled Extremity Severity Score (MESS), the Predictive Salvage Index, and the Limb Salvage Index can assist the team in making a decision for amputation, it must not be used as a sole criterion and the decision to amputate must be individualized for each patient.
- Whether acute or chronic, evaluation of lower extremity wounds and the eligibility for soft tissue reconstruction begins with vascular status evaluation.
- If clinical and diagnostic examination reveals inadequate perfusion and the value of reconstruction is minimal, amputation should be individually decided.
- An amputated or avulsed tissue should never be disregarded, especially in acute traumas, unless severely contaminated or lacking vascular structure.
- The skin harvested from the degloved or amputated part can be utilized as biologic dressings to permanent skin grafts.
- The leg length can be preserved using soft tissue distal from the zone of injury as fillet pedicled or free flaps.

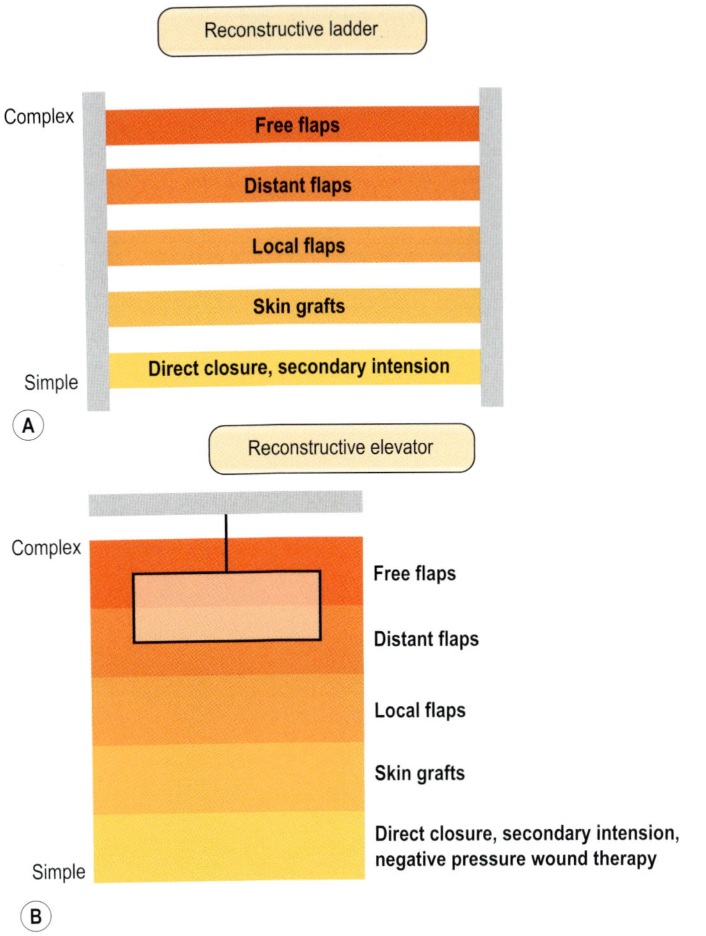

Figure 10.1 The reconstructive elevator requires creative thoughts and considerations of multiple variables to achieve the best form and function rather than a sequential climb up the ladder. This paradigm of thought does not eliminate the concept of reconstructive ladder but replaces it as a ladder of wound closure and makes its mark in the field where variety of advanced reconstructive procedures and techniques are not readily available. Based on the reconstructive elevator, method of reconstruction should be chosen based on procedures that result in optimal function as well as appearance.

- Amputated bones can be banked or used as a flap to reconstruct the leg.
- Once the wound is evaluated to have good vascular supply, stable skeletal structures and a relatively clean wound, soft tissue coverage is then considered.
- The concept of reconstructive ladder was proposed to achieve wounds with adequate closure using a stepladder approach from simple to complex procedures *(Fig. 10.1A)*.
- Although still valued and widely taught, in the era of modern reconstructive surgery, one must consider not only adequate closures but form and function.
- Thus a simpler reconstructive option may not necessarily produce optimal results, which is especially true for lower extremity coverage, where consequences of inadequate coverage will lead to complications such as additional soft tissue loss, osteomyelitis, functional loss, increased medical cost and even amputation.
- The reconstructive elevator requires creative thoughts and considerations of multiple variables to achieve the best form and function rather than a sequential climb up the ladder (Fig 10.1B).
- Based on the reconstructive elevator, method of reconstruction should be chosen based on procedures that result in optimal function as well as appearance.
- The initial evaluation of the lower extremity wound involves visual and manual examination. Neurological evaluation as well as vascular and skeletal evaluation is made to develop a plan for reconstruction.
- After the decision is made to reconstruct the lower extremity, the first preoperative evaluation should start with vascular status.
- Physical examination of palpable pulse, color, capillary refill, and turgor of the extremity allows assessment of initial status and Doppler examination can provide additional information.
- The use of preoperative arteriography for lower extremity reconstruction is considered when physical/Doppler exam reveals inconclusive vascular status or chronic vascular disease is suspected.
- The use of computed tomographic angiography may obtain vascular information of the recipient region without the risk of complications from arterial puncture of the groin and also can provide vascular information of the donor flap facilitating the planning and the surgical procedure.
- Nerve injuries that are irreversible may require special considerations.
- Peroneal nerve injuries result in foot drop and loss of sensation of the dorsum of the foot. Thus lifelong splinting or tendon transfers may be required.
- Complete loss of tibial nerve function results in loss of plantar flexion and is an absolute contraindication for reconstruction.
- The loss of plantar sensation can be devastating and may hinder the need for reconstruction although it is not an absolute contraindication.
- An algorithm of approach is outlined in ***Figure 10.2***.

Anatomical/technical pearls

Skin grafts and substitutes

- Autologous skin grafts are used in a variety of clinical situations.
- The split-thickness grafts are usually used as the first line of treatment where wounds cannot be closed primarily or undue tension is suspected.
- In the extremity often with complex wounds, bone exposure and/or avascular beds, infected wounds, wound with dead space and poorly coagulated beds, skin grafts should be avoided.
- A skin substitute is defined as a naturally occurring or synthetic bioengineered product that is used to replace the skin in a temporary, semi-permanent or permanent fashion.
- Temporary epidermal replacements may be beneficial in superficial to middermal depth wounds.

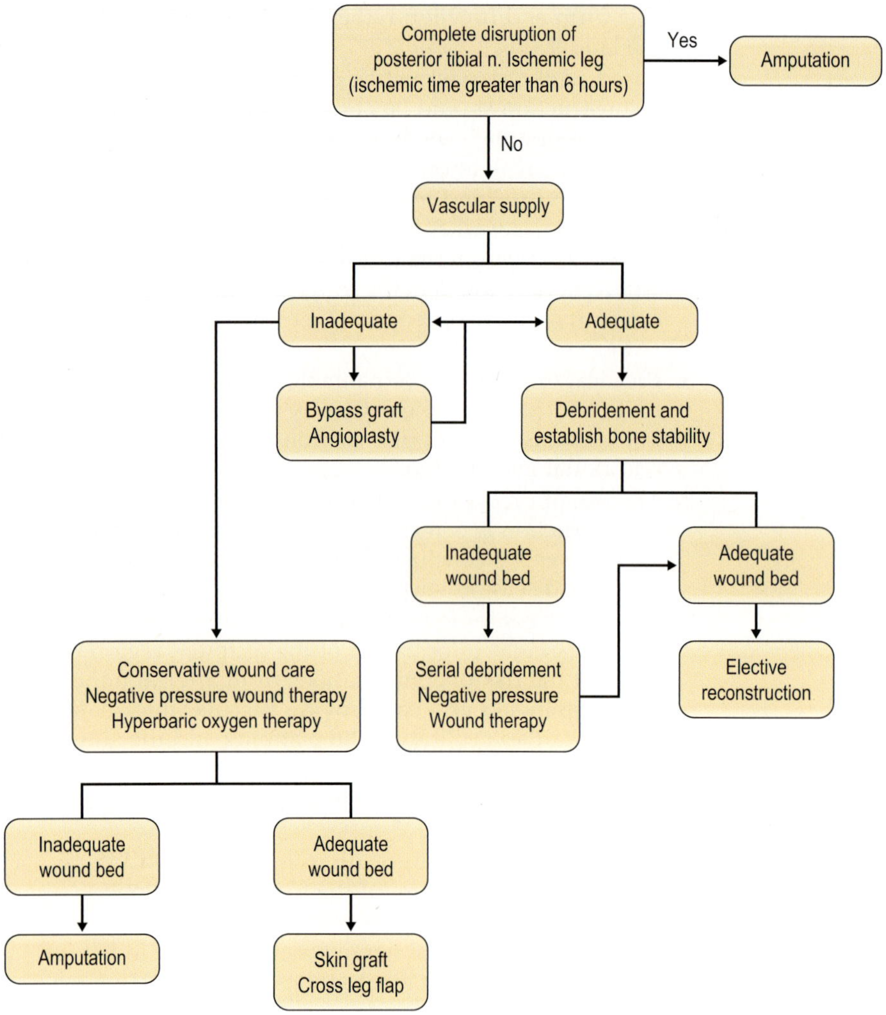

Figure 10.2 Algorithm of approach for soft tissue reconstruction of lower extremity.

- Examples: EZ-derm and Mediskin (Brennen Medical-LLC, St Paul, MN), and Biobrane (UDL Laboratories Inc, Rockford, Illinois)
- In deeper wounds, dermal replacements are of primary importance.
- Examples: Allograft, Alloderm (Life Cell Corporation, Woodlans, TX), Integra (Integra Life Sciences, Plainsboro, NJ), and Apligraf (Organogenesis Inc, Canton, MA).

Approach by location (local flaps)

Thigh

- The thigh can be divided into three parts: the proximal thigh, midthigh, and the distal thigh (supracondylar knee) regions.
- The medial portion of the proximal thigh can be especially challenging due to the location of vital structures and the likely formation of dead space.
- Local lower extremity muscle or myocutaneous flap options include:
  - Using the flaps based from the lateral circumflex femoral artery such as tensor fascia lata, vastus lateralis, and rectus femoris flaps.
  - Vertical rectus abdominis muscle or myocutaneous flap using the deep inferior epigastric artery.
  - The gracilis muscle or myocutaneous flap based on the medial femoral circumflex artery may lack muscle bulk but is a good option when the dead space is not extensive.
- Now with increased knowledge of perforator and perforator based flaps, basically any perforator can be chosen as a source of vascular supply to the skin flap and be rotated to cover a defect.
- When the use of local flaps is not feasible due to the complexity of the wound, free tissue transfer is indicated.
- The midthigh wound, due to the anatomical character where femur is surrounded by a thick layer of soft tissue, rarely requires reconstruction using free tissue transfer and often is sufficiently reconstructed by skin graft or local flap.
- Local muscle or musculocutaneous flaps based on the lateral or medial femoral circumflex artery can be used when available.
- Any perforator can be chosen as a source of vascular supply to the skin flap and rotated to cover a defect.
- If the patient has undergone massive resection or has special considerations such as postoperative radiation therapy, it may warrant free tissue coverage.

- The wounds of the distal thigh (supracondylar knee) can be very difficult due to the limit of rotation from previously described local muscle or musculocutaneous flaps from the thigh.
- Pedicled medial gastrocnemius muscle or musculocutaneous flap from the lower leg can be extended to cover this region.
- Extensive or complex defects may require free tissue transfer or coverage using a perforator based rotation/ advancement skin flap.

Lower leg

- The traditional planning for reconstruction of the lower extremity has been approached according to the location of the defect.
- Divided into thirds, gastrocnemius muscle flap for proximal third, soleus muscle flap for middle third and free flap transfer for the distal third of the leg.
- Like the reconstructive ladder concept, this traditional approach can be useful but the surgeon must individualize each wound and choose the initial procedure that can yield the best chance of success and avoid morbidity.

Microvascular free tissue transfer

- Workhorse flaps for soft tissue coverage include muscle or musculocutaneous flaps such as latissimus dorsi, rectus abdominis, and gracilis.
- The perforator flap, where a skin flap is based on a single or multiple perforators, such as the anterolateral thigh flap or thoracodorsal artery perforator flap have been added on to the list.
- Whichever flap you select, the guidelines for lower extremity reconstruction using free flaps remain the same:
  - Anastomose the vessel outside the zone of injury.
  - Make end-to-side arterial anastomosis and end-to-side or end-to-end venous anastomosis.
  - Reconstruct the soft tissues first and then restore the skeletal support.

Primary limb amputation

- Absolute indications include: anatomically complete disruption of the posterior tibial nerve in adults and crush injuries with warm ischemia time greater than 6 h.
- Relative indications include: serious associated polytrauma, severe ipsilateral foot trauma, and anticipated protracted course to obtain soft tissue coverage and tibial reconstruction.
- In these cases where limb salvage is not possible, attempts should be made to salvage as much limb length as possible.
- Every effort should be made to save the functional knee joint as below-knee amputation results in far superior ambulatory outcome and up to 2–3-fold more full mobility compared to above knee amputation.
- The energy consumption is far less for below-knee amputation and this allows these patients to walk significant daily distances, thus maintaining good quality of life.
- Though the ideal stump length below the knee is more than 6 cm, any length of tibia should be preserved.
- If adequate soft tissue exists, the stump may be closed primarily and where local tissue is inadequate, microsurgery allows preserving maximal length of the stump.
- If the tissue distal to the amputation is usable, a fillet flap can be performed.
- Other flaps such as muscle, musculocutaneous, fasciocutaneous and perforator flaps can be used.
- Muscle flaps may have a tendency to heal slowly and to shrink due to muscle atrophy, while skin flaps may provide better contour and sensibility.

Debridement

- Bony stability is first established using external or internal fixation devices.
- An external device is usually preferred if there is significant bone loss or bone devascularization and may facilitate coverage procedure.
- Debridement must cover devitalized soft tissue and bone and be performed until fresh bleeding is noted.
- Multiple stages of debridement may be needed to achieve adequate wound bed prior to soft tissue coverage.
- The vacuum-assisted closure can be used to optimize the wound bed and minimize dressing changes until definitive reconstruction.

Timing of reconstruction

- Regardless of the degree of contamination and extent of injury when indicated for salvage, there is no need to delay definitive coverage provided that the general condition of the patient and the status of the wound allow it.
- General consensus favors early aggressive wound debridement and soft issue coverage.
- Ideally, the wound is covered in the first 5–6 days after injury at the acute phase of the wound.
- Godina further demonstrated that radical debridement and coverage within 72 h results in best outcome where only 0.75% of flaps fail, 1.5% are infected, and 6.8 months are needed for union of the bone.
- The common idea behind early intervention is that it minimizes the risk for increasing bacterial colonization and inflammation leading to complications.
- Acute coverage by day 5–7 is generally accepted as having a good prognosis in terms of decreased risk of infection, flap survival, and fracture healing.

Selection of recipient vessel

- Many lower extremity wounds resulting from trauma are high-energy injuries with a substantial "zone of injury."
- This thrombogenic zone is known to extend beyond what is macroscopically evident, and failure to recognize the

true extent of this zone is cited as a leading cause of microsurgical anastomotic failure.
- Isenberg and Sherman demonstrated that clinical presentation of recipient vessel (vessel wall pliability and the quality of blood from transected end of vessel) was more important than the distance from the wound.
- Based on these findings, one of the most important factors in selecting the recipient vessel may be the vascular quality itself.

Special considerations

Osteomyelitis

- Osteomyelitis often follows severe open leg fractures with massive contamination or devascularized soft tissue and bone. Inadequate debridement or delayed coverage of the wound increases the chance for osteomyelitis and early debridement remains to be the key to prevention.
- To achieve the goal of infection control and the restoration of function, treatment principles for chronic osteomyelitis are debridement including the complete resection of involved bone, flap coverage with vascularized tissue, and brief course of antibiotic treatment.
- Although there has been controversy in selecting the type of flap for coverage, muscles have shown experimentally to have increased blood flow and antibiotics delivery, increased oxygen tension, increased phagocytic activity, and decreased bacterial counts in wounds reconstructed with muscle flaps rather than fasciocutaneous flaps.
- Clinically, complete debridement and obliteration of dead space are the most important steps to treat osteomyelitis and the type of flap seems less crucial.
  - Bone defects can be managed with vascularized bone flap, secondary bone grafting, bone distraction lengthening or a combination of these techniques.
  - Not all chronic osteomyelitis can be salvaged. As with the indication for amputation, legs with nerves too damaged after osteomyelitis should not be salvaged.

Diabetes

- Patients with diabetes require additional concerns from chronic renal failure, nutrition to blood sugar control and are best approached by a multidisciplinary team.
- Patients will frequently have chronic bacterial colonization, osteomyelitis, complex wounds, bone deformity, local wound ischemia and vascular disease.
- When patients with diabetes are required to undergo a reconstructive procedure of the extremity, vascular status must be evaluated to ensure success.
- Any vascular problems must be addressed first and corrected. If not correctable, the surgeon may be faced with a high risk of failure.
- One must consider the probability of successful reconstruction, based on eliminating the underlying problems of the diabetic wound and also take into account long-term ambulation after reconstruction *(Fig. 10.3)*.

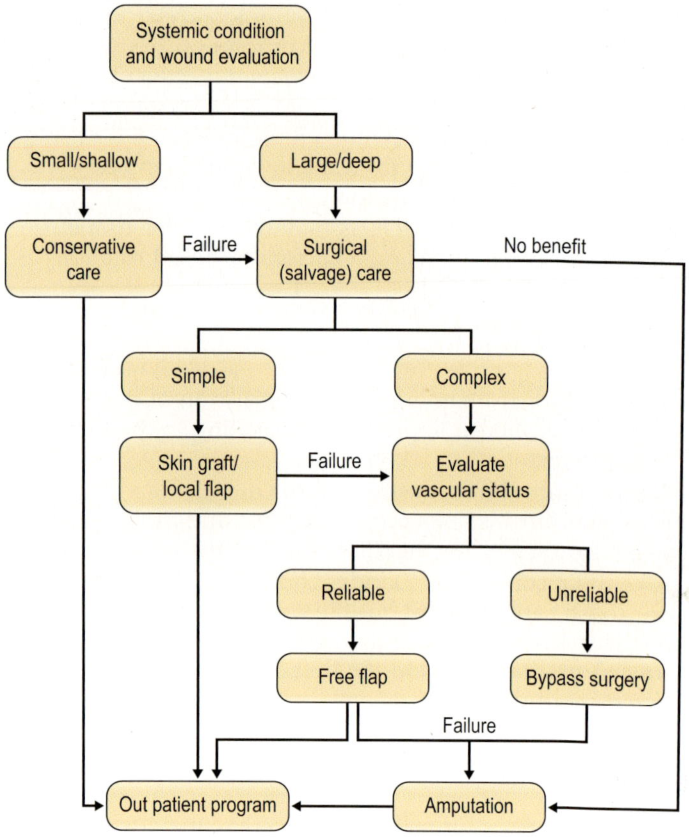

Figure 10.3 Algorithm for diabetic foot reconstruction.

- Large and composite diabetic wounds must be aggressively debrided, including the necrotic bone, and covered with well-vascularized tissue.

Coverage after tumor ablation

- As with any reconstructive procedure, the aim of reconstruction after tumor ablation is to maintain quality of life by preserving function and achieving acceptable appearance.
- In addition, coverage must be able to withstand adjuvant therapy with radiation therapy and/or chemotherapy and play a role in achieving long-term local control of disease.
- Skin grafts are always an option especially for very extensive defects where flap coverage is not available.
- For wounds scheduled for postoperative radiation therapy or located over joints and high friction regions, skin graft should be avoided and be reconstructed with a durable flap.
- Special consideration should be made to preoperative radiation therapy where skin would become fibrotic and ischemic around the cancer and thus will not allow local coverage.
- Various flaps from omentum, muscle with skin graft, musculocutaneous, and perforator flaps can be used for reconstruction depending on location, size, depth, adjuvant therapy, function, and cosmetic appearance *(Fig. 10.4)*.

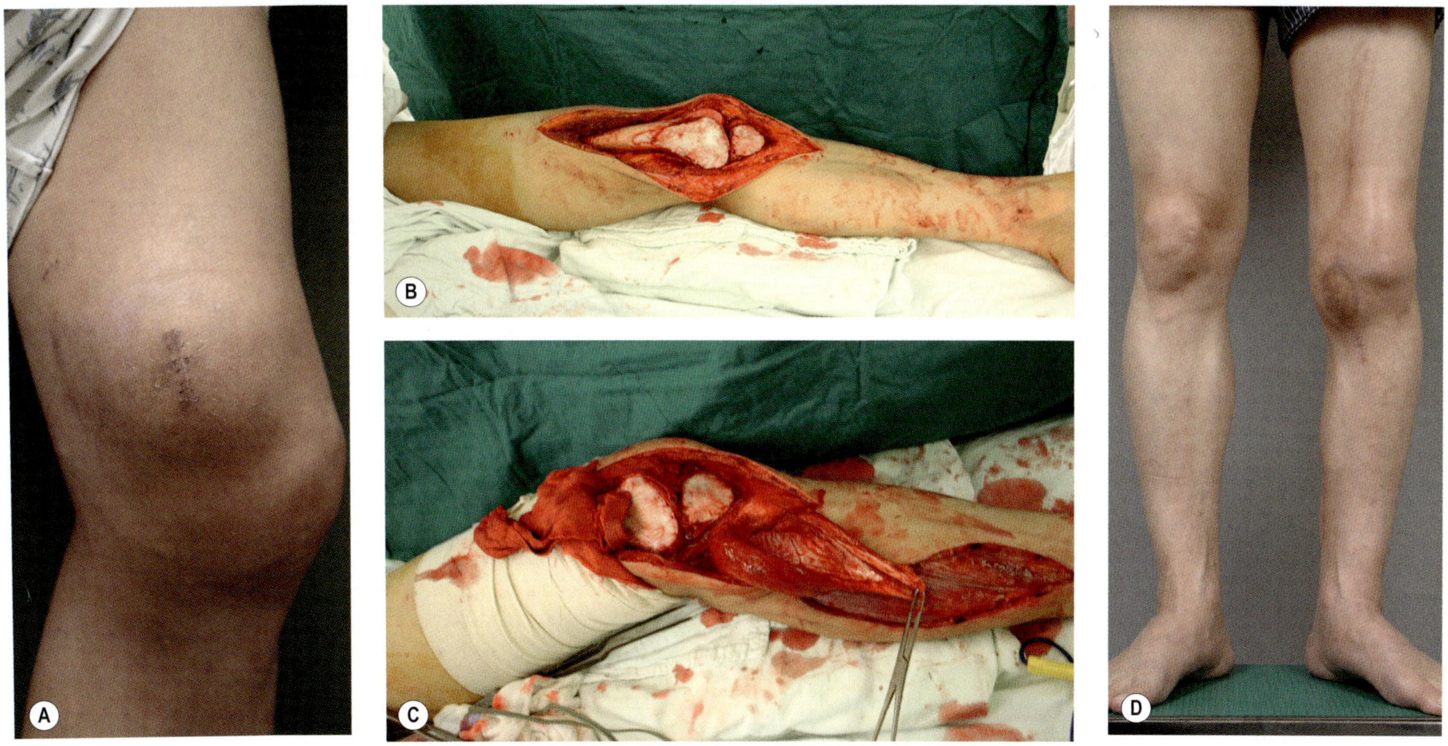

Figure 10.4 **(A)** A patient with soft tissue sarcoma of the knee region was noted. **(B,C)** After wide excision including the bone, a hemi-gastrocnemius muscle was elevated to resurface the knee joint. **(D)** Long-term results show good contour with acceptable function and appearance.

Exposed prosthesis

- The traditional method to manage exposed hardware includes irrigation, debridement, antibiotics, and likely removal of hardware.
- Factors such as location of the hardware, infection (type of bacteria and duration of infection), duration of exposure of hardware, and hardware loosening should be considered as important prognostic factors for successful management of exposed hardware.
- If hardware is clinically stable, time of exposure is less than 2 weeks, infection is controlled, and the location of the hardware is for bony consolidation, then it may increase the likelihood of salvage of hardware using surgical soft tissue coverage.
- Exposed vascular grafts present life- and limb-threatening complications. It should be managed with early debridement and muscle flap coverage to salvage the graft.
- Local muscle flaps such as gracilis, sartorius, and tensor fascia lata are very useful in providing adequate coverage for exposed groin synthetic vascular prosthesis.
- If the defect is extensive and inferiorly based, a vertical rectus abdominis musculocutaneous flap can be considered.

Soft tissue expansion

- The use of tissue expansion in the lower extremity has not been successful as in other areas of the body, such as the breast and scalp.
- The potential advantages of using expanded skin in the lower extremity include improved contour, coverage with like tissue, and improved aesthetic result.
- However, use in the lower extremity has been associated with high rate of infection and extrusion of the implant.
- The technique can be reserved for unstable soft tissues or scars of moderate size.
- The implant is placed suprafascially in the subcutaneous pocket in the lower extremity and application on the ankle and foot region must be avoided.
- Transverse expansion has a lower failure rate compared to longitudinal advancement.
- For avoidance of wound dehiscence, neurapraxia, and fat necrosis, expansion should proceed slowly, stopping before the onset of pain or, if it is measured, before intraexpander pressure exceeds 40 mmHg.
- Flap prefabrication with tissue expansion may have a role in select reconstructions of the lower extremity.

Operative techniques

Muscle/musculocutaneous flaps

Tensor fascia lata

- The tensor fascia lata is a small, thin and short muscle with a long fascial extension from the iliotibial tract of the facia lata to the lateral aspect of the knee.

- The muscle originates 5–8 cm anterior of the external lip of the anterior superior iliac crest immediately behind sartorius and inserts to the iliotibial tract.
- It abducts, medially rotates, and flexes the hip, acting to tighten the fascia lata and iliotibial tract but is an expendable muscle.
- Its flat shape, excellent length, and reliable type I circulation pattern (dominant pedicle is the ascending branch of the lateral femoral circumflex artery and venae comitantes) make it useful in many reconstructive scenarios, both as a pedicled flap for local and regional coverage and as a free, composite unit that incorporates skin, muscle, and iliac bone.
- Motor innervation is from the superior gluteal nerve entering the deep surface between the gluteus medius and gluteus maximus. Sensation is derived from T12 which innervates the upper skin territory and the lateral femoral cutaneous nerve of the thigh (L2–3) innervates the lower skin.
- When based on the dominant pedicle, located 8–10 cm below the anterior superior iliac spine, the anterior arc of location will reach the abdominal areas, groin, and perineum while the posterior arc can reach the greater trochanter, ischium, perineum, and sacrum ***(Fig. 10.5)***.
- The flap can also be advanced superiorly as a V-Y flap to cover trochanteric wounds.

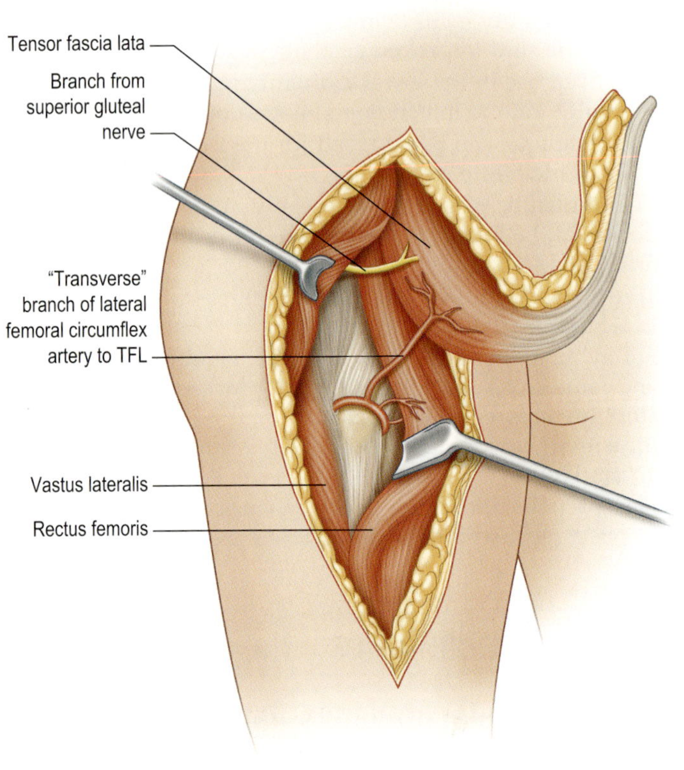

Figure 10.5 Tensor fascia lata flap elevation. When based on the dominant pedicle, located 8–10 cm below the anterior superior iliac spine, anterior arc of location will reach the abdominal areas, groin, and perineum while the posterior arc can reach the greater trochanter, ischium, perineum, and sacrum.

- The skin overlying the muscle and fascia lata can be harvested as a unit with the flap and can extend to within 10 cm above the knee.
- The marking begins by identifying the major landmarks: the anterior superior iliac spine, lateral condyle of femur, and the pubic tubercle.
- A line from the anterior superior iliac spine straight down the thigh to a point 10–12 cm above the knee joint, presents the anterior border of the flap and a parallel line 12–15 cm posterior to the first line is drawn straight down the thigh, curving anteriorly as it crosses posterior to the lateral epicondylar area to meet at the same point.
- The skin island can be designed within this long strip, according to the needs and distance to the recipient defect.
- The distal margin of the flap is entered, carrying the incision through the fascia lata and dissecting deep to the fascia lata and iliotibial tract.
- The pedicle is located approximately 10 cm below the anterior iliac spine along the line drawn.
- One must modify the flap when composite tissues are taken for reconstruction.

Rectus femoris

- The rectus femoris is located superficially on the middle of the anterior thigh, extending between the ilium and patella.
- It is a central muscle of the quadriceps femoris extensor muscles group and acts to extend the leg at the knee.
- The muscle originates with two tendons, one from the anterior inferior iliac spine and one from the acetabulum and inserts to the patella.
- It is a thigh flexor and a leg extensor important in stabilizing the weight-bearing knee, thus is not considered expandable.
- It has a type II pattern of circulation (the dominant pedicle is the descending branch of the lateral circumflex femoral artery with minor pedicles from the ascending branch of the same vessel as well as from muscle branches of the superficial femoral artery) and can reach to cover the inferior abdomen, groin, perineum and ischium.
- Motor innervation is from the femoral nerve, and muscle branches enter adjacent to the dominant pedicle.
- This motor innervation and the adequate dimension of the flap allow it to be used as a functional muscle flap ***(Fig. 10.6)***.
- The intermediate anterior femoral cutaneous nerve (L2–3) provides sensation. The skin perforators are most reliable over the midanterior two-thirds of the muscle itself in the central strip up to 12 × 20 cm.
- A longitudinal incision is marked from 3 cm below the anterior superior iliac spine to just above the superior margin of the patella.
- With the anterior thigh muscle contraction, the lateral border of the vastus medialis and the medial border of the vastus lateralis is visualized, creating a depression of skin.

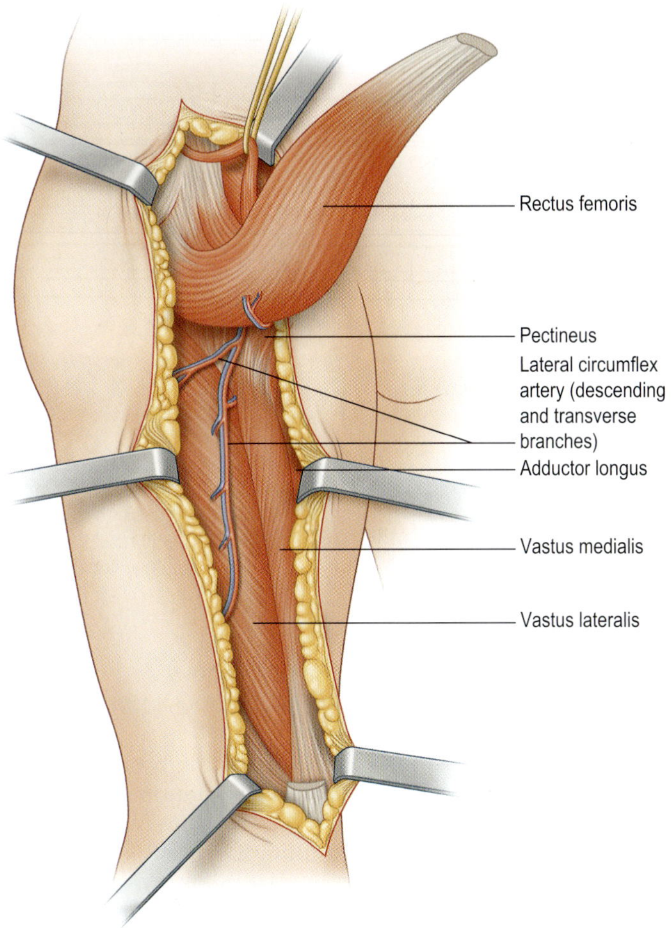

Figure 10.6 Rectus femoris muscle flap elevation. It is a type II pattern of circulation (the dominant pedicle is the descending branch of the lateral circumflex femoral artery with minor pedicles from the ascending branch of the same vessel as well as from muscle branches of the superficial femoral artery) and can reach to cover the inferior abdomen, groin, perineum and ischium.

- The tendon of the rectus femoris can be easily noted below the depression and above the patella.
- The skin island should be designed on the middle-third of the thigh as the majority of the perforators are located in this region.
- Incision at the distal edge of the skin island, along the axis allows the rectus femoris muscle to be identified and separated from the vastus medialis and lateralis.
- The skin island is then incised circumferentially down to the fascia of the muscle.
- The rectus is elevated from distal to proximal and from medial to lateral so that the pedicle and nerve can be identified and protected medially along the underside of the muscle.
- The dominant pedicle enters the posterior medial muscle at a variable distance of 7–10 cm below the symphysis pubis and care must be given to preserve the motor branches from the femoral nerve to the adjacent vastus lateralis and tensor fascia lata.
- The donor area should be repaired by careful suturing of the tendinous fascia of the vastus medialis and lateralis together above the patella in an effort to preserve full knee extension.

Biceps femoris

- This large, well-vascularized posterior muscle of the mid and lateral thigh is useful for the coverage of ischial pressure sores.
- The muscle has two heads: the long head originates on the ischial tuberosity and the short head originates on the linea aspera of femur and both insert onto the head of fibula.
- The long head extends the hip, and both heads flex the leg at the knee and thus is not expandable.
- The pattern of circulation is type II (the long head has dominant and minor pedicles from the first and second perforating branches of the profunda femoris artery, respectively, and the short head receives the second (or third) perforating branch of the profunda and a minor source from the lateral superior geniculate artery) and can be turned over to cover the ischial regions based on the dominant pedicle.
- The long head derives its motor innervations from the tibial division of the sciatic nerve, the short head from the peroneal division of the sciatic nerve. The postcutaneous nerve of the thigh (S1–3) supplies the sensation.
- The entire skin of the posterior thigh can be elevated and advanced in V-Y fashion as a musculocutaneous unit.
- The upper base of the skin flap is horizontally marked along the buttock crease and the apex just above the popliteal fossa.
- The relatively short pedicles make the flap unsuitable for wide rotation flaps but serve well in sliding the muscle proximally along the femur towards the pelvis.
- The medial thigh skin may also be left uncut, preserving skin as a rotation advancement modification of the flap.
- With the skin island isolated, the tendon is divided distally and the dissection proceeds from the distal thigh towards the ischium, freeing the muscle on its deep aspect from the femur and from the adductor group of muscles medially, until enough mobility is attained so that the defect can easily be filled.
- The flap should be inset and sutured with the patient in a jack-knife position and the hips flexed to prevent dehiscence of the flap.

Gracilis

- Located on the medial thigh extending between the pubis and the medial knee, it is a thin and flat muscle which lies between the adductor longus and sartorius muscle anteriorly and the semi-membranous posteriorly.
- It originates on the pubic symphysis and inserts into the medial tibial condyle.
- The gracilis function is a thigh adductor but is expandable from the compensation made from abductor longus and magnus muscle.
- The muscle has a type II circulation pattern (the dominant pedicle is the terminal branch of the medial circumflex femoral artery and one or two minor pedicles arise as branches of the superficial femoral artery) and

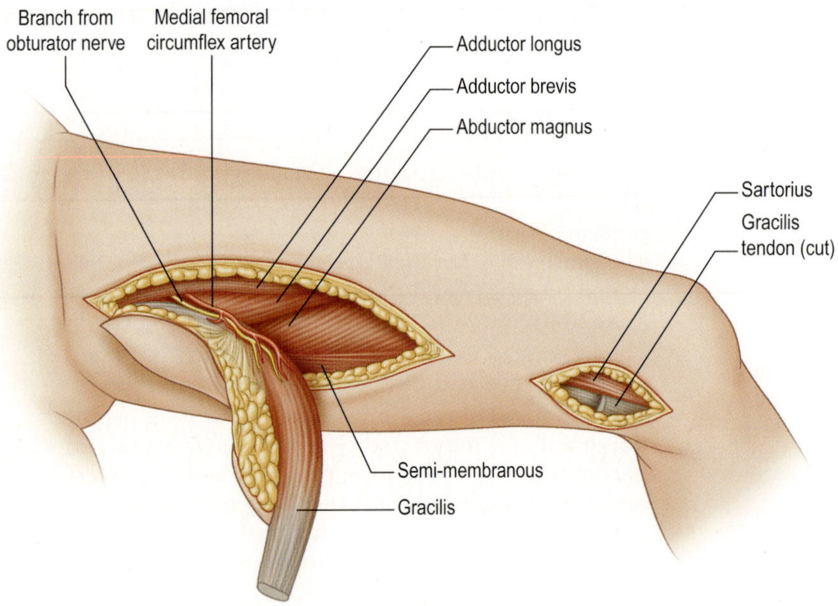

Figure 10.7 Gracilis muscle flap elevation. It is a type II circulation pattern (the dominant pedicle is the terminal branch of the medial circumflex femoral artery and one or two minor pedicles arise as branches of the superficial femoral artery) and can reach to cover the abdomen, ischium, groin, and perineum as a muscle or musculocutaneous flap.

can reach to cover the abdomen, ischium, groin, and perineum as a muscle or musculocutaneous flap ***(Fig. 10.7)***.

- Motor innervation is from the anterior branch of the obturator nerve and enters the gracilis on its deep medial surface immediately superior to the entry of the dominant pedicle.
- The motor nerve allows gracilis to be used as a functional muscle flap for facial reanimation and upper extremity.
- The sensory innervation is from the anterior femoral cutaneous nerve (L2–3), which provides sensation to the anterior medial thigh.
- When skin is harvested with the gracilis muscle, the flap is generally oriented longitudinally and centered over the proximal third of the muscle, where the majority of the musculocutaneous perforators are located.
- A proximal transversely oriented skin flap is optional and the bulky fat of the medial thigh makes this flap suitable for breast reconstruction.
- The symphysis pubis and the medial condyle of the femur are major landmarks.
- The muscle extends the full length of the medial thigh and averages about 6 cm in width proximally and tapers to about 2–3 cm in the distal third of the muscle.
- Although the width may be narrow, the muscle can be fanned out to provide coverage over larger defects.
- With the patient in lithotomy position and slight extension of the knee allows the gracilis to be seen and felt, and it tends to be more posterior than expected.
- For muscle elevation, an incision is made 2–3 cm posterior to the line drawn connecting the symphysis pubis and medial condyle of the knee.
- The muscle is identified posterior to the adductor longus.
- If a skin flap is planned, the skin territory should be designed on the proximal part of the inner thigh.
- Usually, the dissection is easily approached by distal incision identifying the tendon of the gracilis posterior to the saphenous vein and the distal sartorius muscle.
- Tendinous insertion of semi-membranous and semi-tendinosus muscle can be indentified posterior to the gracilis.
- Traction on the tendon will highlight the proximal outline of the muscle and allow accurate estimation of the location.
- This is an important step to minimize faulty elevation of the skin component, as the medial thigh is mobile and makes it easy to incorrectly predict the skin position over the muscle.
- Dissection of the anterior and posterior skin borders then proceed proximally, approximately half the length of the muscle, whereby the distal tendon is divided and the distal muscle elevated.
- During the elevation of the middle and distal third of the flap, one or two minor perforators from the superficial femoral artery will be identified and ligated.
- Retraction of the adductor longus muscle will expose the major pedicle passing over the deep adductor magnus, approximately 10 cm below the pubic symphysis.

Soleus

- The soleus is a very broad, large bipenniform muscle lying deep to the gastrocnemius muscle.
- The muscle has two muscle bellies, medial and lateral, separated by a midline intramuscular septum in the distal half.
- The lateral belly originates from the posterior surface of the head of the fibula and posterior surface of the body of the fibula and the medial belly originated from the middle-third of the medial border of the tibia.
- Both bellies of the soleus insert into the calcaneus bone through the Achilles tendon.
- It contributes to the plantar flexion of the foot. Soleus is expandable, taken that at least one head of gastrocnemius is intact with function.

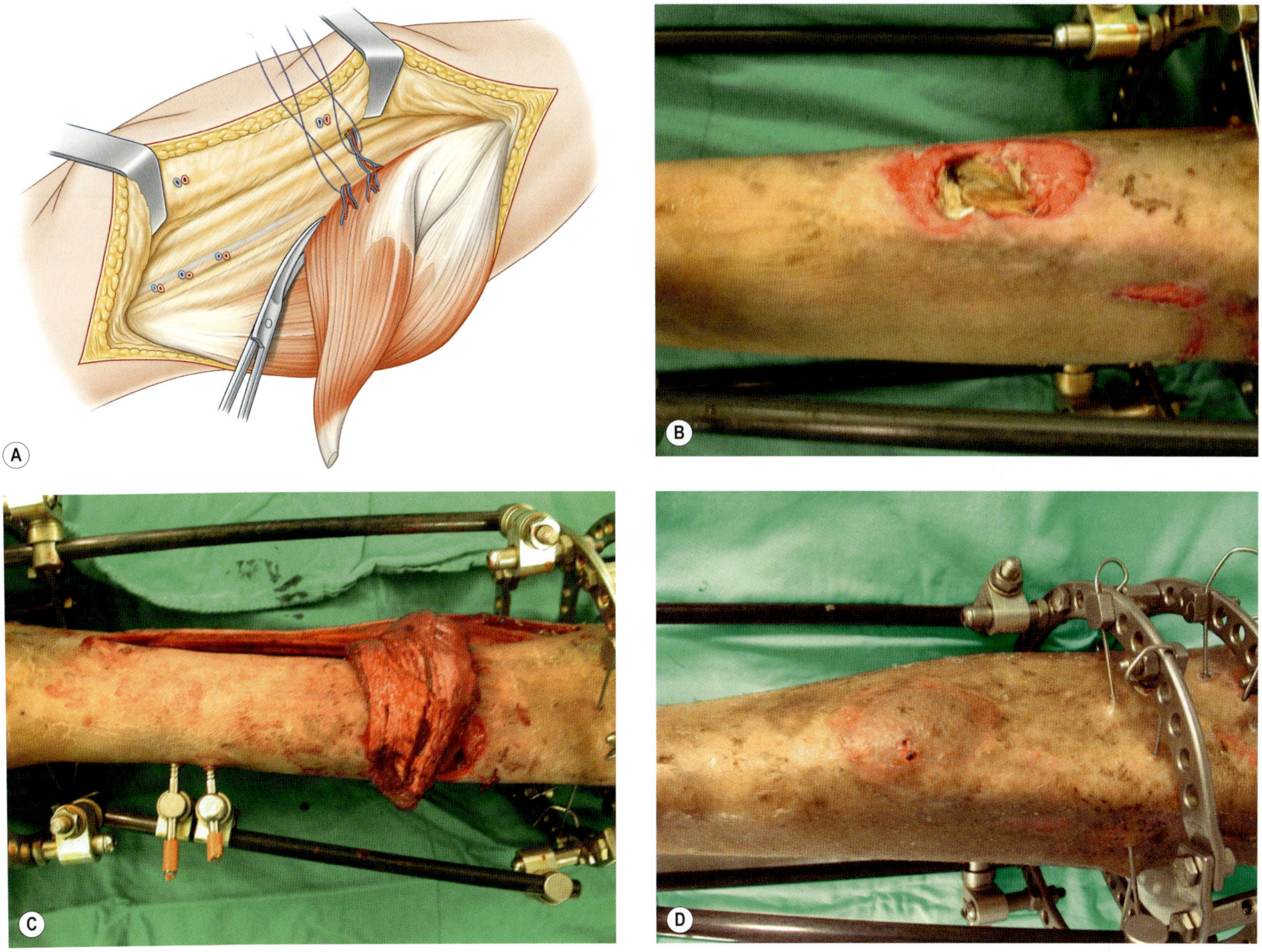

Figure 10.8 Soleus muscle flap elevation. **(A)** It is a type II circulation pattern (with dominant pedicles from the popliteal, posterior tibial, and peroneal arteries and the minor pedicles rise from posterior tibial and peroneal arteries supplying the distal, medial and lateral bellies, respectively) and can cover the middle and lower-third of the leg. **(B–D)** A patient with chronic osteomyelitis of the middle-third of the tibia is reconstructed using a hemi-soleus flap.

- The pattern of circulation is type II (with dominant pedicles from the popliteal, posterior tibial and peroneal arteries and the minor pedicles rise from the posterior tibial and peroneal arteries supplying the distal, medial and lateral bellies, respectively), and can cover the middle and lower-third of the leg *(Fig. 10.8A)*.
- Motor nerve is derived from the posterior tibial and popliteal nerves.
- The arc of rotation for a proximally-based soleus flap after division of minor pedicles and elevation of the distal two-thirds of the muscle can cover the middle-third of the tibia.
- Hemisoleus flaps may improve the arc of rotation and preserve soleus function while sacrificing flap coverage area.
- The medial reversed hemisoleus pivots around the most superior distal minor perforator of the posterior tibial artery, approximately 7 cm above the malleolus.
- The lateral reversed hemisoleus has a tenuous blood supply through minor perforators from the peroneal and a shorter arc of rotation.
- The distal half of the muscle can be reversely transposed based on minor segment pedicles and cover the distal third of the leg.
- The medial border of the tibia is the landmark for medial exposure and the fibula itself is the landmark for lateral exposure.
- A line can be drawn 2 cm medial to the medial edge of tibia or laterally along the fibula.
- Subcutaneous neurovascular structures are identified and preserved, and the posterior compartment fascia is opened.
- The plane between the soleus and gastrocnemius is usually well-defined superiorly, but sharp scalpel dissection is needed to separate the tendons and maintain the gastrocnemius contributions to the Achilles tendon.

- For proximally based flaps, distal perforators are divided in the deep plane, and the tendon is divided distally.
- The dominant pedicle is usually located on the upper third of the muscle for both bellies of the soleus.
- Identification and dissection of the midline raphe allow a hemisoleus flap to be developed (see Fig 10.8B–D).

Gastrocnemius

- The most superficial muscle of the posterior calf, the gastrocnemius has two heads, medial and lateral, which form the distal boundary of the popliteal space.
- Each head can be used as a separate muscle or musculocutaneous unit, based on its own pedicle.
- The medial head originates from the medial condyle of the femur and the lateral from the lateral condyle of the femur and both heads insert to the calcaneus through the Achilles tendon.
- It contributes to the plantar flexion of the foot and either or both heads of the gastrocnemius are expandable if the soleus is intact.
- The pattern of circulation is type I (the medial muscle is supplied by the medial sural artery and the lateral muscle is supplied by the lateral sural artery) and provides reliable coverage to the upper third of the tibia, suprapatellar thigh, and knee regions ***(Fig. 10.9)***.
- Motor innervation derives from branches of the tibial nerve.
- The sensation to the skin overlying the medial head is from the saphenous nerve and that to the lateral and distal skin overlying the lateral head is from the sural nerve.
- The arc of rotation of the medial head after complete elevation can cover the inferior thigh, knee, and upper third of the tibia.
- When origin of the muscle is divided, an extended arc of rotation by 5–8 cm can be achieved to extend to the upper part of the knee.
- The lateral head can be elevated to cover the suprapatellar region, knee and proximal third of the tibia.
- It also can be extended with the division of the muscle origin. Both heads can be inferiorly rotated, based on the vascular anastomosis across the raphe between the two muscle heads to reach the middle third of the leg.
- A skin paddle can be designed based on the perforating vessels with dimension of 10 × 15 cm for the medial and 8 × 12 cm for the lateral head.
- A line is drawn either 2 cm medial to the medial edge of the tibia or along the posterior midleg.
- If the muscle alone is employed, a midline posterior incision affords excellent access to both heads.
- During elevation, care is taken to protect the neurovascular structures, especially the more superficial saphenous and sural nerves.
- In the proximal third, medial surface of the medial head is easily separated from the soleus.

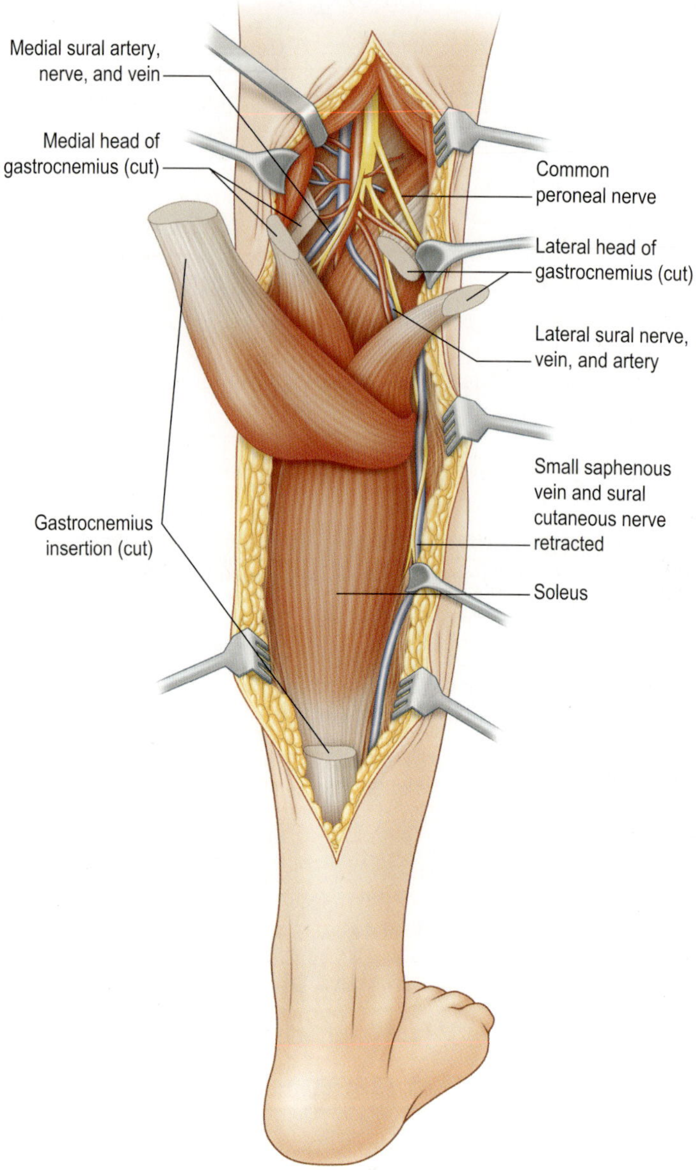

Figure 10.9 Gastrocnemius flap elevation. It is a type I circulation pattern (the medial muscle is supplied by the medial sural artery and the lateral muscle is supplied by the lateral sural artery) and provides coverage to the upper-third of the tibia, suprapatellar thigh, and knee regions.

- The dissection starts at the medial edge of the gastrocnemius muscle and plantaris can be easily noted below the gastrocnemius and above the soleus.
- The midline muscular raphe is located, and with finger dissection, the underlying soleus muscle is separated from the gastrocnemius proximally and distally.
- The musculotendinous raphe is then separated sharply.
- Distally, the thick tendinous layer is sharply dissected free from the remaining calcaneal tendon.
- The transaction of the origin of the muscle allows increased freedom.
- If a tunnel is made over the lateral proximal leg, care must be given not to violate the deep peroneal nerve.

Fasciocutaneous/perforator flap

- A perforator flap is defined as a flap based on a musculocutaneous perforating vessel that is directly visualized and dissected free of surrounding muscles and an adequate pedicle length is achieved.
- This kind of flap that may be based on any perforator, "freestyle free flap", allows the freedom of flap selection from anywhere on the body.
- Although this is a very useful flap, it provides limited coverage.
- Further advancement by Koshima et al. where the flap and the pedicle is taken above the fascia as a perforator flap, truly allows the donor site to have minimal morbidity.
- Anastomosis can be difficult with the vessel's diameter <1 mm, hence this technique is known as supermicrosurgery.
- Hong and Koshima have also stretched the boundary of microsurgery opening the possibility of using perforators as recipient vessels, and introduced the concept of "free style reconstruction".
- Since the basic approach may be similar, the septocutaneous and perforator flaps will be discussed together when necessary.

Groin/SCIP (superficial circumflex iliac perforator)

- The groin flap may be elevated extending between the femoral vessels and the posterior iliac spine.
- The dominant pedicle is the superficial circumflex iliac artery, and venae comitantes and superficial circumflex iliac vein ***(Fig. 10.10)***.
- The pedicle is very short, i.e., up to only 3 cm.
- Koshima defined that the SCIP flap is different from the groin flap in that it is nourished by only a perforator of the superficial circumflex iliac system ***(Fig. 10.11)***.
- The T12 sensory innervation is at the lateral margin of the flap away from the pedicle, precluding use as a sensate flap.
- The long axis of the flap is centered over a line parallel and 3 cm inferior to the inguinal ligament with a flap width of 6–10 cm.
- The flap can be used as a free or pedicled flap.
- For pedicled flaps, the dissection should proceed from lateral to medial and distal to proximal.
- Elevation is begun in a plane superficial to fascia lata and when the sartorius muscle is visualized, the flap is elevated deep to the fascia and superficial to the muscle.
- The perforator flap is elevated suprafascially until a sizable perforator is located and is used either as a pedicled or free flap.
- The groin flap as a septocutaneous flap provides a large amount of skin and soft tissue and may need debulking where excess tissue is not needed.
- The donor site is well tolerated and well hidden, but the pale skin and frequent hair growth of the donor site make for a poor match, particularly with head and neck reconstructions.

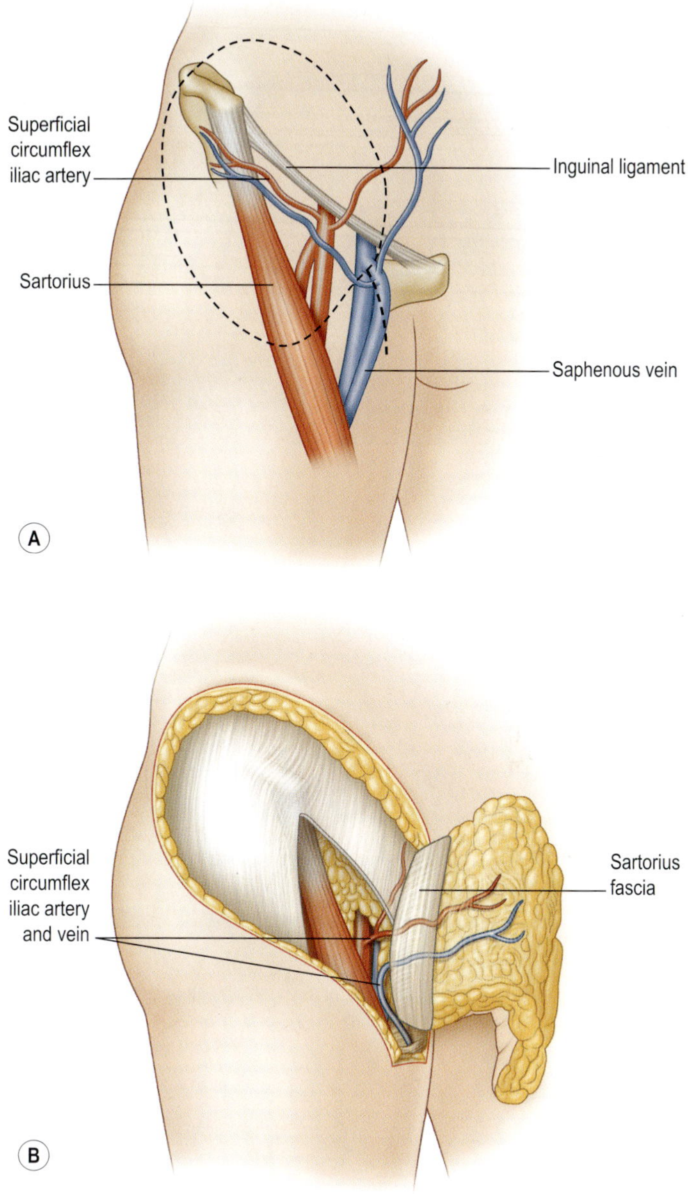

Figure 10.10 Groin flap elevation. The dominant pedicle is the superficial circumflex iliac artery **(A)**, and venae comitantes and superficial circumflex iliac vein **(B)**.

Medial thigh/anteromedial perforator and gracilis perforator

- The medial thigh flap located at the midthigh: the dominant blood supply for this fasciocutaneous flap is the anterior septocutaneous artery and venae comitantes from the superficial femoral artery and vein at the apex of the femoral triangle ***(Fig. 10.12)***.
- The coverage extends to the abdomen, groin, and perineum.
- The saphenous vein may be elevated with the flap for improved venous drainage.
- The sensory innervations are from the medial anterior cutaneous nerve of the thigh (L2–3).

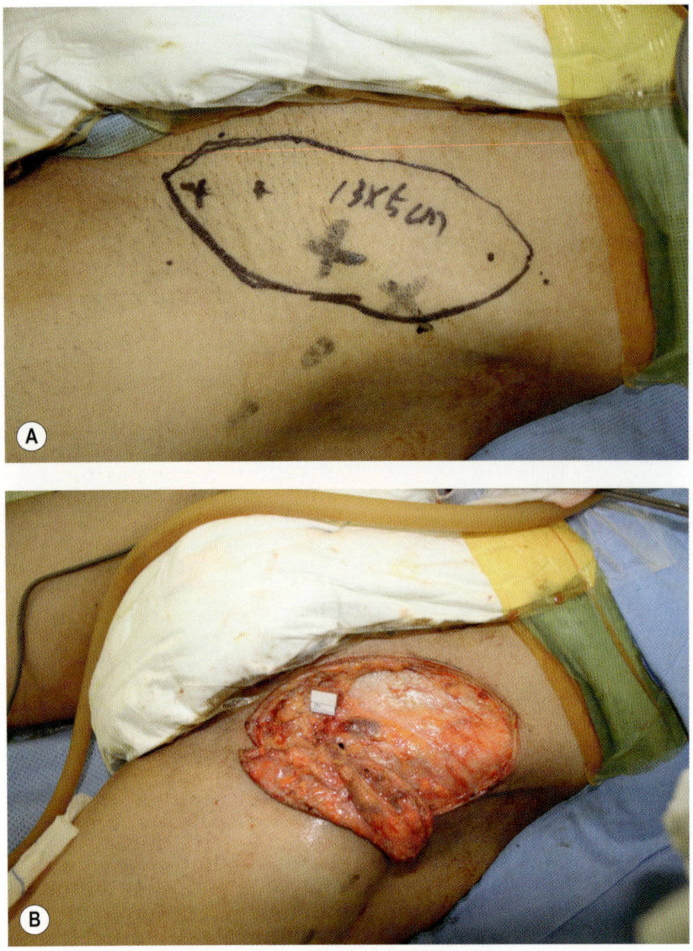

Figure 10.11 The SCIP flap is nourished by only a perforator of the superficial circumflex iliac system. A large dimension of skin from the inguinal region can be sufficiently supplied by a single perforator.

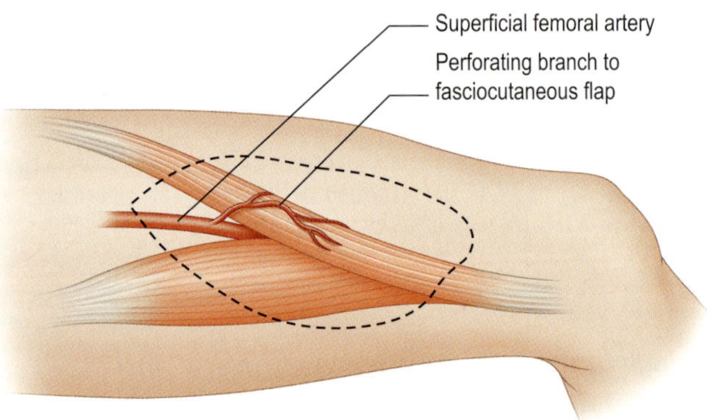

Figure 10.12 The medial thigh flap located at the midthigh. The dominant blood supply for this fasciocutaneous flap is the anterior septocutaneous artery and venae comitantes from the superficial femoral artery and vein at the apex of the femoral triangle.

- When the flap is based more anteriorly, it is termed the anteromedial thigh flap and is based on a branch of the lateral femoral circumflex artery emerging from the lateral border of the sartorius.
- Minor pedicles are contributed by musculocutaneous perforating vessels of the sartorius and gracilis muscles.

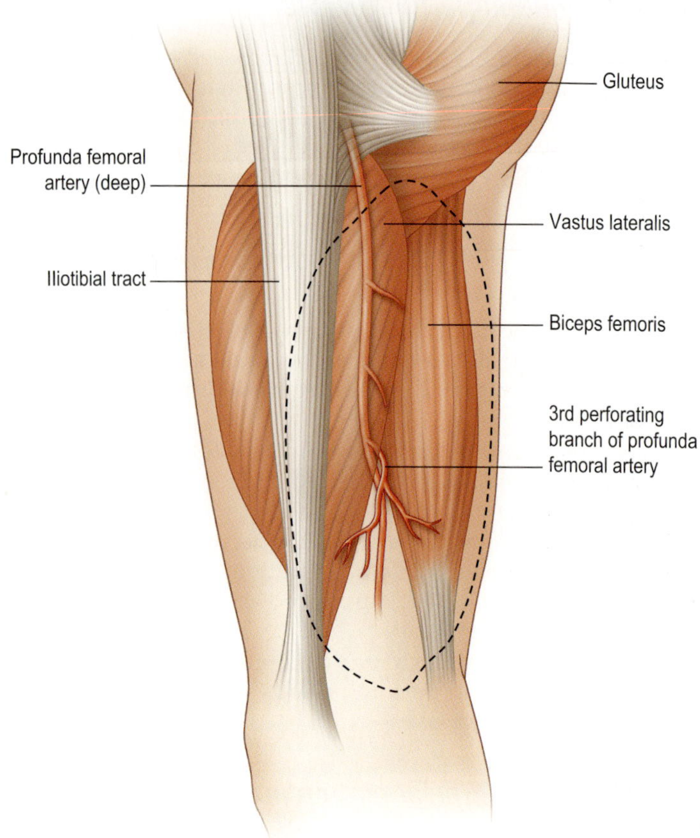

Figure 10.13 The lateral thigh flap. It is located along the lateral aspect of the thigh between the greater trochanter and the knee and can be based on the three perforating branches of the profunda femoris.

- When the flap is moved proximally to the groin, a perforator from the gracilis muscle is found originating from the profunda femoris vessel or the medial femoral circumflex vessel.
- All these flaps can be elevated as a perforator-based flap and named a medial thigh perforator flap, anteromedial thigh perforator flap, and gracilis perforator (medial circumflex femoral artery perforator) flap, respectively.
- For the medial thigh septocutaneous flap, the dominant pedicle is typically located at the apex of the femoral triangle approximately 6–8 cm below the inguinal ligament and is bordered medially by the adductor longus and laterally by the sartorius.
- A proximal incision is made to locate the vessels at the apex of the femoral triangle. The remainder of the flap is then incised and elevated subfascially.

Lateral thigh/profunda femoris perforator

- The lateral thigh flap located along the lateral aspect of the thigh between the greater trochanter and the knee can be based on the three perforating branches of the profunda femoris ***(Fig. 10.13)***.
- The first perforator arises just below the insertion of the gluteus maximus and flaps based on this perforator are

used for proximally based flaps to reach the trochanteric and ischial areas.

- The third perforator arises between the vastus lateralis and biceps femoris muscles, midway between the greater trochanter and lateral condyle of the femur, and the flaps based on the second or third perforator are for use as a microvascular transplantation because of the long pedicle.
- The flap is innervated from the lateral cutaneous nerve of the thigh (L2–3).

Anterolateral thigh perforator (Video 10.1)

Video 10.1

- The anterolateral thigh perforator flap is one of the most widely used perforator flaps.
- The skin can be elevated from a septocutaneous or musculocutaneous perforator.
- Numerous perforators are found along the region of intermuscular septum between the vastus lateralis and rectus femoris.
- These perforators usually drain into the descending branch of the lateral femoral circumflex artery, then proximally to lateral circumflex artery, then to the profunda femoris artery ***(Fig. 10.14)***.
- When perforators are traced to the source vessel, it allows the pedicle to have long length and thicker diameter.
- Innervation of the anterolateral thigh region is from the lateral femoral cutaneous nerve (L2–3).

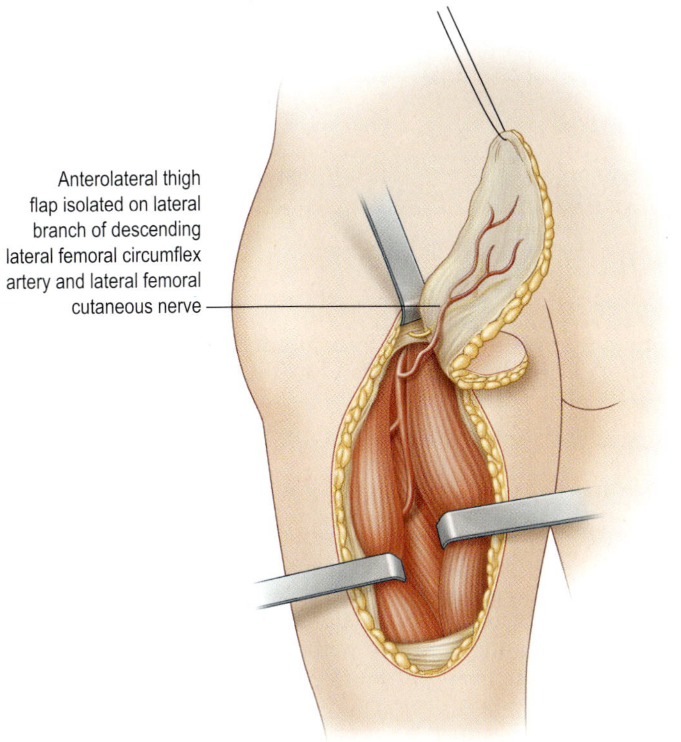

Figure 10.14 The anterolateral thigh flap. Numerous perforators are found along the region of intermuscular septum between the vastus lateralis and rectus femoris. These perforators usually drain into the descending branch of the lateral femoral circumflex artery, then proximally to lateral circumflex artery, then to the profunda femoris artery.

- The perforator frequently dissected is usually located on the midpoint of the line drawn between anterior superior iliac spine and superior lateral border of the patella.
- The perforator branches are identified with Doppler near the midpoint of this line.
- According to our clinical experience, about 90% of perforators are found within 3 cm diameter drawn at the midpoint of the line.
- The skin flap is designed to include the perforator and then elevated from the medial border.
- The flaps can be as large as 35 × 25 cm, based on a single perforator.
- The incision is made through the deep fascia and raised subfascially until the intermuscular septum between the rectus femoris and vastus lateralis muscle is reached.
- Now with increased knowledge of the perforator flap anatomy, flaps can be easily elevated suprafascially taking just a small cuff of fascia.
- At that point, the descending branch of the lateral femoral circumflex is explored along with the perforator to the skin flap.
- The flap can be harvested, either as a perforator flap including only the perforator branch to the skin or combined with the vastus lateralis muscle, as a musculocutaneous flap.
- The skin paddle may be defatted according to the need up to 3–4 mm thickness, except for the portion which the perforator branch enters ***(Fig. 10.15)***.
- The motor branch of the femoral nerve running medial to the descending branch of the lateral circumflex femoral artery should be preserved.
- To elevate as a sensate flap, a branch of the lateral femoral cutaneous nerve should be included. The donor site can be primarily closed depending on the laxity of the skin.

Sural

- The sural flap is located between the popliteal fossa and the midportion of the leg over the midline raphe between the two heads of the gastrocnemius muscle.
- It is one of the longest fasciocutaneous flaps of the lower leg based on the direct cutaneous artery (sural artery branch) in the upper central calf and extending to the Achilles tendon distally.
- The lesser saphenous vein provides venous drainage.
- It can cover defects of the knee, popliteal fossa, and upper-third of the leg.
- When used distally based on a reverse flow through anastomoses between the peroneal artery and the communicating vascular network of the medial sural nerve, it can reach difficult areas of defects in the lower leg and the ankle and heel region ***(Fig. 10.16)***.
- It is innervated by the medial sural cutaneous nerve (S1–2).
- The flap is raised from distal to proximal, in the plane beneath the deep fascia and above the gastrocnemius muscles.
- The sural nerve and lesser saphenous vein are divided distally and elevated with the flap.

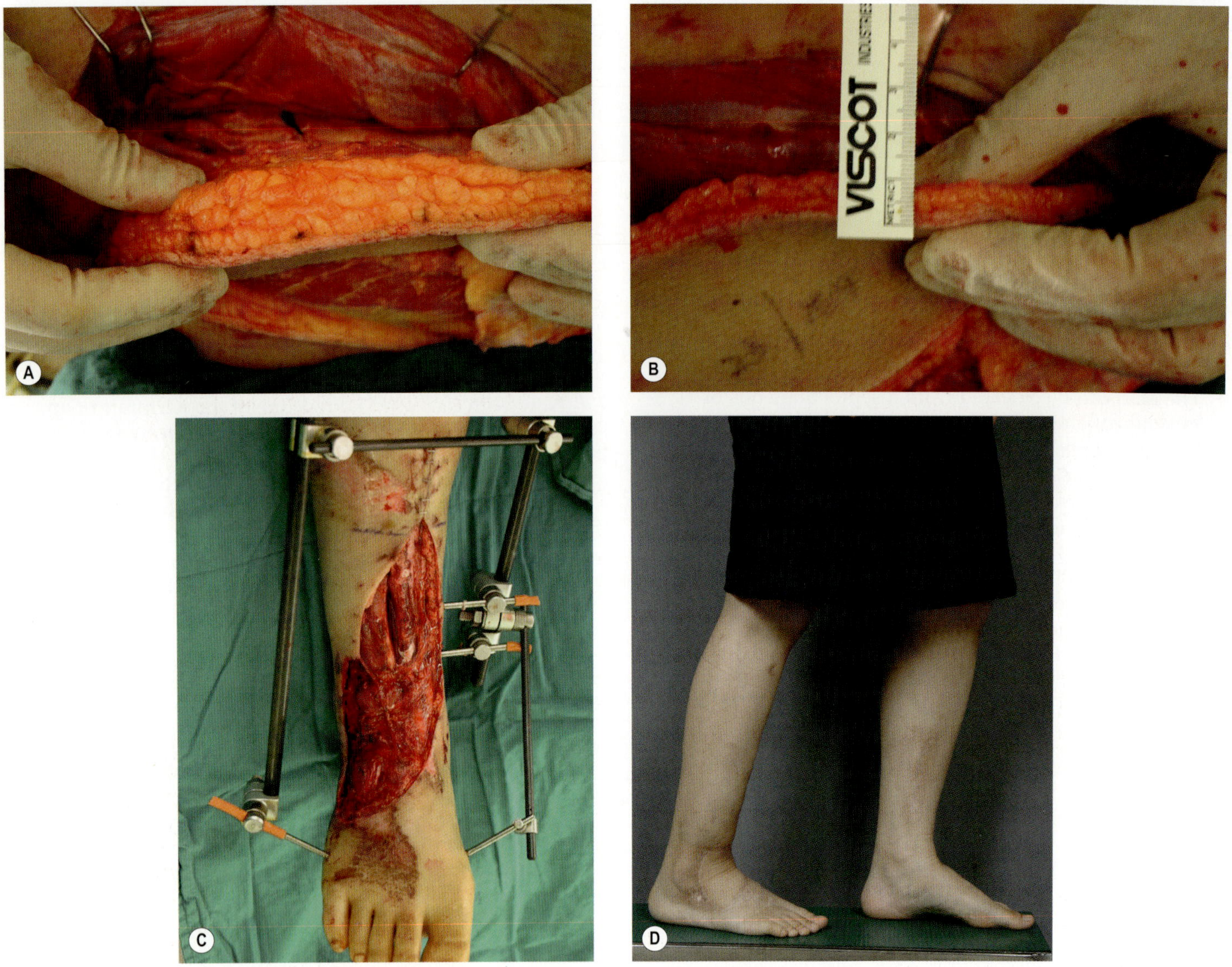

Figure 10.15 (A, B) The deep fat portion of the anterolateral thigh can be debulked to obtain a thinner pliable flap. **(C,D)** The patient with soft tissue defect of the ankle region is seen with excellent contour after reconstruction without further debulking.

- The pedicle should be visualized and protected in the popliteal fossa, with continued dissection of the pedicle for free tissue harvesting.
- For free tissue transplantation, proximal superficial veins should be dissected and preserved for possible anastomosis because the venae comitantes are small.

Tap (thoracodorsal artery perforator)

- The vascular territory lies on top of the latissimus dorsi muscle.
- The main perforators are located along the course of the descending branch of thoracodorsal artery or from the lateral branch.
- The most proximal perforator reaches the subcutaneous tissue in a point located 2 or 3 cm posterior to the lateral edge of the muscle and 8 cm below the posterior axillary fold.
- The patient is positioned in a lateral decubitus position with the upper arm in 90° abduction and 90° flexion at the elbows.
- The lateral border of the latissimus is palpated and marked.
- Doppler can be useful to identify potential perforators for the flap.
- Once perforators are identified, a flap can be designed based on the perforator.
- Although larger flap dimensions have been reported, flap dimensions under 255 cm^2 within its vascular territory should be safe from partial necrosis.
- Incision is made from the anterointerior border of the flap allowing the identification of the anterior border of the latissimus dorsi muscle.
- The dissection is performed between the fat and deep fascia covering the muscle.
- This plane is easy to dissect as it is in a loose areolar plane.

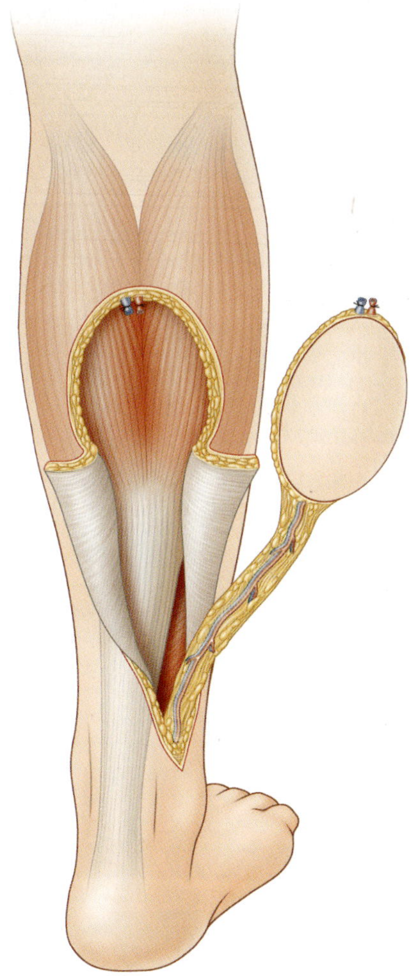

Figure 10.16 The sural flap. It is located between the popliteal fossa and the midportion of the leg over the midline raphe between the two heads of the gastrocnemius muscle. It is one of the longest fasciocutaneous flaps of the lower leg based on the direct cutaneous artery (sural artery branch) in the upper central calf and extending to the Achilles tendon distally.

- While dissecting for the perforator, care should be given when dissecting the proximal portion as direct cutaneous or perforators adjacent to the anterior borders are easily missed.
- After a suitable perforator is identified, the design of the flap, in accordance with the defect and pedicle, can be made.
- Perforators can be isolated or taken with a muscle cuff reaching down to the main pedicle.
- Total pedicle length depends on the location of perforator and the intramuscular course of the pedicle. Pedicle length can be acquired up to 14–18 cm ***(Fig. 10.17)***.

Compound flaps

- A compound flap consists of multiple tissue components linked together in a manner that allows their simultaneous transfer.
- These separate components can be maneuvered and placed in a three-dimensional manner to achieve an ideal one-stage reconstruction.

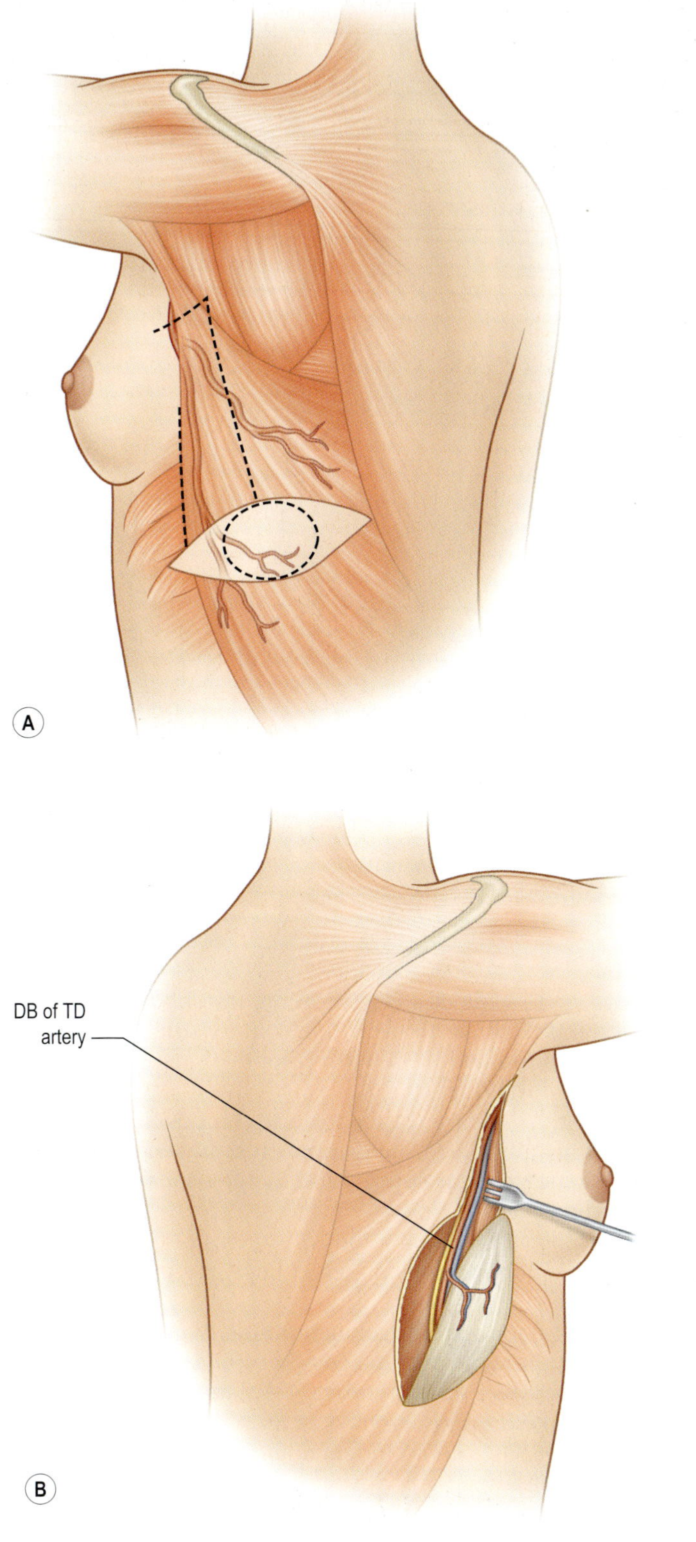

Figure 10.17 Thoracodorsal artery perforator flap. The main perforators are located along the course of descending branch (DB) of thoracodorsal (TD) artery or from the lateral branch. The most proximal perforator reaches the subcutaneous tissue in a point located 2 or 3 cm posterior to the lateral edge of the muscle and 8 cm below the posterior axillary fold.

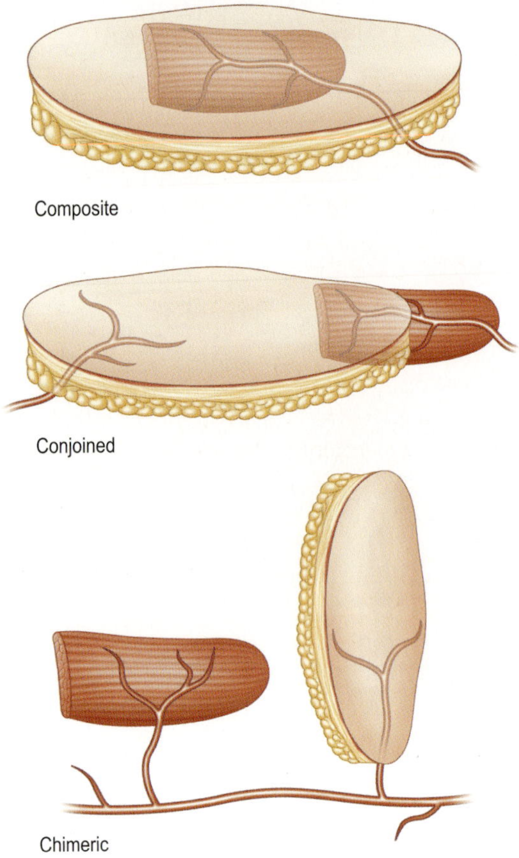

Figure 10.18 Classification of compound flaps.

- According to Hallock's classification, the subdivisions of compound flaps are those with a solitary source of vascularization and those with combinations of sources of vascularization *(Fig. 10.18)*.
- Those with a solitary source include composite flaps, defined as multiple tissue components, all served by the same single vascular supply, and thereby consisting of dependent parts.
- Those flaps with combinations of sources of vascularization include conjoined flaps and chimeric flaps.
- Conjoined flaps are defined as multiple flap territories, dependent because of some common physical junction, yet each retains its independent vascular supply.
- The chimeric flaps are defined as multiple flap territories, each with an independent vascular supply, and independent of any physical interconnection, except where linked by a common source vessel *(Fig. 10.19)*.

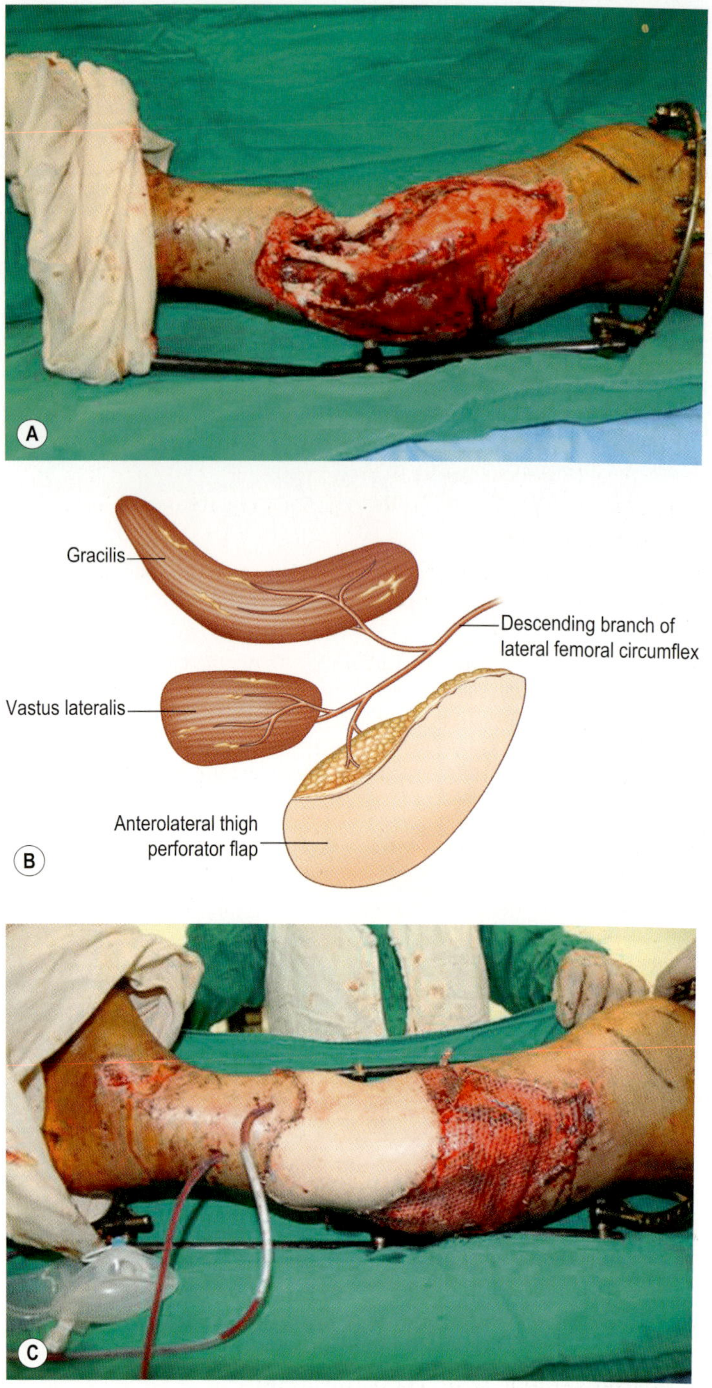

Figure 10.19 The chimeric flaps defined as multiple flap territories, each with an independent vascular supply, and independent of any physical interconnection except where linked by a common source vessel. Example of complex extremity reconstruction is shown using a chimeric approach. The source vessel of the descending branch of the lateral femoral circumflex artery feeding the vastus lateralis and the anterolateral thigh perforator flap. A gracilis is connected using a branch from the source vessel.

Supermicrosurgery

- The supermicrosurgery technique is defined as microsurgical anastomosis of vessels, with a diameter <0.8 mm.
- This technique, although reported frequently on lymphaticovenous shunting to treat lymphedema and sporadically in soft tissue reconstruction with specific indications, is a relatively new concept for lower extremity reconstruction.
- For the lower extremity soft tissue reconstruction, one of the applications can be seen in the perforator-to-perforator anastomosis approach.

- With an evident pulse on the perforating artery, it can be successfully used as a recipient vessel to supply a sizable flap.
- This approach will allow an increase in the selection of recipient pedicles.
- By using a perforator-to-perforator anastomosis approach, less time is consumed to secure the recipient vessel, to elevate the flap by taking just a short segment of the perforator pedicle, and minimizes any risk for major vessel injury or can utilize collateral circulation without apparent flow of major vessels while having acceptable flap survival.

Postoperative considerations

- During the postoperative period, the patient as a whole and the flap should be closely monitored.
- Monitoring flaps, especially free flaps in the first 24 h is essential due to the majority of thrombosis occurring at this time.
- It is also important to monitor hemodynamic and pulmonary function as adequate hydration and oxygenation are critical to flap survival.
- Limiting range of motion may be needed for flaps covering the joints as extension or flexion may increase the tension of the pedicle.
- There is no ideal method of flap monitoring but recent techniques such as tissue oxygen measurement, implantable Doppler device, laser Doppler flowmetry, and fluorescent dye injections may assist the judgment made from clinical evaluation which remains as the "gold standard" of monitoring.
- Emergent re-exploration should be performed once pedicle compromise is noted.
- Although there are no clinical reviews that conclusively show any agents that increase flap survival rate, most microsurgeons use some form of prophylactic antithrombotic treatment such as heparin, dextran and aspirin or in combinations with other agents.
- The routine use of dextran should be carefully approached due to allergic reaction and pulmonary edema.
- Thrombolytics such as urokinase can be used when flow is not immediately re-established after pedicle rearrangement or revision anastomosis.
- Leeches have a role in the postoperative care for a jeopardized flap. By injecting a salivary component called hirudin, which inhibits platelet aggregation and coagulation cascade, leeches can decongest flaps by extracting blood directly and indirectly through persistent oozing after it detaches.
- The use of leeches for 5–7 days can sometimes help salvage the flaps that do not resolve, despite re-exploration of the venous flow.
- Bone grafts are usually placed 6 weeks after soft tissue reconstruction to allow time for transferred tissue to settle in and sterilize the wound.
- Cancellous autografts or vascularized bone transfers can be chosen depending on length of the bone gap.
- Bone transfer mechanism can be an alternative to free bone transfer of bone defects longer than 6 cm.

Complications and outcomes

- Complications of lower extremity reconstruction include flap loss, infection, dehiscence, and wound related complications, wound recurrence, and amputation.
- To achieve optimal motion of tendons of the lower extremity, secondary tenolysis procedure may be needed.
- The risk for adhesion may increase when the skin graft is performed over granulated tissue directly above the tendons and may warrant flap coverage.
- Patients after recovery frequently show scars, depression, bulky flaps, and donor site morbidities.
- Although complete restoration is nearly impossible, a reasonable endpoint should be set and efforts to minimize scars and achieve good contours should be made.
- Debulking by surgical excision or liposuction can improve the contour of the flap and fat grafts can be added to elevate depressed scars.
- Scar revision by Z-plasties or expanders can help to alleviate scars not only physical but psychological.

Further reading

Bosse MJ, MacKenzie EJ, Kellam JF, et al. An analysis of outcomes of reconstruction or amputation after leg-threatening injuries. *N Engl J Med.* 2002;347(24):1924–1931.

The authors from Carolinas Medical Center performed a multicenter, prospective, observational study of 569 patients with severe leg trauma and evaluated the sickness-impact profile, a multidimensional self-reported health status to determine the long-term outcomes after amputation or limb reconstruction. They report that at 2 years, there was no significant difference in scores for the Sickness Impact Profile between the amputation and reconstruction groups. They advise patients with limbs at high risk for amputation may undergo reconstruction and will have results in 2- years equivalent to those of amputation.

Chen KT, Mardini S, Chuang DC, et al. Timing of presentation of the first signs of vascular compromise dictates the salvage outcome of free flap transfers. *Plast Reconstr Surg.* 2007;120(1):187–195.

Chung KC, Saddawi-Konefka D, Haase SC, et al. A cost-utility analysis of amputation versus salvage for Gustilo type IIIB and IIIC open tibial fractures. *Plast Reconstr Surg.* 2009;124(6):1965–1973.

The authors from the University of Michigan Health System evaluated the cost following amputation and salvage using the data presented in a study from the Lower Extremity Assessment Project. The authors extracted relevant data on projected lifetime costs and analyzed them to include discounting and sensitivity analysis by considering patient age. They report amputation is more expensive than salvage, independently of varied ongoing prosthesis needs, discount rate, and patient age at presentation. Moreover, amputation yields fewer quality-adjusted life-years than salvage. Salvage is deemed the dominant, cost-saving strategy.

Godina M. Early microsurgical reconstruction of complex trauma of the extremities. *Plast Reconstr Surg.* 1986;78(3):285–292.

Gottlieb LJ, Krieger LM. From the reconstructive ladder to the reconstructive elevator. *Plast Reconstr Surg.* 1994;93(7):1503–1504.

Hong JP. The use of supermicrosurgery in lower extremity reconstruction: the next step in evolution. *Plast Reconstr Surg.* 2009;123(1):230–235.

Kindsfater K, Jonassen EA. Osteomyelitis in grade II and III open tibia fractures with late debridement. *J Orthop Trauma.* 1995;9(2):121–127.

Lange RH. Limb reconstruction versus amputation decision making in massive lower extremity trauma. *Clin Orthop Relat Res.* 1989;243:92–99.

This study from the University of Wisconsin describes the absolute and relative indications for primary amputation of limbs with open tibial fractures. Absolute indications include: anatomically complete disruption of the posterior tibial nerve in adults and crush injuries with warm ischemia time greater than 6 h. Relative indications include: serious associated polytrauma, severe ipsilateral foot trauma, and anticipated protracted course to obtain soft tissue coverage and tibial reconstruction. However, he states that individual patient variables, specific extremity injury characteristics, and associated injuries must all be weighed before a decision can be reached and further prospective studies are necessary before a well-defined protocol for primary amputation can be properly developed.

Ong YS, Levin LS. Lower limb salvage in trauma. *Plast Reconstr Surg.* 2010;125(2):582–588.

The authors from the Duke University Medical center review the approach to lower limb salvage. They state that the primary goal of limb salvage is to restore or maintain function based on proper patient selection, timely reconstruction, and choosing the best procedure which should be individualized for each patient. Aggressive debridement and skeletal stabilization, followed by early reconstruction, are the current standard of practice and give better results than the more traditional approach of repeated debridements and delayed flap cover. For reconstruction, they state that free tissue transfer remains the best choice for large defects, but local fasciocutaneous flaps are a reasonable alternative for smaller defects and cases in which free flaps are deemed not suitable.

Wei FC, Celik N. Perforator flap entity. *Clin Plast Surg.* 2003;30(3):325–329.

The authors from the Chang Gun Memorial hospital state that the perforator flap is not a new concept in microsurgery but there is still confusion and that studies about the differences between these flaps and the conventional flaps, including donor site morbidity and long-term follow-ups, are increasing in literature. Better accuracy in reconstruction, including the use of only cutaneous tissue, minimization of the morbidity, and preserving the same survival rate in free flaps are reassurances to microsurgeons to perform perforator flaps. They believe that in the near future, with refinements in the techniques and instruments, perforator flaps will be the first choice flap.

Chapter 11

Chest reconstruction

This chapter was created using content from Neligan & Song, Plastic Surgery 3rd edition, Volume 4, Lower Extremity, Trunk and Burns, Chapter 10, Reconstruction of the chest, David H. Song and Michelle C. Roughton.

SYNOPSIS

- Rigid chest wall support may be achieved with mesh, acellular dermal matrix, or autogenous material such as tensor fascia lata. Of these, alloplastic mesh is most prone to infection.
- Soft tissue coverage can be achieved with local muscle flaps.
- Proper treatment of mediastinitis includes debridement, rigid sternal fixation when possible, and soft tissue coverage.
- Pectoralis muscle is the workhorse for sternal and anterior chest wall defects.
- Latissimus muscle is known for its bulk and ability to reach intrathoracic defects. Caution is advised for patients with previous thoracotomy incisions as it may have been divided.
- Serratus muscle supplies less bulk than the latissimus but will function to cover lateral chest wall defects and some intrathoracic needs.
- Rectus abdominus is an excellent choice for sternal and anterior chest wall defects, especially the lower two-thirds. Furthermore, it can be used to fill space within the mediastinum.
- The omentum can reach almost any chest wall defect. Its greatest advantage is its pedicle length, which can be extended by dividing the arcades. It does, however, require a laparotomy for harvest.

Brief introduction

- Common etiologies for chest wall defects include tumor resection, deep sternal wound infections, chronic empyemas, osteoradionecrosis and trauma.
- Mediastinitis occurs in 0.25–5% of patients undergoing median sternotomy.
- Historically, mortality approached 50% in these patients.
- Sternal wound infections may be classified into three distinct types as described by Pairolero and Arnold (Table 11.1).
  - Type 1: wounds that occur in the first several postoperative days and are usually sterile.
  - Type 2: infections which occur in the first several weeks postoperatively.
  - Consistent with acute deep sternal wound infection, including sternal dehiscence, positive wound cultures, and cellulitis.
  - Type 3: infections that present months to years later.
  - Represent chronic wound infection and uncommonly represent true mediastinitis.
  - Usually confined to the sternum and overlying skin and may be related to osteonecrosis or persistent foreign body.
- Although each mechanism carries individual nuances, they will all require adequate debridement and, when possible, replacement of like with like.
- Fundamentally, the chest wall must be restored for the protection of underlying viscera, maintenance of respiratory mechanics, and base for the upper limb and shoulder.
- Chest wall reconstruction can be generalized to include skeletal support and soft tissue cover.
- Skeletal support to prevent paradoxic chest wall motion is usually required when the defect exceeds 5 cm in diameter.
- Generally, this corresponds to those defects exceeding a two rib resection. (Table 11.2).
- Posterior chest wall defects may tolerate up to twice the size of those in the anterior and lateral chest due to scapular coverage and support.

- Anecdotally, patients who have undergone radiation and have decreased chest wall compliance will tolerate larger resections without skeletal replacement due to an overall fibrosis of their viscera.
- Options for skeletal support include various mesh products including PTFE (Gore-Tex®), polypropylene, Mersilene (polyethylene-terephthalate)/ methylmethacrylate, and acellular dermal matrix ***(Fig. 11.1)***. Furthermore, use of TFL as both graft and flap reconstruction has been described.
- Chest wall reconstruction almost always requires some form of soft tissue coverage as very few defects will close primarily. Reconstructive goals include wound closure with maintenance of intrathoracic integrity, restoration of aesthetic contours, as well as minimization of donor site deformity.
- Recruitment of local muscles with or without overlying skin is often the first-line of reconstructive offense, including: pectoralis major, latissimus dorsi, serratus anterior, and rectus abdominus. The omentum may also be used.
- Commonly, the ipsilateral latissimus muscle is divided during thoracotomy incisions and the authors encourage early communication between surgeons if there are multiple teams in order to mitigate against routine division. Muscle sparing thoracotomies help to preserve both the latissimus and serratus muscles while providing adequate intrathoracic access ***(Fig. 11.2)***.

Table 11.1 **Classification of infected sternotomy wounds**

Type I	Type II	Type III
Occurs within first few days	Occurs within first few weeks	Occurs months to years later
Serosanguineous drainage	Purulent drainage	Chronic draining sinus tract
Cellulitis absent	Cellulitis present	Cellulitis localized
Mediastinum soft and pliable	Mediastinal suppuration	Mediastinitis rare
Osteomyelitis and costochondritis absent	Osteomyelitis frequent, costochondritis rare	Osteomyelitis, costochondritis, or retained foreign body always present
Cultures usually negative	Cultures positive	Cultures positive

Table 11.2 **Regions of the chest wall**

Anterior	Between anterior axillary lines
Lateral	Between anterior and posterior axillary lines
Posterior	Between posterior axillary lines and the spine

Preoperative considerations

- The importance of a multidisciplinary approach to chest wall reconstruction cannot be underestimated. These patients, whether suffering from malignancy, infection, or trauma, are often also plagued with cardiac or respiratory insufficiency, diabetes, obesity, malnutrition, and generalized deconditioning.
- Acquired chest wall deformities are commonly the result of iatrogenic injury. Usually encountered in conjunction with cardiac or thoracic surgery, wound infections, mediastinitis, osteoradionecrosis, refractory empyema and bronchopleural fistulas, can all necessitate chest wall reconstruction.
- Utilizing the workhorse flaps described below, combined with general principles of thorough debridement and skeletal stabilization, the surgeon is generally well prepared to reconstruct any deficit. Common chest wall reconstructive problems are described below.
- Preoperative risk factors for the development of mediastinitis include: older patients, COPD, smoking, ESRD, DM, chronic steroid or immunosuppressive use, morbid obesity including large, heavy breasts, prolonged ventilator support (>24 h), concurrent infection and reoperative surgery. Other variables include off midline sternotomies, osteoporosis, use of LIMA or RIMA, long cardiopulmonary bypass runs (>2 h), and transverse sternal fractures.
- Empyema is defined as a deep space infection between the layers of visceral and parietal pleura.
- The chest cavity, unlike most other regions in the body, is rigid and non-collapsible. Thus, deep space infections,

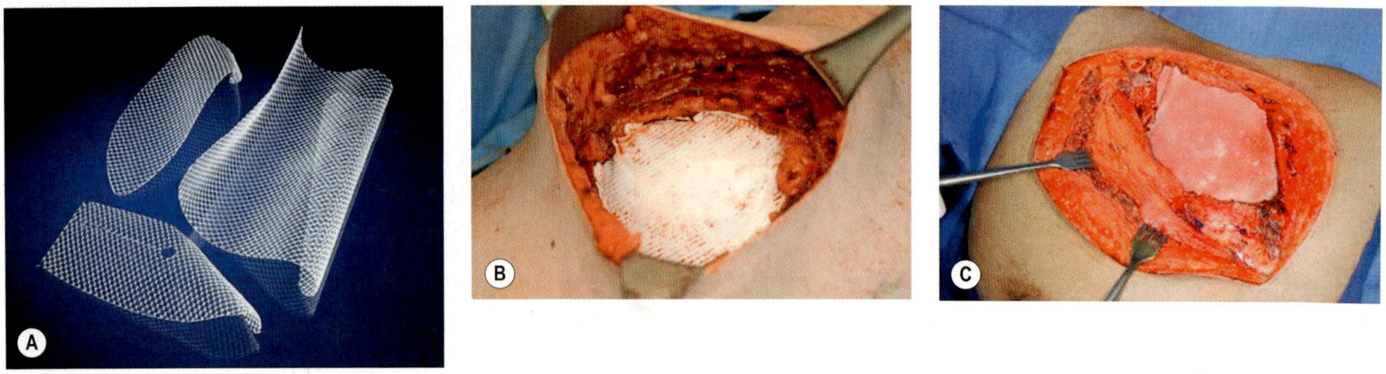

Figure 11.1 Implantable mesh products including polypropylene, PTFE (Gore-Tex®), and acellular dermal matrix.

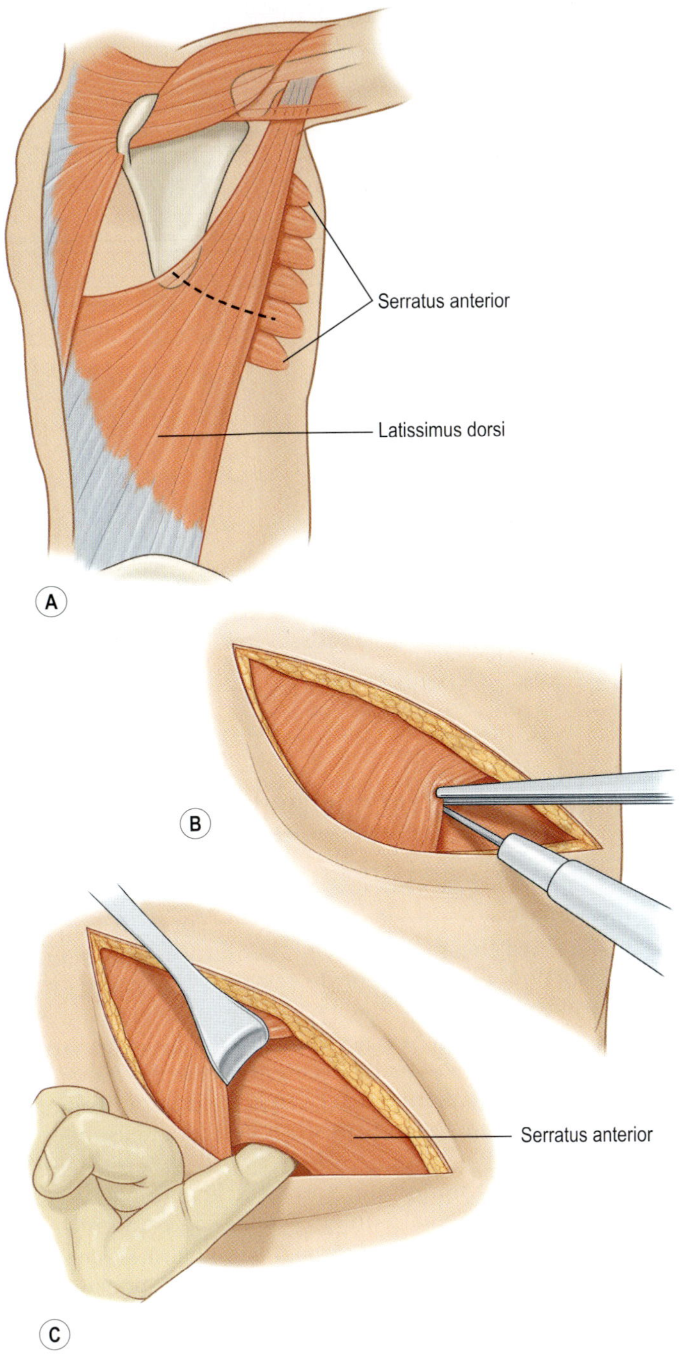

Figure 11.2 Muscle sparing thoracotomy. (From Ferguson MK. *Thoracic Surgery Atlas*. Edinburgh: Elsevier©; 2007.)

such as empyemas, are unlikely to heal without collapse of dead space or filling of the cavity.

- As adjuvant radiation therapy is becoming increasingly common in the treatment of both breast and lung cancer, osteoradionecrosis (ORN) of the ribs is becoming an increasing problem for reconstructive surgeons.
- Management of ORN of the chest wall consists of surgical excision and reconstruction.
- Again, should more than two ribs be resected from the anterior chest wall, skeletal support will traditionally be required.
- Radiation damage also affects overlying soft tissues, creating hyperpigmentation, decreased pliability, and even ulceration. Thus, recruitment of healthy tissue in the form of local myocutaneous flaps is recommended.

Operative techniques

Mediastinitis/sternal wound infection

- If tissue culture is positive, >10^5 organisms/cm^3 of tissue, indicating deep sternal wound infection rather than early sternal dehiscence, early debridement is encouraged and should be performed urgently.
- A thorough debridement includes:
  - Removal of sternal wires and extraneous foreign bodies including any unnecessary pacing wires and chest tubes ***(Fig. 11.3)***.
  - Debridement of necrotic and/or purulent tissue until remaining tissue appears healthy and bleeding.
  - Radical sternectomy is not indicated and sternal salvage should be attempted if the bone is viable. This may be determined by bleeding from the marrow and the presence of hard, crunchy cortical bone. Topical antimicrobials such as silver sulfadiazine and mafenide creams are employed to gain and maintain bacteriologic control of the wound.
- Subatmospheric pressure wound therapy (e.g. V.A.C.™) may be utilized to increase wound blood flow and expedite granulation tissue, thereby decreasing dead space.
- This has been shown to decrease the number of days between operative debridement and definitive closure of sternal wounds, from 8.5 to 6.2 days, as well as the number of flaps required per patient, 1.5–0.9.
- It is now standard practice for the treatment of mediastinitis at many institutions.
- Fixation of the sternum or residual sternal bone is crucial for bony healing, preventing paradoxic motion of the anterior chest wall, and improvements in chest wall pain and/or sternal rubbing or clicking sensations ***(Fig. 11.4)***.
- Sternal dehiscence occurs early in the postoperative course, consistent with type 1 sternal wound infections, and is secondary to mechanical failure of wire closure rather than infection.
- The wounds are sterile and surgeons should proceed to immediate rigid sternal fixation.
- Once rigid fixation is achieved, soft tissue closure must be addressed.
- When the wound involves the upper two-thirds of the sternum, pectoralis major muscle advancement or turnover flaps are easily harvested and are the first-line therapy for wound closure ***(Fig. 11.5)***.
- Caution is advised for turnover flaps when the ipsilateral internal mammary artery (IMA) has been harvested for CABG.
- When the lower sternal pole lacks coverage, the pectoralis may be inadequate, based on its limited arc of rotation.

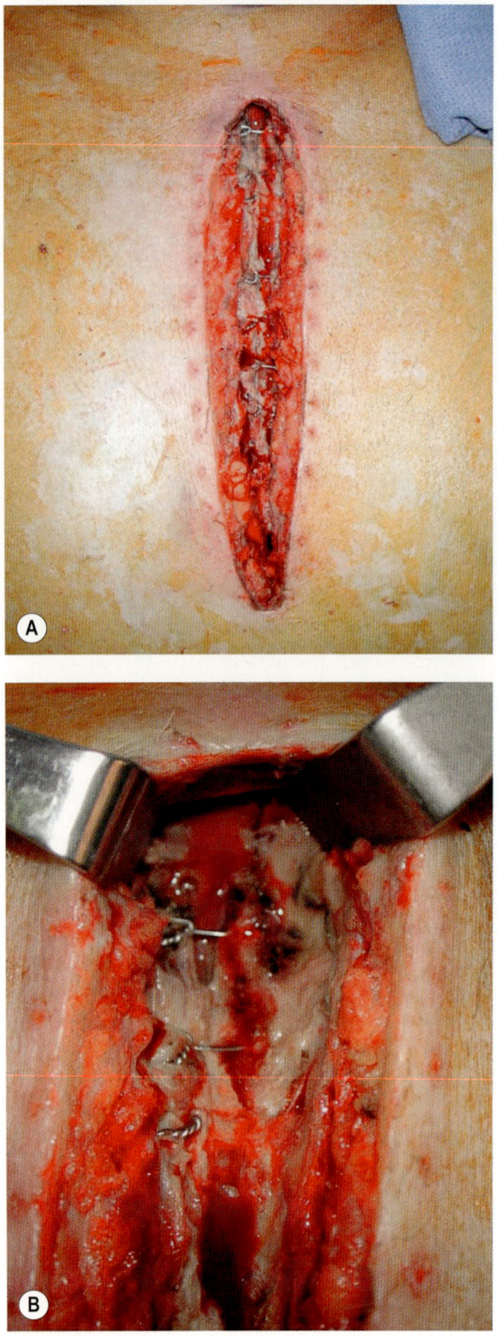

Figure 11.3 Thorough debridement requires removal of necrotic tissue and foreign bodies.

For these cases, the rectus abdominus muscle flap is a better choice.

- It may be used despite LIMA or RIMA harvest based upon the 8th intercostal artery, its minor pedicle.
- If the rectus is unavailable secondary to previous surgery, a pedicled omental flap should be considered for soft tissue sternal coverage.
- Finally, if the omentum has been previously resected or the patient has had multiple prior abdominal operations, the latissimus dorsi flap can be used.

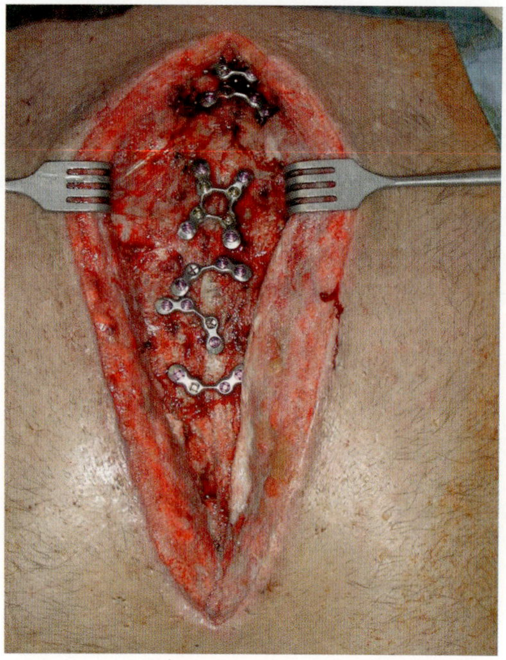

Figure 11.4 Rigid fixation is crucial for sternal union.

Common flaps for reconstruction

Pectoralis major

- Pectoralis major, a muscle overlying the superior portion of the anterior chest wall, is the workhorse for chest wall reconstruction, especially for defects of the sternum and anterior chest.
- Main function is to internally rotate and adduct the arm. Additionally, it serves as the foundation for the female breast and when absent, such as in Poland's syndrome, reconstruction may be indicated for aesthetic reasons ***(Fig. 11.6)***.
- Originates from the sternum and clavicle and inserts along the superomedial humerus in the bicipital groove.
- Dominant pedicle is the thoracoacromial trunk which enters the undersurface of the muscle below the clavicle at the junction of its lateral and middle third.
- Segmental blood supply is derived from IMA perforators.
- Based on the thoracoacromial blood supply, it will easily cover sternal and anterior chest wall defects as an island or advancement flap.
- Division of the pectoralis major muscle insertion can also aid in advancing the muscle flap into a properly debrided mediastinal wound.
- The muscle can also be turned over based on the IMA perforators and with release of its insertion, cover sternal, mediastinal, and anterior chest wall defects.
- Importantly, when used as a turnover flap, the internal mammary vessels and their perforators must be examined and deemed intact particularly in the setting of post-sternotomy mediastinitis.
- This vessel may be absent (left more commonly used than right) due to harvest for coronary artery bypass

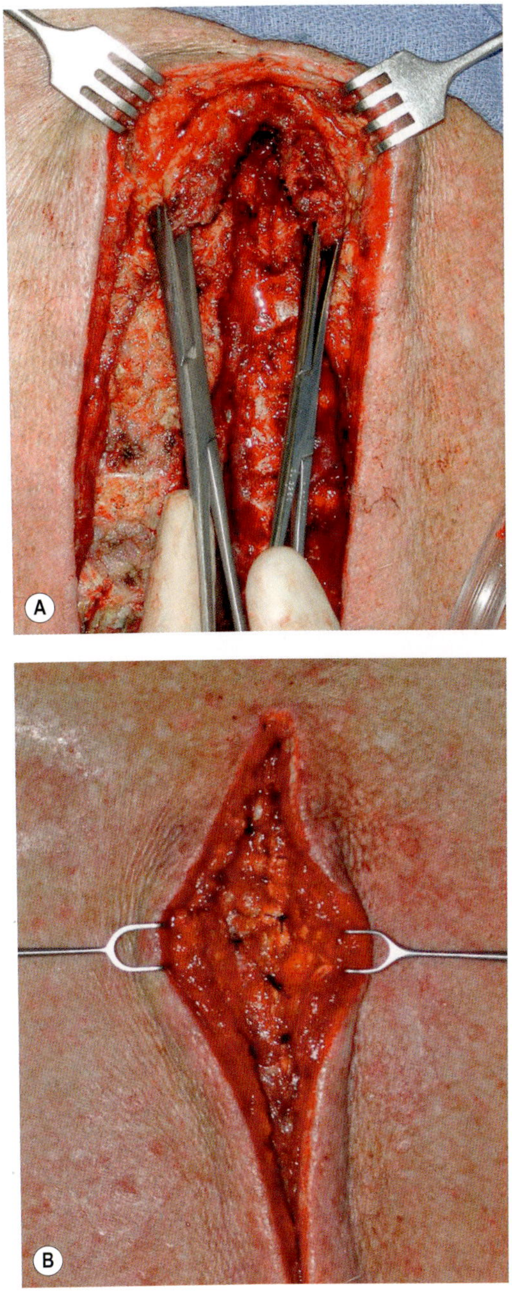

Figure 11.5 Bilateral pectoralis advancement flaps. Allis clamps on pectoralis muscle. Muscle sutured together in midline. (Courtesy of Dr David Song.)

grafting or damaged during wide debridement of a post-sternotomy wound.

- The muscle may also be placed intrathoracically; however, this will necessitate resection of a portion of the 2nd, 3rd, or 4th rib ***(Fig. 11.7)***.
- May be harvested with or without a skin paddle.
- Donor site deformity including scar placement and loss of anterior axillary fold may be aesthetically displeasing.

Latissimus dorsi

- Latissimus dorsi, a large, flat muscle covering the mid and lower back is often recruited for chest wall

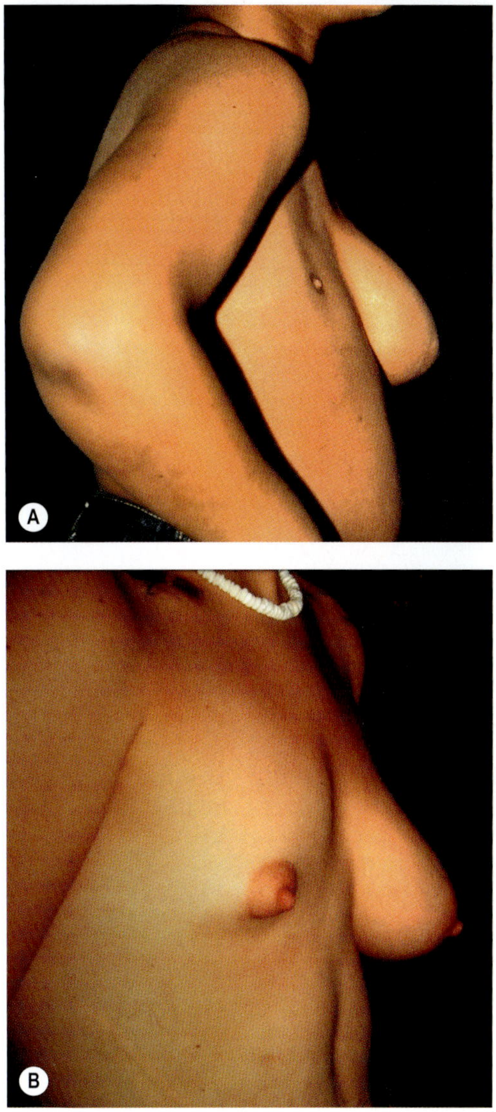

Figure 11.6 Pectoralis major serves as the foundation for the female breast and when absent, such as in Poland syndrome, reconstruction may be indicated for aesthetic reasons.

reconstruction especially when significant bulk and mobility is required. It is easily placed into the chest for intrathoracic space-filling.

- Main function is to adduct, extend, and internally rotate the arm.
- Originates from the thoracolumbar fascia and posterior iliac crest and inserts into the superior humerus at the intertubercular groove. Superiorly, it is attached to the scapula and care must be taken to carefully separate this muscle from the serratus at this point to avoid harvesting both muscles.
- Dominant blood supply is the thoracodorsal artery which enters the undersurface of the muscle 5 cm from the posterior axillary fold.
- Segmental blood supply is derived from the posterior intercostal arteries as well as the lumbar artery.
- Based upon its thoracodorsal pedicle, the muscle can easily reach the ipsilateral posterior and lateral chest

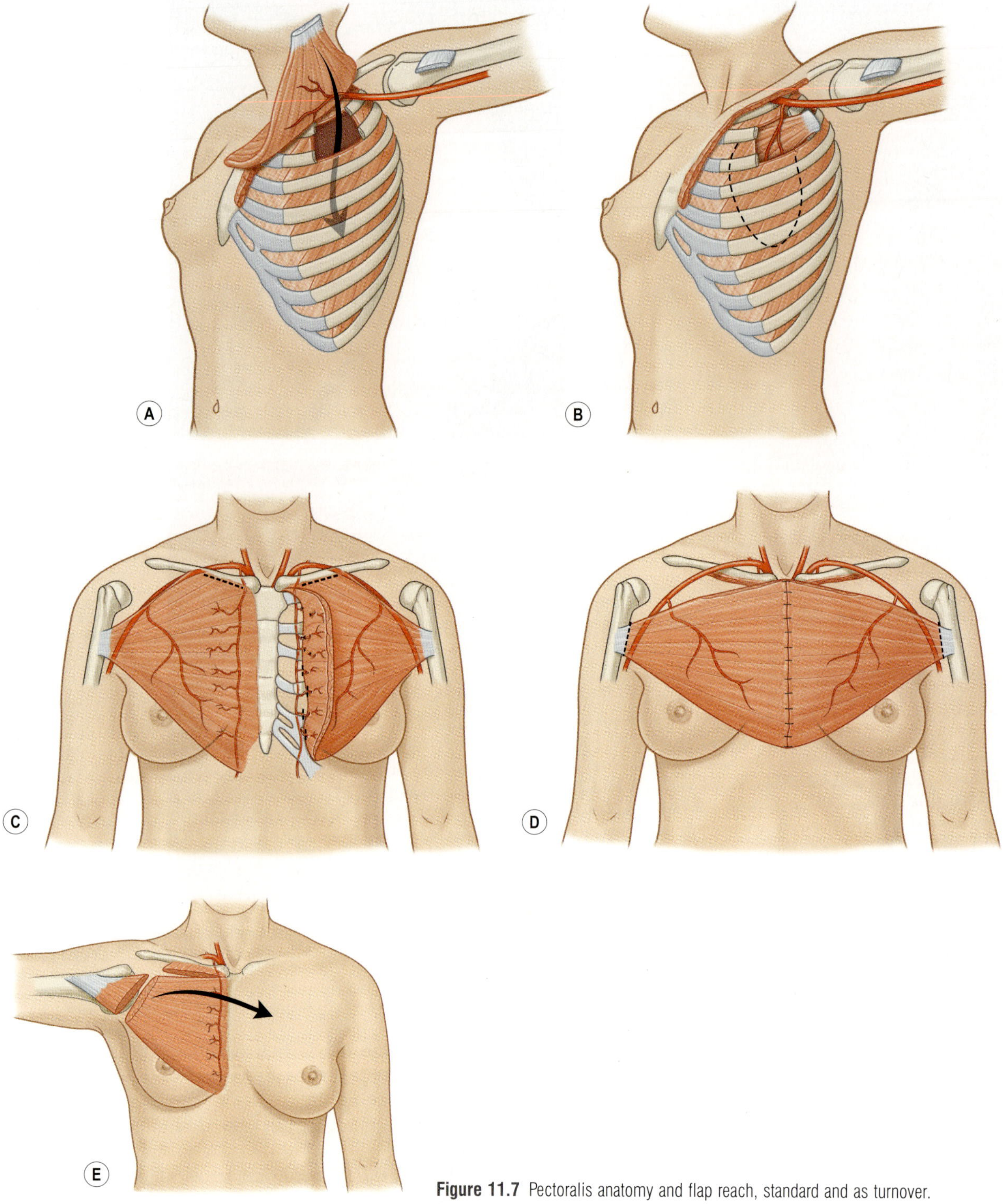

Figure 11.7 Pectoralis anatomy and flap reach, standard and as turnover.

wall, including those defects involving either the anterior chest wall, sternum, or mediastinum.

- It can also be turned over and based upon the lumbar perforators and can cross the midline of the back
- Donor site morbidity can include shoulder dysfunction, weakness and pain, as well as unattractive scarring.
- Also, transposition of this muscle can blunt or obliterate the posterior axillary fold, resulting in some asymmetry ***(Figs 11.8, 11.9)***.
- Care must be taken to properly drain the donor site, as seromas are common. Quilting or progressive tension sutures may mitigate against seroma formation.

Serratus anterior

- Serratus anterior is a thin broad multi-pennate muscle lying deep along the anterolateral chest wall.

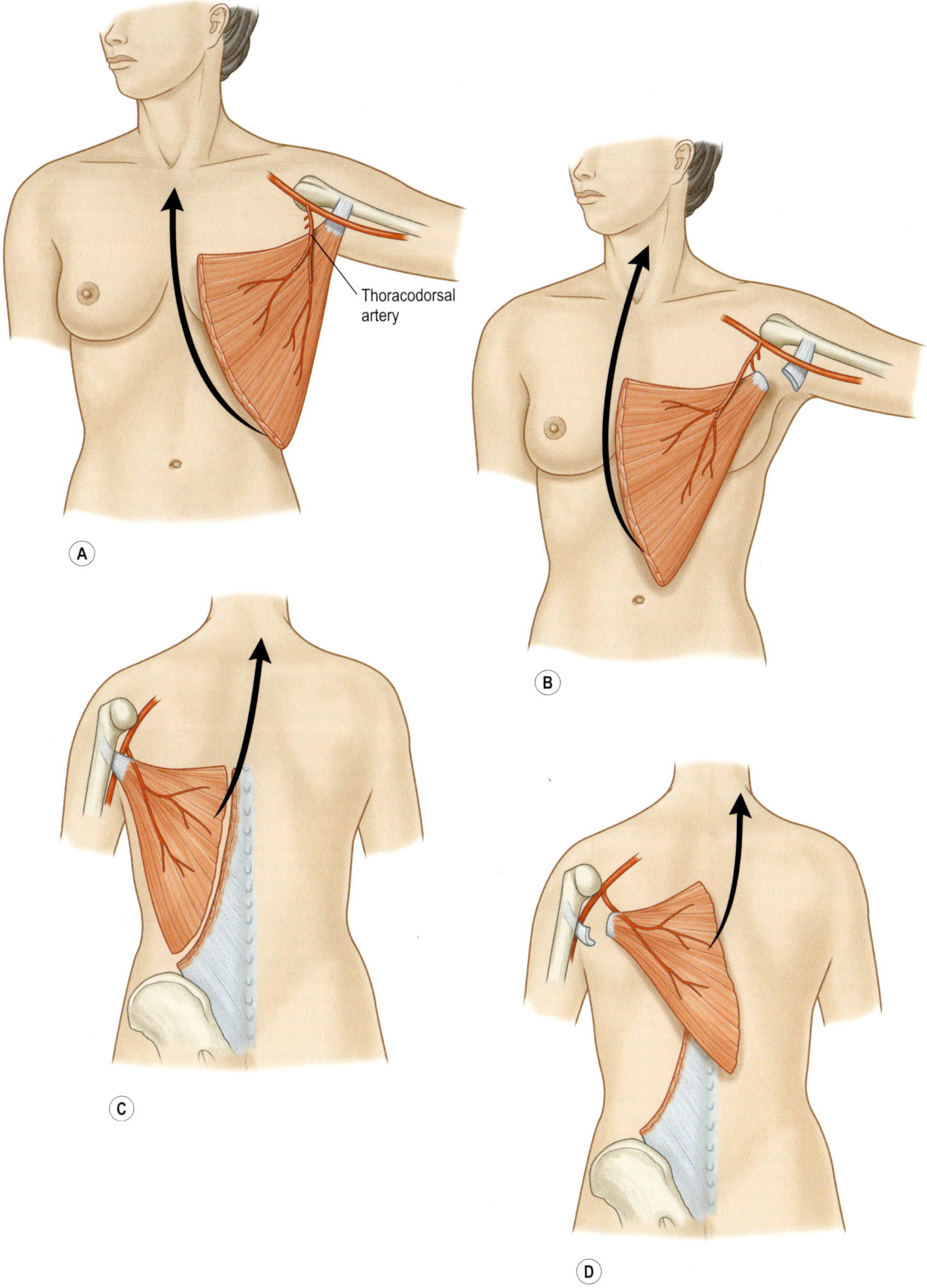

Figure 11.8 Latissimus dorsi, anatomy and standard arc of rotation.

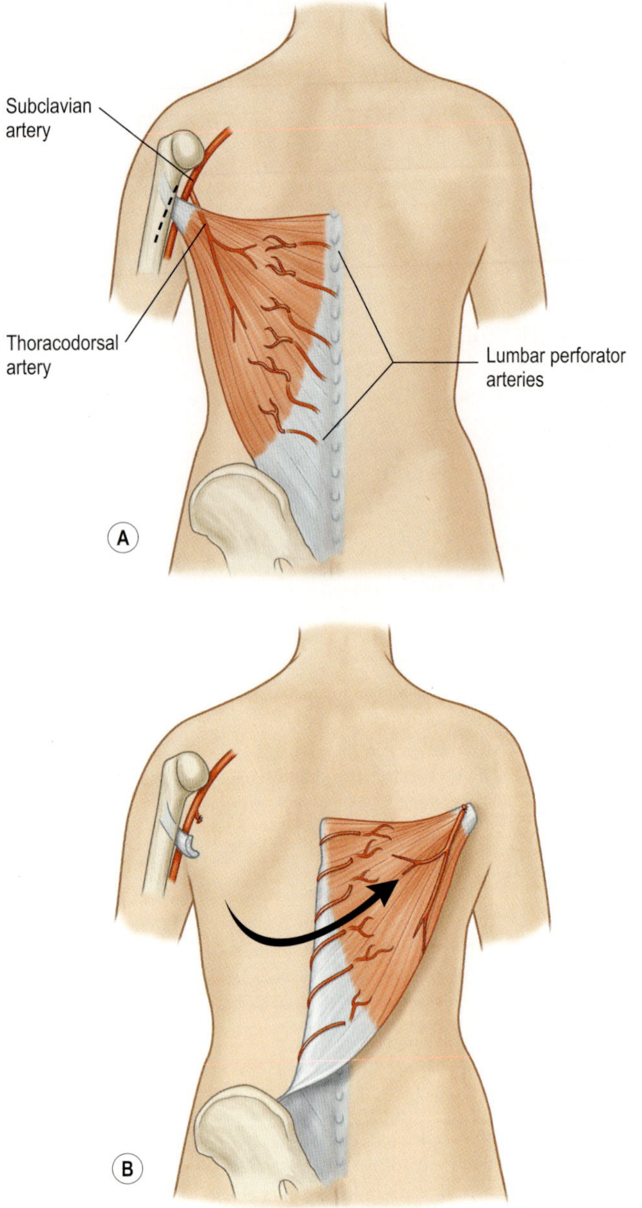

Figure 11.9 Latissimus turnover flap. Thoracodorsal pedicle ligated, muscle turned over based upon thoracolumbar perforators. Provides coverage of contralateral posterior chest wall.

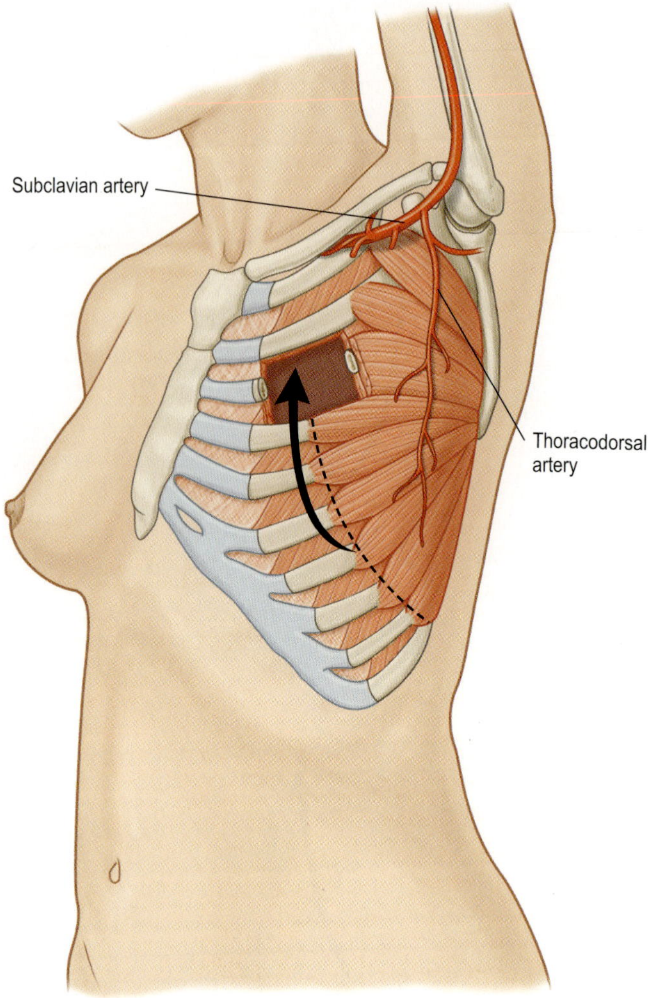

Figure 11.10 Serratus anatomy and arc of rotation.

- Main function is to stabilize the scapula and move it forward on the chest wall such as when throwing a punch.
- Originates from the upper 8 or 9 ribs and inserts on the ventral-medial scapula.
- Two dominant pedicles include the lateral thoracic and the thoracodorsal arteries.
- Division of the lateral thoracic pedicle will increase the arc posteriorly and similarly division of the thoracodorsal will increase the arc anteriorly.
- The muscle will reach the midline of the anterior or posterior chest. More commonly, however, it is used for intrathoracic coverage, again requiring rib resection.
- An osteomyocutaneous flap may be harvested by preservation of the muscular connections with the underlying ribs.
- Donor site morbidity is related to winging of the scapula and can be avoided if the muscle is harvested segmentally and the superior five or six digitations are preserved ***(Fig. 11.10)***.

Rectus abdominus

- Rectus abdominus is a long, flat muscle which constitutes the medial abdominal wall.
- Main function is trunk flexion.
- Originates from the pubis and inserts onto the costal margin. It can easily cover sternal and anterior chest wall defects and can also fill space within the mediastinum.
- Two dominant pedicles, the superior and inferior epigastric arteries.
- It may be utilized despite previous IMA harvest based upon its minor pedicle, the 8th intercostal artery.
- With division of the inferior pedicle, the muscle will cover the mediastinum and the anterior chest wall.

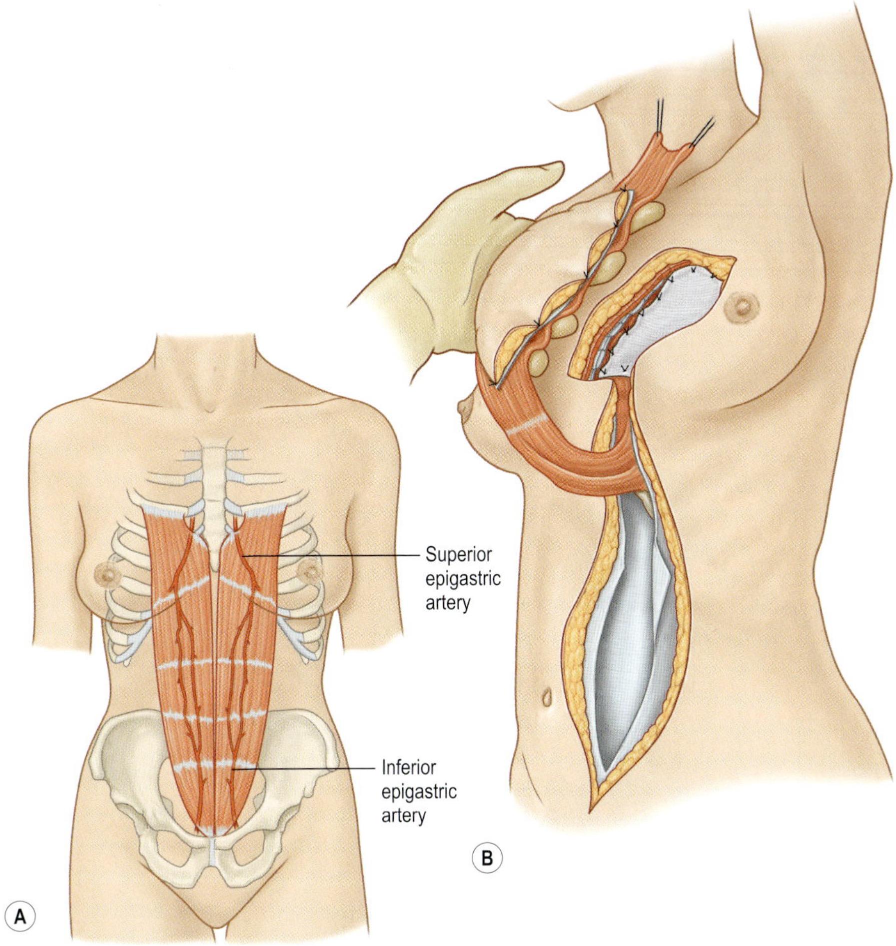

Figure 11.11 Rectus anatomy and arc of rotation.

- When taken with overlying fascia, there is a risk for resultant hernia, and at times, mesh reinforcement of the abdominal wall is necessary. Caution is also advised for patients with prior abdominal incisions as the skin perforators or intramuscular blood supply may have been previously violated ***(Fig. 11.11)***.

Omentum

- The omentum is comprised of visceral fat and blood vessels and arises from the greater curve of the stomach and is also attached to the transverse colon.
- This flap can easily cover wounds in the mediastinum, anterior, lateral and posterior chest wall.
- Two dominant pedicles, the right and left gastroepiploic arteries.
- The greatest benefit of this flap is the pedicle length, which can be easily elongated with division of internal arcades.
- The flap is mobilized onto the chest or into the mediastinum through the diaphragm or over the costal margin.
- Ideally, the flap is mobilized through a cruciate incision in the right diaphragm as the liver helps to buttress the incision and prevent diaphragmatic hernia.
- Right-sided transposition obviates the need to navigate the flap around the heart.
- Care must be taken when interpolating the omentum as it is often of very little substance and can easily be avulsed during passage through the diaphragm.
- Strategies to protect the omentum during transposition include placing the omentum into a bowel bag. The empty bag can be passed from the mediastinum into the abdomen via the diaphragm incision, past the left lobe of the liver. The omentum is then gently packed into the bowel bag with tension transferred to the bowel bag rather than the omentum during interpolation.
- Caution is again advised for patients with prior laparotomy incisions as the omentum may have significant intra-abdominal adhesions or have been previously resected ***(Figs 11.12–11.14)***.

Postoperative considerations

- As with most reconstructive surgeries, after chest wall reconstruction, the patient should limit physical activity for several days. In particular with sternal reconstruction, upper extremity use should be limited and patients

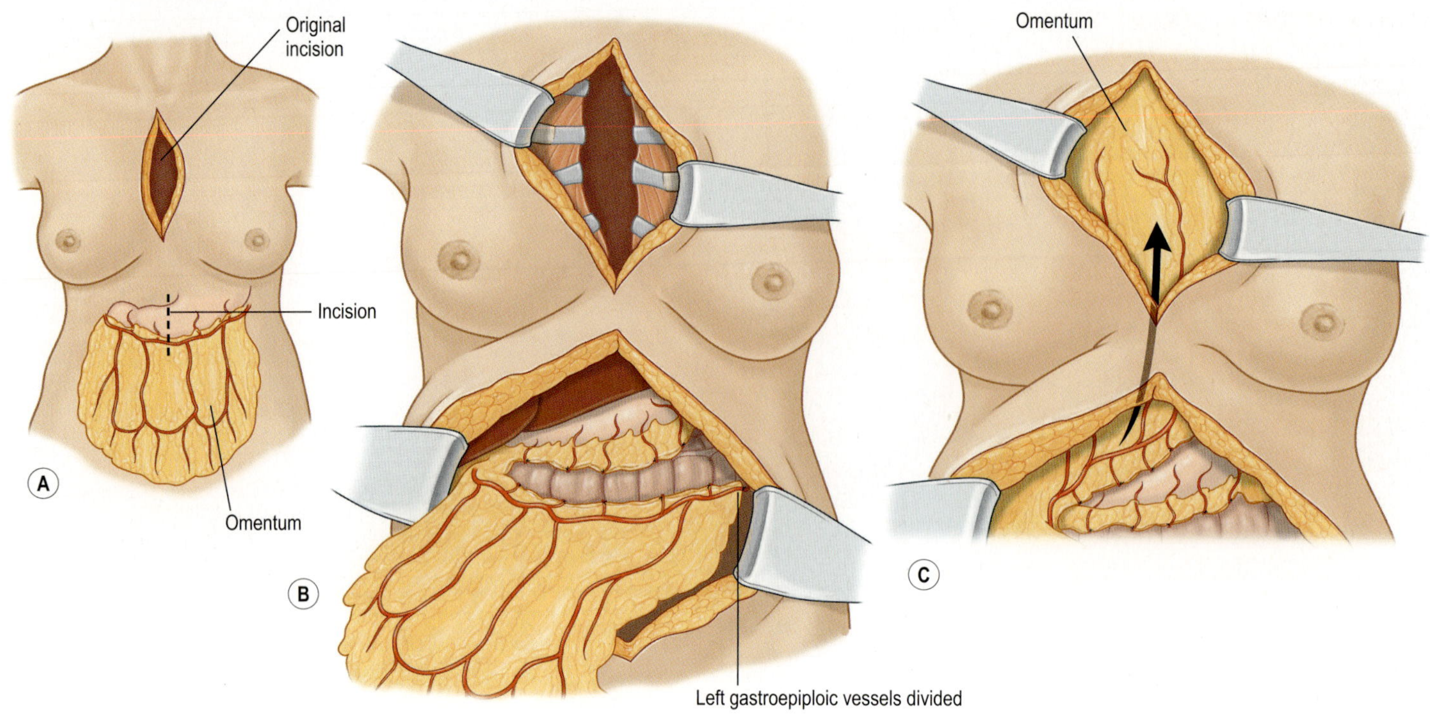

Figure 11.12 Omentum anatomy.

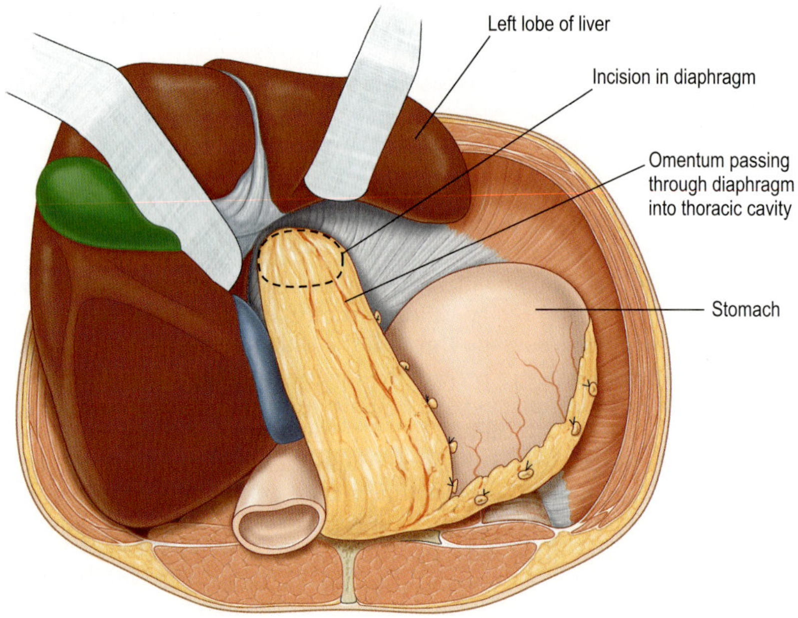

Figure 11.13 Omentum is passed through cruciate incision in the diaphragm under the left lobe of the liver.

instructed to avoid lifting, reaching for objects, and/or raising arms above their heads to avoid undue tension on the reconstruction.

- Flap monitoring should be employed where appropriate.
- Patients will likely require postoperative monitoring in an intensive or acute care unit postoperatively to monitor pulmonary function.

Complications and outcomes

- Chest wall reconstruction has been, over the last three decades, very successful.
- Cases of failure commonly result from inadequate control of infection or residual tumor burden.

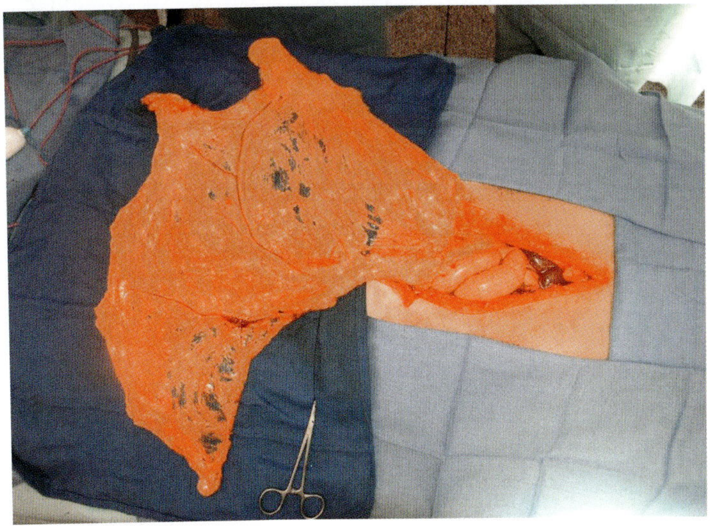

Figure 11.14 Omentum arc of rotation.

- In either case, an aggressive resection is often indicated and use of a second flap.
- An unfortunate complication of skeletal chest wall reconstruction is the potential for infection of alloplastic mesh products or implanted hardware.
- In these cases, removal of the infected prosthesis/ hardware is required.
- In cases of mesh removal, use of acellular dermal matrix or autologous fascia or even contralateral ribs may be indicated.
- At least 50% of patients undergoing sternal debridement and muscle flap reconstruction will complain of persistent chest and shoulder pain.
- And of these patients, 43% will complain of sternal instability which is thought to result from irritation of intercostal nerves when the residual sternal edges abut one another.
- Strength, following use of popular muscle flaps (i.e., pectoralis major, latissimus dorsi, and rectus abdominus), has been both surveyed and objectively measured and is somewhat decreased following sternectomy and muscle flap reconstruction.
- Patients' abilities to perform activities of daily living (ADLs) and return to preoperative activities was found to be no different when compared to their peers with uneventful healing poststernotomy.
- Pulmonary function following sternectomy and reconstruction with pectoralis muscle flaps has been measured pre- and postoperatively and seems to be nearly unchanged following reconstruction.
- When patients were surveyed regarding their general condition following sternal osteomyelitis and reconstruction, 83% of patients reported improvement in quality of life following their chest wall reconstruction.
- Outcomes following muscle flap transposition for empyema or bronchopleural fistula reconstruction are reported as quite successful, with 73% resolution or prevention of infection in Arnold and Pairolero's retrospective review of 100 patients with severe intrathoracic infections.
- Rib plating has been shown to reduce ventilator-dependence and ICU stay as well as incidence of pneumonia in patients with flail chest.

Further reading

Arnold PG, Pairolero PC. Intrathoracic muscle flaps. An account of their use in the management of 100 consecutive patients. *Ann Surg*. 1990;211(6):656–660.

The authors detail a 73% success rate with treatment and prevention of intrathoracic infection following muscle transposition into the chest of high risk patients.

Deschamps C, et al. Early and long-term results of prosthetic chest wall reconstruction. *J Thorac Cardiovasc Surg*. 1999;117(3):588–592.

The authors review their experience with nearly 200 patients requiring chest wall reconstruction over 15 years. Mesh is utilized (polypropylene and polytetrafluoroethylene) for skeletal support and over half of the patients required muscle transposition for soft tissue coverage. Wound healing was complete for 95% of patients, although 24% experienced local cancer recurrence.

Dickie SR, Dorafshar AH, Song DH. Definitive closure of the infected median sternotomy wound: A treatment algorithm utilizing vacuum-assisted closure followed by rigid plate fixation. *Ann Plast Surg*. 2006;56(6):680–685.

This paper contains a treatment algorithm for mediastinitis emphasizing debridement, the use of subatmospheric pressure, rigid fixation, and soft tissue coverage.

Mathes SJ, Nahai F. *Reconstructive Surgery. Principles, Anatomy, and Technique*. Edinburgh: Churchill Livingstone; 1997.

This textbook detailing nearly all commonly-used flaps in plastic surgery continues to be an excellent reference for relevant anatomy, flap selection, and arc of rotation.

Song DH, Lohman RF, Renucci JD, et al. Primary sternal plating in high-risk patients prevents mediastinitis. *Eur J Cardiothorac Surg*. 2004;26:367–372.

This is a case-controlled study of prophylactic sternal plating in high risk patients. The group who were plated experienced no mediastinitis, while 14.8% of the control group, closed with wire, developed mediastinitis.

12 Chapter

Back reconstruction

This chapter was created using content from Neligan & Song, Plastic Surgery 3rd edition, Volume 4, Lower Extremity, Trunk and Burns, Chapter 11, Reconstruction of the soft tissues of the back, Gregory A. Dumanian.

SYNOPSIS

- Reconstruction of the soft tissues of the back at first may seem to be a daunting task compounded by large wounds, unfamiliar and segmental anatomy, radiation, hardware, and difficulties with postoperative positioning.
- Many of the conditions treated require significant coordination with surgical colleagues.
- Many of the conditions are unfamiliar to the plastic surgeon and without parallel conditions elsewhere in the body, an example being pseudomeningoceles filled with cerebrospinal fluid (CSF).
- The goal of this chapter is to provide the reader with real-life solutions to difficult problems involving back wounds.

Brief introduction

- The back is 18% of the total body surface area, yet it is an area commonly neglected in older texts of plastic surgery. However, with advancements in spine instrumentation and surgery, and subsequent wound related complications, surgical procedures to close the back reliably have been developed.
- Spine teams have noted the efficacy of muscle flap closure of open spine wounds, and this has led to the introduction of prophylactic use of muscle flaps at the time of spine surgery. The same algorithms described in the chapter below are used, but now at the time of the back procedure, rather than only when there is a complication.
- It is difficult, if not impossible, to define exactly who should need a prophylactic soft tissue reconstruction of the back.
  - Patients with previous hardware infections, a woody feel to the soft tissues at the time of surgery, prior back surgery, long reconstructions greater than six vertebral bodies, CSF leaks, and a radiation history to the area all seem to be appropriate candidates to receive a soft tissue reconstruction.
  - In our center, we limit prophylactic closures to patients with prior infections, when the muscles will not close in the midline due to tissue loss or prior surgery, a history of radiation with a woody feel to the tissues, and CSF leaks.
- Chronic hardware exposures, those which occur 6 months after placement, act differently from acute exposures. From experience, long-term coverage of chronically exposed hardware is not successful.
- When patients present with small areas of drainage and by palpation a piece of hardware can be reached, this defines a hardware infection. Similarly, patients with fluid collections or "fluid cysts" in association with hardware have chronic infections.
- These infections can be present for months or years and yet not suppurate, nor make the patient overly ill and are undoubtedly due to the low virulence of the organism, such as *Staphylococcus epidermidis*.
- Debridement, irrigation, and soft tissue coverage of these chronic exposures may be initially successful, but eventually fail. Thus, for most patients the involved hardware should be removed.
- The question is whether all of the hardware needs to be removed, or if just a local portion (such as a large bolt) should be removed and the soft tissues closed. These are decisions made in the operating room.
  - All hardware in association with exudative fluid should be removed.

- Well-incorporated hardware encased in bone can be allowed to remain.
- No flaps are typically required for closure when all of the hardware is removed.
- Patient outcomes depend more on the structural stability of the spine than on any soft tissue work.
- The soft tissues are simply approximated over drains, and complete healing is the rule rather than the exception. Antibiotics are not needed for prolonged periods in these situations.

Preoperative considerations

Midline back wounds

- When a spine surgeon calls to discuss new drainage from a midline spine wound, the thought process for treatment should be methodical and thorough. A review of operative details, and thorough history and physical examination are critical.
- A complete history should include operative details, the presence, visibility, and/or palpability of hardware, any history of postoperative complications and/or dural injury with associated CSF leak, and a review of imaging demonstrating hardware position relative to areas of wounds or drainage.
- An evaluation of patient co-morbidities and potential wound healing issues is also necessary, including a history of malnourishment, diabetes, obesity, dead-space management problems, and/or prior radiation.
- A thorough examination should note wound characteristics including the presence of persistent drainage and dieback of wound edges commonly seen with deep fluid collections, new pressure points as a result of new postoperative spinal alignment.
- The time course of the presentation is critical.
- Early postoperative episodes of drainage less than 4–6 weeks after the spine surgery are typically successfully treated with repeat surgery and soft tissue reconstruction with hardware preservation.
- However, drainage that has been only partially treated with a small debridement or treated solely with intravenous antibiotics, only to resurface months later, is more difficult to treat.
- A chronic hardware infection, defined as bacteria in association with hardware greater than 6 months after placement, is typically not a situation that plastic surgery can definitively treat without hardware removal.
- Much can be learned with the simple examination of a patient's chest X-ray in terms of the existence and location of hardware. Otherwise, plain films of the spine are obtained to reveal the length of the construct when present, degenerative spine disease, and the presence or absence of fusion.
- CT scans and magnetic resonance imaging (MRI) are helpful to look for fluid collections, pseudomeningoceles, and inflammation of the soft tissues.
- A key issue is if fluid collections are above or below the standard back muscle closure. If fluid or hematoma is seen deep to the musculature, a deep hardware infection is more likely.

Non-midline back wounds

- While midline wounds are either due to pressure sores or spine procedures, non-midline wounds represent a much more heterogeneous collection of etiologies and therefore require a wide range of solutions.
- Much like acquired wounds elsewhere in the body, wounds of the non-midline back are due to poor wound healing after access incisions of the chest cavity or retroperitoneum, necrotizing infections, or after tumor excision.
- For these patients, a more standard thought process often suffices in the absence of hardware, deep wounds, and CSF leaks.
- The wounds are typically flat, and often allow skin grafting.
- When flaps are needed to cover bone or prosthetic material, the muscles that are used to cover the midline spine are often available and even easier to mobilize to the lateral back due to the lateral placement of their pedicles.
- The lateral tissues, being more mobile than the midline tissues, are easier to transpose for adjacent tissue transfers.
- Free flaps are facilitated by having larger inflow vessels available, such as the axillary artery, than exist for midline reconstructions.

Technical pearls

Flap selection by region

Cervical region

- The cervical spine area is more often instrumented from the anterior than the posterior approach.
- Wounds of the anterior cervical spine are uncommon, and when they occur can be in association with esophageal injuries. Wounds of the posterior cervical spine are more common.
- Soft tissue defects without spine involvement are treated depending on the size and location of the defect either with skin grafts or adjacent tissue transfers. Pressure sores tend to be treated conservatively with pressure relief. Laminectomies are performed for spinal cord pressure from metastases, and the wound beds are typically radiated.
- Trapezius pedicled flaps are the preferred treatment for patients who have received radiation following laminectomy and oncologic tumor resection.

Thoracic region

- Soft tissue defects without spine involvement are treated depending on the size and location of the defect either with skin grafts or adjacent tissue transfers.

- The scapular and parascapular flaps can be helpful in closing some of these soft tissue defects without spine involvement, and the donor site should be oriented perpendicular to the long axis of the wound to facilitate closure.
- Latissimus flaps based on the paraspinous perforators are ideal in radiated wounds to allow the muscle to be "dropped in" these defects, and thereby not manipulate the radiated and stiff erector spinae muscles. Myocutaneous latissimus flaps have easier insets with the overlying skin paddle sewn to the adjacent midline back skin.
- Wounds of the thoracic back after spine surgery and placement of hardware are best treated with erector spinae flaps. There is no need for a "double muscle" closure with further mobilization of a latissimus flap if the erector spinae muscles come together normally.
- Rarely, in extremely deep wounds, the pedicled omental flap is ideal to fill the defect and to help achieve closure. These unusual circumstances often also require either erector spinae flaps or latissimus flaps to aid in the closure.

Lumbar region

- The high lumbar area is the optimal area for reclosure with erector spinae flaps. The muscles are largest in this area, and exist in a lordotic area of the back that is protected from pressure.
- Other flaps are also possible for the lumbar area and include turnover latissimus flaps, which can reach this area, but only with some difficulty. Sliding of myocutaneous latissimus flaps elevated from the lower lumbar area and transposed medially provides thick coverage of the spine, but only at the expense of a skin-grafted donor site. The omentum will also reach this area with some ease.
- The inferior region of the lumbar spine is best covered with superior gluteal artery-based flaps.
- Often, a gluteal flap will be combined with erector spinae flaps for coverage of a longer lumbar and lumbosacral defect.

Lumbosacral region

- The recess between the sacrum and the inferior aspect of the spine is best filled with a superior gluteal artery-based flap as the erector spinae muscles are thin and laterally displaced in this area, precluding their use.
- Omental flaps are possible but require position changes in the operating room and bowel dissection. Random-pattern skin flaps of the lumbar tissue or perforator-based flaps are also possible, but are difficult to inset and control in an area that is subjected to high shear forces with position changes. Finally, while latissimus flaps can be mobilized to reach this area, there are many wounds that are simply too big to have the latissimus muscle both reach and fill the entire cavity.
- Patients undergoing a full sacrectomy for tumor can undergo bilateral gluteus myocutaneous flaps if the superior and/or inferior gluteal arteries are preserved during the sacrectomy. Closure of the gluteus muscles in the midline, like a pressure sore, can be done with V-Y advancement of the skin paddles if necessary.
- For low rectal tumors with invasion into the sacrum, a transabdominal flap using a flap based on the inferior epigastric artery is also feasible.
  - The oblique rectus abdominis musculocutaneous flap, using a skin paddle based in an oblique direction off the periumbilical perforators and using only the lower aspect of the rectus muscle, can easily bring non-radiated skin to the lumbosacral area.
  - The vertical rectus abdominis musculocutaneous flap is another common design to achieve wound closure, but requires the harvest of more muscle.
  - These abdominal flaps need to be parked adjacent to the sacrum and the abdomen closed. After sacrectomy, the flap can be retrieved from the posterior approach into the abdomen.
- For the majority of patients with lumbosacral defects, the tissue near the trochanter can be elevated with the blood vessels in continuity with the superior gluteal artery for soft tissue coverage ***(Fig. 12.1)***.
  - This can be done as a pure perforator flap, or else with a strip of gluteus muscle under the skin paddle (which is de-epithelialized).
  - As the flap is typically flipped 180°, the skin paddle will rest over the dura. To re-emphasize, this is a different design than for superior gluteal artery perforator flaps done for sacral pressure sores.

Wounds of the lateral back

- Soft tissue reconstruction of the lateral back has certain special characteristics.
- In the thoracic area, if the ribcage is intact, then most wounds would be closeable with local wound care, latissimus flaps, parascapular/scapular flaps, serratus flaps, or posterior movement of a perforator flap from tissues in the anterior axillary line area.
- If the ribs are involved, then a decision about possible reconstitution of the pleural line needs to be made. Most authorities recommend that three or more ribs be reconstructed with a prosthetic patch, and this patch would then need to be covered with soft tissues. However, when the rib defect is located under the scapula, then the scapula serves to protect and camouflage any defect, and so larger rib resections are tolerated.
- The lateral lumbar area in adults typically is protected by its lordotic shape, and the only structure that needs to be reconstructed is the posterior aspect of the abdominal wall. All other wounds can be closed with local wound care, skin grafts, or transfer of the latissimus muscle.

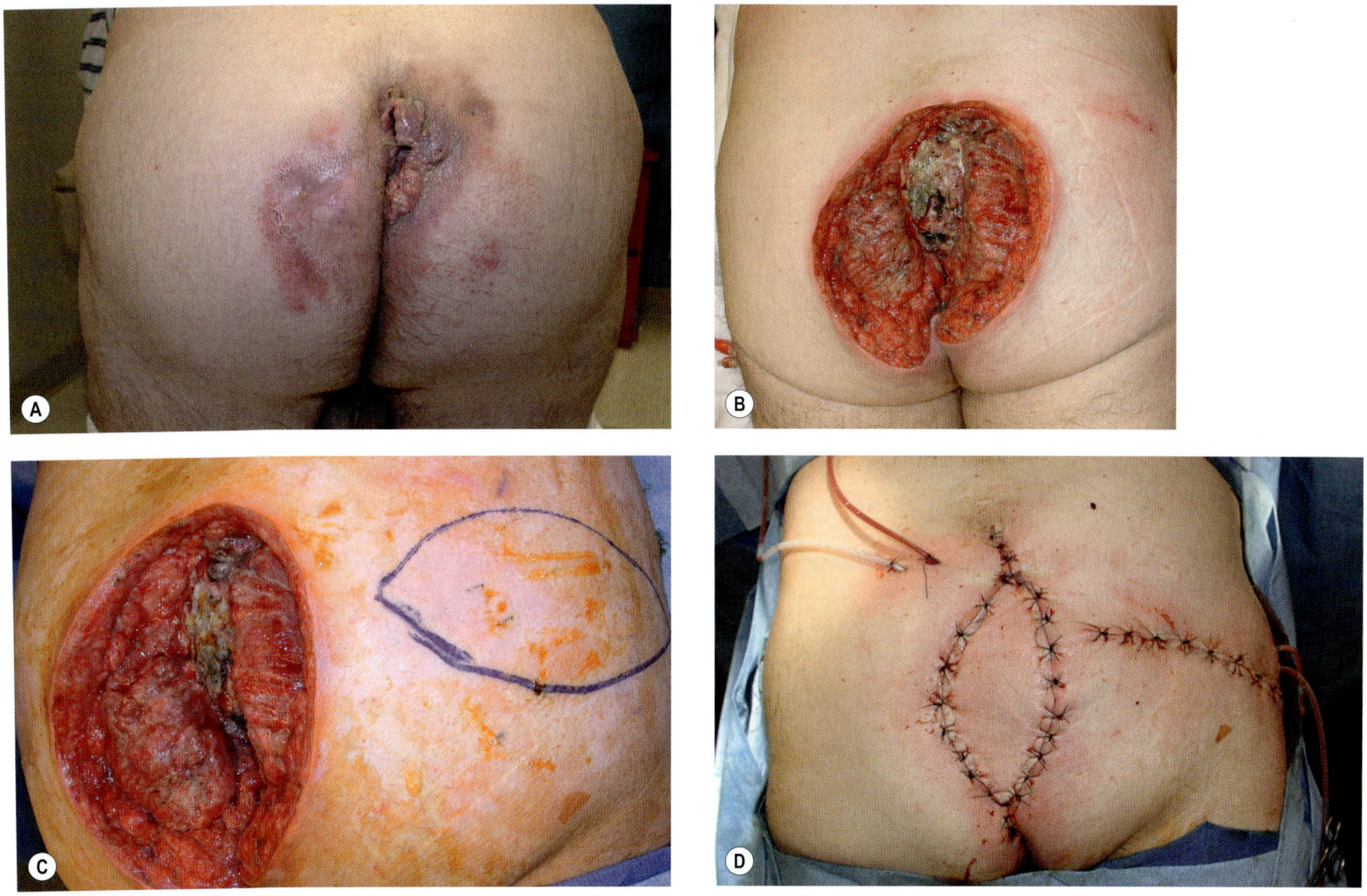

Figure 12.1 **(A)** Large Marjolin's ulcer found in a chronic pilonidal cyst in an ambulatory patient. **(B)** Tumor excision. **(C)** A superior gluteal artery perforator flap is drawn out. The long axis of the skin paddle is perpendicular to the long axis of the defect to facilitate closure. The tumor excision and the final closure were staged to allow for definitive pathologic clearance of the margins. **(D)** Flap inset into defect.

Operative techniques

Local wound care

- For superficial, relatively painless wounds without exposed hardware, local wound care with dressings is a relatively risk-free way to achieve wound closure.
- Draining midline incisions tend to have wide areas of undermining along the length of the closure. These tunnels can typically be opened in the office with local injection of anesthesia and finger fracturing of the incision.
- A long wound without tunnels with a saucer shape typically heals faster than small wounds with a fishbowl-shaped internal wound; therefore, tunnels should be opened along old incision lines.
- All necrotic tissue should be debrided. All non-absorbable sutures such as braided polyester should be removed.
- Patients are often unaware of the real size of the wound, and must be prepared for the resulting appearance of the surgical site after opening of tunnels.
- Dressings can be simple wet-to-wet saline dressings, with twice-a-day showers to cleanse the surface of the wound. Subatmospheric-pressure dressings can be employed, but the tubing is sometimes difficult to place under back-bracing devices.
- After a wound has granulated, or if it is painful, then delayed primary closure or skin grafts can be performed if the wound is sizeable.

Operative debridement

- Patients with persistently draining wounds after spine surgery associated with hardware should be evaluated critically for an operating room debridement.
- Secondary indications for a debridement include unexplained fevers and fluid collections seen on imaging scans.
- The maneuvers in the operating room are a critical step in the treatment of patients with postsurgical back wounds.
- A thorough incision and drainage should be performed for patients with unexplained or purulent drainage through their incision.
- The entire length of the incision should be opened as widely as necessary to explore for purulence and drain fluid collections.

- The erector spinae muscle closure should be reopened for cultures and to evaluate for liquefying hematomas.
- The surgeon should be knowledgeable at the beginning of the debridement if a laminectomy had been performed at the original spine surgery in order to prevent injury to the spinal cord and dura during the incision and drainage.
- After adequate exposure, the surgeon will need to make a decision as to the quality of the tissues.
- Non-purulent benign fluid collections in the subcutaneous tissues with no purulence deep to the musculature can be reclosed over drains, or else closed secondarily with a subatmospheric-pressure dressing.
- Purulent and deep collections require additional decisions.
- If the local wound is so purulent as to preclude an immediate reclosure, then all non-viable tissue should be debrided, the wound irrigated and left open for local wound care.
- Alternatively, a subatmospheric-pressure dressing may be applied, but this often involves a return trip to the operating room for its next exchange.
- For those deep wounds judged amenable to reclosure, a radical incision and drainage are performed. This should involve the surgical excision of scarred tissues where possible to reveal supple soft tissues with pulsatile bleeding.
- Pulsatile bleeding at wound margins has been shown to correlate with wound healing in problematic incisions, such as distal foot amputations.
- Tissues with a pseudobursa should be excised, as this too represents scar. Tissue that is stiff is unyielding and does not conform well, and so the tissues should be removed until they are soft to palpation.
- An interesting issue is the removal of non-viable elements such as hardware and bone graft.
- Hardware that is well fixed should remain in place in early hardware infections. This is done both to stabilize the wound for improved healing as well as to avoid the surgery involved with removal and later replacement of hardware.
- Long-term maintenance of the hardware as well as clinical and radiographic evidence of fusion are well documented in patients who were returned to the operating room for washouts within 6–8 weeks of placement.
- In the absence of definitive studies, it seems reasonable to remove non-incorporated and easy-to-remove graft, but to leave in place graft that has in any way begun to stick to the local tissues due to inosculation.
- In the treatment of wounds of the spine, the three-dimensional shape should be evaluated and converted as much as possible to a two-dimensional wound.
- Prominent hardware should be exchanged for something with a lower profile.
- Patients with incomplete corrections of the spine deformities should be revised to recreate better the natural contours.
- The deeper the hole, the more a flap should be "dropped into" the defect, rather than tissue simply slid towards the midline. This requires a more redundant soft tissue flap such as an omentum to fill the defect appropriately.

Flap closure

Principles

- The first step in reconstruction is a timely debridement.
- The second step is local wound control with a radical debridement of all stiff and scarred tissue.
- Finally, the reconstruction should be performed to do the "maximum for the minimum."
- The procedure with the highest chance for success and with the lowest morbidity should be selected for the patient.
- Central questions to be answered include the presence or absence of a fusion, and the vertebral levels involved.
- When an instrumented fusion has been performed, then the erector spinae musculature function is no longer necessary, and the muscles are completely expendable in terms of a reconstruction. The fusion rods prevent postoperative motion, and so when the erector spinae muscles are reapproximated in the midline, they tend to stay there.
- Spine patients without fusions still require the function of the erector spinae musculature when healing is completed for flexion and extension of the spine. These patients do better with flaps that are "dropped into the hole," rather than with erector spinae muscles that are closed side to side and that would dehisce with back flexion.
- Local wound care often suffices for superficial wound problems above the erector spinae.

Possible flap choices for spine closure

Erector spinae muscle flaps

- The erector spinae muscles, also called the paraspinous muscles, are expendable after a previous spine fusion and no longer are functional for spine extension and flexion.
- This flap is appropriate from the high cervical area to the low lumbar area, but it will not adequately cover an occipitospinal fusion, and nor will it be sufficient for lumbosacral soft tissue coverage.
- One must be careful in its use when a lateral approach to the spine has been made, because the muscle can be transected for access.
- First, skin flaps are elevated superficial to the thoracolumbar fascia ***(Fig. 12.2)***.
- The latissimus muscle and trapezius muscle should stay attached to the skin and skin flap.
- The dissection is easiest inferiorly in the lumbar area where the muscle is round and large, and most confusing superiorly where the muscle is thinnest and becomes attached to the undersurface of the trapezius.
- The erector spinae muscles have a convex shape, and there is a rounded aspect of the muscle that then descends laterally towards the more lateral neck, thoracic, and lumbar areas.

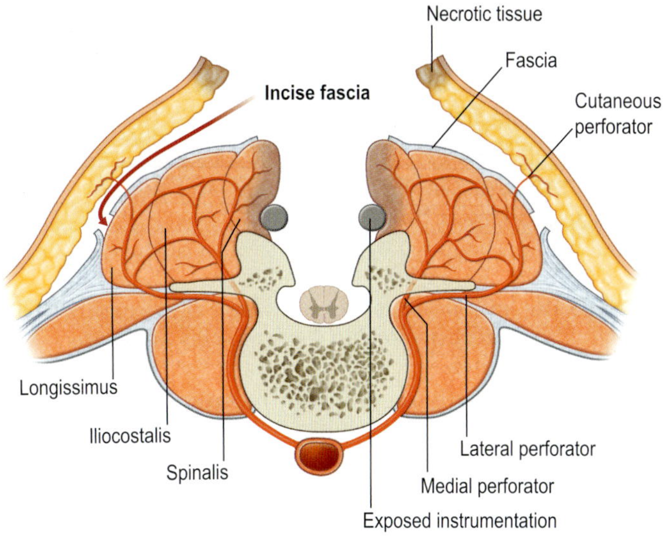

Figure 12.2 Cross-section of lumbar spine area. Skin flaps are elevated to expose the thoracolumbar fascia and to reach the region of the lateral pedicle entering the erector spinae muscles. The thoracolumbar fascia is incised to allow a medial movement of the muscles.

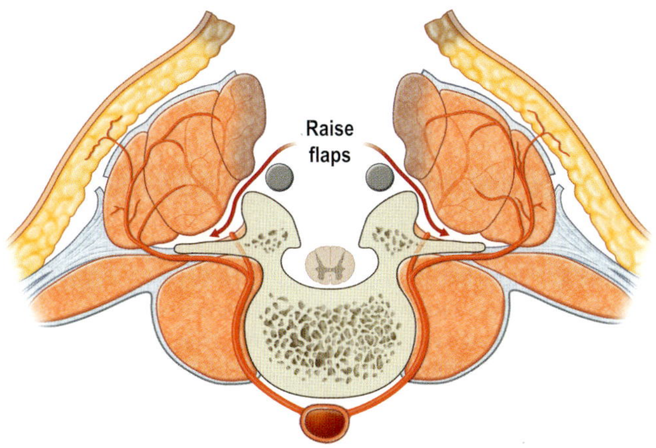

Figure 12.3 A dissection is then performed to release the medial and deep attachments of the erector spinae muscles to the spine and transverse processes. The lateral blood supply is approached from the deep aspect of the muscle.

- It is in this groove that segmental blood vessels enter the lateral and deep aspects of the longissimus and iliocostalis muscles. Continuation of these blood vessels continues more superficially to the skin and to the latissimus muscle in the thoracolumbar area.
- While the surgeon is elevating the skin flaps, the perforators and dorsal sensory nerves going up to the skin often can be identified and preserved to maintain skin vascularity.
- The thoracolumbar fascia is incised much like the development of any standard bipedicled flap in order to mobilize the erector spinae muscle and/or overlying skin to the midline.
- The dissection up until this point is rather easy and bloodless, but only moves the muscle an estimated 30% of its potential.
- Complete mobilization of the muscle requires a dissection along the deep aspect of the erector spinae ***(Fig. 12.3)***.

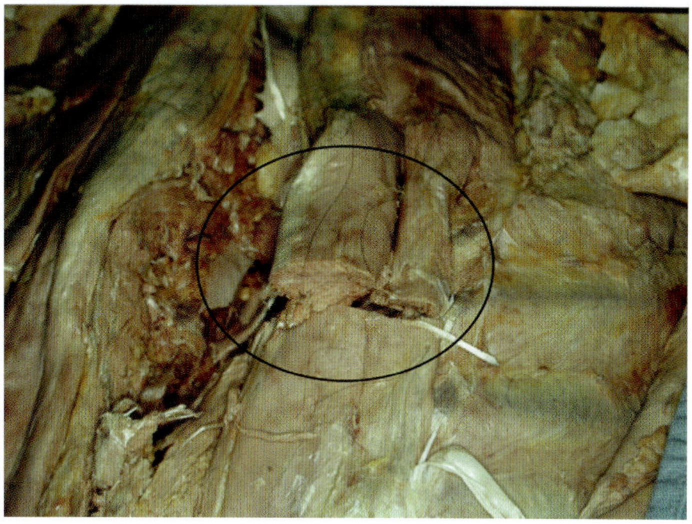

Figure 12.4 Cadaver dissection of the erector spinae muscles at the lumbar level.

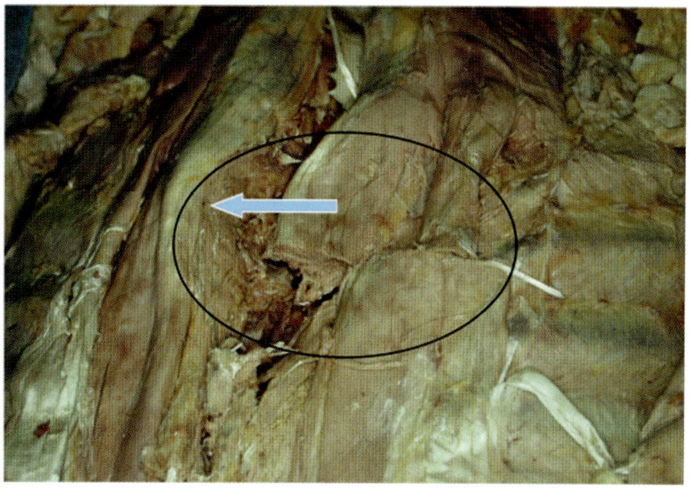

Figure 12.5 Release and medial movement of the muscles.

- Again with tension applied on to the tissue with retractors, cautery dissection of the deep and medial attachments of the erector spinae will mobilize the muscle and detach it from the lateral aspects of the transverse processes of the spine.
- This move will by necessity divide the medial row of blood vessels entering the paraspinous muscles, but the prior dissection to identify the lateral vessels entering the muscle will suffice to preserve vascularity.
- The medial muscle elevation is a powerful means to allow the paraspinous muscles to "unfold" like an accordion to be advanced toward the midline ***(Figs 12.4, 12.5)***.
- The medial aspect of the skin, subcutaneous tissue, and paraspinous muscles is sharply debrided. The muscles are brought together in the midline ***(Fig. 12.6)***, and any extra tissue can be imbricated to help fold the soft tissue into crevices between vertically oriented hardware bars ***(Fig. 12.7)***.

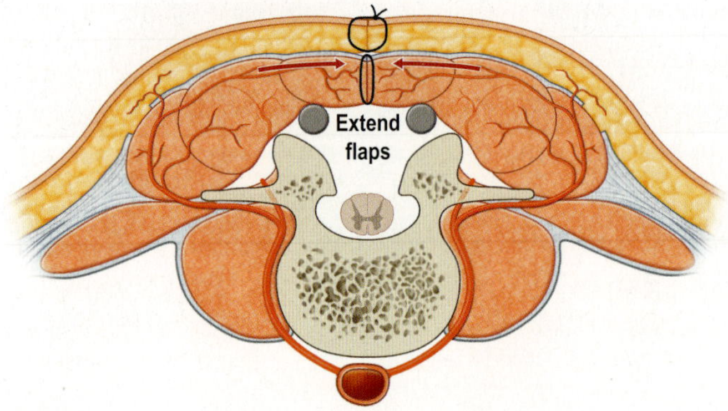

Figure 12.6 The muscles are approximated in the midline. The erector spinae muscles unfurl, changing shape from circular to elliptical.

- Drains are left both deep and superficial to the erector spinae closure, and are left in until the drainage is minimal.
- When the erector spinae muscle closure is of good quality, there is no need for a second overlying muscle flap using the trapezius or the latissimus muscles.

Latissimus muscle or myocutaneous flap

- The latissimus muscle is a well-known and understood flap. Based on the thoracodorsal pedicle, the muscle can be moved superiorly up to the level of the top of the scapula. Based on its minor perforators that also supply the paraspinous muscles, the latissimus can reach the lower lumbar area.
- An advantage to the latissimus is being able to be "dropped in" to a hole, and so it is useful for patients who have not been fused, or for more lateral defects.
- The muscle can reliably carry a skin paddle, and this often helps in the inset of the flap.
- Caution should be taken in patients who have had thoracotomy incisions, as the muscle is often divided.
- The latissimus muscle is a good but still second-line flap for the coverage of midline back wounds. In comparison to the paraspinous flaps, the latissimus flap can only cover a spine wound 10–12 cm in length, while the erector spinae flaps can cover practically the entire length of the spine.
- The latissimus muscle is a good choice for a radiated non-fused wound of the midback, where the patient has not been fused, and the erector spinae musculature is in the field of radiation ***(Fig. 12.8)***.
- The orientation and design of the skin paddle should be done carefully.
- For flaps based on the thoracodorsal pedicle, a skin paddle oriented with its long axis perpendicular to the midline will result in the skin paddle vertically oriented. Closure of the donor site initially oriented perpendicular to the spine does not make the midline spine any more difficult to close due to added tension.
- Another helpful skin paddle design is a V-Y design. The donor site for the skin is in the midaxillary line. The latissimus muscle is elevated and the skin paddle moved medially, rather than turned 90°. This flap can be re-elevated and moved a second time if necessary.

Trapezius muscle flap

- The trapezius flap is useful for high cervical wounds because the paraspinous musculature is of limited mobility and size at that level.
- The dissection begins with identification of the distal and inferior triangular aspect of the trapezius where it just overlaps the latissimus muscle, because the crossing muscle fiber directions of the two muscles are quite distinct in this area.
- A skin paddle overlying this inferior muscle can be taken to help with the inset. The more cephalad and larger the skin paddle, the better in terms of reliability ***(Fig. 12.9)***.
- The inclusion of the superficial dorsal scapular artery on the lateral border of the trapezius also helps skin flap viability.
- Further cephalad and lateral to the elevated skin paddle, the upper back skin is elevated off the trapezius. The main pedicle is the transverse cervical artery and it enters the muscle approximately 7–8 cm lateral to the midline and at the level of the spinous process of C7 on its deep aspect.
- The deep dissection is then performed, with the muscle elevated off the paraspinous musculature and the rhomboids.
- The main pedicle is encountered, and with this vessel under direct view, the lateral aspect of the muscle is divided.
- Movement of the flap is tested, and the lateral muscle division is extended if greater mobility is required for wound coverage. The higher the dissection continues, the higher the morbidity due to shoulder drop, but the greater the arc of rotation of the muscle.
- Because of its sizeable donor site morbidity to the shoulder, the indication for the trapezius flap is in a non-fused patient with a radiated deep back wound where the erector spinae have been involved in the field of radiation.
- As the muscle is typically turned 90° for inset, the length of midline coverage of the trapezius is typically short, and so either a combination of two trapezius flaps, or else the trapezius flap with erector spinae flaps, should be planned for long wounds.

Superior gluteal artery

- The superior gluteal artery flap technique is the most challenging of all of the reconstructive soft tissue procedures for the spine, but it is a necessary and useful procedure.
- A line is drawn between the superior lateral aspect of the sacrum and the posterior superior iliac spine.
- From a point that bisects this line, a second line is drawn toward the greater trochanter.
- This second line represents the path of the superior gluteal artery, and is the long axis of the flap.
- A skin paddle is designed that encompasses the Doppler signal of the perforator of the superior gluteal artery and

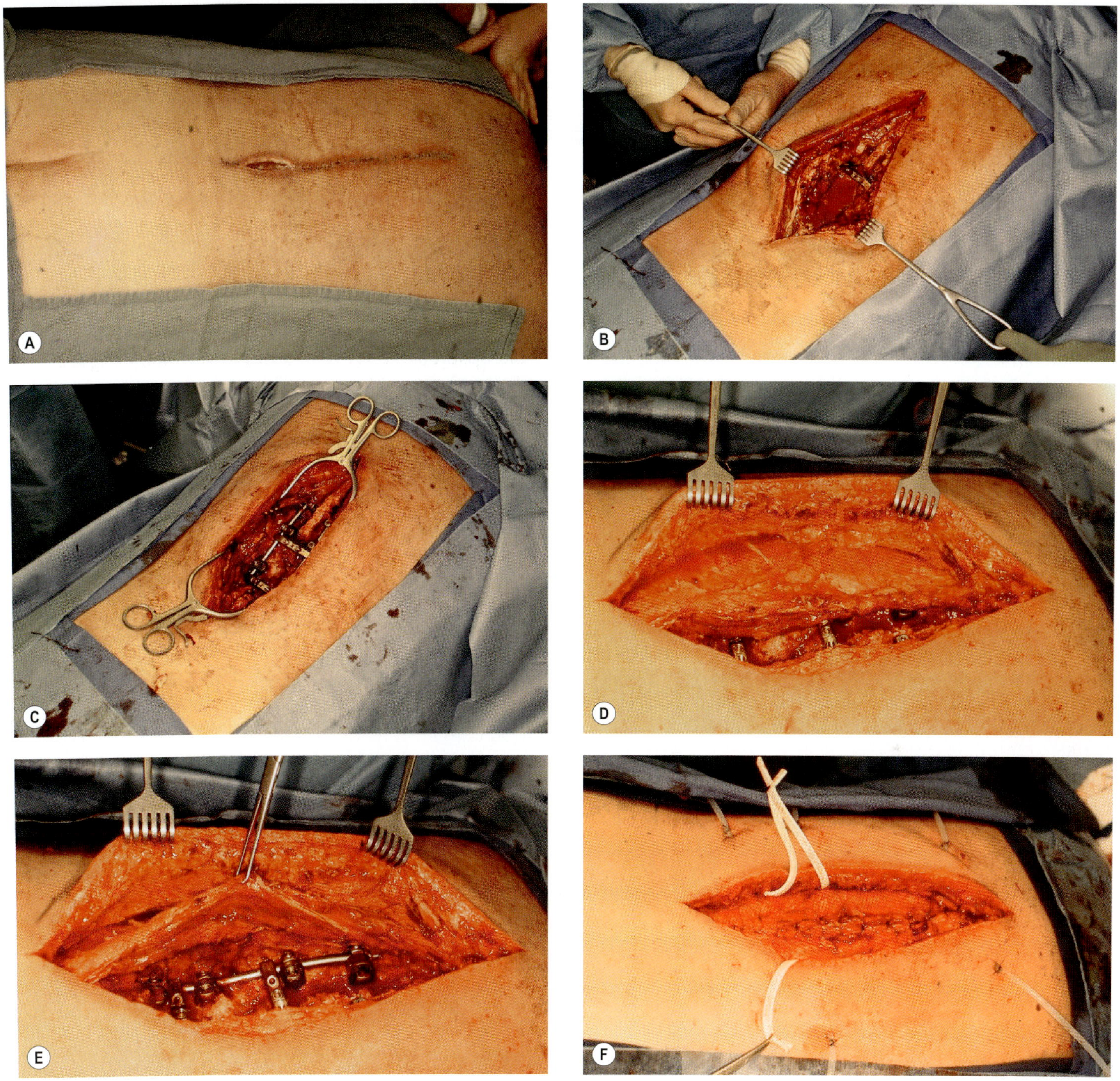

Figure 12.7 **(A)** Patient with a long thoracolumbar fusion with drainage 3 weeks after a posterior spinal fusion. Note the erythema of the staple line. **(B)** Complete opening of the superficial and deep tissues reveals an infected fluid collection surrounding the hardware. A crossbar is visible. **(C)** The wound is radically debrided to reveal the entire spinal hardware construct. The hardware seems solidly fixed to the bone. **(D)** Dissection deep to the thoracolumbar fascia to the lateral border of the erector spinae muscles. A large nerve traveling through the muscle to the overlying skin is spared. **(E)** Dissection on the deep aspect of the erector spinae muscles to the level of the lateral perforators. **(F)** Erector spinae muscles closed in the midline.

is oriented laterally towards the greater trochanter *(Fig. 12.10)*. This is a different orientation than the skin paddle used for closure of sacral pressure sores, where extra skin is taken medial to the Doppler signal.

- To improve the reliability of the tissue, a strip of gluteus muscle oriented underneath the skin paddle can be taken along with the perforator.
- The superior border of the skin is incised, and the skin flap elevated until the perforator from the superior gluteal artery is seen to be entering the skin paddle.
- Medial to this, the gluteus muscle is split to aid in the dissection of the pedicle.
- With the pedicle under full view, the remainder of the skin paddle can be incised and the flap dissection completed.

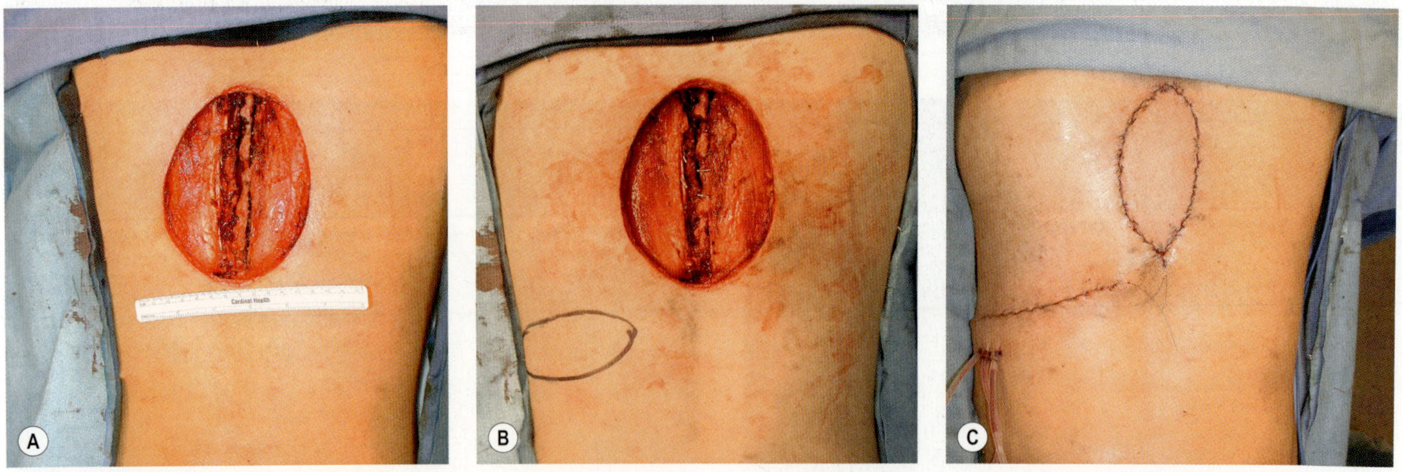

Figure 12.8 **(A)** A 26-year-old man had a recurrent desmoid tumor removed from his thoracic spine area. There is exposure of the spinous processes. There is no hardware present. **(B)** A skin paddle slightly less wide than the defect and oriented at a right angle to the long axis of the wound is drawn out. **(C)** Final inset of the flap. The flap donor site is oriented perpendicular to the long axis of the defect, so that closure of the donor site will not make the recipient site more difficult to close.

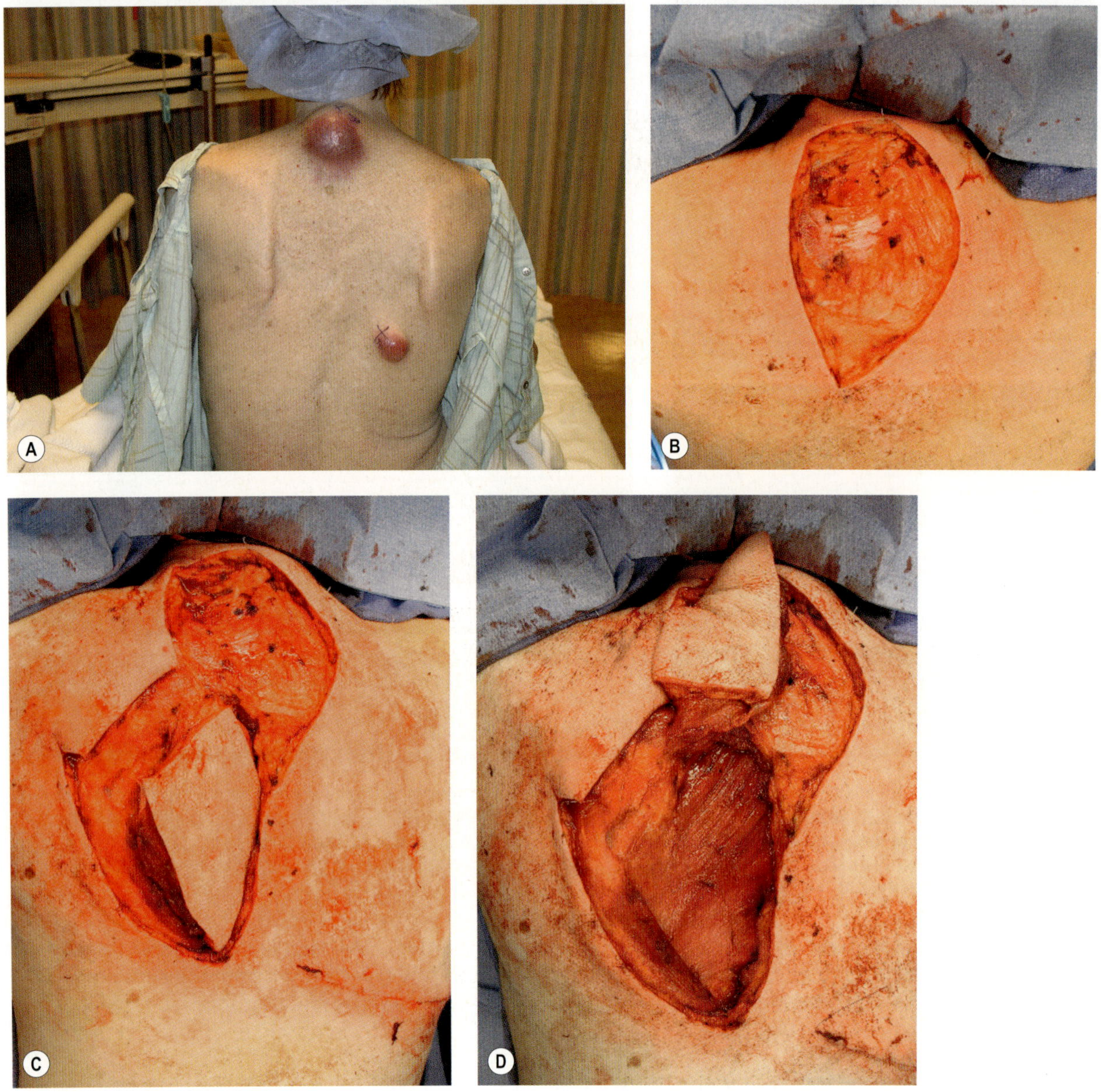

Figure 12.9 **(A)** A 60-year-old patient with painful metastatic neuroendocrine tumors to the cervical spine area. The tumors have been radiated, precluding closure with skin grafts. **(B)** Wound after tumor excision. **(C)** Incised myocutaneous trapezius flap. The skin paddle was oriented at the inferior aspect of the muscle. **(D)** Trapezius flap during inset with 180° twist. The superficial dorsal scapular artery was not included with this flap, resulting in mild hypoperfusion of the skin paddle. The donor site was closed in the vertical midline.

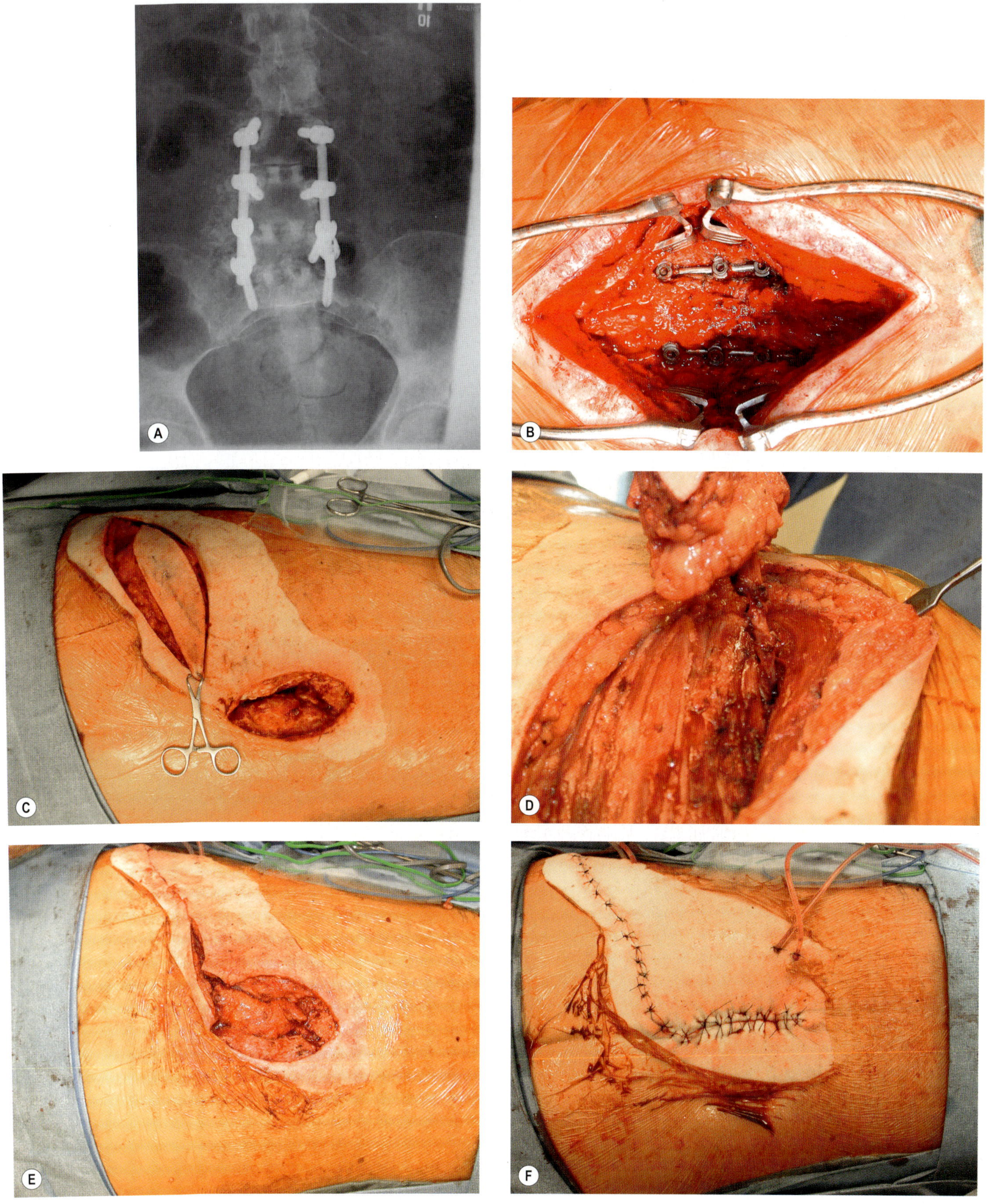

Figure 12.10 (A) Radiograph of low lumbar fusion of a patient with drainage 3 weeks after spinal fusion. **(B)** Intraoperative view after debridement of fusion site. **(C)** Incised skin paddle for left superior gluteal artery perforator (SGAP) flap. The staple marks the audible Doppler signal of the SGAP perforator to the skin. **(D)** Vascular pedicle to the superior gluteal artery perforator flap. Muscle around the pedicle must be minimized to allow for a facile flip of the flap to the midline. **(E)** The skin paddle is de-epithelialized and placed to fill the lumbosacral recess. **(F)** Closed incisions.

- If there is difficulty with identification of the superior gluteal artery perforator, additional muscle should be elevated with the skin paddle, or a decision made to dissect the other buttock.
- Medially, any muscle along the pedicle will resist the 180° flip required of the pedicle for the flap to reach the midline.
- Muscle found around the pedicle that impedes this 180° turn should be excised so that there is no tension on the flap to reach the lumbosacral spine.
- The skin paddle is de-epithelialized and will be able to cover the dura.
- The donor and recipient sites are closed over drains.
- Both buttocks should be prepped into the field, in case there is an injury to the pedicle.
- In patients with buttock weakness preoperatively, the stronger side should be used.
- Caution should be taken in patients who are markedly obese, and those with prior pressure sore procedures.
- A complete pressure relief bed is necessary for 10–14 days after the procedure to prevent pressure on the pedicle as it runs from the lateral sacrum towards the midline.

Omentum

- The primary criteria for using a pedicled omental flap include scarred, irradiated, divided, and otherwise unusable back musculature suitable for local flap transfer in a patient in need of soft tissue coverage of thoracolumbar spinal instrumentation ***(Fig. 12.11)***.
- Secondary criteria include extremely deep wounds, such as for those patients with coverage needs of both anterior and posterior instrumentation, and for patients in whom the abdominal cavity is already entered for exposure.
- Absolute contraindications to the use of a pedicled omental flap include a history of intra-abdominal malignancy and a previously resected omentum.

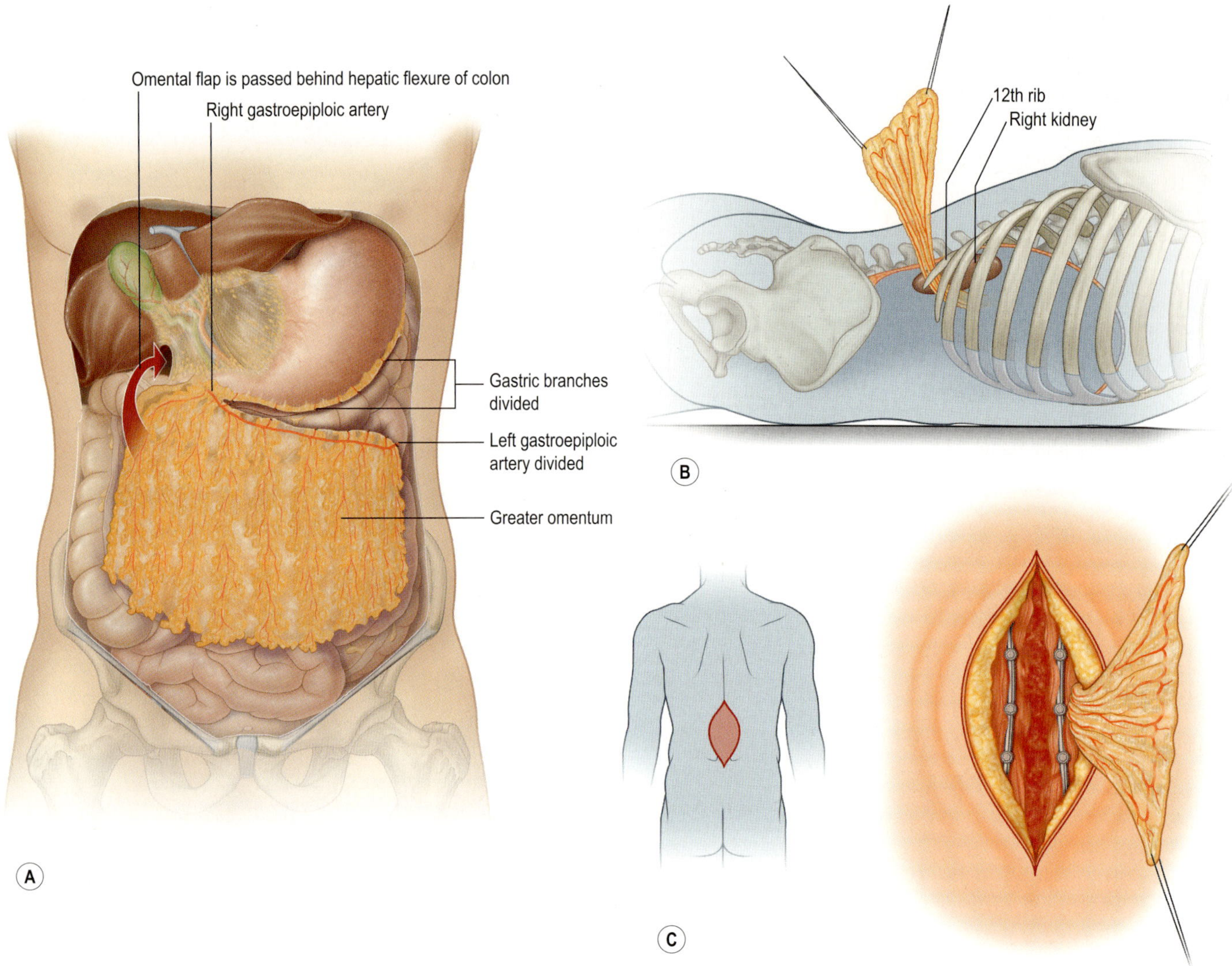

Figure 12.11 (A–C) Diagram of a pedicled omental flap for coverage of the spine.

- Relative contraindications include morbid obesity and the potential for intra-abdominal adhesions from previous laparotomies.
- The zone of coverage for an omental flap is from the lumbosacral recess inferiorly up to the level of the midscapula superiorly.
- Typically, a posterior spinal instrumentation for stabilization has been performed before the omental flap is harvested and the abdomen is entered either through an upper midline incision, a Kocher, or a right paramedian incision.
- After entering the peritoneal cavity and identifying the omentum, dissection begins by liberating the omentum and transverse colon such that they can be lifted out of the abdominal cavity. The omentum can be dissected from its attachments to the transverse colon. Performed correctly, the entire colon from the hepatic flexure to the splenic flexure can be mobilized away from the omentum and stomach.
- Next, a decision is made regarding whether to base the flap on the right or left gastroepiploic (gastro-omental) artery.
  - The right-sided vessel is usually larger; the left is used when the spine exposure includes a left-flank incision.
- The omentum is mobilized off the stomach by taking down the short gastric vessels between snaps and ties. One should not attempt to travel great distances for each tie, as this tends to shorten the reach of the flap.
- The stomach should be decompressed with a nasogastric tube, and this tube should remain in place for several days so that gastric distension will not cause any of the vessel ligatures on the greater curve to pull off.
- After complete mobilization of the gastroepiploic vessel off the stomach, it can be followed to the area where it emerges as the gastroduodenal artery (a branch off the hepatic artery/celiac plexus just inferior to the pylorus and still superior to the transverse colon mesentery).
- The artery and vein should not be skeletonized, so that the surrounding soft tissue will help to prevent unexpected tension on the vessels during the tunneling process.
- The passage of the omentum toward the spinal column requires creativity and knowledge of anatomy of the gastroduodenal artery and its relationship to the attachments of the colon to the retroperitoneum.
  - The most straightforward means to tunnel the omentum to the spine is to mobilize the hepatic flexure and right colon toward the midline. This is an avascular plane, and the mobilization of the colon is greatly simplified by the prior elevation of the omentum off the colon. The line of lateral peritoneal reflection (the white line of Toldt) is incised, exposing the retroperitoneum.
  - The omental flap is then positioned behind the colon in the right paracolic gutter. The right kidney and Gerota's fascia are mobilized medially, and the omentum is "parked" on top of the 12th rib, which is confirmed by palpation. The abdomen is then closed in standard fashion and the patient reprepped in the prone position.
  - The 12th rib is identified by palpation after elevating the latissimus muscle and skin off the ribcage. Lateral to the paraspinous muscles, the 12th rib is excised, the periosteum opened, and the omental flap will be immediately identifiable.
  - When skin is not available for coverage of the omentum, a negative-pressure suction dressing is applied immediately on to the flap, and a delayed skin graft performed.

Adjacent tissue transfers/perforator flaps

- Adjacent tissue transfers without a defined blood supply and perforator flaps are two ends of a spectrum of possible reconstructions of the soft tissues of the back.
- In adjacent tissue transfers such as V-Y flaps, transposition flaps, and rotation flaps, the thick soft tissues of the back will create large dog ears; donor sites will typically need to be covered with skin grafts.
- Perforator flaps, on the other hand, will allow transposition and insets in a more facile manner, and are especially useful in the iliolumbar and scapular area. However, the stresses on the soft tissues of the back with movement in and out of bed and with position changes will make the delicate nature of perforator flaps difficult to protect.

External oblique flap

- Patients with huge lower lateral thoracic and lumbar wounds can have these closed with pedicled external oblique turnover flaps.
- These patients will have large radiated wounds where the remaining soft tissues would not be expected to accept a skin graft, or where there was a prosthetic material used for reconstruction of the posterior abdominal wall.
- These large flat flaps can be thought of as an interface to help with healing of skin grafts to the wound bed.
- The muscle is exposed with wide elevation of the abdominal skin, done through an oblique incision paralleling the dermatomes. Then, the insertion of the muscle is divided, just as it fuses with the anterior rectus fascia. Much like a components separation procedure, the external oblique is bluntly elevated towards the posterior axillary line off the internal oblique, to the point where segmental vessels enter the muscle. The muscle is flipped on itself 180° to cover the defect and subsequently to be skin-grafted. When the flap is done unilaterally, the corresponding muscle imbalance of the anterior abdomen may cause an unusual contour of the abdominal wall.

Tissue expansion

- Tissue expansion can be preferable to other solutions for reconstruction of the soft tissues of the back in certain instances. Those situations are more for pediatric cases than for adults, and include the closure of wounds for giant congenital nevi excisions.
- The indication for tissue expansion is scarred local tissues, laterally displaced muscles, and need for spinal instrumentation ***(Fig. 12.12)***.

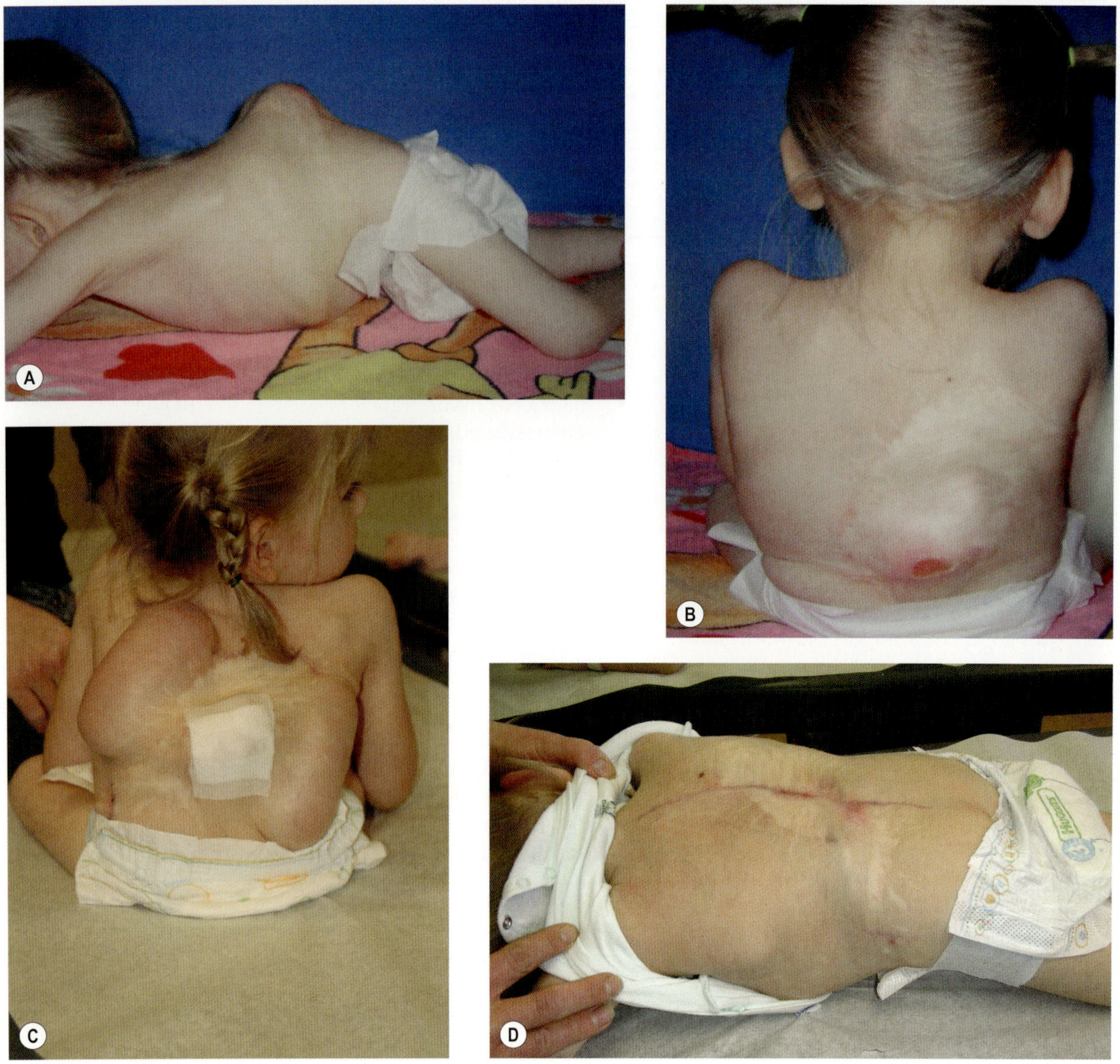

Figure 12.12 **(A)** Lateral photo of a young child with a significant congenital spine defect. **(B)** Previous attempts at correction have produced numerous scars. A well-cared for pressure sore is at the apex of the deformity. **(C)** Bilateral subcutaneous tissue expanders placed on the posterior trunk. **(D)** Healed incision after spine correction and advancement flap closure with expanded skin flaps.

- The largest expanders possible should be placed immediately adjacent to the area that will require coverage, and the long axis of the expander should be oriented in a superior–inferior direction to allow for a medial sliding of the expanded tissue with a minimum of back-cuts and transposition flaps.
- Incisions for placement should be parallel to the axis of the expander to decrease the chance of extrusion of the implant through this newly placed scar.
- Ports should be placed over bony prominences to facilitate their palpability.

Free flap coverage of the back

Soft tissues

- In patients with scarred erector spinae muscles from previous advancements or neuromuscular conditions such as polio, patients who have received wide-field radiation with defects longer than 12 cm precluding transposition flaps, or when an omental flap is not possible, free flaps may be required.
- The difficulties with free flap coverage of the spine is finding a suitable donor vessel. Possibilities include the superior gluteal artery pedicle and intercostal vessels. A long saphenous vein graft anastomosed to the common femoral artery can provide both inflow and outflow when divided for a lower trunk defect, and a long cephalic vein graft tied to the external carotid can bring inflow for an upper trunk flap.

Bone

- The vertebral bodies of the spine are typically reconstructed with cages and bone grafts when corpectomies are performed, and with good results.

- Certain patient subpopulations exist where vascularized bone is preferable. In these patients, more rapid incorporation of the bone graft due to its viable osteocytes reduces the chance of construct failure and infection.
- It is difficult to define exactly who should receive vascularized bone flaps, as the success rates of non-vascularized autograft and allograft are high.
- Fusions longer than three vertebral bodies in length, previous failed reconstructions, a history of radiation, esophagocutaneous fistula on to the fusion site, and active osteomyelitis may all be indications for a free fibula flap to the anterior spinal column.
- In the thoracic area, vascular inflow is either end-to-end from a segmental lumbar vessel, or off a saphenous vein patch of the aorta fashioned by vascular surgery.

Vascularized bone reconstruction of the spine

- A straightforward means of bringing vascularized bone to the anterior aspect of the thoracic spine is with a pedicled rib flap.
- For patients undergoing both anterior and posterior fusion of the spine with an associated thoracotomy for access, a pedicled rib based on its intercostal neurovascular bundle can be harvested.
- Unlike vascularized fibula flaps, the vascularized rib brings viable osteocytes but no structural support to the spine. The rib graft can either be placed next to or within the metal cage that is used for structural replacement of the vertebral body.

Special clinical situations

Esophageal fistula after spine procedures

- A small number of patients undergoing cervical spine fusion will suffer a traumatic injury to the esophagus, causing drainage and contamination of the fusion site. Another group of patients will develop a pressure sore of the cervical spine hardware into the esophagus, and so the hardware can be seen during an esophagoscopy.
- Everything depends on the timing of the esophageal leak with the placement of the hardware.
  - If the esophageal injury occurred at the time of hardware placement, then the spinal fusion is not solid, and the hardware is still needed.
    - Simple repair of the esophageal defect is problematic even without the spine issues, as the standard treatment by otolaryngology is to drain fluid collections and let the wounds heal by secondary intention.
    - Improvement of the soft tissues between the spinal hardware and the cervical esophageal repair is important and local flaps from the neck, the pectoralis flap, and the omental free flaps are all thin flaps that can be interposed into this space. The omentum is perhaps best able to deal with the contaminated drainage, and it easily conforms to the space crevices. Pectoralis flaps are perhaps best avoided in spinal cord patients who use their accessory chest muscles to breathe.
  - Patients who develop pressure sores of the hardware into the cervical esophagus are often found months after the cervical fusion, and the hardware can often be removed.
    - Repair of the esophagus if possible and interposition of the soft tissue flap are much easier in the absence of hardware and when the bone is fused.
    - Replacement of the esophageal wall using a radial forearm flap is possible in these situations of a fused cervical spine and a persistent leak.

"Tethered cord surgery" or "lipomas of the spine"

- Infants will sometimes receive procedures in their infancy for closure of their spinal canal or removal of large "lipomas of the spine". After these procedures, the spinal cord can become adherent to the spinal canal, and with growth and age, the spinal cord can be unusually stretched. Management of this tethered cord involves opening of the dura and freeing the spinal cord from scar attachments, which typically allows the cord to slide cephalad.
- Some patients with just thick fat over the lumbosacral recess have done well with preoperative liposuction. Patients with thick scars can be resurfaced with tissue expanders prior to the spine exploration. Others with pseudomeningoceles and need for cord re-exploration do best with superior gluteal artery-based soft tissue reconstructions, as described below.

Pseudomeningocele repair and cerebrospinal fluid leaks

- Pseudomeningoceles are contained leaks of CSF through dura into the soft tissues of the back, while CSF leaks of the spinal cord exit through drains or through the skin. The former situation typically requires treatment due to pressure of the fluid on the spinal cord with worsening motor and sensory function. The latter situation must be addressed to prevent an ascending meningitis.
- Typically, the hole in the dura must be repaired or patched by the neurosurgeon and it is up to the plastic surgery team to improve the soft tissue envelope for the dural reconstruction to heal.
- Important adjuncts to the above procedures are a temporary or permanent decompression of the CSF pressure on the flap, which can include:
  - Flat patient positioning on a pressure relief air-fluidized sand bed for a week after the procedure.
  - A lumbar or head drain of CSF monitored by the neurosurgery team to keep the pressure low on the reconstruction.
  - The CSF pressure is probably more important than the quality of the soft tissue reconstruction long-term for pseudomeningocele recurrences.

Postoperative considerations

- There are two critical components to postoperative care following reconstruction of back wounds: closed suction drainage and pressure relief.
  - Closed suction drainage between the base of the wound and the flap should be maintained until less than 30 cc/day emerges in the bulbs. The more drains the better, and for large procedures even 6–8 bulbs have been required.
  - Postoperative placement on a pressure relief air-fluidized bed will allow the patient to lie directly on the flap and yet not cause a pressure injury to the tissues. It is suspected that compression of the flap directly on to the wound bed has beneficial effects in helping the wound to seal.

Further reading

Duffy FJ, Weprin BE, Swift DM. A new approach to closure of large lumbosacral myelomeningoceles: The superior gluteal artery perforator flap. *Plast Reconstr Surg.* 2004;114:1864–1868.

Dumanian GA, Ondra SL, Liu J, et al. Muscle flap salvage of spine wounds with soft tissue defects or infection. *Spine.* 2003;28:1203–1211.

Long-term results of successful salvage of posterior hardware with soft tissue reconstruction of the back are presented.

Erdmann D, Meade RA, Lins RE, et al. Use of the microvascular free fibula transfer as a salvage reconstruction for failed anterior spine surgery due to chronic osteomyelitis. *Plast Reconstr Surg.* 2006;117:2438.

Garvey PB, Rhines LD, Dong Wenli, et al. Immediate soft-tissue reconstruction for complex defects of the spine following surgery for spinal neoplasms. *Plast Reconstr Surg.* 2010;125:1460–1466.

Large series of prophylactic flaps from the MD Anderson group demonstrates improved outcomes.

Glass BS, Disa JJ, Mehrara BJ, et al. Reconstruction of extensive partial or total sacractomy defects with a transabdominal vertical rectus abdominis myocutaneous flap. *Ann Plast Surg.* 2006;56: 526–530.

Lee MJ, Ondra SL, Mindea SA, et al. Indications and rationale for use of vascularized fibula bone flaps in cervical spine arthrodeses. *Plast Reconstr Surg.* 2005;116:1–7.

Mathes DW, Thornton JF, Rohrich RJ. Management of posterior trunk defects. *Plast Reconstr Surg.* 2006;118:73e–83e.

Mitra A, Mitra A, Harlin S. Treatment of massive thoracolumbar wounds and vertebral osteomyelitis following scoliosis surgery. *Plast Reconstr Surg.* 2004;113:206–213.

Nojima K, Brown SA, Acikel C, et al. Defining vascular supply and territory of thinned perforator flaps: Part II. Superior gluteal artery perforator flap. *Plast Reconstr Surg.* 2006;118:1338–1348.

O'Shaughnessy BA, Dumanian GA, Liu JC, et al. Pedicled omental flaps as an adjunct in complex spine surgery. *Spine.* 2007;32:3074–3080.

Small series illustrating the use of pedicled omental flaps in spine reconstruction surgery.

Said HK, O'Shaughnessy BA, Ondra SL, et al. Integrated titanium and vascular bone: A new approach for high risk thoracic spine reconstruction: P34. *Plast Reconstr Surg.* 2005;116:160–162.

Wilhelmi BJ, Snyder N, Colquhoun T, et al. Bipedicle paraspinous muscle flaps for spinal wound closure: An anatomic and clinical study. *Plast Reconstr Surg.* 2000;106:1305–1311.

This is an early description of paraspinous muscle flaps for repair of soft tissue defects after spine surgery. This paper illustrates the performance of superior gluteal artery flaps that can then be used for spine reconstruction.

Chapter 13

Abdominal wall reconstruction

This chapter was created using content from Neligan & Song, Plastic Surgery 3rd edition, Volume 4, Lower Extremity, Trunk and Burns, Chapter 12, Abdominal wall reconstruction, Navin K. Singh, Marwan R. Khalifeh and Jonathan Bank

SYNOPSIS

- Abdominal wall reconstruction techniques are indicated for hernia repair, reconstruction of tumor defects, congenital defects, and correction of traumatic defects (e.g., from damage control laparotomies).
- Patients may be complicated by fistulae, adhesions, infections, scarring from previous injury or surgery, and presence of dehisced prior mesh.
- Preoperative optimization of patients is requisite – smoking cessation, weight loss if indicated, and nutritional restitution.
- Autologous techniques are ideal in reconstruction, utilizing muscle and fascia – utilizing separation of components and fascia lata grafts.
- Prosthetic meshes and bioprosthetics may be utilized in addition to, or in lieu of, flaps for recalcitrant cases.
- Advanced techniques may include tissue expanders, laparoscopic methods, free flaps, and even abdominal wall transplantation.
- Postoperative management begins in the intensive care unit (ICU) and continues into postoperative rehabilitation.

Brief introduction

- Hernias and abdominal wall defects may be asymptomatic or symptomatic, and range from the minor cosmetic inconvenience to major destructive processes of the abdominal wall.
- Narrow-neck hernias are at greater risk for incarceration and strangulation of bowel, whereas large-neck hernias, although more dramatic, are less likely to cause bowel trauma.
- Risk factors for postoperative infection and repair failure include co-morbidities of smoking, diabetes mellitus, chronic obstructive pulmonary disease (COPD), coronary artery disease, poor nutritional status/low serum albumin, immunosuppression, chronic corticosteroid use, obesity, and advanced age.
- Some hernias begin as multiple small "Swiss cheese" defects, and when one defect is repaired, the other unrepaired defect(s) can enlarge.
- Rectus diastases are not true abdominal wall fascial defects but are pathological stretching to the linea alba either congenitally or, most frequently, postpartum.
- Functionally, a diastasis is analogous to an aneurysm – wherein the adventitia (fascia) and intima (peritoneum) are intact but the muscular layer is absent ***(Fig. 13.1)***.
- In techniques for abdominal wall reconstruction that do not centralize muscle, or cases in which the abdominal muscles have retracted beyond the possibility to be reapproximated, a functional diastasis remains, in lieu of the tendinous fusion of the paired rectus abdominis muscles.
- This diastasis can enlarge over time from intra-abdominal pressure, even to the point of requiring repair.
- Repair is achieved without intraperitoneal entry, by plicating or imbricating the defect so that the rectus abdominis muscles are returned to the midline ***(Fig. 13.2)***.

Preoperative considerations

- Hernias should be treated as a chronic disease process – a conglomeration of collagen disorders, excess mechanical loads, co-morbidities, and outdated surgical techniques, and other poorly understood factors.

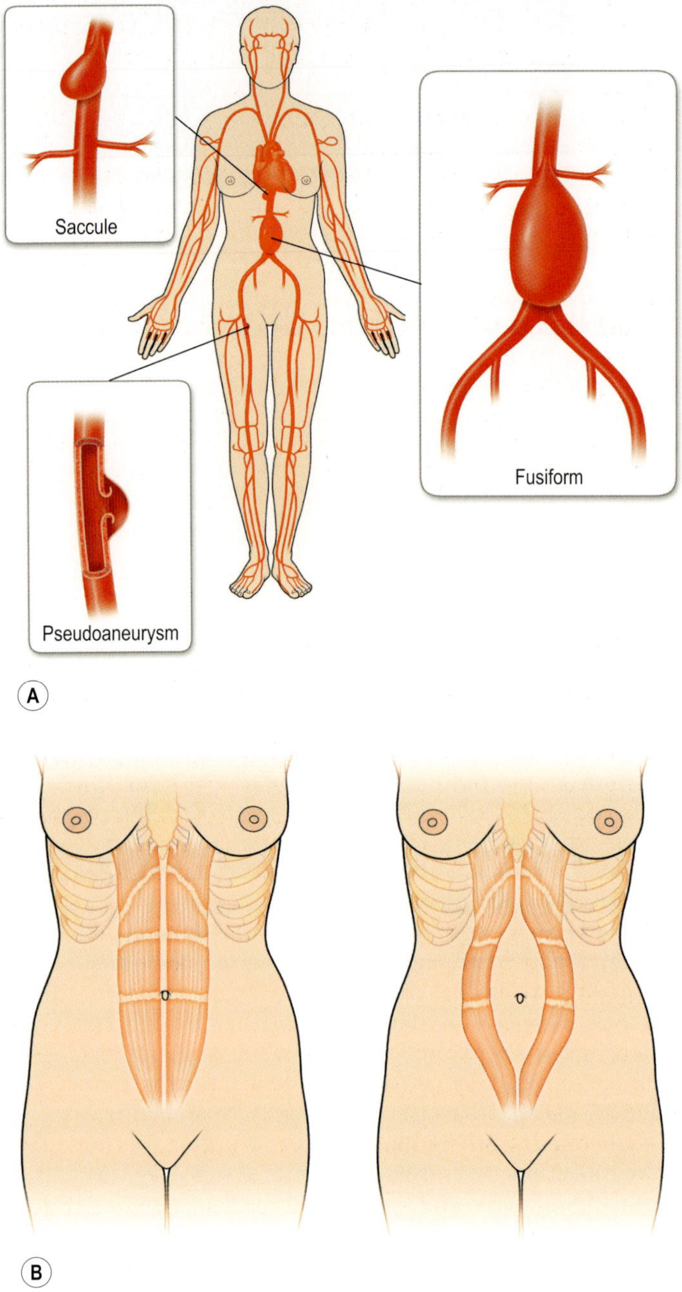

Figure 13.1 Rectus diastases are not true abdominal wall fascial defects but are pathological, stretching to the linea alba. **(A)** A diastasis is analogous to an aneurysm – here the adventitia (fascia) and intima (peritoneum) are intact but the muscular layer is absent. **(B)** Diastases can enlarge over time to the point of requiring repair. Repair is achieved without intraperitoneal entry, by plicating or imbricating the defect and restoring midline approximation of the rectus abdominis muscles.

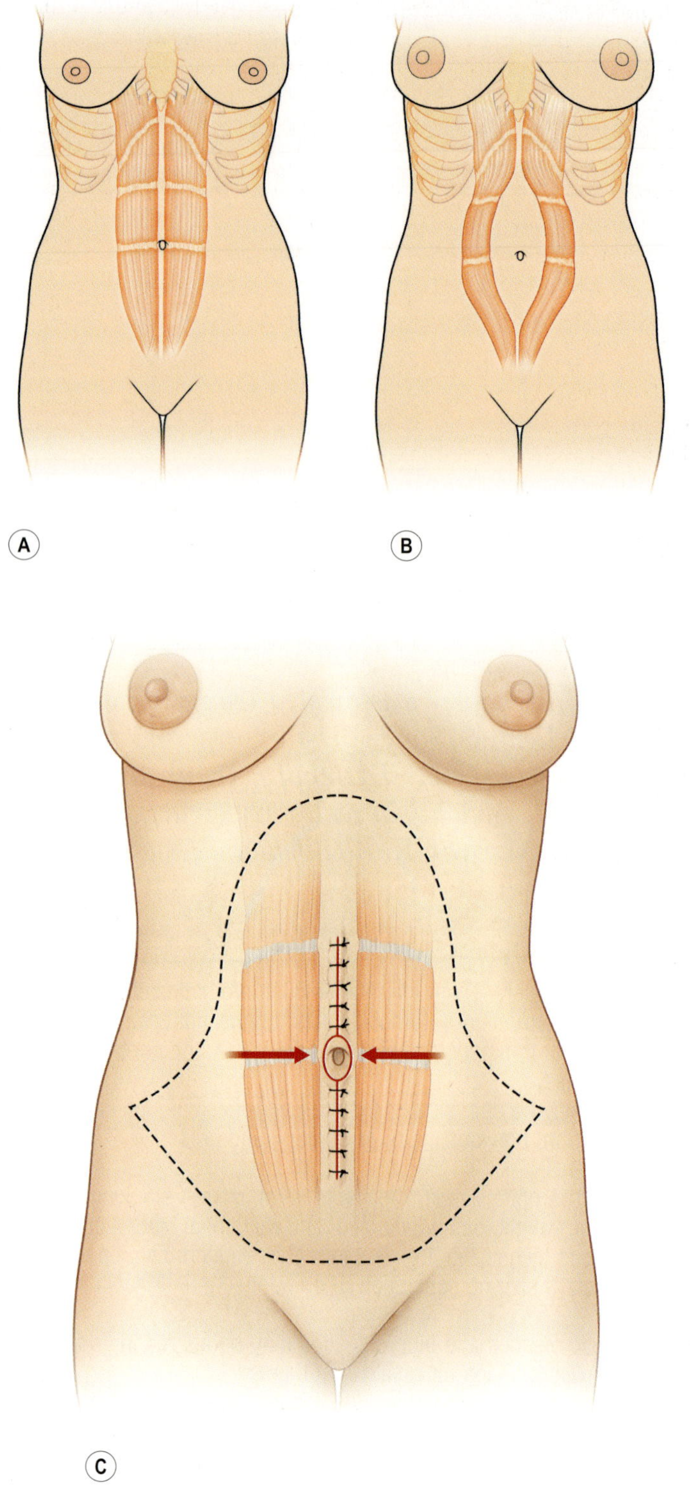

Figure 13.2 **(A)** Normal lay of the rectus abdominis muscles on either side. **(B)** Diastasis recti. **(C)** Schematic representation of the extent of subcutaneous dissection with reapproximation at the midline and fascial plication.

- Success is predicated on a systematic approach from understanding the etiology of prior failure, risk factors, metabolic status, the biology and biomechanics of repair materials, employment of an appropriate surgical technique (i.e., open or laparoscopic), to postoperative vigilance.
- Diagnosis is made on physical exam and confirmed by CT scan.
- Loss of domain occurs when muscle, fascia, and/or skin have necrosed or retracted and have become contracted over time and abdominal viscera extrude into the hernia sac.
- The only absolute contraindication to abdominal wall reconstruction is if the patient is medically unsuitable for surgical clearance.

- Patients with ascites are extremely likely to have a poor outcome and should be referred to a hepatologist for management of cirrhosis or hepatic failure prior to attempt at a repair.
- Metastatic disease (hepatic, abdominal, or distant) is a relative contraindication.
- Postoperatively, patients may develop weakness in the abdominal wall and/or donor sites, acute and chronic pain, respiratory problems, or chronic disability.
- A preoperative discussion of the different implant choices should be held (synthetic mesh, human and non-human bioprosthetics).

Technical pearls

- Halsted's tenets still ring true 100 years later and are applicable to modern hernia surgery:
  - Aseptic technique.
  - Atraumatic handling of tissues.
  - Sharp anatomic dissection.
  - Meticulous hemostasis.
  - Using non-reactive sutures.
  - Minimizing foreign body.
  - Avoiding non-physiologic tension.
  - Obliterating dead space.
- The specific steps in hernia repair are: (1) preparation of the wound by reducing bioburden; (2) realignment of muscles; (3) reinforcing attenuated areas; (4) minimizing foreign body; and (5) controlling dead space to prevent seroma which will delay revascularization ***(Fig. 13.3)***.

Bioburden reduction

- The first step in adherence to surgical principles.
- The wound should be cleansed mechanically if needed by pulse lavage or sharp "oncologic" *en bloc*-type excision.
- Wound preparation should excise any non-vital tissues, indurated and fibrotic tissues likely to become avascular, and any retained prior foreign-body prosthetics and mesh.
- Debridement may necessitate removal of the umbilicus since it is often marginally attached to one of the skin flaps or may be deemed non-viable at the end of the operation. The patient should be prepared for this, and the umbilicus can always be secondarily reconstructed.
- Pre-existing fistulae may be managed by controlling them with surgical drains, percutaneous drainage and diversion of collections, surgical washouts and antibiotic treatment for existing infection or colonization.
- After non-surgical care for a period of 24–72 h, definitive closure can be scheduled. At the time of conclusive repair, any intra-abdominal collections and pathology, such as fistulae and tumors, should be addressed.

Negative-pressure wound therapy

- If, after debridement, the wound still remains unsuitable for immediate closure, it can be temporized with topical antimicrobial creams and dressings to decrease bacterial colony counts.
- For frank infection or gross contamination not adequately addressable by bioburden techniques, the wound may be temporized by using negative-pressure (subatmospheric pressure) dressings.
- The proposed mechanisms by which NPWT works are: (1) compression of tissues creating shear and hypoxia which are signals for angiogenesis/granulation; (2) hypoxia which releases nitric oxide, causing vasodilatation; (3) decrease of third-space fluid; (4) compression of vessel causes, which increases velocity, leading to decrease in hydrostatic pressure by Bernoulli's law and thus less exudate; (5) increased blood velocity, which "aspirates" exudate back into the second space via Venturi effect; and (6) splinting of the wound mechanically.

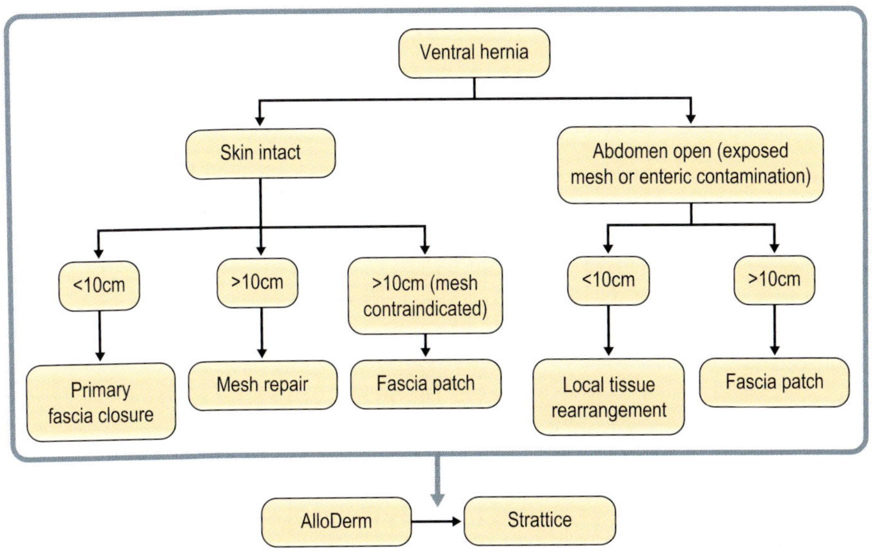

Figure 13.3 Modified algorithm for abdominal wall reconstruction. (After Disa JJ, Goldberg NH, Carlton JM, et al. Restoring abdominal wall integrity in contaminated tissue deficient wounds using autologous fascia grafts. *Plast Reconstr Surg.* 1998;101:979–986.) The expanding usage of biologics such as AlloDerm and Strattice has replaced the use of fascial patches and augments primary fascial closure, and in many instances synthetic meshes.

Operative techniques

Primary suture technique

- The primary suture technique may achieve repair for small defects by mobilizing the edges and primarily suturing them together, much like a postpartum abdomen, when a rectus diastasis is sutured by imbrication to recentralize the rectus abdominis muscles.
- Large sutures such as number 1 or number 2 monofilament sutures are used.
- They may be slowly absorbable sutures such as PDS (polydioxanone) or non-absorbable sutures like nylon or Prolene (polypropylene).
- Faster-absorbing sutures such as chromic (surgical gut) or polyglactin 910 (Vicryl) are not appropriate for suture technique.
- Braided sutures are more prone to be a nidus for infection.
- Permanent sutures provide greater reassurance, but may form suture granuloma or be palpable or visible in thinner patients, potentially requiring surgical removal at a later time.
- The matter of running suture line versus interrupted suture line remains unadjudicated by prospective peer-reviewed publications.

Video 13.1

Component separation method (Video 13.1)

- Component separation is the mobilization of the rectus abdominis muscles bilaterally as a musculofascial, bipedicled, neurotized flap.
- After the initial description by Ramirez et al., several authors have reported favorable outcomes with this technique and have offered improvements and variations which include preservation of peri-umbilical perforators through lateral minimal access incisions.
- In the original description of this technique, the skin and subcutaneous tissues are widely degloved to the anterior or midaxillary line.
- The transition point where the external oblique muscle becomes tendinous and attaches on to the anterior rectus sheath aponeurosis is identified as the linea semilunaris.
- Approximately 10–20 mm lateral to that line, a fasciotomy is made with scissors or electrocautery to separate the external oblique from the rectus abdominis.
- Maneuvers to identify the linea semilunaris include palpation of the rectus abdominis muscle bulk and cautery stimulation can also be used to check the orientation of muscular fibers ***(Fig. 13.4)***.
- Once the fascia is incised, an avascular plane is entered, between the external oblique and the internal oblique directly below it.
- Orientation of the fibers can confirm that the correct plane has been entered since the fibers of the external oblique run superolateral to inferomedial, and the fibers of the internal oblique are orthogonal to the external oblique ***(Fig. 13.5)***.
- The segmental neurovascular bundles emanating from the intercostal vessels and nerves are deep to the internal oblique, and so the plane of dissection is a safe and privileged plane.
- Inadvertent dissection below the internal oblique might damage the innervation, resulting in a patulous and adynamic rectus abdominis muscle segment ***(Fig. 13.6)***.
- The intraperitoneal adhesions of the bowel to the abdominal wall should be regarded as a "component" as well, and must be separated.
- Wide adhesiolysis, freeing the viscera from the abdominal wall undersurface to the bilateral paracolic gutters, is an important step in mobilizing the abdominal wall.
- To gain additional mobility, should it be required, a posterior release of the rectus sheath can be performed a few millimeters lateral to the free edge of the fascia where the hernia is encountered ***(Fig. 13.7)***.
- This posterior release is not always necessary, and it offers an additional 2–3 cm of mobility on each side.
- It also creates a retrorectus space for placing a mesh or biologic, should that option be chosen by the surgeon.
- If a stoma (colostomy, ileostomy, ureterostomy) is present, extra care should be taken in performing component separation on the involved side.
- Component separation should create musculofascial flaps, which advance 6 cm at the epigastrium, 10 cm at the waistline, and 5 cm at the suprapubic region on each side ***(Figs 13.8, 13.9)***.
- Orthopedic-type bone anchors with attached sutures can be used to suture fascia, mesh, or a biologic matrix to the pelvis or ribs.
- A tidy alternative to bone anchors, if unavailable or unfamiliar, is to use a 1 mm wire-passing drill to create tunnels in the bone, through which to pass the suture.
- Most surgeons prefer an underlay as opposed to an onlay mesh reinforcement, but this has not been prospectively shown to be superior.
- The underlay material can be placed intraperitoneally, in which case it should span all the way from external oblique to the contralateral external oblique to reinforce and secure the entire operative field.
- U-sutures are placed full-thickness from the abdominal wall down into the peritoneum, into the mesh or biologic, and back into the abdominal wall.
- The biologic or mesh material used in the underlay technique should be tensioned so that the mobilized muscles passively close in the midline, if possible.
- There will be some instances where the muscles will not come together, and the mesh or biologic will be placed as a "bridging" material.
- As mentioned above, a bridged material will have greater risk for bulging and will not be a dynamic or neurotized portion of the abdominal wall.
- After placement of the underlay, the posterior rectus sheath and then the anterior rectus sheath can each be closed with standard technique ***(Fig. 13.10)***.
- An underlay, alternatively, may be performed in a retrorectus position, where it is superficial to the peritoneal cavity (Rives–Stoppa method).

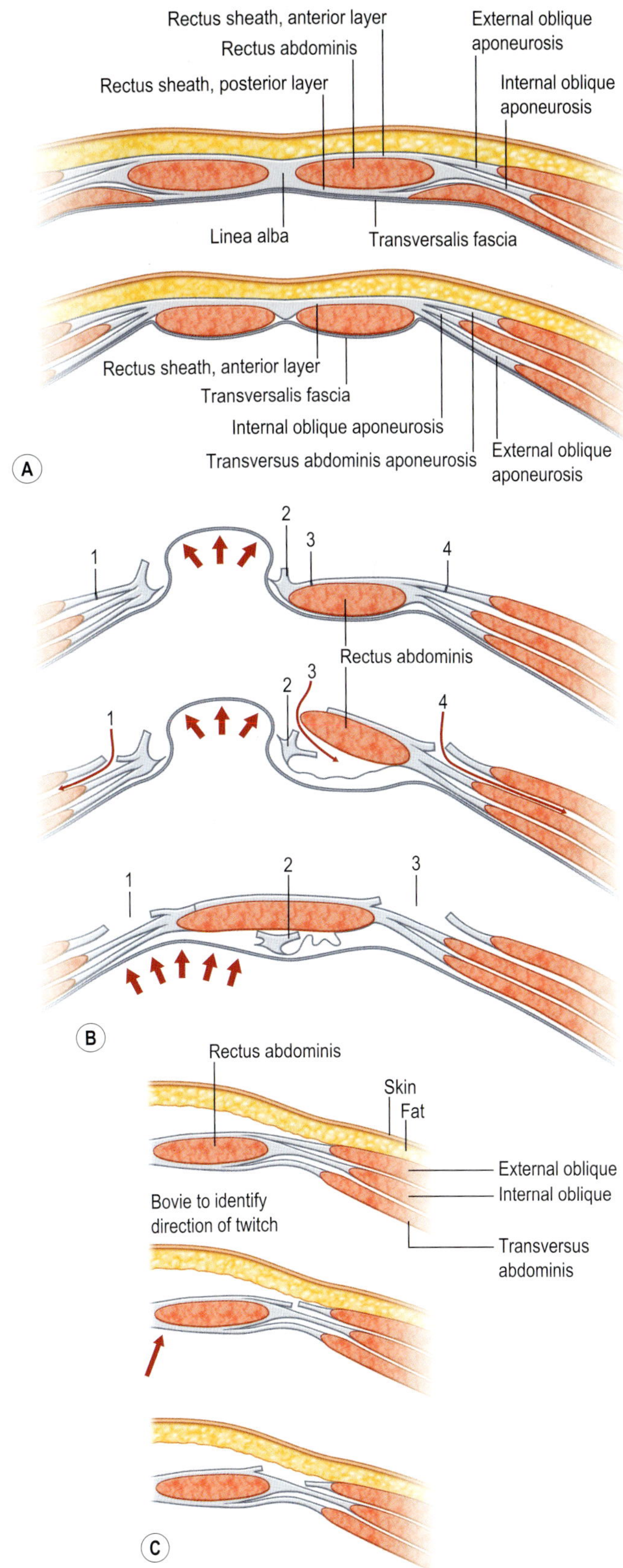

Figure 13.4 **(A)** Normal anatomy above and below the arcuate line. **(B)** Steps in component separation method: the transition point where the external oblique muscle becomes tendinous and attaches on to the anterior rectus sheath aponeurosis is identified as the linea semilunaris. On either side (1, 4), 10–20 mm lateral to the linea semilunaris, a fasciotomy is made, separating the external oblique from the rectus abdominis. Cautery stimulation can also be used to check the orientation of muscular fibers. An avascular plane is entered (between the external oblique and the internal oblique muscles). Orthogonal orientation of the fibers can confirm the correct plane. The segmental neurovascular bundles are protected, coursing deep to the internal oblique muscle. The plane between the rectus abdominis and the posterior rectus sheath may be developed by incising just lateral to the linea alba (2) to gain additional length (3). Flap edges are sutured together. **(C)** Cross-sectional illustration showing external oblique muscle release.

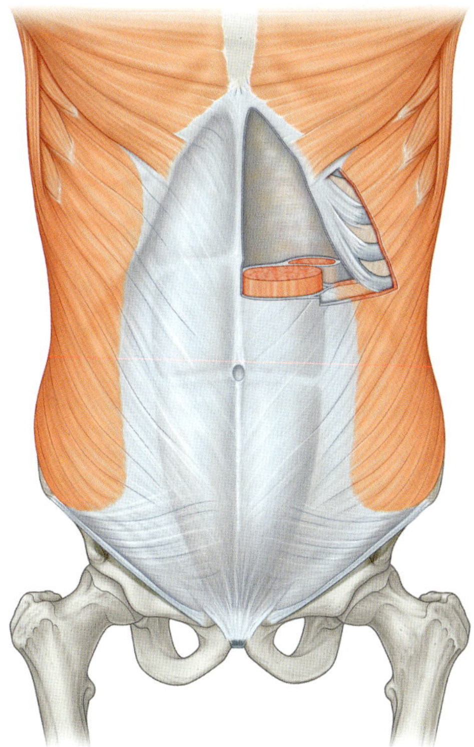

Figure 13.5 Schematic representation of the abdominal musculature and fascial layers above the arcuate line. Note the orthogonal directionality of the oblique muscles.

- The peritoneum and posterior rectus sheath are closed, then a mesh or biologic is placed within the limits of the rectus sheath.
- The advantages include having the strength layer placed in proximity to the muscle sheath and muscle, and having the implant not in communication with the bowel.
- Disadvantages include the fact that it does not resurface the abdominal wall more broadly, and may leave the potential for herniation lateral to the rectus sheath, or through a component separation release site.

- A frequent criticism of the original separation of parts technique is the need for elevation of wide skin flaps that predisposes the skin to edge ischemia and seroma.

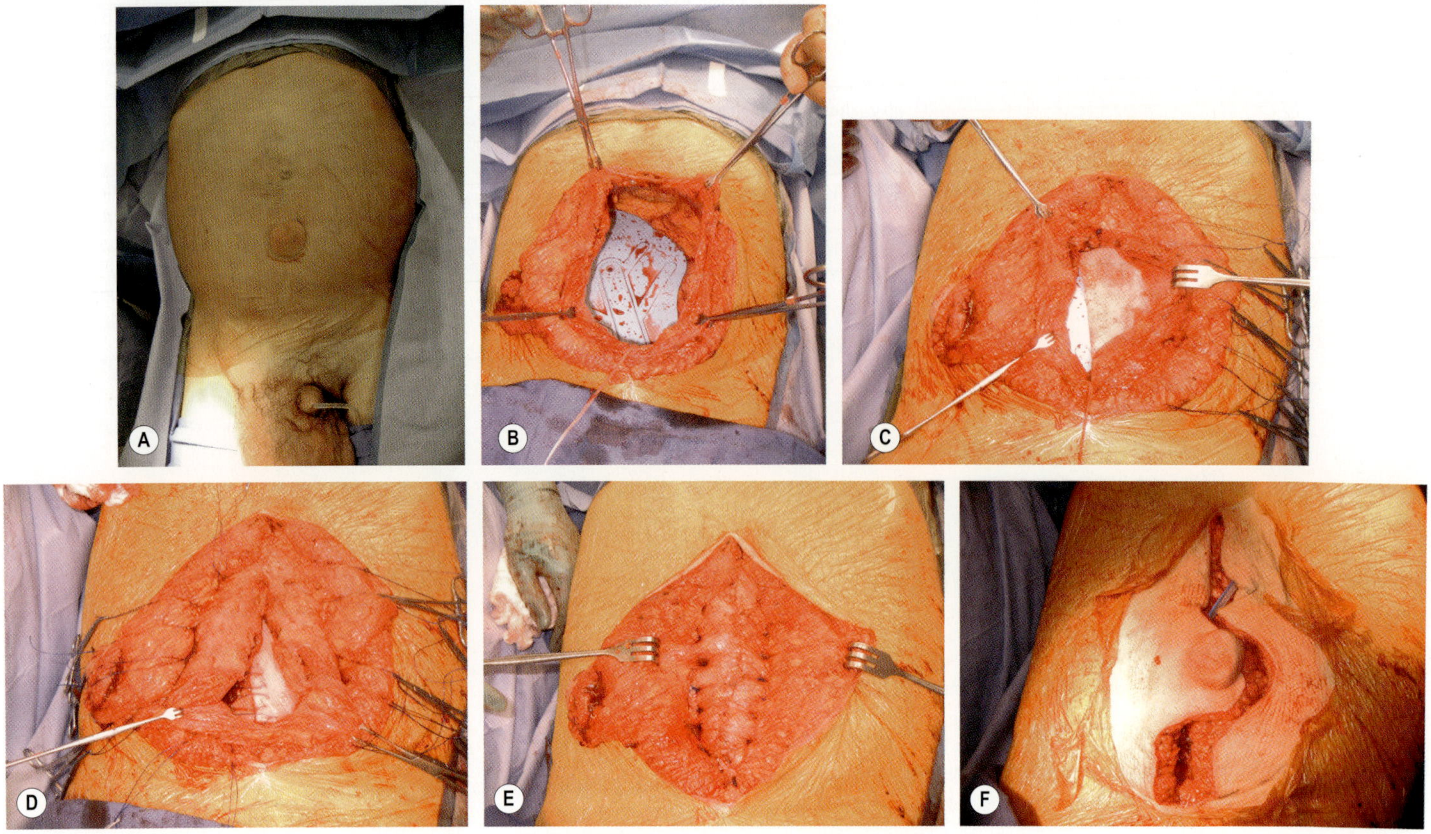

Figure 13.6 Component separation with Strattice underlay. **(A)** Preoperative photo – ventral hernia. **(B)** Hernia sac identified. **(C)** Strattice underlay sutured to one side. **(D)** U-stitches through contralateral side. **(E)** Fascial layers closed above Strattice. **(F)** Drain placement. (Courtesy of Dr David H. Song.)

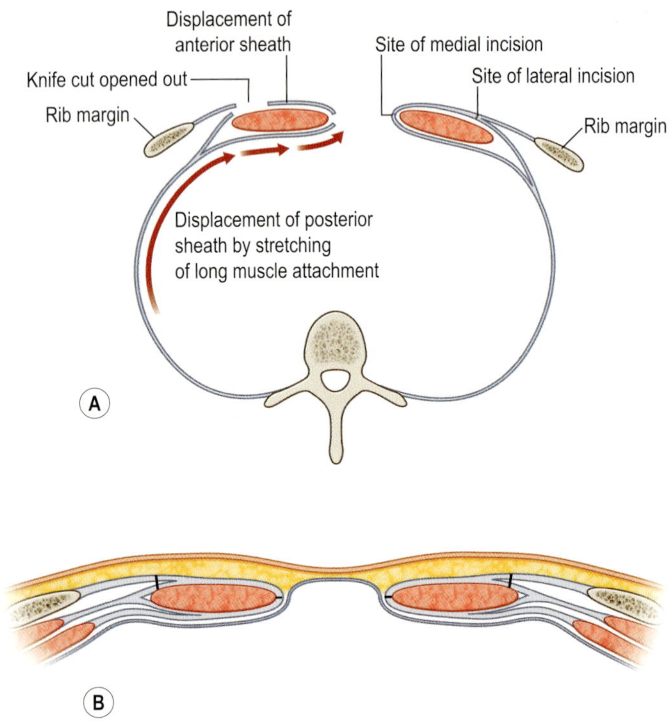

Figure 13.7 **(A)** Cross-sectional diagram demonstrating medial and lateral incisions to initiate the component separation with development of the posterior rectus plane. Detachment from the lower rib margins offers additional length in the upper abdominal region. **(B)** Incision planes in the upper abdomen. Note the lateral incision traverses both components of the anterior rectus sheath.

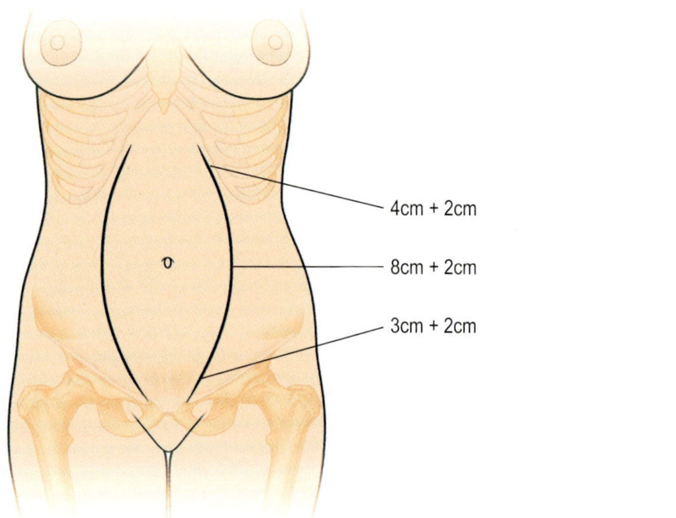

Figure 13.8 As per Shestak et al., maximal unilateral rectus complex mobility in the upper, middle, and lower abdominal levels, by means of component separation of the external and internal oblique muscles to the posterior axillary line. The additional 2 cm of advancement is gained if the rectus abdominis muscle is separated off the posterior rectus fascia.

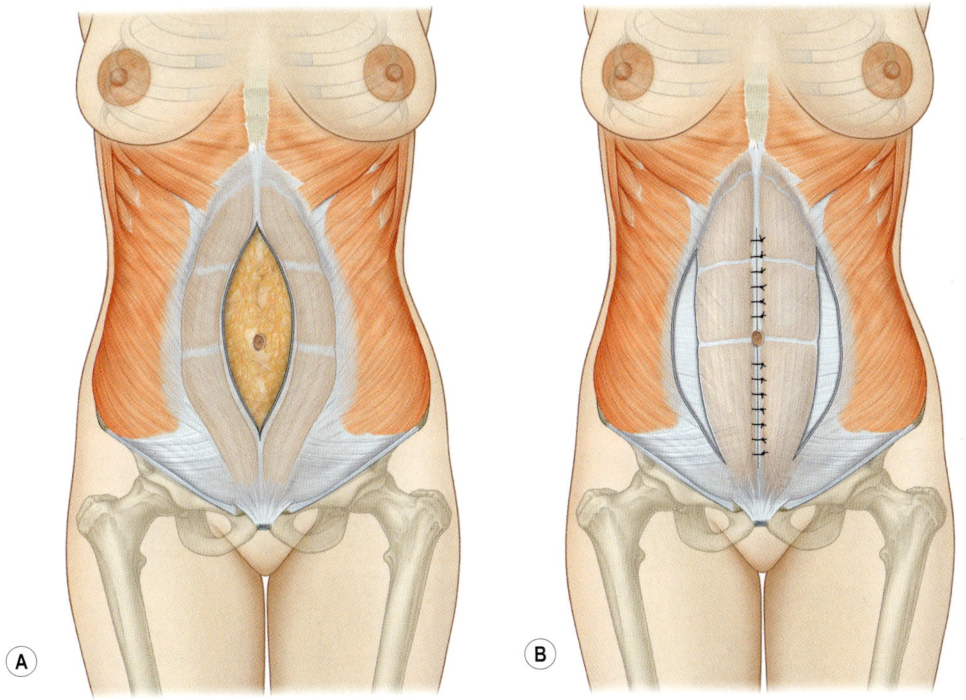

Figure 13.9 **(A)** Preoperative ventral hernia schematic. **(B)** Postoperative illustration showing midline closure at the linea alba. Note the external oblique fascial release. (After Ramirez OM, Ruas E, Dellon AL. "Components separation" method for closure of abdominal-wall defects: an anatomic and clinical study. *Plast Reconstr Surg.* 1990;86:519–526.)

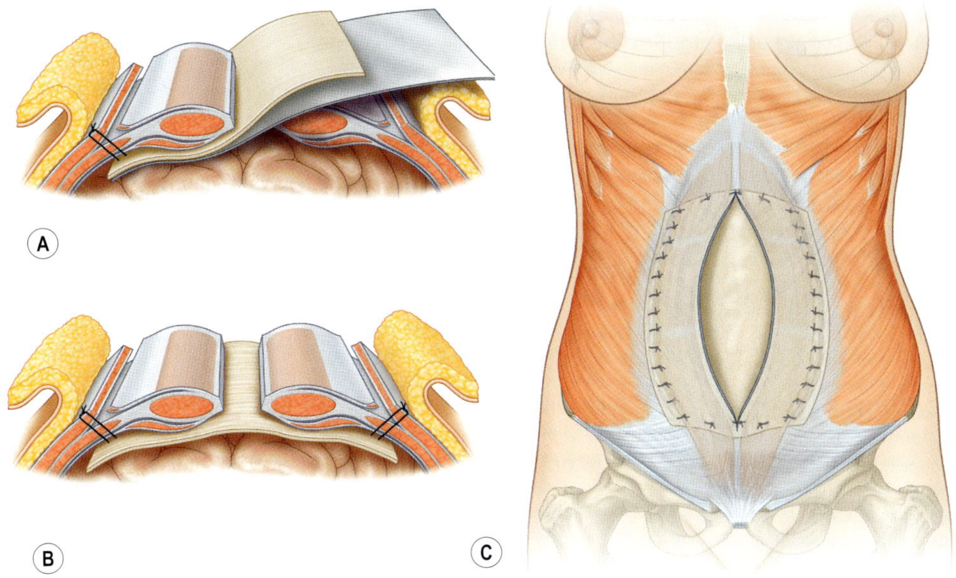

Figure 13.10 Intraperitoneal placement of prosthetic material for ventral hernia repair. **(A)** Cross-sectional view of prosthetic placement, secured initially to one side. After initial separation of components, the underlay material is introduced and secured to the lateral musculature with a full-thickness U-suture. **(B)** If possible, the underlay is tensioned to bring both muscle complexes to the midline. If midline approximation is impossible, the mesh or biologic will be placed as a "bridging" material. This inherently poses a greater risk for bulging and will not be a dynamic or neurotized portion of the abdominal wall. After placement of the underlay, the posterior rectus sheath and then the anterior rectus sheath can each be closed with standard technique. **(C)** Anterior view of underlay suture postioning.

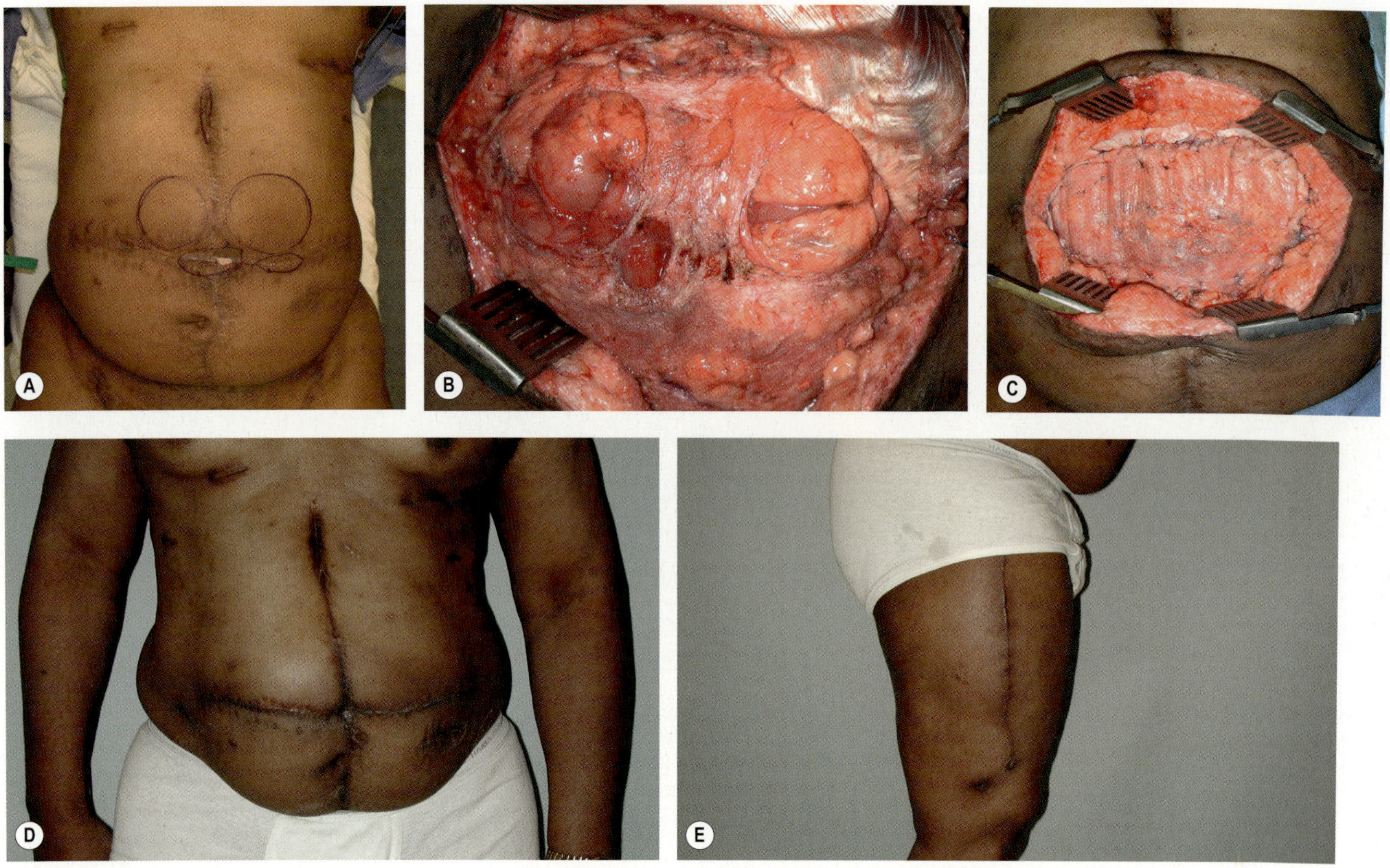

Figure 13.11 Hernia repair with fascia lata graft. **(A)** Preoperative image with markings of multiple fascial defects. **(B)** Intraoperative image of the defects. **(C)** 20 × 15 cm fascia lata graft spanning the defects. **(D)** Postoperative image of abdomen. **(E)** Donor site. (Courtesy of Dr David H. Song.)

- Saulis and Dumanian have championed a perforator-sparing technique in which the release of the semi-lunar lines occurs through separate small lateral access incisions approximately two finger-breadths beneath the costal margin. Using a lighted retractor or a long electrocautery, these access incisions allow for release of the external oblique along its length while sparing several centimeters of soft tissue and fascial perforators near the midline.

Regional and distant autologous tissue repair

- If the surgeon prefers an autologous reconstruction, and does not want to use a biologic matrix or a synthetic mesh, then the established technique of fascia lata grafting can be employed ***(Fig. 13.11)***.
- TFL grafting involves placing a longitudinal incision along the lateral aspect of one or both thighs.
- After dissecting through skin and subcutaneous tissues, the broad and dense fascia of the TFL is identified and mobilized.
- The tensor muscle itself (in the superior portion) is not harvested, but a broad sheet with a longitudinal "grain" of fibers is harvested.
- Five to 10 cm should be left above the knee to prevent lateral knee instability since the fascia lata is part of the iliotibial tract, which provides stability to the lateral knee.
- A graft as large as 28 × 14 cm can be harvested; if needed, two pieces can be sutured together.
- Drains are routinely placed in the donor site, and physical therapy for crutch or cane ambulation is recommended.
- Beyond fascial grafts, a fascial flap can be utilized for closure.
  - Rectus femoris musculocutaneous pedicled flap is one option.
  - A pedicled TFL flap based on the transverse branch of the lateral femoral circumflex vessels, can reach the lower abdomen, and provide skin, subcutaneous bulk, and fascia.
  - A free TFL musculocutaneous fascial flap can also be performed with the anastomoses to intraperitoneal vessels such as the gastroepiploic artery.
  - Free flaps are more commonly utilized for tumor resection than for hernia repair.

Tissue expansion

- Some patients not only have fascial deficiencies but also have skin and soft tissue deficits.
- Tissue expanders can be placed in the subcutaneous space, on top of the fascia and serially expanded over several weeks, recruiting additional skin.

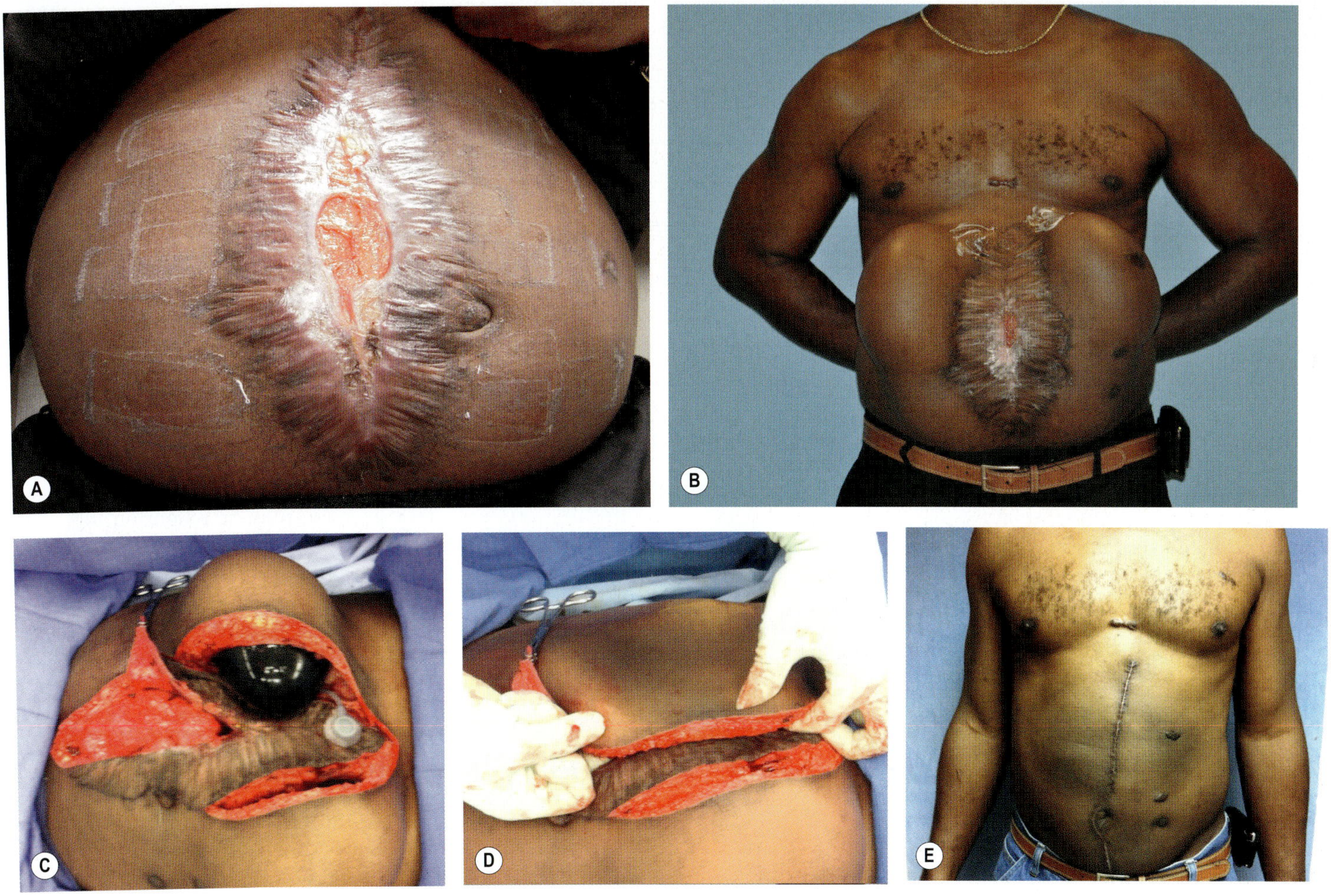

Figure 13.12 Tissue expansion. **(A)** Preoperative image of a poorly healed abdominal skin defect. **(B)** After placement of subcutaneous tissue expanders. **(C)** Expander removal. **(D)** Transposition of expanded skin. **(E)** Postoperative result. (Courtesy of Dr David H. Song.)

- After fascial reconstruction, the tissue expanders are removed, flaps elevated, and closed recruiting the viscoelastic properties of skin – creep and stress relaxation *(Fig. 13.12)*.
- Not commonly done, the fascia itself can be expanded via a technique of placing tissue expanders in the plane between the internal and external oblique.
- Both subcutaneous and interfascial tissue expander techniques are partially limited by the fact that the expander does not rest on a rigid platform (as in the scalp or on the chest wall for breast reconstruction) and the expansion process expands both some tissue outward and some tissue inward, in the path of least resistance.

Parastomal hernia repair

- Parastomal hernias present a notable challenge because the creation of a stoma is *de facto* the creation of a defect in the abdominal wall from which bowel emerges – the very definition of a hernia.
- Attenuation and enlargement of the fascial defect are sadly part of the natural history of a sizeable portion of the stoma-bearing population.
- Repairs may include reinforcing materials such as biologic matrices, since synthetics would be more prone to infection in the setting of stoma.
- Early data suggest a role for the use of a prophylactic placement of material to prevent late herniation, in combination with Sugarbaker keyhole or flap valve technique and/or resiting the ostomy.

Abdominal wall transplantation

Patients undergoing intestinal or multiorgan transplantation may suffer from loss of abdominal domain, requiring reconstruction.

In recent years, abdominal wall transplantation has been described and utilized in the setting of other organ transplants.

The inferior epigastric vasculature is the pedicle typically used.

Like all transplanted tissues, the immunogenicity of the transplanted skin requires lifelong immunosuppression, rendering this reconstructive option to be restricted in cases involving other transplantations.

Postoperative considerations

- DVT prophylaxis. At the very least, sequential compression devices and early ambulation are indicated.
- In the vast majority of cases, chemoprophylaxis is initiated, including heparin, low-molecular weight fractionated heparins, and/or coumadinization postoperatively.
- In many trauma centers or in those patients with an established history of venous thromboembolism, caval filters (permanent and reversible) may be utilized.
- Consideration should be made to keeping the patient intubated on the night of surgery and offering a deeper extubation on the first postoperative day.
- An agitated extubation may create non-physiologic forces of bucking against an endotracheal tube and could disrupt the repair.
- Patients with abdominal wall reconstruction may require ICU care and monitoring to support their fluid requirements since they will sequester fluids in the third space.
- Monitoring for abdominal compartment syndrome via indwelling bladder pressure transducers may be indicated.
- Nutritional support can be provided by total parenteral nutrition (TPN) or early enteral feeds. Enteral feeding is generally not begun until flatus has occurred. If enteral feeding is to be avoided for significant time, TPN can be employed.
- Current state-of-the art data unequivocally indicate that a dose of antibiotics for prophylaxis should be administered intravenously 30–60 min before the case starts and may require redosing depending on the duration of the case and half-life of the antibiotic.
- For clean cases, only the single preoperative dose may suffice, but common usage patterns are for 24 h of antibiotics for prophylaxis.
- A recurrent hernia repair, certainly one with retained prior synthetic mesh, should be treated not only as prophylaxis, but also as therapeutic intent for a longer course.
- Dirty and contaminated cases should be treated with therapeutic intent.
- Cases with violation of the gastrointestinal tract should be offered broader coverage for anaerobic as well as Gram negative bacteria.
- Because of the risk for deep space collections near anastomoses and areas of contamination, and because of the risk for hematomas and seromas in the various dissected layers, the use of drains is essential in abdominal wall reconstruction.
- Abdominal binders can provide compression in the postoperative interval which may help with comfort, minimizing risks for seroma and also supporting the deeper fascial repair.
- One must consider, however, that in the setting of wide subcutaneous flaps, a binder may actually compress marginally perfused tissue and lead to infarction of the tissue and suture line ischemia.
- Proper pain control includes the use of analgesics, pain pumps, and regional anesthetic via epidurals.
- Some centers have reported on use of botulinum toxin at the time of operation into the lateral musculature of the abdominal wall – the external obliques, internal obliques, and transversus muscles – which temporarily attenuates the force of these muscles and decreases spasm and pain, and diminishes the lateral disruptive forces which might disrupt a healing repair.
- Botulinum toxin may be administered a week in advance so that maximal effect is appreciated at the time of surgery.
- Contraindications include neuromuscular disorders such as myasthenia gravis and Guillain–Barré syndrome.
- There is broad consensus that only extremely limited activity should be undertaken for at least the first 6 weeks of convalescence.
- In patients felt to be at higher than average risk, prohibitions for heavy exertion may be extended for months, and for the patient undergoing reconstruction of multiply recurrent hernias, a lifetime of limited physical activity may be indicated.
- Those in physically demanding vocations may need to be retrained or reassigned to different occupations.

Complications and outcomes

- Current data estimate the rate of hernia recurrence in a range from 2% to 54%, depending on the type of repair (mesh 2–36% versus suture repair 12–54%).
- Suture repair of primary ventral has reported recurrence rates of 25–52%.
- The number of prior attempts at abdominal wall herniorrhaphy is predictive of the relative risk of failure.
- In a population-based study of approximately 10 000 patients, the 5-year reoperative rate was 23.8% after the first reoperation, 35.3% after the second, and 38.7% after the third operation.
- Other complications include hematoma, seroma, infection, pain, bulging, and weakness of the abdominal wall, in addition to donor site considerations.
- Skin breakdown leading to exposed mesh or biologic may occur.
- The biologic mesh should be prevented from desiccation with either moist dressings such as NPWT or topical antimicrobials such as silver sulfadiazine.
- Granulation is likely to form through a biologic or lightweight mesh, although the concern for infection is heightened.
- Alternatively, the patient may be returned to the operating room for excision of devitalized skin edges and readvancement closure over drains.
- If synthetic mesh devices are used in the operation, and a periprosthetic infection develops, it will likely necessitate its removal.
- Certain macroporous or lightweight meshes may be able to be treated with local wound care if exposed.

- Biologic meshes may be more resilient under infective or contaminative situations, but they are certainly not resistant to infection or contamination.
- All surgery incites an inflammatory reaction and this reaction can cause adhesions of the intra-abdominal viscera to the abdominal wall.
- During abdominal wall reconstruction, great care should be exercised to interpose omentum between the bowel and the abdominal wall.
- When omentum is not available, Seprafilm (composed of hyaluronic acid and carboxymethylcellulose) may be useful as a barrier to impede adhesion formation.
- Complications of seroma can be managed with serial aspiration with sterile technique, introduction of a sclerosant such as Betadine or tetracycline into the seroma activity, or placement of a percutaneous drain.
- Seromas refractory to these techniques may require operative ablation of the seroma cavity by excising the pseudobursa that has formed, and closing the new space over drains.
- For the seroma requiring operative intervention, additional techniques such as quilting sutures or fibrin glues should be given due consideration.
- Secondary procedures for abdominal wall reconstruction include scar revision, contour improvement, correction of stretch or diastasis, reconstruction of the umbilicus, and amelioration of pain.
- Donor site morbidity must be considered if harvesting autologous grafts for abdominal wall reconstruction.

Further reading

Disa JJ, Goldberg NH, Carlton JM, et al. Restoring abdominal wall integrity in contaminated tissue deficient wounds using autologous fascia grafts. *Plast Reconstr Surg*. 1998;101:979–986.

After conducting animal studies, the authors present their experience with non-vascularized tensor fascia latae autografts in a series of patients in whom prosthetic mesh was contraindicated, or components separation impossible. Recurrence rates, local complications, and donor site morbidity were within acceptable limits. Several patients underwent subsequent laparotomy for other purposes, at which point the transferred fascia was revascularized (concordant with the authors' previous findings in animal experiments). Maximal graft dimension was 28 (14 cm).

Dixon CF. Repair of incisional hernia. *Surg Gynecol Obstet*. 1929;48:700.

Gibson CL. Post-operative intestinal obstruction. *Ann Surg*. 1916;63:442–451.

Hershey FB, Butcher HR Jr. Repair of defects after partial resection of the abdominal wall. *Am J Surg*. 1964;107:586–590.

Luijendijk RW, Hop WC, Van Den Tol MP, et al. A comparison of suture repair with mesh repair for incisional hernia. *N Engl J Med*. 2000;343:392–398.

This landmark prospective multi-institutional European study evaluated 200 cases of primary hernia repair with repair reinforced with mesh. The investigators found that retrofascial preperitoneal repair with polypropylene mesh is superior to suture repair with regard to the recurrence of hernia, even in patients with small defects. However, even with this significant finding, recurrence rates remain high at 10-year follow-up (approximately 30%).

Ramirez OM, Ruas E, Dellon AL. "Components separation" method for closure of abdominal-wall defects: an anatomic and clinical study. *Plast Reconstr Surg*. 1990;86:519–526.

This seminal paper describes 10 cadaver dissections of the abdominal wall with the purpose of determining the amount of mobilization possible by dissecting each layer of the abdominal wall versus the entire complex as a block. The mobility achieved, allowing for functional transfer of abdominal wall components, negates the need for distant muscle flaps. This set the stage for later works by multiple authors and essentially defining today's standard of care for abdominal wall reconstructions applicable in many cases.

Rohrich RJ, Lowe JB, Hackney FL, et al. An algorithm for abdominal wall reconstruction. *Plast Reconstr Surg*. 2000;105:202–216; quiz 217.

This continuing medical education article provides a good overview of abdominal wall anatomy, and provides an additional perspective to the various techniques of reconstructing abdominal wall defects and offers a reconstructive algorithm for partial and complete defects, addressing location of the defect. Autologous tissue transfer sources are discussed (cutaneous, local, and distant flaps), with critique.

Saulis AS, Dumanian GA. Periumbilical rectus abdominis perforator preservation significantly reduces superficial wound complications in "separation of parts" hernia repairs. *Plast Reconstr Surg*. 2002;109:2275–2280; discussion 2281–2282.

Acknowledging the strengths of the "component separation" method, Saulis and Dumanian point out the weaknesses of the method, particularly regarding wound breakdown associated with the wide undermining that is part and parcel of the technique. By preserving the periumbilical rectus abdominis perforators, the authors have shown reduction in wound complications while enabling similar advancement distances and maintaining acceptable hernia recurrence rates.

14 Chapter

Breast augmentation

This chapter was created using content from Neligan & Grotting, Plastic Surgery 3rd edition, Volume 5, Breast, Chapter 2, Breast augmentation, G. Patrick Maxwell and Allen Gabriel.

SYNOPSIS

- Breast augmentation is the most common aesthetic procedure performed in the United States, and perhaps in the world.
- In preparing for a breast augmentation, one must understand each patient's goals and expectations and see if they can be achieved.
- Three important variables have to be addressed prior to surgery: (1) *incision length and placement* (inframammary, periareolar, transaxillary, transumbilical); (2) *pocket plane* (subfascial, subglandular, submuscular, subpectoral with dual plane 1,2,3); (3) *implant choice*: (saline vs silicone, round vs anatomic, smooth vs textured).
- Biodimensional planning may be utilized for optimal preoperative examination.

Brief introduction

- Glandular hypomastia may occur as a developmental or involutional process and affects a significant number of women in the United States.
- Developmental hypomastia is often seen as primary mammary hypoplasia, or as a sequela of thoracic hypoplasia (Poland syndrome) or other chest wall deformity.
- Involutional hypomastia may develop in the postpartum setting and may be exacerbated by breast-feeding or significant weight loss.
- Underfilling saline-filled implants may lead to:
  - Increased deflation rates due to folding or friction subjected to the implant shell, and is not recommended.
  - Wrinkled appearance or *rippling* with the breast in certain positions.
- Aggressive overfilling of saline implants may lead to a more spherical shape and *scalloping* along the implant edge with knuckle-like palpability and unnatural firmness.
- The first generation silicone gel-filled implant (Cronin–Gerow implant):
  - Anatomically shaped with Dacron fixation patches, composed of a thick, smooth silicone elastomer shell that contained a seam, filled with a moderately viscous silicone gel.
  - Had high contracture rates.
- The second-generation silicone implants:
  - Round, without fixation patches, composed of a thinner, seamless shell and filled with a less viscous silicone gel to promote a *natural feel*.
  - Had high rates of diffusion or *bleed* of small silicone molecules into the periprosthetic intracapsular space.
- The third-generation silicone gel-filled implants:
  - Developed in the 1980s, focused on improving the strength and integrity of the shell to reduce bleed and rupture. Despite reducing bleed rates to near zero, the FDA required temporary removal from the American market in 1992.
- The fourth-generation gel-filled implants:
  - Manufactured for market re-introduction.
  - Wider variety of surface textures and implant shapes.
- The *fifth-generation* silicone gel implant:
  - Anatomically-shaped and available with a range of volumes and any of the twelve combinations of low, moderate, and full *height* with low, moderate, full and extra *projection*.

Preoperative considerations

- Preoperative mammography is recommended for patients over 35 years of age or patients of any age with significant risk factors for breast cancer.
- The ideal breast should have the nipple-areola complex (NAC) centered over the most projecting portion of the breast mound ***(Fig. 14.1)***.
- Physical examination should include observation and documentation of:
  - Chest wall deformity or spinal curvature.
  - Asymmetries.
  - Quantity and compliance of the parenchyma and soft tissue envelope.
  - Palpation of all quadrants of the breast and axilla to rule out any dominant masses or suspicious lymph nodes.
  - The soft tissue pinch test: in general, a pinch test result of <2 cm will often indicate a need for subpectoral placement of the implant ***(Figs 14.2–14.4)***.

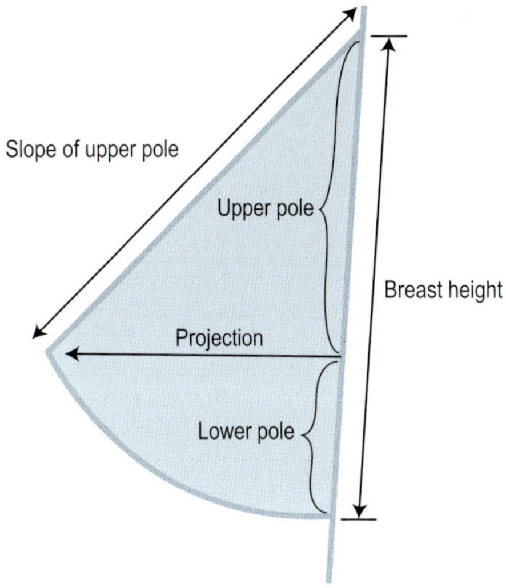

Figure 14.1 The aesthetic breast form is composed of measurable parameters. The resultant breast form desired after surgical augmentation is determined by the dynamic interaction between the character and compliance of the soft tissue envelope; the quality, volume, and consistency of the breast parenchyma; and the dimensions, volume, and characteristics of the breast implant. This form can be attained by the careful planning and surgical performance of a breast augmentation.

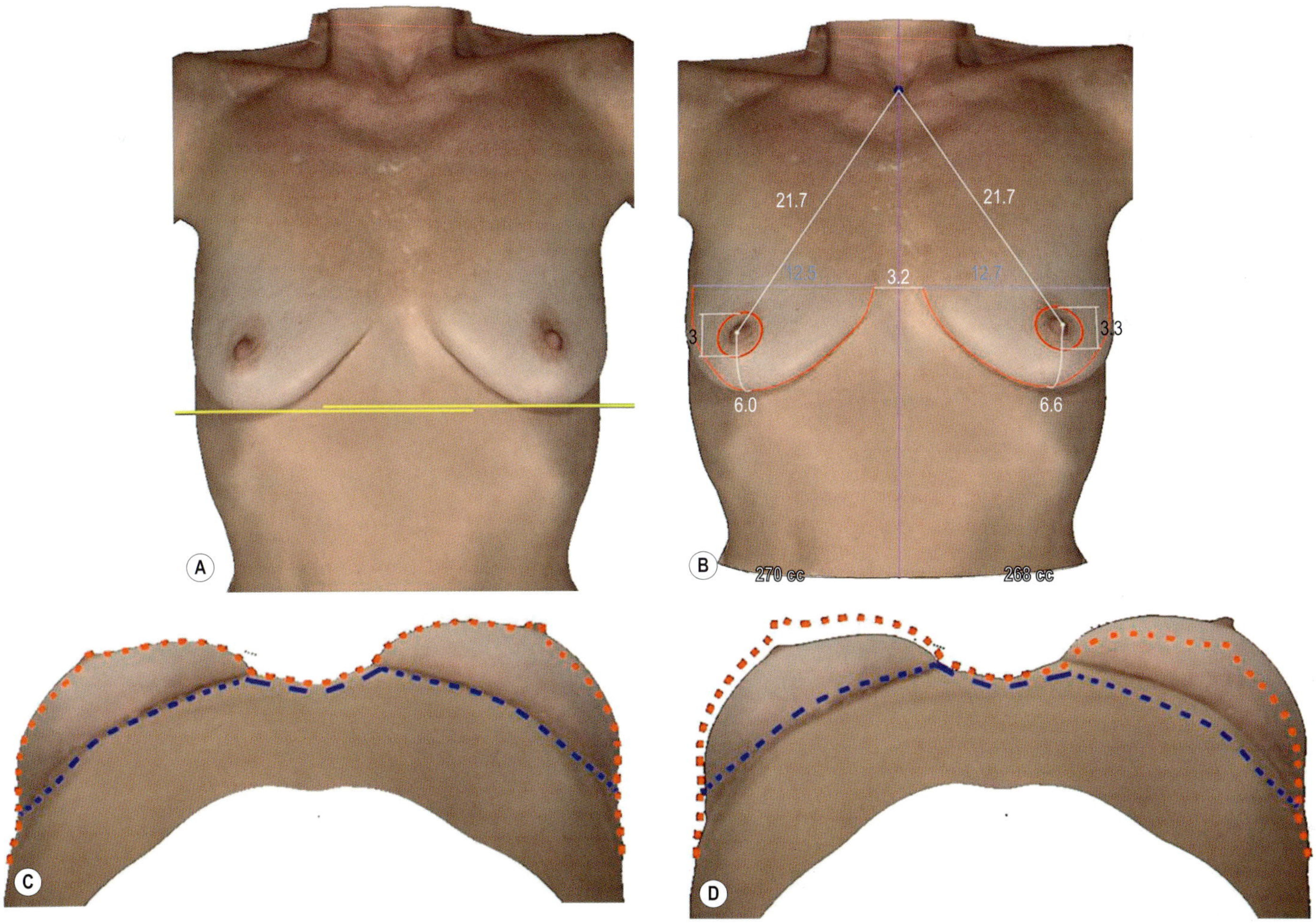

Figure 14.2 Example of hard tissue asymmetry. **(A)** Patient's AP view. **(B)** Patients AP view following automated biodimensional measurements and volume characterization. **(C)** Bird's eye view of patient's chest. Red line delineating the soft tissue envelope, and blue line the chest wall. **(D)** Bird's eye view of patient's chest with superimposed soft tissue and chest wall outlines as mirror images with identification of chest wall asymmetry. Even though the volume is identical, the presenting anatomy is very different.

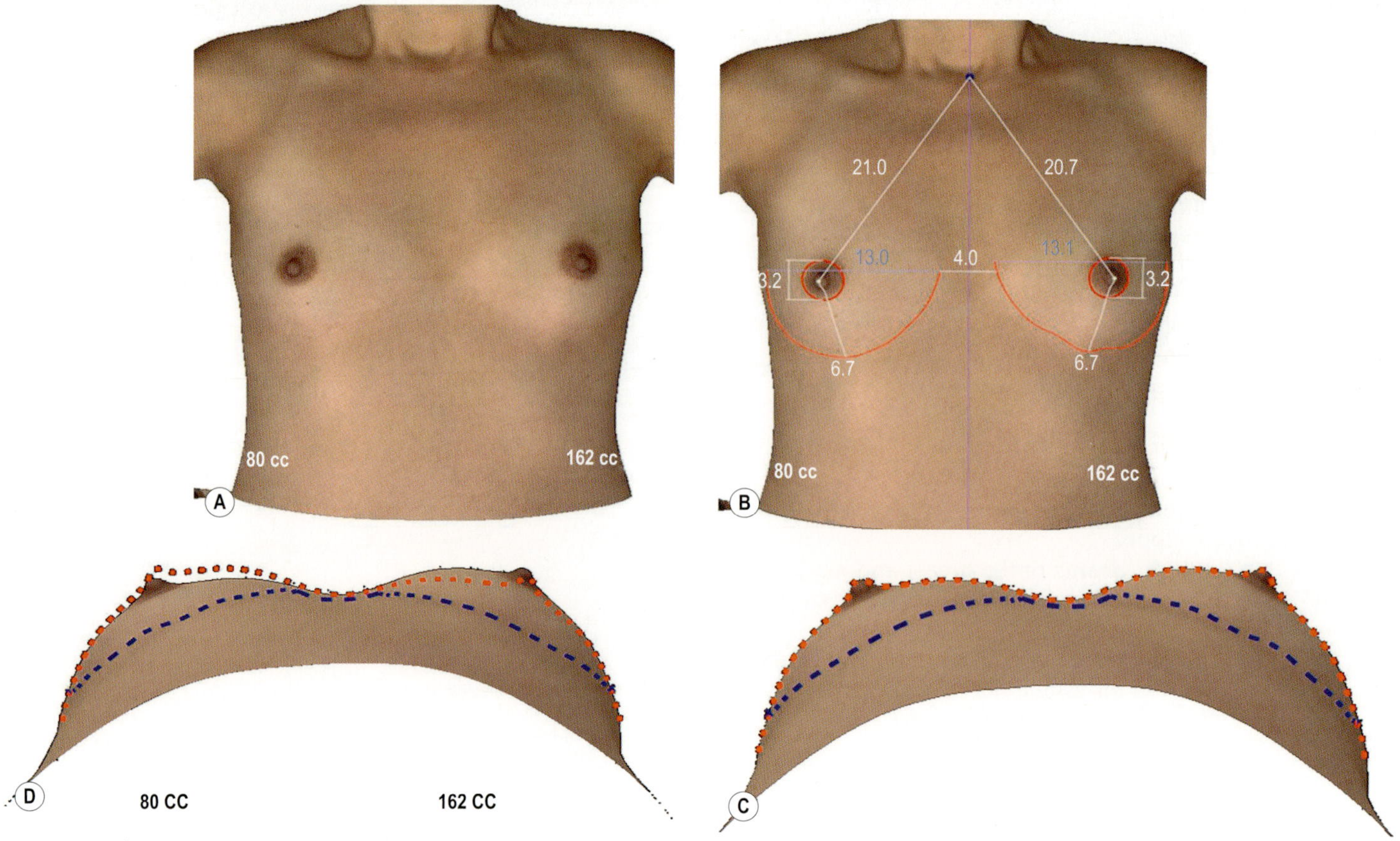

Figure 14.3 Example of soft tissue asymmetry. **(A)** Patient's AP view. **(B)** Patients AP view following automated biodimensional measurements and volume characterization. Bird's eye view of patient's chest. Red line delineating the soft tissue envelope, and blue line the chest wall. **(C,D)** Bird's eye view of patient's chest with superimposed soft tissue and chest wall outlines as mirror images with identification of soft tissue asymmetry.

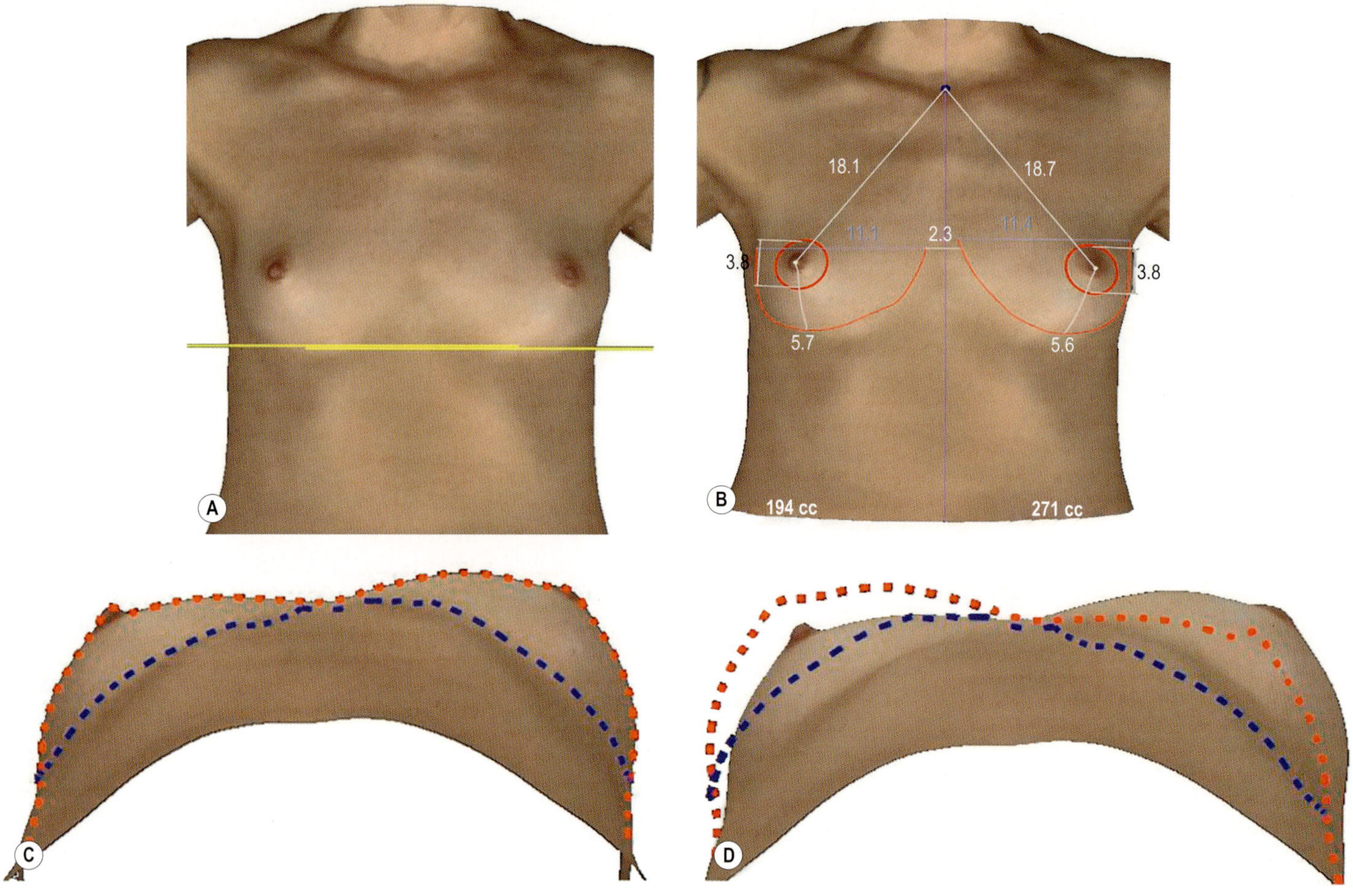

Figure 14.4 Example of hard and soft tissue asymmetry. **(A)** Patient's AP view. **(B)** Patients AP view following automated biodimensional measurements and volume characterization. **(C,D)** Bird's eye view.

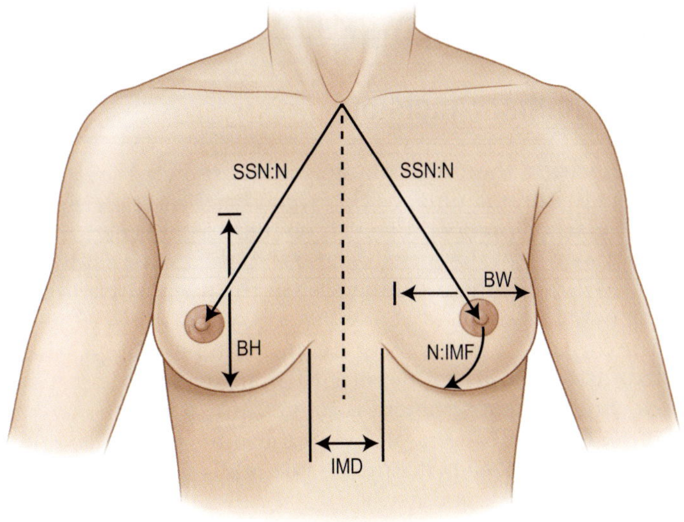

Figure 14.5 Preoperative measures (taken before breast augmentation) include SSN:N (suprasternal notch to nipple); N:IMF (nipple to inframammary fold); BW (breast width); BH (breast height), and IMD (intermammary distance).

- Precise measurements must be taken using the inframammary fold (IMF), the nipple-areola complex, and the suprasternal notch as key landmarks ***(Fig. 14.5)***. Measurements include:
  - Breast width (BW) , the breast height (BH), the distance from the nipple-areola complex to the inframammary fold (N:IMF), the distance from the suprasternal notch to the nipple areola complex (SSN:N), and the intermammary distance (IMD).

Anatomical/technical pearls

- The *inframammary* incision permits complete visualization of either the prepectoral or subglandular pocket and allows precise placement of virtually all implants.
- Smaller incisions (<3 cm) can be used for saline-filled implants, but silicone gel implants often require incisions up to 5.0 cm in length.
- Should be placed in the projected inframammary fold rather than in the existing fold to avoid visibility and widening of the subsequent scar.
- The *periareolar* incision is placed at the areolar-cutaneous juncture and generally heals inconspicuously in light pigmented patients.
- Disadvantages include limited exposure of the surgical field, transection of the parenchymal ducts (which are often colonized with *Staphylococcus epidermidis*), potentially increased risk of nipple sensitivity changes, and visible scarring on the breast mound.
- Should not routinely be used on patients with an areola diameter <40 mm and may not allow introduction of larger gel or enhanced cohesive gel implants.
- The *transaxillary* approach can be performed either bluntly or with the aid of an endoscope.
- Disadvantages include difficulty with parenchymal alterations and the probable need for a second incision on the breast mound for revisionary surgery, and difficulty with precise implant placement.
- *Transumbilical* breast augmentation has the obvious advantage of a single, well-hidden, remote incision.
  - Only saline implants.
  - Hemostasis can be difficult from the remote access port.

Pocket position

- The decision of subglandular/subfascial or subpectoral implant placement depends on implant selection (fill and texture) and tissue thickness ***(Fig. 14.6)***.
- In patients with a pinch test result of >2 cm, the implant can safely be placed in the subfascial plane.
- Textured implants are the preferred implant for subfascial placement due to lower risk of capsular contracture when compared to smooth gel implants.
- When using subpectoral pockets, the origin of the pectoralis major muscle can be divided just above the inframammary fold to allow better projection in the lower pole of the augmented breast and to maintain a natural inframammary fold ***(Fig. 14.7)***. This places the superior portion of the implant in a subpectoral position while the inferior portion is subglandularly located – the so-called "dual-plane".

Implant selection basics

- The base width of the breast is related to the width of the patient's chest and is proportional to the overall body habitus. It is imperative that this dimension is respected during augmentation in order to maintain the normal anatomical landmarks such as the lateral breast fold in the anterior axillary line and the intermammary distance (IMD).
- Generally, the surgeon should select an implant that is slightly less wide than the existing breast.
- The choice between textured and smooth-walled implants is based primarily on minimizing capsular contracture:
  - For subpectoral augmentation, either implant can probably be used with comparable results. When the device is placed in the subfascial pocket, a textured implant is preferred to minimize capsular contracture. ***(Fig. 14.8)***.
- The typical round shaped breast implant has its greatest projection centrally with the remainder of the volume distributed evenly along the base of the implant. While anatomically shaped breast implants have a flatter upper

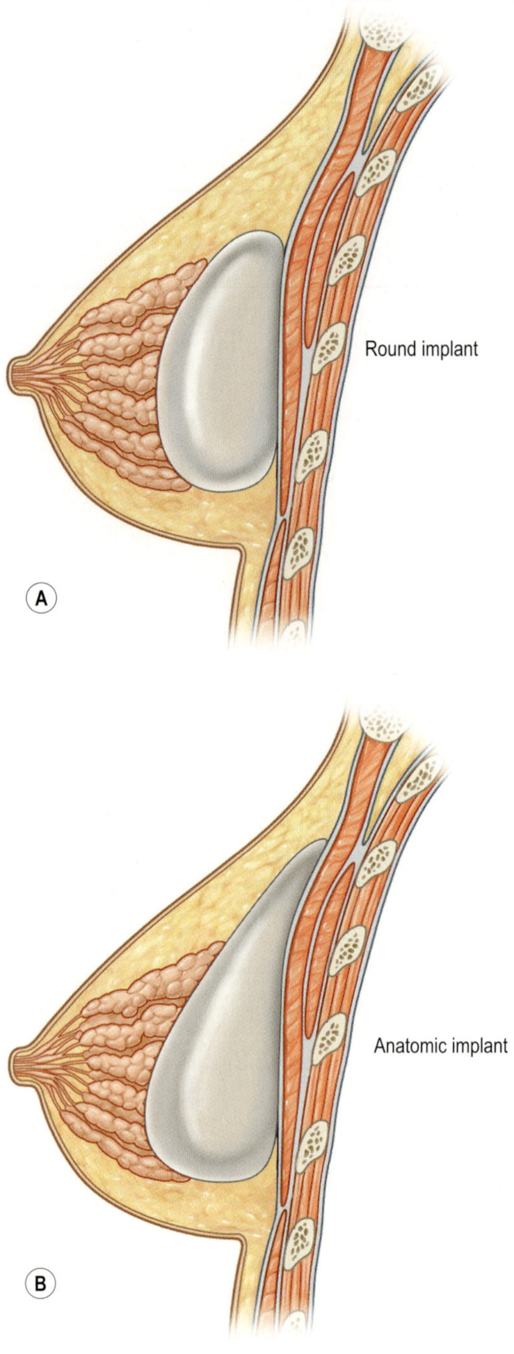

Figure 14.6 (A,B) When ample soft tissue is present, implants may be placed in the subglandular position or subfascial position. When there is soft tissue inadequacy, the subpectoral position is generally preferable.

pole with the majority of the volume and projection in the lower pole ***(Fig. 14.9)***.

- The anatomically shaped implant of a given base width and volume will produce less upper pole convexity than a round implant of the same base width and volume ***(Fig. 14.10)***. This characteristic of anatomically shaped implants can be extremely useful when the patient desires a significant volume augmentation but has a relatively narrow breast width.

Operative techniques

Inframammary incision

- The incision should be placed in the predicted location of the new inframammary fold which has been determined and marked preoperatively. It should be designed with the majority of the incision lateral to the breast midline as this will place the resulting scar in the deepest portion of the new IMF.
- The incision is made along the proposed markings, and the dissection is continued with an insulated electrocautery instrument through Scarpa fascia.
- If the implant is to be placed in the subfascial pocket, the dissection proceeds below the pectoralis fascia but above the pectoralis major fascia.
- For smooth-walled implants, a larger pocket is dissected to allow mobility of the implant.
- For anatomic implants, the pocket is precisely dissected to snugly accommodate the implant.
- Care should be taken to preserve the lateral intercostal cutaneous nerves, especially the fourth intercostal, which contains the primary sensory innervations of the nipple-areola complex.
- If a subpectoral pocket is chosen, the dissection is initially carried out laterally to identify the lateral border of the pectoralis major muscle. The muscle edge can be lifted by forceps to allow easy entry into the submusculofascial plane.
- The inferior origin of the pectoralis major is released from lateral to medial at the level of the inframammary fold and continues medially to the sternal border.
- Exact implant "sizers" (gel or saline) are used when available to evaluate the pockets and resultant breast form.
- After the sizers are in place, the patient is placed in a 90° upright position and evaluated from various perspectives. Any asymmetry or under-dissected areas are marked, and the patient is placed back in the supine position.
- Once adequate hemostasis is obtained and pocket dimensions are finalized, the pocket is irrigated with an antibiotic-containing solution, and the implants are carefully placed by a minimal-touch technique.
- The final results are assessed, again with the patient in a sitting position, and a multilayer closure is performed.

Periareolar incision

- The periareolar incision is placed along the inferior portion of the areolar-cutaneous juncture from the 3-o'clock and 9-o'clock positions.
- After the incision is made, the wound edges are elevated directly up from the chest wall with an opposing pair of small sharp retractors.
- An insulated electrocautery unit is used to dissect straight down through the breast parenchyma to the

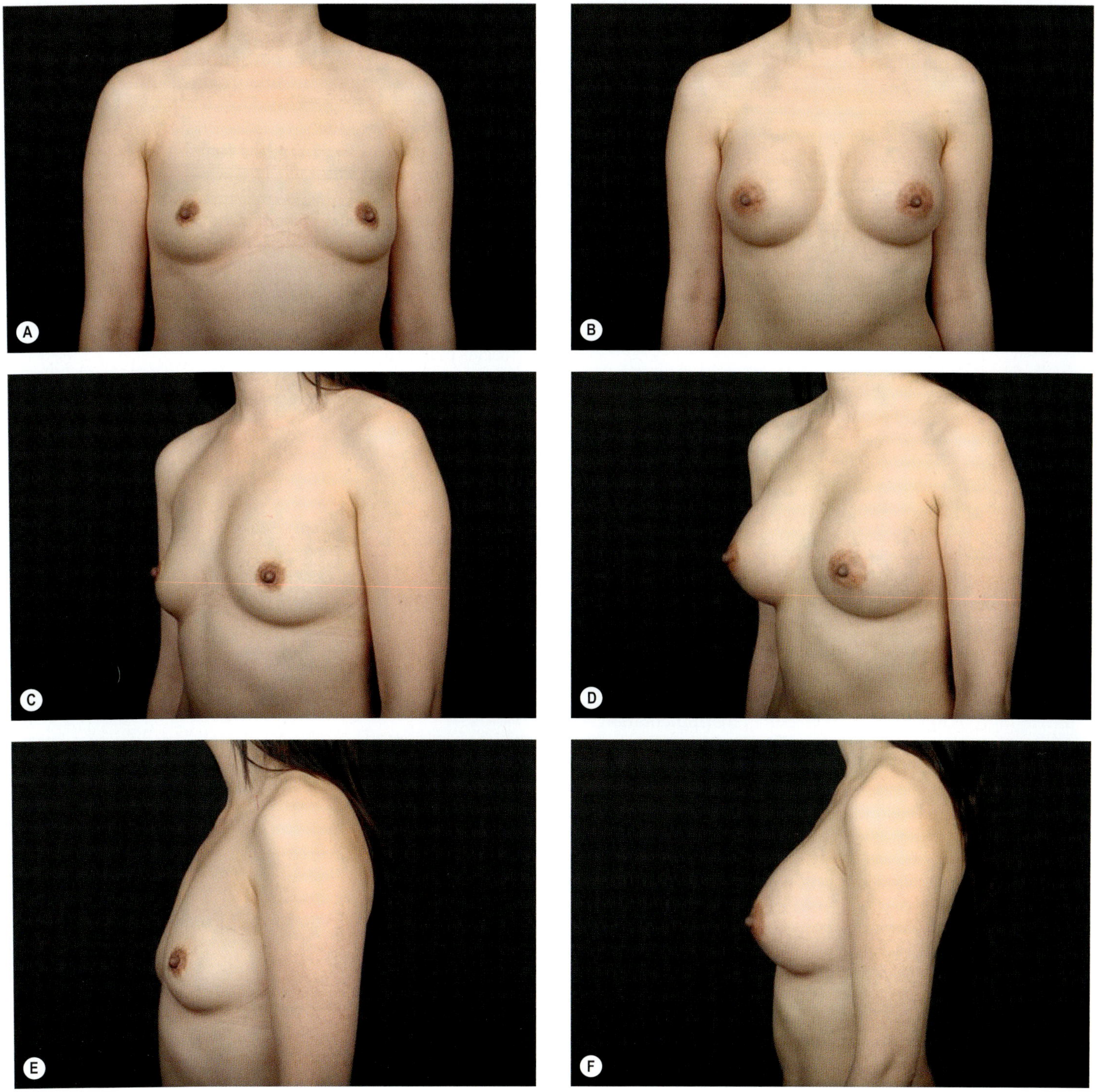

Figure 14.7 **(A–F)** Preoperative and postoperative views of a 36-year-old female with Style 20 implants at 12 months: R, 400 cc; L, 400 cc in a subpectoral position.

pectoralis major fascia. The dissection is the same as described through the inframammary incision.

- If the inferior pole of the breast is constricted (tuberous breast deformity), radial scoring of the gland in the inferior pole can allow proper redraping of the soft tissue over the implant to correct the deformity.
- The gland must be precisely reapproximated and closed with several layers of interrupted absorbable sutures to prevent distortion of the nipple-areola complex.

Transaxillary incision (Video 14.1; Video 14.2)

Video 14.1

Video 14.2

- This procedure can be performed either bluntly using the Montgomery dissector, or using an endoscope for precise visualization, and dissection of the implant pocket.
- To locate and mark the incision, the patient's arm is placed in complete adduction and the most anterior aspect of the axilla is marked. The incision should not extend beyond this line. The arm is then abducted

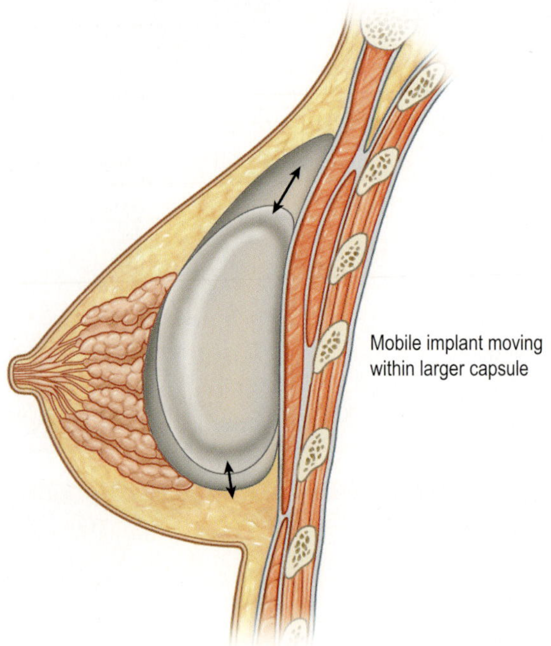

Figure 14.8 Large pocket for smooth-surfaced implants to allow tissue redraping and encourage implant mobility to minimize capsule contracture which is different for textured devices (including anatomic), where a precise pocket is created that is either the same or slightly larger than the base and height of the implant to help maintain implant position.

approximately 45°, and a prominent axillary crease is identified. Any fold may be used, but preference is given to one high in the axilla, which aids in instrumentation during the procedure. For saline-filled implants, the incision should generally be 2.5–3.5 cm. Silicone implants require larger incisions.

- The incision is made, and small sharp retractors are used to elevate the medial aspect of the incision. Superficial subcutaneous dissection to the lateral border of the pectoralis major prevents injury to the intercostobrachial nerve.
- The fascia of the pectoralis major muscle is visualized at the lateral edge of the muscle, and the dissection is carried deep to this for a subfascial placement or deep to the muscle for subpectoral placement.
- For an endoscopically assisted augmentation, the endoscope is passed into the transaxillary tunnel, and the subpectoral space is seen under direct vision. This allows a more controlled release of the pectoralis major origin with a long insulated electrocautery instrument.
- The remaining steps follow those above. On closure, the pectoralis muscle fascia is repaired with a single absorbable suture, and the incision is closed in one or two layers.

Transumbilical

- While the markings are similar to those for a standard inframammary fold approach, an additional mark is made with the patient supine: a line is drawn from the umbilicus to the medial border of the areola bilaterally.
- An incision is made within the umbilicus, large enough to easily accommodate an index finger.
- An endotube with a blunt obturator is passed just above the rectus fascia along the line from the umbilicus to the areola.
- Constantly palpate the progress of the obturator with the other hand, always keeping the force up and away from the abdominal and thoracic cavities.
- The endotube is advanced over the costal margin. For subglandular implant placement, the force applied to the endotube is directed upward at the inframammary fold to prevent the obturator from slipping beneath the pectoralis major. The tunnel ends just cephalad to the nipple. Subpectoral positioning is possible by careful technique with use of special instruments to enter the fascial plane high laterally.
- The obturator is then removed, and an endoscope may be used to verify correct pocket identification.
- An expander is rolled up and placed within the incision and "milked" up the tunnel by manual external pressure. The expander is filled with saline to 150% of the final volume of the implant. Pocket adjustments can be made manually during filling.
- When the expansion is complete, the expander is drained and removed from the pocket by traction on the fill tube. The implant is placed and filled in exactly the same manner as the expander.
- The incision is closed with a single layer of absorbable suture. An abdominal binder is used for compression on the abdominal tunnels.

Postoperative considerations

- If smooth (non-textured) implants were used, initiation of implant mobility exercises is recommended at first follow-up visit.
- If the patient is at risk for superior implant displacement, a circumferential elastic strap may be used to apply continuous downward pressure during the early postoperative period.
- Patients are usually able to return to work a few days after surgery, but are not permitted to resume rigorous exercise for 2–3 weeks. Additional follow-up visits are scheduled at 4–6 weeks, 3 months, and 1 year.

Complications and outcomes

- Alterations of nipple sensitivity after augmentation are thought to result from traction injury, bruising, or transection of the lateral intercostal cutaneous nerves.
- Periprosthetic seroma fluid is usually resorbed by the soft tissues within the first week of surgery, and use of topical antibiotics intraoperatively has been shown to decrease the rates.
- Hematoma after breast augmentation has several deleterious effects in both the early and late postoperative period including pain, blood loss, disfigurement, and capsular contracture.

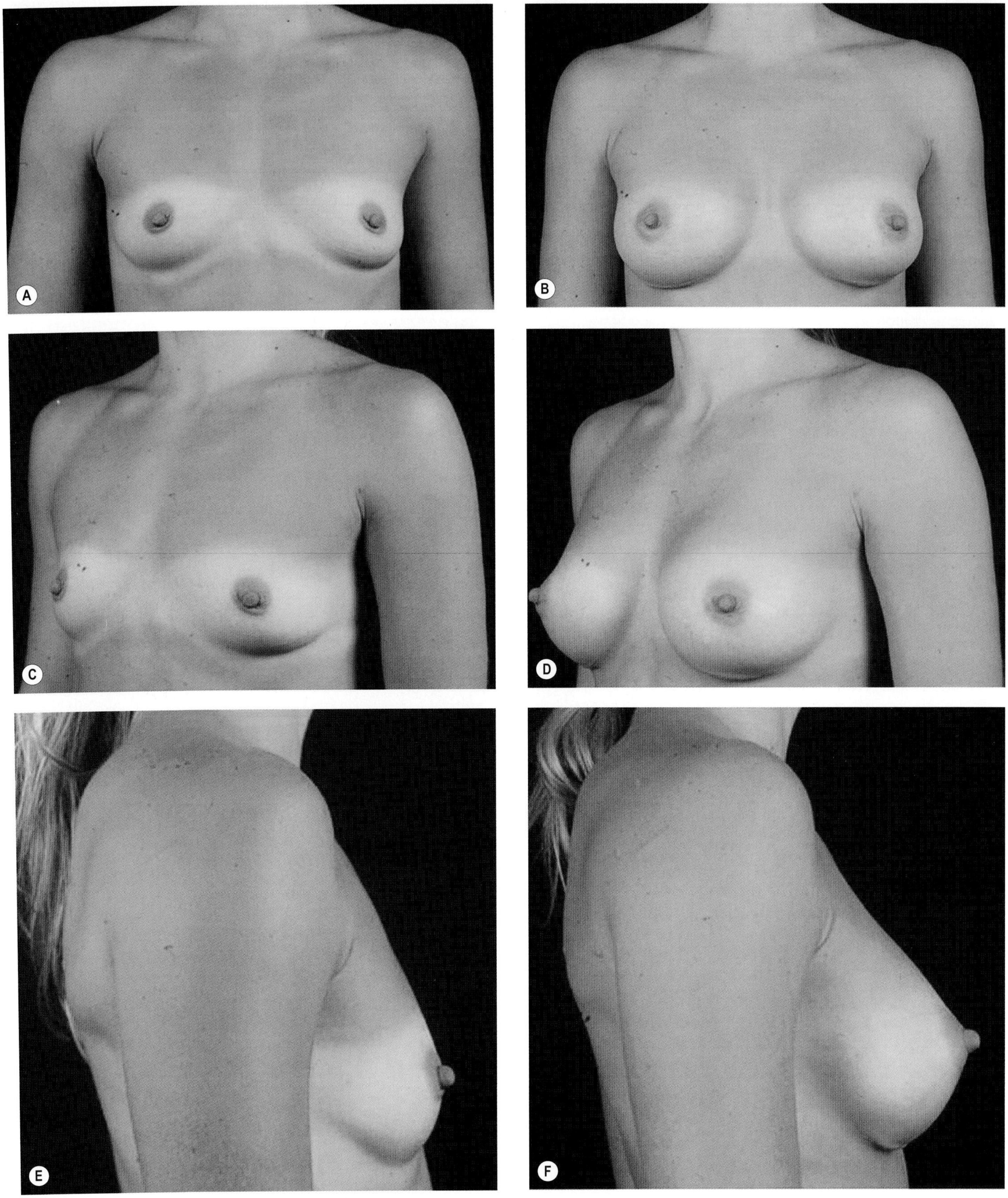

Figure 14.9 (A–F) Preoperative and postoperative views of a 29-year-old female with CPG 332 implants at 12 months: R, 350 cc; L, 350 cc in a subpectoral position.

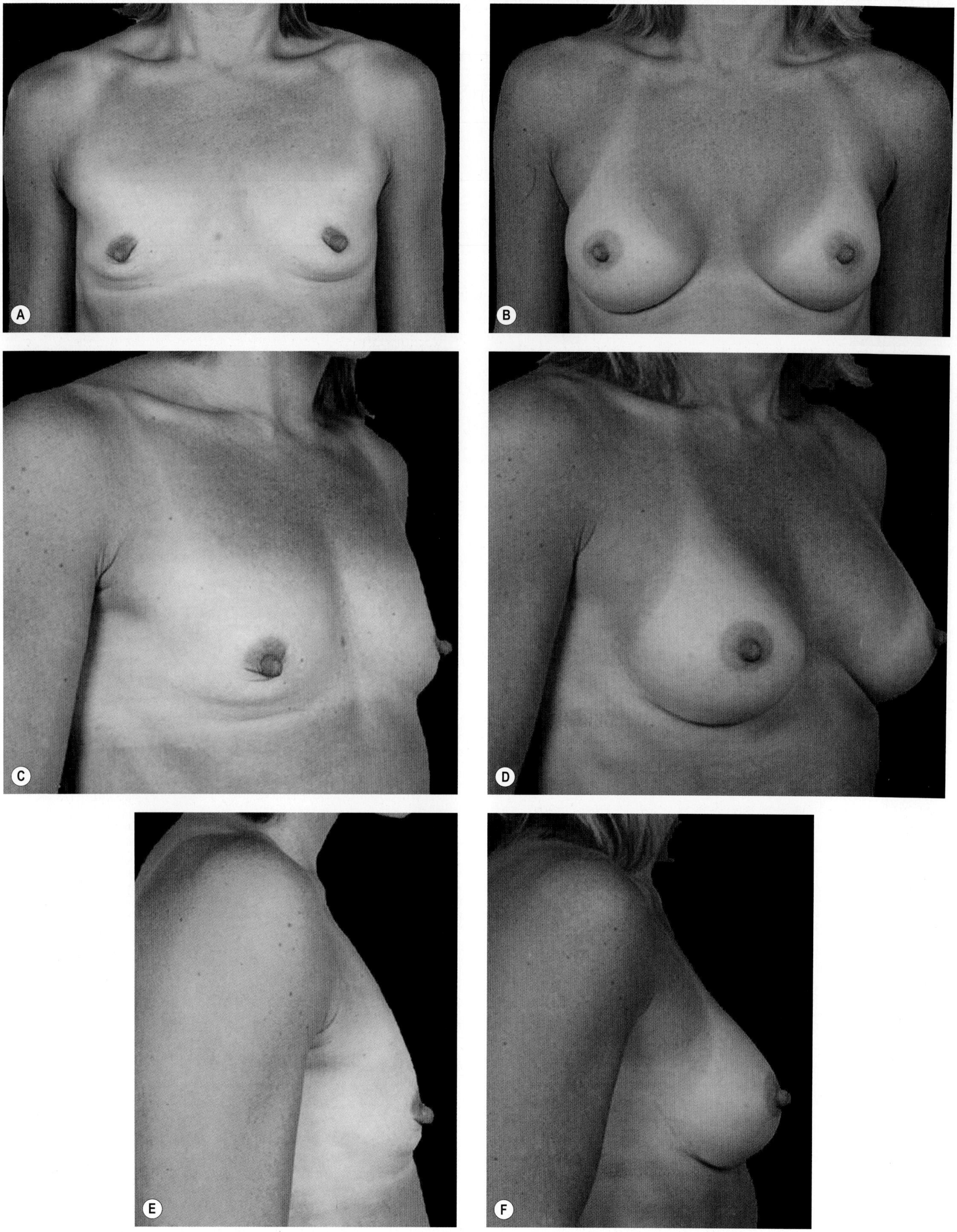

Figure 14.10 (A–F) Preoperative and postoperative views of a 33-year-old female with Style 410 MM implants at 12 months: R, 280 cc; L, 245 cc in a subpectoral position.

Table 14.1 The grades of capsular contracture are divided into the following four types

Grade	Description
I	Capsular contracture of the augmented breast feels as soft as an unoperated breast
II	Capsular contracture is minimal. The breast is less soft than an unoperated breast. The implant can be palpated but is not visible
III	Capsular contracture is moderate. The breast is firmer. The implant can be palpated easily and may be distorted or visible
IV	Capsular contracture is severe. The breast is hard, tender, and painful, with significant distortion present. The capsule thickness is not directly proportional to palpable firmness, although some relationship may exist

Reproduced with permission from Spear SL, Baker JL Jr. Classification of capsular contracture after prosthetic breast reconstruction. *Plast Reconstr Surg.* 1995;96(5):1119–1124.

- Immediate evacuation of all hematomas is recommended.
- Postoperative wound infection may present with a spectrum of severity ranging from a mild cellulitis of the breast skin to a purulent periprosthetic space infection. *Staphylococcus epidermidis* is the most frequently identified pathogen in postoperative wound infections.
- Most infections will respond to oral or intravenous antibiotics if therapy is initiated very early in the course of the infection.
- If the infection persists or progresses, then the implant should be removed and the wound should be allowed to heal over a drain or in severe cases by secondary intention.
- Once the infection has totally cleared, a secondary augmentation and scar revision should be planned in 6–12 months.
- Mondor's disease is a superficial thrombophlebitis of the breast that may occur in up to 1–2% of augmentation patients.
- Usually affects the veins along the inferior aspect of the breast and occurs most frequently with the inframammary approach.
- Self-limiting process that usually resolves with warm compresses over a period of several weeks.
- Clinically significant periprosthetic capsular contracture is characterized by excessive scar formation that leads to firmness, distortion, and displacement of the breast implant.
- Histological examination reveals circumferential linear fibrosis, which is especially severe when formed in response to smooth shell implants.
- In 1975, Baker proposed a clinical classification system of capsular contracture after augmentation that is still commonly used to describe periprosthetic contractures (Table 14.1).
- Risk factors for capsular contracture: periprosthetic hematoma, seroma, silicone gel bleed, other foreign body particles such as glove powder, lint, or dust, and infectious etiologies (subclinical infection and biofilm).
- Strategies to prevent capsular contracture: the creation of a large implant pocket, and maintenance of this oversized pocket with implant displacement exercises; the use of textured implants; meticulous hemostasis and sterility.
- Treatment of established capsular contractures usually requires operative intervention.
- Very thick fibrous capsules, or those heavily calcified containing silicone granulomas often require either a partial or complete capsulectomy
- Any defect in the silicone elastomer shell of a saline-filled breast implant will ultimately result in *deflation* of the implant. The saline filling material leaks out of the implant and is harmlessly absorbed by the surrounding tissues.
- Magnetic resonance imaging (MRI) of the breast is considered the state-of-the-art technique for evaluating breast implant integrity.
- For gel-filled implants, the recommendation is initial MRI 3 years after the augmentation, followed by imaging every 2 years.
- Modern fourth generation silicone gel is substantially more cohesive than the second- and third-generation gel, and less likely to leak into the surrounding tissues, even when the implant shell is ruptured.

Further reading

Adams WP Jr, Rios JL, Smith SJ. Enhancing patient outcomes in aesthetic and reconstructive breast surgery using triple antibiotic breast irrigation: six-year prospective clinical study. *Plast Reconstr Surg.* 2006;117(1):30–36.

The authors show the clinical importance of the use of triple antibiotic breast irrigation. This study shows the lower incidence of capsular contracture compared with other published reports, and its clinical efficacy supports previously published in vitro studies. Application of triple antibiotic irrigation is recommended for all aesthetic and reconstructive breast procedures and is cost-effective.

Bengtson BP, Van Natta BW, Murphy DK, et al. Style 410 highly cohesive silicone breast implant core study results at 3 years. *Plast Reconstr Surg.* 2007;120 (7 Suppl 1):40S–48S.

Cunningham B. The Mentor study on contour profile gel silicone MemoryGel breast implants. *Plast Reconstr Surg.* 2007;120(7 Suppl 1):33S–39S.

Cunningham B, McCue J. Safety and effectiveness of Mentor's MemoryGel implants at 6 years. *Aesthet Plast Surg.* 2009;33(3):440–444.

The authors update on the post-approval study for the Mentor Corporation. The study shows that Mentor MemoryGel silicone breast implants represent a safe and effective choice for women seeking breast augmentation or breast reconstruction following mastectomy.

Gabriel SE, O'Fallon WM, Kurland LT, et al. Risk of connective-tissue diseases and other disorders after breast implantation. *N Engl J Med.* 1994;330(24):1697–1702.

The authors conducted a population-based, retrospective study to examine the risk of a variety of connective-tissue diseases and other disorders after breast implantation. No association between breast implants and the connective-tissue diseases and other disorders that were studied was found.

Magnusson M, Hoglund P, Johansson K, et al. Pentoxifylline and vitamin E treatment for prevention of radiation-induced side-effects in women with breast cancer: a phase two, double-blind, placebo-controlled randomised clinical trial (Ptx-5). *Eur J Cancer.* 2009;45(14):2488–2495.

Nelson N. Institute of Medicine finds no link between breast implants and disease. *J Natl Cancer Inst.* 1999;91(14):1191.

Spear SL, Baker JL Jr. Classification of capsular contracture after prosthetic breast reconstruction. *Plast Reconstr Surg.* 1995;96(5):1119–1124.

Spear SL, Murphy DK, Slicton A, et al. Inamed silicone breast implant core study results at 6 years. *Plast Reconstr Surg.* 2007;120(7 Suppl 1):8S–18S.

The authors update on the post-approval study for Allergan Corporation. The study demonstrates the safety and effectiveness of Natrelle (formerly Inamed) silicone-filled breast implants through 6 years, including a low rupture rate and high satisfaction rate.

Tebbetts JB. Dual plane breast augmentation: optimizing implant-soft-tissue relationships in a wide range of breast types. *Plast Reconstr Surg.* 2001;107(5):1255–1272.

This article describes specific indications and techniques for a dual plane approach to breast augmentation. Indications, operative techniques, results, and complications for this series of patients are presented. Dual plane augmentation mammaplasty adjusts implant and tissue relationships to ensure adequate soft tissue coverage, while optimizing implant soft tissue dynamics to offer increased benefits and fewer tradeoffs compared with a single pocket location in a wide range of breast types.

Chapter 15

Mastopexy

This chapter was created using content from Neligan & Grotting, Plastic Surgery 3rd edition, Volume 5, Breast, Chapter 1, Anatomy for plastic surgery of the breast, Jorge I. de la Torre and Michael R. Davis, Chapter 7, Mastopexy, Kent K. Higdon and James C. Grotting.

SYNOPSIS

- Breast ptosis is a common problem caused by several different factors: pregnancy, weight changes, aging, delayed effect of breast implants and developmental deformities.
- Mastopexy and augmentation-mastopexy techniques are varied and can be applied to different breast shape deformities.
- Mastopexy techniques can be periareolar, vertical or based on the inverted-T techniques, as well as being performed in some instances by liposuction alone.
- Preoperative deflation prior to mastopexy or augmentation-mastopexy is a safe and effective technique that offers the patient and surgeon many benefits.

Brief introduction

- Mastopexy is a parenchymal reshaping that may or may not require a small parenchymal reduction, whereas reduction mammaplasties always require parenchymal reduction.
- The difference between mastopexy and reduction mammoplasty, is whether the patient truly exhibits symptoms of macromastia.
- Typically, the ptotic breast has a paucity of breast parenchyma in relation to a lax, excessive skin envelope while the cardinal finding of the hypertrophic breasts seen in cases of macromastia and gigantomastia is a predominance of parenchyma without skin excess.
- The pathophysiology of breast ptosis is the result of the combination of expansion and aging, or separately as a result of a congenital deformity.
- Breast ptosis in its various degrees is defined by its anatomic relationship to the inframammary fold (IMF). In 1976, Regnault described degrees of breast ptosis ***(Fig. 15.1)***.
  - Grade I ptosis (mild): the nipple is within 1 cm of the IMF, and above the lower pole of the breast.
  - Grade II (moderate): the nipple is 1–3 cm below the IMF, but still above the lower pole of the breast.
  - Grade III (severe): the nipple is more than 3 cm below the IMF and is below the lower breast contour.
  - Grade IV (psuedoptosis): the nipple rests above the IMF but the majority of breast parenchyma is below it, giving the appearance of ptosis.
- An additional caveat to the Regnault classification was submitted by Brink, which takes into account other causes of the ptotic breast, such as parenchymal maldistribution, and posits an algorithm by which they can be surgically addressed (Table 15.1, ***Fig. 15.2***).

Preoperative considerations

- One of the most helpful questions that can be posed to a patient is "can you make your breasts look the way you want them to in a bra?"
  - If the answer is yes, then perhaps a mastopexy alone is the best recommendation.
  - If the answer is no, and the patient relies on adding volume by stuffing or padding, then adding an implant may be necessary.

Table 15.1 Procedural specifics for forms of breast ptosis

	Inframammary fold position	Parenchymal position	Nipple–areola position	Nipple to fold distance	Clavicle to nipple distance	Clavicle to fold distance
True ptosis	Fixed normal	Fixed rotated	Low downward pointing	Unchanged normal	Elongated	Unchanged normal
Glandular ptosis						
Common	Mobile descended	Mobile descended	Low forward pointing	Elongated	Elongated	Elongated
Uncommon	Fixed normal	Mobile descended	Low relative to fold	Elongated	Normal to elongated	Unchanged
	Normal					Normal
Parenchymal maldistribution	Fixed high	Fixed high	Normal downward pointing	Short	Normal	Short
Pseudoptosis[a]	Variable, usually low[a]	Mobile re-descended	Surgically fixed	Elongated	Surgically fixed	Variable, usually elongated[a]

[a]Pseudoptosis is most common after corrective procedures for glandular ptosis where the fold has descended preoperatively. (From Brink RR. Management of true ptosis of the breast. *Plast Reconstr Surg.* 1993;91:657–662.)

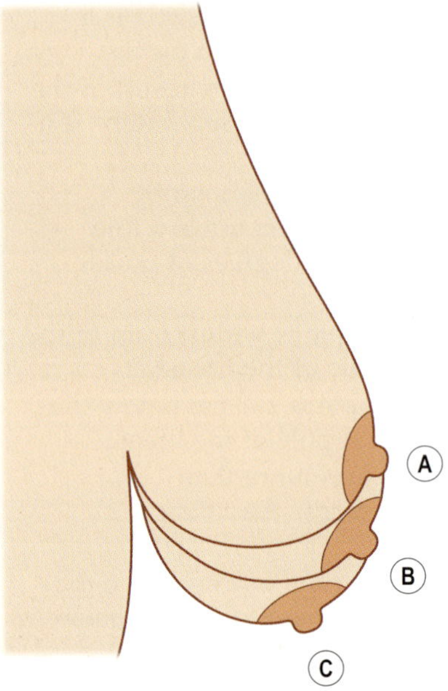

Figure 15.1 Breast ptosis classification as described by Regnault. **(A)** Minimal ptosis: the nipple is at the level of or just inferior to the inframammary crease. **(B)** Moderate ptosis: the nipple is 1–3 cm below the inframammary crease. **(C)** Severe ptosis: the nipple is >3 cm below the inframammary crease. (Redrawn from Georgiade GS, Georgiade NG, Riefkohl R. Esthetic breast surgery: In: McCarthy JG, ed. *Plastic surgery.* Philadelphia: WB Saunders; 1991:3839.)

- The plastic surgeon must take into account the degree of skin laxity, the excess amount of skin in relation to the parenchyma, the position or malposition of the parenchyma, and degree of nipple-areolar complex elevation anticipated.
- Measurements are a key component to the diagnosis and treatment of the patient with breast ptosis. These measurements offer guidelines for altering the breast, which must be individualized, based on proportionality, variances in chest wall anatomy, posture and patient preference. Important measurements and their reported statistical standards ***(Fig. 15.3)*** include:
  - The sternal notch to nipple distance: 19–21 cm.
  - The nipple to IMF distance: 5–7 cm.
  - Nipple to midline distance: 9–11 cm.
  - The breast base diameter.
  - The degree of ptosis: based on Regnault Classification.
- The majority of patients presenting for mastopexy procedures typically fall into three categories. The analysis of the quality and amount of skin in relation to the mass and anatomic distribution of the breast parenchyma usually dictates which procedure is necessary.
  - Patients who indeed would benefit from mastopexy. Normal volume of breast parenchyma and a minimal-to-moderate excess of skin that is of good quality.
  - Patients who need an augmentation with mastopexy. Minimal glandular mass and breast ptosis.
  - Patients who need a formal reduction mammaplasty. Overabundance of parenchyma and ptosis.
- Any history of breast changes/masses, nipple-areolar changes or discharge, mammography, previous breast surgery, pregnancies and breast-feeding, radiation therapy to the chest or breast, and personal or family history of breast cancer must be explored with the patient in detail.
- Most agree that patients over 35 years of age should obtain a recent mammogram, unless a normal one has been documented in the year prior, before proceeding with surgery.

Anatomical/technical pearls

- Knowledge of the breast anatomy is critical for optimizing outcomes following mastopexy. ***(Figs 15.4–15.11)***.

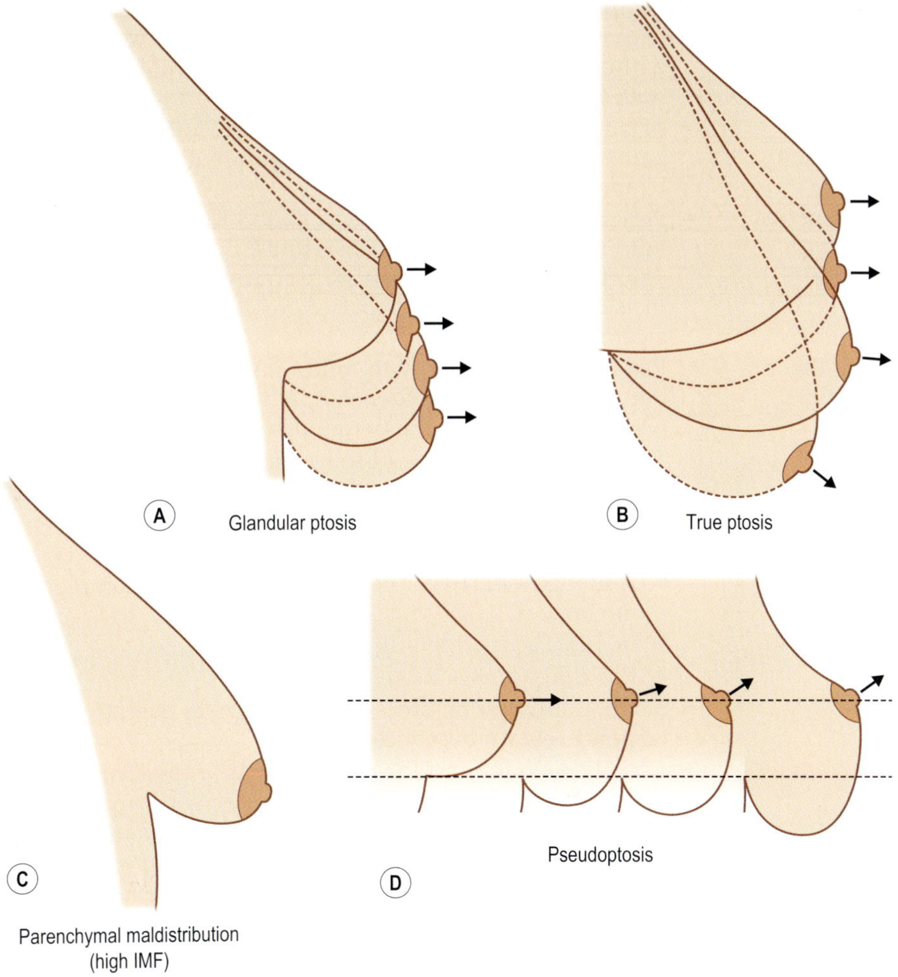

Figure 15.2 (A–D) Different types of breast ptosis. IMF, inframammary fold. (Redrawn after Brink RR. Management of true ptosis of the breast. *Plast Reconstr Surg.* 1993;91:657–662.)

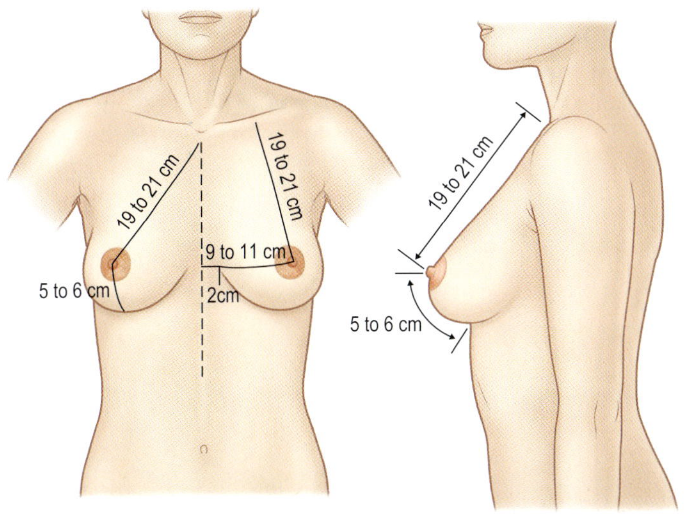

Figure 15.3 Statistical standards for the dimensions of the breast.

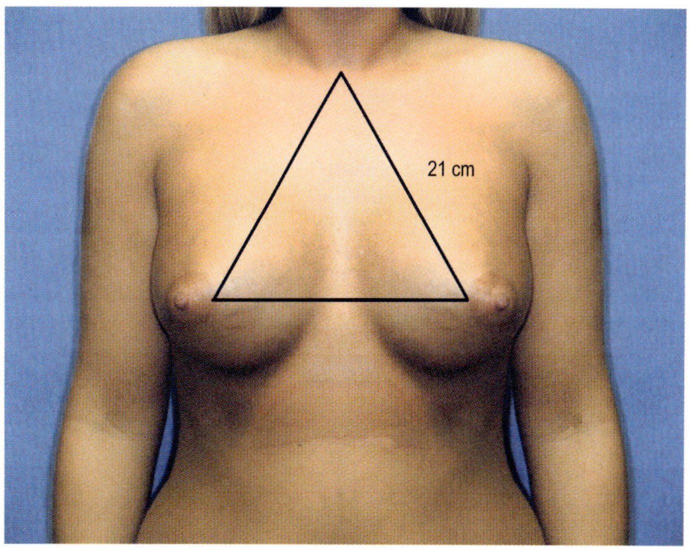

Figure 15.4 AP image: ideal breast dimensions demonstrating symmetry and projection.

- The vascular supply to the breast and nipple-areolar complex is rich and redundant and includes contributions from the internal mammary perforator, lateral thoracic perforators, and the intercostal perforators from both the anterolateral and anteromedial origins.
- Branches of the lateral division of the fourth intercostal nerve provide the primary innervation of the nipple. Contributions from the third and fifth anterior cutaneous intercostals, as well as the fifth lateral cutaneous intercostals, may also provide some sensation of the nipple.
- Cooper's ligaments run from the pectoralis muscular fascia, through breast parenchyma, and insert into the dermis ***(Fig. 15.12)***. Parenchymal changes with aging, weight changes in the obese, and pregnancy, are accompanied by specific alterations in the integrity of Cooper's ligaments, as well as the breast's fascial components, and the overlying skin. The breast parenchyma, once held in place on the chest wall by and within these structures, becomes mobile and descends with the constant pull of gravity.
- Mastopexy techniques are often described by the scar pattern from the skin reduction: periareolar, vertical, J or L, and inverted-T.
- Periareolar techniques are best suited for patients with mild to moderate breast ptosis and in whom the parenchyma is adequate from a volume standpoint. Incisions range from a superior crescent of excised skin to a complete donut.
- Patients who present with mild to moderate breast ptosis, but with inadequate parenchymal volume can be treated with an implant via the periareolar technique.
- The greatest advantage of the periareolar technique is that the incision is camouflaged in the aesthetic transition from breast skin to the skin of the nipple-areola.
- Disadvantages of periareolar techniques include:
  - A limited degree of cephalic nipple-areolar complex movement.
  - Possible scar widening.
  - Possible decreased breast projection.
- Small, mildly ptotic breasts with adequate parenchyma respond best to these techniques.
- Excising skin around the nipple-areola at the same operative setting elevates the nipple-areolar complex to a more aesthetic location and completes the periareolar mastopexy. Usually, the amount of lift obtained is limited to 1–2 cm.
- In an effort to limit complications associated with periareolar mastopexy techniques, Spear et al. designed a series of rules to follow.
  - Rule 1: $D_{outside} \leq D_{original} + (D_{original} - D_{inside})$. The amount of non-pigmented skin excised should be less than the amount of pigmented skin excised. In doing so, there will be no undue tension on the new areola that could cause subsequent widening. The distance from the edge of the areola to the outer diameter located on the normal breast skin should roughly equal the distance to the inner diameter, which should be located within the areola.
  - Rule 2: $D_{outside} < 2\times D_{inside}$. The design of the outside diameter should be no more than two times the inside

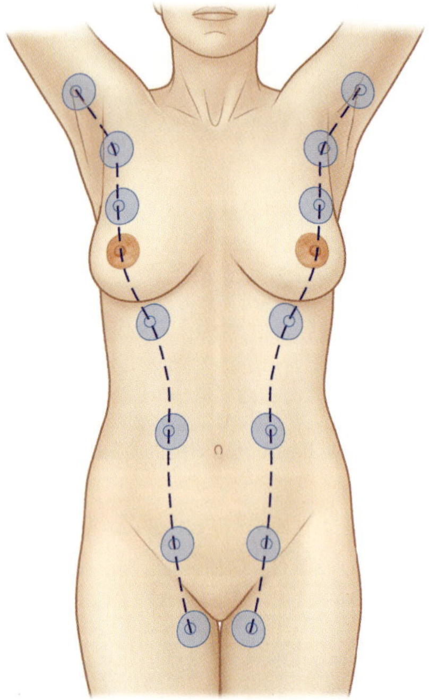

Figure 15.5 The milk lines. (Reproduced with permission from Standring S, ed. *Gray's anatomy.* 40th ed. London: Churchill Livingstone; 2008.)

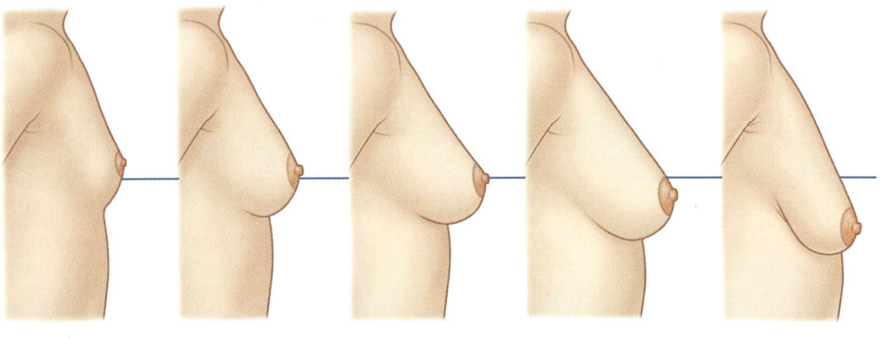

Figure 15.6 Stages in breast development. Pre-and post-pubertal development and structure of the female breast, demonstrating changes in the contour of the breast. (Reproduced with permission from Standring S, ed. *Gray's anatomy.* 40th ed. London: Churchill Livingstone; 2008.)

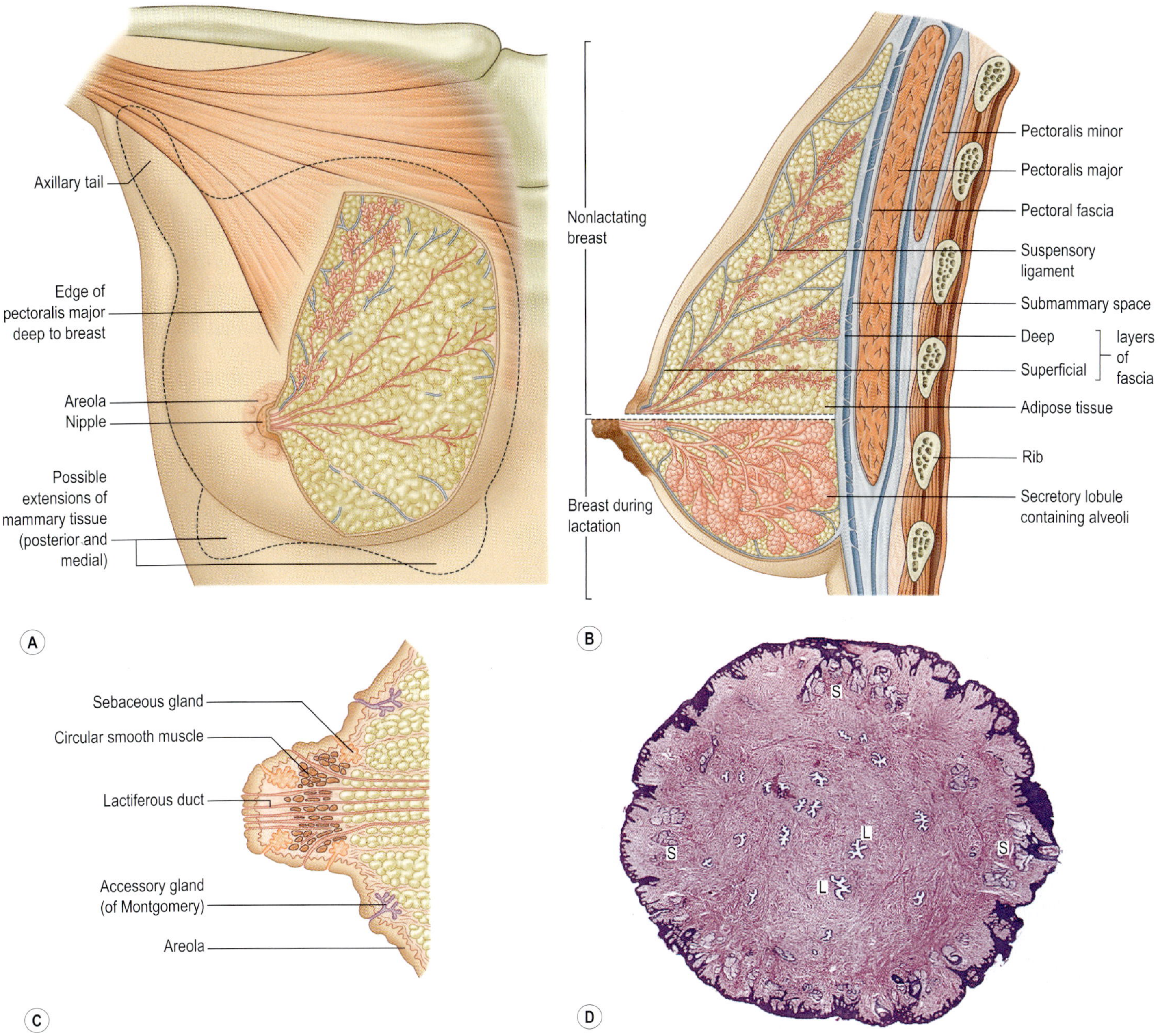

Figure 15.7 (A) Structure of the breast. **(B)** Changes in the breast during lactation. **(C)** Section of the nipple. **(D)** Cross-section of the nipple. There is a corrugated layer of stratified squamous keratinized epithelium over the nipple surface; 20 or more lactiferous ducts (L) open onto the surface; sebaceous glands (S) are deep to the epidermis. (**A–C,** Reproduced with permission from Standring S, ed. *Gray's anatomy.* 40th ed. London: Churchill Livingstone; 2008; **D,** from Kerr JB. *Atlas of functional histology.* London: Mosby; 1999, with permission from Dr JB Kerr, Monash University.)

diameter in order to minimize the discrepancy in circle sizes, thereby reducing tension on the closure.

- Rule 3: $D_{final} = \frac{1}{2}(D_{outside} + D_{inside})$. This final rule helps predict the final areolar size, which is particularly useful in asymmetry cases, as well as those in whom no round block suture is employed *(Fig. 15.13)*.

- As the degree of the breast ptosis increases, so does the total length of the incision necessary to correct it. The logical extension of the periareolar scar is the addition of a vertical component.
- Lassus and other vertical mastopexy techniques combine four principles:
  - (1) a central wedge resection to reduce the size of the breast, if needed; (2) transposition of the areola on a superiorly-based flap; (3) no undermining of the skin; (4) addition of a vertical scar component.
- Vertical mastopexy techniques are best for young women with good skin elasticity, a firm, glandular breast, and breasts that are not excessively large or ptotic.
- Advantages of vertical techniques: almost no risk of skin, nipple, or glandular necrosis; preservation of most of the

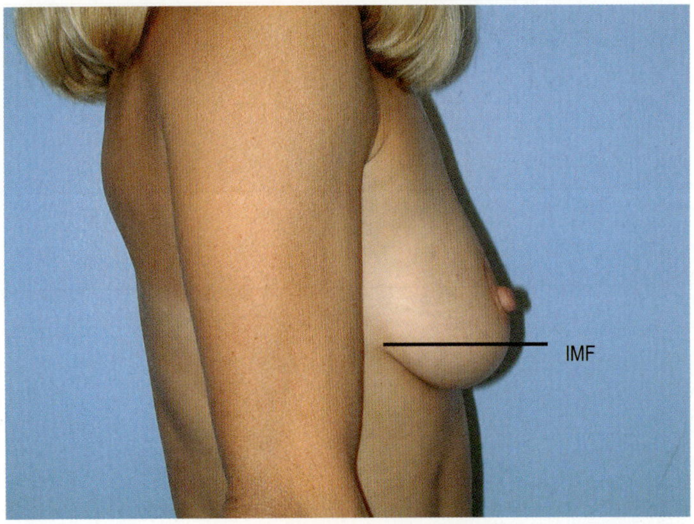

Figure 15.8 Lateral pseudo ptosis. IMF, inframammary fold.

neurovascular supply to the areola, long-lasting results from cicatricial healing, drains are usually not necessary.

- Disadvantages of vertical techniques: a visible vertical scar, less than ideal early postoperative breast shape that may take several months to settle, and an "adjust as you go" approach to reshaping.
- The advantages and disadvantages of the mastopexy techniques remain the same; however, the added benefits and risks of augmentation mammaplasty must now be considered.
- Advantages include: improved fill of the skin envelope by virtue of the implant.
- Risks include: wound problems and dehiscence because of the added weight of the implant, the inherent risks of the implants (malpositioning, leakage, rupture, capsular contracture), potential risk of devascularizing the nipple-areolar complex.

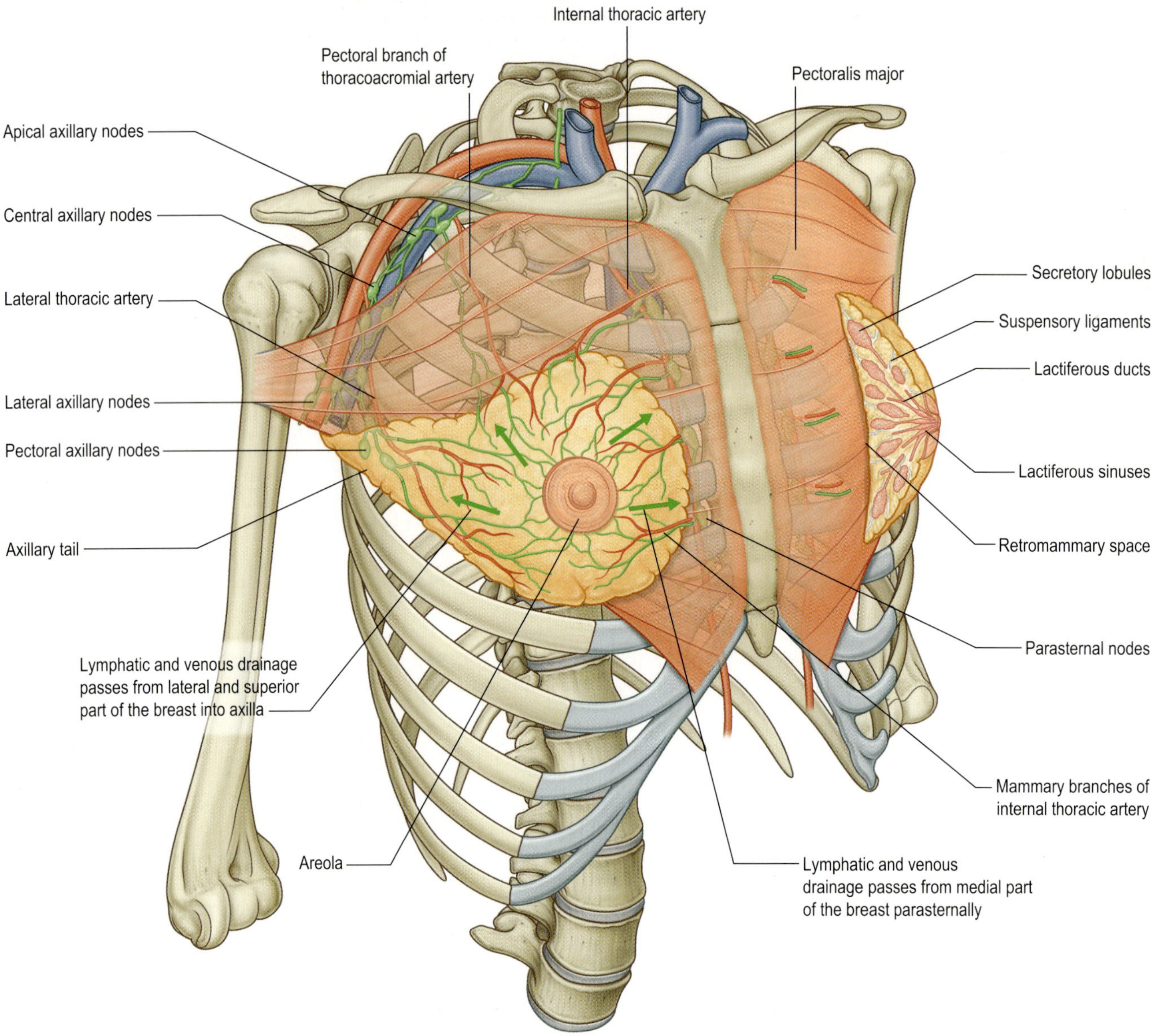

Figure 15.9 The relations of the breast. (Reproduced with permission from Drake et al. *Gray's anatomy for students.* London: Churchill Livingstone; 2005.)

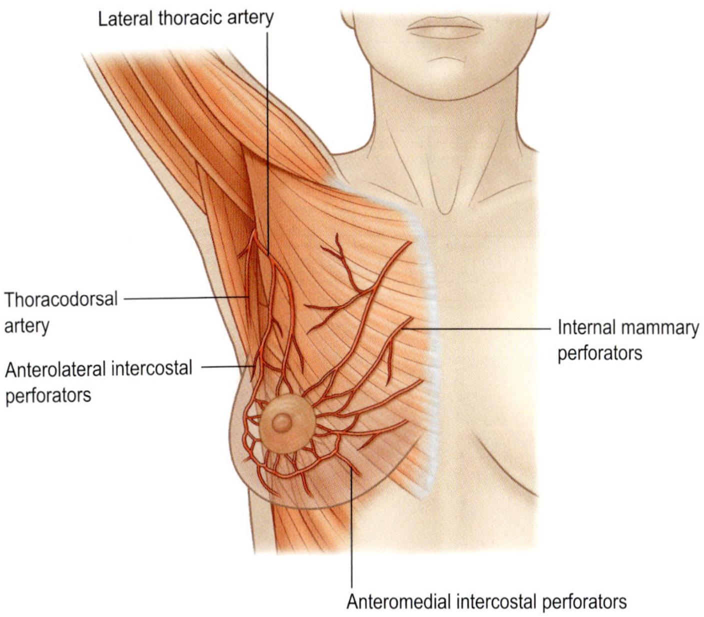

Figure 15.10 Blood supply to the breast.

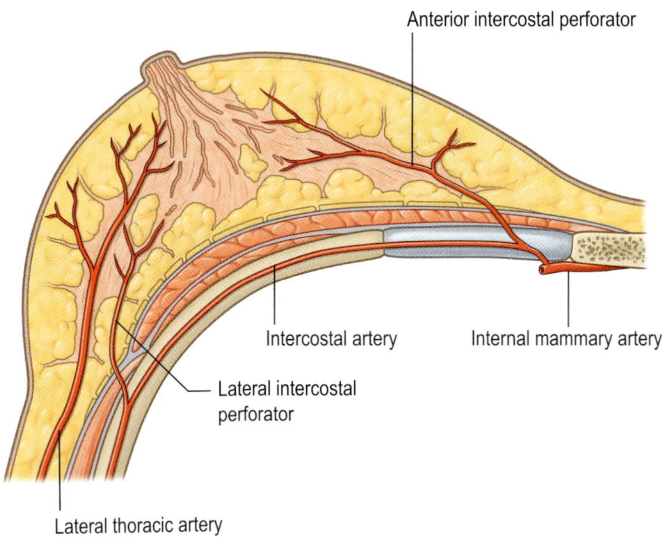

Figure 15.11 Blood supply to the breast – cross-sectional view.

- In general, the base diameter and projection of implants chosen for augmentation-mastopexy procedures are smaller than in implants chosen for standard augmentation procedures.
- Textured implants may assist in avoiding malposition, especially when the subglandular plane is selected. If the parenchymal volume is deficient in the upper pole (<3 cm pinch thickness), then we prefer a subpectoral placement.
- The inverted T-scar technique is reserved for those women with moderate to severe breast ptosis with a large excess of skin and a moderate amount of glandular tissue.
- Advantages: ability to excise all excess skin, ability to see the final shape of the breast while the patient is still on the operating table leading to a decreased chance for revision.

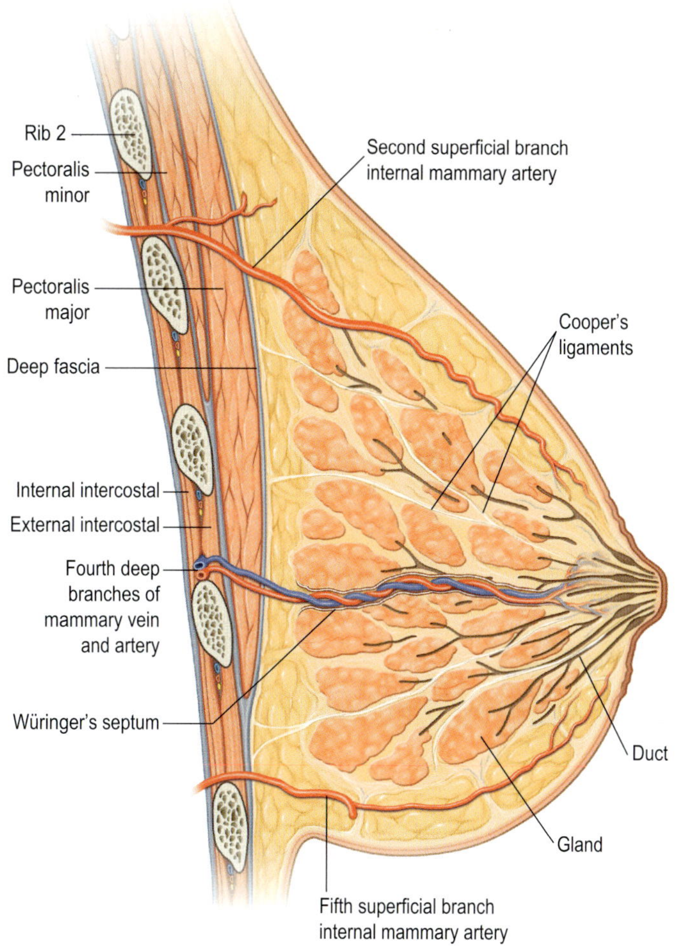

Figure 15.12 Profile anatomic view of the hemisected human breast. The ligaments described by Sir Astley Cooper are clearly demonstrated to run from the posterior, or deep, breast fascia, which is intimately associated with the pectoralis major muscle fascia, to the anterior, or superficial, breast fascia, and insert into the dermis. The parenchyma, which is encapsulated within these fascial borders, changes with aging, implants, weight changes, and pregnancy. These types of parenchymal changes result in alterations to the integrity of Cooper's ligaments, the breast's fascial components, and the overlying skin and fat.

- Disadvantages: Increased length of the incisions/scars; the breast shape is supported mainly by the skin envelope which increases the chance of recurrent ptosis during the subsequent months and years.

Operative techniques

Concentric mastopexy without parenchymal reshaping

- The amount of skin to be excised is determined by the position of the nipple-areola complex.
- Excise only the amount of skin necessary to raise the nipple-areola complex to the proper level for correction of the ptosis.
- The lines of excision are marked on the breast with the patient in a sitting or standing position in the preoperative area.

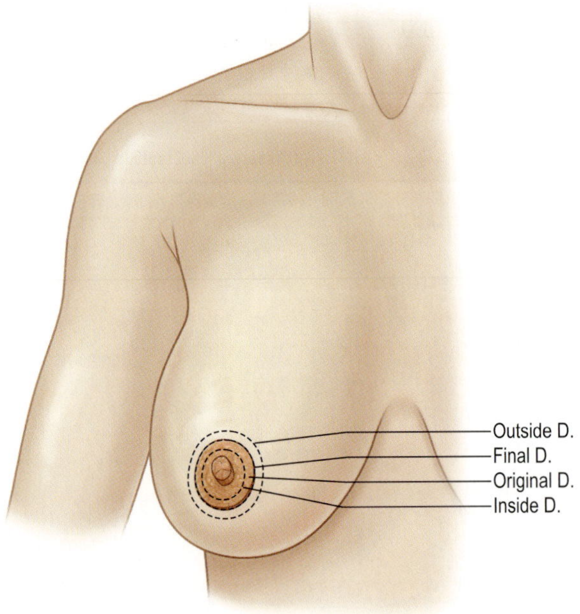

Figure 15.13 Periareolar design guides as described by Spear et al. D, diameter. (Modified from Michelow BJ, Nahai F. Mastopexy. In: Achauer BM, Erikson E, Guyuron B, et al., eds. *Plastic surgery: indications, operations and outcomes.* Vol. 5. St Louis: Mosby; 2000.)

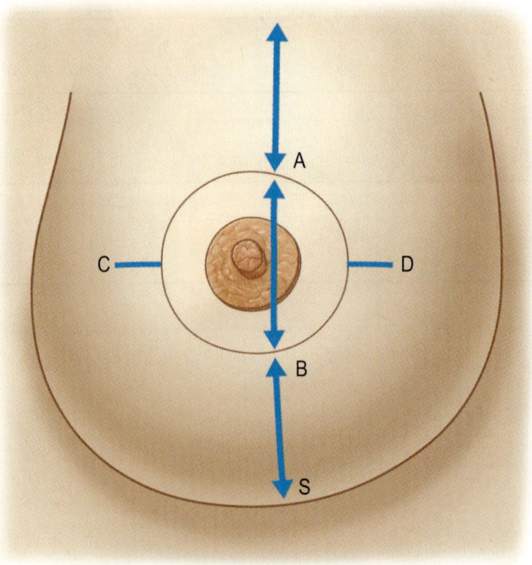

Figure 15.14 Markings for Benelli mastopexy. **(A)** Future superior point of the nipple; **(B)** future inferior point of the nipple; **(C)** medial limit of the nipple; **(D)** lateral limit of the nipple. Point C averages 8–12 cm from the midline. S is the point where the breast meridian intersects the inframammary fold. (Redrawn after Benelli L. A new periareolar mammaplasty: the "round block" technique. *Aesthetic Plast Surg.* 1990;14:93–100.)

- Symmetry is checked by comparing sternal notch to nipple distance and sternum to nipple distance.
- In the operating room, the amount of the areola that is to remain is marked on the stretched breast with an areolar marker or "cookie-cutter".
- The skin between these two marks is infiltrated with 0.5% lidocaine with 1:200 000 epinephrine to facilitate de-epithelialization.
- Once the skin is removed, the edge of the dermis can be elevated. At the same time, the remaining skin around the exposed dermis can be elevated off the gland for a short distance superiorly.
- A purse string suture of 4-0 Gore-Tex or Mersilene is then placed in the deep dermis of the skin edge. This is then cinched to the approximate size of the areola and tied.
- The areola is then approximated to the skin with half-buried horizontal mattress sutures, followed by a running, subcuticular 4-0 Monocryl or polydioxanone closure.

Periareolar Benelli mastopexy

- The Benelli mastopexy technique is an extension of the donut mastopexy with modifications that allow the periareolar techniques to be used on larger breasts with increasing degrees of ptosis.
- The fundamental concept behind the Benelli mastopexy is treatment of the skin and the gland as two separate components.
- Preoperative markings:
  - Mark the midline and the estimated meridian of the newly shaped breast.
  - The new meridian is often medial to the breast meridian approximately 6 cm from the midline.
  - Mark the future superior border of the areola, point A, on the meridian approximately 2 cm above the anterior projection of the inframammary fold.
  - Mark the future inferior border of the areola, point B, approximately 5–12 cm above the inframammary fold on the basis of the estimated final breast volume and the expected skin retraction.
  - Mark the medial and lateral limits of the new areola, points C and D, on the basis of estimates of the final breast volume. These limits are equidistant from the previously-marked meridian, and point C averages 8–12 cm from the midline ***(Fig. 15.14)***.
  - The opposite breast is marked with reference to the already marked breast.
  - The preoperative markings are verified by pinching together the superior and inferior points and then the medial and lateral points, ensuring that enough skin will remain to adequately cover the breast tissue without tension.
- The desired areolar diameter is marked, and the periareolar ellipse is de-epithelialized. The de-epithelialized dermis is incised from the 2 o'clock to the 10 o'clock position. The dissection is extended toward the inframammary fold in the subcutaneous plane ***(Fig. 15.15)***. The dissection continues to the upper outer quadrant of the breast and becomes more superficial to preserve the vessels coming from the lateral thoracic artery.
- Glandular dissection is initiated with a semicircular incision approximately 3 cm from the inferior areola edge to preserve innervation and blood supply to the areola.

Dissection is continued to the prepectoral space in the avascular central space, preserving the peripheral blood supply.

- The inferior glandular flap is then cut vertically beyond the breast meridian up to the fascia.

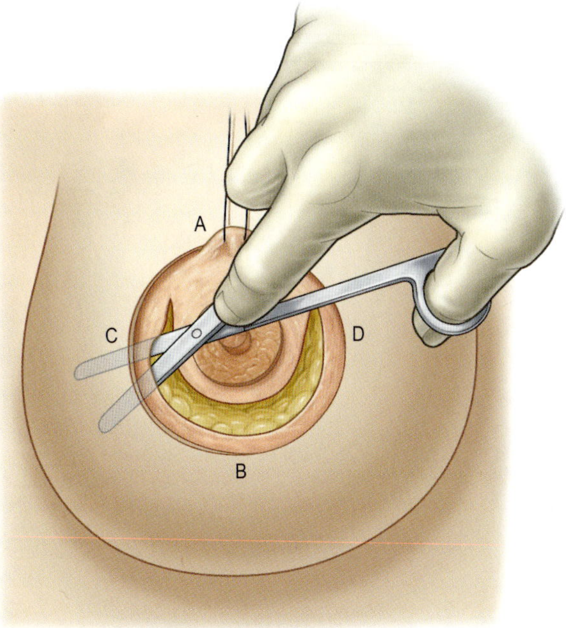

Figure 15.15 Dissection of the breast during Benelli mastopexy. Incision of dermis from the 2 o'clock to the 10 o'clock position with dissection to the inframammary fold subcutaneously. (Redrawn after Benelli LC. Periareolar Benelli mastopexy and reduction. In: Spear SL, ed. *Surgery of the breast: principles and art.* Philadelphia: Lippincott-Raven; 1998:685.)

- Four flaps will have thus been created: a superior dermoglandular flap supporting the areola, a glandular medial flap, a glandular lateral flap, and the detached skin flap ***(Fig. 15.16)***.
- The glandular flaps will be reassembled and repositioned to decrease the base of the breast, thus promoting the lifted appearance. If necessary, these flaps can be trimmed to reduce unwanted fullness. Volume reduction should be performed at the distal ends of the flaps to limit their length.
- Once the appropriate resection is complete, the gland is lifted and reshaped:
  - A stitch is placed in the glandular tissue of the superior flap and fixed to the pectoralis fascia ***(Fig. 15.17)***, elevating the areola and causing an exaggerated convexity in the superior pole of the breast ***(Fig. 15.18)*** that will eventually disappear within a few weeks secondary to gravity and the weight of the breast.
  - The medial and lateral flaps are folded over one another and sutured in place. Because most ptosis involves a lateral migration of the breast, the goal here is to medialize the breast. Therefore, the crisscross mastopexy is begun by rotating and folding the medial flap behind the areola, fixing its distal portion to the pectoralis muscle with superficial stitches ***(Fig. 15.19)***. The lateral flap is then crossed over and fixed to the medial flap ***(Fig. 15.20)*** thereby reducing the breast base and forming a glandular cone on which the areola is placed ***(Fig. 15.21)***.
  - The areola is fixated to the superior border of the ellipse through a 1 cm dermal incision made near the superior skin edge ***(Fig. 15.22)***.

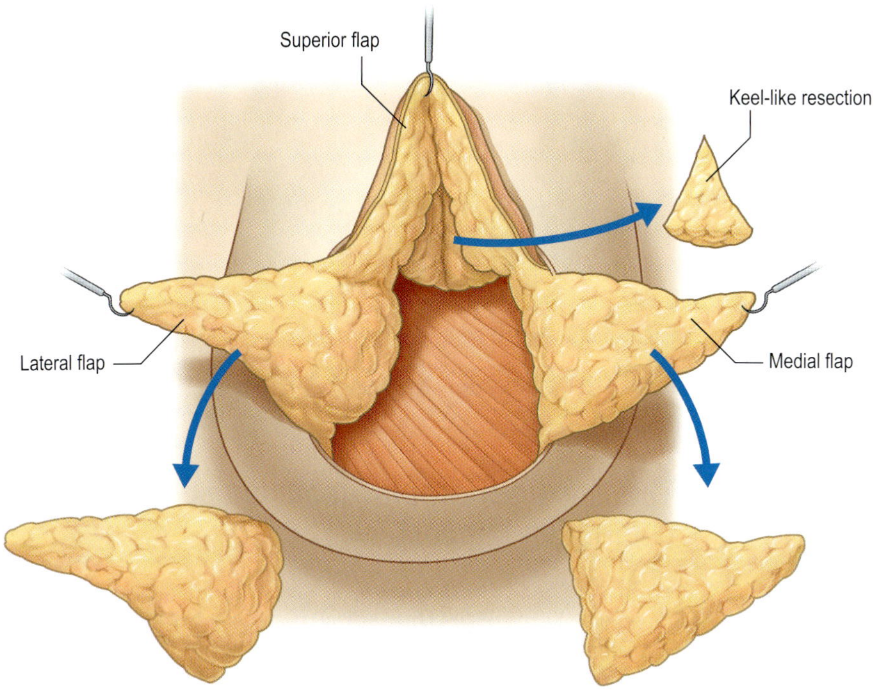

Figure 15.16 Four flaps of the Benelli mastopexy: superior dermoglandular flap supporting glandular medial and lateral flaps, and detached skin flap. (Redrawn after Benelli LC. Periareolar Benelli mastopexy and reduction. In: Spear SL, ed. *Surgery of the breast: principles and art.* Philadelphia: Lippincott-Raven; 1998:685.)

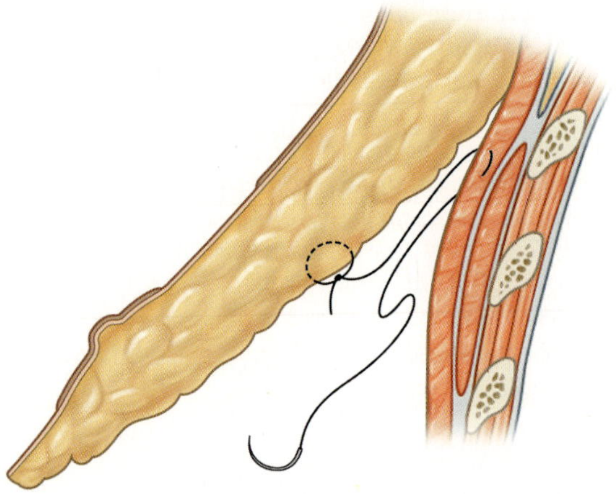

Figure 15.17 Benelli mastopexy. Attachment of the superior flap to the chest wall by the pectoralis fascia. (Redrawn after Benelli LC. Periareolar Benelli mastopexy and reduction. In: Spear SL, ed. *Surgery of the breast: principles and art.* Philadelphia: Lippincott-Raven; 1998:685.)

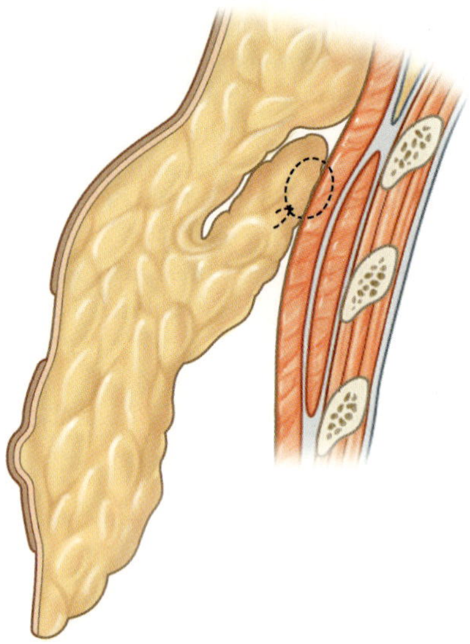

Figure 15.18 Benelli mastopexy. Superior flap attached to the chest wall demonstrating areolar elevation and exaggerated convexity of superior pole. (Redrawn after Benelli LC. Periareolar Benelli mastopexy and reduction. In: Spear SL, ed. *Surgery of the breast: principles and art.* Philadelphia: Lippincott-Raven; 1998:685.)

- Support for the breast shape is achieved by full-breast lacing in which braided polyester suture on a long straight needle is used to place inverted sutures along the underside of the gland. These sutures should be applied without tension, as overly tight sutures can result in glandular necrosis.
- The skin is redraped over the breast, and a round block cerclage stitch is passed in the deep dermis in pursestring fashion ***(Fig. 15.23)*** and cinched around a tube of the desired diameter.
- A diametrical transareolar U suture is placed to serve as a barrier and help prevent areola protrusion ***(Fig. 15.24)***. It can also be used to give a circular shape to the areola in those patients in whom it tends to be ovoid.

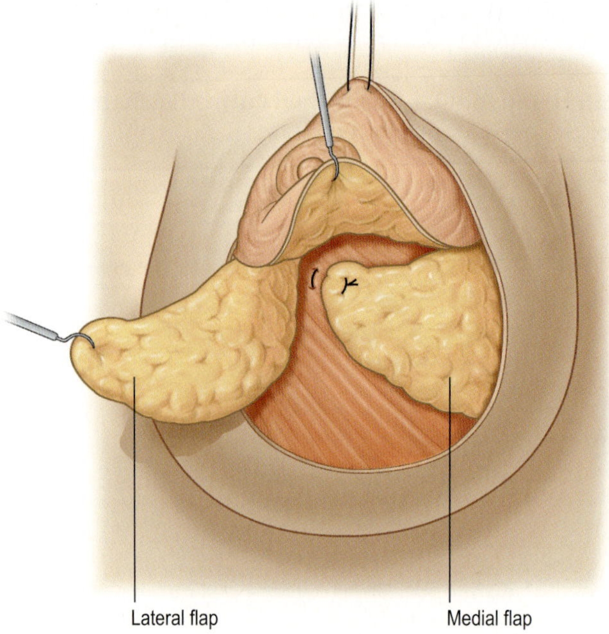

Figure 15.19 Benelli mastopexy. Medial glandular flap affixed to the underlying pectoralis muscle. (Redrawn after Benelli LC. Periareolar Benelli mastopexy and reduction. In: Spear SL, ed. *Surgery of the breast: principles and art.* Philadelphia: Lippincott-Raven; 1998:685.)

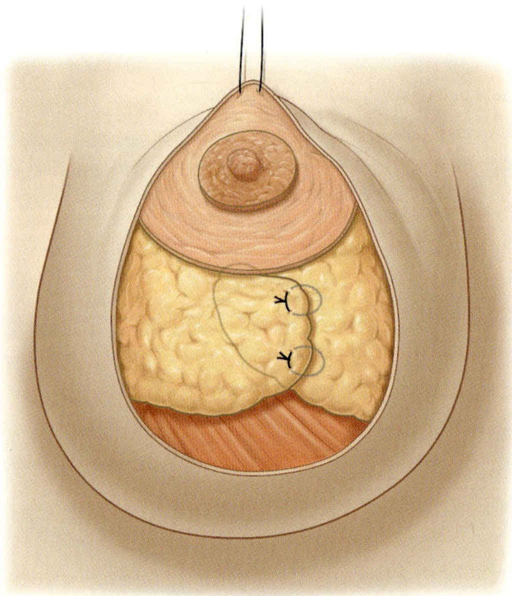

Figure 15.20 Benelli mastopexy. Lateral flap is affixed to the medial flap. (Redrawn after Benelli LC. Periareolar Benelli mastopexy and reduction. In: Spear SL, ed. *Surgery of the breast: principles and art.* Philadelphia: Lippincott-Raven; 1998:685.

The Goes periareolar technique with mesh support

- Also called the "double skin" technique, the basic principle involves formation of a resistant lining of the breast by the use of a layer of prosthetic mesh which acts as an internal brassiere to provide increased breast

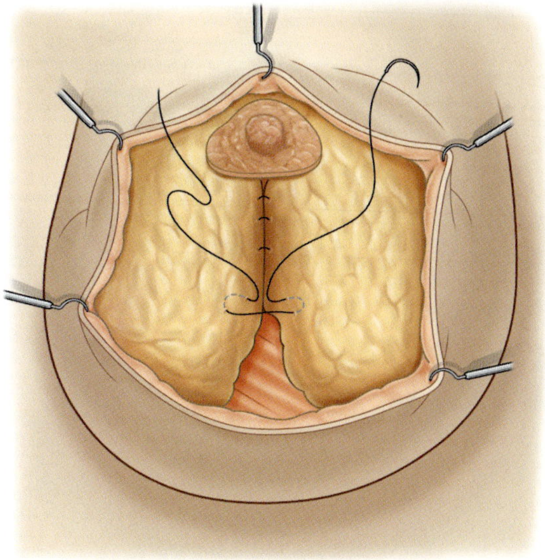

Figure 15.21 Benelli mastopexy. Plication invagination of the gland to form a conical shape. (Redrawn after Benelli LC. Periareolar Benelli mastopexy and reduction. In: Spear SL, ed. *Surgery of the breast: principles and art.* Philadelphia: Lippincott-Raven; 1998:685.)

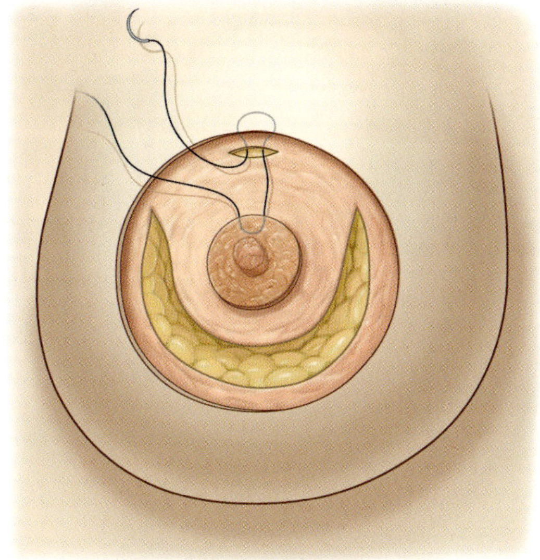

Figure 15.22 Benelli mastopexy. Fixation of areola to the superior border of the ellipse. (Redrawn after Benelli LC. Periareolar Benelli mastopexy and reduction. In: Spear SL, ed. *Surgery of the breast: principles and art.* Philadelphia: Lippincott-Raven; 1998:685.)

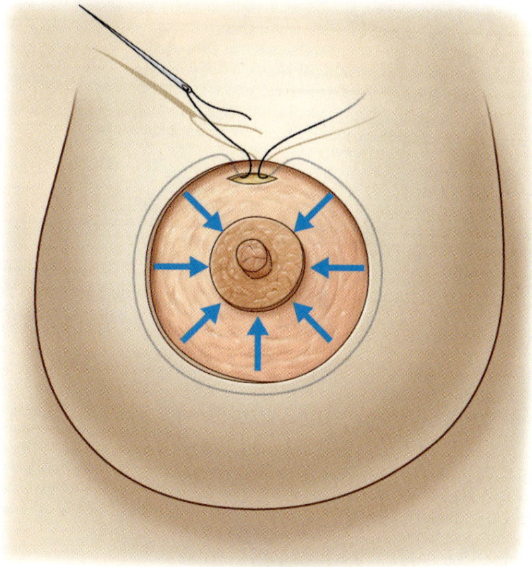

Figure 15.23 Benelli mastopexy round block suture. (Redrawn after Benelli LC. Periareolar Benelli mastopexy and reduction. In: Spear SL, ed. *Surgery of the breast: principles and art.* Philadelphia: Lippincott-Raven; 1998:685.)

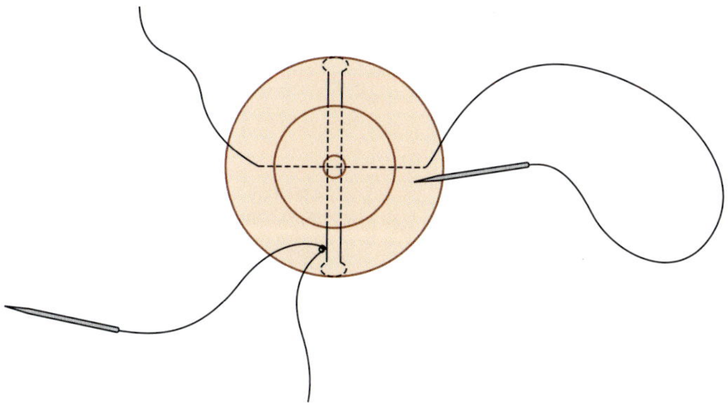

Figure 15.24 U stitches to help prevent areolar herniation and aid in producing a round shape in the Benelli mastopexy. (Redrawn after Benelli LC. Periareolar Benelli mastopexy and reduction. In: Spear SL, ed. *Surgery of the breast: principles and art.* Philadelphia: Lippincott-Raven; 1998:685.)

support during the healing and skin contraction processes.

- The primary indication for this method is the correction of ptosis or a slight reduction of hypertrophy with or without ptosis. Reductions from each breast ideally should be no more than 500 g.
- Preoperative markings include four cardinal points ***(Fig. 15.25)***:
  - Point A is the level of the top of the new areola.
  - Point B marks the distance from the inframammary fold to the bottom of the new areola (average 7 cm).
  - Point C is the distance from the medial breast border to the medial aspect of the new areola at the level of the nipple (average 9 cm).
  - Point D is the distance from the anterior axillary line to the lateral aspect of the new areola at the level of the nipple (average 12 cm).
- The area between the areola and the skin marking is de-epithelialized.
- An incision is made along the outer ellipse, and the skin flap is developed.
- The superior dissection proceeds along the base; the thickness of the subcutaneous fat tissue is progressively increased as one gets closer to the base of the breast and undermining continues over the pectoral fascia for approximately 5 cm superiorly and then inferiorly under the gland approximately one-third of the way into the retromammary space.
- Care should be taken to identify and preserve all perforating vessels ***(Fig. 15.26)***.

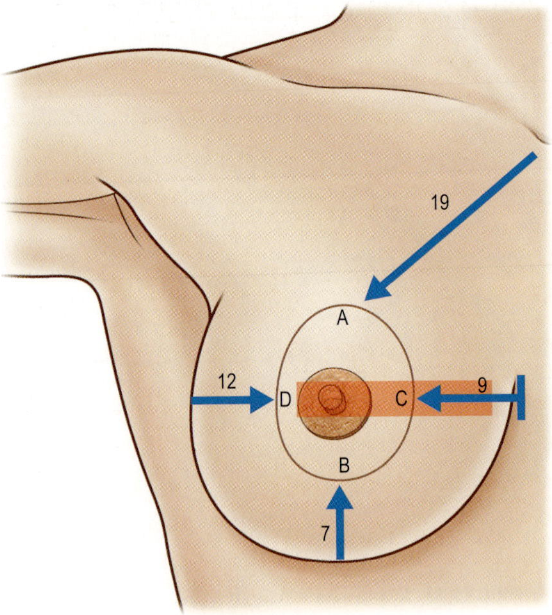

Figure 15.25 Four cardinal points for the Goes mammaplasty. (Redrawn after Goes JC. Periareolar mastopexy and reduction with mesh support. In: Spear SL, ed. *Surgery of the breast: principles and art.* Philadelphia: Lippincott-Raven; 1998:697.)

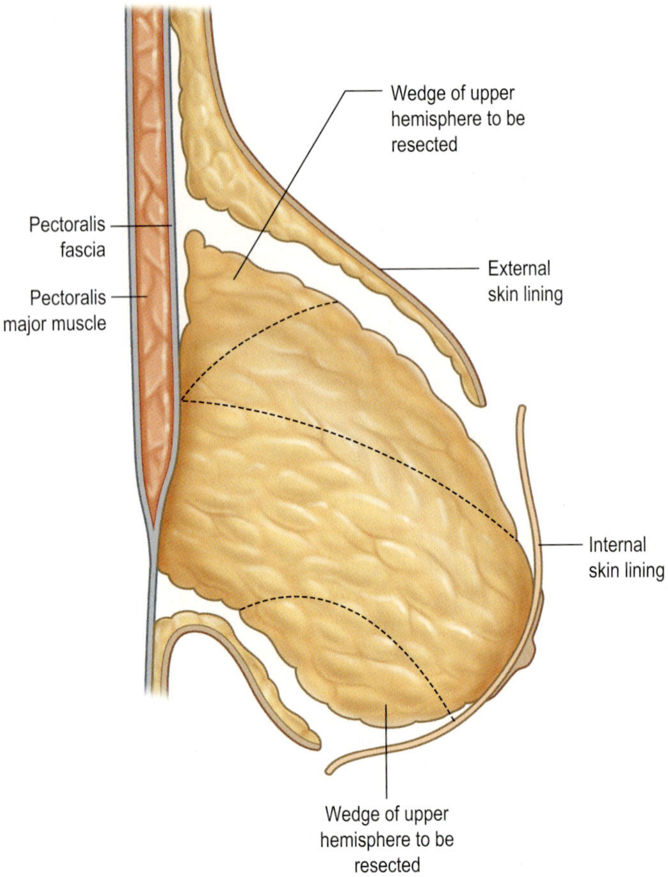

Figure 15.26 Goes technique. Dissection of the gland to separate it from the skin along with lines of excision of the gland. Note the formation of the internal skin lining. (Redrawn after Goes JC. Periareolar mastopexy and reduction with mesh support. In: Spear SL, ed. *Surgery of the breast: principles and art.* Philadelphia: Lippincott-Raven; 1998:697.)

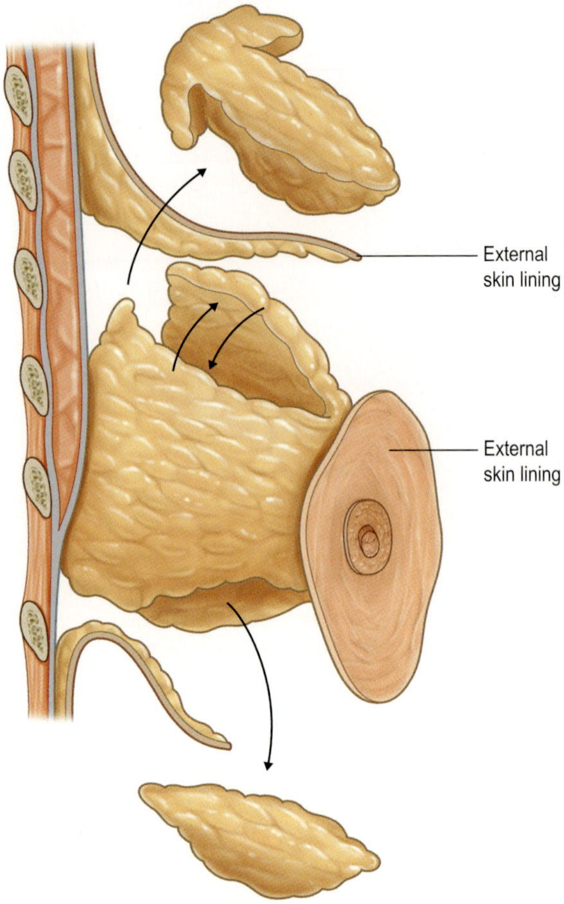

Figure 15.27 Goes technique. Lines of resection from the superior and inferior hemispheres to narrow the base. Note that mastopexy alone, these regions can simply be imbricated rather than resected. (Redrawn after Goes JC. Periareolar mastopexy and reduction with mesh support. In: Spear SL, ed. *Surgery of the breast: principles and art.* Philadelphia: Lippincott-Raven; 1998:697.)

- Once the skin and the gland are separated, wedges of tissue can be removed superiorly and inferiorly to accomplish any needed reduction of breast tissue. The base of the mammary gland should not be disturbed.
- To reassemble the gland, any superior excisional defect is closed, and the gland is fixed to the thorax in a way that fills and elevates the upper pole of the breast ***(Fig. 15.27)***. The lower hemisphere excisional defect is then closed and secured to the intramammary connective ligaments and the anterior pectoral fascia.
- The dermal flap, which has been undermined to the areola, is gently stretched over the gland; it is attached inferiorly to the anterior pectoral fascia when possible and superiorly to the connective ligaments. This dermal component is the so-called internal skin lining ***(Fig. 15.28)***.
- Next, the mixed mesh (polyglactin mesh with Dacron filaments), woven mesh (polyglactin/polypropylene), or biologic mesh is applied over the dermal flap as a brassiere. It is used to give an ideal shape to the parenchymal cone and to elevate the breast slightly. It is sutured to the anterior pectoral fascia.

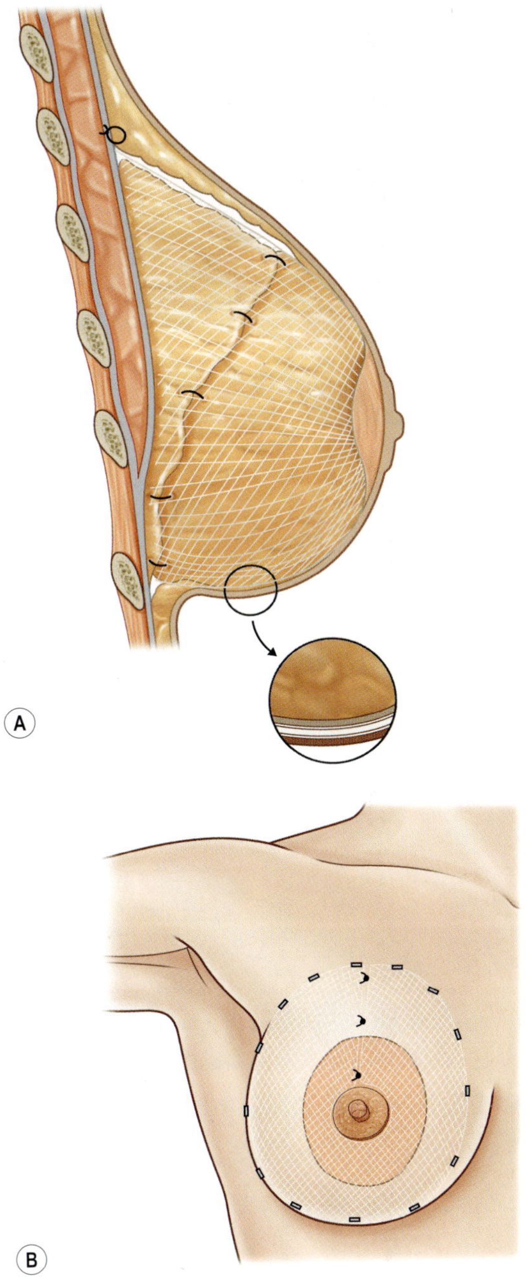

Figure 15.28 Goes technique. **(A)** The breast projects anteriorly and superiorly after formation of the cone and reinforcement of the breast with mesh. **(B)** Schematic for the placement of mesh. The polyglactin–Dacron composite mesh of Goes' original description is replaced with a Vicryl–Prolene composite. (Redrawn after Goes JC. Periareolar mastopexy and reduction with mesh support. In: Spear SL, ed. *Surgery of the breast: principles and art.* Philadelphia: Lippincott-Raven; 1998:697.)

- The external skin lining is brought up over the breast mound and closed around the areola with a circular continuous deep intradermal suture of Mersilene 2-0 on a straight needle. A continuous, intradermal Monocryl 4-0 suture is used to fix the areola skin to the external skin lining.
- Dressings consist of triangular pieces of Micropore tape covering the whole gland, which is left in place for 20 days. Tegaderm also works well for this purpose. Suction drains are removed after approximately 5 days.

Grotting sculpted vertical pillar mastopexy (Video 15.1)

Video 15.1

- Modification of the Lassus technique that allows resection of glandular tissue, if desired, and/or also the insertion of an implant in either the subglandular or the subpectoral plane if more volume is required.
- Preoperative markings include:
  - The IMF.
  - The future nipple position – determined by many reference points including transposition of the IMF onto the anterior surface of the breast, pinching/gathering of the lower breast to simulate the mastopexy in order to determine if the nipple elevates to the mark, cross-checking against the midhumeral line, and measuring the notch to new nipple position (typically 20–23 cm) ***(Fig. 15.29)***.
  - If parenchymal volume asymmetry exists, it is often necessary to mark the superior border of the nipple position, the A point, a centimeter or so lower on the larger side than the smaller side, in order to account for skin recoil after tissue resection.
- The next mark is the breast meridian, marked on its anterior surface. The midpoint of the inframammary fold is measured and will be the reference point for creating the marks for the medial and lateral pillars that will approximate at this point after completing the vertical closure.
- It is preferable to use the standard superior pedicle for the nipple-areolar complex, but if the density of the gland or distance of elevation appears restrictive, the superomedial pedicle recommended by Elizabeth Hall-Findlay is used.
- The medial and lateral pillar lines are drawn by manually distracting the breast tissue medially and laterally. These marks are joined inferiorly by a parabolic line whose lowest-point of the curve is approximately 2–3 cm above the inframammary fold ***(Fig. 15.30)***.
- Superiorly, the vertical lines are curved up to the new nipple point. Small inflections of the lines to create a mosque-dome effect can be used to accentuate the future 6 o'clock position on the areolar closure if desired.
- The top of the vertical closure at this point is pinched approximated to ensure adequate skin will remain for closure.
- From the top of the vertical closure, one measures down 5–6 cm and makes another mark that will represent the approximate position of the new inframammary fold.
- The breast tissue below that point will comprise the bottom of the future superiorly-based dermoglandular flap (if the intention of the surgeon is to autologously-augment the patient) or be resected (as in small reductions, with or without an implant).
- Preaxillary fullnesses and lateral chest rolls may need liposuction to contour and should be marked.
- The nipple areola is marked with an appropriate sized nipple marker, and then lidocaine 0.5% with epinephrine 1:200000 is infiltrated in the intended lines of incision, areas to be de-epithelialized, as well as beneath the gland.

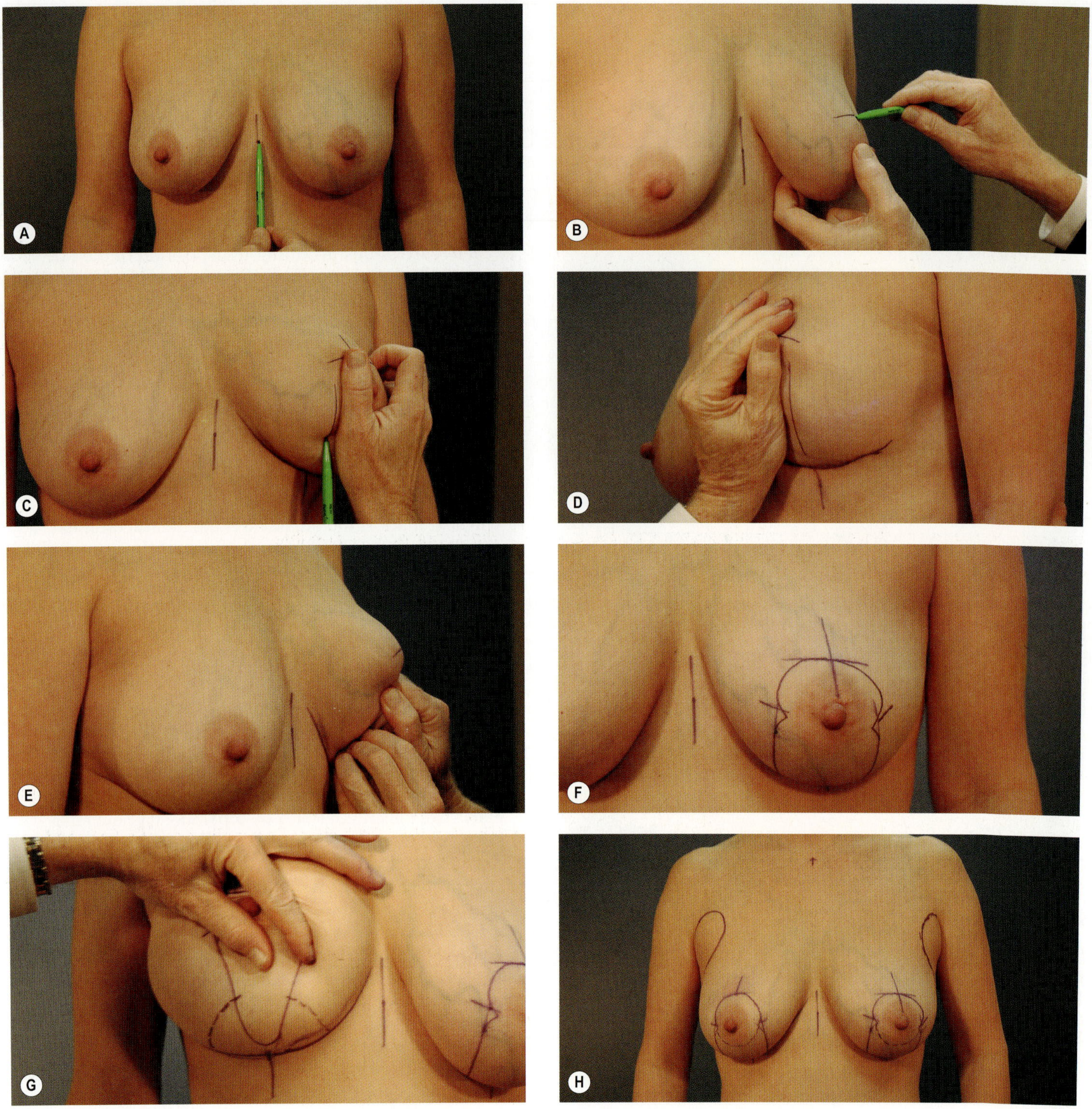

Figure 15.29 (A–H) Authors' preferred modification of vertical technique, preoperative markings. The midline and inframammary folds are marked. Point A, the transposed location of the inframammary fold, is marked on the breast anteriorly, as is the breast meridian. The breast is then manually distracted laterally and then medially to estimate and mark the medial and lateral vertical limbs, respectively. Points C and D are the cephalic extents of these vertical limbs and will become the bottom of the new areola. Often the vertical limbs can be manually approximated to simulate the mastopexy. The upper curved line represents the new areola boundary and is usually 12–14 cm in length.

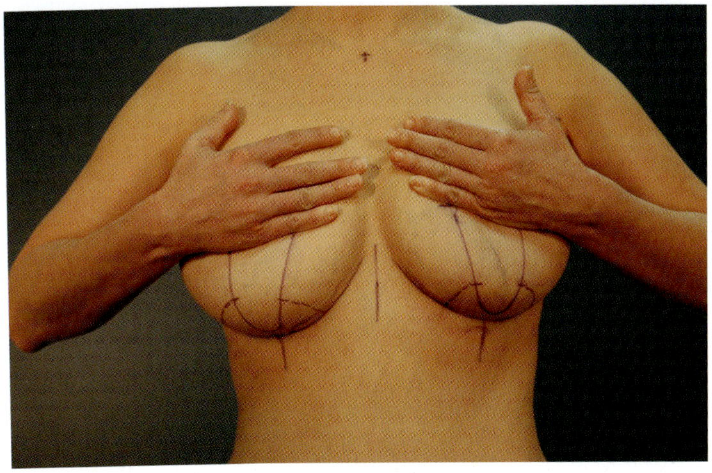

Figure 15.30 Note the bottom of the incision line coming to a V approximately 2 cm above the inframammary fold (point B). The hatched lines show the location of the glandular resection at the bases of the medial and lateral pillars. A superiorly-based flap can be created from the tissues between the marked medial and lateral pillars, rotated retro-areolarly, and then sutured to the pectoralis fascia to improve upper pole fill.

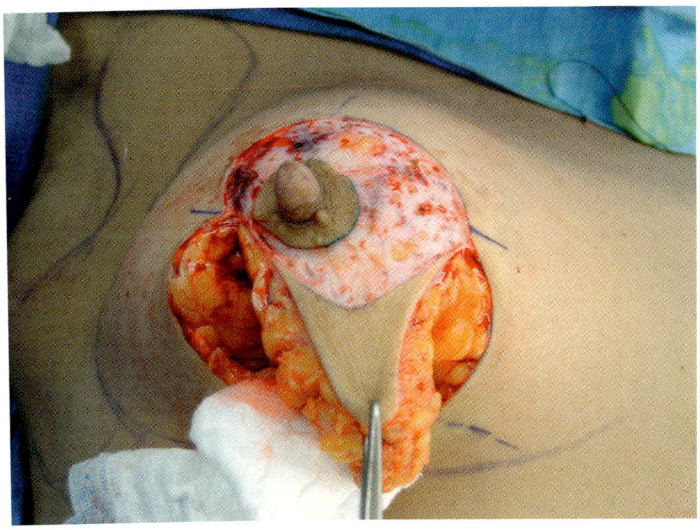

Figure 15.31 The lower pole of the breast has been detached. The resulting flap may be transposed into the retro-areolar location to augment the upper pole or resected in cases such as a small reduction or when an implant is to be added (addition–subtraction concept).

- After de-epithelialization of the periareolar skin and that between the medial and lateral pillar marks, the lower pole of the breast is undermined in the subcutaneous plane over that portion of the breast to be resected inferiorly, if any ***(Fig. 15.31)***.
- The gland is then undermined at the level of the pectoralis fascia from the inframammary fold inferiorly to the superior pole to establish space into which to fold the superiorly based inferior flap.
- At this point, the bases of the pillars can be trimmed if needed.
- The flap is sutured into an appropriate position. However, if no flap is used and the tissue is resected between the medial and lateral pillars, then a suture is used from the undersurface of the gland beneath the nipple-areola complex to the pectoral fascia as high up in the upper pole as possible.

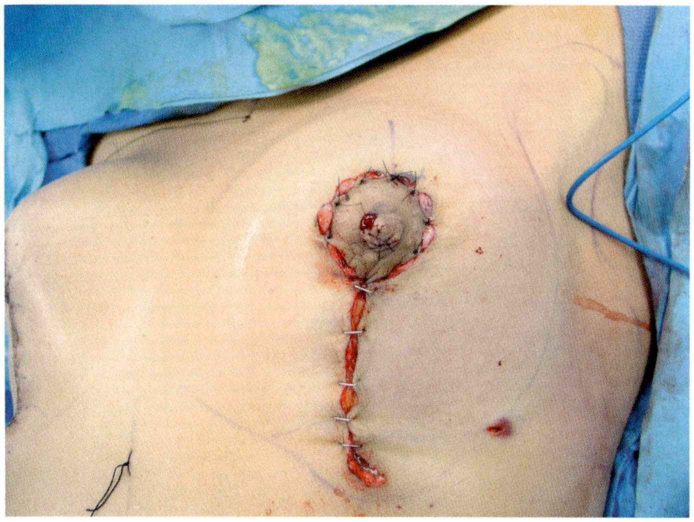

Figure 15.32 Temporary closure of the breast.

- In cases where no implant is planned, a "lateral shaping suture" is used to bring the lateral parenchyma at the anterior axillary fold toward the midline of the breast to form an aesthetic curve to the lateral portion of the breast.
- The medial and lateral pillars are then simply reapproximated with 2-0 Vicryl sutures in the parenchyma and 3-0 polydioxanone as a layered and running skin closure.
- The nipple-areola complex is exteriorized in its virtual position with the patient sitting up in the operating room ***(Fig. 15.32)***.
- The "on the table" shape is usually one of a flattened lower pole and a rounded upper pole with the nipple pointing slightly inferiorly, creating the so-called "upside-down breast" ***(Fig. 15.33)***.

Augmentation mastopexy

- Any of the previously discussed mastopexy techniques can be combined with augmentation.
- In general, this technique is most useful for those women with a deficit of glandular tissue regardless of the size of the skin envelope.
- Another good indication is asymmetry when one breast is hypoplastic and the other is ptotic.
- Augmentation mammaplasty proceeds with marking and incisions according to the mastopexy technique chosen. Once the breast tissue or muscle is exposed, the pocket for the implant, either submuscular or subglandular, can be formed and the implant inserted. The mastopexy can then be completed.
- It is critical to insert the implant prior to performing the mastopexy to avoid over-resection and undue tension on the closure, and provide better control to nipple areolar complex positioning.

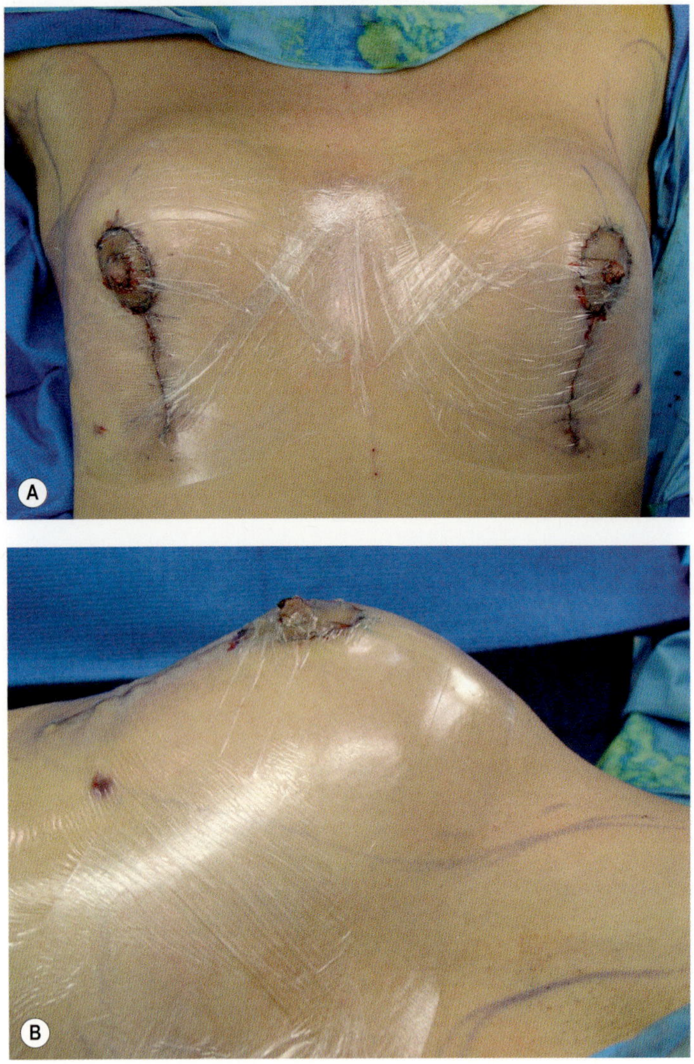

Figure 15.33 (A,B) Authors' preferred technique. Rounded superior pole, flat lower pole, and slightly downward pointing nipple.

- If there is the suggestion of nipple or skin flap compromise at the conclusion of the procedure, the following steps can be taken:
  - Removing the periareolar skin sutures.
  - Removal of the implant *(Fig. 15.34)*.

Mastopexy postexplantation

- When an implant is removed, the breast may assume an excessively lax and ptotic position. The potential for this postexplantation result should be included when the explantation procedure is discussed with a patient.
- A particularly useful technique in the case where mastopexy is planned postexplantation of saline-filled implants is the intentional deflation of the implants preoperatively, which can be performed in the office using a sterile 18 G needle *(Fig. 15.35)*.
- As with mastopexy procedures in general, the most important component in determining the ability to reshape the gland is the amount of glandular tissue available.
- The next issue that needs to be addressed is whether to perform capsulectomy or capsulotomy.
- In general, capsulectomy should be performed in patients with ruptured silicone gel implants, in patients with severe capsular contracture, or when the capsule contains large amounts of calcium deposits. Otherwise, the capsule, with or without additional capsulotomy incisions, may be left in place to add bulk to the glandular reconstruction.
- Before removal of the implant, the new areolar border is marked.
- De-epithelialization is performed on the basis of the mastopexy technique and any of the previously discussed mastopexy procedures may be used.
- It is usually easier to perform the initial mastopexy maneuvers with the implant in place.
- An incision is usually made in the inframammary fold, but a periareolar incision can occasionally be used to gain access to the implant or capsule.
- The capsule can be dissected and removed if necessary at this time, otherwise it is entered to allow removal of the implant.
- Reshaping of the gland can then be accomplished.
- Drains are placed, the skin envelope is closed and the nipple is repositioned and sutured into place.

Inverted-T technique

- Markings proceed with the standard Wise pattern:
  - The meridian line of the breast is marked.
  - The new position of the nipple is marked along this line at the anterior projection of the IMF.
  - A wire keyhole pattern is spread to allow it to just encompass the original areola.
  - The superior aspect of the pattern is placed approximately 2 cm above the location of the projected nipple position.
  - The vertically-oriented keyhole markings are extended laterally and medially on the breast to converge with the IMF.
- The portion of the areola to be preserved is marked with an appropriate diameter.
- The area within the preoperative marks is de-epithelialized.
- Transdermal incisions are made along the upper portion of what would be the vertical bipedicle flap of a reduction mammoplasty on either side of the nipple-areola complex.
- If planning to perform an auto-augmentation, and there is an abundance of de-epithelialized breast tissue below the inframammary fold, dissection of the gland off the pectoralis muscle is undertaken starting from the inframammary fold and proceeding upward to establish a superiorly based dermoglandular pedicle.
- The dissection continues until the pocket can accept the excess inferior glandular tissue. This tissue is folded behind the breast and attached to the pectoralis fascia

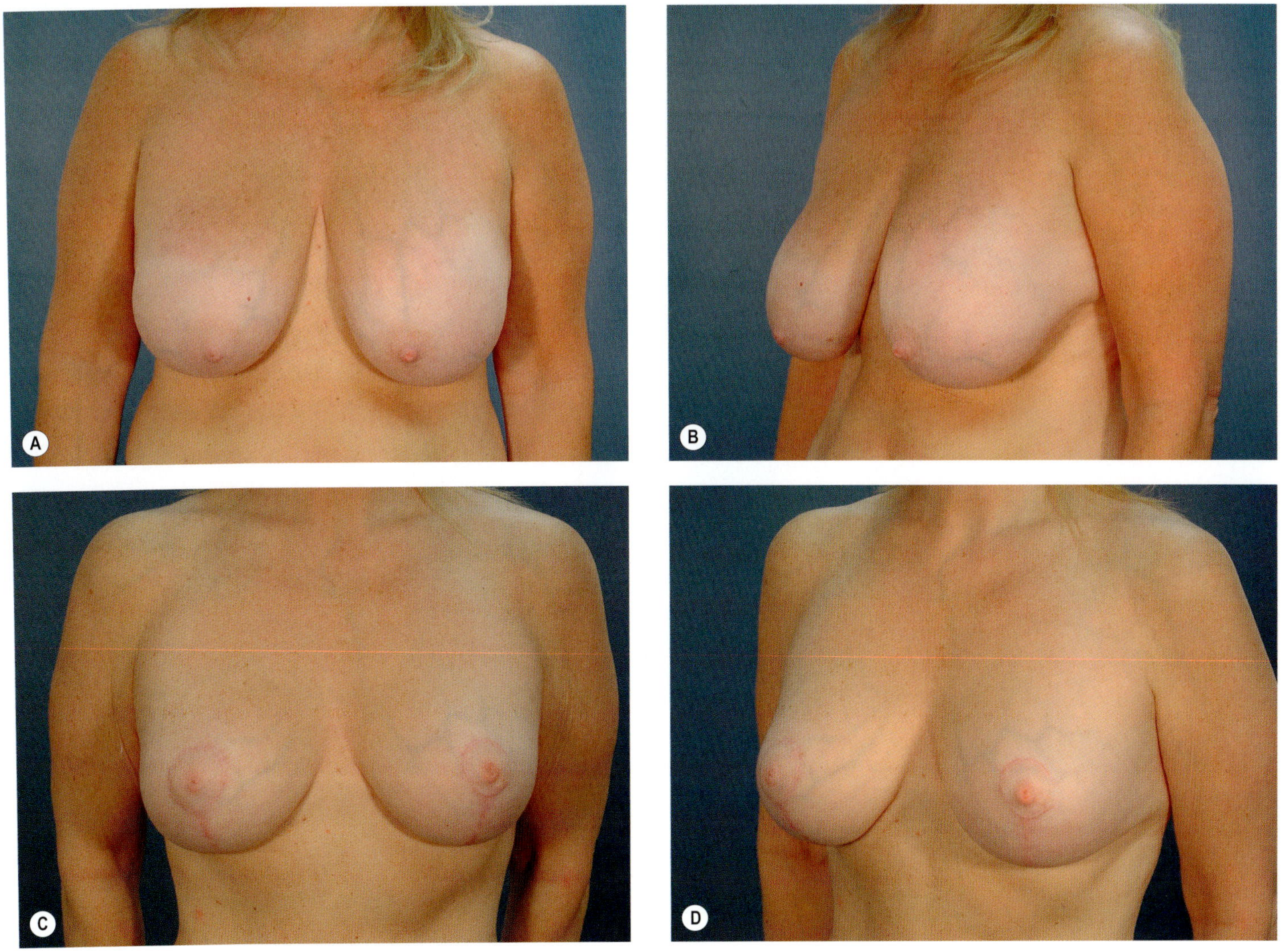

Figure 15.34 (A,B) Preoperative views of a 44-year-old female postlapband and a 60 lb weight loss. She had previously-placed oversized subpectoral implants. **(C,D)** Postoperative views after bilateral removal of implants and replacement with subglandularly-placed silicone gel implants in combination with parenchymal resection (addition–subtraction concept).

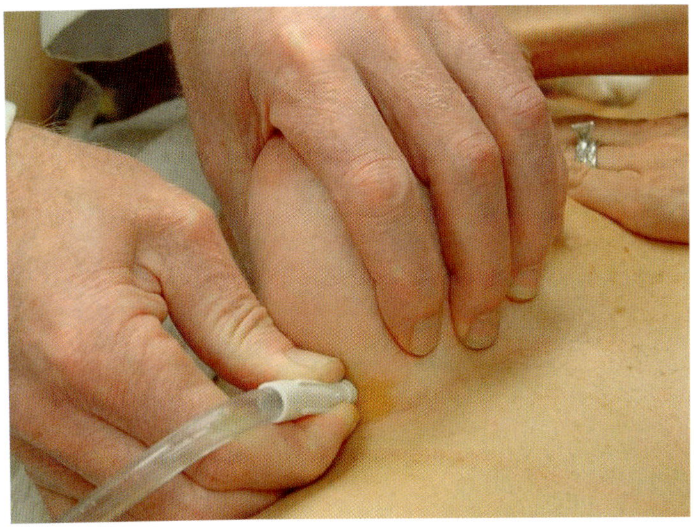

Figure 15.35 Preoperative saline implant deflation. The right hand guides the needle, holding it in place within the implant cavity, while the left hand compresses the implant and displaces it inferiorly.

high enough to eliminate gross glandular redundancy creating an auto-augmentation.

- Skin closure is accomplished in standard fashion with little or no further undermining. The nipple-areola complex is positioned and sutured into place *(Fig. 15.36)*.

Postoperative considerations

- Following the vertical mastopexy technique, the use of Tegaderm to support the final shape is an important aspect of postoperative care *(Fig. 15.37)*. It should be left on for up to 2 weeks, at which point a bra should be used day and night for 6–8 weeks *(Figs 15.38, 15.39)*.
- Postoperative brassieres are used for at least 8 weeks after surgery, in an effort to support the new breast as the postoperative edema begins to egress.

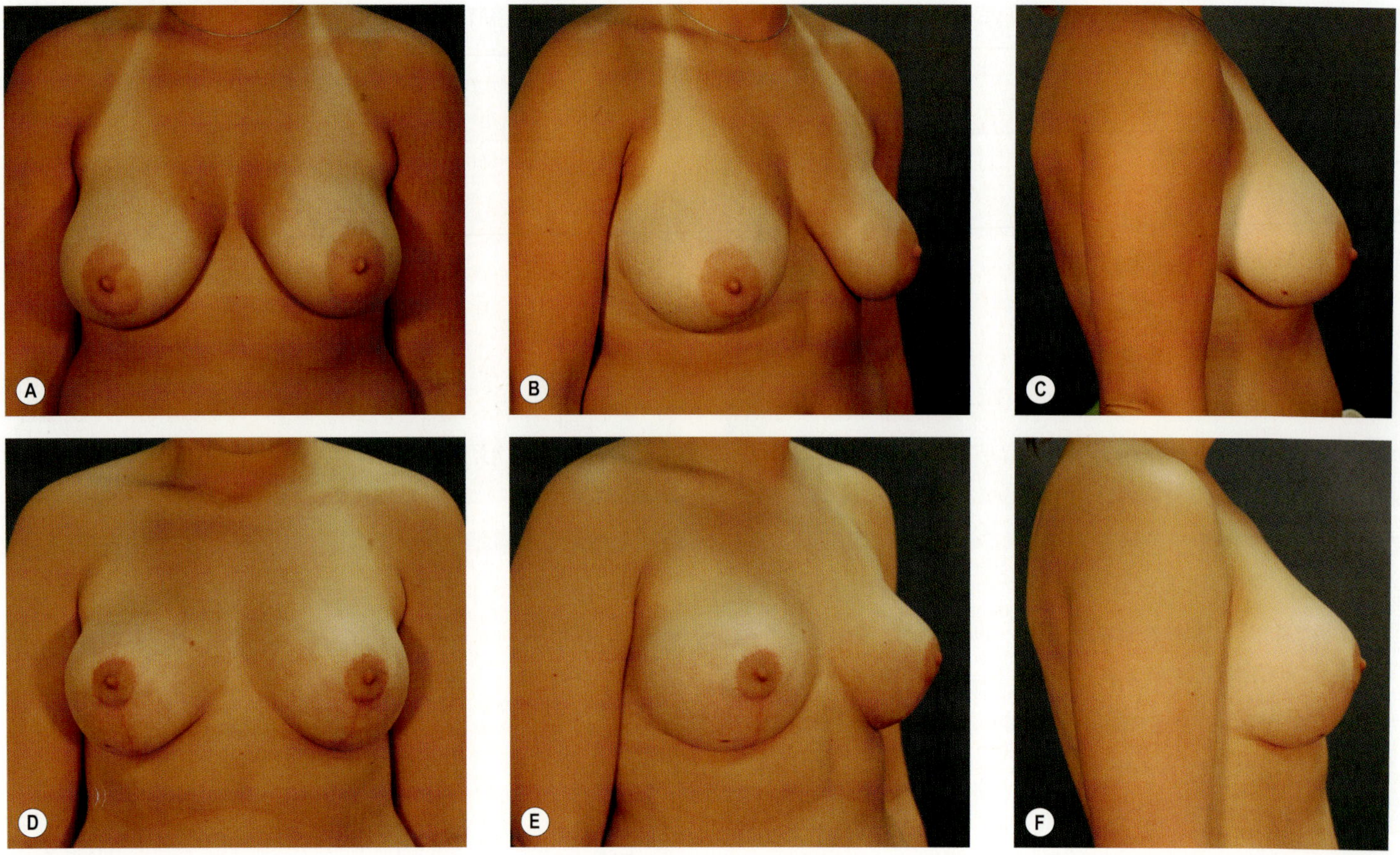

Figure 15.36 (A–C) A 35-year-old patient with bilateral breast pseudoptosis and asymmetry of parenchymal volume. **(D–F),** Postoperative views after inverted-T technique mastopexy and asymmetric small reduction of the inferior pole parenchyma.

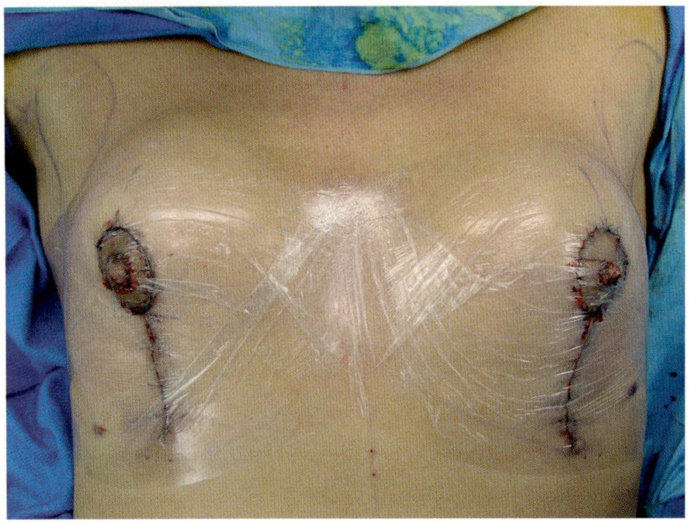

Figure 15.37 Final closure and cover with Tegaderm dressing.

- Full-on running or activities that tend to cause vigorous up and down motion of the new breasts are restricted until 8 weeks postoperatively.

Complications and outcomes

- One of the most devastating complications of mastopexy is nipple loss, with an incidence reported to be less than 10%, usually in the range of 0–5%.
- Risk factors include technical errors, smoking, diabetes, obesity, and hypertension.
- In high-risk patients (smokers, patients with diabetes or obesity, or those with severe ptosis), a free nipple graft technique is an option that can be considered and is also a possibility intraoperatively or postoperatively if the viability of the transposed nipple appears compromised.
- The nipple-areolar complex may be converted to a free nipple graft up until approximately 12 h postoperatively.
- After 12 h, conservative treatment of any nipple necrosis should be undertaken, including release of sutures, topical nitropaste or leeches, greasy dressings, hyperbaric

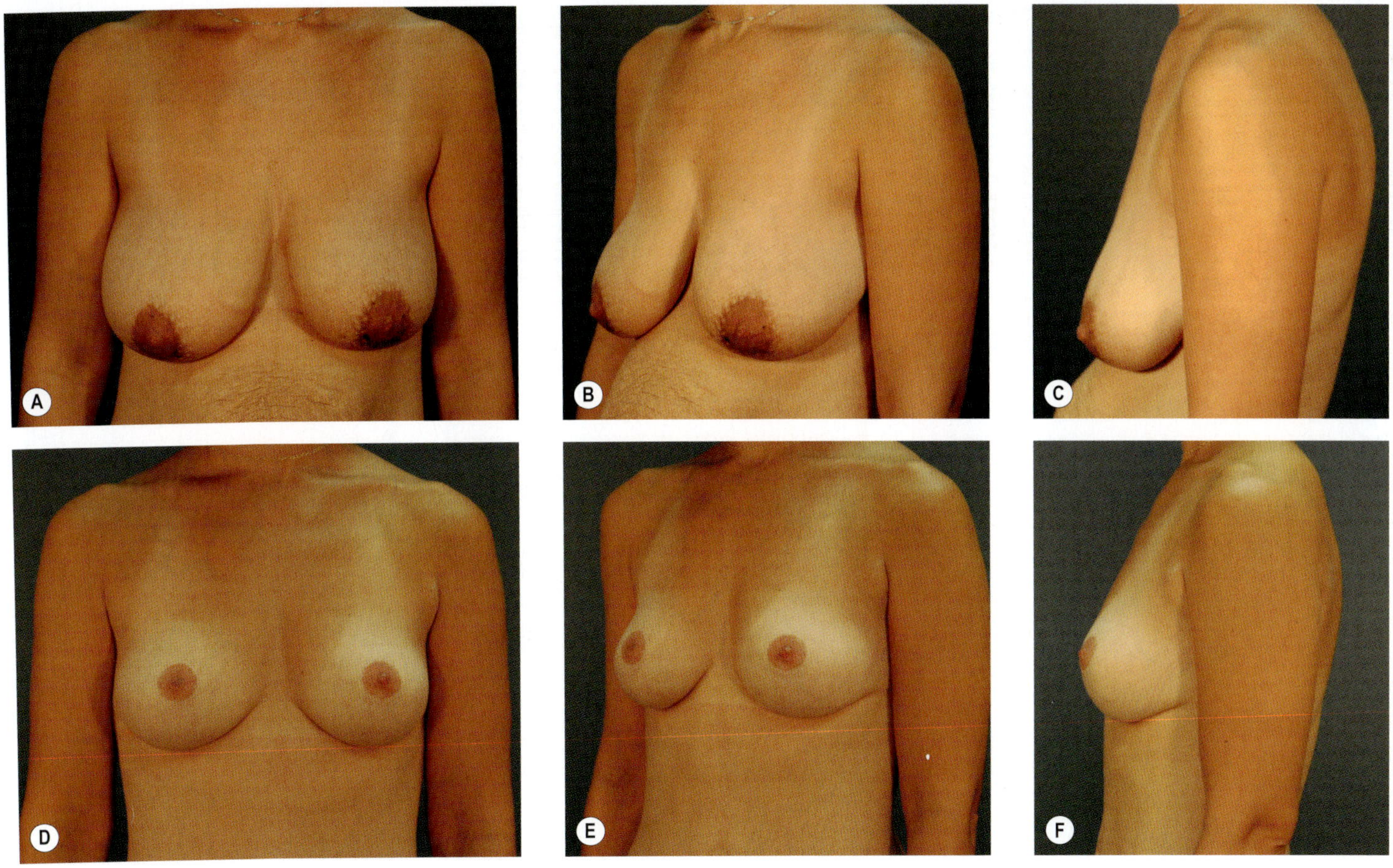

Figure 15.38 (A–C) Preoperative views of a 31-year-old patient with moderate to severe ptosis. **(D–F)** Postoperative views after vertical mastopexy via the authors' technique.

oxygen therapy (if available), and appropriate antibiotic therapy.

- Many times, conservative treatment and closure by secondary intention produce a satisfactory result. If healing does not produce a satisfactory result, the nipple-areola complex can be reconstructed by standard reconstruction techniques ranging from simple tattooing of the areola to flap reconstructions of the nipple itself.
- Prominent scars may first receive a trial of vitamin E, compression with tape or silicone sheeting, laser treatment, or intralesional triamcinolone (Kenalog) injections.
- It is preferable to assess patients for scar revision after 1 year.
- Flap necrosis can occur by virtue of the flaps used, especially when the inverted-T or Wise-pattern mastopexy technique is used.
- Treatment is similar to that of the ischemic nipple: greasy dressings, hyperbaric oxygen, or antibiotics.
- Debridement of large areas of flap necrosis should be undertaken when they are clearly demarcated and delayed closure can be performed, thereby avoiding weeks or months of caring for an open breast wound.
- Small areas of skin necrosis (1–2 cm) may be treated conservatively, especially along the inframammary fold.
- The nipple should be properly situated on the breast, at or near the point of greatest projection, with ample but not an excessive amount of tissue underneath it.
- When malposition of the nipple occurs, one can attempt to reposition it; however, one should wait at least several months to allow complete healing of the breast and nipple-areolar complex.
- It is easier to raise the nipple-areolar complex than to lower it.
- Nipples that appear too high can be caused by one of two situations: bottoming out or incorrect positioning.
- If bottoming out has occurred, simple tissue resection can be performed inferiorly.
- If incorrect positioning has occurred, attempts to lower the nipple include V-Y advancements inferiorly, transposition as a flap, or transfer as a graft.
- Over-resection, under-resection, and healing complications can contribute to cosmetic disappointments.
- Other complications can include infection and hematoma.

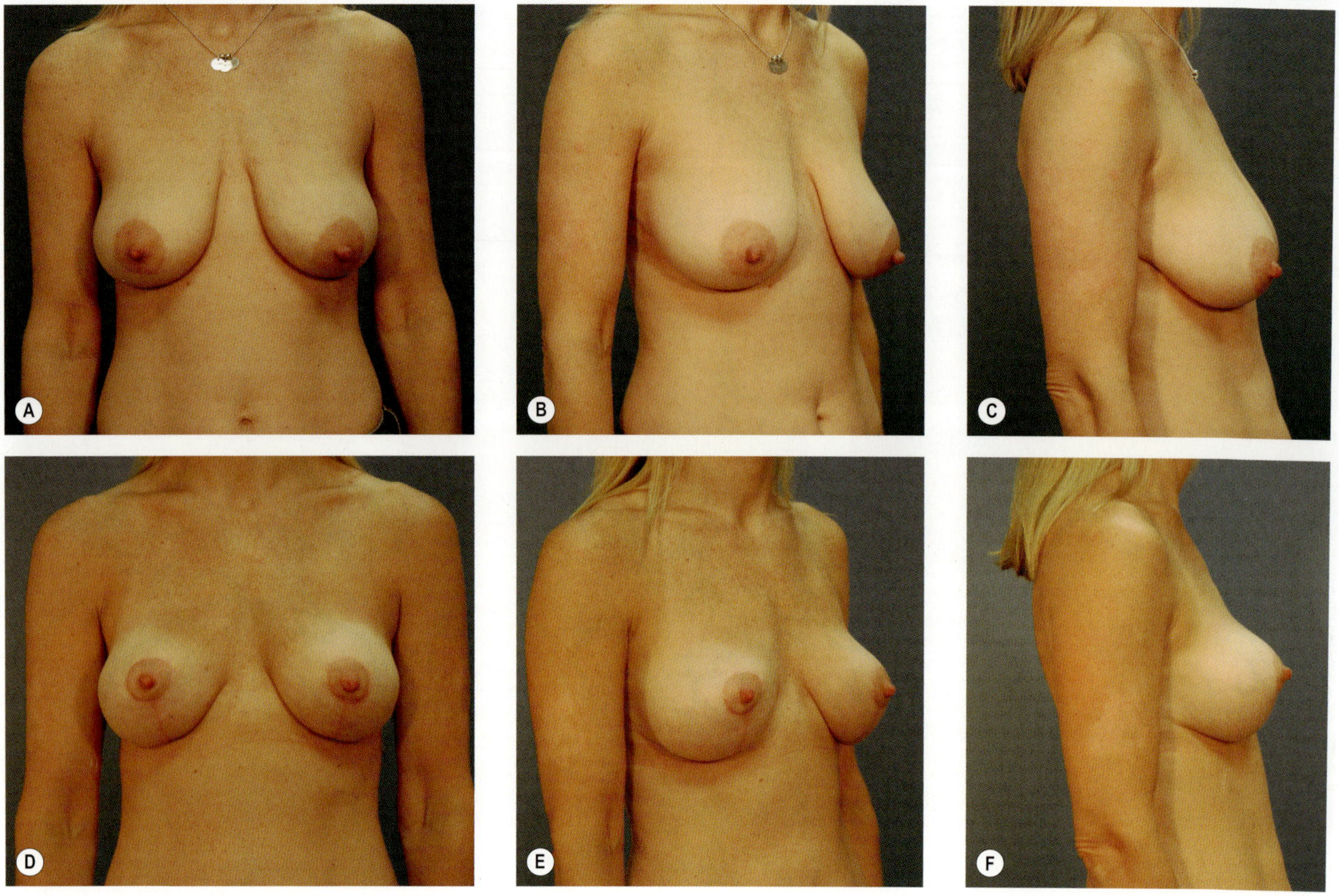

Figure 15.39 **(A–C)** Preoperative views of a 37-year-old female with bilateral breast ptosis with asymmetric nipple position but similar parenchymal volumes. **(D–F)** Postoperative views after bilateral vertical mastopexy via the authors' technique.

Further reading

Benelli L. A new periareolar mammaplasty: the "round block" technique. *Aesthetic Plast Surg*. 1990;14:93–100.

The round block acts as a keystone element to support the reshaped breast. The keystone relies on a crisscross mastopexy and by a circular nonresorbable suture of woven nylon included in the periareolar circular dermal scar. The crisscross mastopexy is achieved via dermis-to-dermis, gland-to-gland, and gland-to-musculoperiosteal unions, all of which are fixed definitively with nonresorbable suture. This technique can be used in many different breast cases, such as that for correction of ptosis, hypertrophy, or hypomastia, among others. In cases of hypomastia, the use of the round block technique permits easy access for insertion of the prosthesis as it simultaneously corrects ptosis. In cases of tumor excision, the round block produces a discrete scar and a more regular breast contour. In all types of mammaplasty, the main goal is to limit the scar.

Góes JC. Periareolar mammaplasty: double skin technique with application of polyglactine or mixed mesh. *Plast Reconstr Surg*. 1996;97(5):959–968.

Hall-Findlay EJ. A simplified vertical reduction mammaplasty: shortening the learning curve. *Plast Reconstr Surg*. 1999;104:748–763.

Hall-Findlay EJ. Pedicles in vertical breast reduction and mastopexy. *Clin Plast Surg*. 2002;29(3):379–391.

Lassus C. Breast reduction: evolution of a technique. A single vertical scar. *Aesthetic Plast Surg*. 1987; 11:107.

Patients had become more critical about the result of a breast reduction operation over the past 20 years. Natural and lasting shape, as well as minimal residual scarring, is now expected by most of the patients undergoing that surgery. In 1969, the author described a vertical technique that achieved reduction and good shape but the end of the vertical scar could be seen below the brassiere line. In 1977, the author modified the technique by adding a small horizontal scar that eliminated the visible part of the vertical scar. In this article, the author demonstrates that the same technique he described in 1969 and modified in 1977 can produce a single residual vertical scar if properly used.

Lejour M. Vertical mammaplasty and liposuction of the breast. *Plast Reconstr Surg*. 1994;94:100–114.

From 1989 to 1994, the author has used vertical mammaplasty without a submammary scar for all breast reductions. Using a technique relying on adjustable markings, an upper pedicle for the areola, and a central breast reduction with limited skin undermining, the author achieves a breast whose shape is created by suturing the gland and does not rely on the skin. A personal series of 100 consecutive patients (192 breasts) operated on from 1990 through 1992 is reviewed, and mastopexy was performed in 39 breasts. Among the 153 breasts that required reduction, liposuction was attempted as a complementary procedure before the surgical reduction in the 120 fattest breasts. Between 100 and 1000 cc of fat (mean 300 cc) was suctioned in 86 breasts. This figure represents 50% of the large breasts in patients under 50 years old and 100% of the breasts in patients older than 50 years. There were few complications, and none required early reoperation. This series proves that vertical mammaplasty can be used in all cases of breast reduction, producing consistently good, stable results with limited scars. The adjunctive use of liposuction in fatty breasts can be considered safe and efficient.

Marchac D, Olarte G. Reduction mammaplasty and correction of ptosis with a short inframammary scar. *Plast Reconstr Surg*. 1982;69:45.

Spear SL, Kassan M, Little JW. Guidelines in concentric mastopexy. *Plast Reconstr Surg*. 1990;85(6):961–966.

In an effort to limit complications associated with periareolar mastopexy techniques, Spear et al. designed a series of rules to follow. Rule 1: $D_{outside} \leq D_{original} + (D_{original} - D_{inside})$*. The amount of nonpigmented skin excised should be less than the amount of pigmented skin excised. This should prevent a postoperative areola larger than the original. Rule 2:* $D_{outside} < 2 \times D_{inside}$*: the design of the outside diameter should be no more than two times the inside diameter in order to minimize the discrepancy in circle sizes, thereby reducing tension on the closure. This should prevent an overly ambitious plan to remove skin, and, as a result, limit the risk of poor scars and overly-flattened breasts. Rule 3:* $D_{final} = \frac{1}{2}(D_{outside} + D_{inside})$*. This final rule helps predict the final areolar size, which is particularly useful in asymmetry cases, as well as those in whom no round block suture is employed.*

Steinberg JP, Braun BI, Hellinger WC, et al. Timing of antimicrobial prophylaxis and the risk of surgical site infections: results from the Trial to Reduce Antimicrobial Prophylaxis Errors. *Ann Surg*. 2009;250(1):10–16.

von Heimburg D, Exner K, Kruft S, et al. The tuberous breast deformity: classification and treatment. *Br J Plast Surg*. 1996;49:339–345.

Wise RJ, Gannon JP, Hill JR. Further experience with reduction mammaplasty. *Plast Reconstr Surg*. 1963;32:12.

In 1955, the senior author (Wise) presented a new technique for reduction mammaplasty using special patterning devices, and this publication demonstrates the further experiences of the authors. The author's technique allows rapid design of skin flaps and predictable size, contour, symmetry, and nipple position, all of which are difficult to achieve using a free-hand design. A four quadrant form is placed after designing and shaping the skin flaps, and the excess breast tissue is removed via wedge-shaped excisions. Care is taken not to remove too much from the central breast axis and the nipple, as well as not to undermine the skin flaps, to maintain perfusion of all these areas. The results allow for correction of varying degrees of ptosis and breast hypertrophy, as evidenced by case examples.

16 Chapter

Reduction mammaplasty

This chapter was created using content from Neligan & Grotting, Plastic Surgery 3rd edition, Volume 5, Breast, Chapter 8.1, Reduction mammaplasty, Jack Fisher and Kent K. Higdon.

SYNOPSIS

- Macromastia, or mammary hypertrophy, is a disease process which can result in physical and psychological symptoms.
- Macromastia symptoms rarely improve without surgical intervention, which typically results in significant improvement in the patient's quality of life.
- Reduction mammaplasty techniques have evolved over millennia, with particularly great strides made in the last 100 years.
- Currently, there exist several well-designed techniques based on sound surgical principles to address macromastia via reduction mammaplasty.

Brief introduction

- Patients with mammary hypertrophy can present with a variety of symptoms.
- Physical complaints include neck and back pain, shoulder grooving from bra-straps indenting the skin, headaches, difficulty finding well-fitted clothes and limited ability to exercise, intertriginious skin maceration and rashes.
- Psychosocial issues include embarrassment, especially teenagers and elderly women.
- Though the symptomatic improvement of patients suffering from mammary hypertrophy is the primary goal of reduction mammaplasty, there is another goal that is nearly as equally important – creating a more aesthetic breast.
- Spear describes the reduction mammaplasty as "the clearest example of the interface between reconstructive plastic surgery and aesthetic plastic surgery."
- This chapter seeks to demonstrate the most popular techniques for reduction mammaplasty. The key point for choosing the reduction mammoplasty technique is finding what works for you, the surgeon, and what gives your patients the best results.
- As breast reduction procedures have evolved, certain goals have been consistent:
  - Aesthetic, natural breast shape.
  - Maintainance of shape long term.
  - Reducing scar length.

Preoperative considerations

- Careful consideration of the factors that compel patients to seek reduction mammaplasty are key in the plastic surgeon's assessment of patients with mammary hypertrophy.
- A thorough history of symptoms associated with mammary hyperplasia should be recorded.
- A personal and family history of breast disease and surgery should be recorded, and the results of any testing, such as mammography, breast ultrasound or MRI, and BRCA testing should be obtained prior to surgical intervention.
- In addition to screening, a thorough physical examination should be performed as well, noting any relevant points of the patient's general condition as well as an examination of the breast. In the USA, only some breast reduction procedures are considered medically necessary.
- Such salient general points relate to the patient's height, weight, and habitus, and these measures are often mandatory for insurers to calculate the amount of breast

tissue they require for the reduction procedure to be covered.
- This amount of tissue can, however, vary from state to state and from insurer to insurer.
- A focal breast exam is mandatory as well, evaluating for any masses of the breast, axilla, and supra- and infraclavicular fossae. The nipple-areolar complex should be assessed for changes or discharge, as well as its preoperative sensitivity.
- Some women have decreased sensitivity due to prior surgery, but often there is decreased sensitivity due to the excess weight of the breast causing traction injury to the cutaneous innervation of the nipple-areolar complex.
- The skin of the breast should be scrutinized to assess for stigmata of previous operations or physiologic changes, such as scars or striae, which should be pointed out to the patient preoperatively.
- Finally, shape and symmetry of the breasts preoperatively must also be assessed and pointed out to the patient, especially in cases of very large breasts, because some degree of asymmetry will virtually always remain postoperatively.
- Breast measurements, such as the sternal notch to nipple distance, the nipple to inframammary fold distance, and the nipple to nipple distance, must be documented preoperatively.

Anatomical pearls

- The pathophysiology of mammary hypertrophy is thought to be the result of an abnormal response of the breast to circulating estrogens, causing breast proliferation which is predominantly fibrous tissue, fat, and, to a lesser degree, glandular tissue.
- Most women with mammary hypertrophy have normal circulating levels of estrogen as well as normal numbers of estrogen receptors in the breast tissue.
- Cases of juvenile virginal hypertrophy of the breast can be seen as early as late childhood and often is present in the age range of 11–14 years of age.
- Gigantomastia is a condition in patients with mammary hypertrophy that is defined by their need to have over 1800 g of tissue resected.
- Increasing sternal notch to nipple distances portend a decreased likelihood for success using a superiorly-based pedicle.
- Vertical short-scar techniques can be performed comfortably if the sternal notch to nipple distance is <38 cm.
- In cases where the sternal notch to nipple distance exceeds 40 cm, plastic surgeons should seriously consider lower pole breast amputation via a Wise pattern skin resection with either free nipple grafting or immediate nipple reconstruction with subsequent tattoo of the areola.
- Longer inframammary fold to nipple distances ultimately may preclude the use of an inferior pedicle technique.
- If the inframammary fold to nipple distance is >22 cm, there may be difficulty with inferior pedicle or central mound techniques.

Operative techniques (Video 16.1; Video 16.2; Video 16.3)

Video 16.1
Video 16.2
Video 16.3

General concepts

- Reduction mammaplasty is performed by combining a skin incision/resection with a parenchymal resection.
- There have been many techniques described for incision placement, parenchymal resection, and dermoglandular pedicled position. And in general, any combination of these techniques can be utilized for a successful reduction.
- Preoperative markings and measurements are placed with the patient standing or seated in an upright position. This includes:
  - The midline from sternal notch to xyphoid.
  - The midclavicular and breast meridian line.
  - The projection of the inframammary crease superimposed onto the midclavicular line.
  - The appropriate skin incision pattern i.e., vertical, Wise, etc.
- The patients are placed in the supine position, under general anesthesia.
- Make certain the patients hips are placed at the break in the bed to allow for the head to be raised during the surgery to assist with determination of symmetry.
- Lidocaine with epinephrine is infiltrated along the incisions and into the planned parenchymal resection.
  - Infiltration of local anesthetic into the dermoglandular pedicle should be avoided.
- Some authors have combined suction lipectomy with reduction mammaplasty techniques to assist with postoperative breast contour and reduction of axillary fullness or lateral chest rolls.
  - Care must be taken to avoid infiltration of tumescent solution or passage of suction cannulas into the planned dermoglandular pedicle.
- A nipple-areolar complex marker or cookie cutter of desired size is used to mark the periareolar incisions.
- The peri-areolar incision is performed first and the surrounding areas of the pedicle are de-epithelialized.
  - Care must be taken to avoid getting too deep as direct injury to the subdermal plexus could lead to vascular compromise of the nipple.
- The remaining skin incisions are made and skin flaps created.
- After parenchymal resection and excess skin is removed, meticulous hemostasis should be obtained.
- Closure often involves a combination of deep shaping sutures within the remaining parenchyma, followed by layered closure of the skin.
- The new nipple areolar complex position is marked using the nipple areolar complex marker of desired size.

- The nipple areolar complex is inset into its new position and secured using a combination of dermal and subcuticular closure.

Specific techniques *(Figs 16.1–16.9)*

Postoperative considerations

- Most patients can be discharged home on the same day following reduction mammaplasty.
- Depending on the size of the parenchymal resection, some authors advocate the use of closed suction drains.
- When used, drains are typically removed on postoperative day 1.
- In Wise pattern skin incision techniques, postoperative brassieres containing underwires should be avoided for 6–8 weeks to prevent direct pressure over incisions.
- Full-on running or activities that tend to cause vigorous up and down motion of the new breasts are restricted until 8 weeks postoperatively.
- Nipple-areolar complex sutures are generally removed on the 10th day.

Complications and outcomes

- One of the most devastating complications of reduction mammaplasty is nipple loss.
- Risk factors include technical errors, smoking, diabetes, obesity, and hypertension.
- In high-risk patients (smokers, patients with diabetes or obesity, or those with severe ptosis), a free nipple graft technique is an option that can be considered and is also a possibility intraoperatively or postoperatively if the viability of the transposed nipple appears compromised.

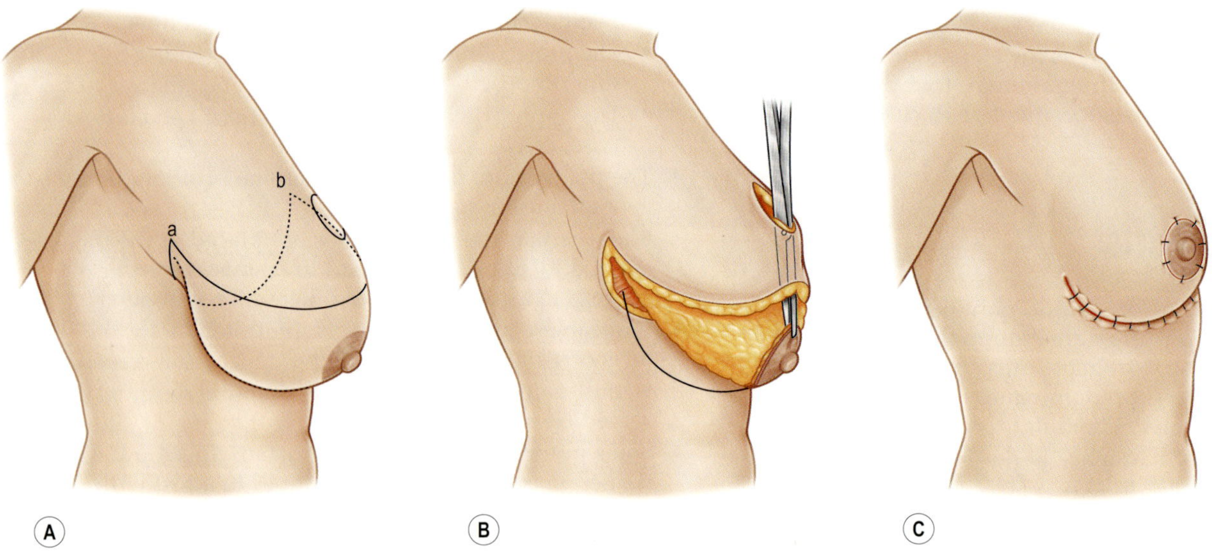

Figure 16.1 (A–C) Passot technique of nipple transposition. (Redrawn after Lickstein LH, Shestak KC. The conceptual evolution of modern reduction mammoplasty. *Operat Tech Plast Reconstr Surg.* 1999;6:88–96.)

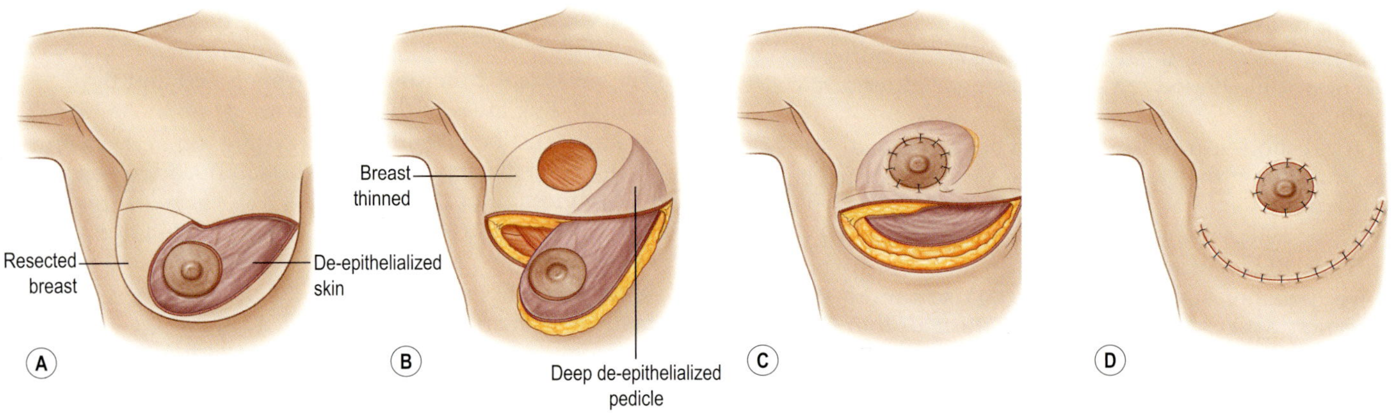

Figure 16.2 (A–D) Schwarzmann reduction with superomedial dermoglandular pedicle. (Redrawn after Lickstein LH, Shestak KC. The conceptual evolution of modern reduction mammoplasty. *Operat Tech Plast Reconstr Surg.* 1999;6:88–96.)

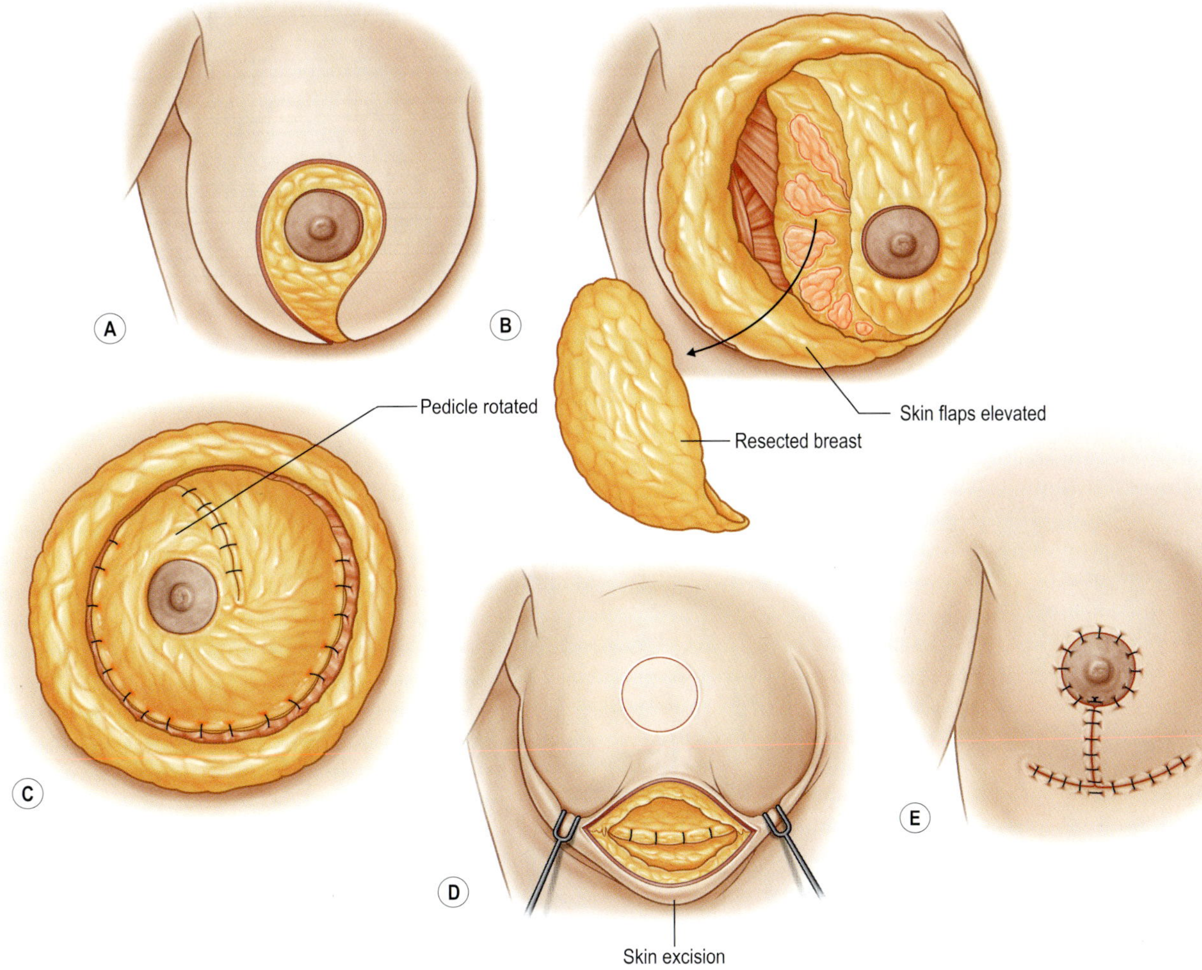

Figure 16.3 (A–E) Biesenberger reduction – degloving the breast with inverted T closure. (Redrawn after Lickstein LH, Shestak KC. The conceptual evolution of modern reduction mammoplasty. *Operat Tech Plast Reconstr Surg.* 1999;6:88–96.)

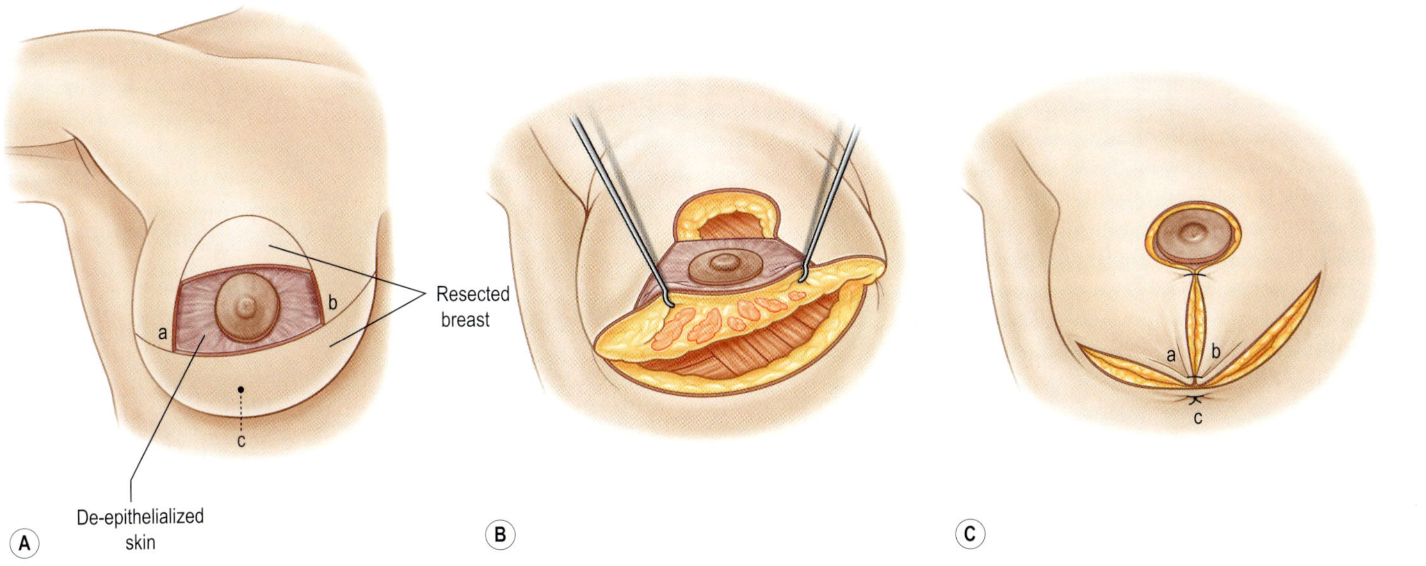

Figure 16.4 (A–C) Strombeck horizontal bipedicle technique. (Redrawn after Lickstein LH, Shestak KC. The conceptual evolution of modern reduction mammoplasty. *Operat Tech Plast Reconstr Surg.* 1999;6:88–96.)

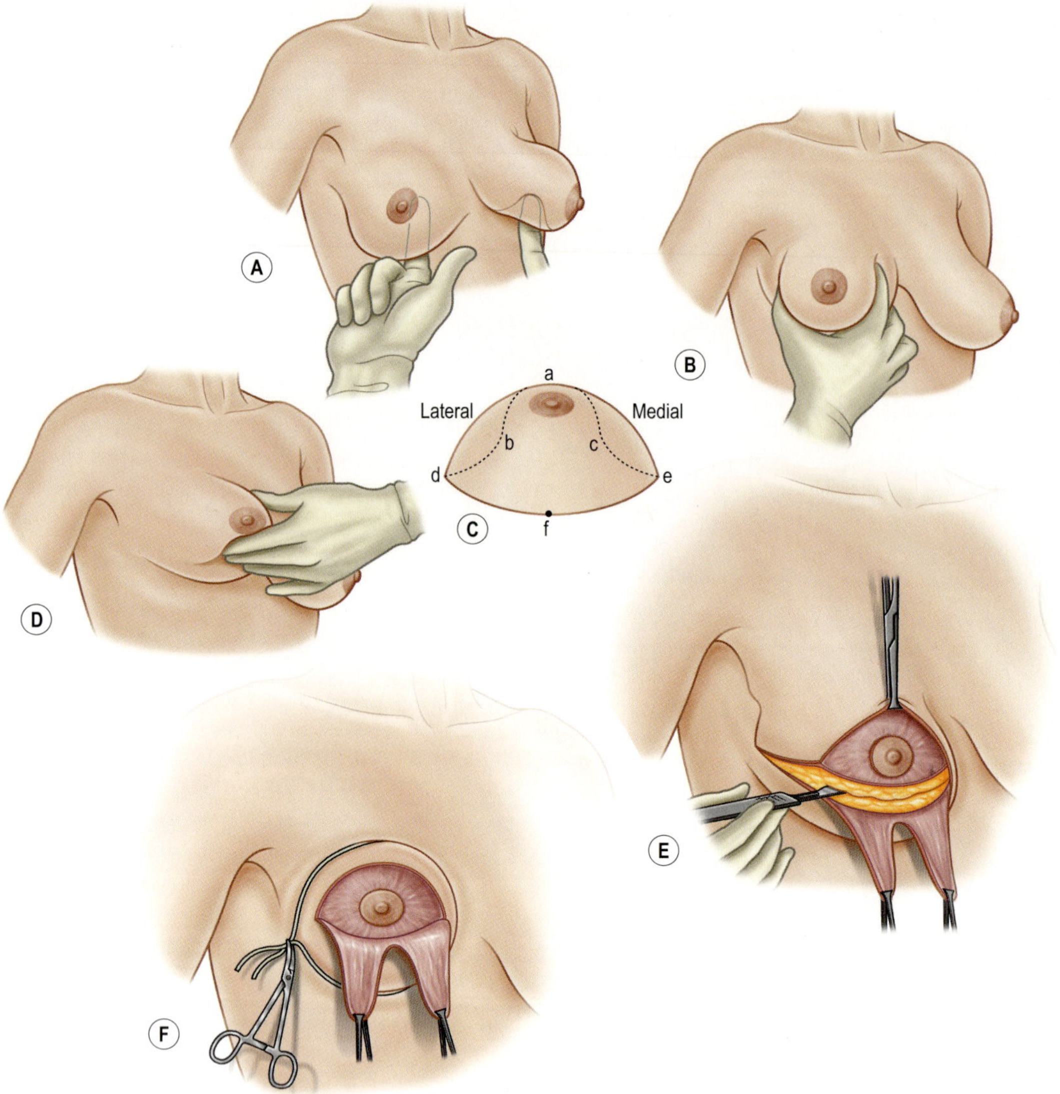

Figure 16.5 (A–N) McKissock vertical bipedicled dermoglandular flap with Wise-pattern skin excision. (Redrawn after Lickstein LH, Shestak KC. The conceptual evolution of modern reduction mammoplasty. *Operat Tech Plast Reconstr Surg.* 1999;6:88–96.)

- The nipple-areolar complex may be converted to a free nipple graft up until approximately 12 h postoperatively.
- After 12 h, conservative treatment of any nipple necrosis should be undertaken, including release of sutures, topical nitropaste or leeches, greasy dressings, hyperbaric oxygen therapy (if available), and appropriate antibiotic therapy.
- Many times, conservative treatment and closure by secondary intention produces a satisfactory result. If healing does not produce a satisfactory result, the nipple-areola complex can be reconstructed by standard reconstruction techniques ranging from simple tattooing of the areola to flap reconstructions of the nipple itself.
- Hypertrophic and/or prominent scars may be treated with compression, silicone sheeting, laser treatment, or intralesional triamcinolone (Kenalog) injections.
- Tension free closure can minimize the risk of hypertophic scarring.
- It is preferable to assess patients for scar revision after 1 year.
- Flap necrosis can occur, especially when the inverted-T or Wise-pattern technique is used.
- Treatment includes vaseline gauze dressings, antibiotics, and selective debridement.
- Small areas of skin necrosis (1–2 cm) frequently occur along the inframammary fold at the T-junction and may be treated conservatively.
- Malposition of the nipple can sometimes be corrected with repositioning; however, one should wait at least several months to allow complete healing of the breast and nipple-areolar complex.
- Over-resection, under-resection, and healing complications can contribute to cosmetic disappointments.
- Other complications can include infection, hematoma, seroma, and fat necrosis.

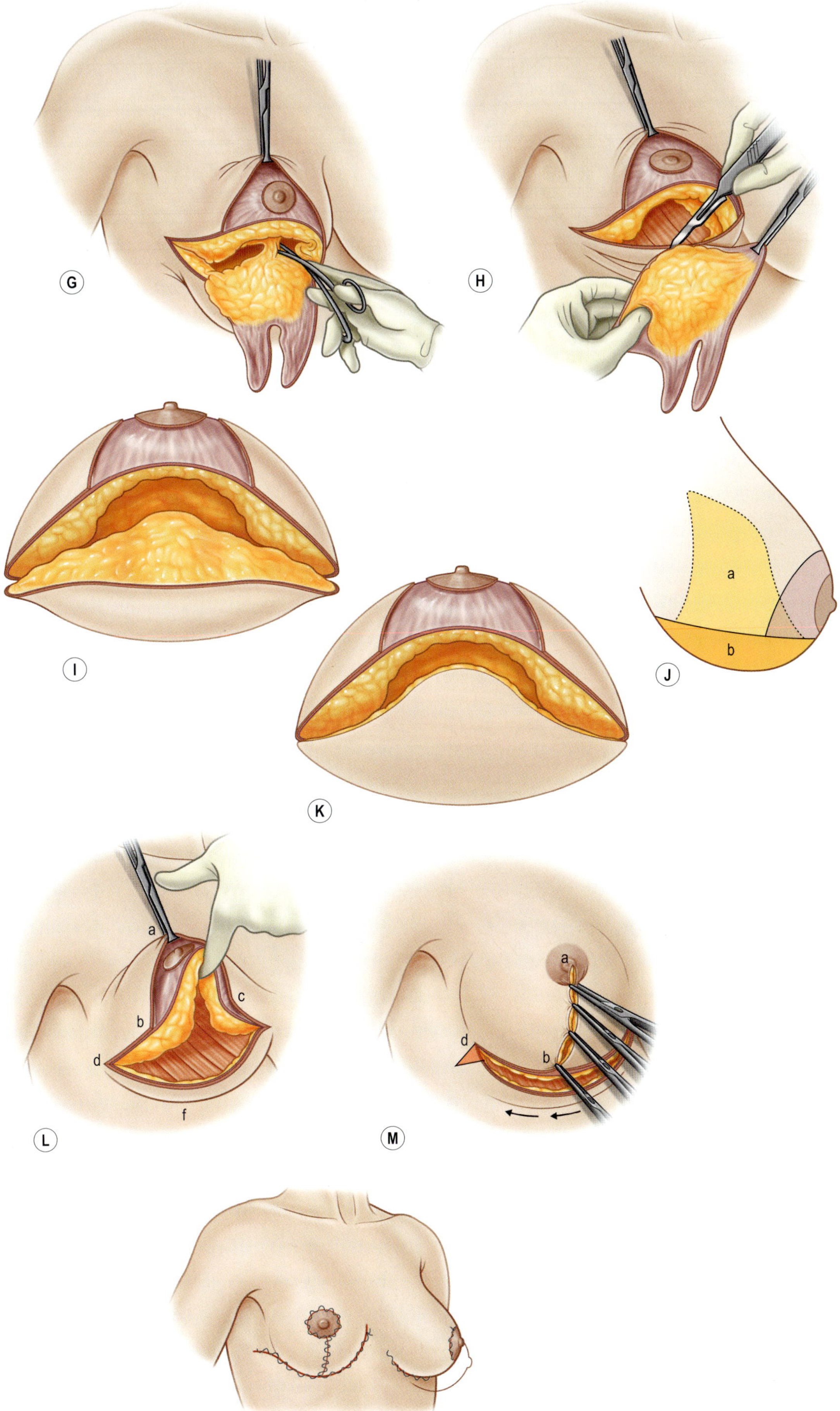

Figure 16.5, cont'd

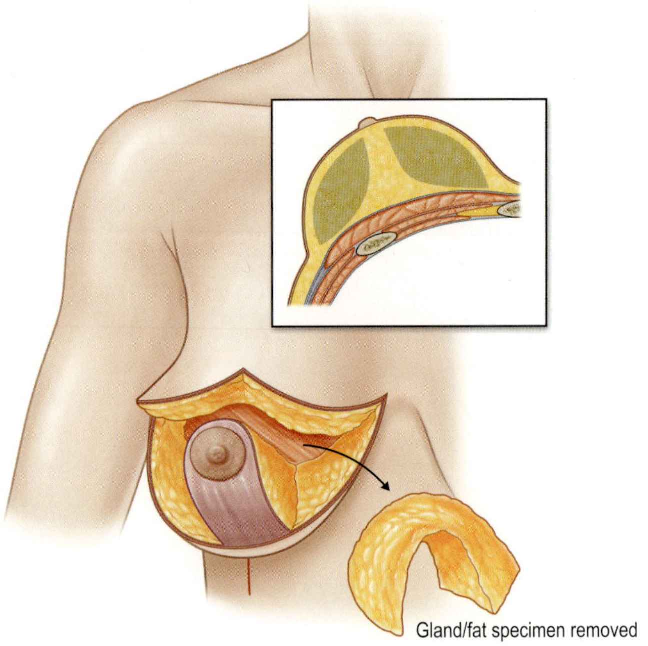

Figure 16.6 Inferior pedicle technique with Wise-pattern skin excision.

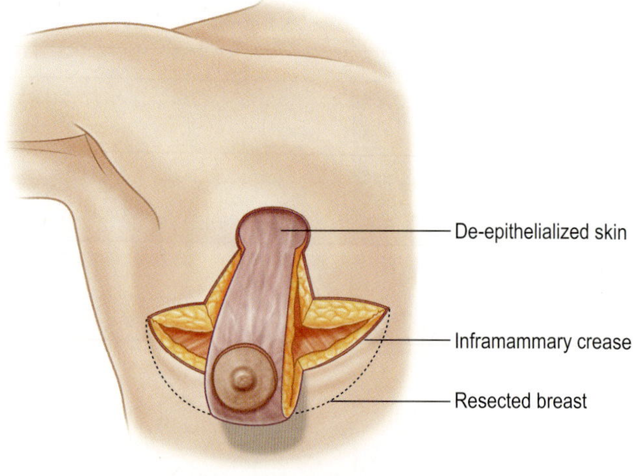

Figure 16.7 McKissock vertical dermoglandular flap with Wise-pattern skin excision. (Redrawn after Lickstein LH, Shestak KC. The conceptual evolution of modern reduction mammoplasty. *Operat Tech Plast Reconstr Surg.* 1999;6:88–96.)

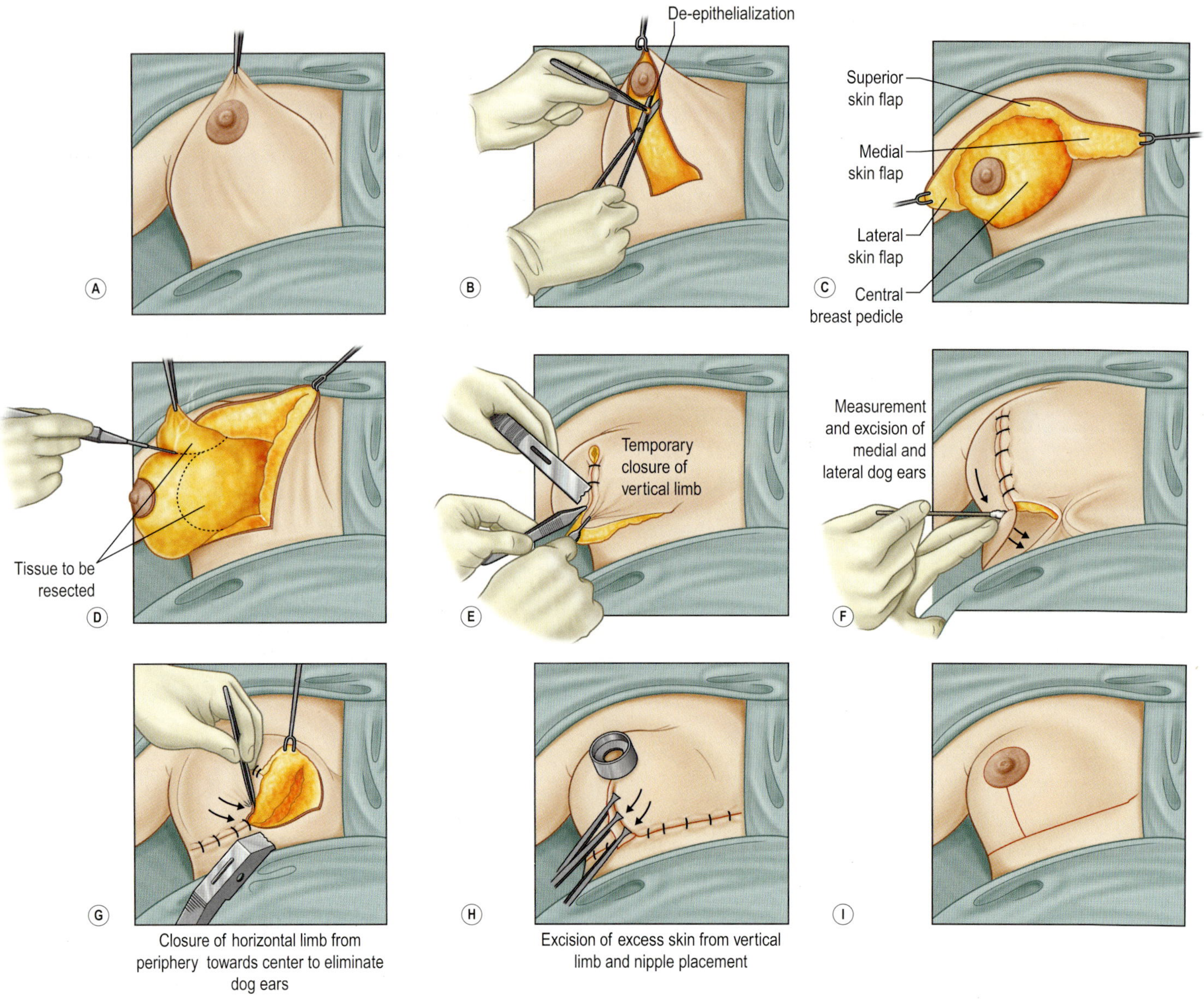

Figure 16.8 **(A–I)** Central mound technique popularized by Hester. (Redrawn from Hester TR Jr, Bostwick J III, Miller L. Breast reduction utilizing the maximally vascularized central pedicle. *Plast Reconstr Surg.* 1985;76:890–900.)

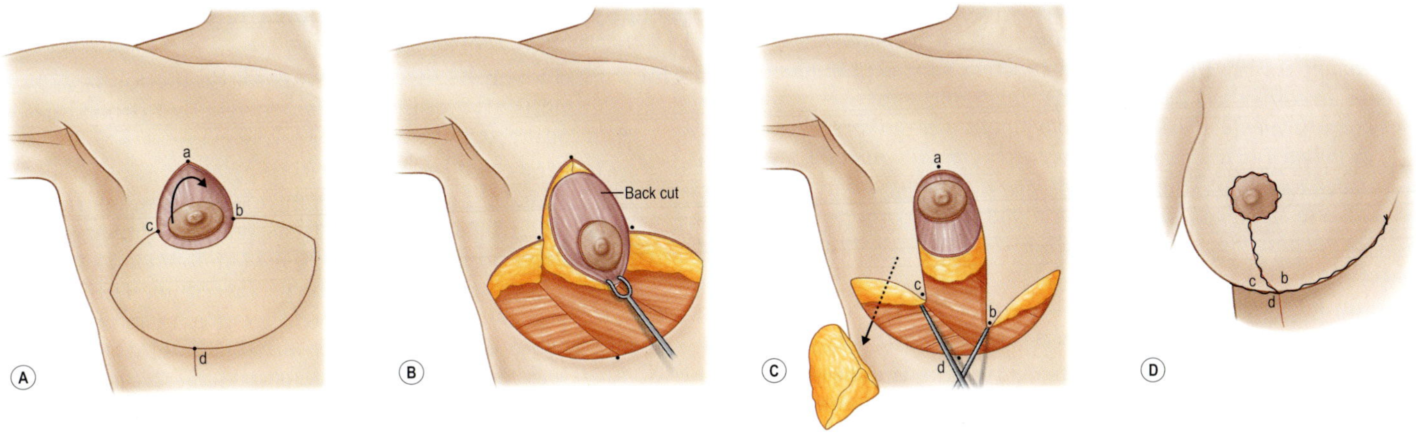

Figure 16.9 **(A–D)** Superomedial pedicle with Wise-pattern skin closure.

Further reading

Adams F. *The seven books of Paulus Aegineta. [Translated from the Greek.] With a commentary embracing a complete view of the knowledge possessed by the Greeks, Romans, and Arabians on all subjects connected with medicine and surgery. Vol 2.* London: Kessinger; 2009;(1844–1847):334–335.

Appel 3rd JZ, Wendel JJ, Zellner EG, et al. Association between preoperative measurements and resection weight in patients undergoing reduction mammaplasty. *Ann Plast Surg.* 2010;64(5):512–515.

Appel et al. performed a retrospective analysis of 348 patients undergoing bilateral reduction mammaplasty (696 breasts) between October 2001 and March 2009. The association between resection weight and sternal notch to nipple distance (SNN), inframammary fold to nipple distance (IMFN), and body mass index (BMI) was assessed. The authors concluded that resection weight correlates strongly with SNN, IMFN, and BMI in patients undergoing reduction mammoplasty and, when considered together, resection weight can be predicted with a great degree of accuracy.

Benelli L. A new periareolar mammaplasty: round block technique. *Aesthetic Plast Surg.* 1990;14:93.

Blomqvist L, Eriksson A, Brandberg Y. Reduction mammaplasty provides long-term improvement in health status and quality of life. *Plast Reconstr Surg.* 2000;106(5):991–997.

Blomqvist et al. investigated the health status and quality of life of patients who underwent reduction mammoplasty. They conducted a prospective four part questionnaire study in 49 women who were ≥20 years, using preoperative and postoperative assessments at 6 and 12 months. The authors found that reduction mammaplasty provided significant reduction of pain in all locations ($p < 0.001$), with an average weight of resected tissue being 1052 g, and the improvements continued up to 12 months postoperatively. Postoperatively, patients reported a significantly improved quality of life. After 1 year, there was no statistically significant difference between the post-reduction patients and the age-matched unoperated women, which suggested those women were normalized in health-related quality of life.

Dieffenbach JF. *Die operative chirurgerie. Vol 2.* Leipzig: Brockhaus; 1848:370.

Eliasen CA, Cranor ML, Rosen PP. Atypical duct hyperplasia of the breast in young females. *Am J Surg Pathol.* 1992;16(3):246–251.

Eliasen et al. demonstrated a predominance of atypical ductal hyperplasia in nine patients with macromastia, who ranged in age from 18 to 26 years (average 21 years). Though unable to find any significant gross abnormalities within the resected breast tissue except for two fibroadenomas, the authors were able to demonstrate that each case had a continuum of microscopic ductal changes, which ranged from partial to complete involvement by micropapillary and lactiform epithelial hyperplasia.

Hall-Findlay EJ. A simplified vertical reduction mammaplasty: shortening the learning curve. *Plast Reconstr Surg.* 1999;104(3):748–763.

Hester Jr TR, Bostwick III J, Miller L. Breast reduction utilizing the maximally vascularized central pedicle. *Plast Reconstr Surg.* 1985;76:890.

Lassus C. Breast reduction: evolution of a technique – a single vertical scar. *Aesthetic Plast Surg.* 1987;11(2):107–112.

Lejour M, Abboud M. Vertical mammaplasty without inframammary scar and with breast liposuction. *Perspect Plast Surg.* 1990;4:67.

Netscher DT, Meade RA, Goodman CM, et al. Physical and psychosocial symptoms among 88 volunteer subjects compared to patients seeking plastic surgery procedures to the breast. *Plast Reconstr Surg.* 2000;105:2366–2373.

Netscher investigated the relationship between macromastia and physical and psychosocial symptoms. A total of 21 augmentation mammaplasty patients and 31 breast reduction patients were graded on their somatic and psychosocial symptoms and compared with a control group of 88 female university students. The study's purpose was to discover which complaints were most common among women presenting for reduction mammaplasty and to determine whether body mass index and chest measurements affected their symptoms. The authors concluded that patients who present with symptomatic macromastia seeking reduction mammaplasty have a disease-specific group of physical and psychosocial complaints that are more directly related to large breast size than to being overweight.

Orlando JC, Guthrie Jr RH. The superomedial pedicle for nipple transposition. *Br J Plast Surg*. 1975;28:42.

Passot R. La correction esthetique du prolapsus mammaire par le procede de la transposition du mamelon. *Presse Med*. 1925;33:317.

Penn J. Breast reduction. *Br J Plast Surg*. 1955;7:357.

Pitanguy I. Surgical correction of breast hypertrophy. *Br J Plast Surg*. 1967;20:78.

Schnur PL, Hoehn JG, Ilstrup DM, et al. Reduction mammaplasty: cosmetic or reconstructive procedure? *Ann Plast Surg*. 1991;27(3):232–237.

In the study by Schnur et al., 92 of 220 plastic surgeons that responded to their survey included information (height, weight, and amount of breast tissue removed) from 600 women regarding the last 15–20 reduction mammaplasties by each surgeon. A second survey followed to estimate percentages of women who sought reduction mammaplasties for purely cosmetic reasons, for mixed reasons, and for purely medical reasons, and 132 of the same 220 surgeons responded.

Wise RJ. A preliminary report on a method of planning the mammaplasty. *Plast Reconstr Surg*. 1956;17:367.

Chapter 17

Implant based breast reconstruction

This chapter was created using content from Neligan & Grotting, Plastic Surgery 3rd edition, Volume 5, Breast, Chapter 14, Expander-implants breast reconstruction, Maurizio B. Nava, Giuseppe Catanuto, Angela Pennati, Valentina Visintini Cividin and Andrea Spano, Chapter 15, Latissimus dorsi flap breast reconstruction, Scott L. Spear and Mark W. Clemens.

SYNOPSIS (IMPLANT-BASED RECONSTRUCTION)

- Implant-based breast reconstructions can be employed in all patients, provided that they have not been previously irradiated.
- Medium size anatomically-shaped permanent silicone implants can be employed to reconstruct virtually all breasts, irrespective of shape and size.
- A contralateral adjustment should be part of the reconstructive project.
- Breast reconstruction in the large breast can be accomplished in one stage ("Skin reducing mastectomy").

SYNOPSIS (LATISSIMUS FLAP RECONSTRUCTION)

- The latissimus flap includes a large well-vascularized flat muscle that is well suited for dealing with poorly-vascularized or radiated defects, contour deformities following breast conservation therapy, or for covering an implant.
- Placement of a tissue expander under the latissimus muscle allows postoperative adjustment of breast volume and ultimately better symmetry with the opposite breast.
- Complete mobilization to reach medial breast defects may require the partial release (90%) of the latissimus dorsi insertion. This helps avoid the displeasing bulge in the low axilla; however, care must be taken to protect the thoracodorsal vessels.
- The extended latissimus dorsi flap is a reliable method for totally autologous breast reconstruction and can be considered a primary choice for breast reconstruction, particularly in women who otherwise are at high risk for a TRAM flap or an implant procedure.

Brief introduction

- With increasing recognition of the value of immediate reconstruction for the mastectomy patient, the option of expander-implant became more practical for incorporation into techniques for reconstruction.
- The first stage is insertion of the expander either at the time of mastectomy or delayed until the patient is referred or presents for reconstruction. If not performed at the time of the mastectomy, it is preferable to delay reconstruction by a minimum of 3 months and until adjuvant treatments are completed.
- Capsular contracture has been widely investigated as the major trade-off of prosthetic reconstructions.
- The beneficial effects of the acellular dermal matrix in the prevention of long-term complications such as capsular contracture or poor morphological results may be hindered by a higher percentage of short-term severe complications, including seroma and infection.
- *Advantages* of the expander-implant technique for breast reconstruction include the following:
  - Minimal morbidity.
  - Reduced operative time.
  - Although there are usually two procedures involved, each is relatively short and may or may not require a hospital stay.
  - No donor site morbidity.
  - If the patient becomes dissatisfied with the result, all pre-existing flaps are still available.
- *Disadvantages* of the expander-implant technique for breast reconstruction include the below.

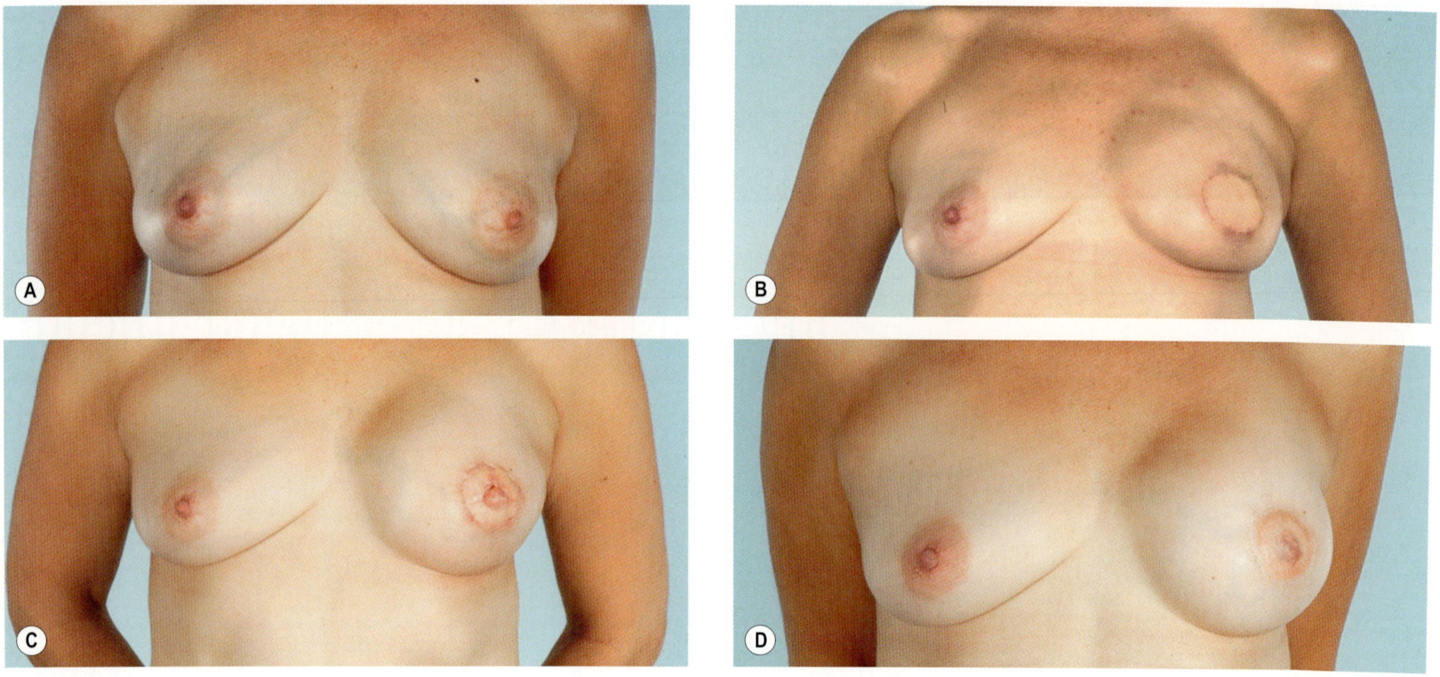

Figure 17.1 **(A)** Preoperative appearance of a 48-year-old female with left breast cancer requiring radiation. **(B)** Postoperative; patient is 2 months post-left mastectomy with reconstruction with a left latissimus dorsi flap and expander. **(C)** Postoperative; patient is 3 months post-left nipple construction and exchange of expander to silicone implant. **(D)** 1-year postoperatively.

- Complications inherent to implant use are:
  - Implant deflation or malfunction.
  - Capsular contracture.
  - Fear of adverse interactions between the patient's immune system and the device.
  - Contour irregularities visible on skin surface due to the underlying implant.
- The implant will not behave like normal vascularized tissue:
  - It will remain cooler than adjacent body parts when ambient temperature is low.
  - The reconstructed breast will not develop natural ptosis with advancing age.
- As the number of breast cancer cases continues to rise, progressively more of these women are receiving adjunctive radiation and may not be candidates for implant alone reconstructions.
- While the main workhorses of autologous reconstructions are abdominal based flaps, the latissimus dorsi myocutaneous flap is an essential reconstructive option and has gained renewed interest due to its reliability, ease of dissection, versatility, and minimal donor site morbidity *(Fig. 17.1)*.

Preoperative considerations

For expander/implant reconstructions

- General criteria for implant-expander reconstruction include an adequate skin envelope to support the expander-implant.
- The patient must be well informed about all options for breast reconstruction.
- The patient must be willing to accept the use of a permanent prosthesis.
- Relative contraindications to implant based reconstructions include previous radiation, skin fibrosis or scleroderma, and smoking as these all portend a higher risk of complications (e.g., infection, capsular contracture, expander/implant failure).
- Postoperative radiotherapy is controversial and the timing of expander-implant exchange with the adjuvant radiotherapy is often site/surgeon specific.

For latissimus flap reconstructions

- Particular attention is given to the amount of skin and subcutaneous tissue obtainable in the dorsal region.
  - A good indication is given by pinching the lateral dorsal pad to estimate the thickness of the adipose layer.
  - It is vital to compare the mass available with that which will be needed to achieve a suitable breast size.
  - It is also important preoperatively to assess the function of the latissimus dorsi muscle.
  - Denervated and non-functional muscle after an axillary dissection increases the risk of damaged thoracodorsal vessels or inadequate circulation.
  - In this instance, the latissimus dorsi must be elevated on an intact serratus collateral pedicle.
  - Functioning muscle is most often a favorable sign for the integrity of the pedicle; however, it does not guarantee intact thoracodorsal vessels.

- Indications for latissimus flap reconstruction include:
  - Breast reconstruction after a skin-sparing mastectomy when a breast prosthesis is part of the plan.
  - Partial mastectomy or lumpectomy deformities.
  - Patients who are not candidates for a TRAM flap.
  - Women who have had a previous abdominoplasty or TRAM flap, women with insufficient abdominal skin or fat, women who smoke, have diabetes, or are obese and may be considered to be too high risk to undergo a TRAM flap.
  - Previous irradiation during breast conservative therapy.
  - Excessively thin or unreliable skin flaps over an implant.
  - After a previous mastopexy or reduction as the skin flaps in these patients may be unreliable.
  - Women who have had breast augmentation previously may select a skin-sparing mastectomy with a latissimus flap over their breast prosthesis.
  - Large ptotic breasts.
  - Contraindications to latissimus flap reconstruction include:
  - Previous posterolateral thoracotomy in which the latissimus muscle had been divided.
  - An atrophic latissimus muscle after division of the thoracodorsal nerve during an axillary dissection.
  - Immediate latissimus reconstruction before radiation therapy.

Anatomical/technical pearls

Expander/implant selection

- The size of the device used is largely based on breast width, size and shape of the contralateral breast. It must also take into account the patient's wishes on contralateral symmetrization procedures.
- The expander should be usually the same height as the contralateral breast.
- The projection of tissue expanders is normally variable and depends on the level of inflation and amount of projection desired.

Latissimus flap anatomy

- The latissimus dorsi muscle is a large, flat, triangular muscle measuring approximately 25 × 35 cm and covering the posterior inferior half of the trunk.
- Origin: the iliac crest, the posterior layer of the thoracolumbar fascia, the lower six thoracic spines, and the lower third to fourth ribs laterally, where it is closely associated with some origins of the external oblique muscle.
- Insertion: intertubercular groove of the humerus.
- Near the tip of the scapula, it converges in a spiral fashion and joins with fibers of the teres major to form the posterior axillary fold.
- Near its insertion, the muscle becomes a 3 cm broad tendon.
- Action: to adduct, extend and internally rotate the upper extremity. It also assists in securing the tip of the scapula against the posterior chest wall.
- It is an expendable muscle because function is preserved by the remaining synergistic shoulder girdle muscles.
- Vascular supply: type V muscle according to the Mathes and Nahai classification.
- Dominant pedicle: the thoracodorsal artery, two venae comitantes, and the thoracodorsal nerve.
- The length of the thoracodorsal artery is 8 cm with a diameter of 2.5 mm.
- Along with the circumflex scapular artery, it is a branch of the subscapular artery arising from the axillary artery.
- Gives off a branch to the serratus muscle shortly after entering the underside of the latissimus muscle in the posterior axilla 10 cm inferior to the muscle insertion into the humerus ***(Fig. 17.2)***.
- Even when the thoracodorsal pedicle has been divided, a reversal of flow through the patent serratus branch can provide adequate blood flow to the flap.
- Secondary segmental pedicles: enter the underside of the muscle through the lateral perforators row off the posterior intercostal arteries 5 cm from the posterior midline and through the medial perforators row off the lumbar artery adjacent to the site of muscle origin.
- These perforators allow the use of the latissimus dorsi as a foldover flap to cover midback defects.
- Once it is in the muscle, the vascular pedicle bifurcates into a large lateral descending branch and a smaller transverse branch.
- This bifurcation makes it possible to split the muscle for use as a double flap or to preserve half of the muscle to maintain function.
- Numerous musculocutaneous perforators extend from the rich intramuscular vascular network into the overlying skin and subcutaneous tissue, allowing skin islands to be safely designed anywhere within the margin of the muscle.
- The largest perforators branch from the lateral branch of the thoracodorsal artery, making safest the skin island located in a lateral vertical orientation.
- At the level of the 10th–11th rib, there is a firm, thick aponeurotic attachment between the serratus anterior and the latissimus.
- These attachments must be divided to prevent inadvertent elevation of the serratus anterior muscle along with the latissimus dorsi flap.

Operative techniques

Expander/implant reconstruction

Video 17.1

Stage I: expander insertion (Video 17.1)

- Dissection starts from the lateral border of the pectoralis major muscle and it follows in the subpectoral plane superiorly, medially, and inferiorly ***(Fig. 17.3)***.

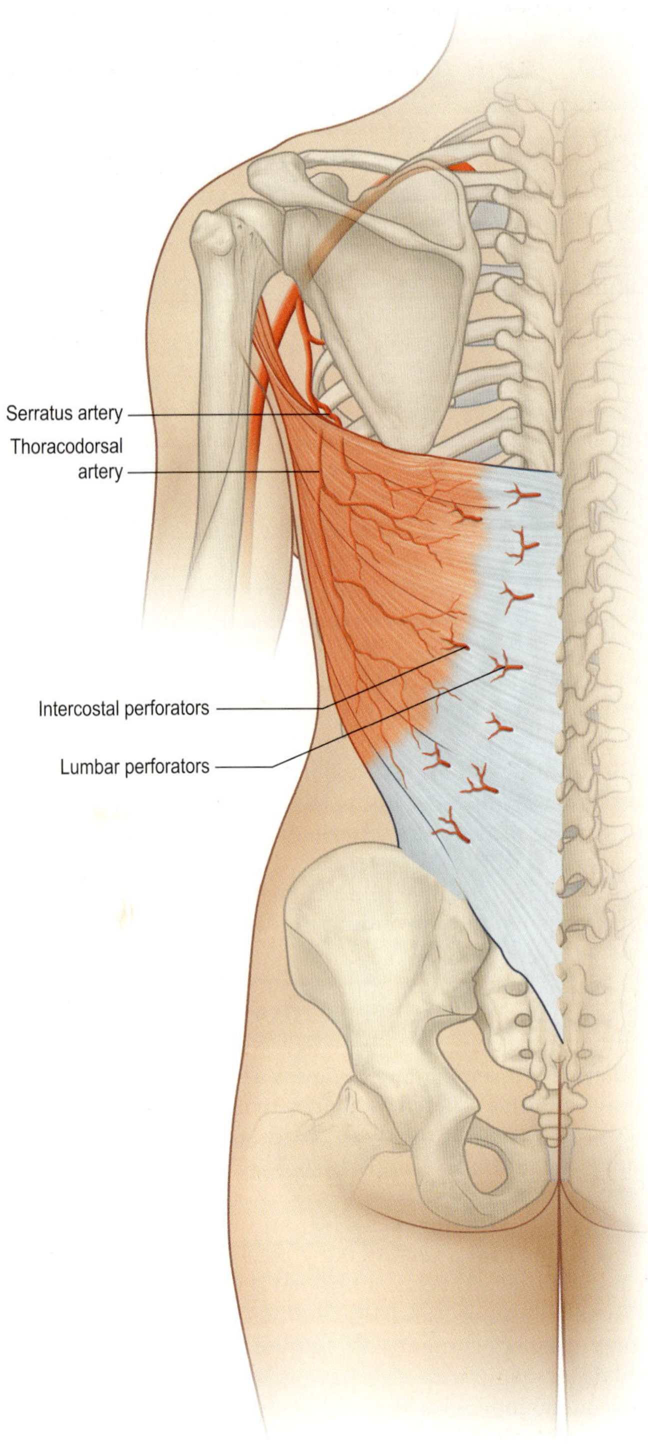

Figure 17.2 The blood supply to the latissimus dorsi muscle.

- The sternal attachments of the pectoralis major are detached from the second intercostal space to the inferior edge of the pocket *(Fig. 17.4)*.
  - The pocket should be completely sub-muscular except at the inframammary fold where, if this has been correctly preserved, it should extend into the deep fascial layer avoiding direct continuity with the mastectomy site *(Figs 17.5–17.7)*.

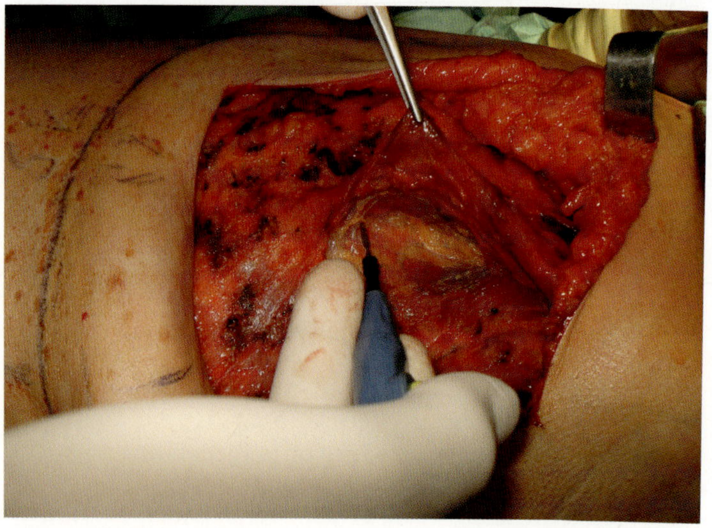

Figure 17.3 Expander positioning: dissection of the lateral border of pectoralis major.

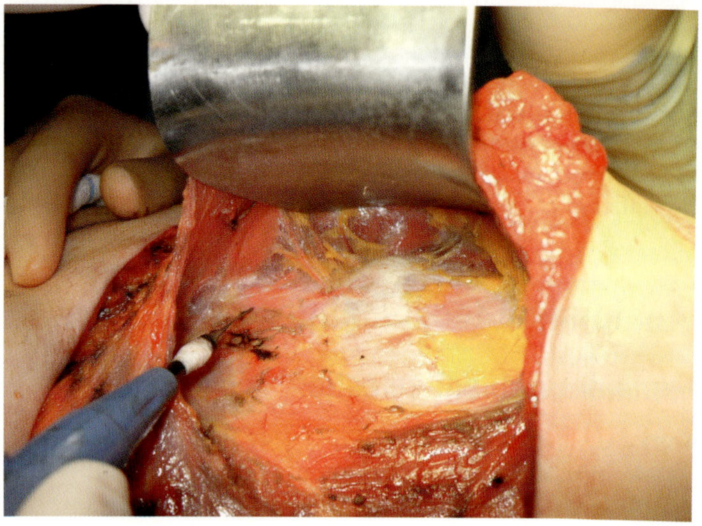

Figure 17.4 Muscular fibers detached from the rib insertion: perforator vessels of pectoralis major muscle can be isolated and diathermized.

  - In circumstances where the muscular fascia is injured, the inferior pectoralis attachments are disrupted, or there is a relative excess of skin which would accommodate greater intraoperative expansion, acellular dermal matrices (ADMs) may be used as an inferior sling to create a larger subpectoral pocket and assist with inferior pole expander coverage.
    - The ADM is secured inferiorly to the rectus fascia, laterally to the serratus fascia, and superiorly to the inferior border of the pectoralis.
- Once the pocket is created and hemostasis obtained, the expander is introduced and correctly oriented *(Figs 17.8, 17.9)*.
- Subcutaneous drains of the mastectomy pocket should be inserted.
- The sub-muscular pouch is closed with absorbable interrupted sutures, and the skin is closed in layers.

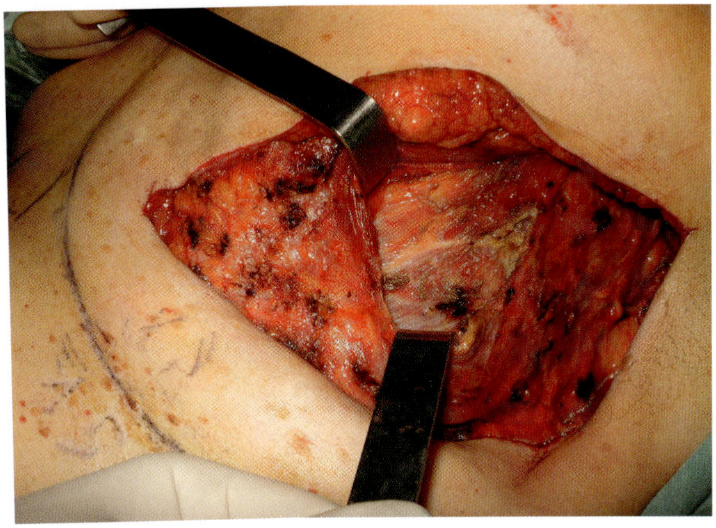

Figure 17.5 The totally submuscular pouch is made up of pectoralis major and serratus.

- The expander can be inflated to the maximal amount without causing undue tension on the skin closure. Typically, one can inflate the expander up to around 50% of the overall volume.

Stage II: expander/implant exchange (Video 17.2)

Video 17.2

- Commonly performed 6 months after the end of tissue expansion which allows tissue stretching and provides an initial degree of ptosis to the reconstructed breast as well as completion of adjuvant therapies when needed.
- The mastectomy scar can often be removed and a new access is created in the same place ***(Fig. 17.10)***.
- The subcutaneous layer is then dissected from the muscular fibers and the muscle is incised and split in the orientation of its anatomical direction.
- The expander is removed and replaced by the permanent implant of choice. In some cases, a total capsulectomy must be performed.

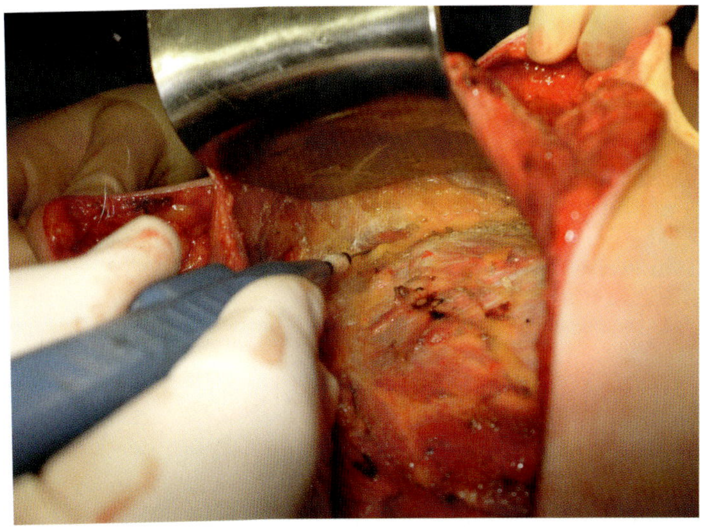

Figure 17.6 Complete dissection of the inferomedial fibers of pectoralis major.

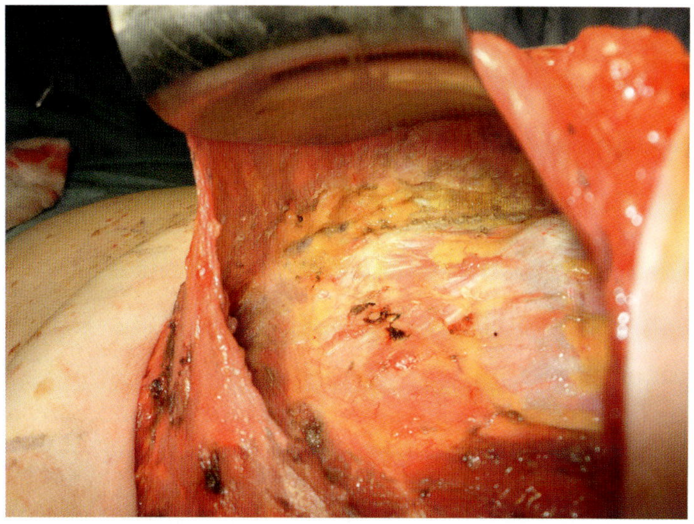

Figure 17.7 Final aspect of the pouch.

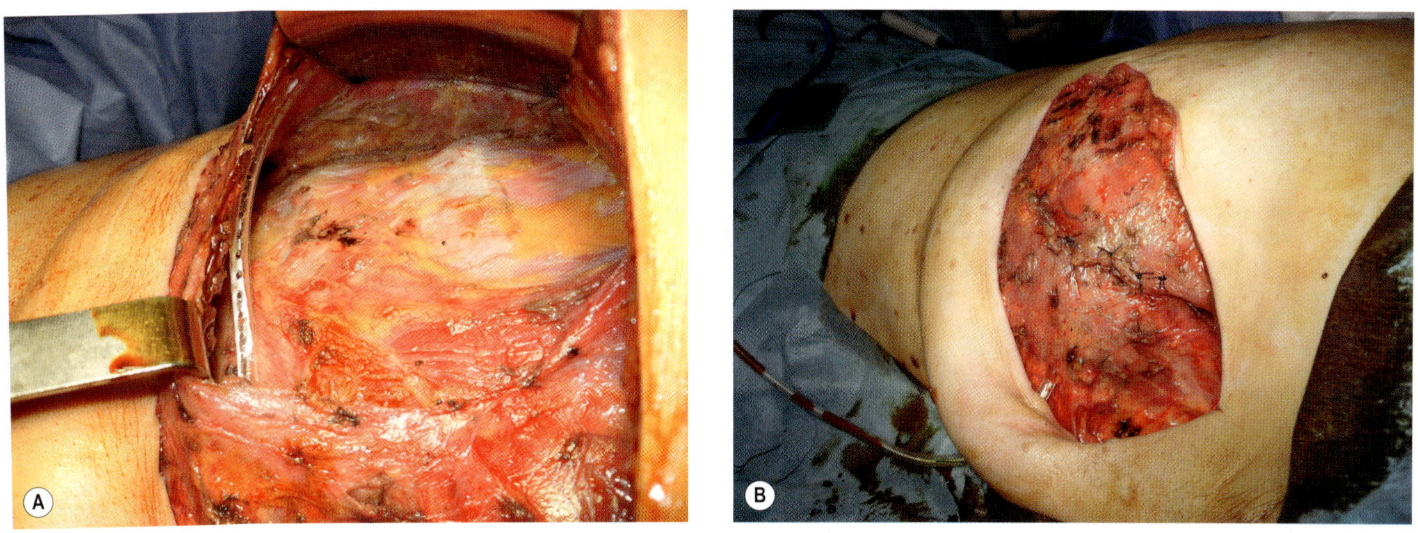

Figure 17.8 A closed suction drain is visible in the pouch.

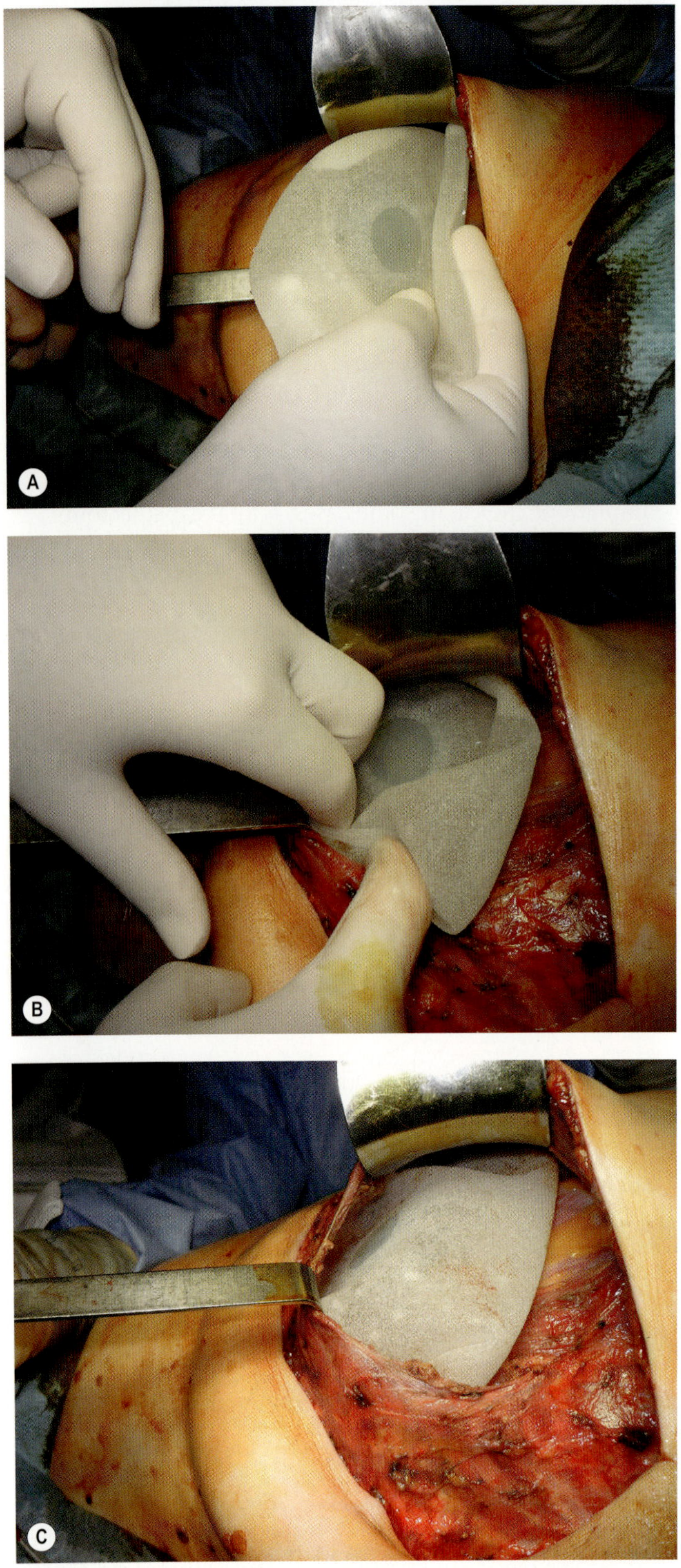

Figure 17.9 **(A)** The expander is partially inflated with saline. **(B)** The expander is correctly positioned. **(C)** The expander is now easily accommodated inside the pouch.

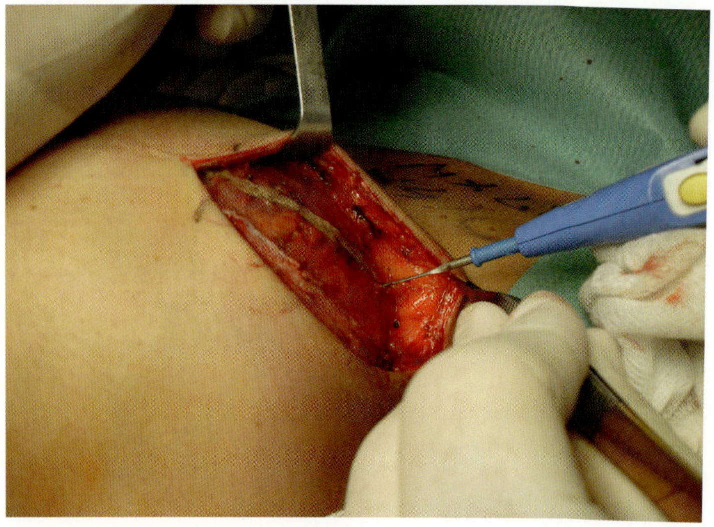

Figure 17.10 Second stage; change of tissue expander for permanent implant. Incision along the previous mastectomy scar.

   - The capsule work can be performed with the expander *in situ* or after expander removal.
- Once the expander is removed, refinements to the capsule/pocket are performed to create a more natural contour.
- The permanent implant is inserted and the wound closed in layers with care to re-approximate the muscular incision using absorbable suture.

Postoperative considerations

Expander implant reconstruction

- Prophylactic antibiotics with activity against staphylococcal bacteria should be routinely administered and therefore postoperative administration is not required without clinical signs of infection.
- A well-fitting sports bra should be worn following reconstruction and contralateral surgery.
- Intensive exercise should be avoided for 2–3 weeks, although arm and shoulder mobilization is important following formal axillary dissection.
- Inflation of the prosthesis should be carried out weekly, beginning only after the initial mastectomy incisions have healed.
- Drains are left until output reaches 30–40 mL per day.
- Most surgeons keep patients on oral antibiotic therapy while drains are in place.
- Expansion usually occurs weekly or every other week in 60–100 cc increments of saline solution.
- In general, the second stage of the operation is not performed until 4–6 months after the initial surgery or following adjuvant radiotherapy.
- Follow-up after the second stage follows the course for traditional augmentations. An ultrasound scan

can be diagnostic in case of implant ruptures. However, the MRI scan is the "gold standard" to diagnose shell ruptures.

Outcomes and complications

Expander/implant reconstruction

- Hematoma incidence ranges from 0% to 5.8%. In the setting of expanding hematomas or hematoma in the vicinity of an expander/implant, operative evacuation and exploration is warranted.
- Stable hematomas or those remote from the expander/implant pocket (i.e., axilla) can sometimes be managed by sterile aspiration.
- Erythema ***(Fig. 17.11)*** is a frequent response of the skin to dissection and it will often resolve spontaneously.
- If erythema is associated with symptoms of infection (malaise, fever, or an increase in drainage through the suction catheters), intravenous antibiotic therapy either on an inpatient basis or via a home-care service, should be provided.
- Failure of cellulitis to resolve indicates peri-implant infection. Expander removal is required with a repeat of stage 1, in 3–6 months.
- Infection rates range from 0% to 15%.
- After 10 days, wound contamination at the drain exit site becomes a real risk.
- If serous accumulation is extensive, reoperation with culture of the expanders, irrigation of the space, and insertion of new drains are appropriate.
- Skin envelope necrosis may occur in the range of 0% to 21%. When necrotic complications occur, the expansion process has to be delayed pending healing of areas of partial or complete skin loss.
- If partial or complete skin necrosis at the suture line is observed, muscle coverage of the expander in this region is generally provided by the pectoralis major muscle or a segmental rectus muscle flap. Thus, for small areas of necrosis, conservative measures or the use of topical antibiotics and local wound care are generally adequate.
- In cases of evident deep skin necrosis, serial debridement can be performed and salvage of the implant sometimes obtained.
- If there is concern about impending expander exposure, options include:
  - Excision of the area of skin necrosis and advancement of the remaining envelope for closure and implant closure and implant coverage.
  - Use of an autologous flap such as the latissimus dorsi flap.
  - Expander removal with plans for delayed reconstruction.
  - Expander-implant reinsertion can be scheduled after a minimum of 3–6 months, depending on the status of the overlying skin envelope.
- Expander failure or malfunction ***(Figs 17.12, 17.13)*** may occur if there has been an injury to the expander wall integrity – expander replacement is required in this instance.
- Late complications primarily involve complications related to the prosthesis including deflations and rupture, capsular contracture, and wrinkling.
- In a study comparing three consecutive study groups, there was no significant difference in major and minor complication rates between autogenous and non-autogenous reconstruction (Table 17.1).
- The total time for expander-implant procedures remains much less than for flap procedures, but the average number of procedures is greater (Table 17.2).
- Implant based two stage breast reconstructions generate high satisfaction rates.
- The Achilles' heel of this strategy is the difficulty in reaching a satisfactory symmetry.

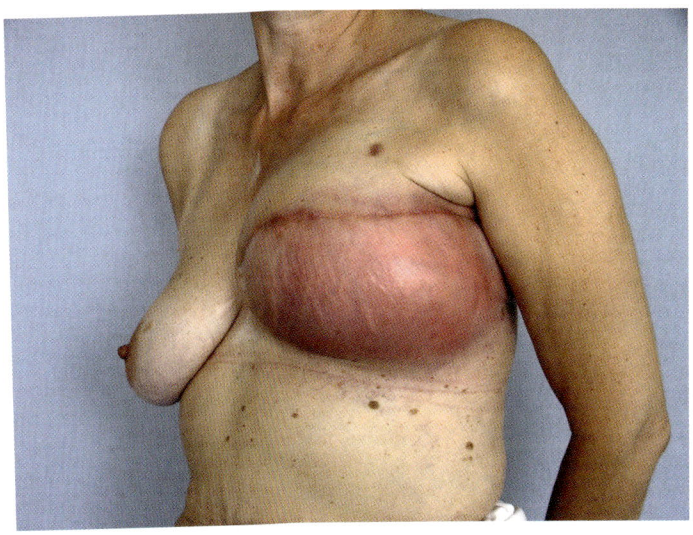

Figure 17.11 Skin cellulitis inflammation.

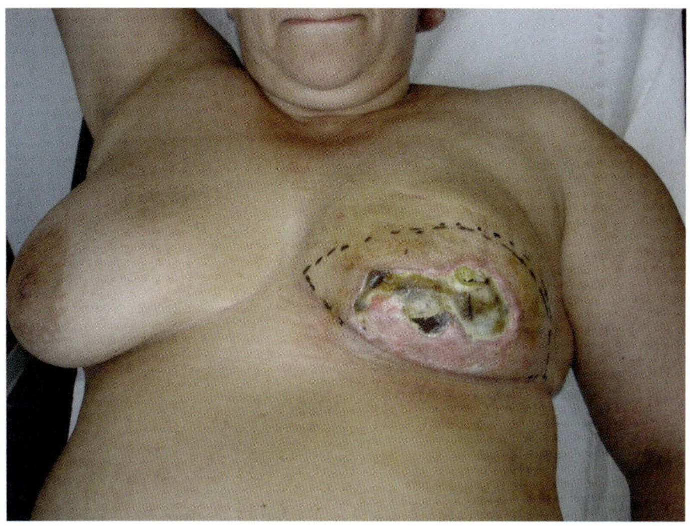

Figure 17.12 Skin necrosis and implant exposure.

Table 17.1 Frequency of complications by type of reconstruction

	Implants		Pedicle TRAM flaps		Free TRAM flaps	
Complication	*n*	(%)	*n*	(%)	*n*	(%)
Back pain	1	1.3	4	2.2	4	6.0
Hernia/abdominal wall laxity	–	14	7	8	8	11.9
Lymphedema	33	8	10	5.6	3	4.5
Capsular contracture	12	15.2	–		–	
Implant shift	1	1.3	–		–	
Wound dehiscence	3	3.8	10	5.6	1	1.5
Partial flap loss (fat necrosis)	5	6.3	29	16	21	14.9
Total flap loss	0	2	1.1	1	1.5	
Anastomotic thrombosis	–		–		4	6.0
Implant failure	3	3.8	–		–	
Infection	28	35.4	21	11.7	12	17.9
Clostridium difficile colitis	0	1	0.5		0	
Hematoma/seroma of the breast	4	5.1	7	3.9	6	9.0
Hematoma/seroma of the abdomen	–		7	3.9	3	4.5
Abdominal wall necrosis	–		3	1.7	0	
Cardiac/pulmonary complications	1	1.3	6	3.4	6	9.0

Reproduced with permission from Wilkins EG, Cederna PS, Lowery JC, et al. Prospective analysis of psychosocial outcomes in breast reconstruction: one-year postoperative results from the Michigan Breast Reconstruction Outcome study. *Plast Reconstr Surg.* 2000;106:1014–1027.

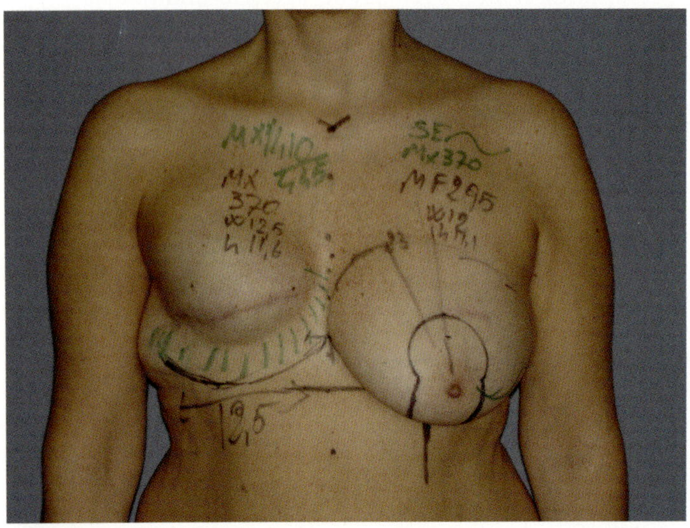

Figure 17.13 Expander malpositioning and rotation.

Table 17.2 Average operative time for each technique and average number of procedures for final result

	Average operative time by technique (h)	Average number of procedures[a] on reconstructed breast by technique
Implant (*n*=82)	1.2	1.8
Staged tissue expander-implant (*n*=142)	3.2	2.4
Latissimus dorsi implant (*n*=107)	3.8	1.7
TRAM flap (*n*=106)	5.5	1.2
Free flap (*n*=12)	9.0	1.2

Operative techniques have improved with experience, and time required for free flaps has been reduced by 3 h on average.
[a]Does not include nipple-areola reconstruction.
(Reproduced with permission from Trabulsy PP, Anthony JP, Mathes SJ. Changing trends in postmastectomy breast reconstruction: a 13-year experience. *Plast Reconstr Surg.* 1994;93:1418–1427.)

Operative technique

Latissimus dorsi flap reconstruction (Video 17.3)

Video 17.3

- Before designing the flap itself, examine the patient's back and mark the lateral margin of the latissimus dorsi muscle along the posterior axillary line down to the posterior iliac crest by supporting the patient's abducted arm and palpating the muscle laterally as the patient pushes downward ***(Fig. 17.14)***. The superior margin of the flap is identified by locating the tip of the scapula, with the patient's arms at their sides ***(Fig. 17.15)***.

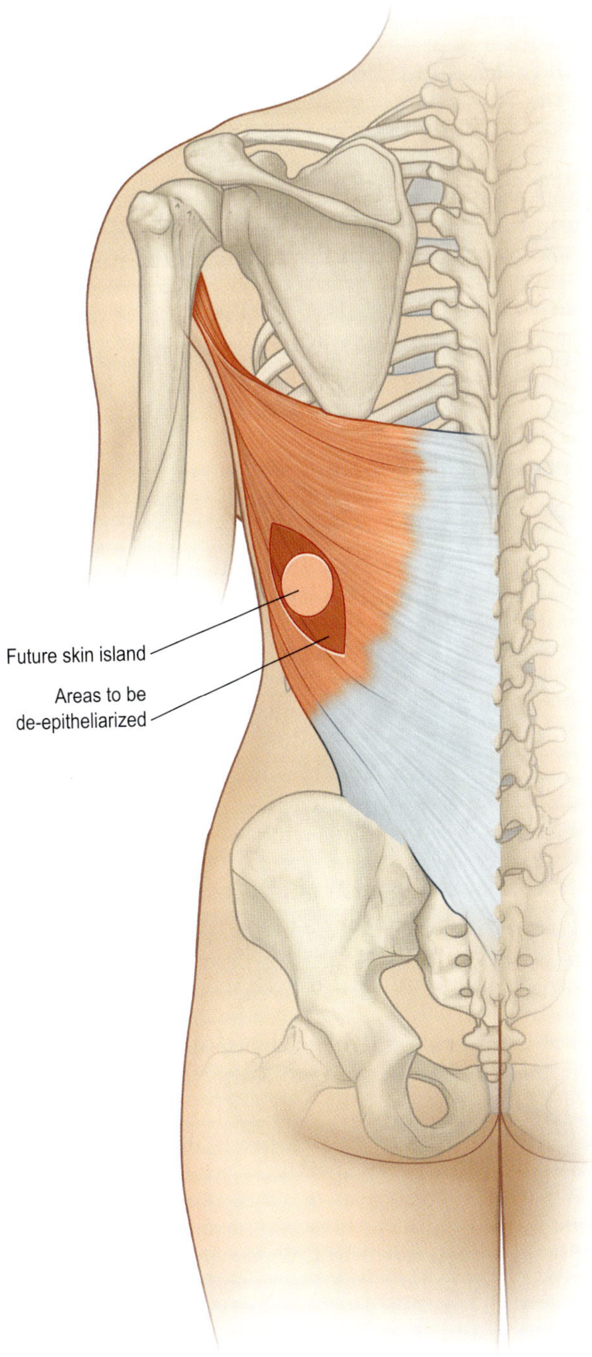

Figure 17.14 Common placement of the skin island in planning of latissimus dorsi flap reconstruction with a prosthesis.

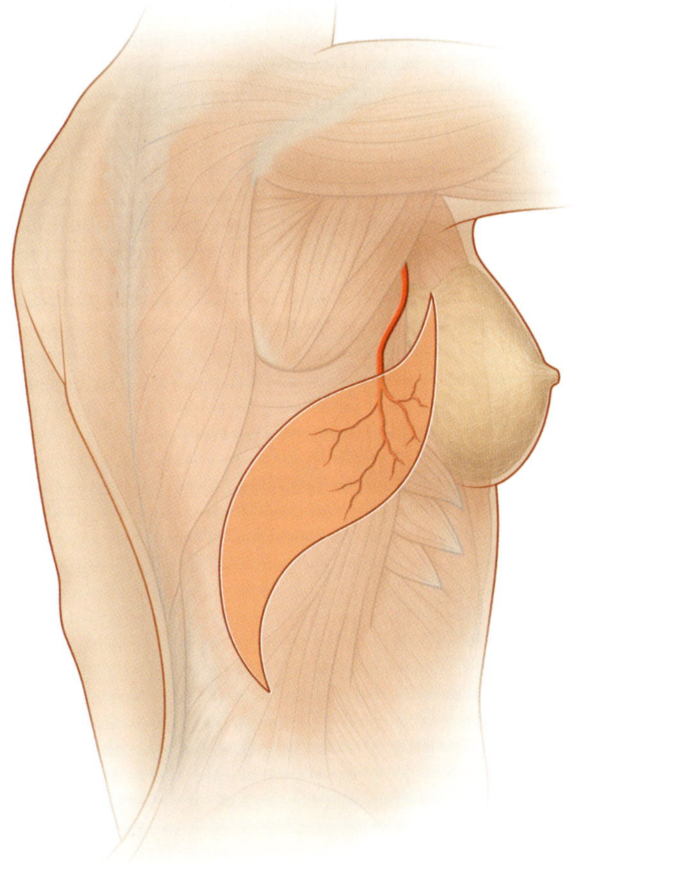

Figure 17.15 When total autogenous latissimus breast reconstruction is planned, the skin island is designed to include all available excess back skin and fat.

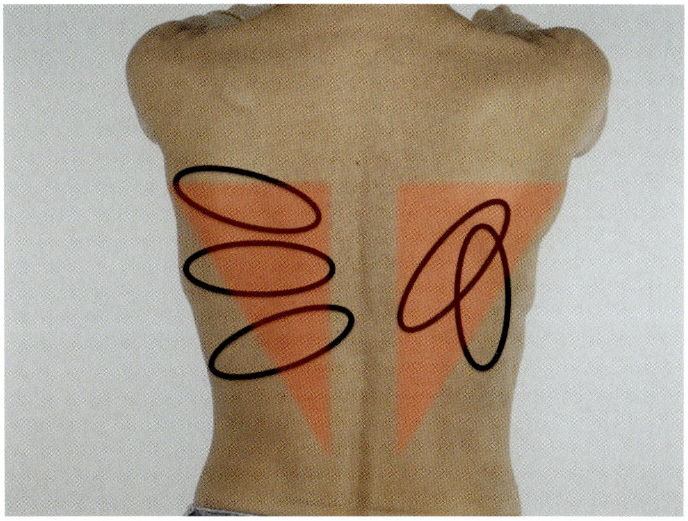

Figure 17.16 The latissimus dorsi skin paddle may be designed transversely (lower, middle, and upper), obliquely, or vertically. Each design has distinct advantages and disadvantages to dissection exposure, amount of harvestable tissue, and final scar contour and location.

- The skin island may be designed laterally, obliquely in a natural skin line along the lower midback, or transversely where the scar can be hidden within the confines of the bra straps *(Fig. 17.16)*.
- Scar location is an important consideration when performing breast reconstruction using the latissimus dorsi flap.
- The low transverse incision (below the level of the inframammary fold) is preferred by most women,

followed by the middle transverse incision (at the level of the inframammary fold), the upper transverse incision (above the level of the inframammary fold), and lastly the vertical and oblique incisions.

- While this is compelling, it must be balanced against the needs of the breast reconstruction.
- Latissimus flap elevation is performed in the lateral decubitus position *(Fig. 17.17)*.
- Dissection is often carried out just beneath the superficial fascia, leaving the deep fat attached to the surface of the muscle *(Fig. 17.18)*.

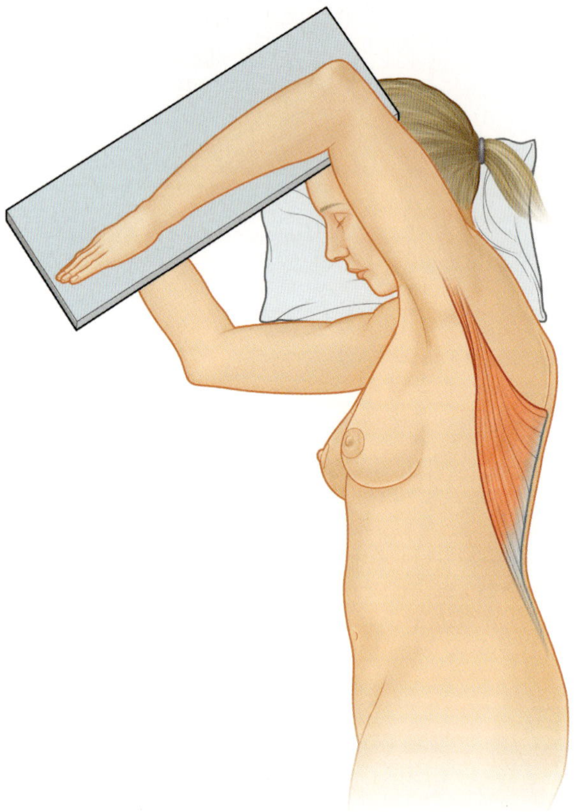

Figure 17.17 The patient is positioned in the lateral decubitus position for latissimus flap elevation. This allows easy access to the entire muscle and its insertion.

- The entire surface of the muscle to be used is exposed in this same plane.
- Dissection then proceeds laterally to identify the lateral border of the latissimus dorsi muscle.
- The latissimus muscle is separated from the serratus anterior, and the flap is elevated along its lateral edge.
- The lumbosacral fascia is divided at the level of the posterior axillary line, then the latissimus fibers of origin are separated from the paraspinous muscle fascia.
- Care must be taken to avoid incising through the paraspinous fascia because this makes identification of the proper plane of dissection difficult.
- The remaining fibers of origin are divided medially from the vertebral column.
- The large intercostal perforating vessels in this region should be carefully controlled to prevent bleeding and postoperative hematoma formation.
- Superomedially, the covering fibers of the trapezius muscle are identified and elevated away from the underlying latissimus muscle.
- After the superior border of the latissimus is identified, dissection is carried out laterally toward the axilla, separating away the fibers of the teres major muscle that diffuse with those of the latissimus.
- The entire muscle flap is then elevated toward the axilla *(Fig. 17.19A)*.
- The thoracodorsal artery and vein are identified at the point of entrance into muscle.
- The serratus branch is easily identified and may be left intact, especially if the patient had axillary dissection in which the thoracodorsal artery may have been injured. The additional blood inflow through the serratus branch may be critical.
- It is desirable in most patients to divide the latissimus dorsi muscle near its insertion at its attachment to the humerus.
- Release of the insertions helps avoid the displeasing bulge in the low axilla that is sometimes seen when the insertion is left intact.
- Care must be taken during this step to preserve the thoracodorsal vessels. A small cuff of muscle, 10–20%, may be preserved to help protect from traction on the pedicle.

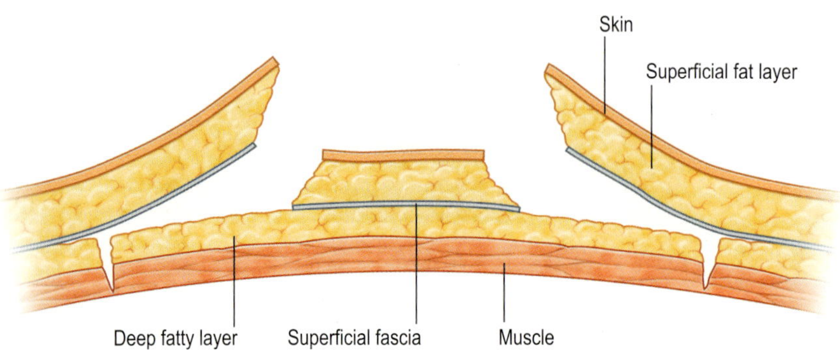

Figure 17.18 In the autogenous latissimus flap, the deep fat is left attached to the muscle as the dissection is carried out just beneath the fascia superficialis. This ensures adequate volume for reconstruction and preservation of the dorsal skin flaps.

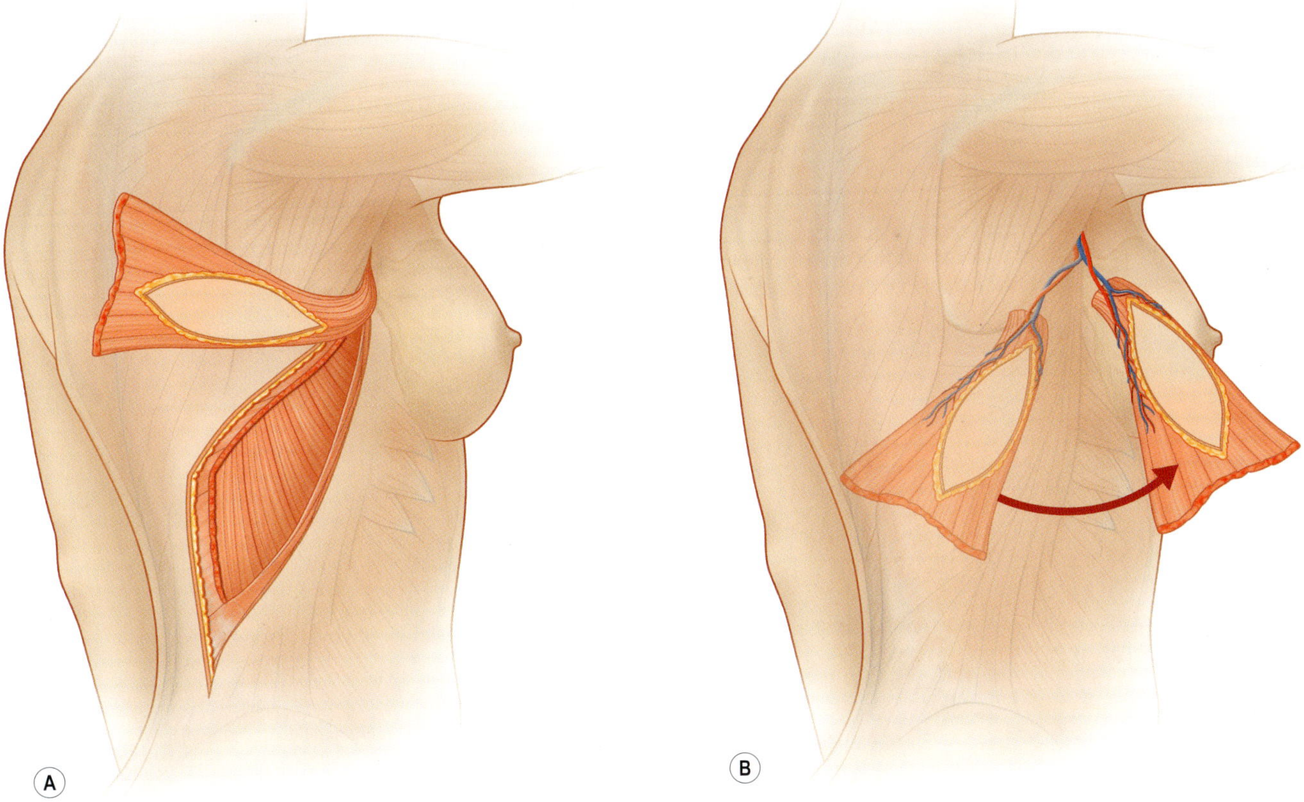

Figure 17.19 **(A)** Elevation of the latissimus dorsi musculocutaneous flap and the underlying anatomy. **(B)** After division of the muscle insertion, the latissimus flap is transposed anteriorly to the mastectomy defect through a subcutaneous tunnel high in the axilla.

- The flap is then transferred to the mastectomy defect through a subcutaneous tunnel high in the axilla to further prevent an unnatural lateral bulge and to fill the axilla (Fig. 17.19B).
- Suturing of the muscle at the anterior axillary line should be performed to prevent lateral migration of the flap and implant and to protect the pedicle from tension.
- The back incision is closed over suction drains. Some surgeons utilize quilting sutures, fibrin sealant adhesives, or barbed sutures during this closure to eliminate or minimize dead space. Skin closure is performed in layers including 2-0 polydioxanone to the fascia superficialis followed by interrupted and running intradermal 3-0 Monocryl to the dermis.
- The inset/placement of the flap depends on the particular circumstances of the reconstruction.

Immediate reconstructions

- When the latissimus flap is used over an expander, it is easier and quicker to leave the pectoralis major muscle intact and to place the expander between the latissimus and pectoralis major muscles ***(Fig. 17.20)***.
- The muscle is typically inset just beneath the upper mastectomy skin flap which helps achieve some soft tissue filling of the upper breast pole.
- The muscle is sutured medially and inferiorly to the underlying muscle and fascia to help establish those borders of the breast.
- Superiorly, marionette half-mattress sutures are used between the overlying breast skin and the edge of the latissimus muscle to help cover the entire mastectomy defect with the latissimus muscle. Not tying these sutures provides access for placement of the expander.

Delayed reconstructions

- The latissimus flap is used both for inferior pole fullness and to cover an expander or implant.
- In most cases, an incision is made at or just above the predetermined inframammary fold along a line from the lateral sternal border to the anterior axillary line.
- The superior chest wall skin flap is elevated, usually in the subcutaneous plane, and the latissimus flap is brought through the tunnel and into the defect.
- Suturing of the muscle at or near the anterior axillary line should be performed to prevent lateral migration of the flap and implant and to protect the pedicle from tension.
- The best projection is achieved when the pectoralis major muscle is left intact and the expander or prosthesis is

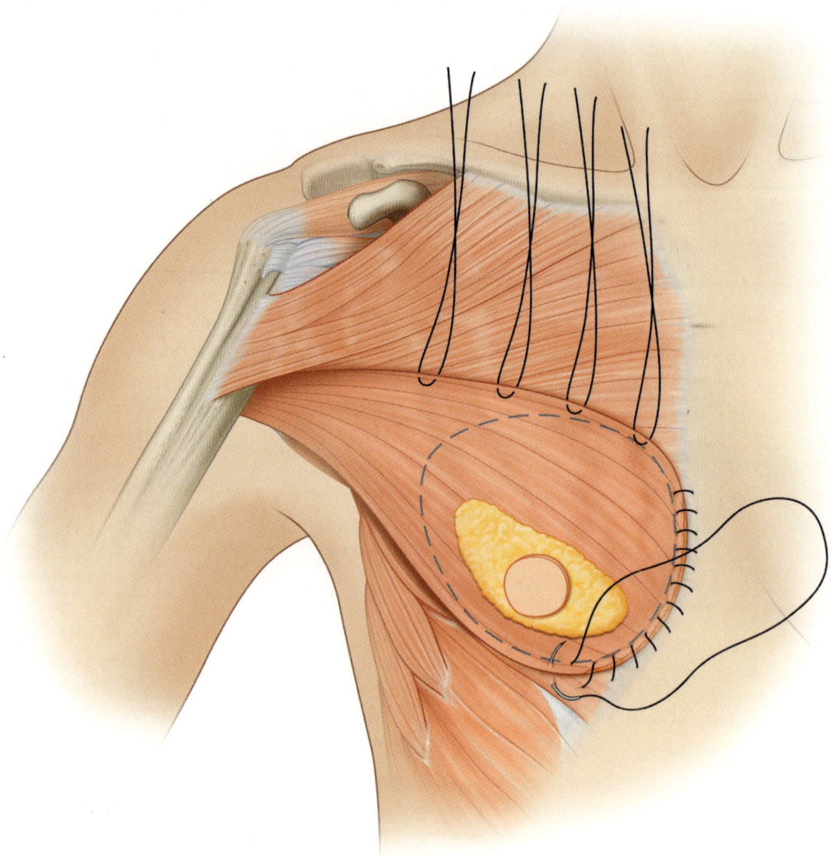

Figure 17.20 When immediate latissimus flap reconstruction is planned with a prosthesis for skin-sparing mastectomy, the skin pattern is designed as a discrete small island. After transposition of the flap, the expander is placed between the latissimus and pectoralis major muscles.

placed between the latissimus and pectoralis major muscles.

- The muscle is sutured medially and inferiorly to the underlying muscle and fascia in such a way as to help form those borders of the breast and superiorly, marionette half-mattress 3-0 Prolene sutures are placed between the overlying breast skin and the edge of the latissimus muscle to help cover the entire mastectomy defect with the latissimus muscle.
- The expander is inserted from above and may be filled with several hundred milliliters of saline because there is generally no tightness to the sub-latissimus pocket.
- Postoperatively, the tissue expander is further inflated until the desired volume is achieved, starting 2 weeks postoperatively or once the wound is healed.
- The second stage (expander/implant exchange) of the reconstruction is typically performed after 4–8 months, allowing adequate healing and settling of the soft tissue.
- When reconstruction is planned with use of the total autogenous latissimus dorsi flap, the cutaneous paddle is molded in the form of an asymmetric U *(Fig. 17.21)*.
- The curved base of the U gives the apex of the breast. The distal part of the muscle and its underlying fat are folded under this breast cone to increase the volume and the projection of the breast.
- Various moldings can be tried until one arrives at a satisfactory shape for the rebuilt breast. This procedure of molding is crucial to the final quality of the result, and one must understand how to achieve the different arrangements necessary for a good morphologic result.

Postoperative considerations

Latissimus flap reconstruction

- Patients will have two back drains and one to two breast drains.
- A loose circumferential dressing or surgical bra may be used with placement of axillary gauze for padding, however, care should be taken to avoid any direct compression over the vessels in the axilla.
- Length of hospitalization is on average three days and patients can expect to return to normal work function from 3–6 weeks.
- Suction drains will remain in place until output is <30 mL/day, with back drains in place up to 3–4 weeks.

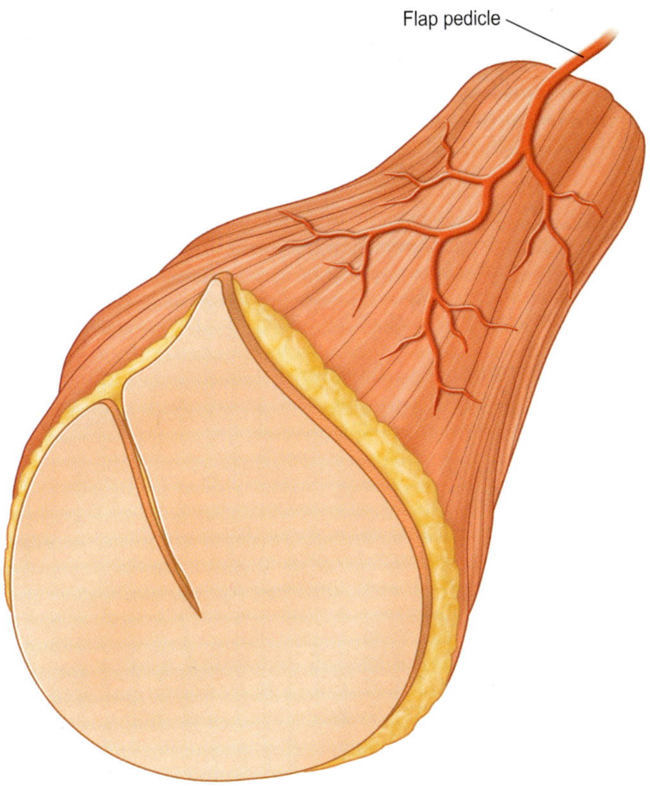

Figure 17.21 For total autogenous latissimus reconstruction, the flap is folded into a cone shape to increase the volume and projection of the reconstructed breast.

- Upper extremity strengthening and range-of-motion exercises are begun 2 weeks postoperatively assuming sufficient progression of healing.

Outcomes and complications

Latissimus flap reconstruction

- Breast reconstruction with the latissimus dorsi musculocutaneous flap has been associated with significant patient satisfaction.
- The latissimus dorsi flap is a hardy flap that has an excellent and reliable circulation with minimal risk of flap necrosis even in smokers and diabetics.
- Significant flap necrosis is unusual and nearly always associated with injury to the vascular pedicle.
- Partial flap necrosis has been noted in up to 7% of patients but is more common when an extended flap has been elevated.
- The most common complication is seroma at the back donor site.
- Other donor site problems include dorsal skin flap necrosis, loss of shoulder mobility, shoulder weakness, winging of the scapula, and dorsal hernia.
- Migration of the expander or implant through the axilla and into the back can occur.
- Should be avoidable by suturing the latissimus muscle to the lateral chest wall.
- Other implant-related complications can occur including capsular contracture, device failure, periprosthetic infection, and device extrusion.

Further reading

Bailey S, Saint-Cyr M, Zhang K, et al. Breast reconstruction with latissimus dorsi flap: Women's preference for scar location. *Plast Reconstr Surg*. 2010;126: 358–365.

Carlson GW, Bostwick 3rd J, Styblo TM, et al. Skinsparing mastectomy. Oncologic and reconstructive considerations. *Ann Surg*. 1997;225:570–575.

This study introduced the basic concepts of skin preservation. Skin incisions for removal of glandular tissue are subdivided into four groups.

Chang DW, Youssef A, Cha S, et al. Autologous breast reconstruction with the extended latissimus dorsi flap. *Plast Reconstr Surg*. 2002;110:751.

The authors present their experience with the extended latissimus dorsi myocutaneous flap for replacement of breast volume without an implant. A total of 75 extended latissimus dorsi flap breast reconstructions were performed in 67 patients (mean age 51.5 years). Flap complications developed in 21 of 75 flaps (28.0%), and donor-site complications developed in 29 of 75 donor sites (38.7%). Mastectomy skin flap necrosis (17.3%) and donor-site seroma (25.3%) were found to be the most common complications. There were no flap losses. The study concluded that patients who are obese are at higher risk of developing donor-site complications.

Cordeiro PG, Pusic AL, Disa JJ, et al. Irradiation after immediate tissue expander/implant breast reconstruction: outcomes, complications, aesthetic results, and satisfaction among 156 patients. *Plast Reconstr Surg*. 2004;113(3):877–881.

The impact of radiation in implant-based reconstruction is investigated in this study. The authors would support this technique as a proper alternative to flap-based reconstructions.

Delay E, Gounot N, Bouillot A. Autologous latissimus breast reconstruction: a 3 year clinical experience with 100 patients. *Plast Reconstr Surg*. 1998;102:1461.

Delay et al. presented their technique of autologous breast reconstruction using the latissimus dorsi flap and studied the results that can be expected. A consecutive sample of 100 patients was studied (average follow-up 20 months). Supplementary volume of the latissimus dorsi was obtained from five fatty zones: fat on the cutaneous paddle, fat taken from the surface of the muscle, the scapular fat pad, the anterior fatty zone, and the supra-iliac fat pad. The authors found the following complications: 1% partial necrosis, 1% total necrosis of the flap, and seroma 79%, most regularly in obese patients. The level of patient satisfaction was high.

Indications for this technique include, when one can bury the cutaneous paddle: cases of skin-sparing mastectomy and cases of conversion of implant reconstruction to an autologous reconstruction.

Delay E, Jorquera F, Lucas R. Sensitivity of breasts reconstructed with the autologous latissimus dorsi flap. *Plast Reconstr Surg*. 2000;106:302–309.

Fraulin FOG, Louie G, Zorrilla L, et al. Functional evaluation of the shoulder following latissimus dorsi muscle transfer. *Ann Plast Surg*. 1995;35:349.

Fraulin et al. looked at the functional effects of latissimus dorsi muscle harvest on shoulder strength and mobility. This was a study of 26 patients (10 males, 16 females) who underwent a pedicled or free vascularized latissimus dorsimuscle transfer. Muscle testing was performed using a Kinetic Communicator machine (Kin Com) and the Baltimore therapeutic equipment (BTE) work simulator. The female unilateral pedicle group (n = 13) showed a significant difference between operated and nonoperated shoulders for both peak torque (power) and work (endurance) measurements of shoulder adduction and extension (mean ratios operated/non-operated shoulders, 55–69%). The male free vascularized group (n = 10) similarly showed a significant deficit of both peak torque and work for shoulder extension and adduction (mean ratios, 74–84%). The paper concluded that dynamic muscle tests demonstrate a deficit of muscle power and endurance of shoulder extension and adduction following latissimus dorsi muscle transfer.

Hammond DC. Latissimus dorsi musculocutaneous flap. *Plast Reconstr Surg*. 2009;124:4.

The author presents his extensive experience with the latissimus dorsi musculocutaneous flap in both immediate and delayed breast reconstruction. Five technical modifications in surgical technique are introduced including orientation of the skin island along the relaxed skin tension lines, harvesting the deep layer of fat with the flap, cutting the thoracodorsal nerve, partially dividing the insertion of the muscle, and using a staged expander/implant sequence. These principles result in a thin line and smooth donor-site scar. The flap advances completely to the breast because of the partial release of the insertion of the muscle, and the volume provided by the flap is increased by keeping the deep layer of fat attached to the flap. Breast animation is minimized as a result of sectioning of the thoracodorsal nerve, and the consistency and quality of the result are improved by using a staged tissue expander/implant strategy.

Handel N, Silverstein MJ. Breast cancer diagnosis and prognosis in augmented women. *Plast Reconstr Surg*. 2006;118(3):587–596.

Herborn CU, Marincek B, Ermann D, et al. Breast augmentation and reconstructive surgery: MR imaging of implant rupture and malignancy. *Eur Radiol*. 2002;12:2198–2206.

Krueger EA, Wilkins EG, Strawderman M. Complications and patient satisfaction following expander/implant breast reconstruction with and without radiotherapy. *Int J Radiat Oncol Biol Phys*. 2001;49:713–721.

Laitung JKG, Peck F. Shoulder function following the loss of the latissimus dorsi muscle. *Br J Plast Surg*. 1985;38:375.

Losken A, Carlson GW, Bostwick 3rd J, et al. Trends in unilateral breast reconstruction and management of the contralateral breast: The Emory experience. *Plast Reconstr Surg*. 2002;110:89–97.

McCraw JB, Papp C, Edwards A, et al. The autogenous latissimus breast reconstruction. *Clin Plast Surg*. 1994;21:279.

Moore TS, Farrell LD. Latissimus dorsi myocutaneous flap for breast reconstruction: long term results. *Plast Reconstr Surg*. 1992;89(4):666–672.

Nava MB, Spano A, Cadenelli P, et al. Extra-projected implants as an alternative surgical model for breast reconstruction. Implantation strategy and early results. *Breast*. 2008;17(4):361–366.

A new reconstructive paradigm is introduced in this paper. Breast reconstructions aim to rebuild a bilateral breast mound of a medium size, with extra-projection and cosmetically pleasing.

Neumann CG. The expansion of an area of skin by progressive distention of a subcutaneous balloon. *Plast Reconstr Surg*. 1957;19:124.

An historical study on tissue expansion.

Papp C, McCraw JB. Autogenous latissimus breast reconstruction. *Clin Plast Surg*. 1998;25:261.

Radovan C. Breast reconstruction after mastectomy using the temporary expander. *Plast Reconstr Surg*. 1982;69:195.

Russell RC, Pribaz J, Zook EG, et al. Functional evaluation of latissimus dorsi donor site. *Plast Reconstr Surg*. 1986;78:336.

Saint-Cyr M, Nagarkar P, Schaverien M, et al. The pedicled descending branch muscle-sparing latissimus dorsi flap for breast reconstruction. *Plast Reconstr Surg*. 2009;123(1):13–24.

Schneider WJ, Hill HL, Brown RG. Latissimus dorsi myocutaneous flap for breast reconstruction. *Br J Plast Surg*. 1977;30:277.

Schwabegger AH, Harpf C, Rainer C. Muscle-sparing latissimus dorsi myocutaneous flap with maintenance of muscle innervation, function, and aesthetic appearance of the donor site. *Plast Reconstr Surg*. 2003;111:1407–1411.

Serra-Renom JM, Muñoz-Olmo JL, Serra-Mestre JM. Fat grafting in postmastectomy breast reconstruction with expanders and prostheses in patients who have received radiotherapy: formation of new subcutaneous tissue. *Plast Reconstr Surg*. 2010;125(1):12–18.

This study investigates the effects of fat grafting in the treatment of radio-induced dermatitis. This is the largest series currently available in literature.

Spear SL, Clemens MW, Boehmler J. Latissimus dorsi flap in reconstruction of the radiated breast. In: Spear SL, ed. *Surgery of the Breast: Principles and Art*. 3rd ed. Amsterdam: Wolters Kluwer; 2010.

The authors reviewed their experience with the latissimus dorsi flap and a prosthesis in reconstruction of the previously irradiated breast. Twenty-eight patients all had soft breasts at follow up, with no evidence of capsular contracture. Donor-site complications included five donor-site seromas. The majority of patients (65%) underwent a planned two-stage reconstruction, and the majority of the revision operations were for exchanges to smaller implants. The overall satisfaction rating was 8.8 of 10. The authors concluded that although purely autologous reconstructions may be the best choice for many irradiated breasts, it has been shown in this study that a cosmetically acceptable reconstruction with manageable risk can be performed using a prosthesis combined with a latissimus dorsi flap. The study concluded that with advancements in surgical technique and improvements in tissue expander and implant design, outstanding results can be obtained using the latissimus dorsi flap in breast reconstruction.

Tobin GR, Moberg AW, DuBou RH, et al. The split latissimus dorsi myocutaneous flap. *Ann Plast Surg*. 1981;7:272–280.

18 Chapter

Autologous breast reconstruction using abdominal flaps

This chapter was created using content from Neligan & Grotting, Plastic Surgery 3rd edition, Volume 5, Breast, Chapter 16, The bilateral pedicled TRAM flap, L. Frankyn Elliot, John D. Symbas and Hunter R. Moyer, Chapter 17, Free TRAM breast reconstruction, Joshua Fosnot, Joseph M. Serletti, Chapter 18, The deep inferior epigastric artery perforator (DIEAP) flap, Phillip N. Blondeel, Colin M. Morrison and Robert J. Allen.

SYNOPSIS (PEDICLED TRAM)

- The pedicled TRAM flap is still the most popular way of transferring abdominal tissue to the breast.
- This technique, introduced by Dr Carl Hartrampf, is consistently successful if it is performed properly.
- The muscle and fascial sparing technique ensures abundant vascularity to the TRAM flap, while allowing secure and complication free closure of the abdominal wall.
- The shaping of the breast using the pedicled TRAM flap is enormously simplified in the immediate reconstructive setting.
- We recommend utilizing the pedicled TRAM flap for bilateral reconstruction and the free TRAM flap for unilateral reconstruction.

SYNOPSIS (FREE TRAM)

- The free TRAM is one tool in an entire armamentarium used for breast reconstruction.
- Although controversial, the free TRAM likely limits donor site morbidity and ischemic complications when compared with the pedicled TRAM.
- Free TRAM reconstruction can be performed safely in an immediate or delayed fashion.
- For the most part, radiation therapy after reconstruction yields more unpredictable results than radiation before reconstruction.
- Free TRAM flap breast reconstruction requires intraoperative attention to detail and postoperative vigilance.
- Although revision is not uncommon, the free TRAM provides for excellent, predictable aesthetic results with a high degree of patient satisfaction.

SYNOPSIS (DIEAP)

- The deep inferior epigastric artery perforator (DIEAP) flap provides a large volume of soft, malleable tissue that resembles the natural consistency of the breast.
- DIEAP flap dissection is comparable to conventional myocutaneous free flap surgery, once the initial learning curve is overcome.
- The main advantage of the DIEAP flap is the preservation of full rectus abdominis muscle function translating into less donor site morbidity.
- In experienced hands, the DIEAP flap loss rate is less than 1%.
- The DIEAP flap is the perforator flap of choice for autologous breast reconstruction.

Brief introduction

- While the free technique utilizing the inferior epigastric vessels undoubtedly provides additional blood flow to the transferred abdominal tissue, it carries with it the need for advanced microsurgical training and, in most hands, a significantly longer operative time.
- Abdominal tissue based breast reconstructions (pedicled TRAM, free TRAM, DIEAP) can be safely performed in either an immediate or delayed fashion with respect to the mastectomy.

- Immediate reconstruction has several advantages:
  - Patients benefit from only needing one operation.
  - Most surgeons find that immediate reconstruction is easier to perform.
  - The mastectomy skin flap envelope is more predictable.
  - Skin sparing or nipple sparing mastectomy techniques are options in some patients to minimize the loss of the native envelope.
- Many patients present in a delayed fashion, either because they did not undergo any reconstruction at the time of mastectomy or because they had prosthetic reconstruction which subsequently failed.
- Generally speaking, delayed reconstruction should not be undertaken sooner than 6 months following mastectomy due to immature scar formation; however, there is no temporal limit.
- Delayed reconstruction requires re-elevation of the skin flaps which are often scarred and less compliant. The mastectomy scar should be completely excised and if radiation injury is evident, this should be excised as well. Scarred or radiated skin can result in inadequate ptosis and poor symmetry over time.
- When designing a DIEAP flap, the main factor is the amount of viable tissue that can be harvested on a particular perforator.
- The most accurate indicator of this is preoperative localization of the dominant source of blood inflow by duplex Doppler or CT imaging.
- In addition to defining the "safe" flap territory, these techniques provide a degree of reassurance by avoiding intraoperative surprises and considerably reduce operative time.

The pedicled versus free TRAM/DIEAP

- The main issues at stake when comparing these two techniques are: the technical aspects of the operation, the long-term results, and the donor site morbidity.
- The pedicled TRAM requires complete dissection of the rectus muscle up to the level of the xiphoid. Because the flap and pedicle are turned over, there is the risk of twisting; thus, the insetting of the flap itself can be quite challenging.
- The free TRAM or DIEAP on the other hand requires the additional expertise of a microanastomosis; however, once the pedicle is created, the insetting of the flap tends to be less problematic.
- Aside from the technical aspects of the two operations, one must compare the long-term results weighed against the donor site morbidity.
- Due to the reliance on "choke" vessels for flap survival in the pedicled TRAM, there is a theoretical increased risk of ischemic complications such as partial or total flap loss and fat necrosis.
- For free TRAMs, there have been various muscle sparing (MS) iterations described, and surprisingly, much of the literature has suggested that as the degree of muscle sparing increases, so does the rate of fat necrosis.
  - MS0: complete transection of the muscle.
  - MS1: transection of most of the muscle.
  - MS2: harvest of only the central portion of the muscle.
  - MS3: complete muscle sparing (DIEAP).
- Although sacrificing the rectus muscle will not leave a patient completely disabled, patients may notice a considerable difference in flexion strength and abdominal contour when the rectus muscles are sacrificed.
- Objective measures of abdominal wall strength after pedicled or free TRAM reconstruction have consistently shown a deficit in strength which may persist long term; however, multiple head to head studies have not shown a significant difference in long-term abdominal wall function.

Preoperative considerations

- Given that most women undergoing mastectomy and reconstruction are young and healthy without significant co-morbidities, it is exceedingly rare for a woman to be considered too high risk for surgery. However, it is important to know the risk factors for poor postoperative outcomes.
- There is an increased risk of wound infection, mastectomy flap necrosis, abdominal flap necrosis and fat necrosis in smokers.
- Obese patients are more likely to experience wound related complications including mastectomy flap necrosis.
- Peripheral vascular disease is a risk factor for wound infection.
- Prior abdominal operations have been shown to increase the risk of complications associated with TRAM flap reconstruction.
- Techniques for minimizing risk include skewing the abdominal flap away from the previous scar, using hemiflaps, minimizing flap undermining, and supercharging.
- A prior abdominoplasty is generally considered an absolute contraindication to TRAM flap reconstruction because the prior skin flap sacrifices all perforating vessels.
- Patients should not only be made aware of the inherent risks of the surgery including the possibility of complications, they should be educated as to the limitations of reconstructions as well.
- It is helpful to point out asymmetries preoperatively.
- Scarring is an unfortunate phenomenon of which patients should have expectations postoperatively.
- Patients should be told of the likelihood of significant sensory loss – although some sensation may return most women never achieve a fully sensate mound.

Procedure selection

- Reconstruction of a breast mound using autologous tissue can be performed using multiple techniques, but there is no one perfect flap which can be used in all circumstances. Ultimately, deciding whether to use a pedicled versus a free TRAM or DIEP mostly has to do with surgeon training, preference and hospital resources such as an operating microscope and microsurgical instruments.

- There are certain circumstances where the free flap techniques should be considered superior.
  - Smoking increases the risk of wound related complications and fat necrosis. Therefore, smokers (even if they quit) should probably be offered a free TRAM rather than pedicled TRAM or DIEP flap.
  - When a larger volume flap is needed for reconstruction, this pushes the vascular supply of the pedicled TRAM and DIEP to its limits. As a result, the free TRAM is likely the better choice.
  - Any patient with a history of previous upper abdominal surgery which may have created a scar in the rectus sheath or destroyed the superior epigastrics should be offered a free flap preferentially.
  - The DIEP and SIEA flaps are excellent options utilizing the same lower abdominal island of tissue – the benefits being less abdominal wall invasion and resultant long-term abdominal wall function. The downside of course is the more tenuous blood supply.

Anatomical pearls

- The anatomy of the abdominal wall is critical to a complete understanding of the differences between various forms of abdominal based breast reconstruction such as the pedicled TRAM, free TRAM, deep inferior epigastric perforator (DIEP), and superficial inferior epigastric artery (SIEA) flaps *(Figs 18.1, 18.2)*.
- The TRAM flap is based on the blood supply from the perforating vessels through the rectus abdominis muscle and the deep epigastric system.
- The arcuate line marks a critical landmark as it represents the point where the inferior epigastric vessels perforate the rectus muscle.
- The anatomy of the perforating vessels is somewhat variable and may be predominantly along the lateral third of the muscle, in the central third of the muscle, or even in the medial third *(Fig. 18.3)*.
- There are generally three basic arterial schemata:
  - Type I pattern: a single intramuscular vessel extends from the superior epigastric artery to the deep inferior epigastric artery.
  - Type II (majority): the inferior epigastric artery branches into two vessels at the arcuate line and communicates with the superior epigastric through anastomosing choke vessels.
  - Type III: exhibited three branches of the inferior epigastric at the arcuate line. On average shows an even greater number of anastomoses with the superior epigastric artery.
- Perforators through the rectus muscle cross the anterior rectus sheath generally in two rows, one medial and one lateral.
- The rectus abdominis muscle is a type III muscle, in addition to the superior and inferior epigastric vessels, circulation includes branches of the 8th, 9th, 10th, 11th, and 12th intercostal vessels which penetrate the posterior rectus sheath just medial to the linea semilunaris.
- The circulation from either rectus muscle across the lower abdomen is divided into four zones. The circulation is best in zone I, somewhat variable in zones II and III, and usually poor in zone IV, particularly with a pedicled TRAM flap *(Fig. 18.4)*.
  - Zone I: zone immediately overlying the rectus muscle.
  - Zone II: zone immediately across the midline.
  - Zone III: ipsilateral zone just lateral to the rectus muscle border.
  - Zone IV: contralateral zone lateral to the contralateral rectus border.
  - Blood supply is improved to some degree in each zone after a delay procedure.

Operative techniques

Pedicled TRAM *(Fig. 18.5; Video 18.1)*

Video 18.1

- The patient is marked in the preoperative area. The abdominal flap is designed with the lower transverse incision located two fingerbreadths above the pubic symphysis and the upper incision usually just at the upper border of the umbilicus.
- The lower incision extends out laterally and crosses over the anterior superior iliac spine and angles cephalad.
- The upper incision is essentially level extending laterally until it meets the rising lower incision *(Fig. 18.6)*.
- The superior skin incision is made first and the dissection continues through the fat, beveled superiorly to recruit additional fat into the flap.
- Once the fascia is reached, the upper abdominal flap is elevated suprafascially up to and over the costal margins bilaterally for about 2 cm while the dissection in the midline continues up to the xiphoid.
- The subcutaneous tunnel (or tunnels in bilateral cases) is then created to allow transfer of the flaps into the mastectomy defects *(Fig. 18.7)*. These tunnels should be made at the 5 o'clock and 7 o'clock positions through the right and left inframammary folds respectively.
- On average, each tunnel needs to accommodate approximately four fingers to allow passage of each hemiflap.
- Once the superior flap is elevated, it can be pulled inferiorly to confirm the position of the appropriate inferior incision line. This maneuver will help determine whether the original incision marking is appropriate to allow abdominal closure without undue tension.
- Once confirmed, the lower incision is then made, straight down to the underlying fascia.
- No attempt is made to bevel inferiorly as the fat in the prepubic region is probably not as reliable based on the superior epigastric system as we would like to think.
- The umbilicus is circumscribed and left in position with some surrounding fat.

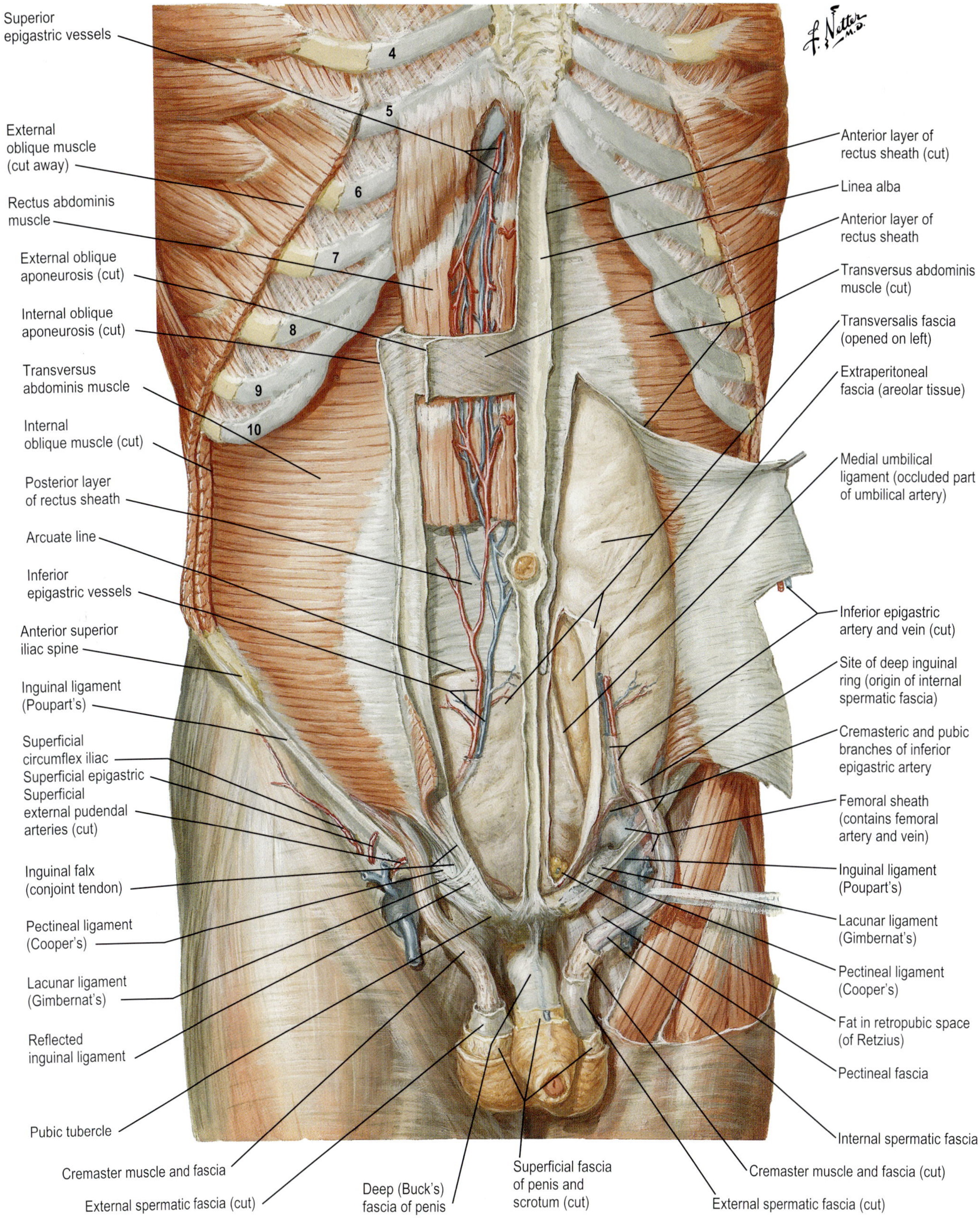

Figure 18.1 The anatomy of the abdominal wall. In particular, note the parallel nature of the rectus abdominis muscles with their dual blood supply from both the inferior and superior epigastric vessels. Multiple layers of muscle and fascia contribute to the overall strength of the abdominal wall. (Netter illustration from www.netterimages.com. ©Elsevier Inc. All rights reserved.)

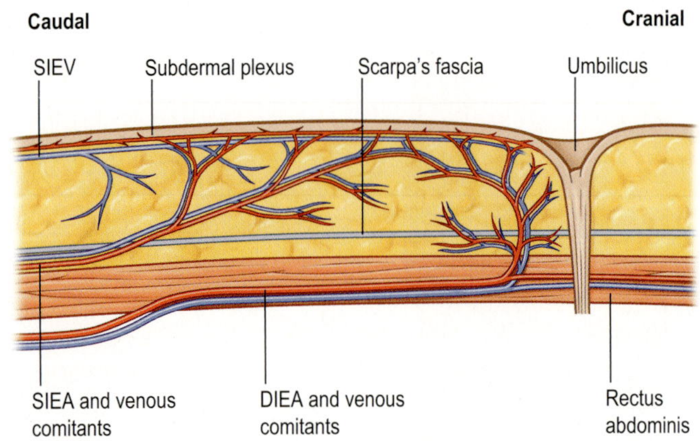

Figure 18.2 The same anatomical structures as explained in Figure 18.1 but seen in a paramedian sagittal view.

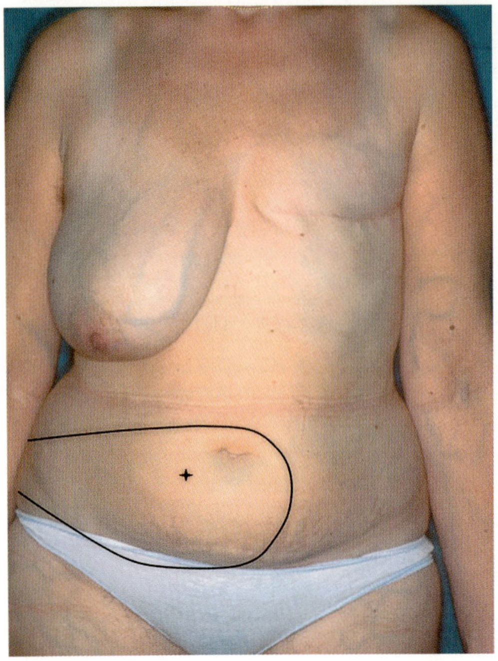

Figure 18.3 The different types of perforators that can be found at the lower abdominal wall. (1) The branches of the superficial inferior epigastric artery are direct perforators that vascularize the subcutaneous fat and skin after perforating the deep and superficial fascia. All other perforators are indirect perforators; (2) perforators that have a predominant vascularization of the subcutaneous fat tissue and skin with few muscular branches; (3) perforators that branch off of side branches that have a predominant goal of nourishing the muscle; (4) perforators that pass through the rectus abdominis muscle without branching; (5) perforators that pass through the septum or around the rectus abdominis muscle with the sole goal of vascularizing the subcutaneous tissues.

- If bilateral pedicled TRAM flaps are being performed, the flap is split in the midline down to the deep fascia to aid in dissection.
- In unilateral pedicled TRAM procedures, the midline should not be incised.
- In unilateral cases, the dissection proceeds from lateral to medial until the lateral row of perforators is encountered.
- In bilateral cases, the dissection can proceed from medial to lateral on each side until the medial row of perforators is encountered.

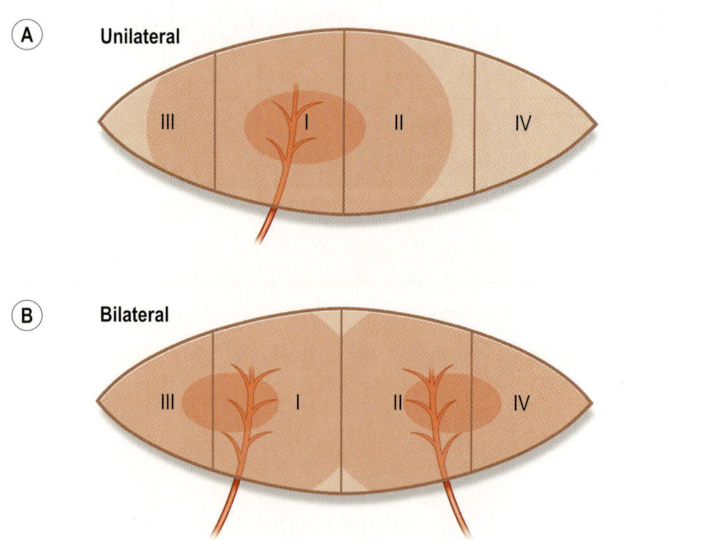

Figure 18.4 The standard elliptical design of a TRAM flap with Zones I through IV. **(A)** Zone I lies directly over the vascular pedicle and is the most reliable. Zones II and III are generally reliable; however, zone IV should be approached with caution due to its distance from the vascular pedicle. **(B)** In bilateral reconstruction, the majority of each hemiflap is used.

- Proposed markings of the boundaries of the left and right rectus sheaths, as well as the costal margin can be made in the superior epigastrium using methylene blue.
- One must carefully observe the degree of the diastasis recti ***(Fig. 18.8A)***.
- The sterile Doppler is now used to locate the position of the superior epigastric artery as it passes from deep to the costal margin. This location is important as it should become the center of the muscle portion that is harvested superiorly (see Fig. 18.8B).
- The proposed muscle and fascial harvest is drawn in using methylene blue incorporating the emanation of the superior epigastric vessels superiorly and harvesting approximately one-third to one-half of the central rectus fascia as the proposed muscle and fascial flap pedicle (see Fig. 18.8).
- Dissection begins at the costal margin laterally and extends through the fascia for 2–3 cm caudal to the costal margin.
- At this point, the anterior fascia is elevated laterally to confirm the position in the muscle relative to its lateral border. We try to leave 1–2 cm of muscle and, more importantly, fascia laterally. One must confirm though that the dissection is not too far lateral or too far medial high up before the dissection continues inferiorly ***(Fig. 18.9A)***.
- The dissection then continues using the cautery on the blend setting. It is important to be sure that the patient has complete muscular paralysis during this intramuscular dissection.
- The dissection can then continue expeditiously through the overlying fascia and underlying muscle down to and below the level of the umbilicus.
- Small oblique vessels will be noted but are only perineural vessels accompanying the lower abdominal wall nerves to the rectus segments reminiscent of intercostal nerves more cephalad.

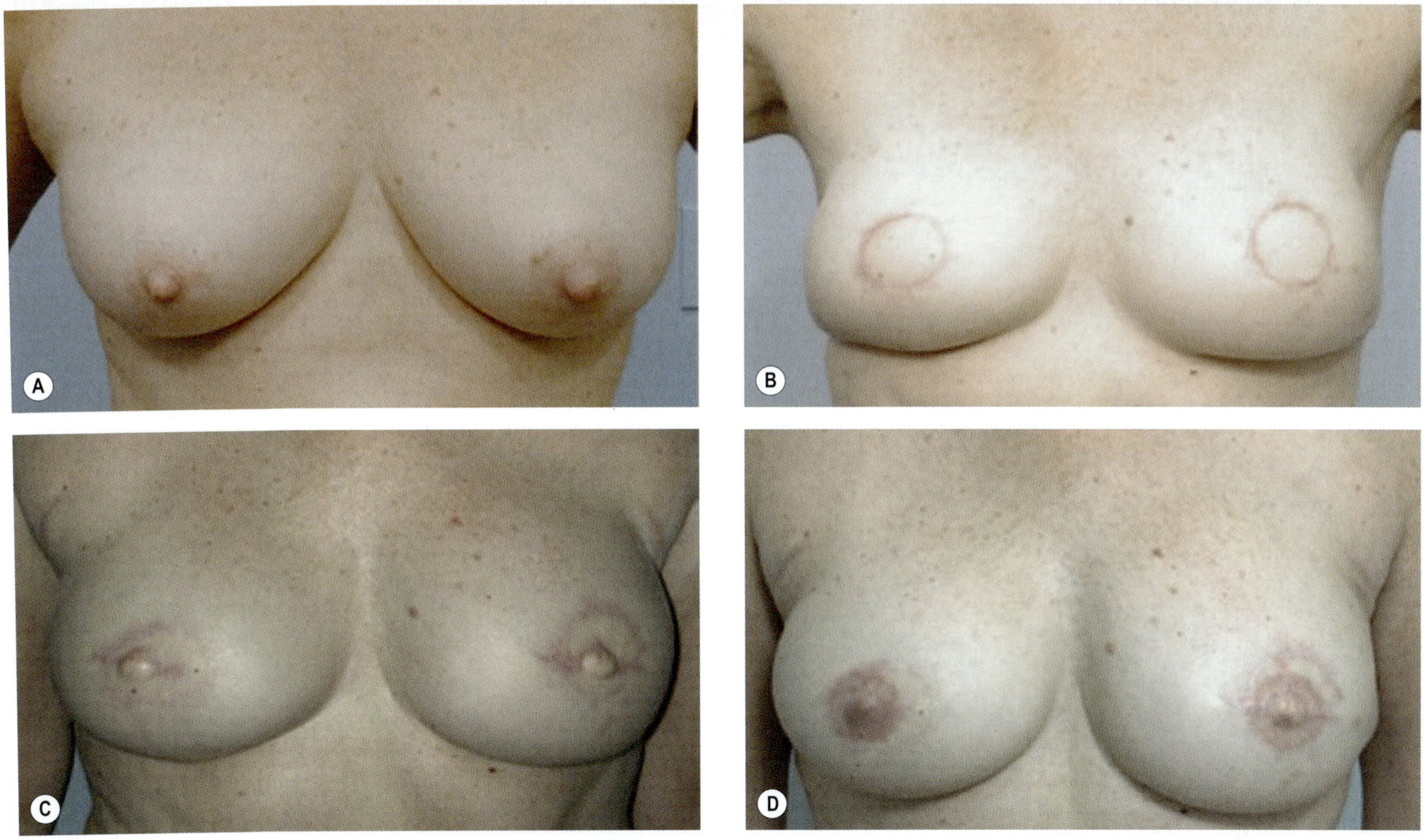

Figure 18.5 (A–D) Pre- and postoperative photographs of a patient who underwent bilateral pedicled TRAMs.

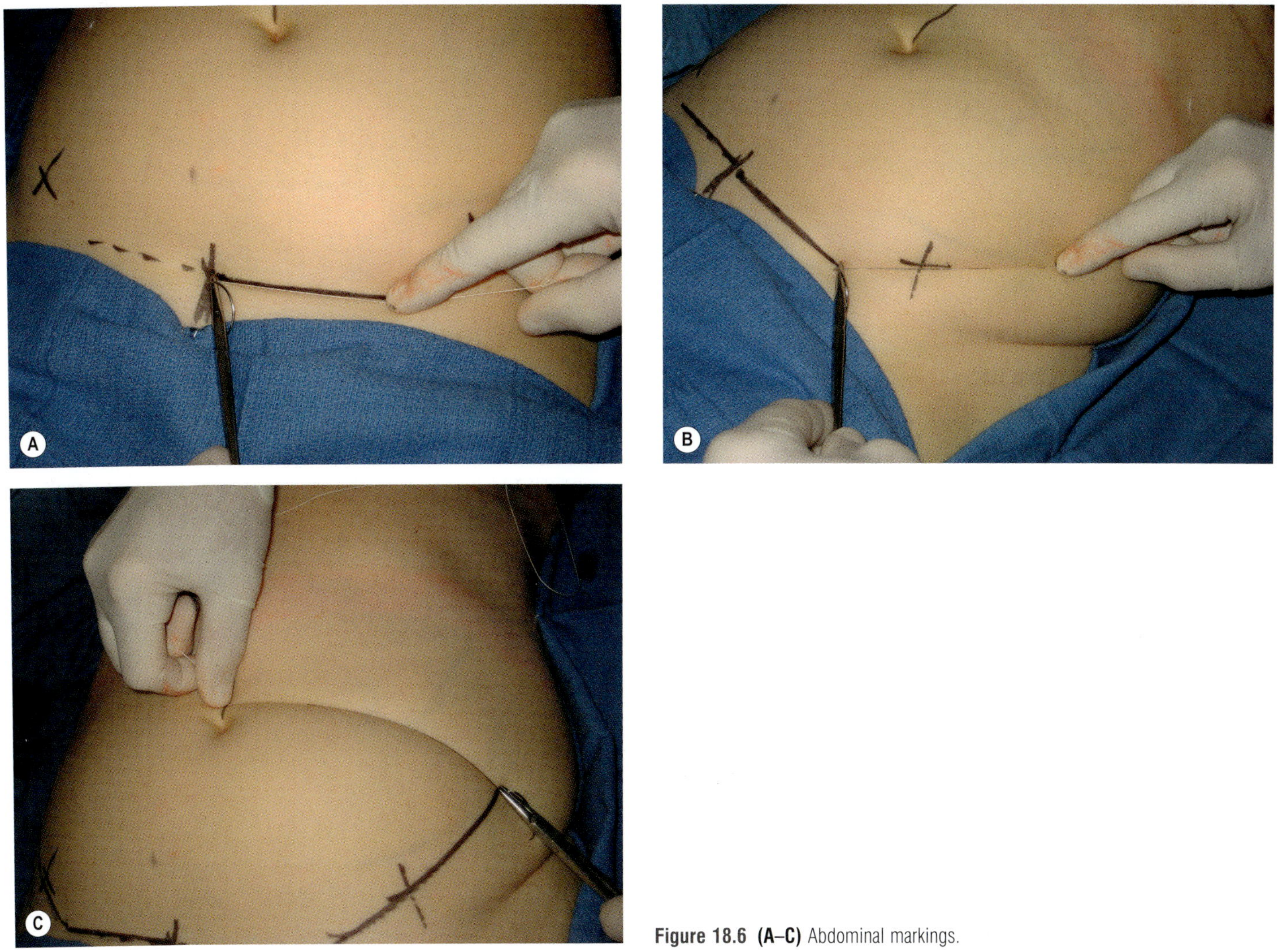

Figure 18.6 (A–C) Abdominal markings.

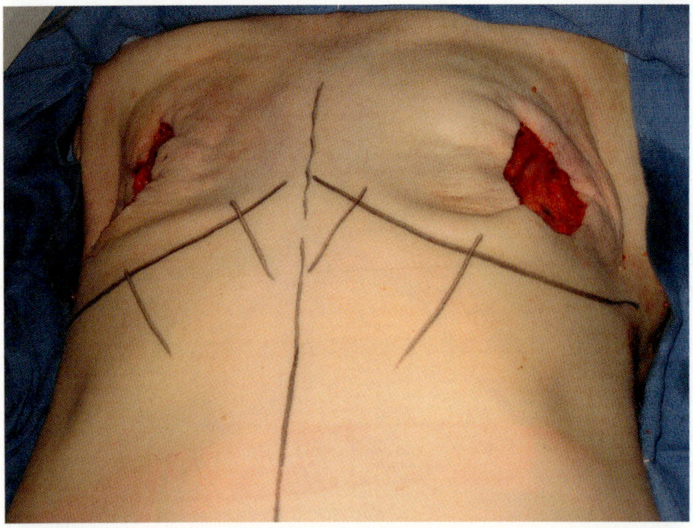

Figure 18.7 Tunnel locations.

- The location of the inferior epigastric vessels is in a relatively constant position two-thirds of the way caudad from the umbilicus to the pubic symphysis. Dissection through the muscle proceeds more cautiously until the inferior epigastric vessels are located (see Fig. 18.9B).
- The muscle can also be elevated from lateral to medial and the vascular hilum of the inferior epigastric vessels entering into the muscle might be noted prior to seeing the inferior epigastric vessels inferiorly (see Fig. 18.9C,D).
- As the central segment of the muscle is elevated out of its bed inferiorly it can also be elevated superiorly and the superior epigastric vessels can also be visibly identified.
- The muscle is now well mobilized, and the inferior epigastric vessels are identified. They are clipped and transected with a medium clip applier or ligature.
- The medial dissection on the fascia and muscle can now be performed. With one hand behind the muscle, one can

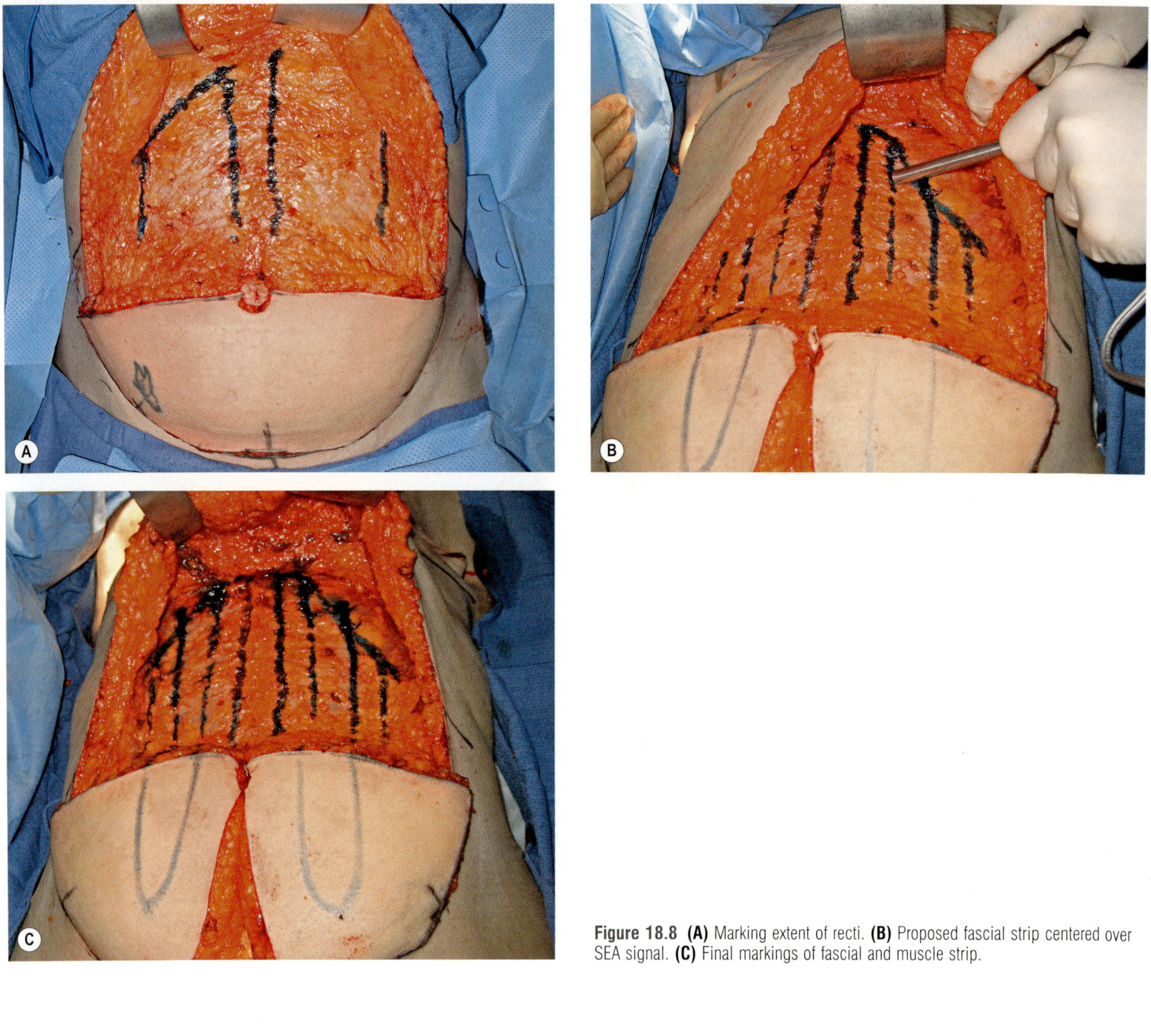

Figure 18.8 **(A)** Marking extent of recti. **(B)** Proposed fascial strip centered over SEA signal. **(C)** Final markings of fascial and muscle strip.

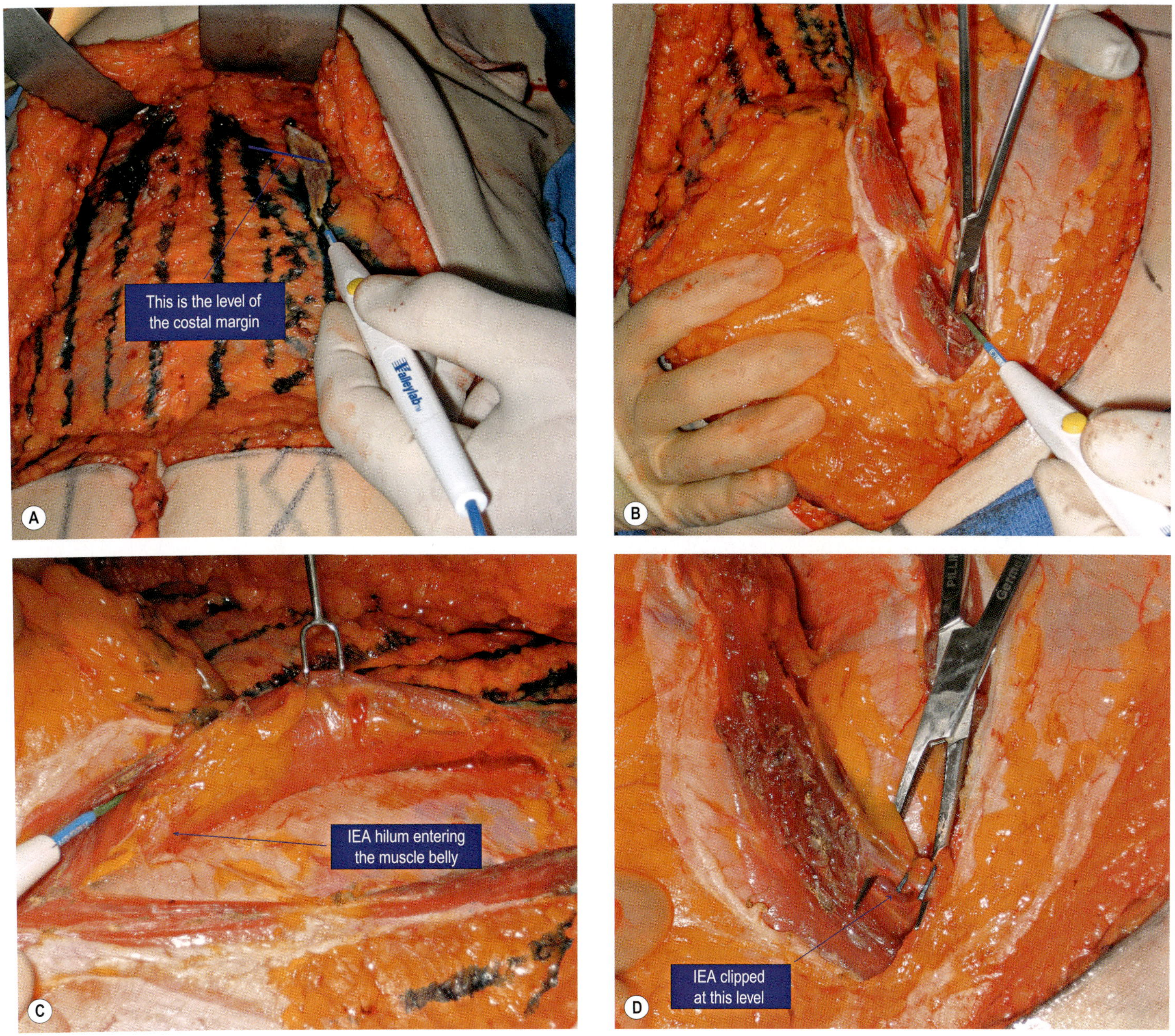

Figure 18.9 Lateral muscle dissection. **(A)** Identifying lateral extent of rectus muscle as a landmark. **(B)** Careful intramuscular dissection around DIEA. **(C)** Identifying DIEA hilum entering inferolateral edge of muscle. **(D)** Clipping the DIEA.

establish the location of the medial border of the muscle. Once again, we shift laterally for 1–2 cm where an incision in the fascia and underlying muscle is made. This is usually first performed at the level of the umbilicus *(Fig. 18.10)*.

- Dissection then continues vertically inferiorly and is curved just below the level of the inferior epigastric vessels to meet the lateral dissection.
- The muscle and overlying flap must be controlled at all times by the surgeon as he conducts the fascial and muscle dissection *(Fig. 18.11)*. At this point, the flap is freed up inferiorly essentially up to the level of the umbilicus.
- The superior dissection medially is now completed by a vertical incision up towards the costal margin. The superior epigastric vessels have been visualized as well as located using the sterile Doppler so this dissection continues up without threat of injury to these vessels. This intramuscular dissection is facilitated by controlling the muscle and fascial pedicle with one hand, placing hemostats on the medial fascia for counter-traction and performing the medial intramuscular dissection with cautery *(Fig. 18.12)*.
- The incision in the fascia continues up over the costal margin and meets the original lateral incision in the fascia; however, muscle is left intact for about 1–2 cm

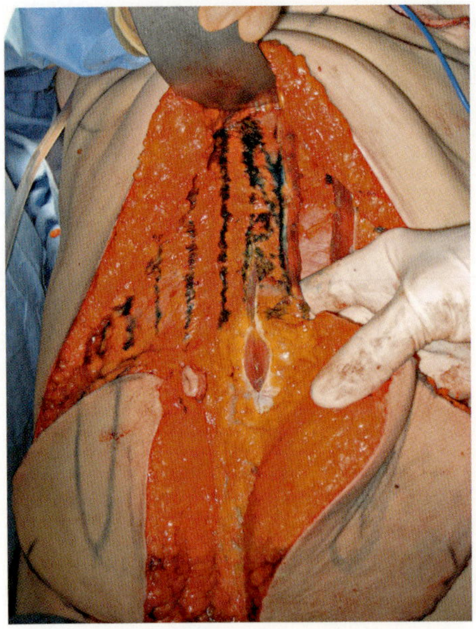

Figure 18.10 Medial dissection maintaining control of flap at all times with opposite hand.

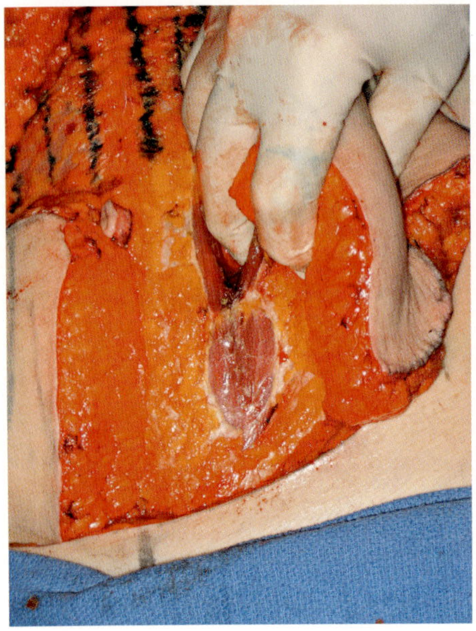

Figure 18.11 Inferomedial dissection to meet inferolateral dissection.

caudal to the costal margin medially which thins the muscle proximally at the costal margin to 1–2 cm in width. This is safe because the presence and location of the superior epigastric pedicle is confirmed with the sterile Doppler, direct vision, and/or palpability.

- This creates a muscular-fascial pedicle length of usually ≥8–9 cm ***(Fig. 18.13)***.
- The distance from the costal margin to the inframammary line of the breast is only about 5–6 cm, so 8–9 cm is more than an adequate length of muscle pedicle to easily reach the chest area (Figs 18.13B***, 18.14***).
- The flap skin is moistened and the flap is gently passed through the preformed tunnel.

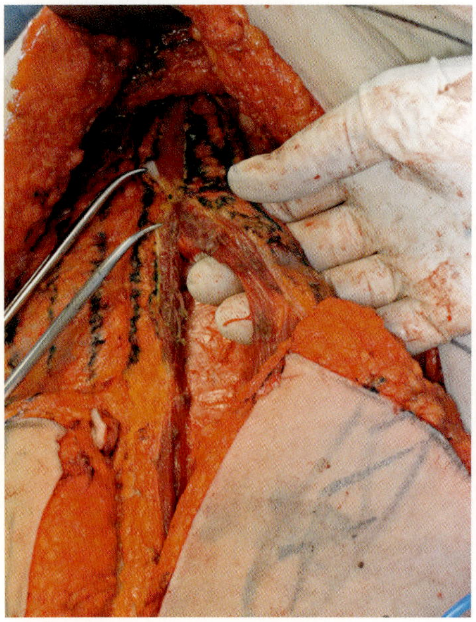

Figure 18.12 Control of muscle and fascial pedicle and use of countertraction on the fascia during superomedial dissection.

- Ipsilateral transfer is often preferred in bilateral cases and avoids crossing the pedicles in the midline.
- In unilateral cases, use of the contralateral flap may be more beneficial to allow a more gentle rotation of the pedicle. However, it is probably safe to use either technique.
- It is helpful to use a towel clip on the lateral tip of the TRAM flap which passes through the tunnel first. It is also helpful then to either work the superior corner or the inferior corner first through the tunnel, the other corner then follows easily.
- Once the flap is in the chest pocket the pedicle is carefully adjusted at the costal margin so that it turns around the costal margin and does not flip over the costal margin.
- If the pedicle flips over the costal margin it causes two major twists in the pedicle which are unnecessary if the gentle turning of the pedicle is instead employed ***(Figs 18.15–18.17)***.
- The flap is secured to the chest using skin staples and attention is turned to abdominal wall closure. This will allow time for any vascular compromise to the flaps to occur and be observed.

Abdominal closure

- After the TRAM flap is harvested, a fascial defect remains in the lower abdominal wall. Depending on the amount of fascia sacrificed, various techniques may be employed for closure.
- An MS-3 or MS-2 flap typically has a very small resultant fascial defect which may be closed primarily without tension.
- A pedicled TRAM, MS-1 or MS-0 free TRAM defect on the other hand, may preclude apposition of the free fascial edges. In this case, mesh is routinely employed.

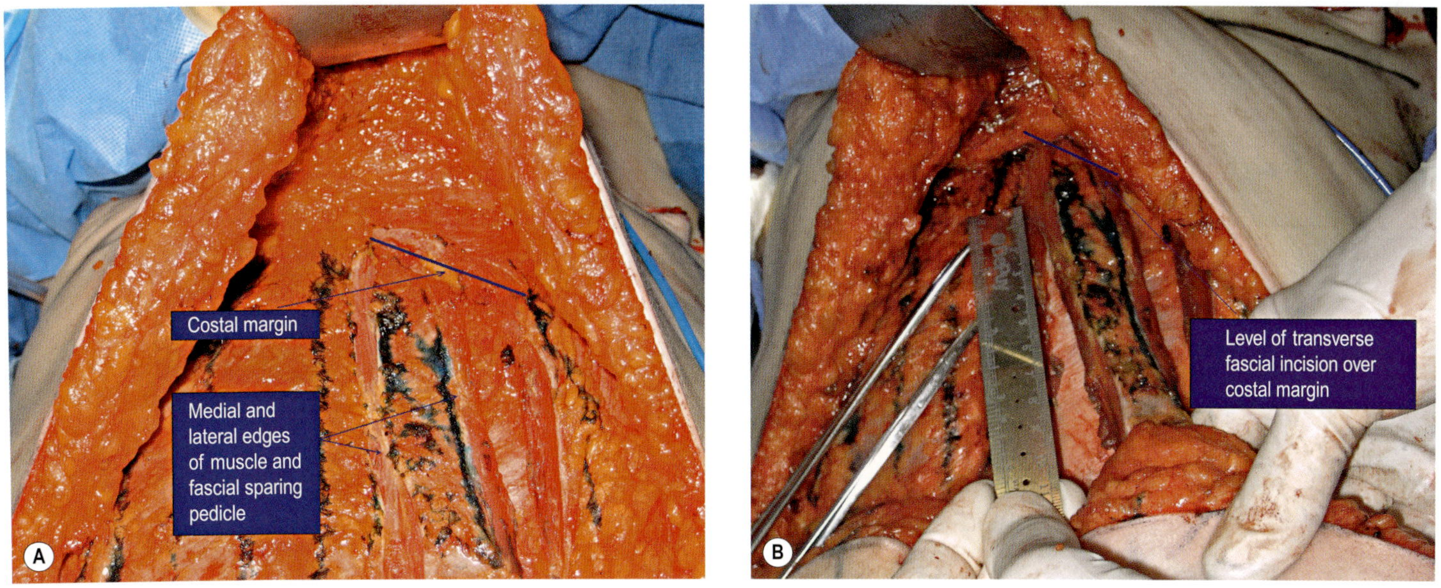

Figure 18.13 (A,B) Demonstrating width and length of fascial and muscle strip and extent of dissection up over costal margin.

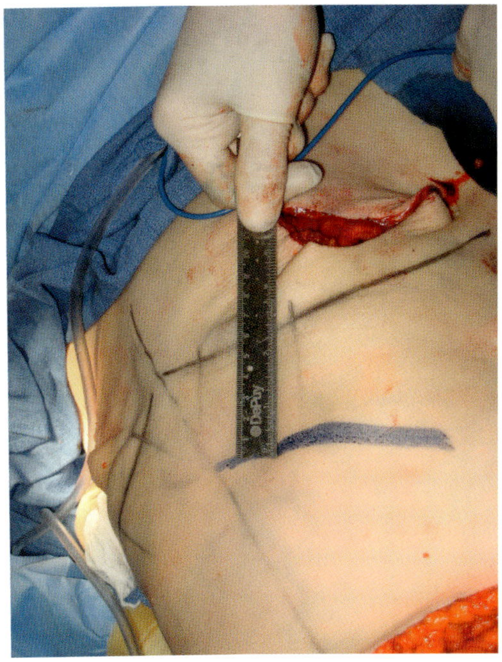

Figure 18.14 Further demonstrating that pedicle length is more than adequate to reach chest wall defect.

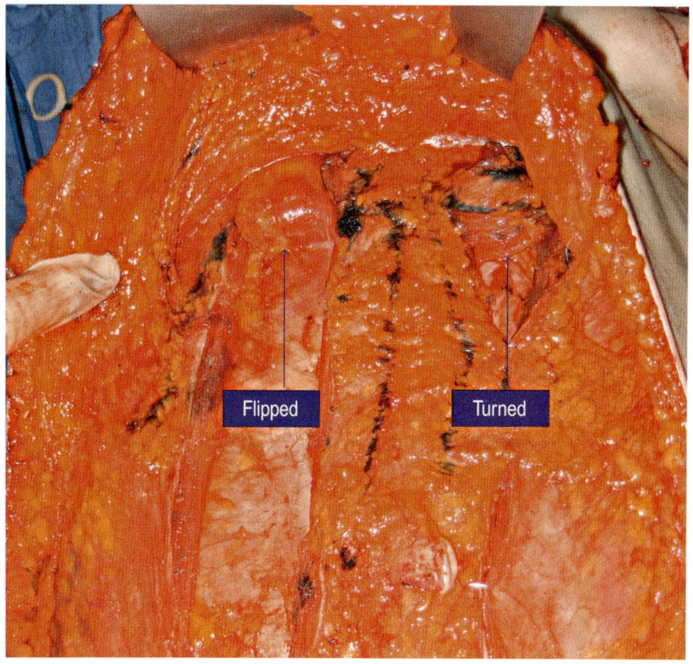

Figure 18.15 Gently turning the pedicle around the costal margin avoids two kinks which result if the pedicle is flipped.

- Polypropylene mesh remains the most common subtype employed for fascial closure in a clean wound *(Fig. 18.18)*.
- In unilateral reconstruction, after closure of the fascia, the abdominal wall and midline may no longer be symmetrical. As a result, some surgeons recommend plication of the fascia on the contralateral side. Care must be taken, however, to not add to the tension of the fascial repair.
- The closure typically begins superiorly using double stranded 0-nylon sutures. The double stranded suture is looped and avoids a knot superiorly. The closure then proceeds inferiorly in tandem being careful to include both the external and internal oblique components of the anterior rectus sheath. These two components become very obvious at and below the level of the umbilicus *(Fig. 18.19)*.
- It is extremely important to include both of these components, particularly the internal layer which probably accounts for the most important strength of the closure.
- The most difficult part of the abdominal closure is below the umbilicus and attention to detail must be stressed here to be sure that the closure is sound. Each bite is at

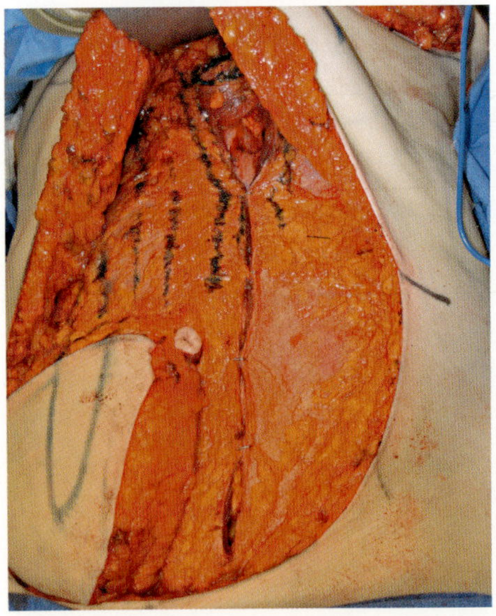

Figure 18.16 Note the distortion of the lines towards the side of closure.

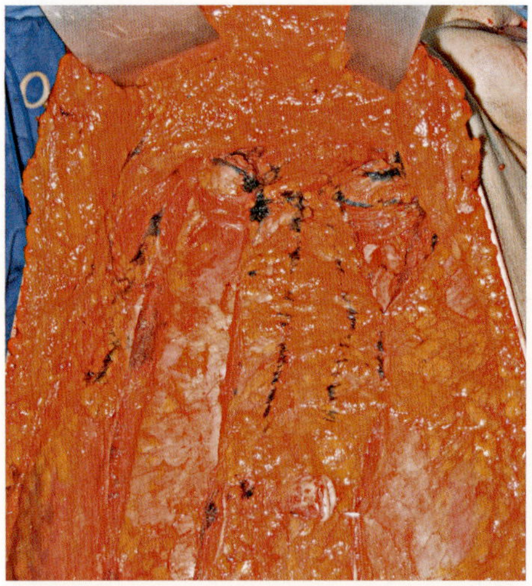

Figure 18.17 Seen here on one side only, staples were used identically on the contralateral side. Also note the turning of the pedicle around the costal margin.

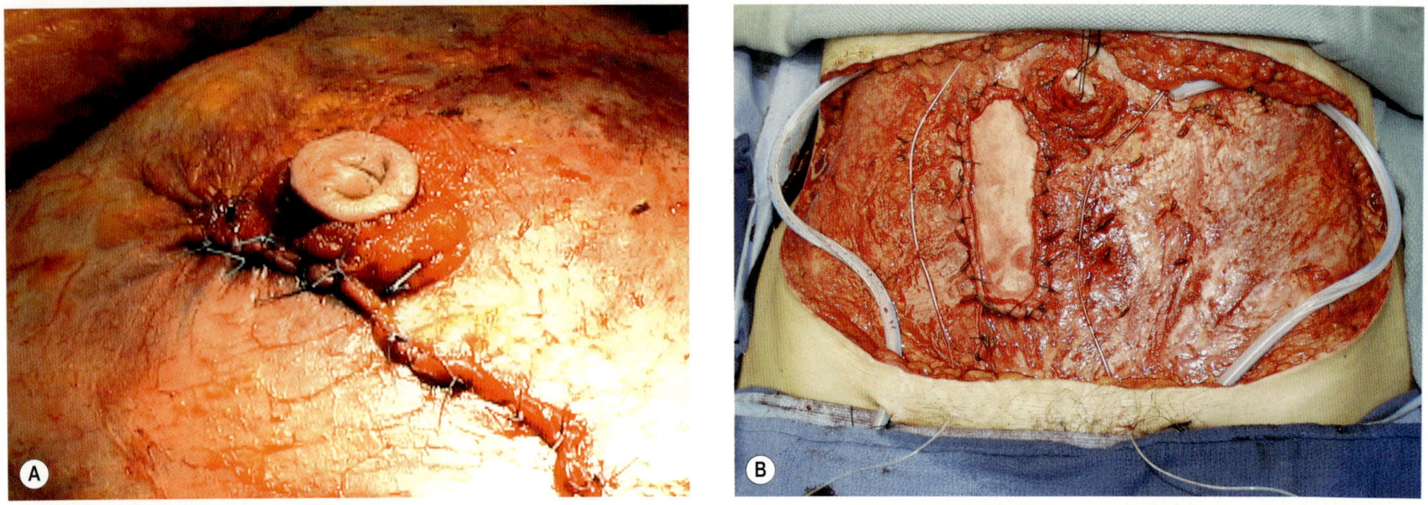

Figure 18.18 Abdominal wall closure. **(A)** Standard primary closure without mesh. **(B)** In this case, the abdominal wall fascial defect was insufficient to allow primary closure. Polypropylene mesh was used to span the gap and provide added strength. On-Q infusion catheters (I-Flow Corporation, Lake Forest, CA) are placed for pain control and JP drains are left for drainage. The umbilical stalk is reset in an appropriate position as the superior flap is draped over the donor site.

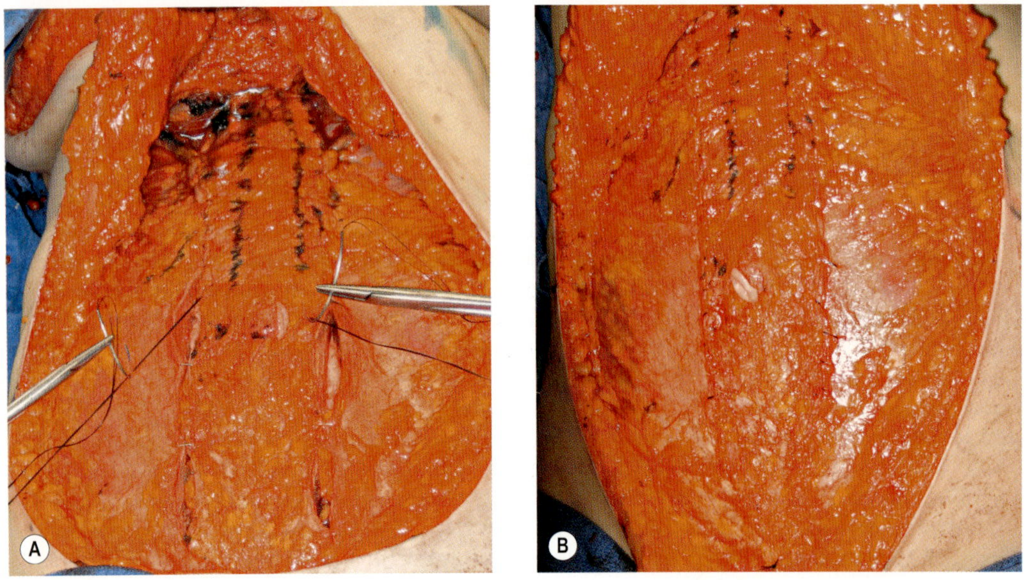

Figure 18.19 **(A,B)** Simultaneous fascial closure distributes tension across the abdomen and aids in primarily closing the fascial defects.

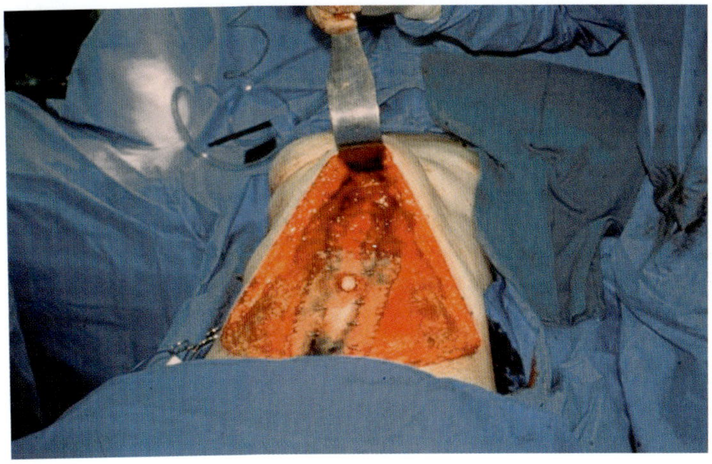

Figure 18.20 Double layer prolene mesh.

least 1 cm back on the fascia, and each bite advances 1–2 cm inferiorly on the fascia. The closure is completed with the double stranded suture, and fascial staples are added on both sides over the suture line for additional support.

- If there is any concern about the abdominal wall closure, Prolene mesh support is added over the closure once it is completed.
- The Prolene mesh, if used, is used in a double layer and is sutured in place using 0-Prolene in a running and interrupted manner ***(Fig. 18.20)***.
- The abdominal skin is closed in layers over closed suction drains in similar fashion to that performed during aesthetic abdominoplasty procedures, including umbilicoplasty.

Flap inset/breast shaping

- After closure of the abdominal wall, adequate time will have passed to observe any vascular compromise. The flap should have good pink color at this time.
- If any significant duskiness is noted, one may release the clips on one or both inferior epigastric veins to decompress the flap. Additionally, the tunnel width should be re-evaluated.
- By the time the flap is de-epithelialized, red healthy bleeding should be observed from the dermis. If not, the pedicle should be examined visibly for undue twisting and with the sterile Doppler for arterial inflow.
- Shaping of the TRAM in the immediate setting is significantly assisted by the presence of native skin on the chest. While there are many variations of remaining skin after skin sparing mastectomies, the idea is to leave a remaining skin envelope which will cover the TRAM flaps with mild but not undue tension.
- The TRAM flap is sutured internally in the pocket medially, superiorly and laterally to stabilize the flap on the chest wall so that the skin closure will effect the final shaping.
- It is important to adequately fill any deficit in the infraclavicular location (superior pole), as this is an extremely important aesthetic subunit of the breast.
- Laterally, the TRAM flap should be tacked to the chest wall to define the lateral contour of the breast as sharply as possible. However, any sutures placed through TRAM tissue for positioning purposes should be tied down relatively loosely to avoid localized areas of fat necrosis (see Fig 18.5).
- The flap is inset in layers using absorbable deep dermal sutures and a running subcuticular skin closure.

Video 18.2

Free TRAM *(Fig. 18.21; Video 18.2)*

- The dissection of the free TRAM flap begins in similar fashion to that described above for the pedicled TRAM through creation of the superior abdominal flap ***(Fig. 18.22)***.
- Of course, in free TRAM techniques, the IMF tunnel is not necessary.
- While making the inferior incision, the superficial inferior epigastric vessels are encountered bilaterally in the midinguinal region. At this point, if sufficient for use (palpable arterial pulse, large vein), one should consider the possibility of performing an SIEA flap (Video 18.3). If insufficient for use, they may be ligated and divided, although preserving a large vein for additional or alternate drainage should be considered even if performing a TRAM. Video 18.3
- The dissection is carried down to the fascia and the lateral apices of the flap may be dissected off the fascia.
- The dissection is carried from lateral to medial up to the point of the identification of the lateral row of perforators projecting through the rectus fascia into the subcutaneous tissue of the flap.
- If performing a unilateral reconstruction, the side of the flap opposite the vascular pedicle (zones II and IV) may be completely dissected off the abdominal wall and carried up to the point of the medial row of perforators on the pedicle side (across the midline).
- If a bilateral flap is being performed, division of the flap in the midline will aid in the medial row dissection on either side.
- A decision is made at this point to use either the medial perforators, lateral perforators, or both.
- The fascia is incised vertically and circumferentially to incorporate the chosen perforators, creating an island of excised fascia as part of the flap. The size of this excised fascia depends on the number of perforators chosen.
- Next, the surgeon identifies the vascular pedicle posterior to, and at the lateral edge of the rectus muscle.
- It should be followed as far down to the external iliac vessels as possible, but should not be divided until the recipient site is ready for anastomosis and insetting.
- After division of the pedicle, the rectus muscle is divided inferiorly to the perforators, allowing for tension free release of the pedicle.
- Lastly, the superior muscle is divided; however, care must be taken to identify and oversew the superior pedicle to prevent bleeding.

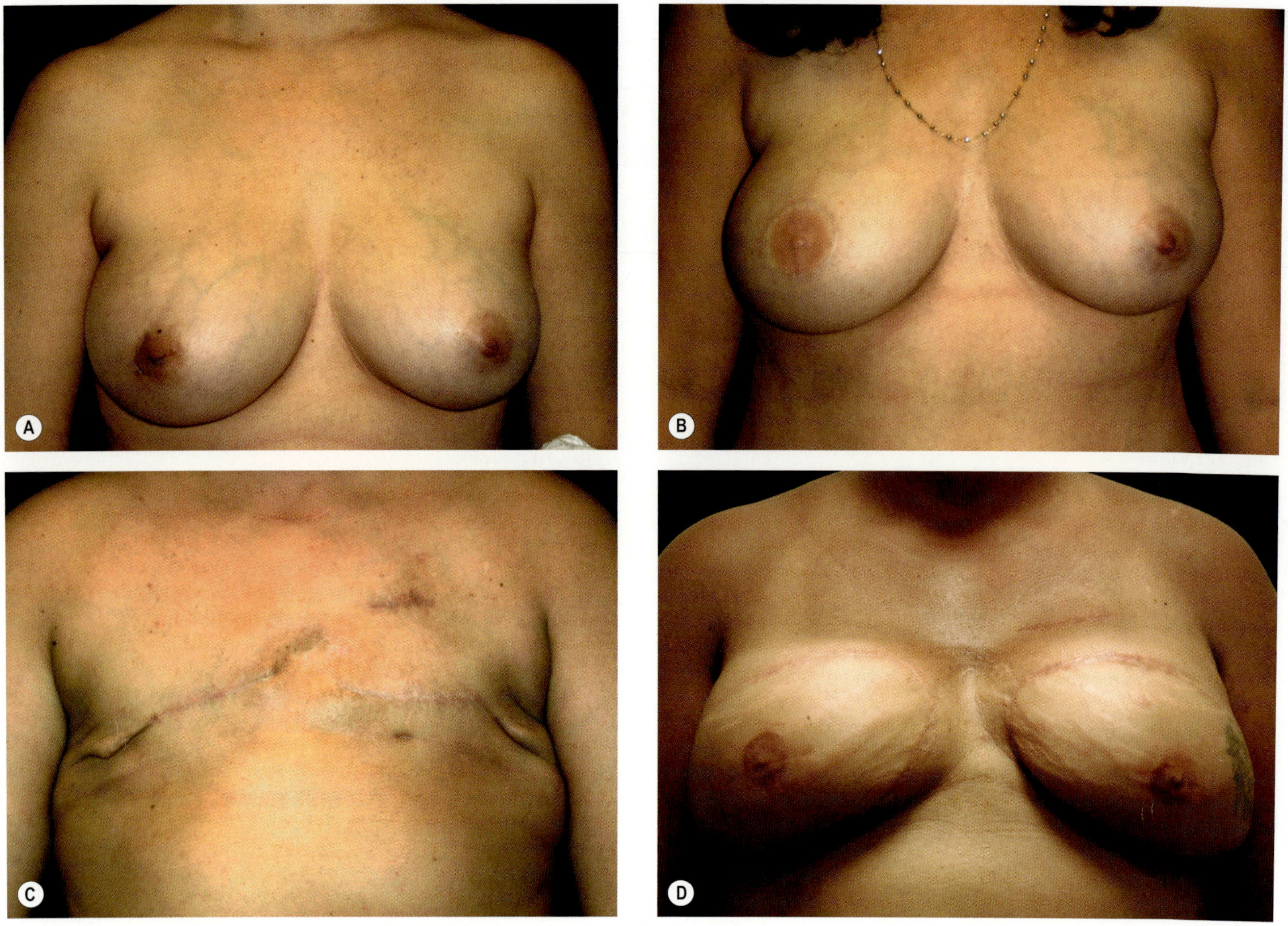

Figure 18.21 The final results. **(A)** Preoperative photograph, note the patient has a recent periareolar incision for a breast biopsy. **(B)** Postoperative following a right free TRAM flap and subsequent NAR reconstruction with tattooing for color. **(C)** Preoperative photograph of a patient with previous bilateral mastectomies. **(D)** Postoperative following a bilateral muscle sparing free TRAM with subsequent NAR and reconstruction with tattooing for color. Note there is a significantly higher utilization of the skin from the flap for creation of an envelope.

- The degree of muscle sacrificed is dependent on the anatomic variability of the perforators and can range from no muscle sacrifice (DIEP or MS-3), central excision only (MS-2), medial or lateral excision (MS-1), or to complete transection of the lower rectus (MS-0) ***(Fig. 18.23)***.
- The two most common recipient vessel sites in free tissue reconstruction of the breast are the thoracodorsal vessels and the internal mammary vessels ***(Fig. 18.24)***.
- In immediate breast reconstruction following a modified radical mastectomy, the thoracodorsal vessels are either fully or partially exposed.
- The thoracodorsal vessels are usually chosen as long as the autologous flap for reconstruction has a sufficiently long donor pedicle.
- End-to-end anastomoses are performed using either interrupted 8-0 or 9-0 nylon sutures for both the artery and vein or using sutures for the artery and a coupler for the vein.
- In the setting of delayed breast reconstruction, some surgeons choose the thoracodorsal recipient vessels because of their familiarity with flap insetting and because of the proven efficacy of these vessels in delayed reconstruction. But, for many surgeons, the internal mammary vessels are the recipient vessels of choice.
- Advantages of internal mammary recipient vessels:
  - Avoidance of surgery within the axilla that has been scarred from previous surgery.
  - Allows a more medial positioning of the flap for improved symmetry and aesthetics.
  - The internal mammary vessels have also been used preferentially when mastectomy combined with sentinel node biopsy is performed.
- The internal mammary vessels are first approached by separating the fibers of the pectoralis muscle overlying the third costal cartilage ***(Fig. 18.25)***.

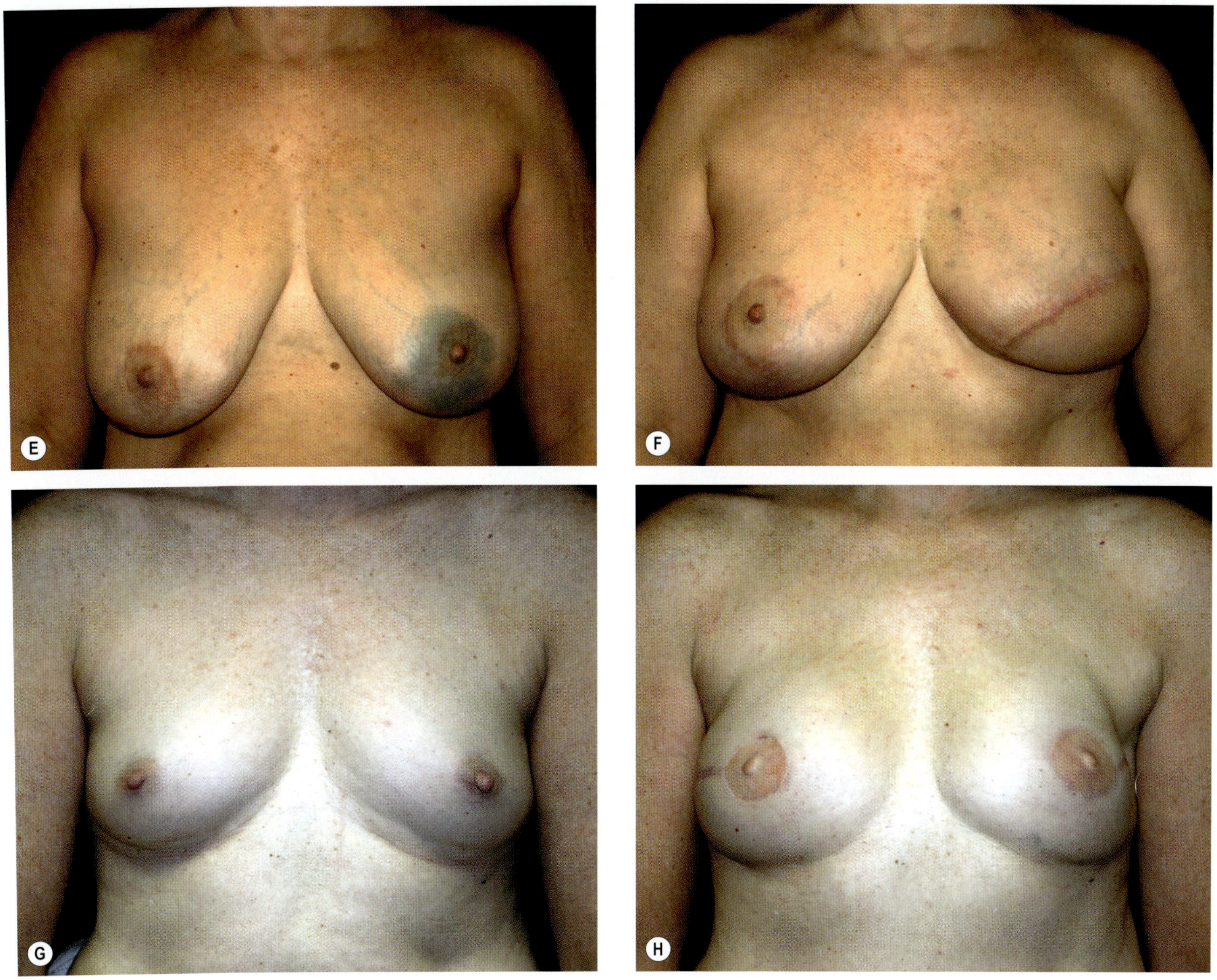

Figure 18.21, cont'd **(E)** Preoperative photograph in a patient with a recent left axillary sentinel lymph node biopsy and significant ptosis. **(F)** Postoperative following a left free TRAM via a Wise pattern with concomitant balancing right mastopexy. She has yet to undergo NAR. **(G)** Preoperative photograph of a patient with bilateral malignancies. **(H)** Postoperative following bilateral skin sparing mastectomy with free TRAM reconstruction.

- Self-retaining retractors are placed perpendicularly, exposing the cartilage and intercostal musculature.
- The perichondrium is incised along the midanterior surface from the junction of the sternum to 1–2 cm medial to the costochondral junction and separated off of the cartilage, first on the anterior surface and then extending to its posterior surface. Complete separation of the posterior perichondrium can be difficult and is unnecessary.
- Once the perichondrium is partially separated on the upper and lower edges of the costal cartilage, a rongeur is used to remove the cartilage.
- The deep perichondrium is then incised lateral to the internal mammary vessels and reflected lateral to medial. Care must be taken to avoid transection of the small intercostal vessel branches coming off the internal mammary system.
- Once the vessels are identified and separated from the internal mammary lymphatics, the length of dissection is extended by dividing the intercostal musculature from the top of the fourth rib to the bottom of the second rib; this is done by staying lateral to the internal mammary vessels.
- As compared with most other recipient vessels throughout the body, the internal mammary artery is more susceptible to injury and thrombosis during its dissection. Minimal use of vascular forceps is recommended.
- The internal mammary vein tends to be larger on the right side than on the left side. Although the third cartilage is currently recommended, the second cartilage can be similarly removed for access to a recipient vein of greater diameter.

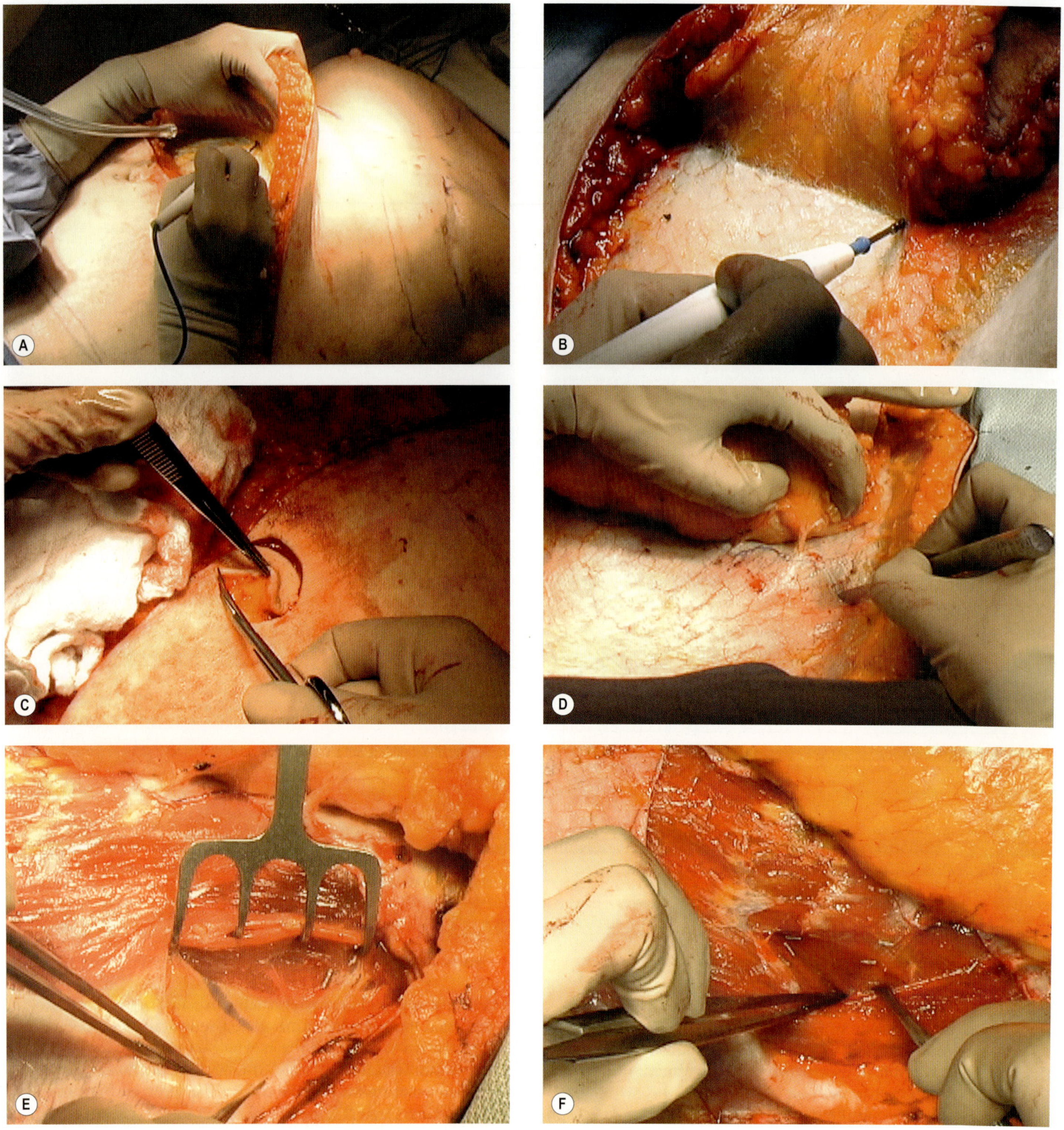

Figure 18.22 Dissection of the free TRAM flap. **(A)** A superior abdominal flap is raised to allow for eventual tension free closure. The height of the TRAM flap is dependent on the mobility of this flap. **(B)** The lateral flaps of the TRAM are raised to the point of the lateral perforators. **(C)** The umbilicus is preserved. **(D)** An anterior rectus sheath fasciotomy is made above and below the perforators. **(E)** Within the rectus sheath, the muscle is reflected medially to allow for visualization and dissection of the inferior epigastric vessels. **(F)** The perforators are identified and preserved as they traverse the muscle. This allows for preservation of at least the lateral aspect of the rectus muscle for a muscle sparing free TRAM.

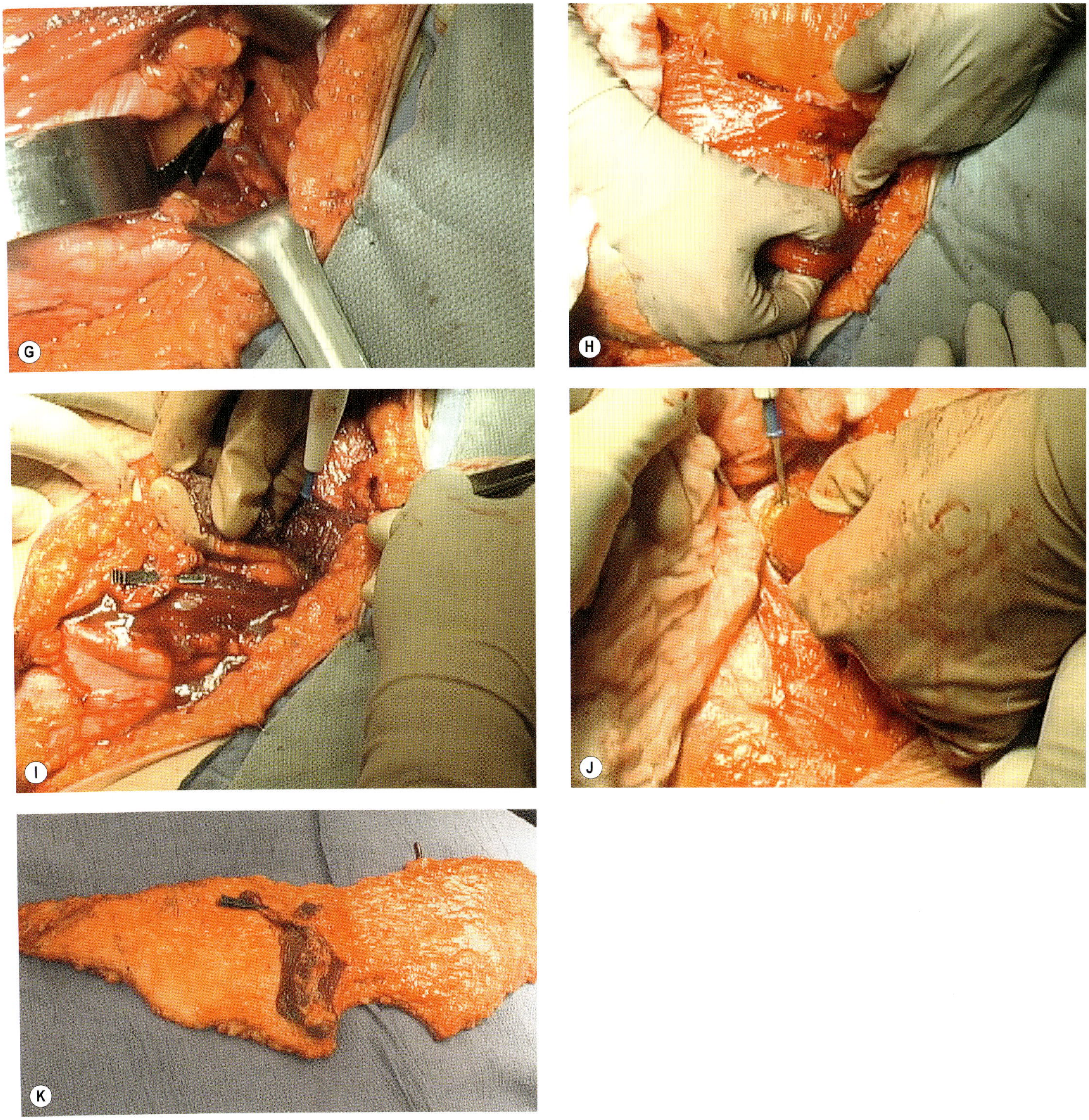

Figure 18.22, cont'd **(G)** After the recipient site is prepared, the vascular pedicle is clamped and divided inferiorly to allow for ample pedicle length. **(H)** The pedicle is passed through the middle of the rectus muscle in the plane of the perforators. **(I)** The inferior muscle is divided. **(J)** The superior muscle is divided. **(K)** The flap is ready for anastomosis.

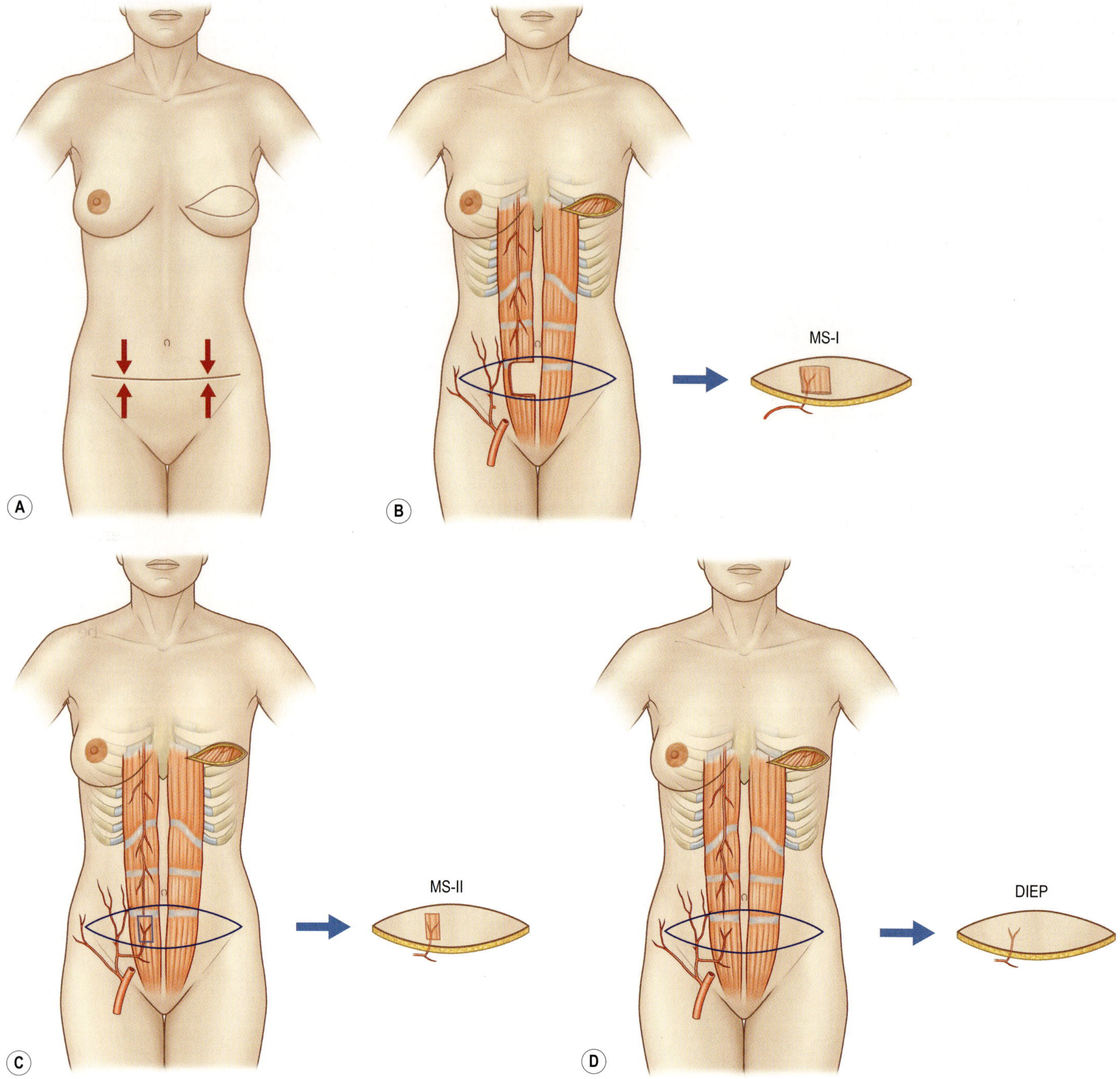

Figure 18.23 The variations of a free TRAM. **(A)** The MS-0 flap in which the rectus muscle is completely transected. **(B)** The MS-I spares the lateral band preferably (as opposed to the medial band) of muscle with the goal of preserving the innervation of the muscle. **(C)** In an MS-II flap, only a small central portion of the rectus muscle around the perforators is transected. **(D)** The MS-III, otherwise known as a DIEP, preserves the entire rectus muscle.

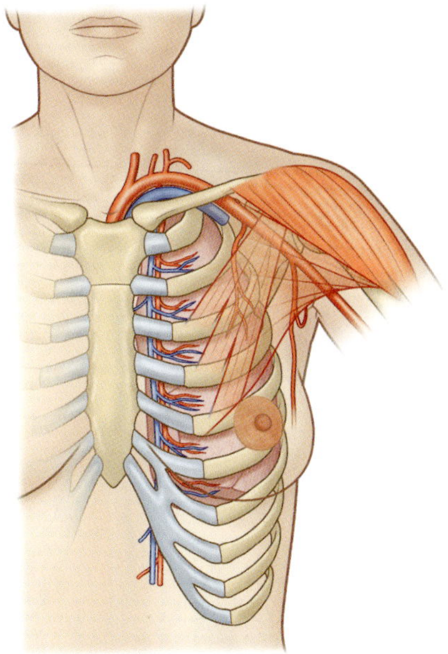

Figure 18.24 The vascular anatomy of the chest wall. The two most common sites for recipient vessel harvest and subsequent vascular anastomoses are the internal mammary vessels and the thoracodorsal vessels.

- Once fully dissected, the internal mammary artery and vein are divided at the level of the fourth rib and supported on their deep surfaces by a neurosurgical sponge ***(Fig. 18.26)***.
- The free flap is temporarily positioned to allow easy performance of the anastomoses. Sutures of 9-0 nylon may be used for both anastomoses; however, the internal mammary artery is at times quite large, requiring 8-0 nylon. The vein is usually amenable to use of the coupler device.
- Other potential recipient vessels include the scapular circumflex vessels, the thoracoacromial vessels, and the axillary artery and vein. These are rarely used as the planned primary recipient vessel site; rather, they are used when problems have occurred during surgery at one of the two routine recipient vessel sites.

Flap insetting

- A decision as to whether to use an ipsilateral or contralateral free flap has usually been made preoperatively, based on the shape of the contralateral breast, the timing of reconstruction and the planned recipient vessels ***(Fig. 18.27)***.
- In general, when the thoracodorsals are used, a narrow ptotic breast is reconstructed with an ipsilateral flap which has been rotated 90° with the umbilicus positioned in an inferomedial orientation.
- A less ptotic, but wide breast is reconstructed with a contralateral free flap with the flap rotated approximately 140° such that the lateral aspect of the initial flap design becomes the tail of the neo-breast mound. This may be rotated up to 180° for increased width.
- If the internal mammary vessels are used, the concept is the same except that the exact opposite is performed – a contralateral flap is used for a narrow, pendulous breast whereas an ipsilateral flap is used to construct a wider breast mound.
- Once the anastomosis is complete and orientation established, the buried portions of the flap are de-epithelialized.
- The goal is to remove the epidermis and a portion of the dermis; however, care should be exercised not to injure the subdermal vascular plexus which likely helps with more uniform perfusion of the edges of the flap.
- The flap is secured in place in multiple layers and the skin closed with running 4-0 absorbable monofilament.
- If there is a question about the viability of the mastectomy flaps prior to conclusion of the case, the TRAM may be "banked" under the mastectomy flaps without de-epithelialization. The patient returns to the operating room 72 h later, after the skin flaps have fully demarcated, at which time the TRAM flap can be formally inset.
- Abdominal closure proceeds similarly to that described in the pedicled TRAM technique

DIEP flap *(Figs 18.28, 18.29; Video 18.4)*

Video 18.4

- Flap dissection is similar to that of the free TRAM described above.
- While making the inferior incision, care is taken to preserve the superficial epigastric vessels.
- If the venous drainage of the flap is insufficient or thrombosis of the perforating vein(s) occurs after the anastomosis, the superficial epigastric veins can be used as an additional venous conduit.
- Two or three veins may be present but they commonly unite further down the abdominal wall. The veins are dissected over a length of 2–3 cm and ligated with clips to make them easily retrievable later, if needed.
- If the caliber of the superficial epigastric artery is noted to be large enough, a similar skin island to the DIEAP flap can be harvested on these two vessels.
- Dissection of the vascular pedicle of a DIEAP flap can be divided into three different technical stages; suprafascial, intramuscular and submuscular dissection. The most demanding stage is the intramuscular dissection of the vascular pedicle.
- Suprafascial dissection is carried out similar to free TRAM procedures and proceeds laterally to medially up to the lateral row of perforators ***(Fig. 18.30A,B)***.
- If the caliber of one vessel is estimated to be insufficient, an adjacent perforator located on the same vertical line can also be dissected.
- The abdominal wall muscles must be relaxed at all times and the perforating vessels kept moist with normal saline.
- When dissecting a perforator from the lateral side, it is important to realize that a side branch may be located more medially. Extra care must be taken when dissecting the full circumference of a vessel, but complete dissection helps prevent vessel damage when raising the flap from the contralateral side (see ***Fig. 18.31C,D***).

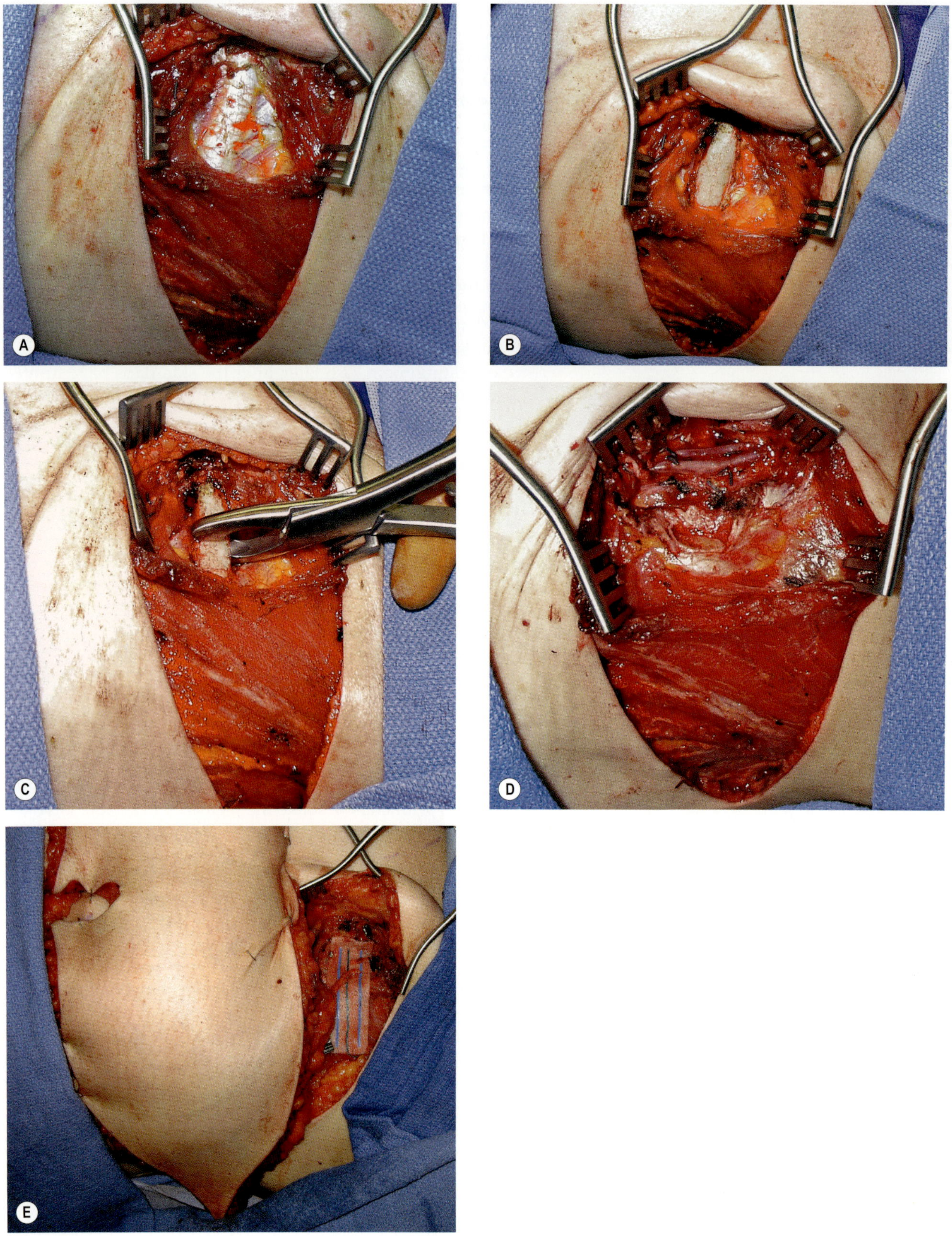

Figure 18.25 The vascular anastomosis to the internal mammary vessels. **(A)** The third rib is cleaned off, followed by **(B)** incision of the anterior perichondrium. **(C)** The costochondral junction is removed with a rongeur. **(D)** Further dissection allows for exposure of the internal mammary vessels. **(E)** The anastomoses are performed.

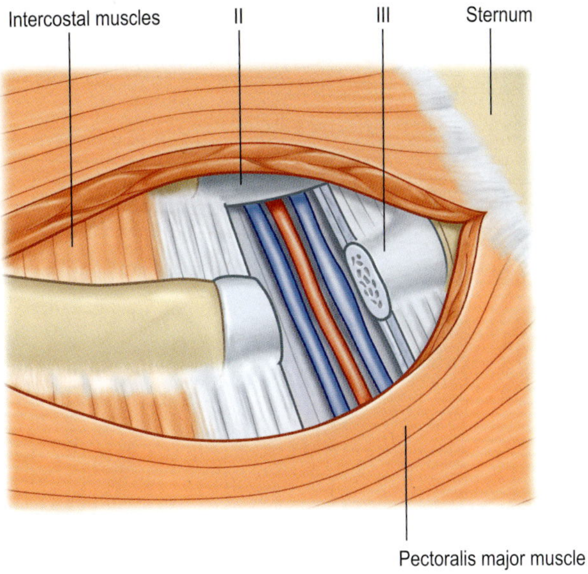

Figure 18.26 The internal mammary artery and two common veins on the right side after removing a small part of the costal cartilage of the third rib.

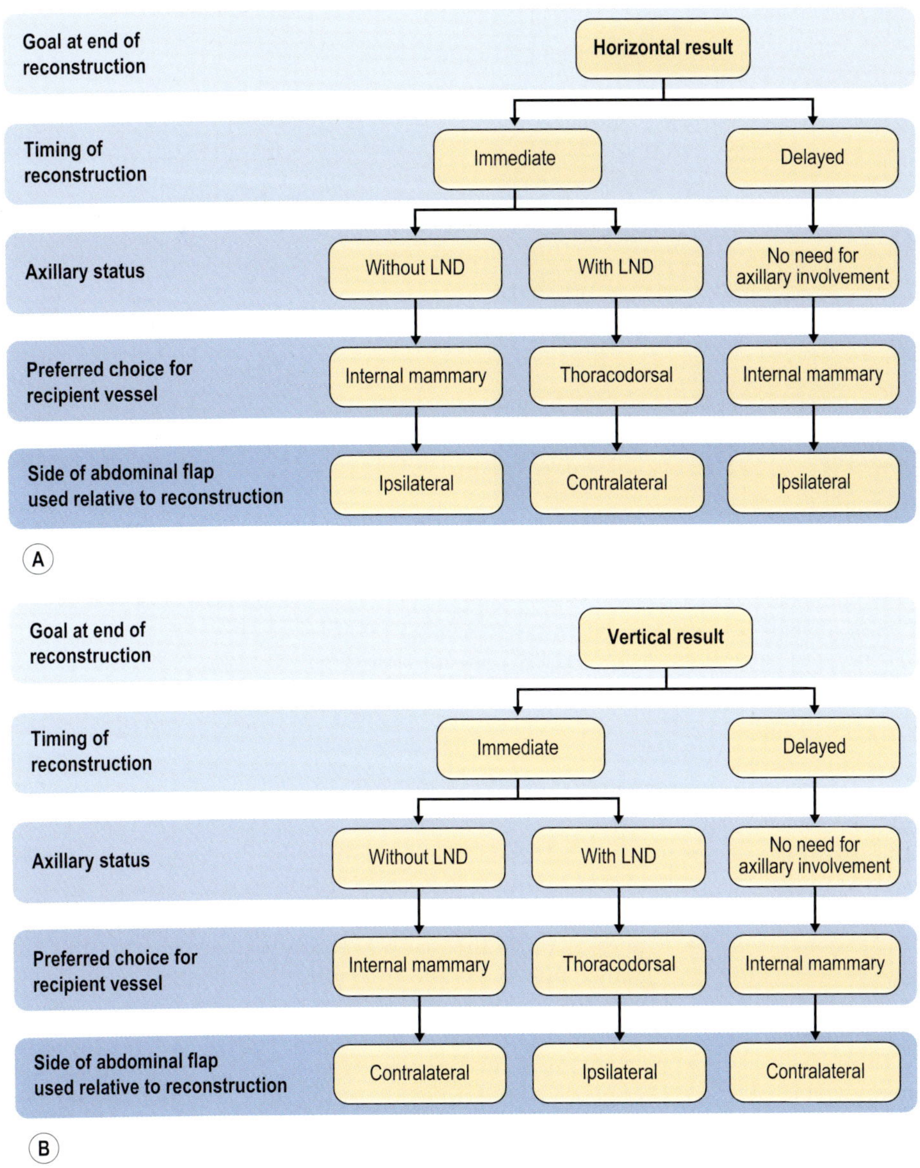

Figure 18.27 Whether unilateral or bilateral, the standard approach to insetting is shown in this algorithm and takes in to consideration the overall goal, the timing of reconstruction, node status, choice of recipient vessels and the laterality of the flap. The goal of a wider, more horizontal breast mound is shown in **(A)**; whereas, **(B)** depicts a more vertical, pendulous breast.

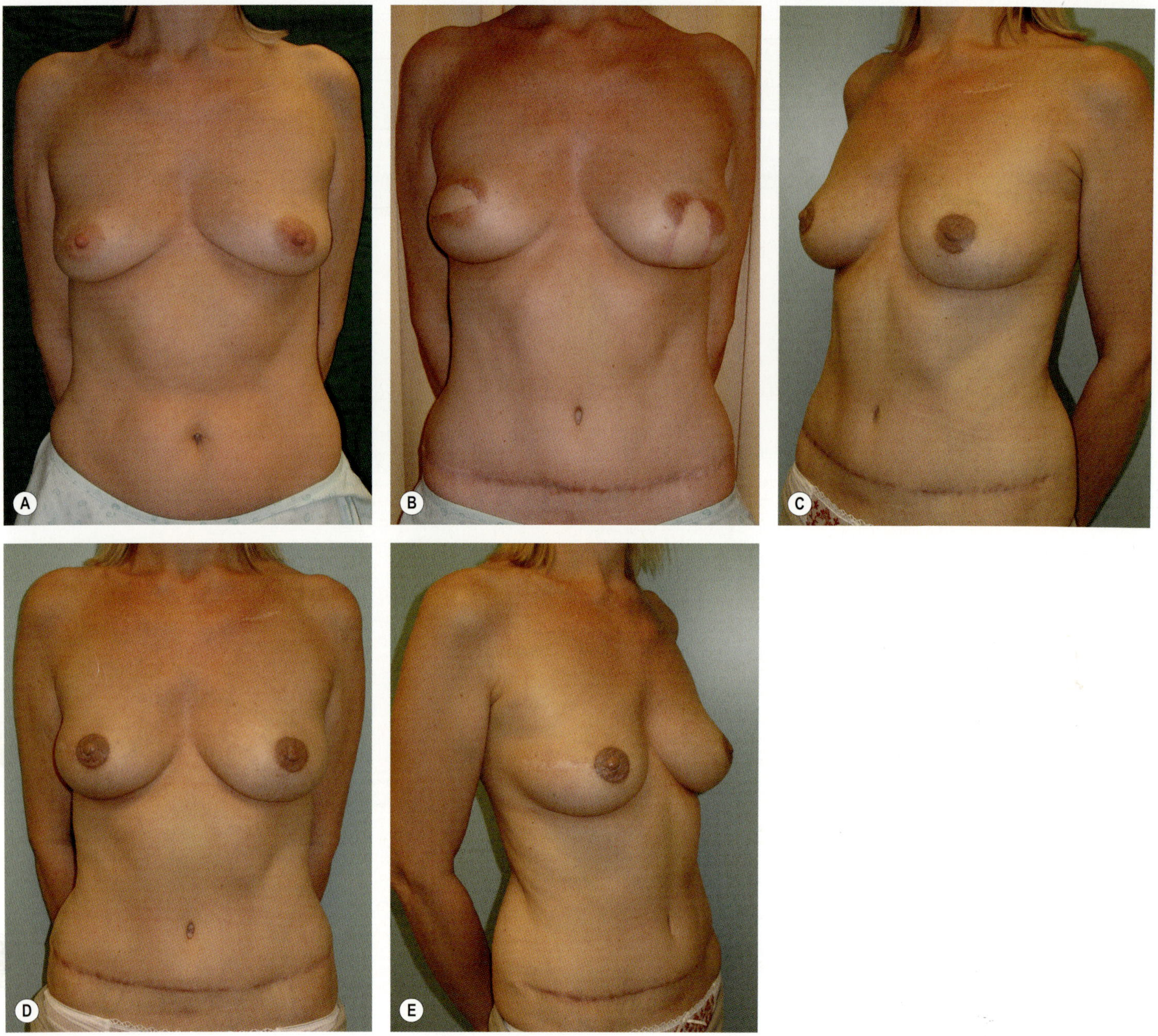

Figure 18.28 (A) Preoperative image of a 46-year-old-woman, carrier of a BRCA-2 mutation, following tumorectomy through a horizontal racquet incision at the right breast. **(B)** Intermediate phase after bilateral areola-sparing mastectomy, using the same scar on the right breast and a more conventional vertical scar on the left breast, and bilateral autologous reconstruction by means of a bilateral free DIEAP flap. **(C–E)** A 2-year-postoperative image after bilateral nipple reconstruction using the interposed skin island of the flap and bilateral tattoo.

- The anterior rectus fascia is then incised with a pair of scissors following the direction of the rectus abdominis muscle fibers at the rim of the tiny gap in the fascia through which the perforating vessel passes (see Fig. 18.30E).
- If more than one perforator is dissected, the different gaps can be connected with each other. A small cuff of fascia may be left around the perforator if the vessel is small or if the surgeon feels more comfortable doing so.
- Lifting the fascia helps mobilize the perforator, which can be freed by blunt dissection, gently pushing away the loose connective tissue.
- The division of the fascia is continued superiorly for a distance of 3–4 cm and inferiorly to the lateral border of the rectus abdominis muscle in an oblique line towards the inguinal ligament (see Fig. 18.30F).
- At this point the direction of the division of the fascia is changed into the direction of the fibers of the external oblique muscle.

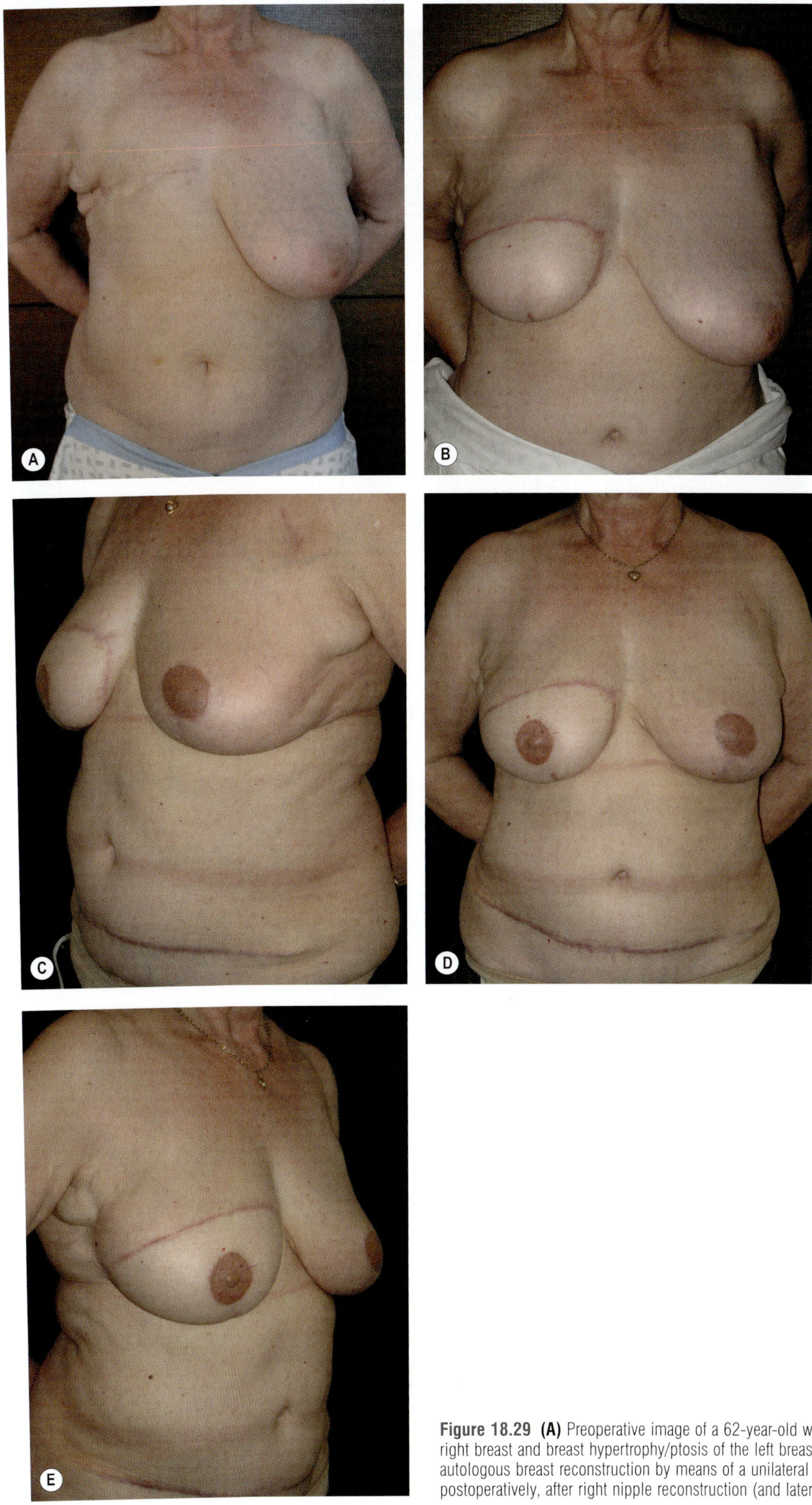

Figure 18.29 **(A)** Preoperative image of a 62-year-old woman following modified radical mastectomy of the right breast and breast hypertrophy/ptosis of the left breast. **(B)** Intermediate phase after secondary autologous breast reconstruction by means of a unilateral free DIEAP flap. **(C–E)** Final result, 1 year postoperatively, after right nipple reconstruction (and later tattoo) and left breast reduction.

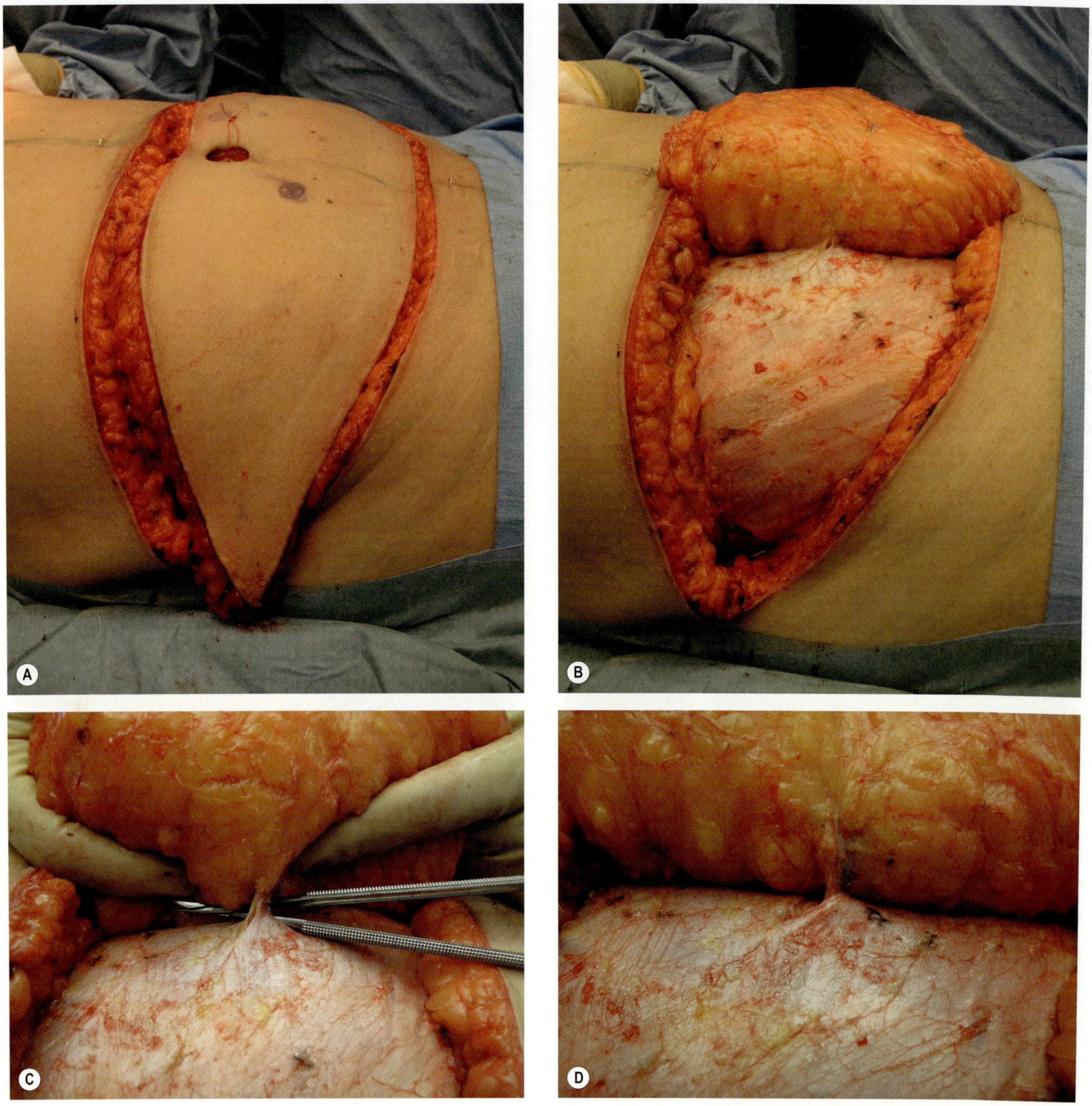

Figure 18.30 (A) Incision of skin and subcutaneous tissue is extended towards the flanks if additional tissue is needed. The dominant perforator on the right side is marked with an "x" on the flap. (B) The flap is laterally undermined towards medial until the area around the preoperatively marked perforator is reached. Undermining of the fat is continued proximal and distal of the perforator. (C) Undermining continues around the perforator for a distance of about 2 cm. Lifting up the subcutaneous tissue is easier at this point when the deep fascia is still closed. (D) Access to the perivascular loose connective tissue is sought by incising the gap in the deep fascia and the tissues surrounding the vessels.

- It is important to emphasize that the vessels must be protected at all stages and complete muscle relaxation is necessary until donor site closure is obtained. As dissection progresses, the DIEAP flap should be secured to the abdominal wall with the aid of staples.
- For the intramuscular dissection, the rectus abdominis muscle should be split in a longitudinal direction in the perimysial plane through which the perforating vessel traverses. Splitting the muscle fibers makes dissection easier as the vessel becomes larger (see Fig. 18.30G).

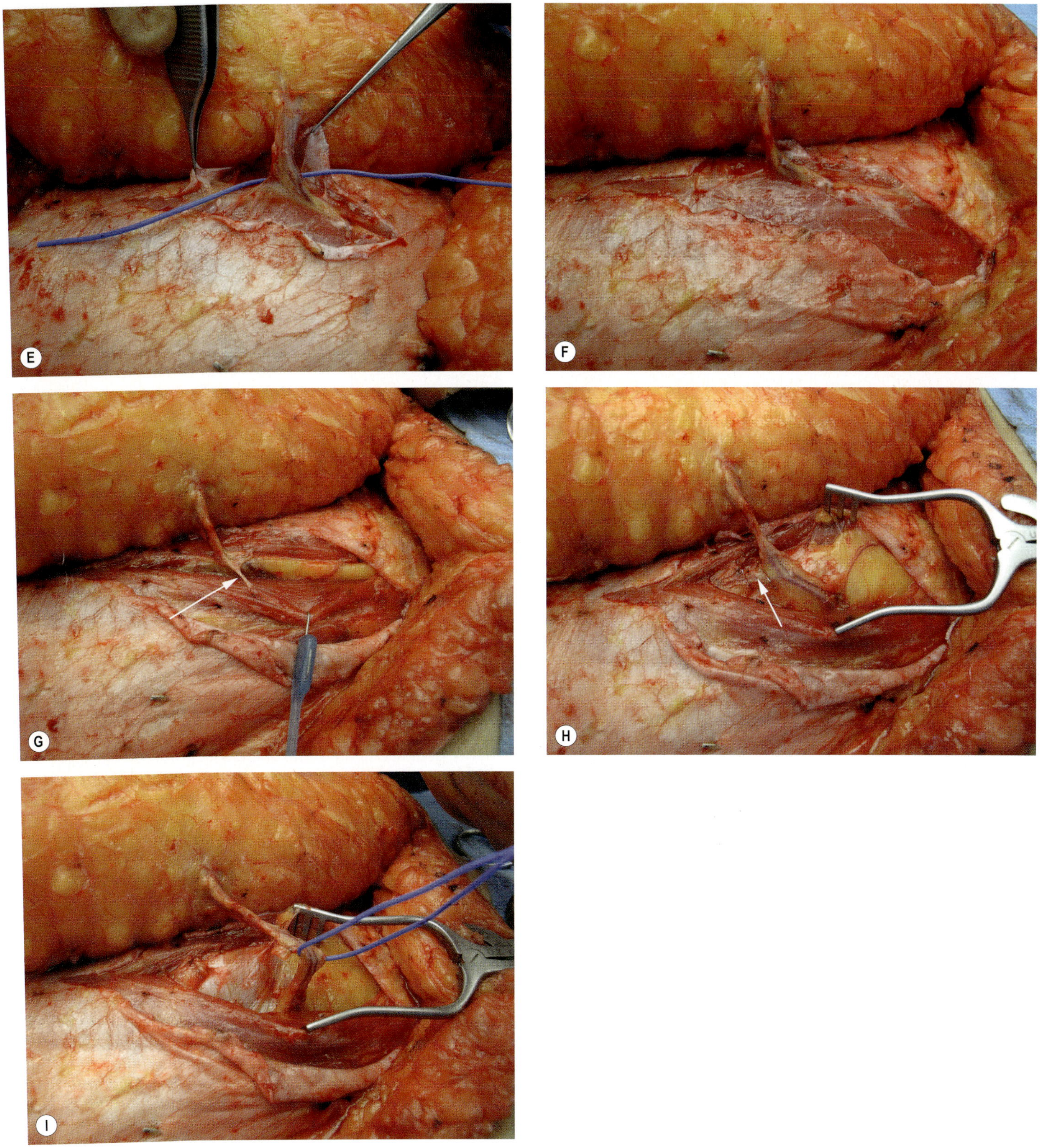

Figure 18.30, cont'd (E) The deep rectus fascia is incised vertically following the fibers of the rectus abdominis muscle both cranially and distally. The perforator is freed in its supra-muscular parts. **(F)** In a next step, the deep fascia is opened all the way down to the infralateral border of the rectus muscle and further distally along its lateral border to create exposure of the deep inferior epigastric artery and vein. **(G)** The rectus abdominis muscle is split following the muscle fibers until the posterior fascia or the peritoneum can be seen. Sensory nerves come here from lateral and following the perforator can be transected. Motor nerves are left intact (white arrow). **(H)** Wide exposure is achieved with a self-retaining retractor. A bloodless field allows perfect control of the dissection. The main axis of the deep inferior epigastric artery and its veins is clipped proximal to the perforators (white arrow). **(I)** Once the entire course of the perforator and the main vessels is clear, the posterior part of the perforator and the main vessels is dissected off the surrounding tissues. The distal part of the deep inferior epigastric vessels can be dissected either through the same incision through the rectus muscle or continued from lateral by pulling the rectus muscle medially.

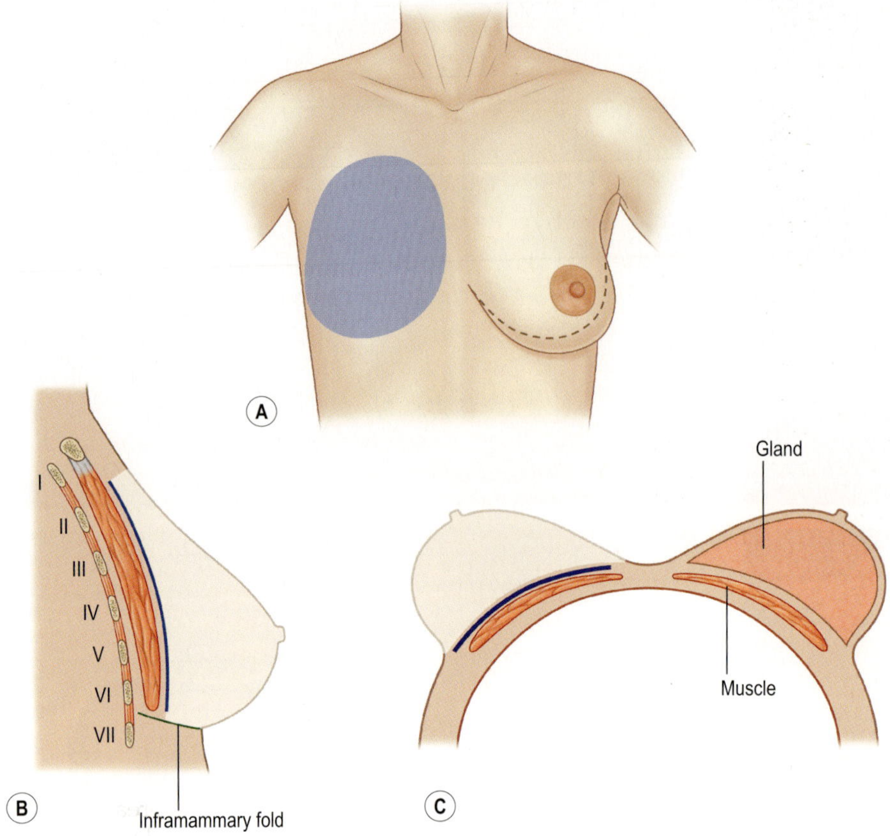

Figure 18.31 **(A)** Coronal, **(B)** sagittal and **(C)** transverse view of the footprint of the breast.

- The perforator is again liberated by blunt dissection, staying close to the vessel at all times, as it remains covered by a thin layer of loose connective tissue.
- As a general rule, if resistance to dissection is encountered, a side branch or a nerve will be identified. Different muscular branches must be ligated with care and hemoclips are placed 1–2 mm away from the main vessel so that if one inadvertently comes off, it can easily be replaced.
- Placing a vessel loop around the vascular pedicle allows additional retraction without any unnecessary tension being placed on the vessel.
- Using bipolar coagulating diathermy and small hemoclips, one continues to ligate all the side branches until the origin of the perforator on the major branch of the deep inferior epigastric vessel is reached at the posterior surface of the rectus abdominis muscle (see Fig. 18.30H).
- If two perforators have been selected, the rectus abdominis muscle must be widely separated. If the perforators run in two adjacent perimysial planes, the fibers may have to be cut. However, trans-section of large parts of the rectus abdominis muscle or division at the level where a motor nerve crosses from the lateral to the medial side should be avoided.
- For the submuscular dissection, the lateral border of the rectus abdominis is raised using non-crushing tissue forceps.
- Special care is taken not to injure the mixed segmental nerves entering the muscle laterally. The sensory nerve branch can be dissected by epineural splitting. In this way, an additional 5–9 cm can be obtained, facilitating neural suturing at the recipient site.
- Between the mixed segmental nerves, the plane posterior to the rectus abdominis muscle is opened, exposing the main deep inferior epigastric vessel. Side branches of the main stem are ligated and the dissection is continued by retracting the rectus abdominis muscle medially until the proximal part of the pedicle is completely liberated.
- The length of the pedicle can be tailored to meet the needs of different recipient sites or the demands of the shape of the flap (see Fig. 18.30I).
- The more distal the perforator is located in the flap, the further the deep inferior epigastric vessels need to be dissected into the groin.
- If one is certain that the blood flow through the deep inferior epigastric vessel is sufficient (an ultrasonic flow meter can be used) the remainder of the flap can be raised.
- In cases of midline scars, or when a large flap is needed, the same vascular dissection can be performed on the contralateral side. Otherwise, all the remaining perforators are ligated, the umbilicus is released and the entire skin flap is raised.
- The pedicle is finally transected when the recipient vessels have been prepared. A hemoclip can be placed on the lateral comitant vein to help orientate the pedicle.
- After division of the pedicle, the flap is turned over and the vessels placed carefully onto its undersurface. One has to be meticulous about the position of the pedicle, as it tends to rotate very easily, especially if only one perforator has been harvested.

Hints and tips

10 golden rules in perforator flap surgery

1. Map the perforators preoperatively: identify the most dominant vessels on each side.
2. Start dissection on one side of the flap: leave the contralateral side intact until you have finished the entire dissection of the pedicle.
3. Preserve every perforator until you encounter a larger one: discard only the smaller ones that you are sure you will not use. Select one or two perforators with the largest diameter that correspond with your preoperative mapping.
4. Consider the best location of the perforator within the flap: the more centrally located, the better the blood flow to the outer parts of the flap.
5. Consider the easiest dissection through the muscle: long intramuscular dissections are more tedious, contain more risk for damaging the vessels and are more time-consuming.
6. Dissect close to the vessels, remaining within the perivascular loose connective tissue, thereby guaranteeing an absolute bloodless field.
7. Ensure sufficient and wide exposure by splitting the muscle along its fibers (avoid digging into a small hole).
8. Carefully ligate every side-branch at a distance of about 2 mm away from the main pedicle.
9. Avoid any traction on the perforator: intima rupture is a frequent cause of unexplained clotting of the perforator.
10. Trans-sect the other perforators after the entire pedicle is dissected.

Abdominal closure

- Unlike TRAM techniques, since no fascia has been resected, primary tension-free closure of the fascia with a running, non-absorbable 1-0 suture is always possible. The remainder of the wound is closed in similar fashion to aesthetic abdominoplasty.

Flap inset

- DIEP flap inset is similar to that of TRAM techniques. A systematic approach is applied to be able to create easy and reproducible results in shaping of autologous tissue by using the "3-step principle".
- Recreating a 3-dimensional organ from a flat piece of abdominal fat and skin is broken down into three essential steps:
  1. Redefining and recreating the basis and borders of the footprint of the breast (the interface of the posterior surface of the breast gland and the thorax) at the right location on the chest wall (Fig. 18.31).
  2. Molding the flap into a drop-shape like conus on top of the footprint by means of specific suturing ***(Fig. 18.32)***.
  3. Redraping the skin envelope ***(Fig. 18.33)*** and the nipple areolar complex ***(Fig. 18.34)*** over the conus with the right tension.
- While the position of the borders of the new breast footprint are at a mirror position of the contralateral footprint, the new inframammary fold position needs to be placed 2–3 cm higher than the contralateral inframammary fold depending on the laxity of the

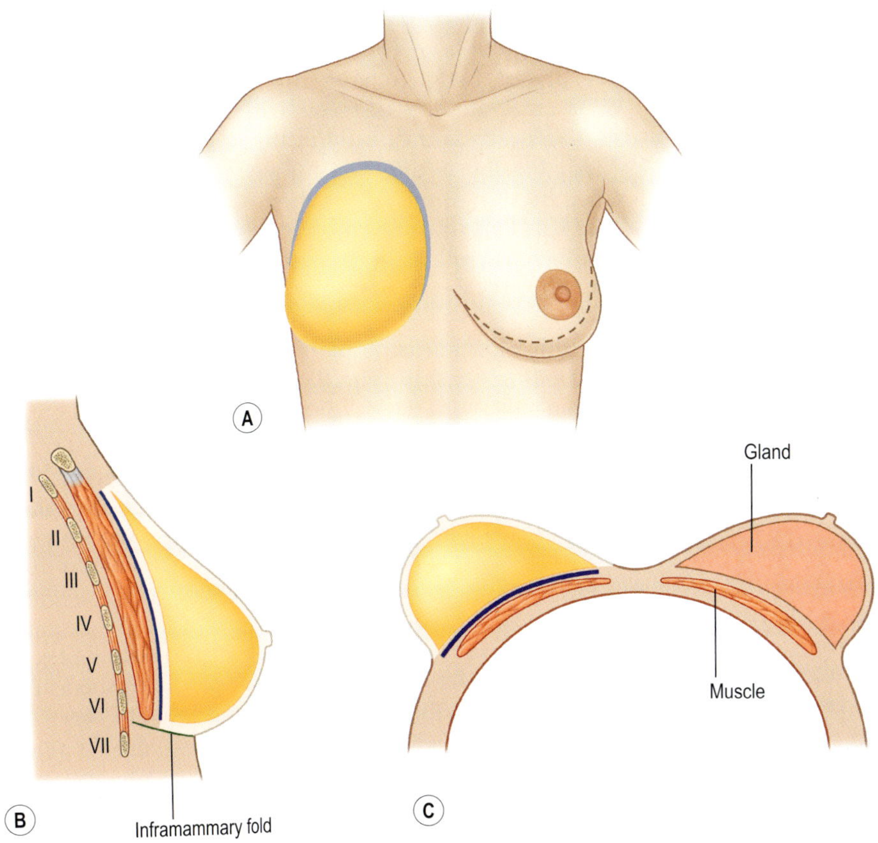

Figure 18.32 (A) Coronal, **(B)** sagittal and **(C)** transverse view of the conus of the breast.

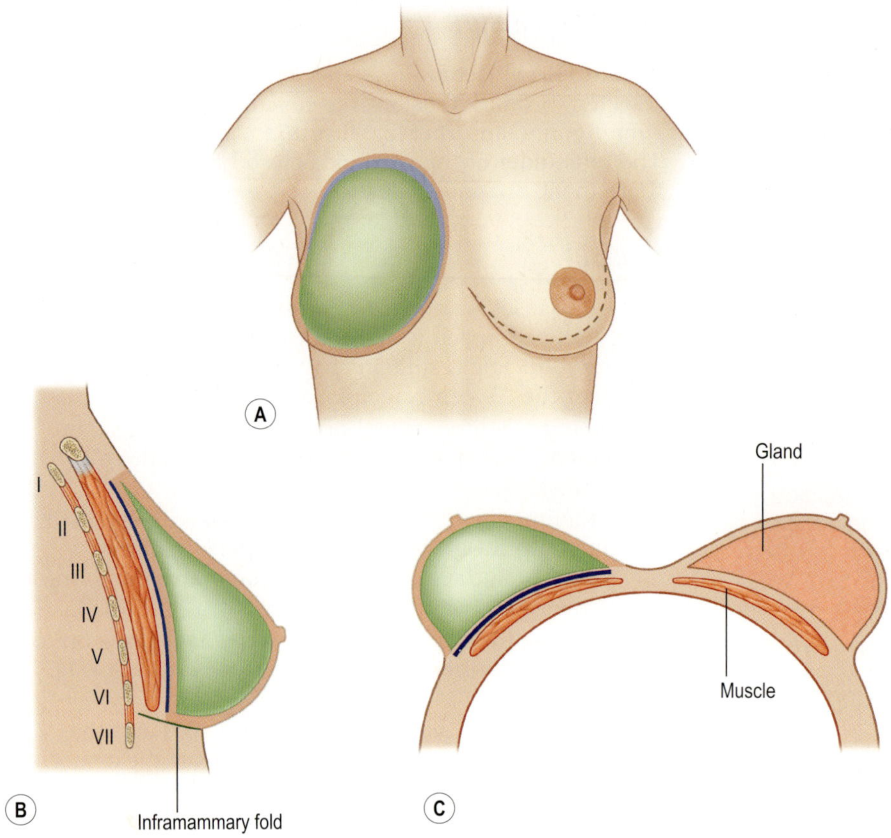

Figure 18.33 **(A)** Coronal, **(B)** sagittal and **(C)** transverse view of the envelope of the breast.

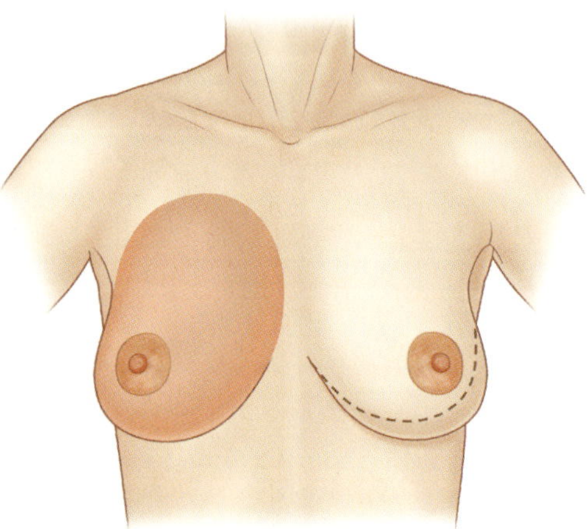

Figure 18.34 The nipple areola complex is an integral part of the envelope of the breast.

mastectomy flap skin and tension exerted on the abdominoplasty flap later in the procedure.

- To recreate the breast cone, three key sutures are utilized:
  - The tip of the DIEAP flap is fixed just below the pectoralis tendon by suturing Scarpa's fascia to the pectoralis fascia 2–3 cm medial to the lateral pectoral muscle border. This first key suture recreates the anterior axillary fold ***(Fig. 18.35A,B)***.
  - The transition from the lateral pectoral border into the lateral portion of the flap also recreates a natural lazy-S shape along the lateral border of the breast. The exact position of the second key suture is determined by moving the flap along the inframammary fold while assessing the lazy-S contour.
  - It is always better to have minimal fullness in this location at the time of reconstruction, as the flap will shift laterally and distally in the postoperative period.
  - Medial to the second key suture, in the midclavicular line, the skin of the flap is then bunched up (see Fig. 18.35C). This dramatically increases flap projection. It also helps create a sharp angle between the skin of the flap and the abdominal skin below the inframammary fold.
  - The third key suture is placed at the medial end of the inframammary fold. The flap is not bunched in this location to avoid overfilling of the inferomedial quadrant of the new breast.
- Overfilling of the superomedial regions of the breast is recommended (see Fig. 18.35D), as gravity will be pulling the flap caudally over the ensuing 6 months. Excessive fat can easily be removed later, whereas a depression in this area can be very disturbing for the patient.
- Once the final volume of the flap is determined, one can make a rough estimate of how much skin overlying the DIEAP flap will be required. The flap can be pushed up into the pocket or pulled down, leaving more or less vertical skin height, respectively, on the skin paddle of the flap.
- The more skin that is left, the more ptosis that can be achieved.

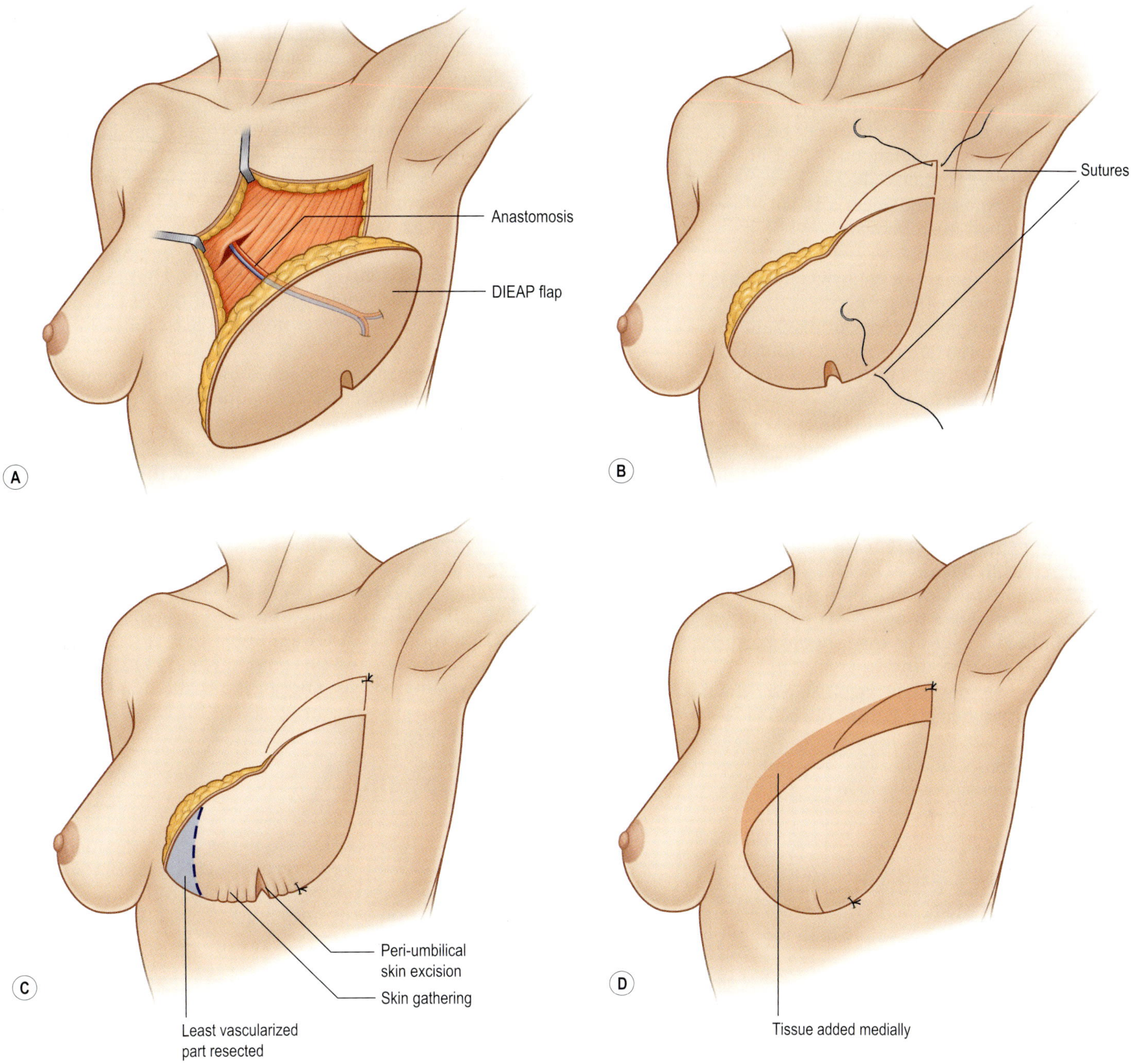

Figure 18.35 **(A)** The diep flap is turned 180° after performing the microsurgical anastomosis of the vessels and then **(B)** sutured with two key sutures to the pectoral fascia at the anterior axillary fold and the lateral part of the new inframammary fold making sure to avoid any fullness of the inferolateral quadrant of the new breast. **(C)** A triangular excision of skin around the umbilical area and gathering of the skin at the inframammary fold around the midclavicular line will create projection of the flap and a sharp angle between the lower part of the breast and the abdominal wall. **(D)** The least vascularized part of the flap is then resected making sure to preserve enough tissue to fill the upper medial quadrant of the breast.

- The more skin resected in the lateral part of the flap, the more the flap will be pushed medially.

Postoperative considerations

- For pedicled TRAM procedures, patients generally spend an average of 3 days in the hospital. Anticoagulation protocols are not utilized.
- For free TRAM/DIEP patients, the patient is extubated, transferred to the PACU and subsequently admitted to either the ICU or a step-down type unit that has the capability for frequent nursing flap checks and Doppler evaluations.
- Our practice pattern is to continue Doppler checks every hour for the first 48 h, then every 4 h until discharge which typically is postoperative day (POD) 3 or 4.

- Pain control is best managed with a patient controlled analgesic pump for the first 48 h at which point patients can usually be transferred over to an oral regimen.
- The patient remains NPO until the morning of POD 1 at which point they start clear liquids.
- Patients are encouraged to get out of bed to a chair on POD 1 and to fully ambulate on POD 2 at which point the Foley catheter is removed.
- Sequential compression devices are placed preoperatively and are continued postoperatively while in bed until discharge.
- Anticoagulation remains a controversial subject following free flap breast reconstruction.
- At our institution, all surgeons utilize subcutaneous heparin immediately after surgery both for DVT prophylaxis and to maintain a mildly hypocoagulable state following microanastomosis.
- The use of aspirin varies, with the goal of decreasing the thrombosis rate without adding additional risk of hematoma postoperatively.
- The use of prophylactic antibiotics for the prevention of surgical site infection (SSI) is another area of controversy.
- We recommend at the very least, preoperative dosing of Cefazolin within 30 min of incision, with re-dosing as needed intraoperatively in prolonged reconstruction. The data on postoperative prophylaxis while drains are in remain limited and at this time should be at the discretion of the operating surgeon.
- The drains are removed in the office over the next several weeks, usually when the output of each is less than 30 cc/day.
- Extensive exercises and heavy lifting are limited until the patient is 6 weeks postoperative.

Complications and outcomes

- Patient satisfaction is extremely high for abdominal based breast reconstruction procedures.
- Autologous breast reconstruction creates a more natural appearing and feeling breast when compared to implant reconstructions.
- Secondary procedures are commonly performed for contour irregularities, nipple-areolar complex reconstruction.
- It is preferable to wait 2–3 months after the initial procedure to perform a secondary procedure.
- If radiation is required postoperatively, it is preferable to wait at least 6 months after the radiation has been completed before performing any secondary procedures.
- Common complications included mastectomy flap necrosis and fat necrosis.
- If native skin loss is encountered in the early postoperative period, it is probably best treated with early excision and closure.
- The incidence of fat necrosis is reportedly 9% and greater in pedicled TRAM flaps when compared to free TRAM or DIEP flaps.
- If small areas of fat necrosis exist, they may be best treated by excision because they could create concern for cancer recurrence by any subsequent examining physician.
- Other potential complications include: dog ears of the abdomen, contour deformities, seromas, partial flap loss, or total flap loss.
- Significant (>25%) or total flap loss in pedicled TRAM cases is exceedingly rare (incidence <1%). Total flap loss for free flap techniques occurs 0.2–4.7% of the time.
- Intuitively, the risk of abdominal bulge or abdominal hernia should be directly related to the amount of rectus muscle harvested/violated, such that the risk is greatest for pedicled TRAM procedures and least for DIEP flap procedures.
- Due to the microvascular anastomosis and operative manipulation in free flap techniques, the artery and vein are both subject to thrombosis.
- Delayed thromboses confer a more clinically detrimental outcome; therefore, close observation of these flaps is paramount in the immediate postoperative period.
- Venous congestion postoperatively can be treated with leech therapy; however, sudden changes in flap character or Doppler signal warrant exploration.
- In inexperienced hands, the DIEAP flap dissection will require a longer operating time than a conventional myocutaneous flap. After a number of cases, operating time will fall back and be comparable to myocutaneous flap harvesting or even shorter if a limited pedicle length is needed.

Further reading

Alderman AK, Kuhn LE, Lowery JC, et al. Does patient satisfaction with breast reconstruction change over time? Two-year results of the Michigan Breast Reconstruction Outcomes Study. *J Am Coll Surg*. 2007;204(1):7–12.

The Michigan Breast Reconstruction Outcomes Study was a well designed prospective analysis of patients undergoing breast reconstruction. This project resulted in several papers which contributed a plethora of prospective data comparing tissue expander, pedicled TRAM and free TRAM reconstruction. In this article, long-term patient satisfaction data are presented. Overall, patients undergoing free or pedicle TRAM have higher satisfaction rates than tissue expander/implant reconstruction at 1 year as measured by survey quantifying overall satisfaction and aesthetic satisfaction. At 2 years, although the difference in overall satisfaction between treatment groups diminished, women who underwent autologous reconstruction had higher aesthetic satisfaction when compared with tissue expander/implant reconstruction. This entire series of papers is worth reading for anyone interested in breast reconstruction.

Allen RJ, Treece P. Deep inferior epigastric perforator flap for breast reconstruction. *Ann Plast Surg*. 1994;32:32–38.

Andrades P, Fix RJ, Danilla S, et al. Ischemic complications in pedicle, free, and muscle sparing transverse rectus abdominis myocutaneous flaps for breast reconstruction. *Ann Plast Surg*. 2008;60(5):562–567.

This was a retrospective review at one institution comparing ischemic complications between pedicled TRAM and MS-0 through MS-3 free TRAM reconstructions. Their data follow theoretical predictions based upon anatomy: there is a higher rate of fat necrosis in pedicled TRAMs when compared with free TRAM. There is a trend toward higher complication rates as the degree of muscle preservation increases. The bulge and hernia rates were, however, no different between groups. Although limited by a retrospective design, this is one of many articles which gives credence to improved outcomes with free versus pedicled TRAM.

Baldwin BJ, Schusterman MA, Miller MJ, et al. Bilateral breast reconstruction: conventional versus free TRAM. *Plast Reconstr Surg*. 1994;93:1410–1416.

Pedicle versus free TRAMs and differences in perfusion.

Blondeel PN. One hundred free DIEP flap breast reconstructions: a personal experience. *Br J Plast Surg*. 1999;52(2):104–111.

The transverse rectus abdominis myocutaneous (TRAM) flap has been the gold standard for breast reconstruction until recently. Not only autologous but also immediate reconstructions are now preferred to offer the patient a natural and cosmetically acceptable result. This study summarizes the prospectively gathered data of 100 free DIEP flaps used for breast reconstruction in 87 patients. Primary reconstructions were done in 35% of the patients. Well known risk factors for free-flap breast reconstruction were present: smokers 23%, obesity 25%, abdominal scarring 28% and previous radiotherapy 45%. Mean operating time was 6 h 12 min for unilateral reconstruction and mean hospital stay was 7.9 days. These data indicate that the free DIEP flap is a new but reliable and safe technique for autologous breast reconstruction. This flap offers the patient the same advantages as the TRAM flap and discards the most important disadvantages of the myocutaneous flap by preserving the continuity of the rectus muscle.

Blondeel PN, Boeckx WD. Refinements in free flap breast reconstruction: the free bilateral deep inferior epigastric perforator flap anastomosed to the internalmammary artery. *Br J Plast Surg*. 1994;47(7):495–501.

Besides the enormous advantages of reconstructing the amputated breast by means of a conventional TRAM flap, the main disadvantage remains the elevation of small (free TRAM) or larger (pedicled TRAM) parts of the rectus abdominis muscle. In order to overcome this disadvantage, the free deep inferior epigastric perforator (DIEP) skin flap has recently been used for breast mound reconstruction with excellent clinical results. After achieving favorable results with eight unilateral DIEP-flaps, we were challenged by an abdomen with a midline laparotomy scar. By dissecting a bilateral DIEP flap and making adjacent anastomoses to the internal mammary artery, we were able to achieve sufficient flap mobility for easy free flap positioning and breast shaping. Intraoperative segmental nerve stimulation, postoperative functional abdominal wall tests and CT-scan examination showed normal abdominal muscle activity. On the basis of a case report, the technical considerations and advantages of anastomosing the bipedicled DIEP flap to the internal mammary artery are discussed.

Blondeel PN, Hijjawi J, Depypere H, et al. Shaping the breast in aesthetic and reconstructive breast surgery: an easy three-step principle. *Plast Reconstr Surg*. 2009a;123(2):455–462.

Blondeel PN, Hijjawi J, Depypere H, et al. Shaping the breast in aesthetic and reconstructive breast surgery: an easy three-step principle. Part II. Breast reconstruction after total mastectomy. *Plast Reconstr Surg*. 2009b;123(3):794–805.

This is Part II of four parts describing the 3-step principle being applied in reconstructive and aesthetic breast surgery. Part I explains how to analyze a problematic breast by understanding the three main anatomical features of a breast and how they interact: the footprint, the conus of the breast and the skin envelope. This part describes how one can optimize his/her results with breast reconstructions after complete mastectomy. For both primary and secondary reconstructions, we explain how to analyze the mastectomized breast and the deformed chest wall before giving step-by-step guidelines on how to rebuild the entire breast with either autologous tissue or implants. The differences in shaping unilateral or bilateral breast reconstructions with autologous tissue are clarified. Regardless of timing or method of reconstruction, it is shown that by breaking down the surgical strategy in three easy (anatomical) steps, the reconstructive surgeon will be able to provide more aesthetically pleasing and reproducible results.

Edsander-Nord A, Jurell G, Wickman M. Donor-site morbidity after pedicled or free TRAM flap surgery: a prospective and objective study. *Plast Reconstr Surg*. 1998;102(5):1508–1516.

Greco III JA, Castaldo ET, Nanney LB, et al. Autologous breast reconstruction: The Vanderbilt Experience (1998 to 2005) of independent predictors of displeasing outcomes. *J Am Coll Surg*. 2008;207(1):49–56.

Grotting JC, Urist MM, Maddox WA, et al. Conventional TRAM flap versus free microsurgical TRAM flap for immediate breast reconstruction. *Plast Reconstr Surg*. 1989;83(5):828–844.

Hartrampf CR, Scheflan M, Black PW. Breast reconstruction with a transverse abdominal island flap. *Plast Reconstr Surg*. 1982;69:216–224.

The seminal article on TRAM flaps.

Koshima I, Soeda S. Inferior epigastric artery skin flaps without rectus abdominis muscle. *Br J Plast Surg*. 1989;42(6):645–648.

The rectus abdominis musculocutaneous flap has many advantages, but its disadvantages are also well known. These are the possibility of abdominal herniation and, in certain situations, its bulk. To overcome these problems, an inferior epigastric artery skin flap without rectus abdominis muscle, pedicled on the muscle perforators and the proximal inferior deep epigastric artery, have been used in two patients. A large flap without muscle can survive on a single muscle perforator.

Koshima I, Moriguchi T, Soeda S, et al. Free thin paraumbilical perforator-based flaps. *Ann Plast Surg*. 1992;29(1):12–17.

Kroll SS, Baldwin B. A comparison of outcomes using three different methods of breast reconstruction. *Plast Reconstr Surg*. 1992;90:455–462.

Kronowitz SJ, Robb GL. Radiation therapy and breast reconstruction: a critical review of the literature. *Plast Reconstr Surg*. 2009;124(2):395–408.

Radiation therapy can have dramatic effects on both the surgical field and overall outcomes in breast reconstruction. In particular, post-reconstruction radiation therapy has been shown to lead to aesthetic and wound related complications. This excellent review article summarizes the current indications for radiation therapy and the existing literature on its effects on reconstruction. Although no cancer outcomes are presented showing a clinical impact, this article summarizes existing literature showing that reconstruction can compromise radiation delivery. In addition, the article discusses the "delayed-immediate" reconstructive algorithm.

Komorowska-Timek E, Gurtner GC. Intraoperative perfusion mapping with laser-assisted indocyanine green imaging can predict and prevent complications in immediate breast reconstruction. *Plast Reconstr Surg*. 2010;125(4):1065–1073.

Massey MF, Spiegel AJ, Levine JL, et al. Perforator flaps: recent experience, current trends, and future directions based on 3974 microsurgical breast reconstructions. *Plast Reconstr Surg*. 2009;124:737–751.

Perforator flap breast reconstruction is an accepted surgical option for breast cancer patients electing to restore their body image after mastectomy. Since the introduction of the deep inferior epigastric perforator flap, microsurgical techniques have evolved to support a 99% success rate for a variety of flaps with donor sites that include the abdomen, buttock, thigh, and trunk. Recent experience highlights the perforator flap as a proven solution for patients who have experienced failed breast implant-based reconstructions or those requiring irradiation. Current trends suggest an application of these techniques in patients previously felt to be unacceptable surgical candidates with a focus on safety, aesthetics, and increased sensitization. Future challenges include the propagation of these reconstructive techniques into the hands of future plastic surgeons with a focus on the development of septocutaneous flaps and vascularized lymph node transfers for the treatment of lymphedema.

Mathes SJ. A rectus abdominis myocutaneous flap to reconstruct abdominal wall defects. *Br J Plast Surg*. 1977;30:282–283.

Originally described the epigastric artery as the pedicle source.

Mathes SJ, Logan SE. The use of a rectus abdominis myocutaneous flap to reconstruct a groin defect. *Br J Plast Surg*. 1984;37:351–353. 5.

Mehrara BJ, Santoro TD, Arcilla E, et al. Complications after microvascular breast reconstruction: experience with 1195 flaps. *Plast Reconstr Surg*. 2006;118(5):1100–1111.

Moon HK, Taylor GI. The vascular anatomy of rectus abdominis musculocutaneous flaps based on the deep superior epigastric system. *Plast Reconstr Surg*. 1988;82:815–831.

Describes the epigastric arteries as they relate to the TRAM flap.

Newman MI, Samson MC. The application of laserassisted indocyanine green fluorescent dye angiography in microsurgical breast reconstruction. *J Reconstr Microsurg*. 2009;25(1):21–26.

Selber JC, Kurichi JE, Vega SJ, et al. Risk factors and complications in free TRAM flap breast reconstruction. *Ann Plast Surg*. 2006;56(5):492–497.

In this retrospective review of 500 free TRAM flap reconstructions performed by a single surgeon, the authors summarized the most common complications of TRAM reconstruction and worked backwards to find risk factors for poor outcomes. Overall, smoking was the most influential factor, leading to increased rates of wound infection, skin flap necrosis and fat necrosis. Obesity was an independent risk factor for mastectomy flap necrosis. Although limited by a retrospective design, this article offers nice data to help predict poor outcomes.

Spear SL. *Surgery of the breast: principles and art*. Philadelphia: Lippincott-Raven; 1997.

Describes matching procedures that are available for the contralateral breast to help with symmetry.

Taylor GI, Daniel RK. The anatomy of several free flap donor sites. *Plast Reconstr Surg*. 1975;56(3):243–253.

Uppal RS, Casaer B, Van Landuyt K, et al. The efficacy of preoperative mapping of perforators in reducing operative times and complications in perforator flap breast reconstruction. *J Plast Reconstr Aesthet Surg*. 2009;62(7):859–864.

Wu LC, Bajaj A, Chang DW, et al. Comparison of donor-site morbidity of SIEA, DIEP, and muscle-sparing TRAM flaps for breast reconstruction. *Plast Reconstr Surg*. 2008;122(3):702–709.

In this study, the authors combined a patient survey with a retrospective review to assess overall outcomes with donor-site morbidity following SIEA, DIEP and free TRAM flap reconstruction. This article suggests decreased abdominal wall morbidity of the SIEA flap in comparison to the free TRAM. Although more studies are needed, this article highlights one of the limitations of the free TRAM compared with more contemporary options – the donor site. Although sparing muscle likely limits the effect, by sacrificing muscle fibers of the rectus, patients are likely to experience some degree in overall decline of abdominal wall function which may never return to baseline.

Chapter 19

Essential anatomy of the upper extremity

This chapter was created using content from Neligan & Chang, Plastic Surgery 3rd edition, Volume 6, Hand and Upper Extremity, Chapter 1, Anatomy and biomechanics of the hand, James Chang, Francisco Valero-Cuevas, Vincent R. Hentz and Robert A. Chase.

SYNOPSIS

- Introduction – history to anatomy and biomechanics of the hand
- Skin, subcutaneous tissue, and fascia
- Bones and joints
  - Hand elements
  - The wrist
  - Joint motion
  - The thumb
- Muscles and tendons
  - Extrinsic extensors
  - Pronators and supinators
  - Extrinsic flexors
  - The retinacular system
  - Intrinsic muscles
- Blood supply
- Peripheral nerves

Skin, subcutaneous tissue, and fascia

- Dorsal skin of the hand is thin and pliable and anchored to the deep investing fascia only by loose, areolar tissue.
- Palmar skin has a thick dermal layer and a heavily cornified epithelial surface that is held tightly to the thick fibrous palmar fascia by diffusely distributed vertical fibers.
- The skin of the palm is laden with a high concentration of specialized sensory end organs and sweat glands.
- Palmar skin creases can be used to identify and locate underlying joints and structures to help plan precise skin incision placement.
- Kaplan's cardinal line is an important landmark for critical internal structures within the hand (***Fig. 19. 1***/ Box 19.1).
- To avoid contracture in the palm, Littler outlined imaginary diamond-shaped skin surfaces where a longitudinal scar should be avoided. These diamond surfaces can be visualized by noting each joint axis and the kissing surfaces of the palmar skin in full flexion ***(Fig. 19.2A,B)***.
- The palmar fascia consists of resistant, fibrous tissue arranged in longitudinal, transverse, oblique, and vertical fibers ***(Fig. 19.3)***.
- Longitudinal fibers:
  - Concentrate at the proximal origin of the palmar fascia at the wrist.
  - Originate from the palmaris longus when present (80–85% of patients).
  - Make up the fibrous flexor sheath of the digits.
  - Attach to the volar plate and intermetacarpal ligaments at the level of the metacarpal heads.
- Transverse fibers:
  - Concentrated in the midpalm and the web spaces.
  - Make up the transverse palmar ligament.
  - Act as pulleys for the flexor tendons proximal to the level of the digital pulleys.
- Vertical fibers:
  - Superficial to the longitudinal and transverse fibers, vertical fibers travel to the palm skin dermis ***(Fig. 19.4)***.
  - Deep to the palmar fascia, they coalesce into septae and form eight individual compartments for the flexor tendons to each digit, and the neurovascular bundles together with the lumbrical muscles ***(Fig. 19.5)***.
- In the fingers, there are two important bands of fascia which help contain and protect the ulnar and radial

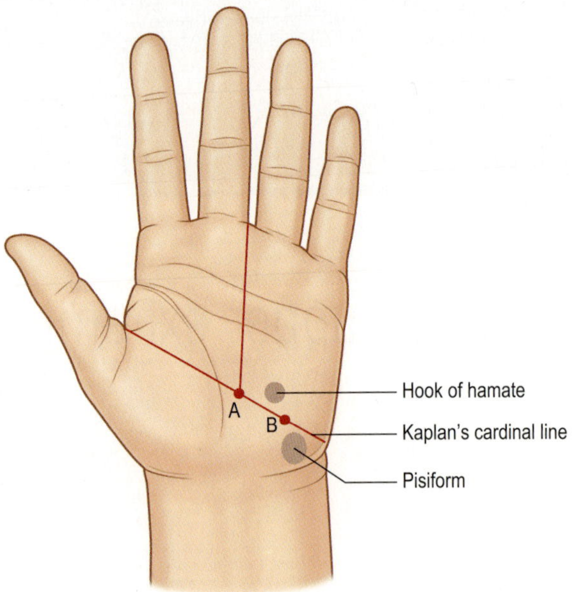

Figure 19.1 Kaplan's cardinal line, along lines from the ulnar aspect of the middle finger and the ulnar aspect of the ring finger. Point A corresponds with the motor branch of the median nerve and point B with the motor branch of the ulnar nerve.

BOX 19.1 **Clinical pearl: Kaplan's cardinal line**

Hand anatomist Emanuel Kaplan described specific surface lines that would aid surgeons in locating key structures in the palm of the hand. The cardinal line has often been misquoted; therefore we refer to Kaplan's classic hand text: *Functional and Surgical Anatomy of the Hand*. Kaplan's cardinal line is drawn from the apex of the first web space to the distal edge of the pisiform bone (Fig. 19.1). Two longitudinal lines are drawn from the ulnar aspect of the middle finger and the ulnar aspect of the ring finger. These will cross the cardinal line. The intersection of the cardinal line and the longitudinal line from the ulnar side of the middle finger corresponds to the motor branch of the median nerve. The intersection of the cardinal line and the longitudinal line from the ulnar side of the ring finger corresponds to the hook of the hamate. The motor branch of the ulnar nerve is found on the cardinal line, equidistant between the hamate and pisiform. See Kaplan's original text for additional surface markings.

digital arteries and nerves: Grayson's ligaments and Cleland's ligaments.

- Grayson's ligaments are volar to the neurovascular bundles and are quite flimsy.
- Cleland's ligaments are dorsal to the neurovascular bundles and are much stouter *(Fig. 19.6)*.

Bones and joints

- The hand skeleton is divisible into four elements:
  - i. The fixed unit of the hand: the second and third metacarpals and the distal carpal row.
  - ii. The thumb and its metacarpal: displays a wide range of motion at the carpometacarpal joint allowed by the joint, ligaments and insertion of five intrinsic and four extrinsic muscles.
  - iii. The index digit: independence of action within the range of motion allowed by its joints, ligaments, and the action of three intrinsic and four extrinsic muscles.
  - iv. The third, fourth, and fifth digits with the fourth and fifth metacarpals: functions as a stabilizing vise to grasp objects for manipulation by the thumb and index finger, or in concert with the other hand units in powerful grasp *(Fig. 19.7)*.
- The distal row of carpal bones forms a solid architectural arch with the capitate bone as a keystone. Together with the 2nd and 3rd metacarpals they form the fixed unit of the hand.
- As a stable foundation, this unit creates a supporting base for the three other mobile units: the first metacarpal, the fourth metacarpal, and the fifth metacarpal.
- The first metacarpal moves through a wide range of motion as a result of loose capsular ligaments and the shallow saddle articulation between it and the trapezium.
- Motion is stabilized by the capsular ligaments, including the volar beak ligament, and by its attachment to the fixed hand axis through the adductor pollicis, the first dorsal interosseous, and the fascia and skin of the first web space.
- The mobile fourth and fifth metacarpal heads move dorsally and palmarly in relation to the central hand axis by limited mobility at their carpometacarpal joints.
- These metacarpal heads are tethered to the central metacarpals by the intermetacarpal ligaments (unite adjacent metacarpophalangeal volar plates).
- The third metacarpophalangeal joint acts as the anatomic center of the hand. With the fingers fully abducted, the tips form radii of equal length from this point. The same radius projected proximally falls at the wrist joint *(Fig. 19.8)*.
- The most important single motor operating the central hand beam at the wrist level is the extensor carpi radialis brevis, which works against gravity, positioning the pronated hand into extension.

The wrist

- The wrist joint has a multi-articulated architecture that creates a potentially wide range of motion in flexion, extension, radial deviation, ulnar deviation, and circumduction *(Fig. 19.9)*.
- The distal radioulnar joint (DRUJ) allows pronation and supination of the hand as the radius rotates around the head of the ulna *(Fig. 19.10)*.
- The proximal row of carpal bones (scaphoid, lunate, triquetrum, pisiform) articulates with the distal radius and ulna, providing the ability to flex and extend the hand and perform radial and ulnar deviation.
- All four of the bones in the distal carpal row present articular surfaces for junction with the metacarpals.
- The principal articulation of the carpus is with the distal surface of the radius at the radiocarpal joint.

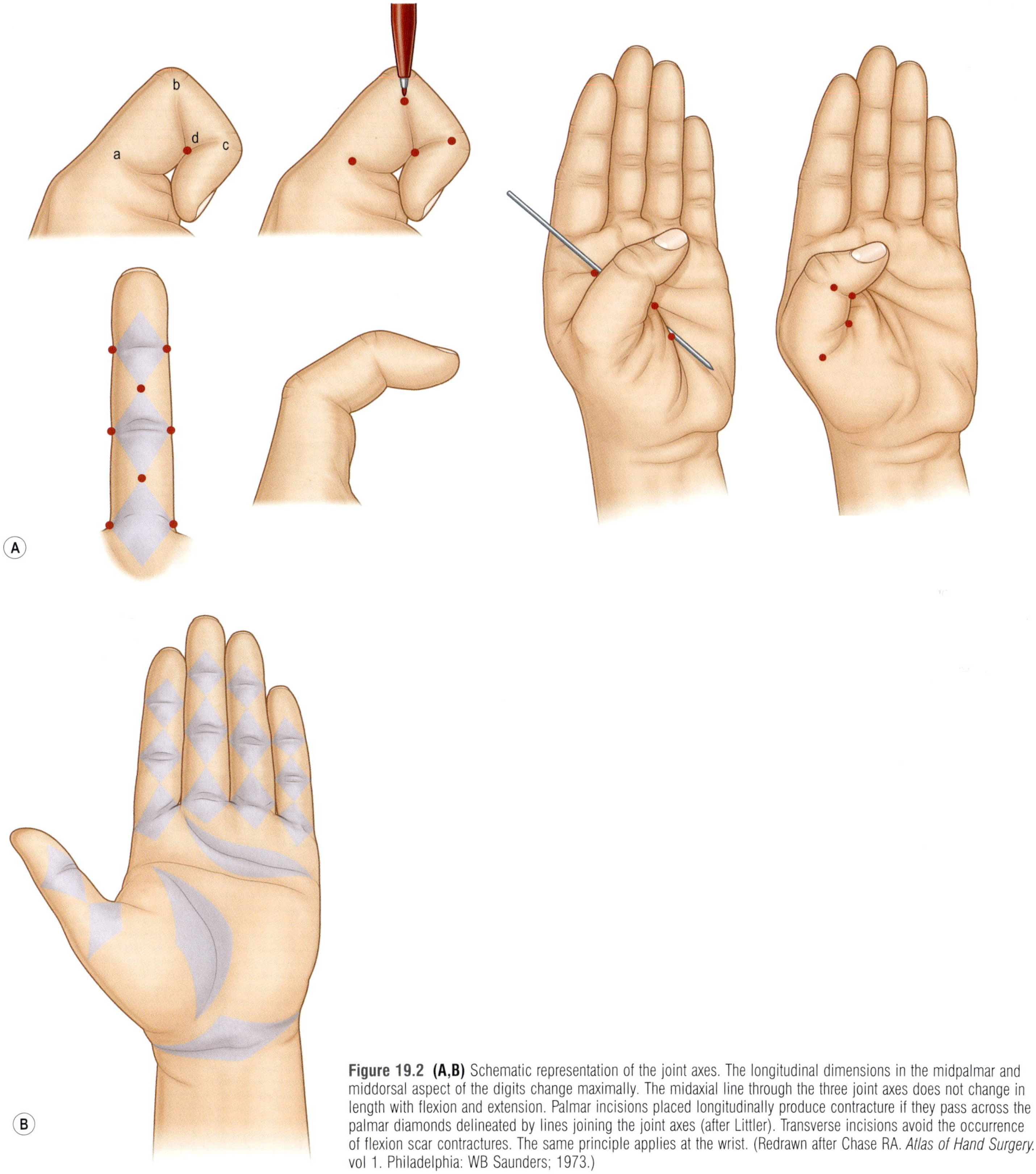

Figure 19.2 (A,B) Schematic representation of the joint axes. The longitudinal dimensions in the midpalmar and middorsal aspect of the digits change maximally. The midaxial line through the three joint axes does not change in length with flexion and extension. Palmar incisions placed longitudinally produce contracture if they pass across the palmar diamonds delineated by lines joining the joint axes (after Littler). Transverse incisions avoid the occurrence of flexion scar contractures. The same principle applies at the wrist. (Redrawn after Chase RA. *Atlas of Hand Surgery.* vol 1. Philadelphia: WB Saunders; 1973.)

- With an articular surface that slopes in several planes, fractures of the distal radius frequently result in a loss of the normal dorsal-to-palmar tilt of the articular surface leading to a change in the biomechanical properties of the wrist joint and degenerative arthritis.
- The relationship of the length of the radius to the length of the ulna is fairly constant in individuals, and is termed ulnar variance.
- Normal ulnar variance: the distal ulna completes the curve of the articular surface of the radius.

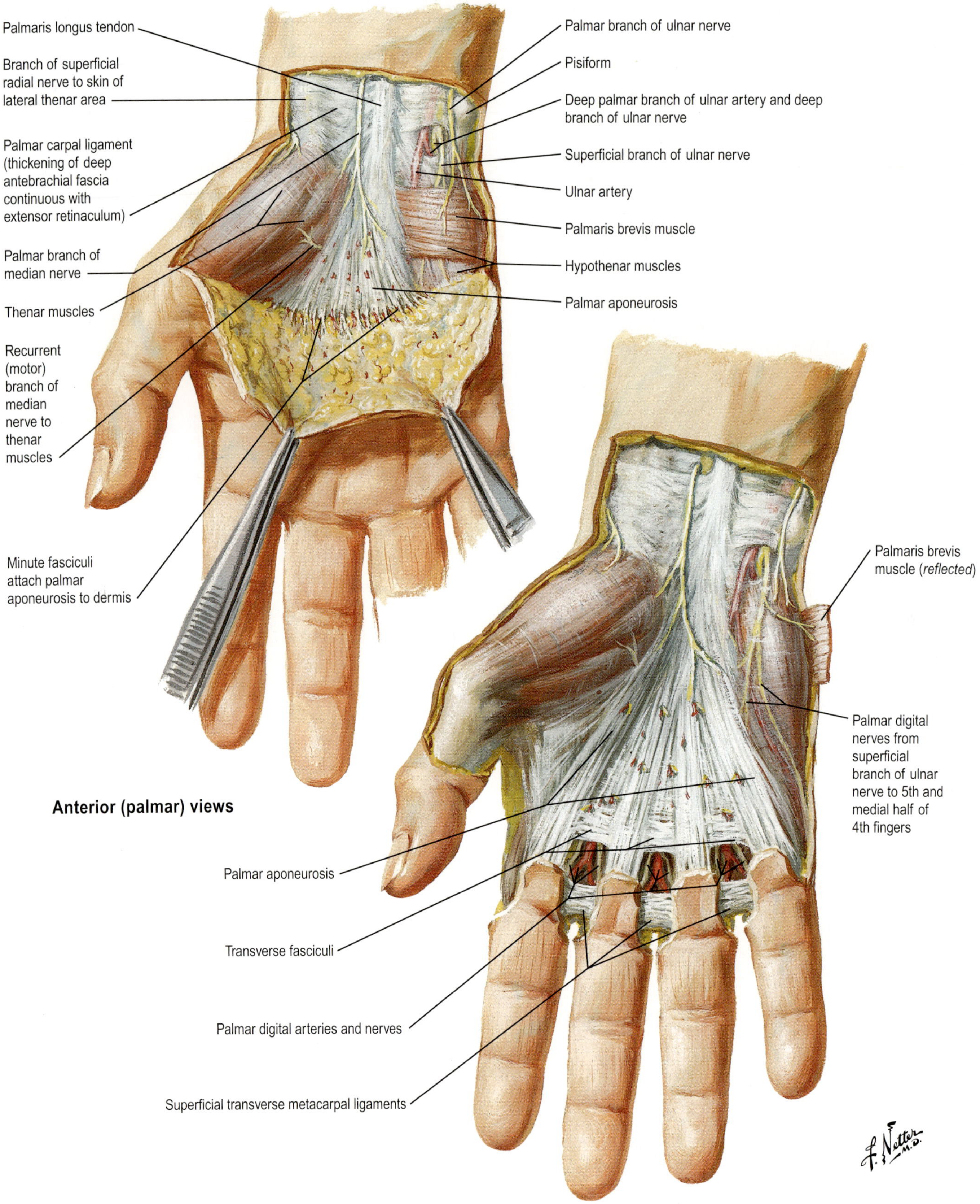

Figure 19.3 Superficial dissection of the palm, showing orientation of the palmar fascia. Reprinted with permission from www.netterimages.com.

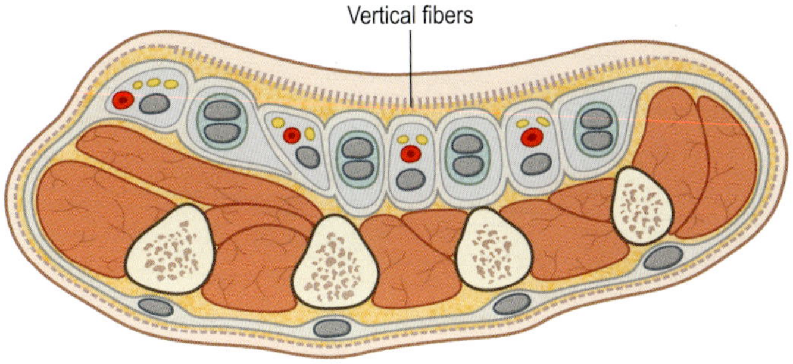

Figure 19.4 The palmar fascia with its longitudinal, transverse, and vertical fibers. The longitudinal fibers take origin in the palmaris longus (when present). Transverse fibers are concentrated in the distal palm supporting the web skin and in the midpalm as the transverse palmar ligament. Vertical fibers extend superficially as multiple, tiny tethering strands to stabilize the thick palmar skin. The deep vertical components concentrate in septa between the longitudinally oriented structures in the fingers. Redrawn after McCarthy JG. *Plastic Surgery.* Philadelphia: WB Saunders; 1990.

- Ulnar negative variance: the end of the ulna falls short of this curvature.
  - Higher incidence of Kienbock's disease (avascular necrosis of the lunate).
- Ulnar positive variance: the ulna extends distal to this imaginary extension.
  - If variance greater than 2–3 mm, associated with ulnar impaction ***(Fig. 19.11)***.
- Gilula's lines: denote normal extracarpal and intracarpal architecture. Any disruption of these lines is a sign of carpal abnormality.
- Greater arc: a line that follows the proximal articular contours of the proximal row of carpal bones circumscribing a smooth arc ***(Fig. 19.12)***.
- Lesser arc: a line between the proximal and distal row of carpal bones circumscribing another smooth arc.
- The scaphoid and lunate form the primary articulation with the distal radius.
- The scaphoid also articulates with the distal carpal row through attachments to the trapezium and trapezoid.
- The triquetrum articulates with the lunate in the proximal row, and with the hamate across the midcarpal joint.
- The pisiform is essentially a floating bone, unimportant for carpal stability.

Wrist motion

- A product of the sums of the movements of the carpal bones in various planes and degrees of rotation relative to one another.
- The motion of any one carpal bone is a consequence of several factors:
- The contour of the bone and the arrangements of its articular surfaces.
- The degree of freedom afforded by the intrinsic ligaments (ligaments originating from one carpal bone and inserting on another carpal bone).
- The degree of freedom afforded by the extrinsic ligaments (ligaments arising from the radius or ulna and attaching to a carpal bone or bones).
- The mechanics of the wrist rely heavily upon the proximal carpal row flexing or extending to accommodate movement of the fixed distal carpus.

Extrinsic carpal ligaments

- Anchor the proximal carpal row to the radius.
- Stout palmar ligaments arise primarily from the radius, and from the ulna and the palmar portion of the triangular fibrocartilage complex (TFCC).
- The TFCC separates the distal end of the ulna from the ulnar-sided carpal bones and serves to suspend the distal ulna to the radius at the distal radioulnar joint.
- The dorsal extrinsic radiocarpal ligament complex is thin and is primarily a condensation of capsular tissues, except for two stout structures: the dorsal intercarpal ligament (joins the distal pole of the scaphoid and the triquetrum), and the dorsal radiocarpal ligament (passes from radius to triquetrum).

Intrinsic carpal ligaments

- Broad structures that link one carpal bone to another, either within the proximal or distal row, or link one carpal row to the other.
- The two most significant intrinsic ligaments are the scapholunate ligament and the lunotriquetral ligament.
- The scapholunate ligament: A U-shaped structure that anchors the scaphoid to the lunate, allowing these two carpal bones to move in synchrony.
  - Subdivided into three regions: dorsal, proximal, and palmar.
  - The dorsal region is thick and controls scapholunate stability.
  - The proximal portion, composed mainly of fibrocartilage, and the palmar region, with thin and obliquely oriented fibers are less important for stability.
- The lunotriquetral ligament: anchors the lunate to the triquetrum.
  - Also composed of dorsal, proximal, and palmar portions.

Hand/joint motion

- Metacarpophalangeal (MCP) joint.
- Motion in the fingers ranges from 0 to 90°.
- Lateral motion is limited by the rein-like collateral ligaments ***(Fig. 19.13)***.
- At the MCP joint, if the collateral ligaments are sacrificed, the interossei remain the sole source of lateral stability.
- The proximal interphalangeal joint (PIP):
  - Can be pushed to 110° of flexion, but extension usually cannot be carried beyond 5° of hyperextension because of the volar plate.
  - The medial and lateral collateral ligaments, also part of the joint capsule, are fixed in a manner that allows no medial or lateral deviation of the joint in any position.
  - Unlike the MCP joints, the collateral ligaments of the PIP and/or DIP cannot be sacrificed without creating a lateral instability that is curable only by fusion.
  - The hinge-shape of the articular joint surface also strongly contributes to this stability in lateral motion.

(cont'd)

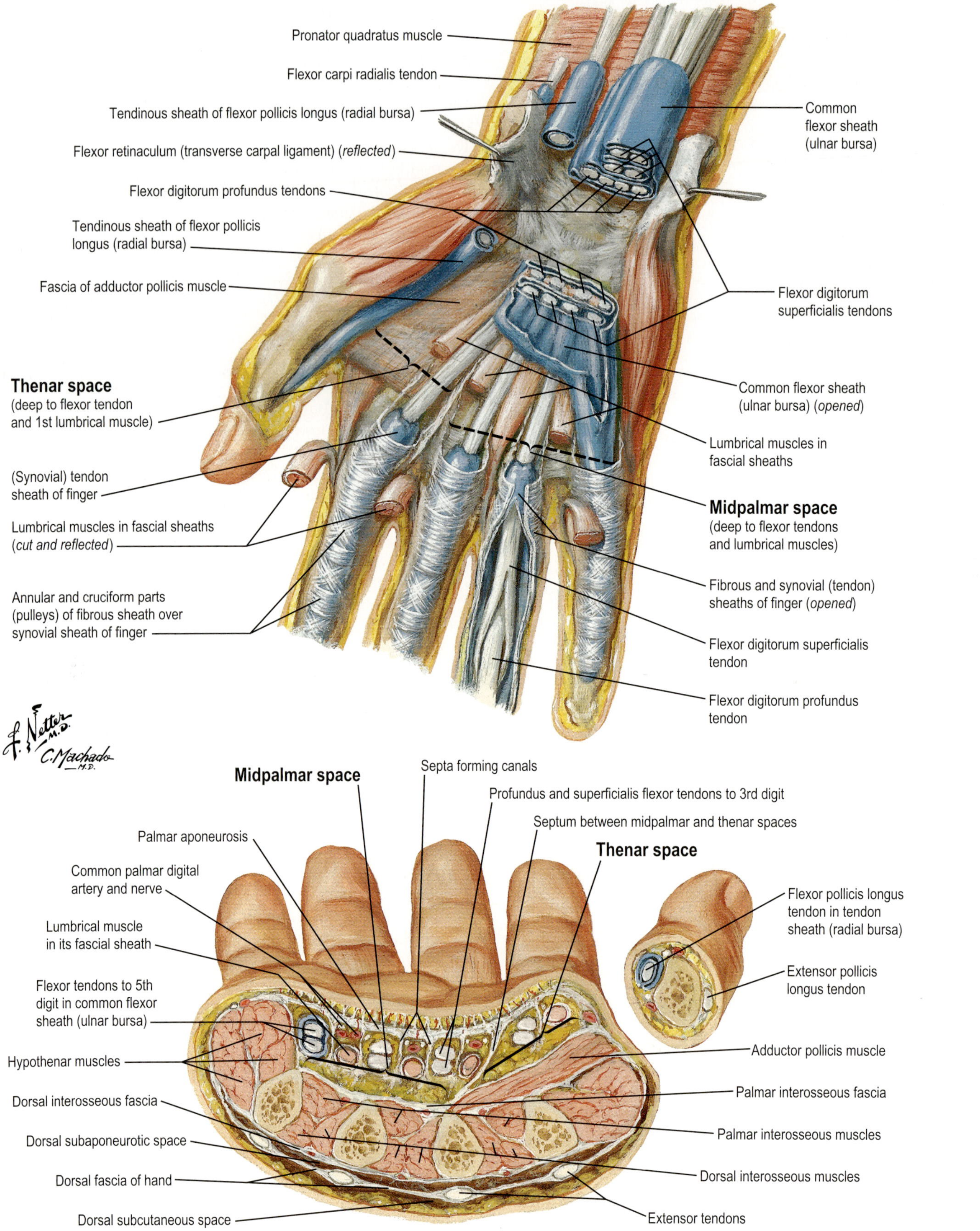

Figure 19.5 These deep palmar and midpalmar axial views of the hand reinforce the concept of distinct anatomic compartments separated by fascia. (Reprinted with permission from www.netterimages.com. © Elsevier Inc. All Rights Reserved.)

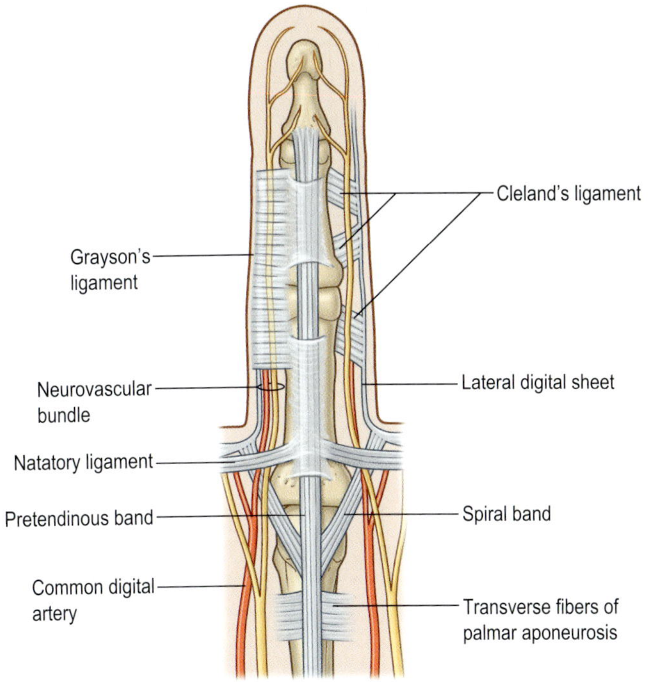

Figure 19.6 The components of the digital fascia that help to anchor the axial plane skin are Grayson's ligaments palmar to the neurovascular bundles and Cleland's ligaments dorsal to the bundles. (Redrawn after McCarthy JG. *Plastic Surgery.* Philadelphia: WB Saunders; 1990.)

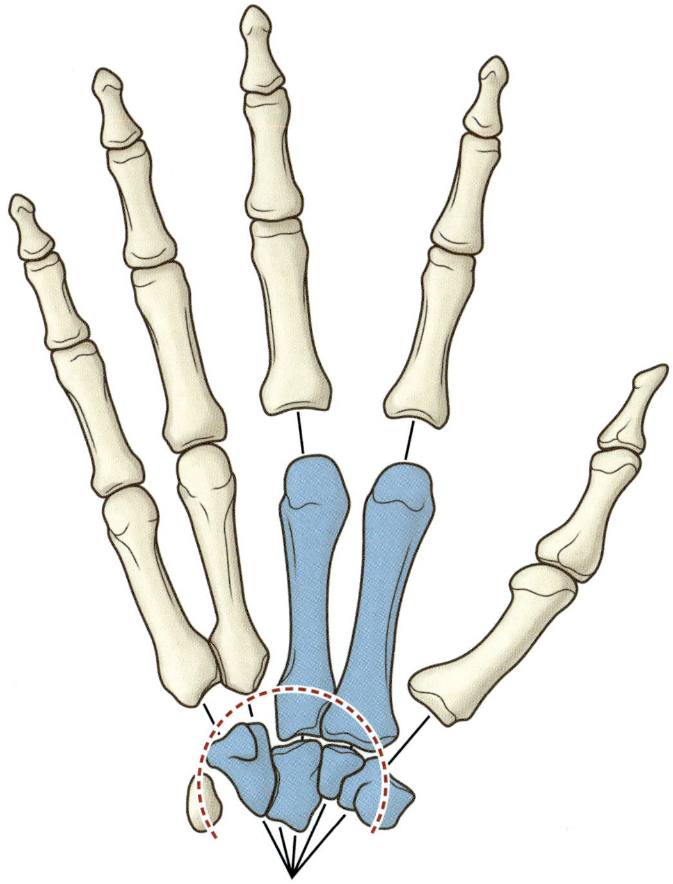

Figure 19.7 Exploded view of the functional elements of the hand: (1) the thumb and its metacarpal with a wide range of motion at the carpometacarpal joint; (2) the index digit with independence of action in several planes; (3) the third, fourth, and fifth digits with the fourth and fifth metacarpals; (4) the fixed unit consisting of the carpals with the fixed transverse carpal arch and the second and third metacarpals forming a fixed longitudinal arch. (Redrawn after McCarthy JG. *Plastic Surgery.* Philadelphia: WB Saunders; 1990.)

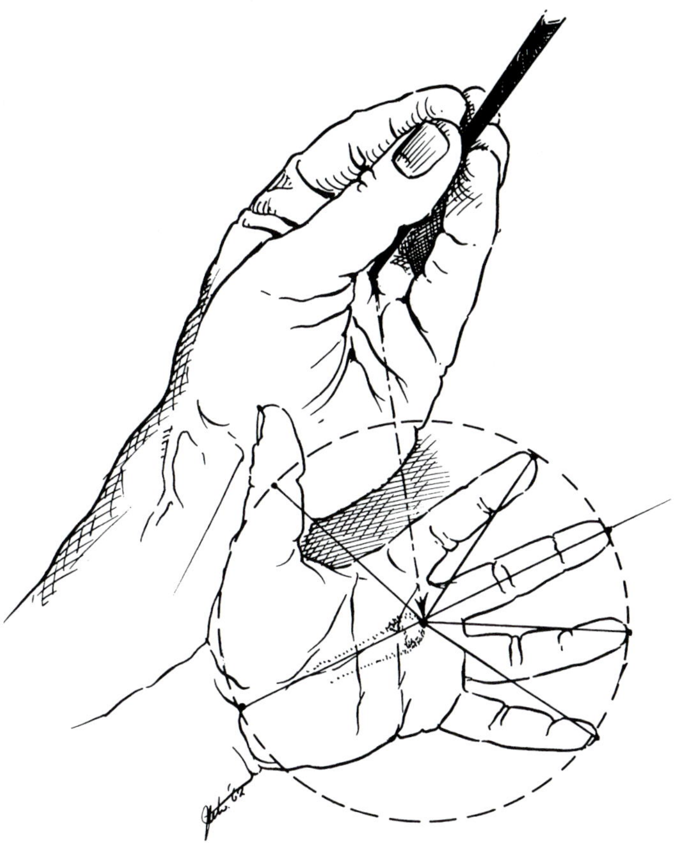

Figure 19.8 When the adaptive arch is semicircular, the fingers converge in a cone over the anatomic center of the hand – the long finger metacarpophalangeal joint. (Redrawn after McCarthy JG. *Plastic Surgery.* Philadelphia: WB Saunders; 1990.)

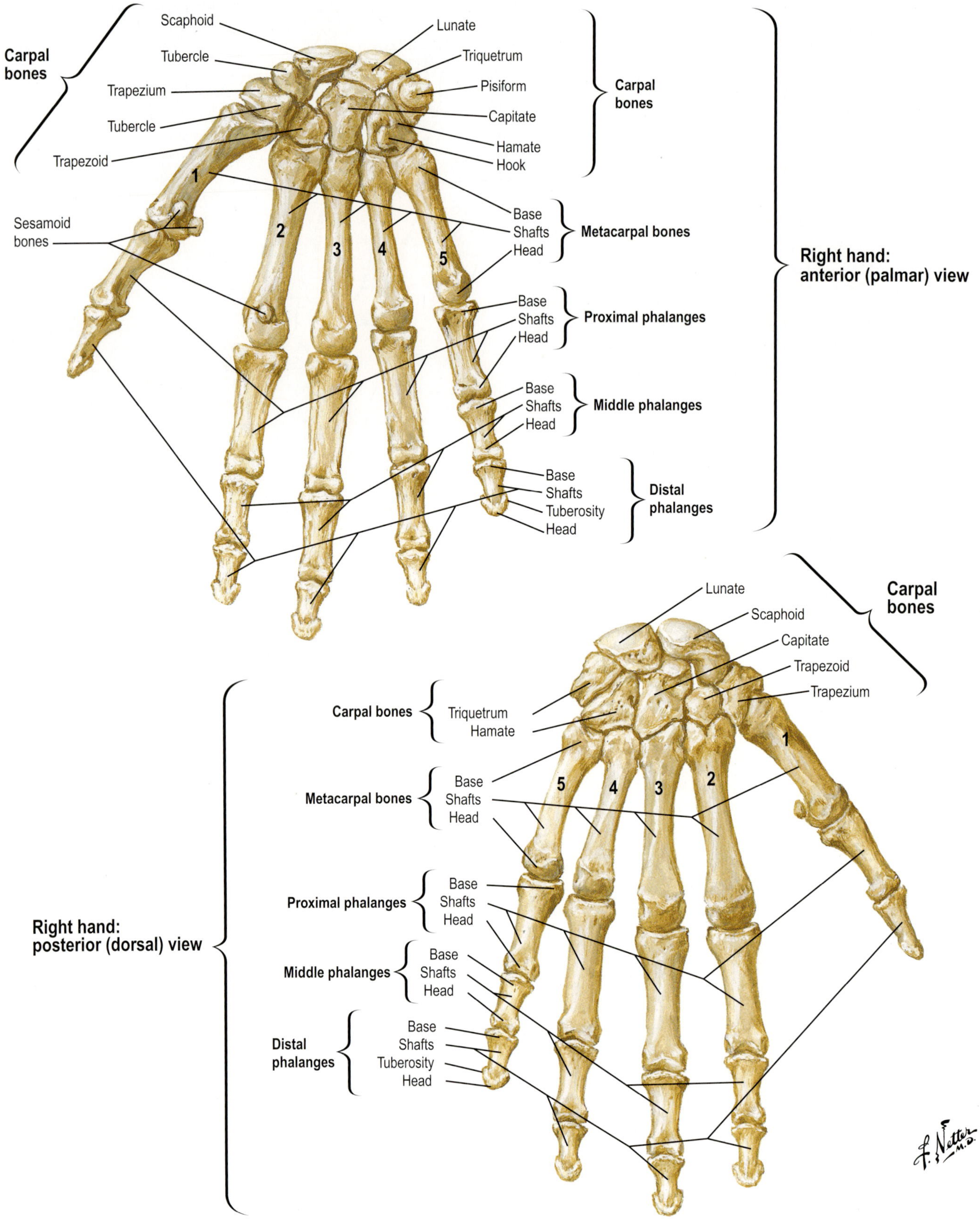

Figure 19.9 Bony anatomy of the wrist and hand. (Reprinted with permission from www.netterimages.com. © Elsevier Inc. All Rights Reserved.)

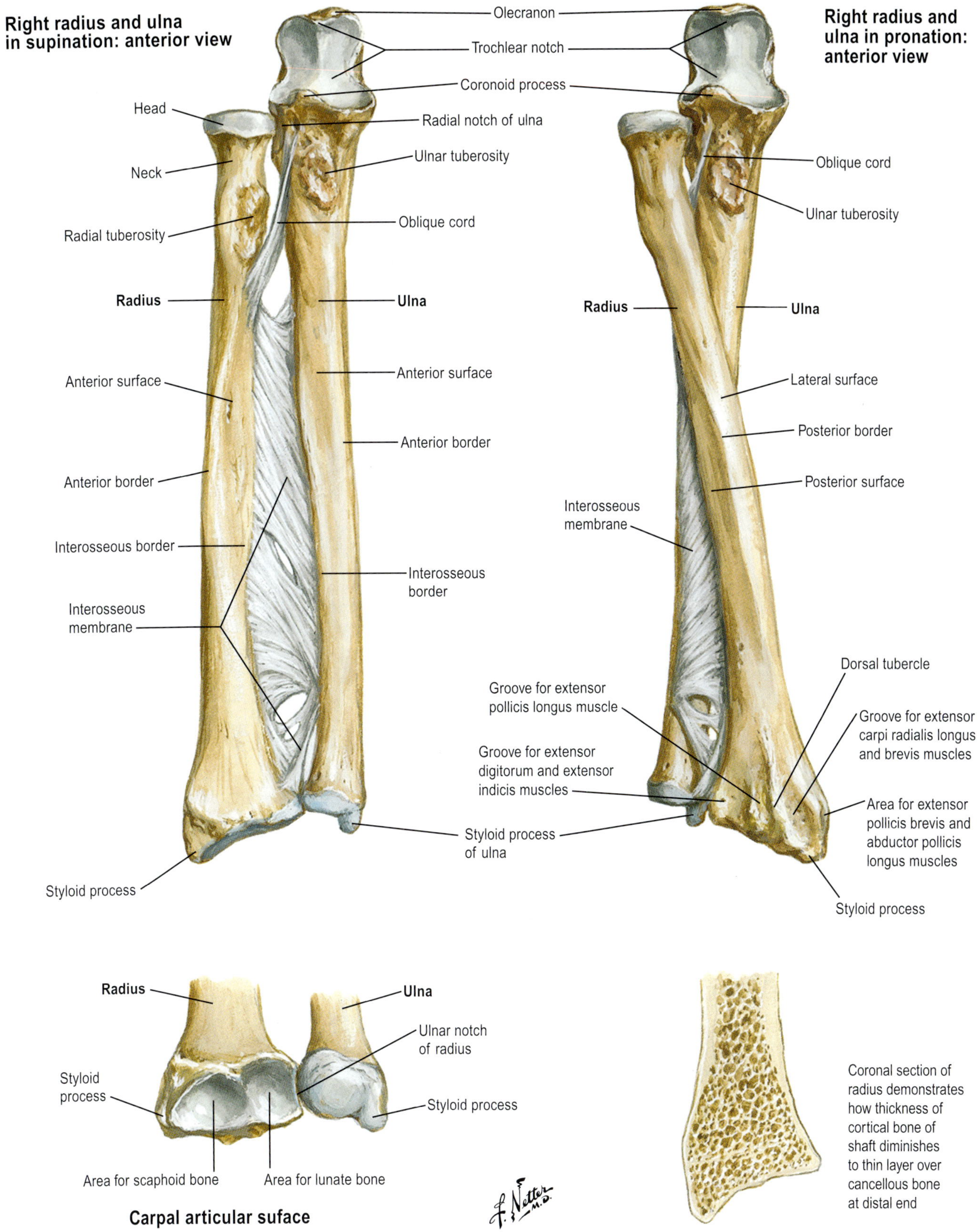

Figure 19.10 Relationship of the radius and ulna at the proximal and distal radioulnar joints. (Reprinted with permission from www.netterimages.com. © Elsevier Inc. All Rights Reserved.)

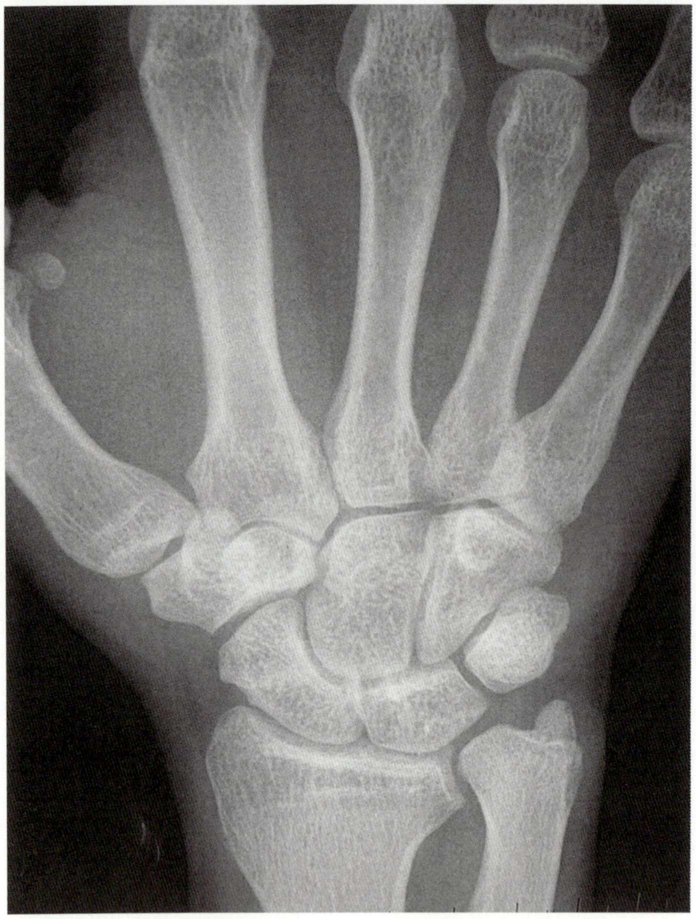

Figure 19.11 X-ray of ulnar positive variance: this patient has ulnar-sided wrist pain due to ulnar impaction syndrome.

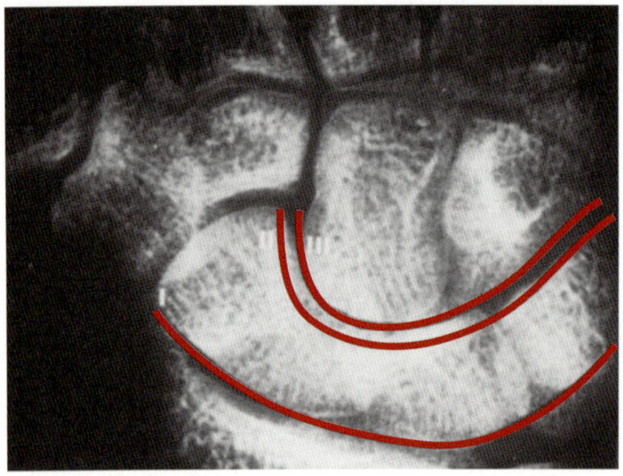

Figure 19.12 X-ray: Gilula's lines showing the greater arc and lesser arc of the carpal bones. (From Hertz VR, Chase RA. *Hand Surgery: A clinical Atlas.* Philadelphia: WB Saunders; 2001.)

- The distal interphalangeal (DIP) joints:
  - Can be pushed into about 90° of flexion before they are limited by the dorsal joint capsule and extensor mechanism.
  - Extend to 30° of hyperextension.
  - As in the PIP joint, there is no lateral mobility in these joints with the collateral ligaments intact.

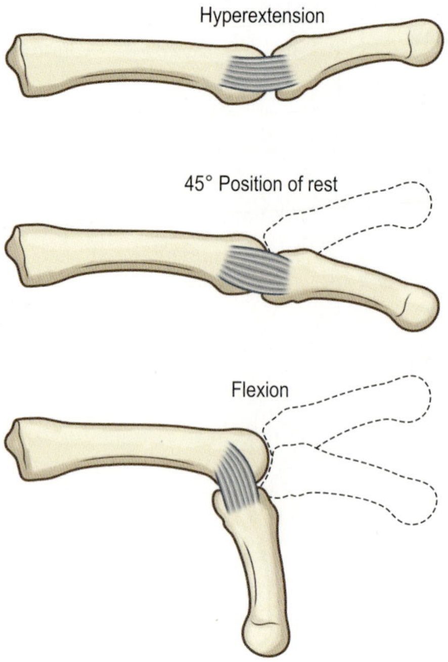

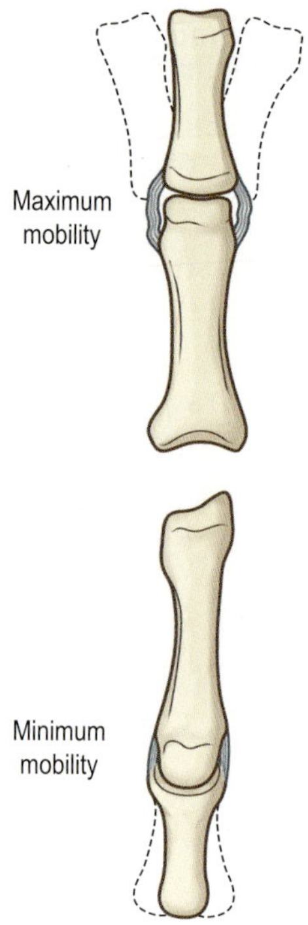

Figure 19.13 The true collateral ligaments of the metacarpophalangeal joint are loose in extension but tight in flexion of the joint as a result of the cam effect of the metacarpal head in relationship to the proximal phalanx. This accounts for the lack of lateral mobility of the joint when it is flexed. (Redrawn after Chase RA. *Atlas of Hand Surgery,* vol. 1. Philadelphia: WB Saunders; 1973.)

The thumb

- Made up of two phalanges, the metacarpal, and the trapezium.
- It differs from the other digits by virtue of its two named phalanges (rather than three).
- From a functional point of view, the thumb metacarpal can be compared to a proximal phalanx and the trapezium to a grossly foreshortened metacarpal ***(Fig. 19.14)***.
- The thumb MCP joint has the greatest degree of freedom of any in the digital rays which is attributable to the double saddle configuration between the base of the first metacarpal and the trapezium which allows three degrees of motion:
  - flexion–extension
  - abduction–adduction
  - medial rotation–lateral rotation.
- The base of the first metacarpal has a concavity that is slightly exaggerated on the ulnar volar side by a protrusion or "beak" for insertion of the anterior oblique carpometacarpal ligament ("volar beak" ligament).
- Volar beak ligament: important in stabilizing the first CMC joint. Clinically, it retains the fragment of bone fractured free from the base of the metacarpal in a Bennett's fracture. Also, in advanced CMC joint arthritis it weakens and attenuates allowing radial subluxation.
- There is also a stout intermetacarpal ligament between the base of the first metacarpal and the adjacent base of

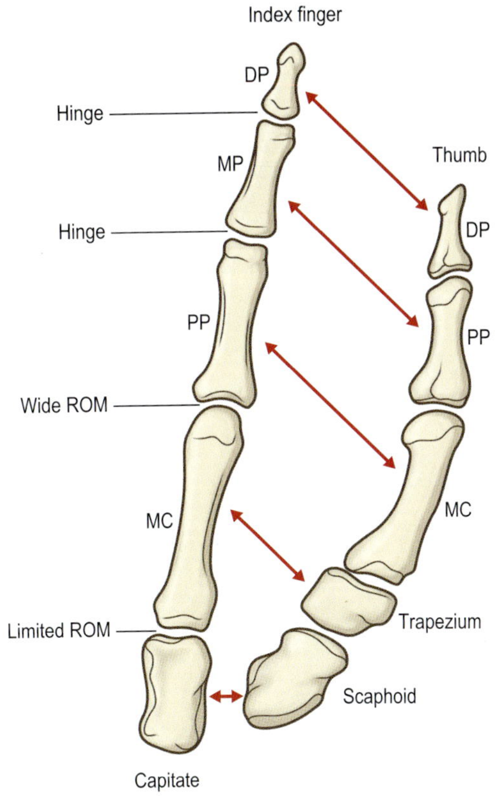

Figure 19.14 The osteoarticular column of the thumb as compared with that of a finger. The trapezium in this comparison is the equivalent of a foreshortened metacarpal, and the metacarpotrapezial joint of the fingers. FDP, flexor digitorum profundus; FDS, flexor digitorum superficialis. (Redrawn after Chase RA. Anatomy of the thumb. In: Strickland J (ed.) *The Thumb*. Edinburgh: Churchill Livingstone; 1989.)

the second metacarpal that is also important to prevention of radial subluxation of the metacarpotrapezial joint.

Muscles and tendons

Extrinsic extensors

- Extensor muscles lie on the dorsum of the forearm and hand and are innervated by the radial nerve ***(Figs 19.15–19.18)***.
- The extensor retinaculum prevents bowstringing of tendons across the wrist ***(Fig. 19.19)***.
- Six extensor compartments exist:
  1. Abductor pollicis longus and extensor pollicis brevis.
  2. Extensor carpi radialis longus and extensor carpi radialis brevis.
  3. Extensor pollicis longus.
  4. Extensor digitorum communis and extensor indicis proprius.
  5. Extensor digiti minimi.
  6. Extensor carpi ulnaris.
- Extension of the phalanges of the fingers and thumb is dependent both on long extensors at the MCP joints and on an interplay between the long extensors and intrinsic muscles at the IP joints.
- The extensor digitorum is a series of tendons with a common muscle belly that enters into the central extensor of each of the fingers. There are intertendinous bridges between these separate tendons over the dorsum of the hand (juncture).
- Independent long extensor power is also supplied to the index finger through the extensor indicis and to the little finger through the extensor digiti minimi.
  - This independent extensor lies ulnar to the extensor digitorum communis tendon.
- Each of the three extrinsic muscles to the thumb on its extensor surface inserts on one of the thumb bones.

Pronators and supinators

- The major pronators and supinators of the hand are the pronator teres, pronator quadratus, and supinator (with assistance from the biceps brachii), respectively ***(Fig. 19.20)***.

Extrinsic flexors

- Flexion of the phalanges into the palm is a complicated motion representing the sum of actions of the long flexors (profundus and superficialis) and long extensors (extensor digitorum, extensor digiti minimi, and extensor indicis), modified and enhanced by the intrinsic muscles (interossei and lumbricals) ***(Figs 19.21–19.25)***.
- The long flexors to the fingers are responsible for flexion of the interphalangeal joints and are supplements to active flexion of the metacarpophalangeal joints and the wrist joint.
- The flexors are located on the volar side of the forearm and wrist and are innervated by the median nerve, except the flexor carpi ulnaris, and the flexor digitorum profundus to the ring and small fingers which are innervated by the ulnar nerve (see Figs 19.21–19.25).
- The flexor digitorum superficialis tendon lies palmar (superficial) to the profundus tendon in the palm. It splits at the level of the proximal phalanx, wraps around and decussates behind the profundus to insert on the middle phalanx.
- The flexor digitorum profundus perforates the flexor digitorum superficialis to run superficial along the length of the proximal and middle phalanges to insert at the base of the distal phalanx.
- The flexor digitorum profundus of the index finger is unique in that it has an independent muscle belly.
- The tendon–muscle unit has an effect on each joint it crosses, which is altered by the positioning of the other joints in the linkage system. Thus, the influence of the tendon on one joint in the system is augmented by the function of its antagonists at each of the other joints it crosses. This is the simplified definition of synergistic function.
- Synergistic and antagonistic groups of muscles in hand function must be considered when functional substitution by tendon transfers is contemplated.
  - Examples of such natural synergism are the united functions of the wrist flexors and digital extensors or the wrist extensors and digital flexors.

(cont'd)

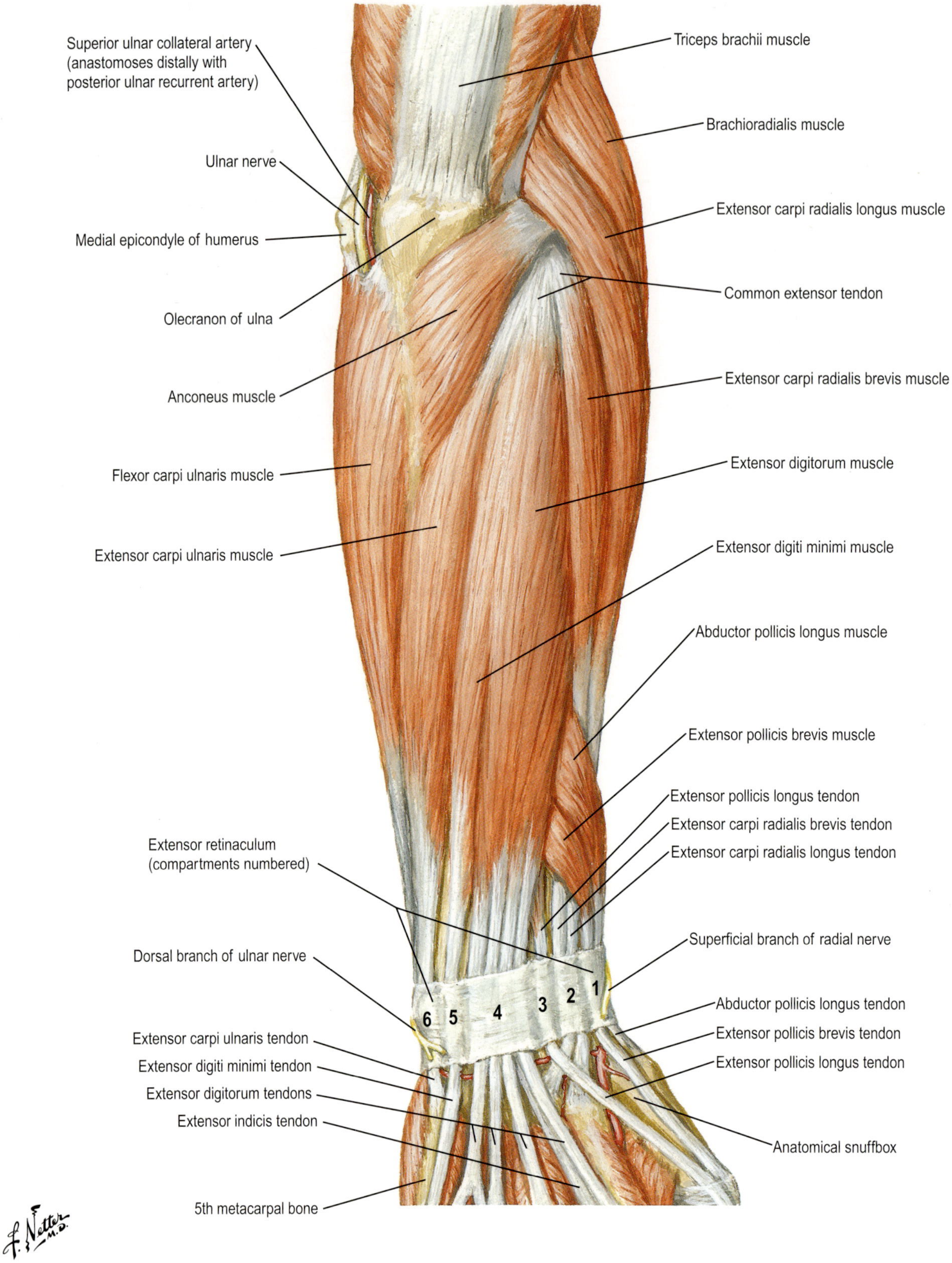

Figure 19.15 The anatomy of the extensor muscles: superficial to deep. (Reprinted with permission from www.netterimages.com. © Elsevier Inc. All Rights Reserved.)

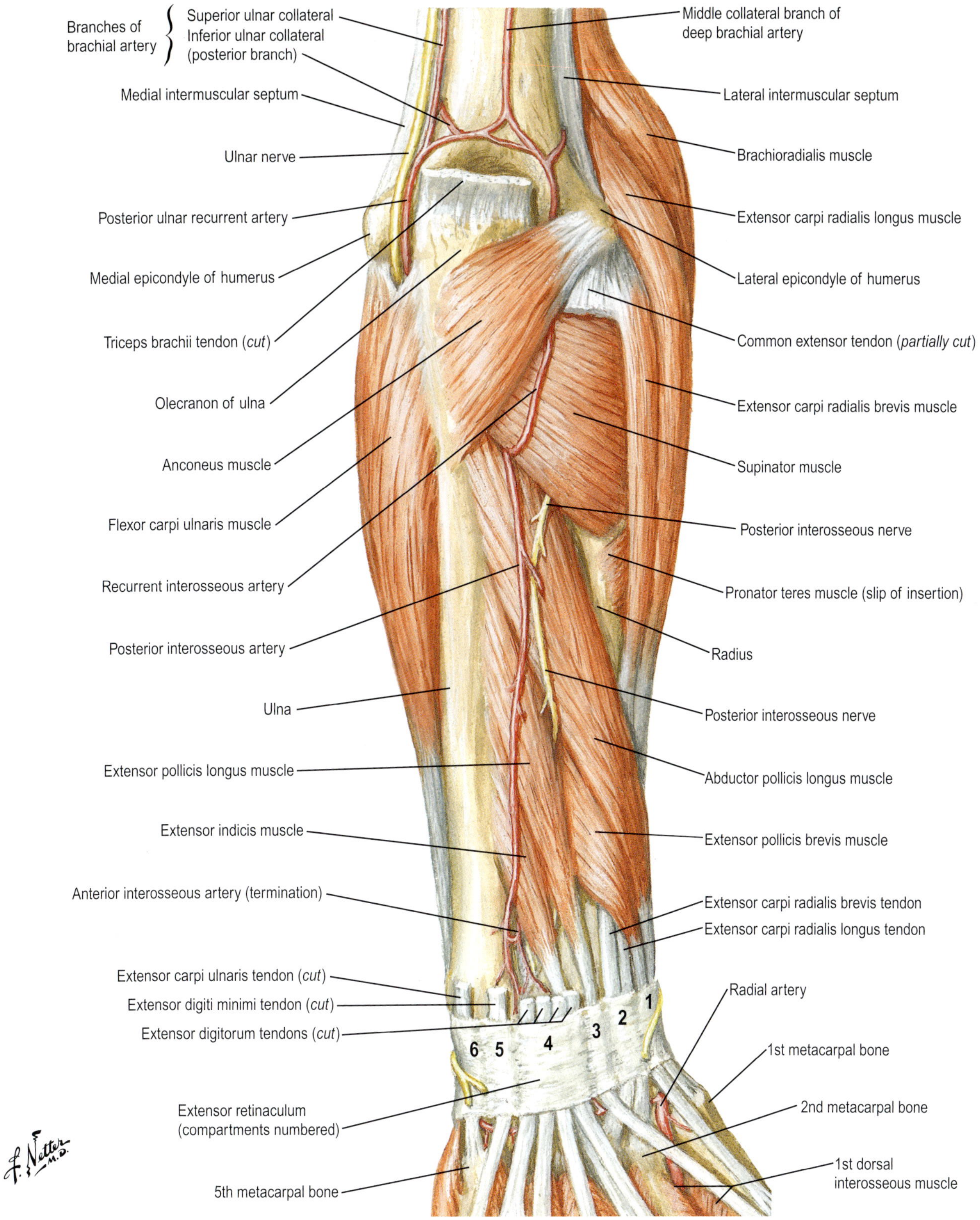

Figure 19.16 The anatomy of the extensor muscles: superficial to deep. (Reprinted with permission from www.netterimages.com. © Elsevier Inc. All Rights Reserved.)

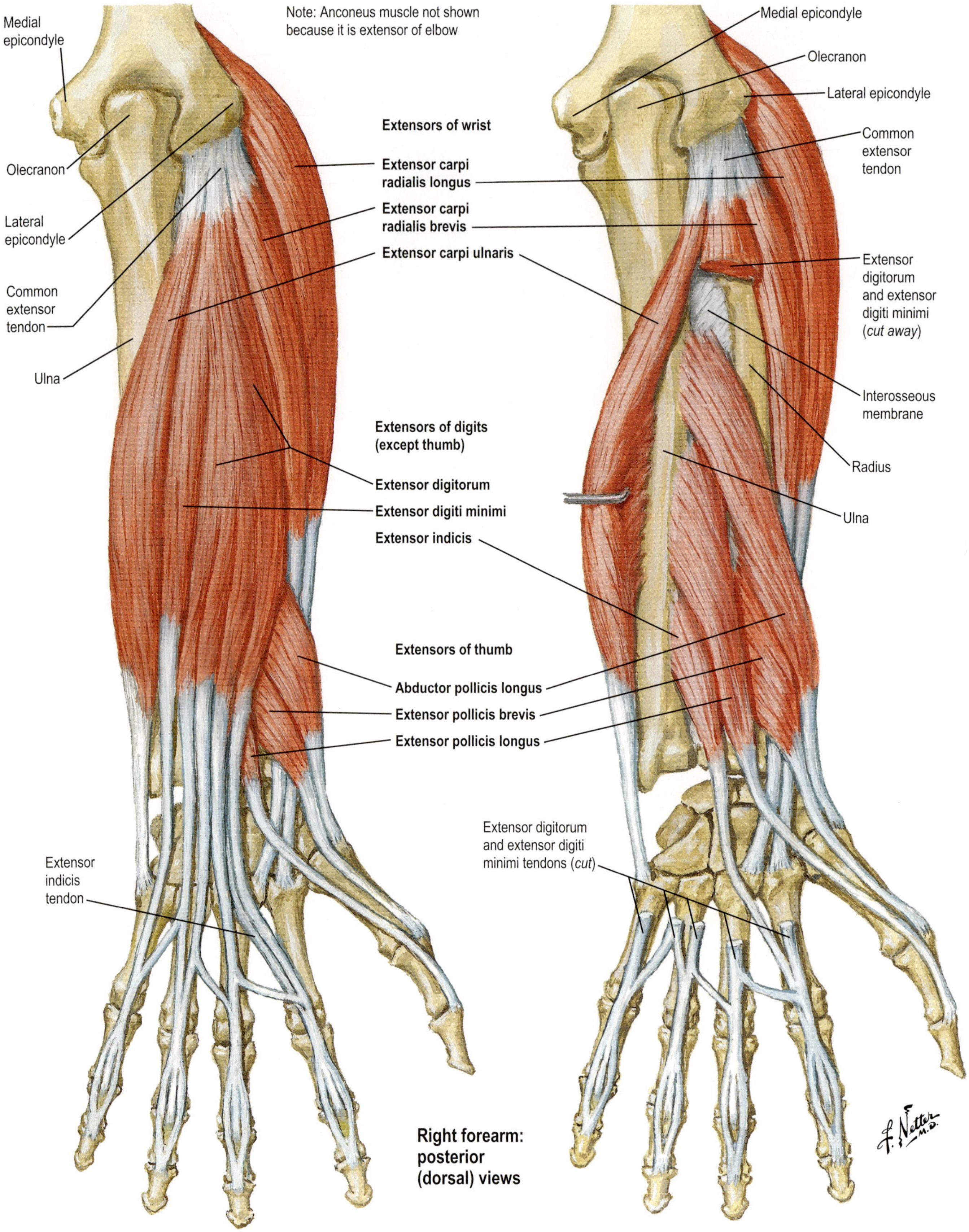

Figure 19.17 The anatomy of the extensor muscles: superficial to deep. (Reprinted with permission from www.netterimages.com. © Elsevier Inc. All Rights Reserved.)

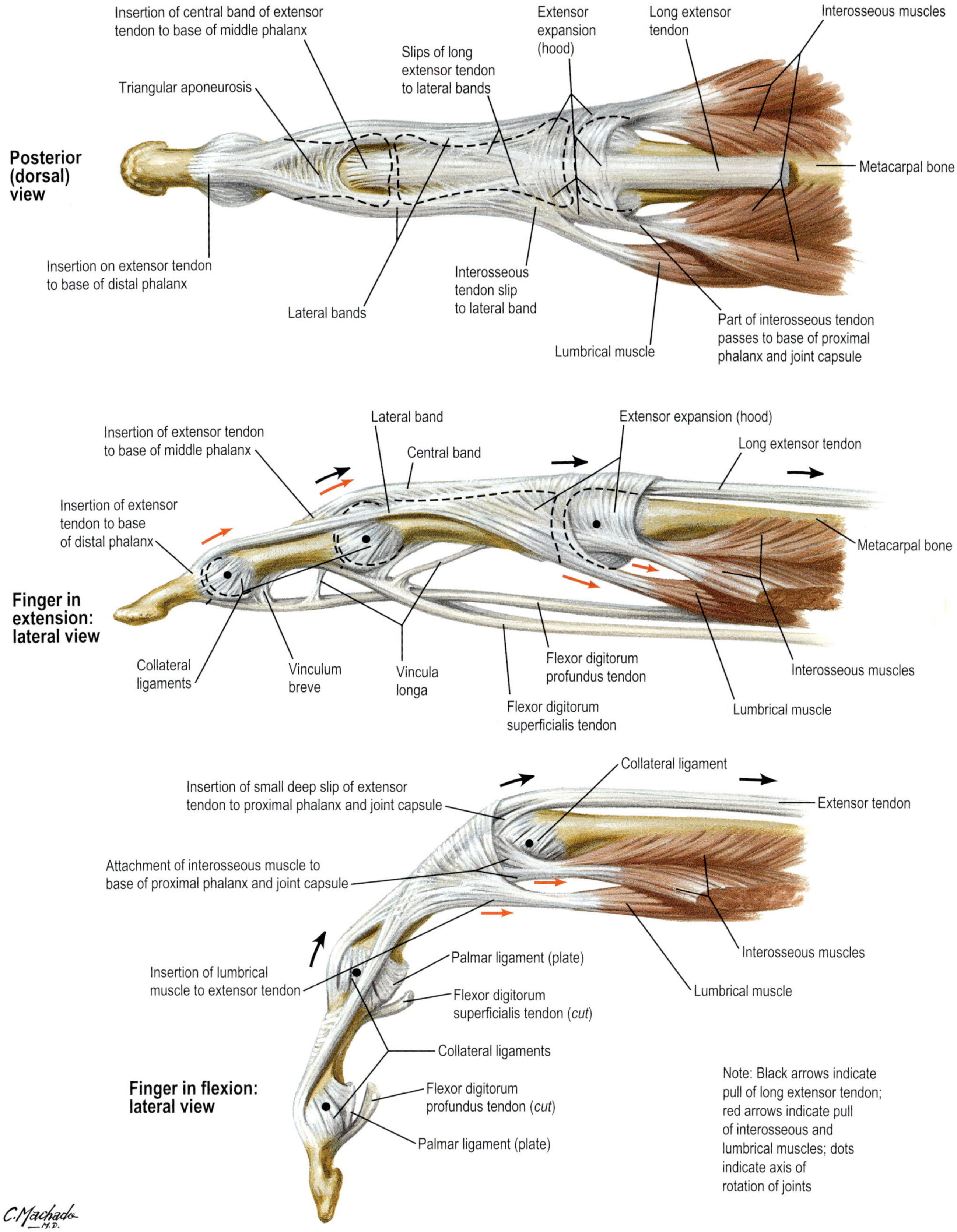

Figure 19.18 The extensor mechanism of the fingers. (Reprinted with permission from www.netterimages.com.)

Posterior (dorsal) view

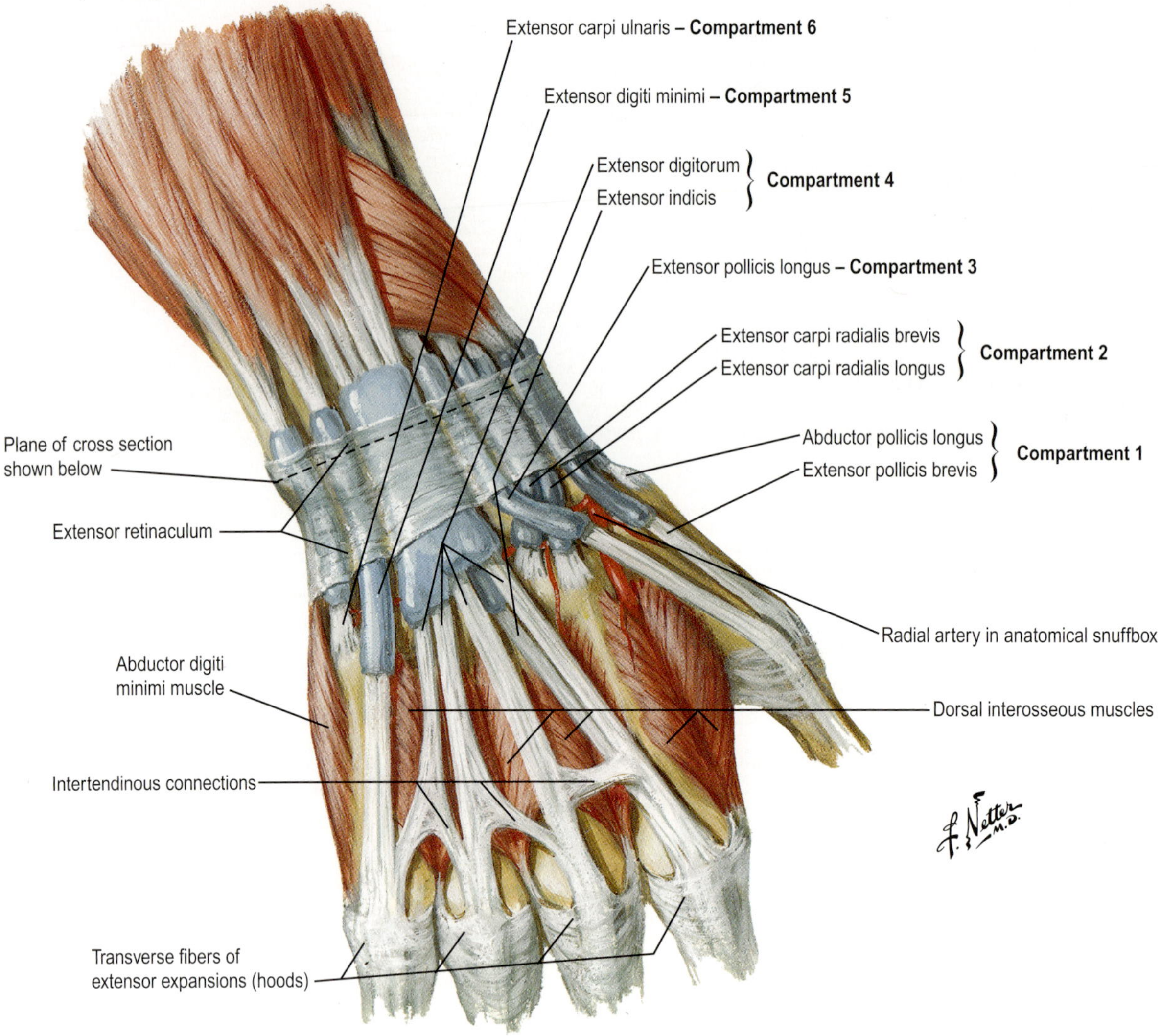

Cross section of most distal portion of forearm

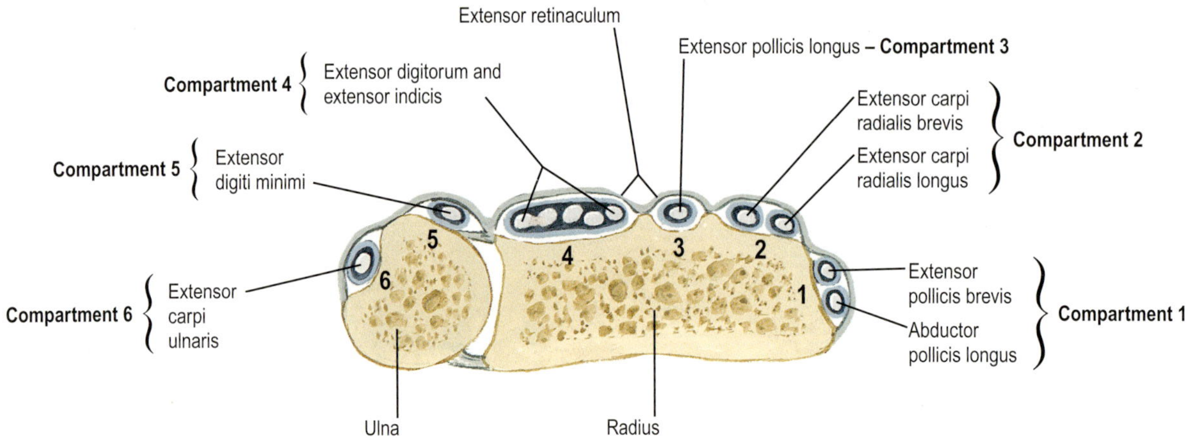

Figure 19.19 The extensor retinaculum and extensor compartments. (Reprinted with permission from www.netterimages.com. © Elsevier Inc. All Rights Reserved.)

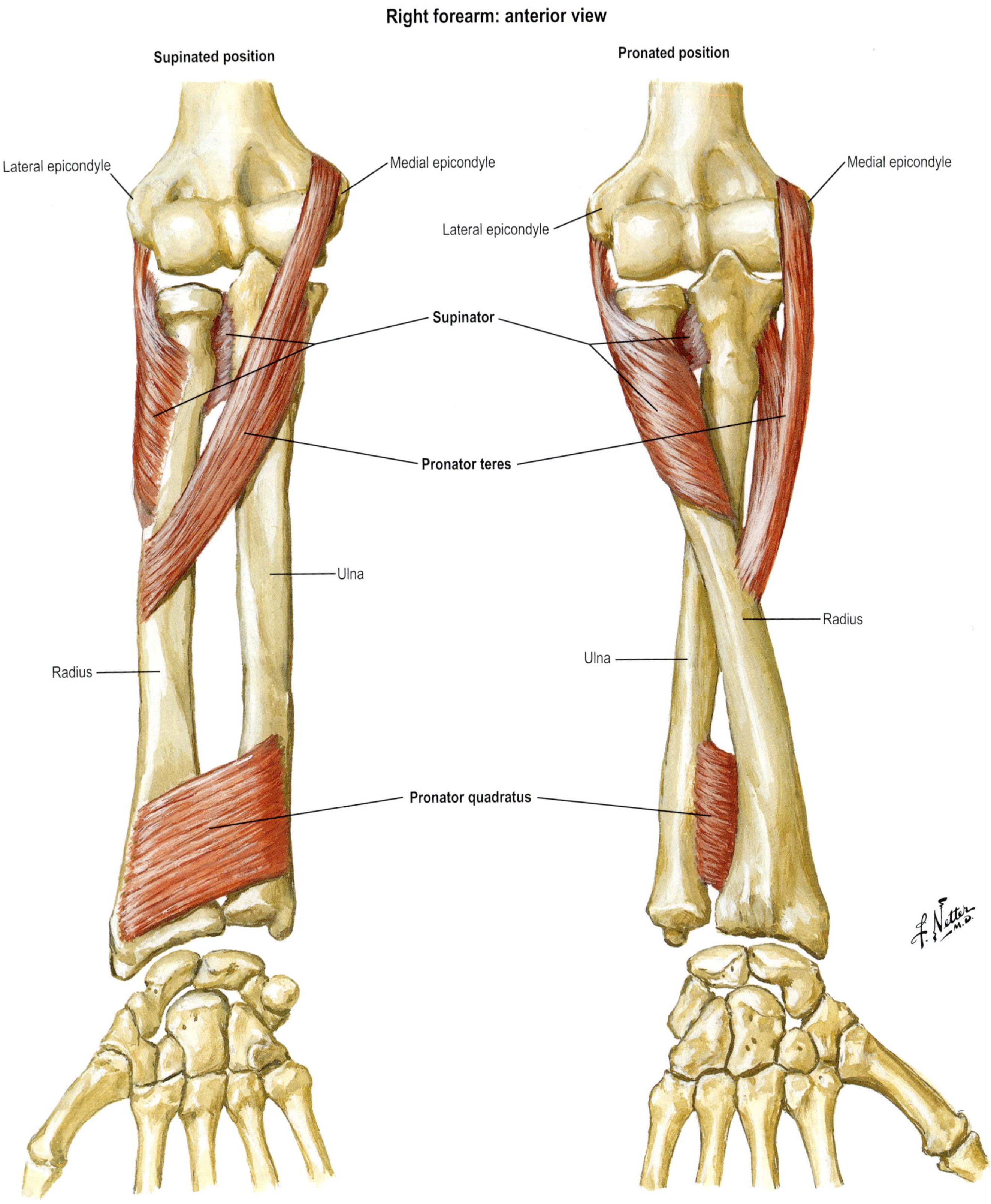

Figure 19.20 The forearm pronators and supinators. (Reprinted with permission from www.netterimages.com. © Elsevier Inc. All Rights Reserved.)

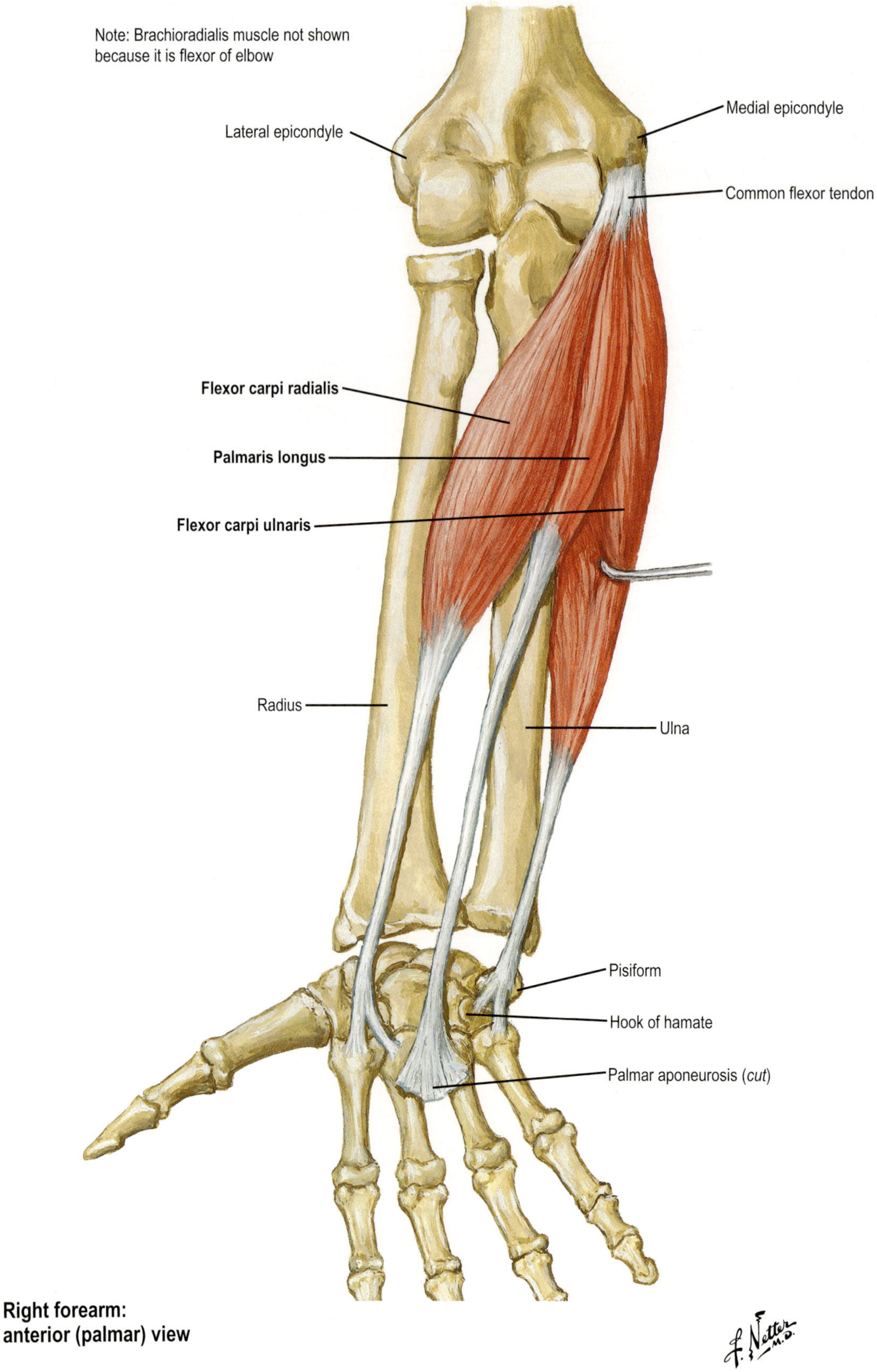

Figure 19.21 The anatomy of the flexor muscles – superficial to deep. (Reprinted with permission from www.netterimages.com. © Elsevier Inc. All Rights Reserved.)

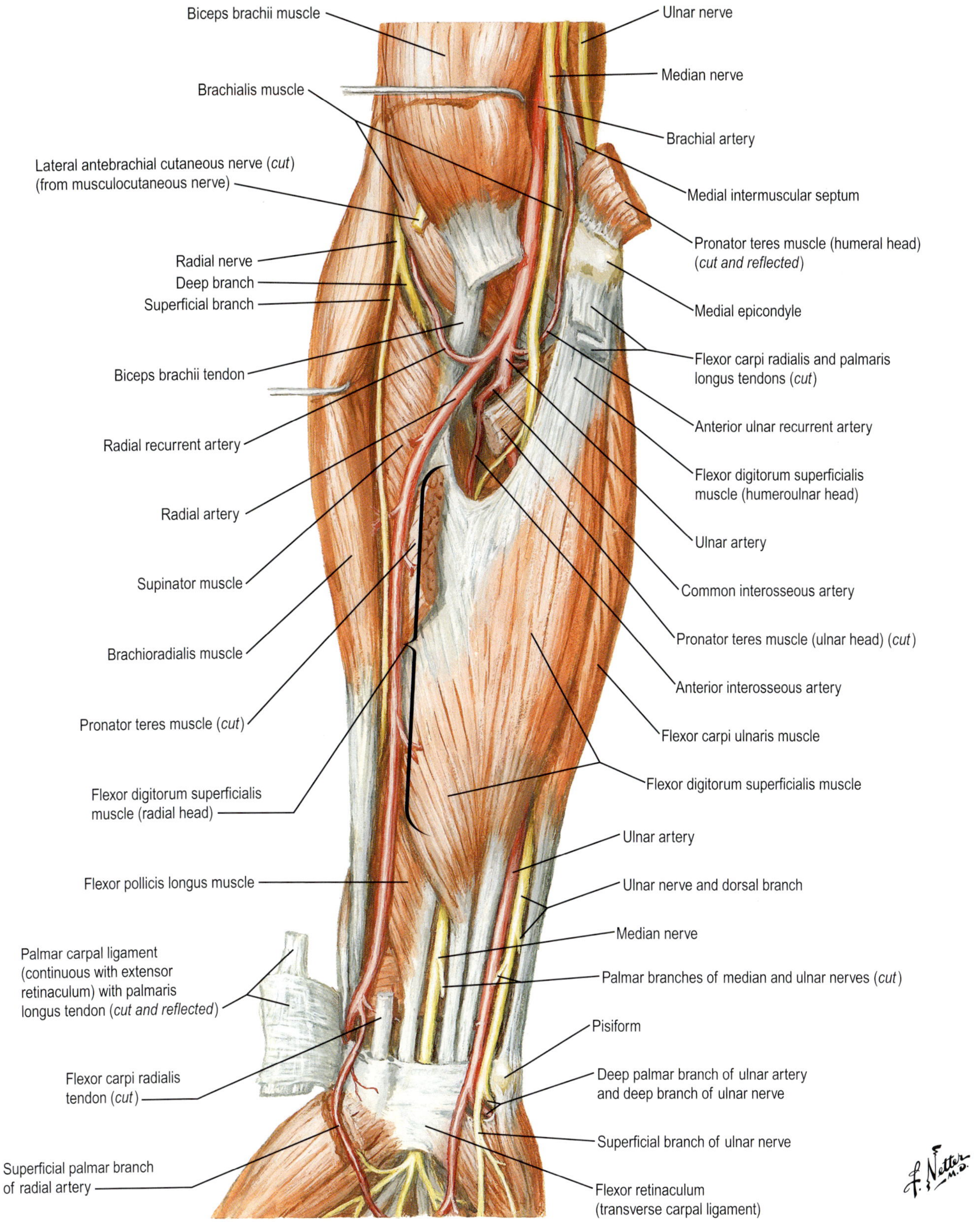

Figure 19.22 The anatomy of the flexor muscles – superficial to deep. (Reprinted with permission from www.netterimages.com.)

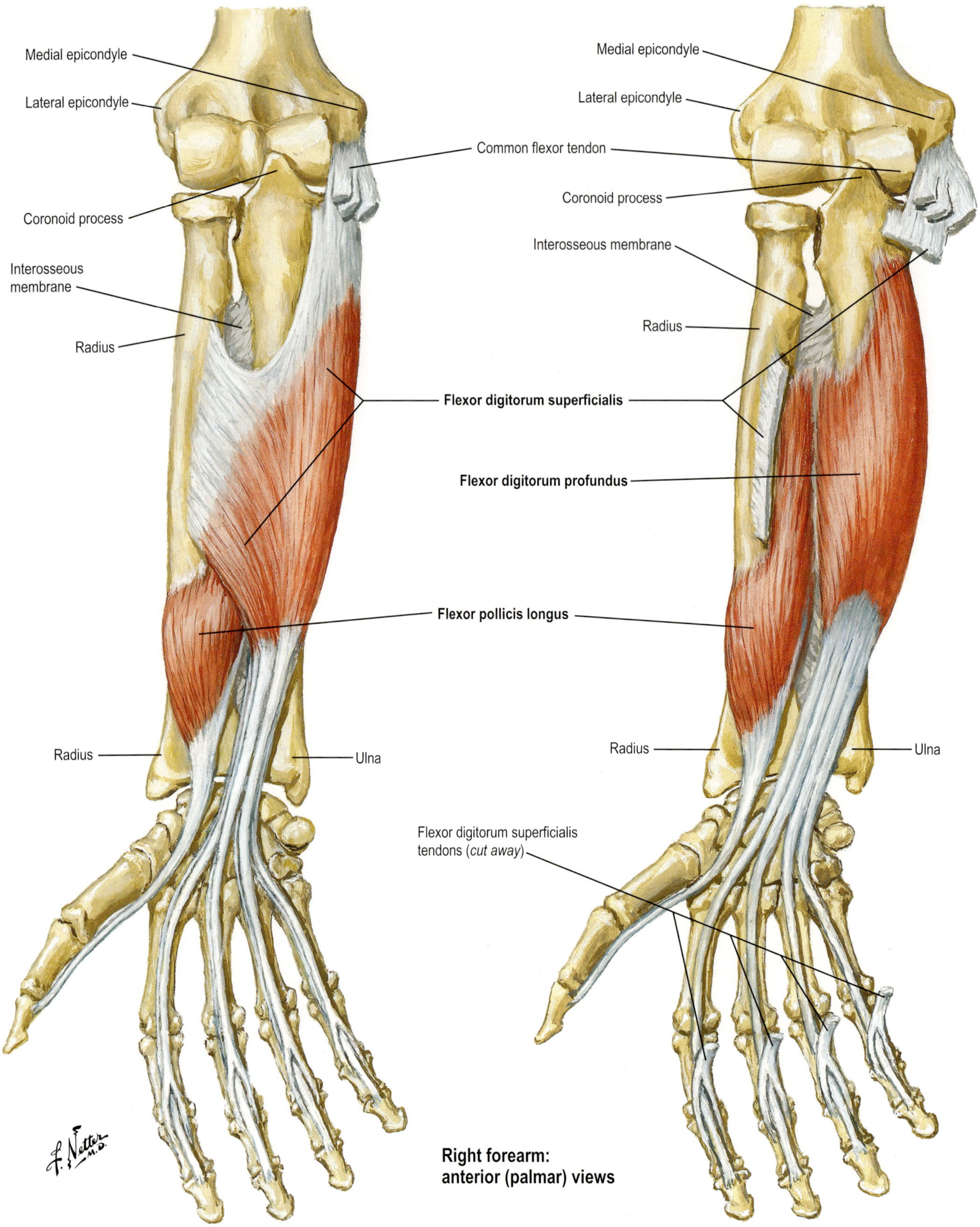

Figure 19.23 The anatomy of the flexor muscles – superficial to deep. (Reprinted with permission from www.netterimages.com. © Elsevier Inc. All Rights Reserved.)

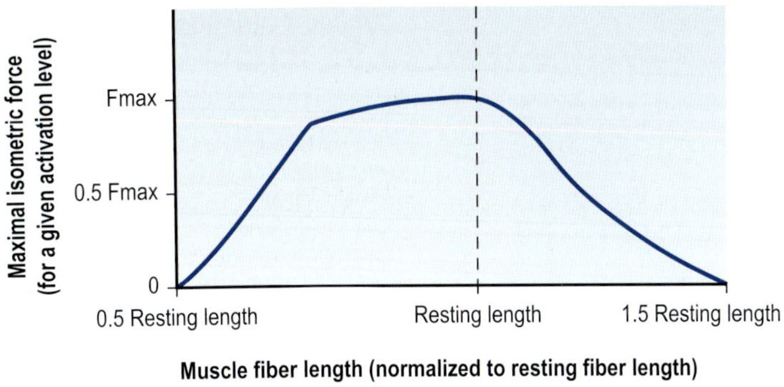

Figure 19.24 The anatomy of the flexor muscles – superficial to deep. (Reprinted with permission from www.netterimages.com. © Elsevier Inc. All Rights Reserved.)

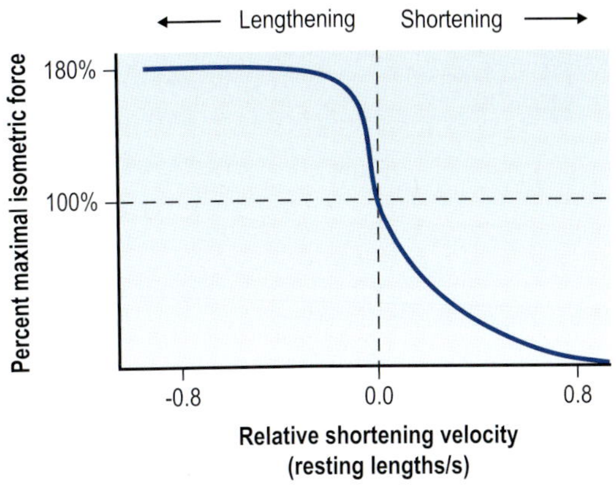

Figure 19.25 The anatomy of the flexor muscles – superficial to deep. (Reprinted with permission from www.netterimages.com. © Elsevier Inc. All Rights Reserved.)

- The relationship of the tendon to the joint axes is maintained by retinacular structures, or pulleys. This prevents the bowstring effect, which would allow the tendon to move away from the joint axis, changing the moment arm and therefore the force exerted at that joint by the flexor tendon.

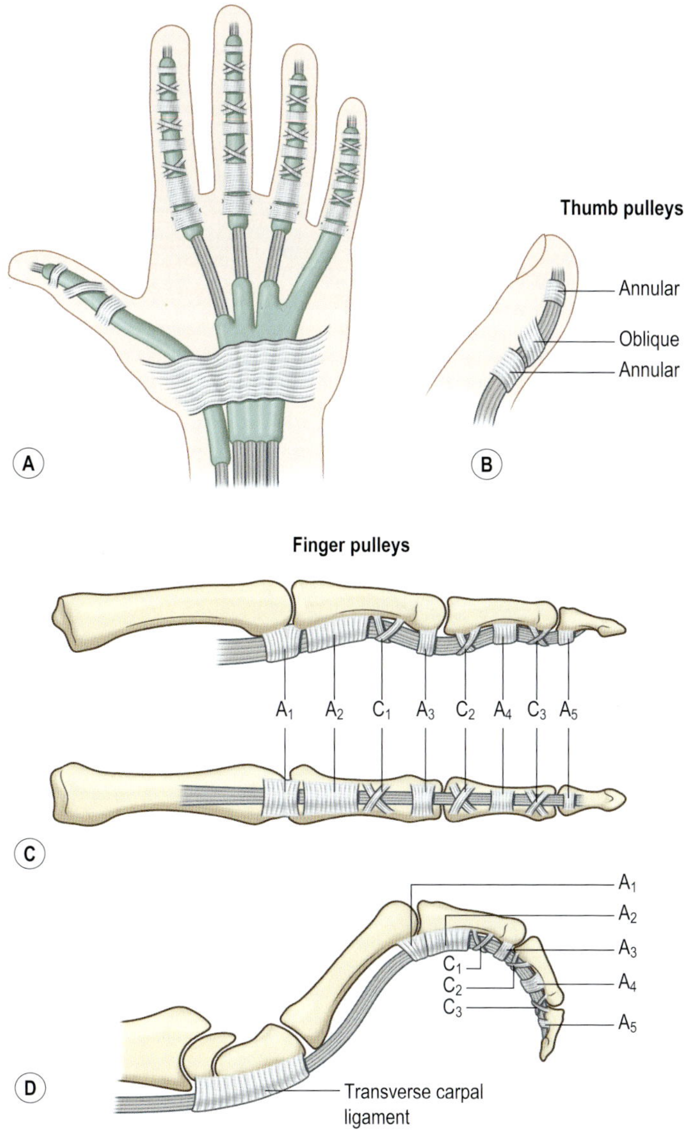

Figure 19.26 The flexor tendon pulley system for fingers and thumb. (Redrawn after Chase RA. *Atlas of Hand Surgery*, vol II. Philadelphia: WB Saunders; 1984.)

The retinacular system

- Transverse carpal ligament ***(Fig. 19.26A–D)***:
  - Bridges the volar surface of the carpals from the pisiform and hook of the hamate ulnarly to the scaphoid tubercle and trapezium radially.
  - Confines the nine extrinsic flexor tendons and the median nerve within the carpal tunnel.
  - Prevents bowstringing of the flexor tendons at the wrist.
- Three pulleys housing the flexor pollicis longus within the thumb are regularly present.
  - The proximal annular pulley: at the level of the MCP joint arising from the volar plate and base of the proximal phalanx.
  - The distal annular pulley: over the volar plate of the interphalangeal joint.
  - Oblique pulley: located between the two, it originates proximally on the ulnar side of the middle phalanx and inserts on the middle one-third of the radial palmar surface of the middle phalanx.
- Four or five discrete annular pulleys and three cruciate bands are ordinarily present in the fingers ***(Fig. 19.27)***.
  - The most proximal pulley (A1) begins 0.5 cm proximal to the MCP joint.
  - A2 is located just distal to A1, is the largest pulley, and extends to nearly the proximal one-half of the proximal phalanx.
  - The first cruciform band (Cl) lies distal to A2 and well proximal to the PIP joint.
  - A3 lies over the PIP joint, arising from its volar plate.
  - The second cruciate ligament (C2) is at the base of the middle phalanx.
  - A4 lies over the middle one-third of the middle phalanx.
  - The third cruciate (C3) is just distal to A4.
  - A5 is often possible to identify as a thickening of the sheath over the DIP joint.

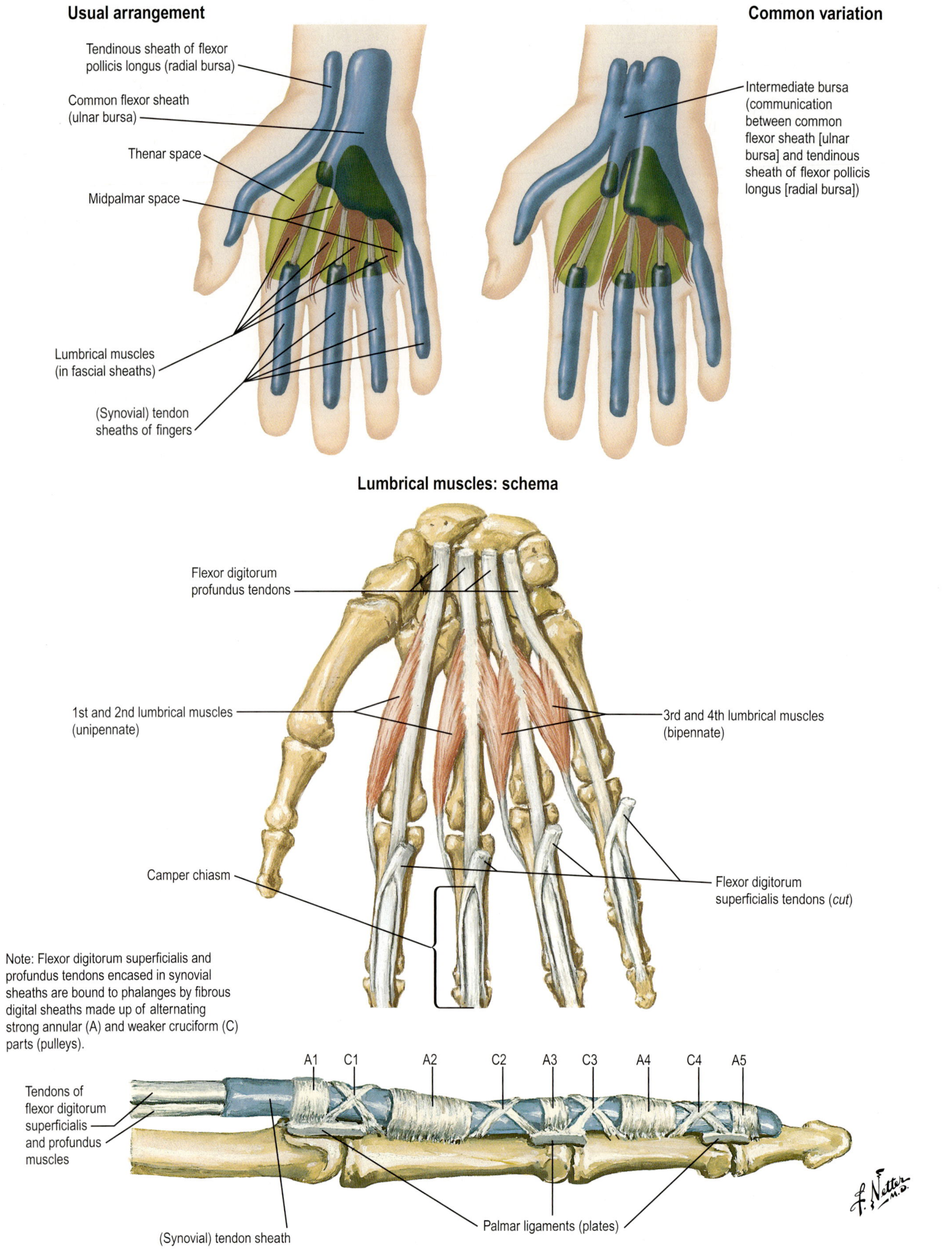

Figure 19.27 Orientation of the flexor tendon sheaths, flexor tendons, and pulleys. (Reprinted with permission from www.netterimages.com. © Elsevier Inc. All Rights Reserved.)

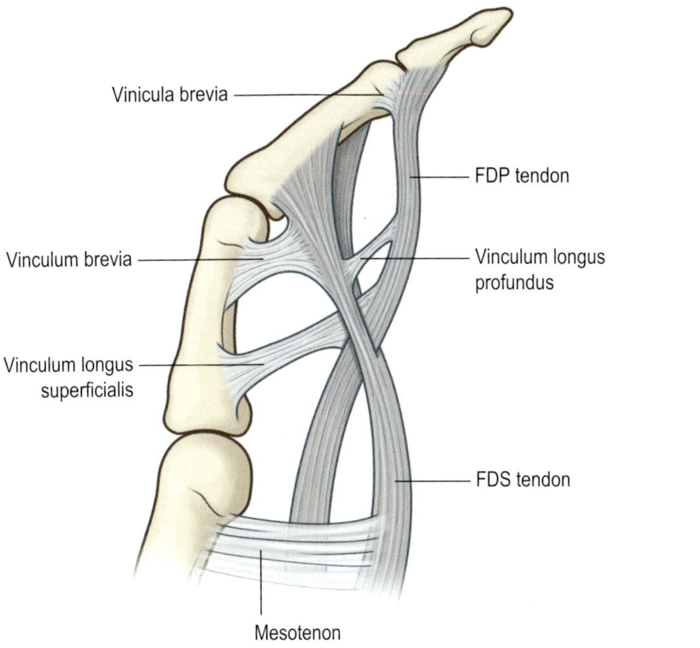

Figure 19.28 The common configuration of the vincula. (From Chase RA. *Atlas of Hand Surgery.* vol II. Philadelphia: WB Saunders; 1984.)

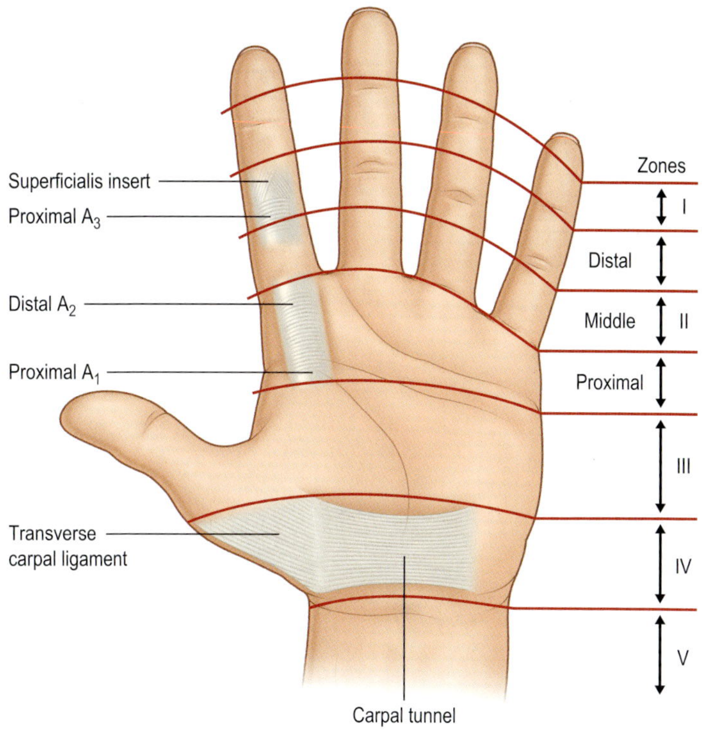

Figure 19.29 Flexor tendon zones are classified for their relevance to flexor tendon injuries. (Redrawn after Chase RA. *Atlas of Hand Surgery,* vol II. Philadelphia: WB Saunders; 1984.)

- The A2 and A4 pulleys are most important for preventing bowstringing in the digits.
- The longitudinal blood supply to a tendon comes from its musculotendinous junction and its insertion site into bone.
- The segmental blood supply derives from the mesotenon and from the vincula within the digital sheaths.
  - The vincula brevia form the residual mesotenon at the sites of insertion of the profundus and superficialis tendons on the phalanges.
  - The vincula longa are the flexible, vessel-carrying bands to each tendon in the area where the complete mesotenon has disappeared ***(Fig. 19.28)***.
- The flexor tendons and the associated synovial and fibrous sheaths are divided into clinically important zones ***(Fig. 19.29)***:
  - Zone 1: The area traversed by the flexor digitorum profundus distal to the insertion of the flexor digitorum superficialis on the middle phalanx.
  - Zone 2: From the proximal end of Zone 1 to the proximal end of the digital fibrous sheath.
  - Zone 3: From the proximal end of the finger pulley system (Al) to the distal end of the transverse carpal ligament.
  - Zone 4: The carpal tunnel.
  - Zone 5: From the proximal border of the transverse carpal ligament to the musculotendinous junctions of the flexor tendon.
- Synovial sheaths are closed sacs around the tendons composed of a visceral layer on the tendon surface and a parietal layer on the fibrous sheath surface.
- Knowledge of the anatomy of the synovial sheaths and potential anatomic spaces in the hand is essential for proper diagnosis and treatment of serious hand infections. Infection starting in the digital synovial sheaths may extend proximally to the deep palmar spaces.

Intrinsic muscles

- Intrinsic muscles arise and insert within the hand ***(Figs 19.30, 19.31)***. They can be divided into four groups:
  - The thenar muscles.
  - Abductor pollicis brevis, flexor pollicis brevis, opponens pollicis brevis and the adductor pollicis brevis.
  - The hypothenar muscles.
  - Palmaris brevis, abductor digiti minimi, flexor digiti minimi brevis, and opponens digiti minimi.
  - The lumbricals.
  - The interossei.
- "Intrinsic plus" posture: results from pull of the interossei resulting in MCP flexion and IP extension ***(Fig. 19.32)***.

Blood supply

- The brachial artery is palpable just medial to the biceps tendon at the level of the elbow.

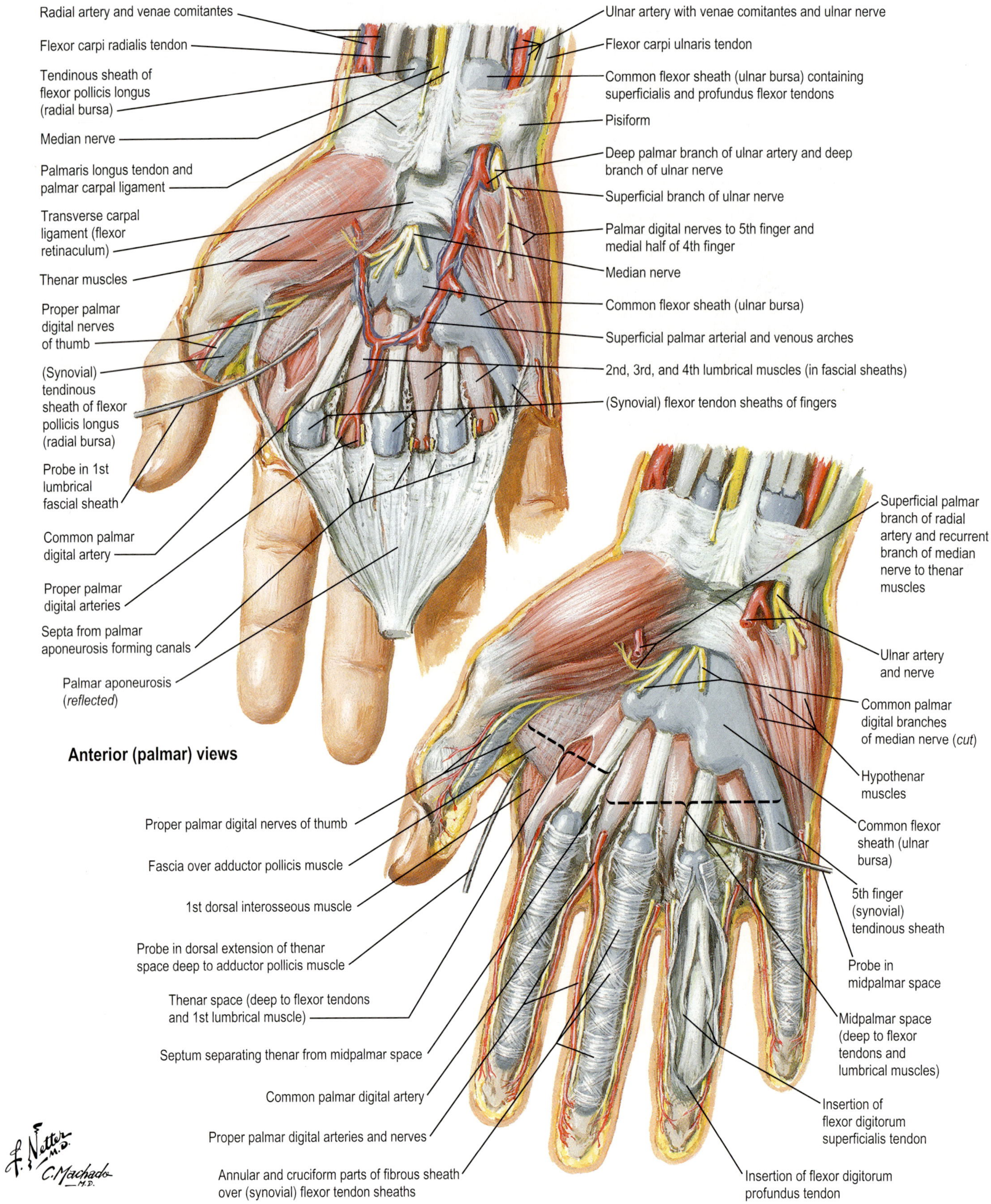

Figure 19.30 Superficial and deep intrinsic muscles in the hand. (Reprinted with permission from www.netterimages.com. © Elsevier Inc. All Rights Reserved.)

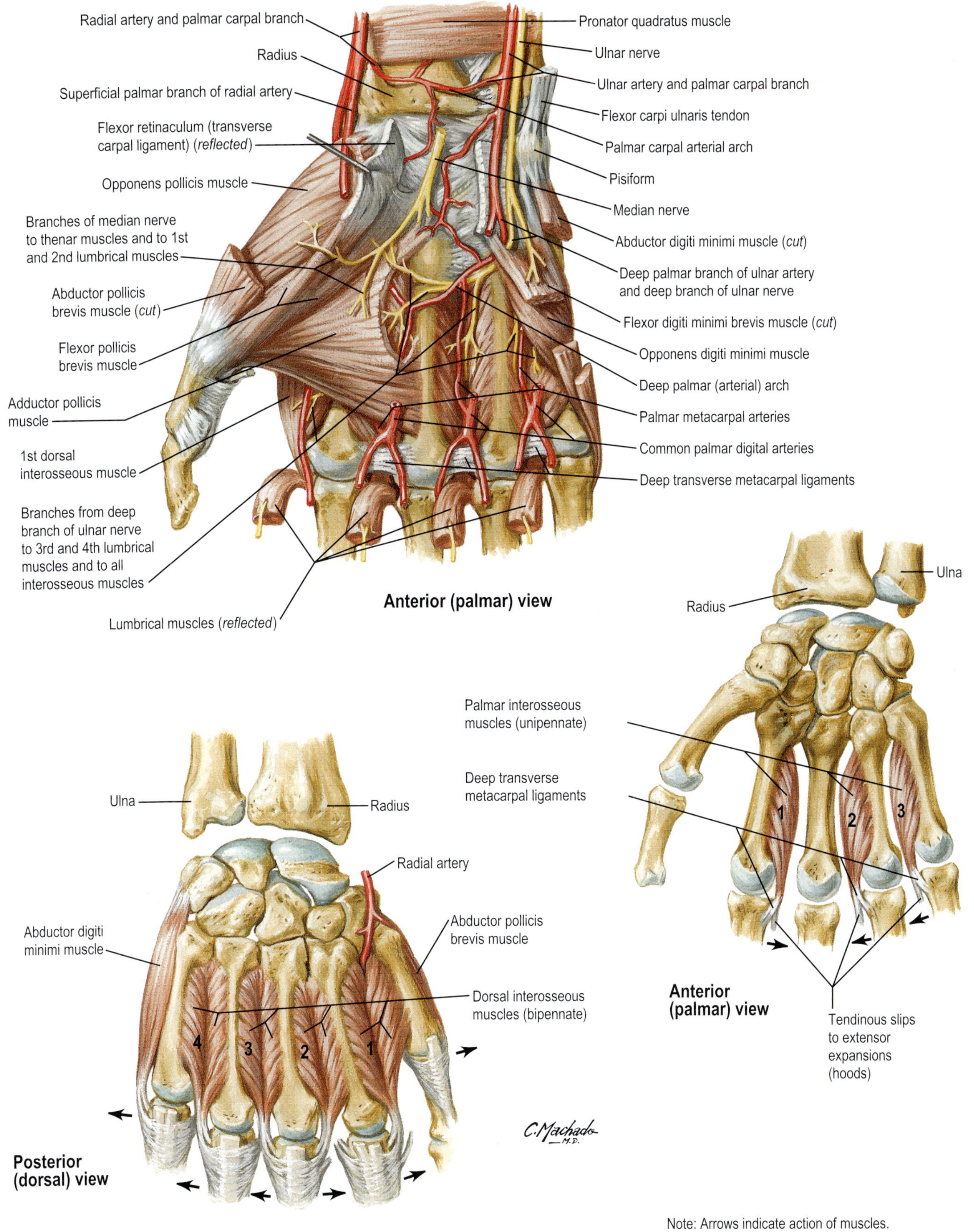

Figure 19.31 Superficial and deep intrinsic muscles in the hand. (Reprinted with permission from www.netterimages.com. © Elsevier Inc. All Rights Reserved.)

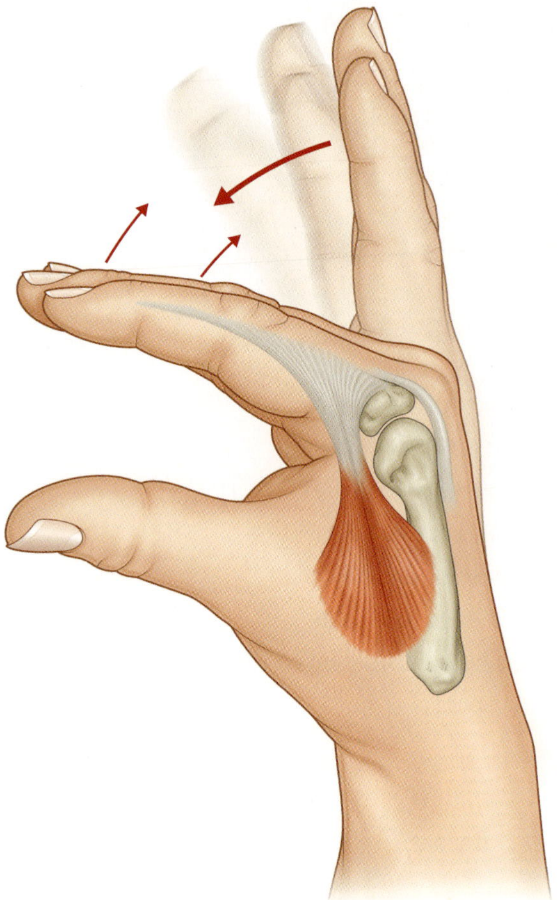

Figure 19.32 All interossei act as prime flexors of the metacarpophalangeal joints since they pass palmar to the joint axis. Extensions into the lateral bands result in extension of the interphalangeal joints. (From Chase RA. *Atlas of Hand Surgery*, vol 1. Philadelphia: WB Saunders; 1973.)

- Branches into the radial and ulnar arteries at the bicipital aponeurosis of the elbow ***(Fig. 19.33)***.
- Supplementary arteries in the forearm include the anterior interosseous artery, the posterior interosseous artery, and the median artery.
- The radial artery continues distally between the brachioradialis and FCR muscles.
  - At the wrist: located near the styloid process of the radius, travels dorsally, crossing the "anatomic snuffbox" deep to the tendons of the APL, EPB, and EPL.
  - In the hand: penetrates between the first and second metacarpal bones, through an arcade in the first dorsal interosseous muscle, to enter the palm and form the deep palmar arch.
  - A superficial branch of the radial artery arises at the level of the distal radius and courses over or through the APB to contribute to the superficial palmar arch.
- The ulnar artery gives off the common interosseous artery soon after its takeoff, which itself branches into the anterior and posterior interosseous arteries.
  - The ulnar artery continues distally under the FCU muscle.
  - At the wrist: it lies radial to the pisiform and ulnar to the hook of the hamate and travels into the hand through Guyon's canal.
  - In the hand: travels deep to the palmaris brevis and the hypothenar fascia where it divides into a deep palmar branch (contributes to deep palmar arch) and a superficial palmar branch (dominant contributor to the superficial palmar arch) ***(Fig. 19.34)***.
  - The superficial palmar arch gives rise to three common digital arteries and multiple branches to intrinsic muscles and skin.
  - The deep palmar arch is the major source of blood supply to the thumb and to the radial side of the index finger.
  - The first metacarpal artery is the prime source of blood supply to the radial and ulnar proper digital arteries of the thumb and the radial proper digital artery of the index finger.
  - After giving its branch to the index finger, the first metacarpal artery becomes the princeps pollicis (the primary source of blood supply to the thumb).
  - A dorsal carpal arch is formed from dorsal arteries (originate proximally from the posterior interosseous artery and a dorsal perforating branch of the anterior interosseious artery), and from branches of the radial and ulnar arteries.
  - Dorsal metacarpal arteries originate from this arch and extend distally to the margins of the fingers. These arteries are joined by branches from the radial and ulnar arteries to form a dorsal carpal arch.

Peripheral nerves

- General peripheral nerve anatomy:
  - The epineurium is the tubular fibrous support structure surrounding the entire nerve; it also courses between the fascicles to create an internal topography.
  - Each fascicle is covered by perineurium.
  - Within each fascicle are separate axons, some myelinated and some unmyelinated. Motor, sensory, and sympathetic fibers are present within each peripheral nerve.
  - Blood vessels are found on the epineurial surface and in the internal supporting structure of the nerve.
- The flexor pollicis longus divides the hand into a median and ulnar-innervated portion from the motor standpoint. The ulnar nerve is far less important from the standpoint of hand sensation but is very important for its motor innervation of all the hypothenar muscles and interossei.
- When there is paralysis of any of the three major motor nerves, thumb stability is compromised.
  - Median nerve palsy results in lost opposition.
  - Ulnar nerve palsy results in adduction weakness.
  - Radial nerve palsy destroys extension and dorsal abduction function.

Radial nerve

- Arises from the posterior cord of the brachial plexus (C6–8) ***(Fig. 19.35)***.
- Divides into terminal deep and superficial branches at the proximal forearm ***(Fig. 19.36)***.

(cont'd)

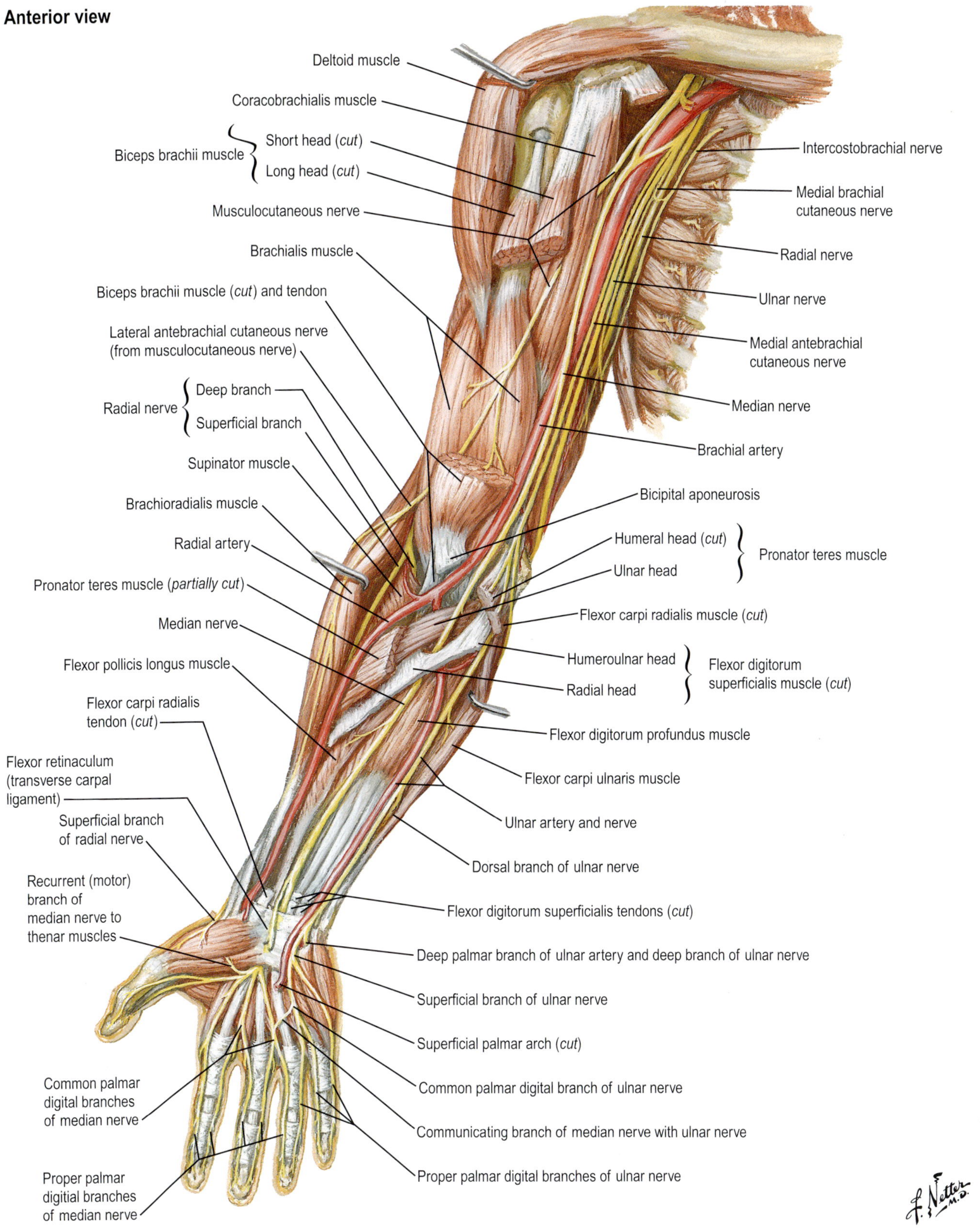

Figure 19.33 Upper arm vascular anatomy and surrounding structures. (Reprinted with permission from www.netterimages.com. © Elsevier Inc. All Rights Reserved.)

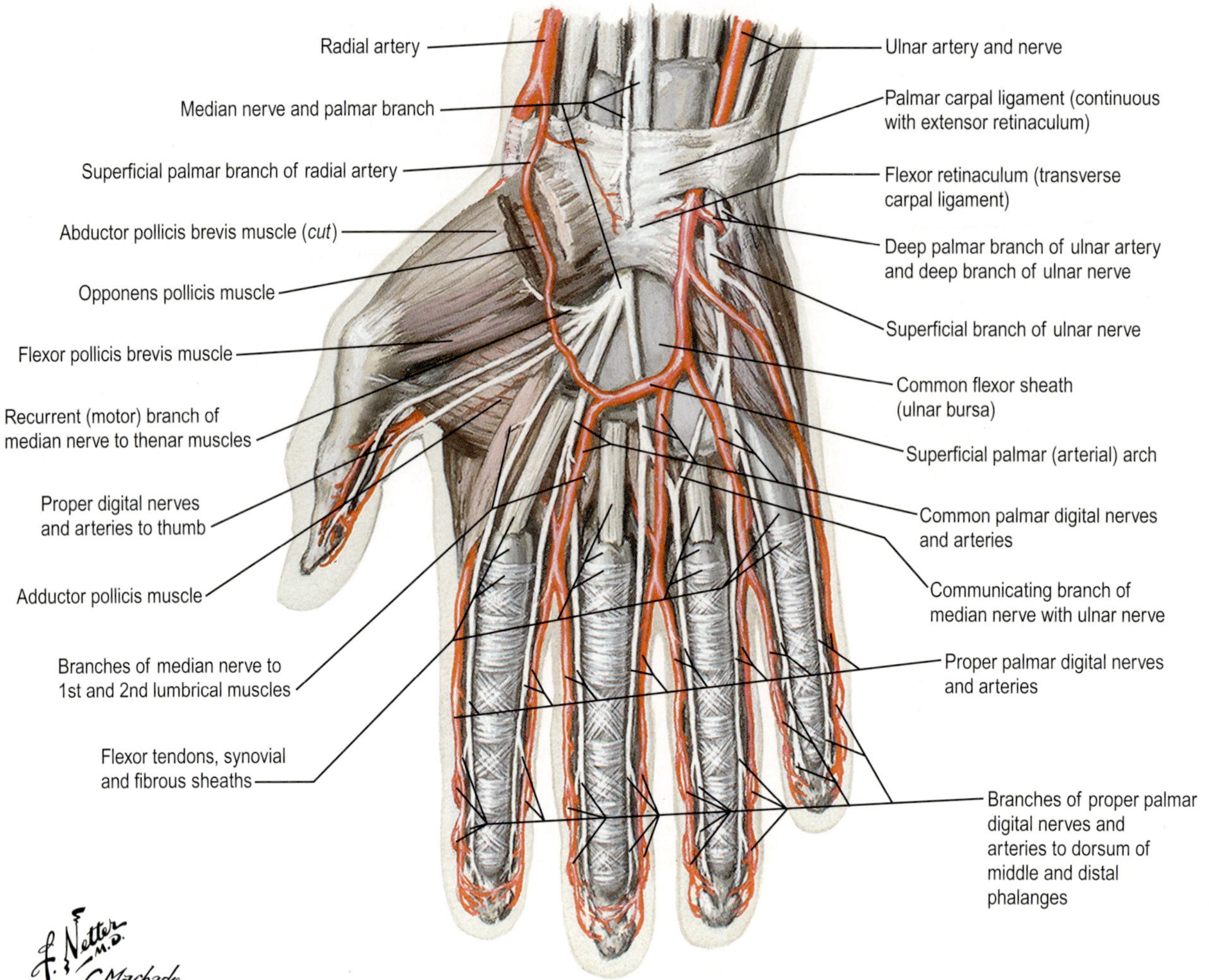

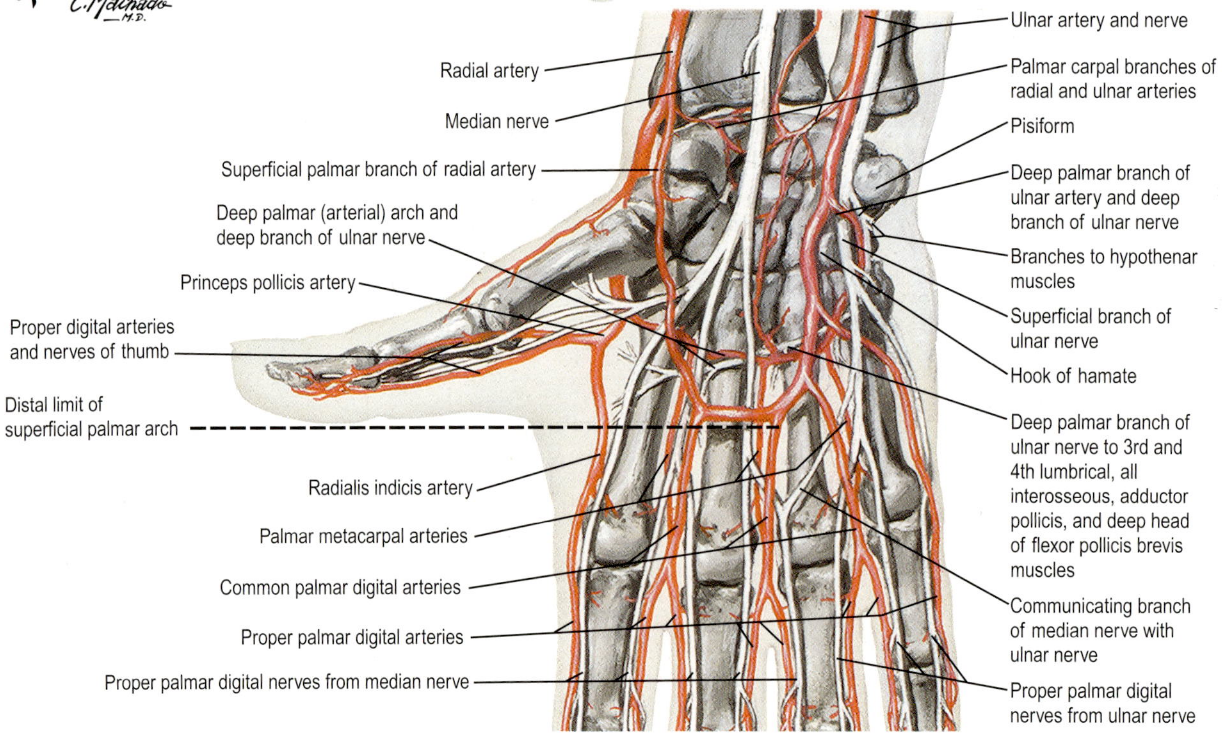

Figure 19.34 Hand vascular anatomy and surrounding structures. (Reprinted with permission from www.netterimages.com. © Elsevier Inc. All Rights Reserved.)

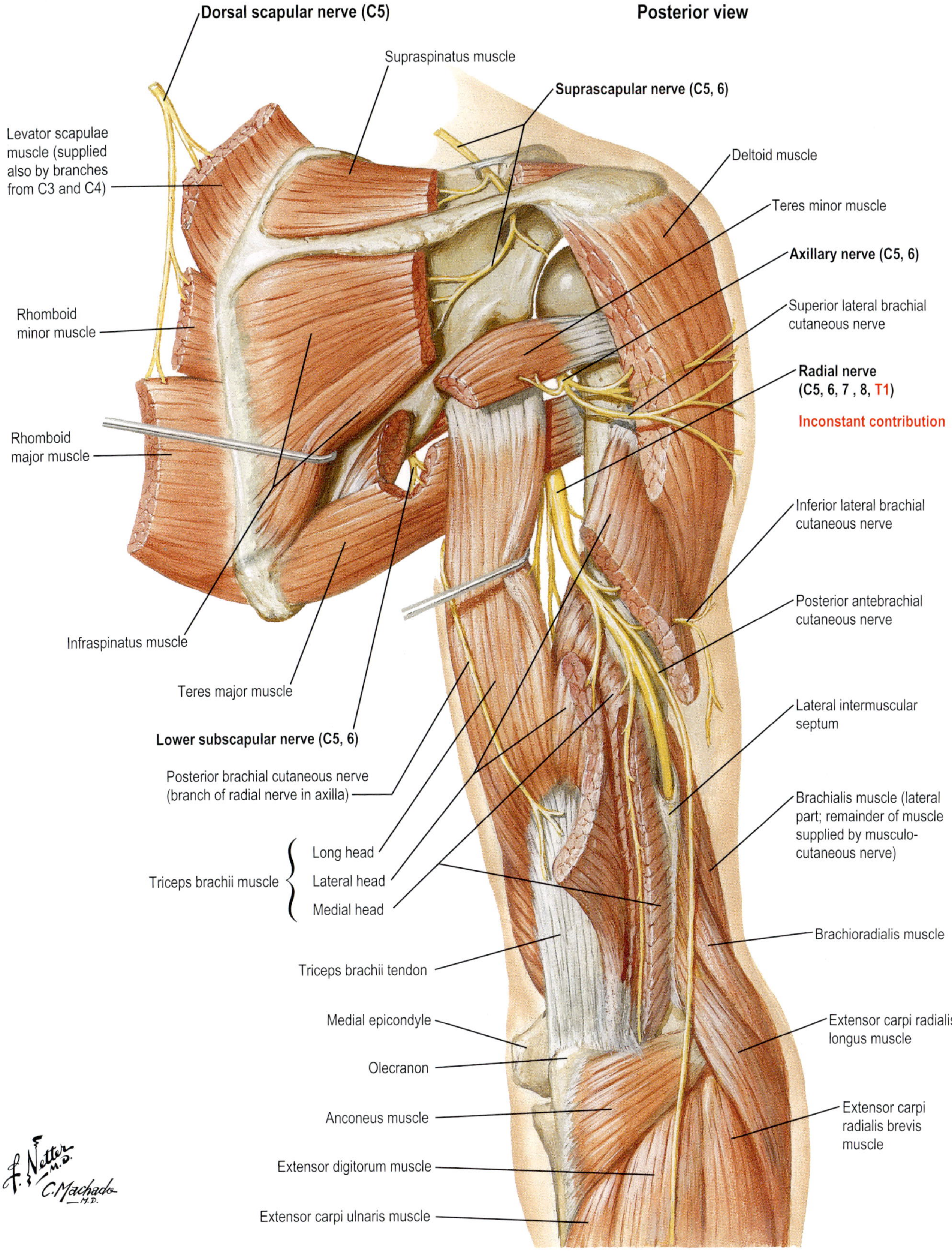

Figure 19.35 The proximal radial nerve wraps posteriorly around the humerus and then proceeds in a dorsal-radial direction distally. (Reprinted with permission from www.netterimages.com. © Elsevier Inc. All Rights Reserved.)

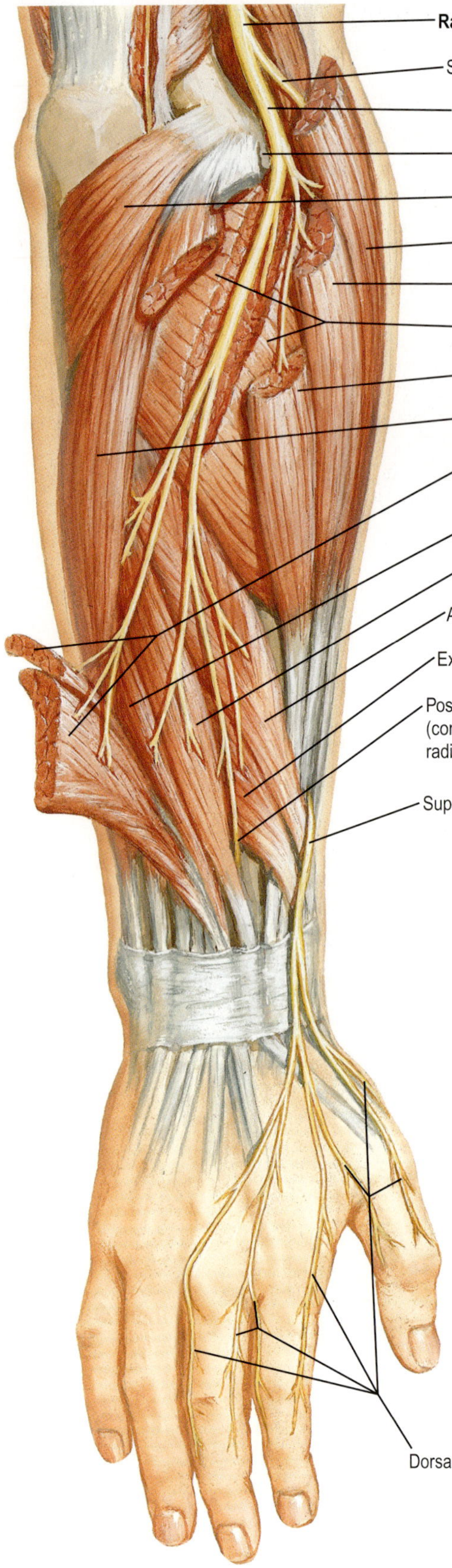

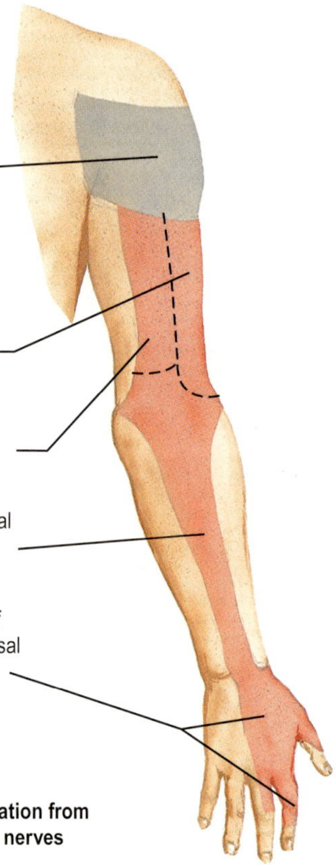

Figure 19.36 The radial nerve in the forearm innervates the extensor muscles and then lends sensibility to the radial dorsal aspect of the hand. (Reprinted with permission from www.netterimages.com. © Elsevier Inc. All Rights Reserved.)

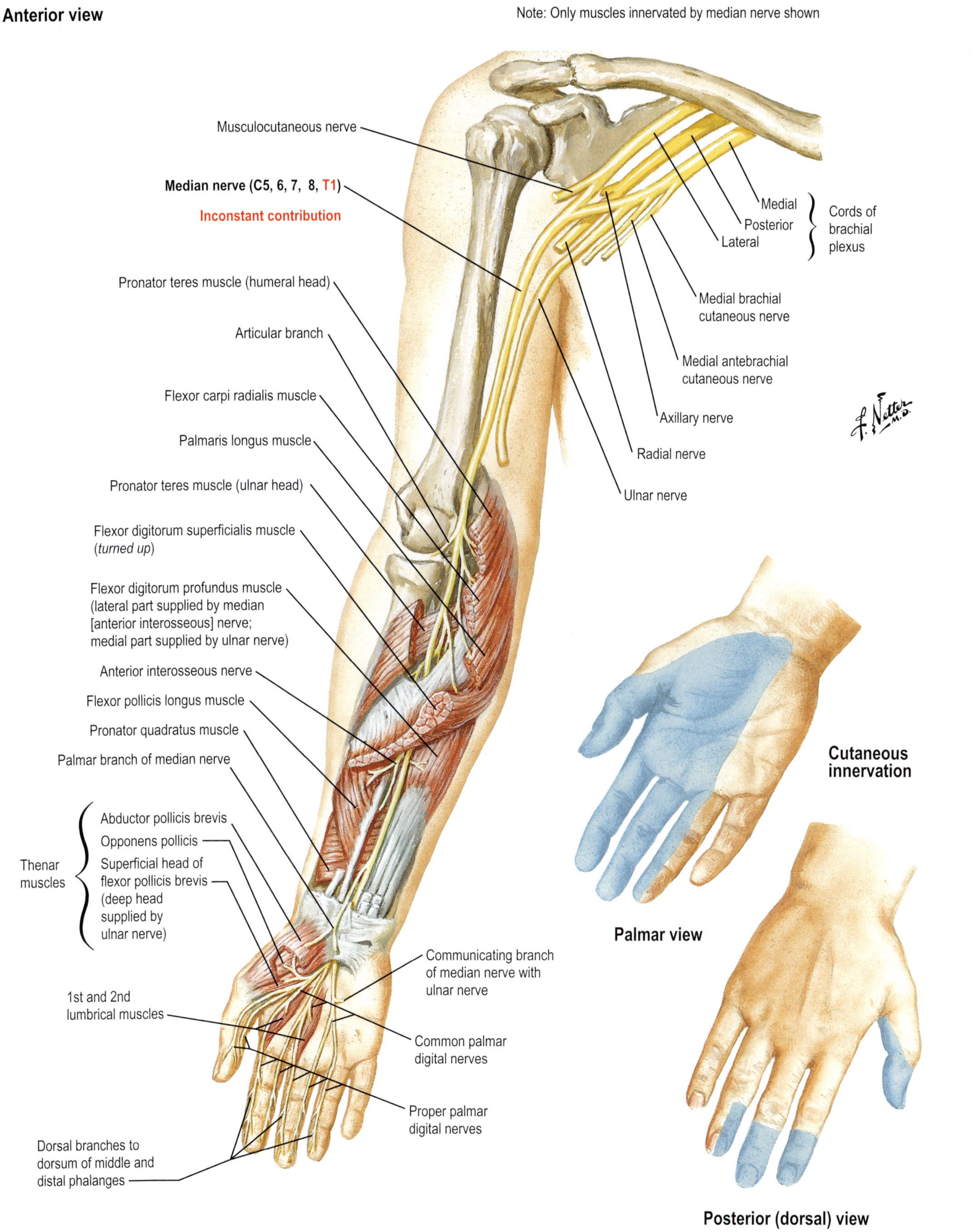

Figure 19.37 The median nerve classically lends sensibility to the palmar aspect and the distal dorsum of the thumb, index, long, and radial half of the ring fingers. Intrinsic muscles radial to the flexor pollicis longus and the two radial lumbricals receive motor innervation from the median nerve. (Reprinted with permission from www.netterimages.com. © Elsevier Inc. All Rights Reserved.)

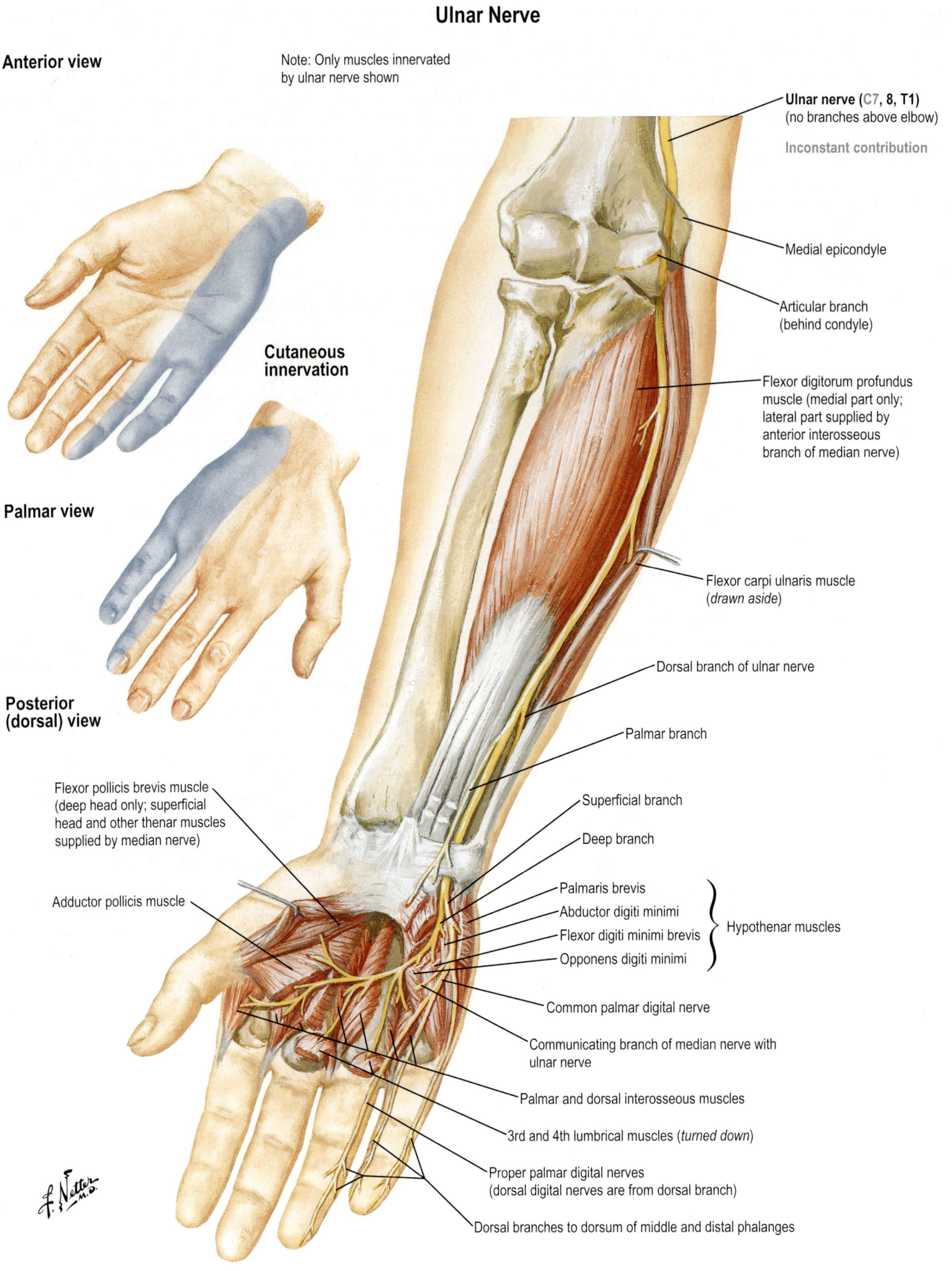

Figure 19.38 The ulnar nerve classically gives sensory innervation to the little finger and the ulnar half of the ring finger. All hypothenar muscles, all interossei, the two ulnar lumbricals, the adductor pollicis, and the ulnar half of the flexor pollicis brevis are usually innervated by the ulnar nerve. (Reprinted with permission from www.netterimages.com.)

- The deep posterior interosseous nerve supplies the supinator as well as muscles in all the extensor compartments: ECRB, EDC, EDM, ECU, EIP, EPL, EPB, and APL. It terminates to supply carpal joint sensation.
- The dorsal or superficial branch of the radial nerve courses through the forearm in relationship to the brachioradialis muscle on the radial side of the arm.
- It crosses the "anatomic snuffbox" between the EPB and the EPL in the loose subcutaneous tissue and divides into multiple branches to supply sensation to the dorsum of the hand over the radial two-thirds, the dorsum of the thumb, and the index, long, and half of the ring finger proximal to the distal interphalangeal joint.

Median nerve

- Arises from the lateral and medial cords of brachial plexus (C5–T1) ***(Fig. 19.37)***.
- The anterior interosseous branch of the median nerve innervates the FPL, FDP (index and middle digits), and the pronator quadratus muscles, and provides wrist sensation.
- Proximal to the wrist and running between the FCR and PL tendons, the palmar cutaneous branch provides lateral palmar sensation.
- As the median nerve passes through the carpal tunnel, the recurrent motor branch innervates the thenar muscles (APB, opponens pollicis, and superficial head of the FPB).
- Sensory branches supply digital nerves to the thumb, index, and middle fingers, as well as the radial aspect of the ring finger.

Ulnar nerve

- Arises as a branch of the medial cord of the brachial plexus (C8–T1) ***(Fig. 19.38)***.
- Muscular branches innervate the FCU and FDP muscles to the ring and small fingers.
- The palmar cutaneous branch of the ulnar nerve provides sensation to hypothenar eminence and medial portion of the palm.
- The dorsal branch of the ulnar nerve courses around the ulnar aspect of the forearm after branching from the main trunk at a variable site in the distal one-third of the forearm.
- It passes from deep to the FCU out through the dorsal fascia to supply sensation to the ulnar portion of the dorsum of the hand, the dorsum of the little finger, and at least part of the dorsum of the ring finger.
- The deep motor branch of the ulnar nerve passes through the pisohamate and opponens tunnel with the deep branch of the ulnar artery and gives off motor branches to the four hypothenar muscles, all the interossei, the two ulnar lumbricals, and the thumb intrinsics ulnar to the flexor pollicis longus – the adductor pollicis brevis and the deep head of the flexor pollicis brevis.

Further reading

Bell C. *The Hand – Its Mechanism and Vital Endowments as Evincing Design*. London: William Pickering; 183.

This treatise by Sir Charles Bell is a literary classic that should be read by any student of hand surgery and anatomy.

Berger RA. The gross and histologic anatomy of the scapholunate interosseous ligament. *J Hand Surg*. 1996;21:170.

In this journal article, Dr Berger clearly describes the unique anatomy of the scapholunate interosseous ligament. He discusses clinical implications of the anatomy for injury patterns and repair/reconstruction.

Bunnell S. *Surgery of the Hand*. Philadelphia: J.B. Lippincott; 1944.

This is the first edition of the first modern textbook in hand surgery, written by Sterling Bunnell, widely regarded as the father of American hand surgery.

Gelberman RH, Menon J. The vascularity of the scaphoid bone. *J Hand Surg*. 1980;5:508.

The authors perform dye injection studies to determine the vascular anatomy to the scaphoid. The relative decreased blood flow to the proximal pole has implications for poor healing of scaphoid fractures in this region.

Legueu F, Juvara E. Des aponèvroses de la paume de la main. *Bull Mem Soc Anat Paris*. 1892;67:383.

In this original manuscript, Legueu and Juvara perform anatomic dissections to outline the palmar aponeurosis of the hand. The vertical fibers that bear the authors' names are described. These vertical fibers separate the neurovascular and flexor tendon compartments within the palm.

20 Chapter

Examination of the upper extremity

This chapter was created using content from Neligan & Chang, Plastic Surgery 3rd edition, Volume 6, Hand and Upper Extremity, Chapter 2, Examination of the upper extremity, Ryosuke Kakinoki.

SYNOPSIS

- Physical examination of the upper extremity starts with a detailed and accurate patient history.
- Physical examination of the upper extremity consists of inspection, palpation, measurement of length, girth and ranges of motion, assessment of stability, and detailed assessment of the associated nerve and vascular systems.
- Thorough understanding of the anatomy, physiology and biomechanics of the upper extremity is essential to perform a physical examination correctly and to make a correct diagnosis of pathologic conditions of the upper extremity.
- Examiners must master correct physical examination techniques based on the anatomic, physiologic and biomechanical rationale.
- Even if a patient's complaint focuses on only the hand, the entire upper extremity should be examined.
- Each technique of physical examination is based on the anatomic, physiologic and biomechanical rationale of the musculoskeletal, nerve or vascular systems.
- Examiners should have their own routine protocol for examination of the upper extremity so as not to leave a part unexamined.
- Comparison of the affected upper extremity with the contralateral unaffected one helps examiners identify pathologic conditions of the affected one.
- Imaging tools such as X-rays, CT or MRI should be used to confirm the diagnosis drawn from the physical examinations or to choose the most possible diagnosis among the several differential diagnoses.

Patient history

- The patient's history can be the most important tool in developing an accurate diagnosis and should include the following components:
  - Patient demographics including age, occupation, hand dominance, hobbies, and history of previous injuries or diseases.
  - Medical history including a history of diabetes, cardiac, pulmonary and/or renal disease or whether the patient has a history of rheumatologic disease.
  - Current complaint including symptoms, and ameliorating or aggravating activities or treatments.
- In trauma cases:
  - The time of the injury and the interval between the injury and the patient's presentation.
  - The environment in which the injury occurred.
  - The mechanism of injury.
  - Any previous treatment associated with the injury.
- In non-trauma cases:
  - The time at which symptoms began and their subsequent progression.
  - The effects of the symptoms on the patient's daily life, hobby or job.
  - Are the symptoms limited to one part of the body.
  - The association between time and the intensity of symptoms.

Physical examination of the hand

Inspection

- When inspecting the upper extremities, it is essential to compare the affected extremity with the contralateral

extremity because the latter can be used as a normal reference if the injury is unilateral.
- Make note of any discoloration, gross deformity, muscular atrophy, trophic changes (e.g., increased hair growth, abnormal perspiration), swelling, and/or changes to skin creases.

Palpation

- Palpation is a powerful maneuver for identifying masses, abnormal skin temperature, areas of tenderness, crepitance, clicking or snapping and effusion.

Range of motion assessment

- Both passive and active ranges of motion should be documented and the range of motion of both the contralateral healthy limb and the affected limb should be measured and compared.
- The passive range of motion is measured by holding the patient's structures proximal and distal to the joint in question and then moving the joint from one limit of motion to the other in the absence of any muscular contraction by the patient. A limited range of passive motion is associated with joint stiffness and soft tissue contracture.
- The active range of motion of a joint is that which occurs when the patient contracts his or her muscles. The active range of motion is affected by tendon excursion, the posture of the hand and fingers, nerve function and muscular strength.

Stability assessment

- The tightness of the ligaments around a joint, morphology of the surface of a joint and musculotendinous balance around a joint are useful indices of joint stability.
- When assessing joint stability, the biomechanical and physiological properties of the ligaments should be taken into consideration and the stress forces applied should be appropriate for the ligament in question.
- The stability of ligaments is tested by holding the portions distal and proximal to the joint and gently moving the joint passively to stress the ligaments that stabilize the joint. It is useful to measure the opening angle of the affected joint under stress using X-rays and to compare the opening angle of the affected joint with that of the corresponding healthy joint of the opposite hand ***(Fig. 20.1)***.
- The stability of the wrist joint is determined by the stability of the radiocarpal, ulnocarpal, distal radioulnar and midcarpal joints. Special tests for assessing the stability of specific ligaments or imaging tools such as X-rays, CT or MRI may be helpful in making a diagnosis.

Musculotendinous assessment

- The integrity of the tendon and the strength of the muscle should be considered when conducting a musculotendinous assessment. The following elements should be evaluated and documented:
  - Posture.
  - Motion: To evaluate muscle function, each muscle should be evaluated in a posture or situation in which the cooperative muscles do not function.
  - Power: Classified according to the Medical Research Council scale, which ranges from zero to five (Table 20.1).
  - Grip strength is a good indicator of the global muscle strength of the upper extremity.

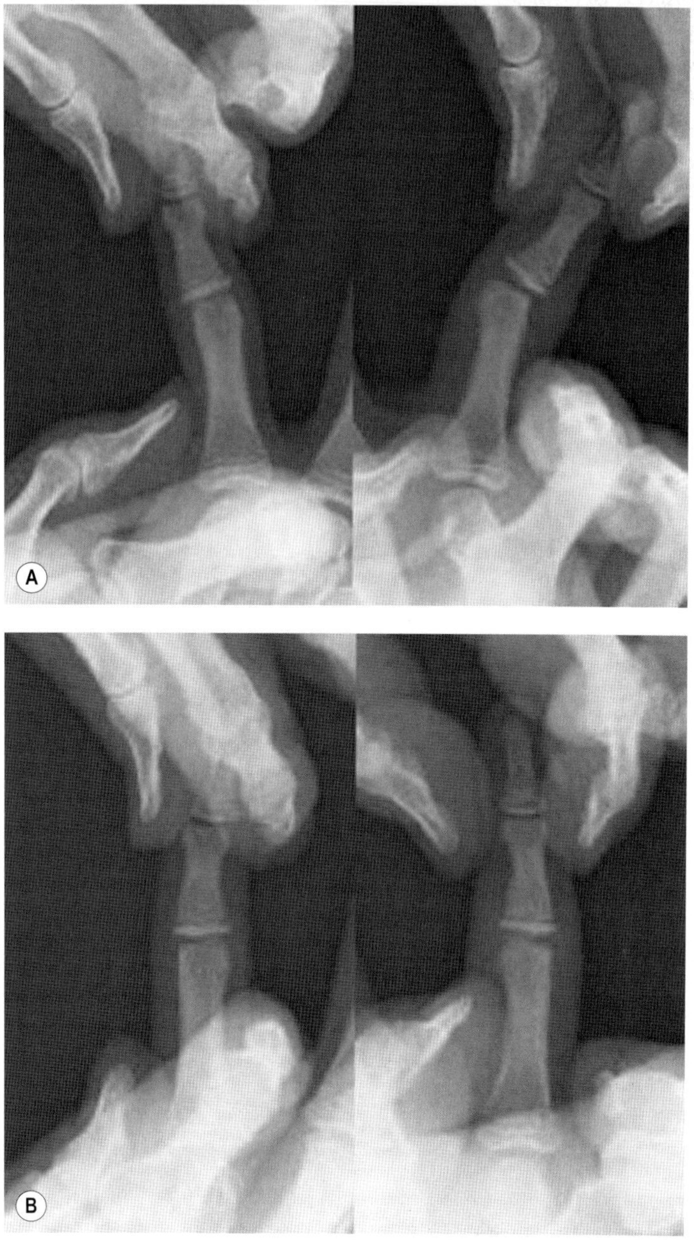

Figure 20.1 Rupture of the radial collateral ligament of the index finger PIP joint. Measure the opening angle of the affected joint under the radial and ulnar stress forces on X-ray films and compare the angle with that of the corresponding normal joint of the opposite hand. **(A)** Affected finger; **(B)** normal opposite finger.

Table 20.1 Medical Research Council scale

Grade	Physical examination findings
0	No contraction
1	Flicker or trace contraction
2	Active movement with gravity eliminated
3	Active movement against gravity
4	Active movement against gravity and resistance
5	Normal power

Reproduced with permission from Seddon HJ. *Peripheral Nerve Injuries. Medical Research Council Special Report Series.* London: 282 Her Majesty's Stationery Office; 1954

Tests for specific muscles

Extrinsic muscles

- The flexor digitorum profundus (FDP) muscle.
  - Flexor profundus test: The patient's hand is placed palm upward on a table. The examiner holds the proximal and middle phalanges of the target finger down to keep the metacarpophalangeal (MP) and proximal interphalangeal (PIP) joints in extension and asks the patient to flex the distal interphalangeal (DIP) joint. The test should be performed on each finger (Video 20.1). The FDP muscles share a common origin, thus holding the DIP joint of a finger in full extension may prevent motion of all FDPs.

Video 20.1

- The flexor digitorum superficialis (FDS) muscle.
  - Flexor sublimis test: Because each FDS tendon has its own muscle belly, its function is independent of the FDS of the adjacent fingers. The patient's hand is placed palm upward on a table. The examiner holds the distal phalanges of all fingers down except that of the finger to be tested to keep the MP, PIP and DIP joints of the other fingers in full extension. The patient is asked to flex the finger to be tested. Each finger is tested individually (Video 20.2).

Video 20.2

- The flexor pollicis longus (FPL) muscle.
  - The FPL can be tested by asking the patient to flex the interphalangeal (IP) joint of the thumb.
- The extensor pollicis brevis (EPB) and the abductor pollicis longus (APL) muscles.
  - Both tendons pass through the first dorsal component at the wrist (the APL tendon lies radial to the EPB in the compartment).
  - When the patient abducts the thumb maximally, the EPB and APL tendons are palpable as taut tendons in the radiopalmar border of the snuffbox.
- The extensor carpi radialis longus (ECRL) and brevis (ECRB) muscles.
  - When the ECRB does not function, extension of the wrist deviates radially because of the intact ECRL tendon.
  - Because the extensor digitorum communis (EDC) tendon also may function as a wrist extensor, to test the ECRL and ECRB only, ask the patient to make a fist and then extend the wrist, which eliminates EDC function.
- The extensor pollicis longus (EPL) muscle.
  - To test the EPL, place the hand palm down on a table with the thumb adducted. The patient is asked to lift only the thumb off the surface of the table, keeping the thumb adducted (Video 20.3). The taut EPL tendon is palpable in the radiodorsal aspect of the wrist.

Video 20.3

- The extensor digitorum communis (EDC) muscles.
  - EDC function is examined by asking the patient to lift the MP joints of four fingers (the index to the small finger) keeping the PIP and DIP joints flexed (Video 20.4).

Video 20.4

- The extensor indicis proprius (EIP) muscle.
  - The EIP is functional if the patient can straighten the index finger completely when the other fingers are flexed in a fist.
- The extensor digiti minimi (EDM) muscle.
  - The EDM is evaluated by asking the patient to straighten the small finger when the other fingers are flexed into a fist.
- The extensor carpi ulnaris (ECU) muscle.
  - The ECU tendon is evaluated by asking the patient to make a fist and to lift and deviate the wrist ulnarly. The tendon is palpable radial to the ulnar styloid process.

Intrinsic muscles

- The thenar muscles (APB, FPB, OP).
  - These muscles are evaluated by asking the patient to place the dorsum of the hand flat on a table and to raise the thumb until it is perpendicular to the palm. The patient is then asked to resist a downward force by the examiner on the thumb (Video 20.5).

Video 20.5

- The adductor pollicis muscle (ADP).
  - Together with the first dorsal interosseous muscle, the ADP approximates the thumb to the second metacarpal.
- The interosseous and lumbrical muscles.
  - Flex the MP joints and extend the PIP and DIP joints of the fingers.
  - Four dorsal interosseous muscles abduct the thumb and the radial three fingers.
  - Three palmar interosseous muscles adduct the fingers.
  - The second and third dorsal interosseous muscles are evaluated by asking the patient to place the hand flat on a table and then to stretch the long finger upward (i.e., to hyperextend it) and to deviate it radially and ulnarly. Patients with ulnar nerve palsy cannot do this because of loss of power in the interosseous muscles (the Pitres–Testut sign).
  - The first palmar interosseous and the second dorsal interosseous muscles are tested by the "crossed fingers" sign. The patient is asked to cross a flexed long finger over the index finger or to cross a flexed index finger over the long finger when the palm and the ring and little fingers are placed flat on a table (Video 20.6).

Video 20.6

- The hypothenar muscles.
  - The hypothenar muscles (ADM, FDM, ODM, palmaris brevis) abduct the small finger, moving it away from the other fingers.

Nerve assessment

- Both motor and sensory nerve assessment is critical.
- When the outcome of a motor assessment does not coincide with that of a sensory assessment, abnormal innervation of muscles or an unusual anastomosis between peripheral nerves should be considered.
- Martin–Gruber connection: An abnormal innervation of the median nerve to the motor branch of the ulnar nerve (e.g., cubital tunnel syndrome with this nerve connection may have a sensory palsy of the ulnar nerve without a motor palsy).
- Comprehensive sensibility evaluation includes:
  - 2 point discrimination (PD) test: Evaluates the tactile sensation of the skin and assesses density of the perception receptors in the skin (Merkel cells – slow-adapting receptors). The normal distance for the fingertips is 6 mm (Video 20.7).
  - Moving 2 PD test: Assesses the density of Meissner corpuscles (quick-adapting receptors) (Video 20.8). The normal distance for the fingertips is 3 mm for the moving 2PD test.
  - The Semmes–Weinstein test: Evaluates the pressure perception of the skin of the fingers and assesses the threshold of the perception receptors in the skin. This test is conducted by touching the fingers with filaments of various diameters (Video 20.9) (Table 20.2).
  - The vibrotactile test: Assesses the threshold of the perception receptors and is performed using two types of tuning fork (30 cycles per second (cps) and 250 cps). The vibrating forks are touched on the area examined and recognition of vibration is recorded (Table 20.3).
  - The cold-heat test: The perception of heat is evaluated by touching the skin with a test tube containing water at 40–45°C and the perception of cold is tested using a test tube containing water at 10°C. Stimuli of the cold–heat test are mainly sensed by free nerve endings of the skin.

Video 20.7

Video 20.8

Video 20.9

Table 20.2 Semes–Weinstein test

Evaluator size	Pressure force (g)	Color	Interpretation
1.65–2.83	0.008–0.07	Green	Normal
3.32–3.61	0.16–0.4	Blue	Normal
3.84–4.31	0.6–2	Purple	Diminished light touch sensation
4.56–4.93	4–8	Red	Diminished protective sensation
5.07–6.45	10–180	Red	Loss of protective sensation
6.65	300	Red	Deep pressure sensation only

Reproduced with permission from Bell-Krotosoki J, Tomancik E. The repeatability of testing with Semmes-Weinstein monofilaments. *J Hand Surg.* 1987;12A:155–161.

Vascular assessment

- Vascular problems are assessed according to the color, capillary refill, pressure (turgor) and temperature of the affected part.
- The Allen's test is helpful for determining if there is an intact circulatory connection between the radial and ulnar arteries in the hand. In this test, the examiner presses down on the radial and ulnar arteries at the wrist to occlude them, while the patient repeatedly makes and releases a tight fist to exsanguinate the hand. The patient then opens the hand and the examiner releases the pressure on one of the arteries at the wrist. If the released artery has an intact circulatory path in the hand, the palm and fingers should turn pink within 2-5 s. The test should then be repeated releasing the pressure on the other artery (see specific tests) (Video 20.10).
- To assess the circulatory connection between the radial and ulnar palmar digital arteries, the same maneuver is performed at the base of the fingers and thumb (digital Allen's test) (Video 20.11). If there is no circulatory connection between the palmar digital arteries, pedicled island flap harvest should be avoided.

Video 20.10

Video 20.11

Additional special provocative tests for the hand

- Intrinsic tightness test (Bunnell): Assesses the contracture of the interosseous muscles.
  - The PIP joint is more easily flexed when the MP joint is flexed than when it is extended (0 degree extended position) if tightness of the interosseous muscles is present ***(Fig. 20.2)***. The test should be performed using radial and ulnar deviation of the finger to

Table 20.3 Specific sensory testing and main receptors

Test	Perception	Main receptor	Type of adaptation	Evaluation of innervation
Static 2PD	Tactile	Merkel cell	Slowly	Density
Moving 2PD	Tactile	Meissner corpuscle	Quickly	Density
Tune fork (250 cps)	Vibration	Pacinian corpuscle	Quickly	Threshold
Tune fork (30 cps)	Vibration	Meissner corpuscle	Quickly	Threshold
S–W test	Pressure	Merkel cell	Slowly	Threshold

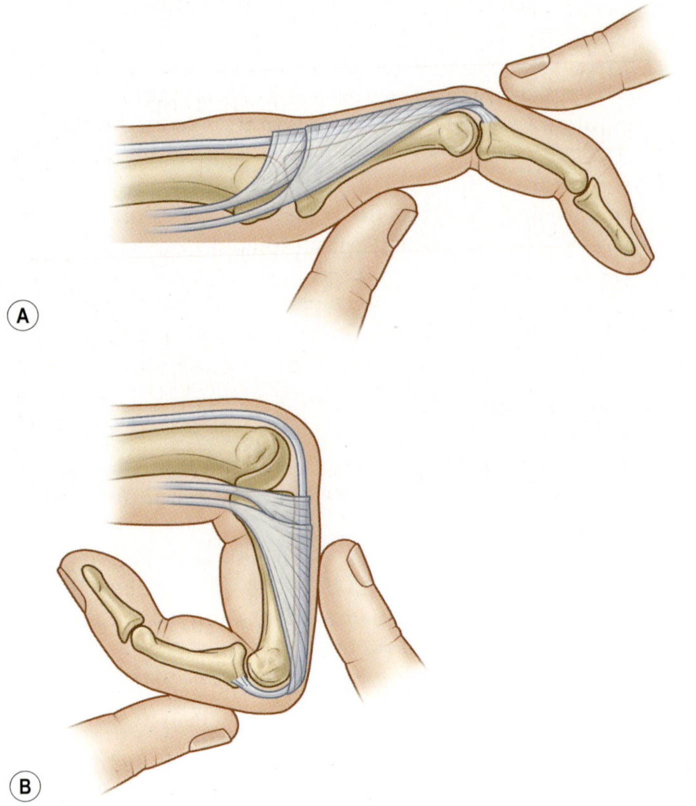

Figure 20.2 Intrinsic tightness test. If there is a tightness of the interosseous muscles, the PIP joint can be more easily flexed when the MP joint is held flexed than when the MP joint is extended. Top: the MP joint is extended. Bottom: the MP joint is flexed.

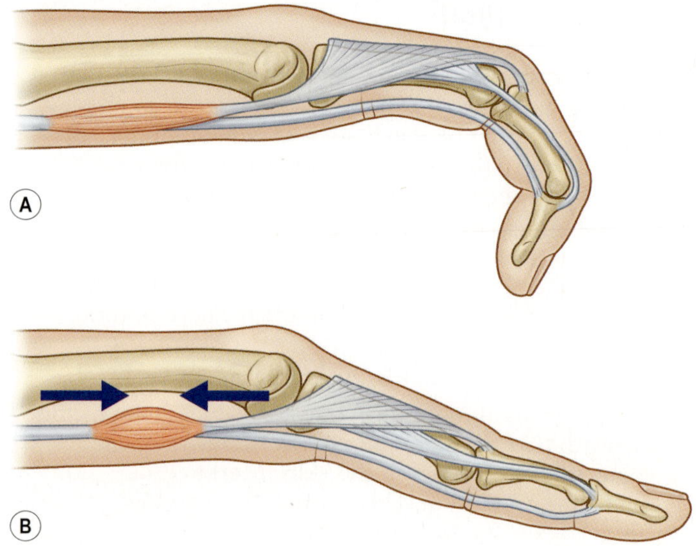

Figure 20.3 Lumbrical muscle tightness test. Because the lumbrical muscle connects the flexor digitorum profundus tendon and the radial lateral band of the extensor tendon, the PIP and DIP joint are apt to be extended when the patient intends to flex the finger (paradoxical movement).

distinguish between tightness of the radial and ulnar lateral bands.

- Extrinsic tightness test: Assesses the contracture of the extrinsic muscles.
  - In contrast to intrinsic tightness, the PIP joint is more easily flexed when the MP joint is kept extended than when it is flexed signifying that tightness of the extrinsic muscles is present.
- Lumbrical muscle tightness test.
  - Because the lumbrical connects the FDP and the radial lateral band of each extensor tendon, in lumbrical tightness the PIP and DIP joints are extended when the MP joint is flexed (paradoxical movement of the finger) ***(Fig. 20.3)***.
- Scaphoid shift test (Watson): Detects loosening or disruption of the scapholunate interosseous ligament, a scaphoid fracture or scapholunate advanced collapse (SLAC) arthritis.
  - When the wrist deviates radially, the scaphoid rotates palmarly (flexes) and the palmar prominence of the scaphoid tubercle becomes evident. However, when the wrist deviates ulnarly, the scaphoid rotates dorsally (extends) and the bony prominence is less evident.
  - The examiner holds the dorsum of the patient's hand with his or her fingers and places his or her thumb onto the radial palmar wrist to palpate the bony prominence of the scaphoid tubercle. When the examiner holds the patient's hand and deviates the wrist radially and ulnarly, he or she will feel the motion of the bony prominence under his or her thumb. When the examiner feels the palmar movement of the bony prominence of the scaphoid tubercle when moving the patient's wrist from the ulnar to the radial deviation, he or she pushes dorsally up on the tubercle against the force of the palmar movement. If scapholunate ligament insufficiency is present, the examiner will feel a clunk on the thumb over the distal tubercle. If the scaphoid tubercle does not move despite deviation of the wrist, the scaphoid may be fractured. If pain is produced by this maneuver, a scaphoid fracture or scapholunate arthritis is indicated (Video 20.12). Video 20.12
- Finger extension test: To detect the pre-dynamic rotary subluxation of the scaphoid (dorsal wrist syndrome).
  - When being asked to extend the DIP and PIP joints of all fingers fully, keeping the wrist and the MP joints of all fingers in a full-flexed position, patients with overloaded scapholunate ligaments (pre-dynamic rotary subluxation of the scaphoid) experience pain around the scapholunate joint in the dorsal wrist.
- Triquetrolunate ballottement test and the lunotriquetral shunk test: To evaluate the stability of the lunotriquetral ligament.
  - The examiner places his or her thumb dorsally over the triquetrum and the index finger palmarly over the pisiform bone to keep the triquetrum–pisiform unit between the thumb and index finger. The examiner then places his or her opposite thumb on the dorsum of the lunate and pushes it palmarly down. If there is triquetrolunate ligament incompetence, the examiner will feel palmar movement of the lunate and the patient will complain of pain in the wrist ***(Fig. 20.4)***. The lunotriquetral shuck test is similar to the

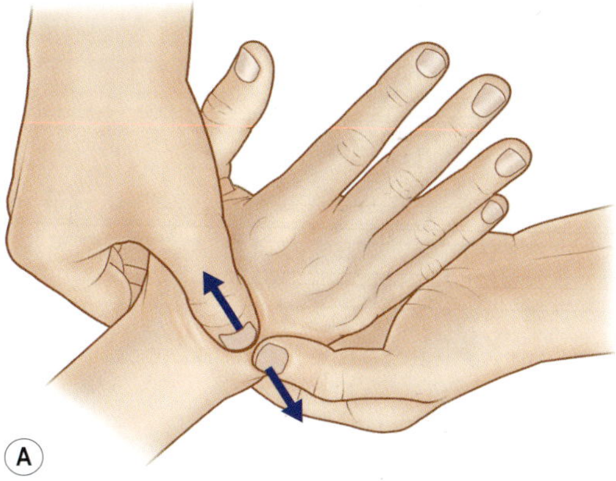

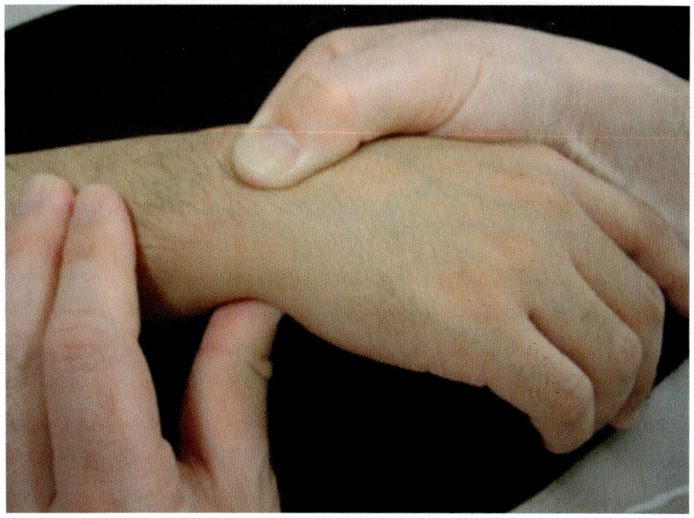

Figure 20.5 Lunotriquetrum shuck test.

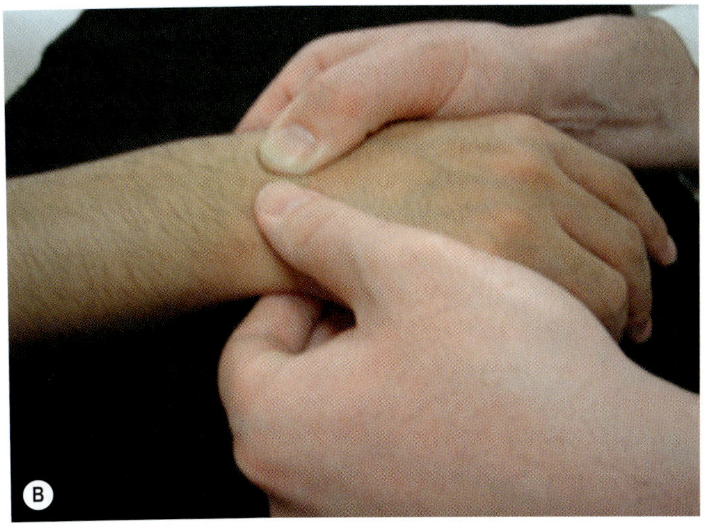

Figure 20.4 Triquetrolunate ballottement test.

triquetrolunate ballottement test. The patient is asked to place the elbow on a table with the forearm in neutral rotation. The examiner's thumb is placed over the dorsal side of the lunate just beyond the radiolunate joint. The examiner's opposite thumb pushes the palmar side of the pisiformis dorsally to load the pisotriquetral joint. In lunotriquetral ligament incompetence, the triquetrum–pisiform unit is moved dorsally and the patient will complain of pain in the lunotriquetral joint *(Fig. 20.5)*.

- Distal radioulnar joint instability test: To evaluate the integrity of the deep layer of the dorsal or palmar distal radioulnar ligaments.
  - The deep layers of the dorsal and palmar ligaments of the distal radioulnar joint (DRUJ) comprise the triangular ligament of the triangular fibrocartilage complex (TFCC) and play a primary role to stabilize the DRUJ. The deep dorsal ligament becomes taut when the forearm is supinated and the deep palmar ligament is taut when the forearm is pronated. The deep layers of the palmar and dorsal ligaments thus restrict dorsal and palmar shift of the ulna head, respectively. The examiner sits opposite the patient at a table. The patient's elbow is flexed 90° and placed on the table. The patient's forearm is fully pronated and the examiner places his or her thumb on the palmar aspect of the ulnar head and pushes dorsally upward. This maneuver should be repeated on the healthy wrist. If abnormal dorsal movement of the distal ulna is felt with the thumb, insufficiency of the deep layer of the palmar distal radioulnar ligament (palmar portion of the triangular ligament of the TFCC) is present. Next, the patient's forearm is fully supinated and the examiner places his or her thumb on the dorsum of the distal ulna and pushes palmarly down. If abnormal palmar movement of the distal ulna compared with that of the opposite wrist is felt with the thumb, insufficiency of the deep layer of the dorsal distal radioulnar ligament (dorsal portion of the triangular ligament of the TFCC) is present *(Fig. 20.6)*.
- Ulnocarpal abutment test: To evaluate TFCC injuries.
  - The examiner places a thumb on the patient's distal ulna and holds the patient's hand with the remaining four fingers. The patient's forearm is stabilized by the examiner's opposite hand. The patient's wrist is fully deviated ulnarly and the forearm is pronated and supinated. A patient with a TFCC injury may complain of ulnar wrist pain and a click or pop may be felt when the examiner's thumb is placed on the ulnocarpal joint *(Fig. 20.7)*.
- Pisiformis gliding test: To evaluate arthritis in the pisotriquetral joint.
  - The examiner palpates the pisiform and pushes it down against the triquetrum and applies shear force between the two bones. If there is arthritis in the pisotriquetral joint, the patient will feel pain in the joint during this procedure *(Fig. 20.8)*.
- Extensor carpi ulnaris (ECU) synergy test: To detect ECU tendinitis.
  - The patient's forearm is held fully supinated. The examiner asks the patient to abduct all fingers and applies a counterforce to the index and small fingers sufficient to prevent abduction of the index and small fingers. A patient with ECU tendinitis will experience pain in the sixth extensor compartment *(Fig. 20.9)*.

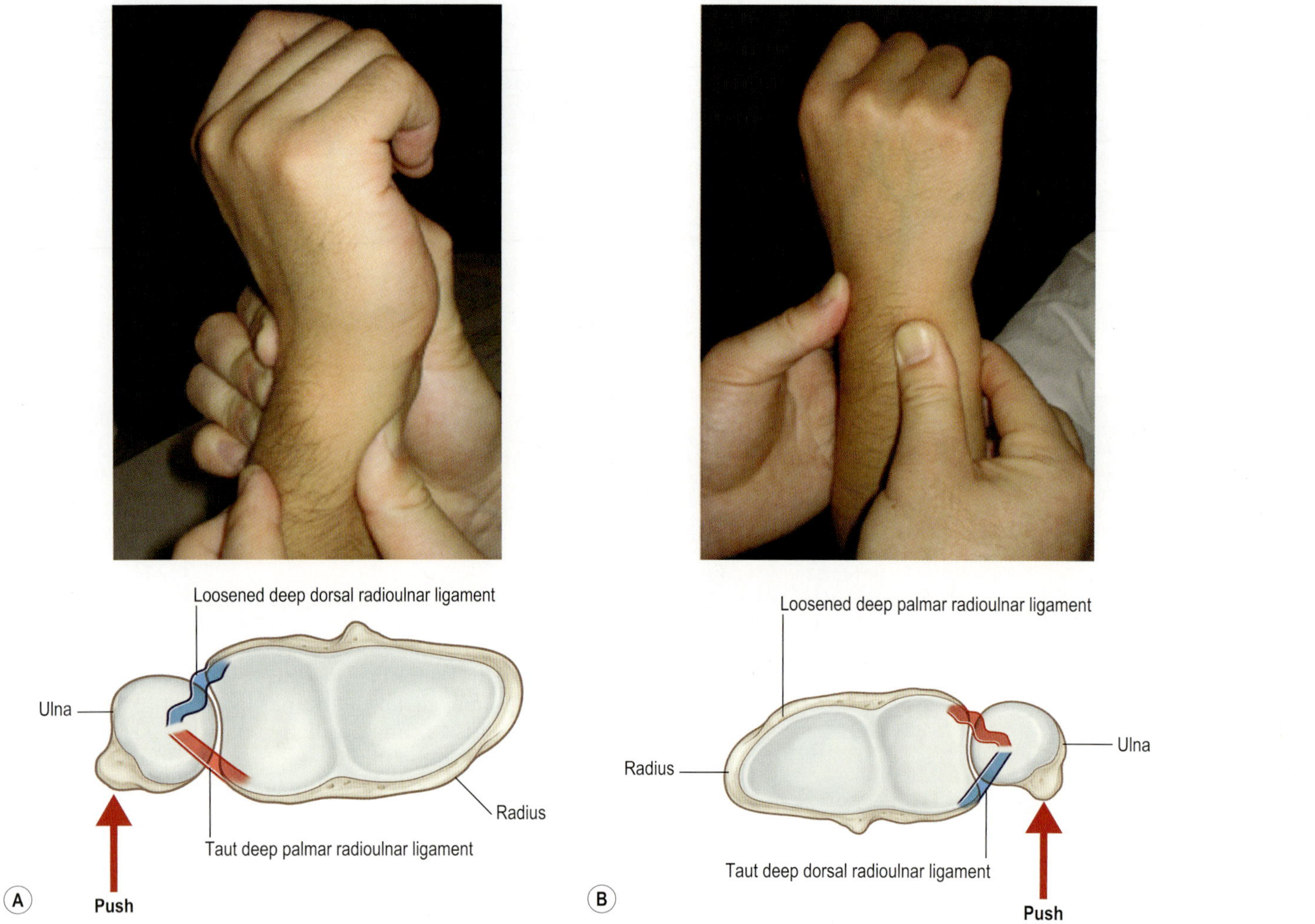

Figure 20.6 Distal radioulnar joint (DRUJ) instability test. **(A)** Examination for the palmar instability of the DRUJ. The examiner pushes the ulna head from the palmar side when the forearm is pronated to examine the deep palmar distal RU ligament. The deep palmar ligament is taut in the forearm pronated. **(B)** Examination for the dorsal instability of the DRUJ. The examiner pushes the ulna head from the dorsal side when the forearm is supinated to examine the deep dorsal distal RU ligament. The deep dorsal ligament is taut in the forearm supinated.

- Midcarpal instability test: To evaluate midcarpal stability.
  - The examiner places a thumb on the dorsal midcarpal joint and holds the patient's affected hand with the remaining four fingers. The patient's forearm is stabilized by the examiner's opposite hand. A patient with midcarpal instability will complain of pain in the midcarpal joint when the wrist is deviated ulnarly or radially. Patients with dorsal intercalary segmental instability (DISI) often complain of pain in the ulnodorsal portion of the midcarpal joint, and a click or pop may be felt when the wrist is deviated ulnarly.
- Dynamic tenodesis effect: To evaluate the continuity and mobility of the extrinsic tendons of the hand.
  - The examiner asks the patient to place an elbow flexed at 90° on a table. If the hand is relaxed, it should flex palmarly and the fingers and thumb should be extended if there are no contractures of the joints and nothing prevents the tendons from sliding in the hand and forearm. When the patient's wrist is held fully extended, the thumb and fingers flex. This phenomenon is called a positive dynamic tenodesis effect. This test is useful for distinguishing nerve palsy from tendon laceration. Because the FPL tendon is intact in patients with anterior interosseous syndrome, it would show the positive dynamic tenodesis effect. However, in patients with FPL rupture, the thumb does not flex when the wrist is held in the extended position (Video 20.13). This maneuver is also used to determine the appropriate tension of transferred or transplanted tendons. Video 20.13
- Milking test of the finger and thumb flexor tendons: To evaluate the continuity and excursion of the extrinsic flexors of the thumb and fingers. This test and the dynamic tenodesis test are useful for distinguishing nerve palsy from tendon rupture.
  - The patient is asked to place the dorsum of the forearm and the hand on a table and to relax. The examiner pushes down on the musculotendinous junctions of the flexor tendons around the palmar aspect of the middle forearm. If the tendons have normal excursion and no adhesions, the fingers and thumb flex as the forearm is pushed down (Video 20.14). Video 20.14

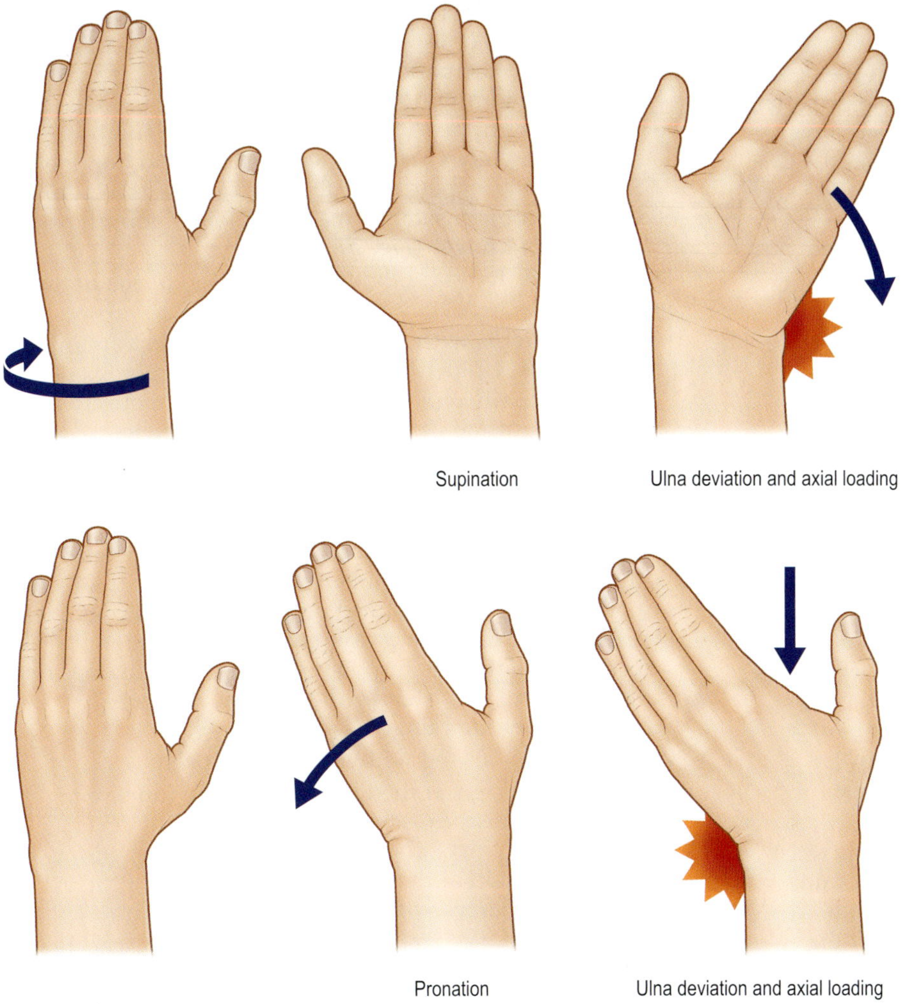

Figure 20.7 Ulnocarpal abutment test. The wrist is subjected to ulnar deviation and axial forces with the forearm fully supinated or pronated.

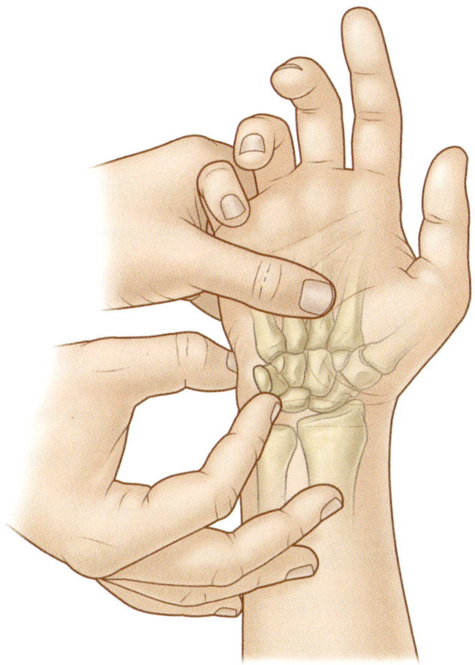

Figure 20.8 Pisiform gliding test.

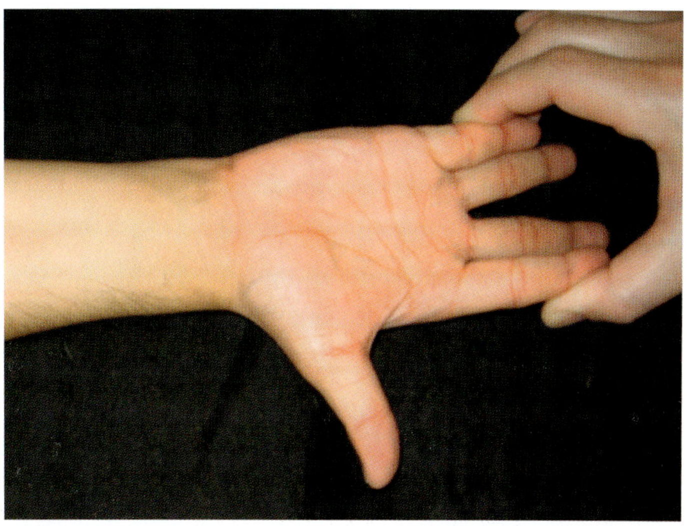

Figure 20.9 Extensor carpi ulnaris synergy test. The patient is asked to abduct the fingers with the forearm fully supinated. The examiner applies counterforce to the index and little fingers.

- Finkelstein test: To detect de Quervain's tendinitis (tendinitis in the first extensor compartment).
  - The patient places their hand on a table with the thumb up. The examiner pushes down on the proximal phalanx of the thumb. A patient with de Quervain's tendinitis will experience pain or discomfort in the first extensor compartment of the wrist.
- Eichhoff test: To detect de Quervain's tendinitis (tendinitis in the first extensor compartment).
  - The patient is asked to hold the thumb with the four flexed fingers of the affected hand. The hand is deviated ulnarly by the examiner. A patient with de Quervain's tendinitis will experience pain or discomfort in the first extensor compartment of the wrist (Video 20.15).

Video 20.15

- Tinel's sign: To detect nerve regeneration.
  - When the examiner taps on a peripheral nerve distal to a nerve injury such as a compression neuropathy or a laceration, the patient will experience tingling that radiates distally along the course of the nerve. This phenomenon is called a Tinel's sign. The most distal point of the pain indicates the site at which axon sprouting has occurred. Peripheral nerve recovery after a nerve injury can be assessed by observing the advancement of Tinel's sign along the nerve (approximately 1 mm per day of advancement).
- Phalen's test: This test is used as a provocative test specific to carpal tunnel syndrome.
  - With the elbow in neutral position, the patient's wrist is held in maximum palmar flexion for up to 2 min. This increases pressure on the carpal tunnel and provokes paresthesia in the area innervated by the median nerve in patients with carpal tunnel syndrome ***(Fig. 20.10)***. Maximum extension of the wrist also increases pressure on the carpal tunnel. This is called the reverse Phalen's test.
- Froment's test: To assess the motor function of the ulnar nerve.
  - The patient is asked to hold a piece of paper between the ulnar tip of the thumb and the radial tip of the index fingers. The examiner slowly pulls the paper away from the patient while encouraging the patient to hold onto it. Patients with normal strength of the first dorsal interosseous and adductor pollicis muscles keep the IP joint of the thumb extended. If the patient has weakness of thumb adduction caused by ulnar nerve palsy, the patient attempts to hold the paper by flexing the thumb IP joint using the flexor pollicis longus and (hyper)extends the thumb MP joint to stabilize it (*Jeanne's sign*). Such patients also flex the PIP joint and hyperextend the DIP joint of the index finger to compensate for weakness of MP joint flexion of the index finger ***(Fig. 20.11)***.
- Jeanne's sign: To assess the motor function of the ulnar nerve.
  - When patients with ulnar nerve dysfunction attempt a lateral or key pinch of the thumb, they hyperextend the thumb MP joint, which locks it to compensate for the lateral instability of the joint secondary to weakness of the thumb adductors (see Fig. 20.11).
- Wartenberg's sign: To assess the motor function of the ulnar nerve.
  - The patient is asked to keep the fingers adducted with the MP, PIP and DIP joints fully extended. If the patient has motor dysfunction of the ulnar nerve, the small finger deviates away from the ring finger because the third palmar interosseous muscle does not function and the extensor digiti minimi muscle abducts the small finger ***(Fig. 20.12)***.
- Other signs associated with ulnar nerve palsy.
  - Duchenne's sign: If the FDP muscles are functioning and the intrinsic muscles are paralyzed (low-level ulnar nerve palsy), the ring and little fingers show hyperextension of the MP joint and flexion of the PIP and DIP joints (claw finger deformity).
  - André–Thomas sign: A conscious effort to extend the fingers by tenodesing the extensor tendons with palmar flexion of the wrist only increases the claw deformity.
  - Bouvier's maneuver: When hyperextension of the MP joint of the ring and little fingers is corrected, the flexion of the PIP and DIP joints of the fingers is reduced.

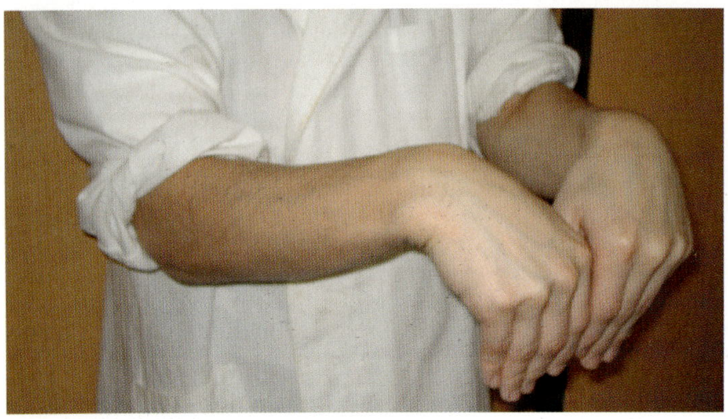

Figure 20.10 Phalen test.

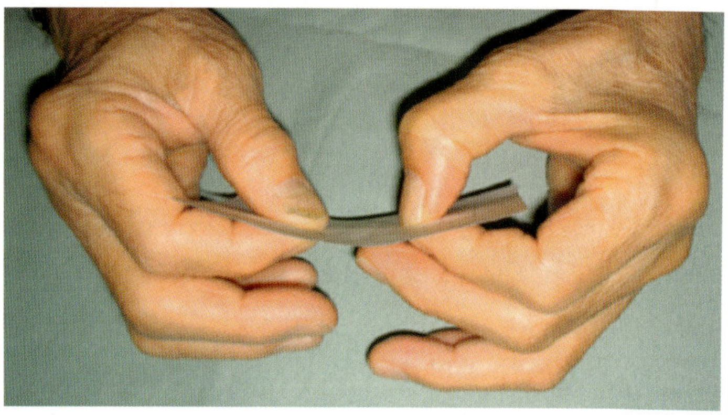

Figure 20.11 Froment's sign. A patient with left ulnar nerve palsy attempts to hold the paper by flexing the thumb IP joint using the flexor pollicis longus and hyperextending the thumb MP joint to stabilize it. He also demonstrates flexion of the PIP joint and hyperextension of the DIP joint of the index finger to compensate for weakness of MP joint flexion of the finger (Jeanne's sign).

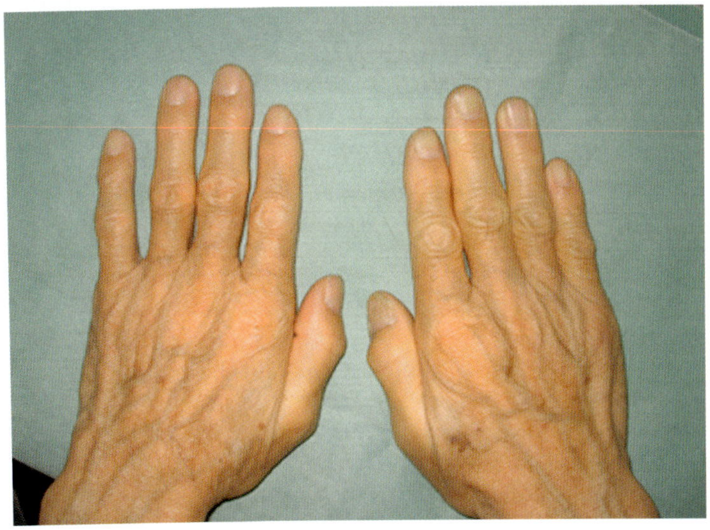

Figure 20.12 Wartenberg's sign. A patient with left ulnar nerve palsy demonstrates inability to perform adduction of the left little finger when attempting to adduct all fingers.

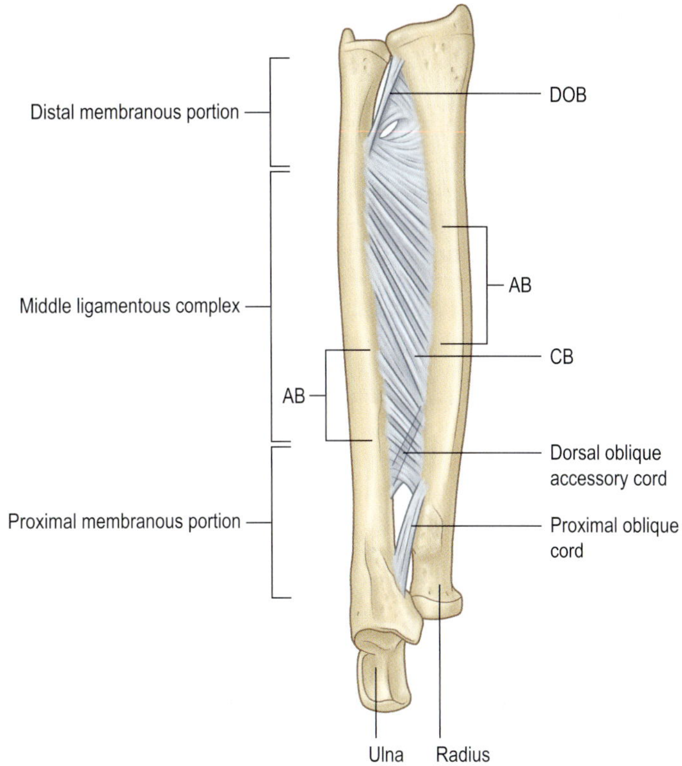

Figure 20.13 Interosseous membrane of the forearm. DOB: dorsal oblique band; CB: central band; DLAB: distal ligament of accessory band; PLAB: proximal ligament of accessory band; DOAC: distal oblique accessory cord; POC: proximal oblique cord.

- The Pitres–Testut sign: This sign reveals the function of the second and third interosseous muscles. The patient is asked to place their hand flat on a table and then to stretch the long finger upward (i.e., to hyperextend it) and to deviate it radially and ulnarly.
- The "crossed fingers" sign: The function of the first palmar interosseous and the second dorsal interosseous muscles is evaluated by this sign. The patient is asked to cross a flexed long finger over the index finger or to cross a flexed index finger over the long finger when the palm and the ring and little fingers are placed flat on a table. See the section on interosseous and lumbrical muscles (Video 20.6).

Video 20.6

- Moberg's pick-up test: To generally evaluate the motor and sensory function of the hand. This test is applied to patients with median nerve injuries or injuries of both the ulnar and median nerves.
  - Small items such as a button, a key and a paperclip are placed on a cloth mat. The patient is asked to pick up each item and put it into a small box as quickly as possible with their eyes open and again with their eyes closed. The times required to finish these tasks are measured.

Physical examination specific to the forearm

- The main functions of the forearm are to transmit force between the elbow and hand and to enable pronation and supination.
  - 80% of an axial load applied to the wrist is transmitted to the radius and 20% is transmitted to the ulna.
  - 60% of the axial force is distributed to the radiocapitellar joint and 40% to the ulnohumeral joints.
  - 20% of an axial force applied to the radius is transferred to the ulna through the interosseous membrane (IOM).
  - After resection of the radial head, 90% of an axial load applied to the forearm is transferred through the IOM.
- The interosseous membrane of the forearm (IOM).
  - Divided into three portions. Each portion contains several fibers that connect the radius and the ulna ***(Fig. 20.13)***.
  - Distal membranous portion.
  - Dorsal oblique band (DOB): This band functions as a stabilizer of the DRUJ, in particular by restricting a palmar shift of the ulna in the supination position.
  - Middle ligamentous portion.
  - Central band (CB): This is the strongest fiber of the IOM and extends from the proximal radius to the distal ulna. When the radial head is removed, the CB carries 71% of the overall mechanical stiffness of the forearm.
  - Distal ligament of accessory band (DLAB).
  - Proximal ligament of accessory band (PLAB).
- Proximal membranous portion.
  - Distal oblique accessory cord (DOAC).
  - Proximal oblique cord (POC): a stabilizer of the proximal radioulnar joint.
- Measurement of forearm rotation.
  - The patient should be seated on a chair with their elbow joints tucked in lateral to their abdomen. The

patient is asked to grasp a pen in each hand and to rotate the forearm. The angle between the pen and a line perpendicular to the floor should be measured.

- Measurement of the muscle strength of the forearm.
  - Supination: The main supinators of the forearm are the supinator muscle and the biceps brachii muscle. The extensor carpi radialis longus (ECRL) and brachioradialis (BR) muscles act as the forearm supinators when the forearm is pronated.
  - Pronation: The main pronators are the pronator teres and pronator quadratus (PQ) muscles. The flexor carpi radialis and palmaris longus muscles also act as forearm pronators. The BR muscle is a forearm pronator when the forearm is in the supinated position.
  - Evaluated with the elbow joint at 90° of flexion. Pronation strength is measured by grasping the wrist with the forearm in a neutral or supination position. To test supination strength, the forearm should be in a neutral or pronation position.

Physical examinations specific to the elbow

- Landmarks of the elbow.
  - The medial epicondyle, lateral epicondyle and the tip of the olecranon are located along a straight line (Hüter's line) when the elbow is extended and form an equilateral triangle (Hüter's triangle) when the elbow is flexed ***(Fig. 20.14)***.
- Lateral/radial:
  - The capitellum of the humerus and the radial head are easily palpable.
  - The extensor muscles originate from the lateral epicondyle.
  - The radial nerve is palpable in the interface between the BR muscle and the brachialis muscle.
- Antero-medial:
  - The cubital fossa is bordered by the BR muscle laterally and the pronator teres muscle medially.

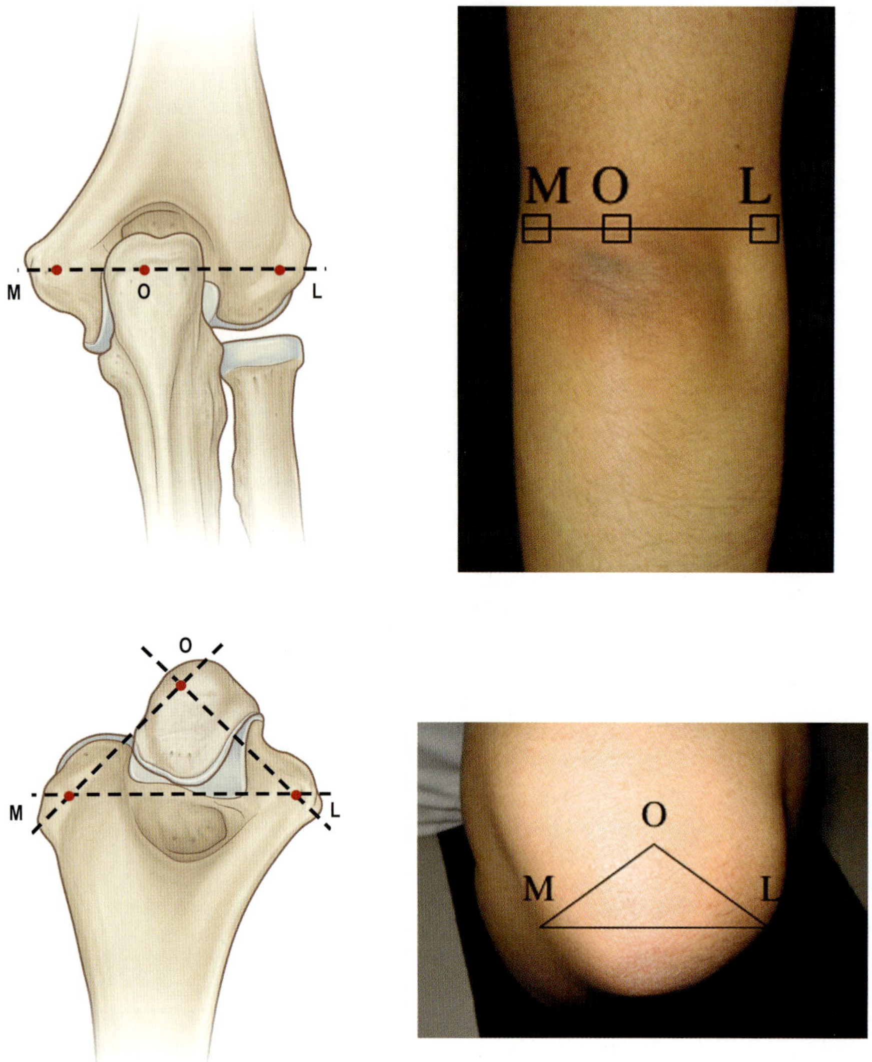

Figure 20.14 Bony landmarks of the elbow. The medial epicondyle, lateral epicondyle, and tip of the olecranon locate on a straight line when the elbow is extended and form an equilateral triangle when the elbow is flexed.

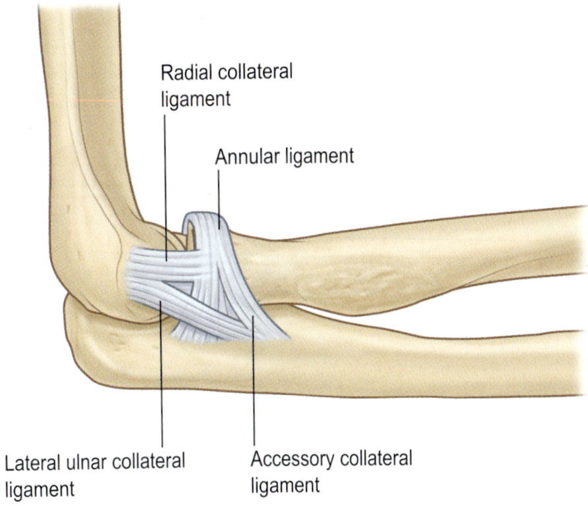

Figure 20.15 Lateral complex of the elbow.

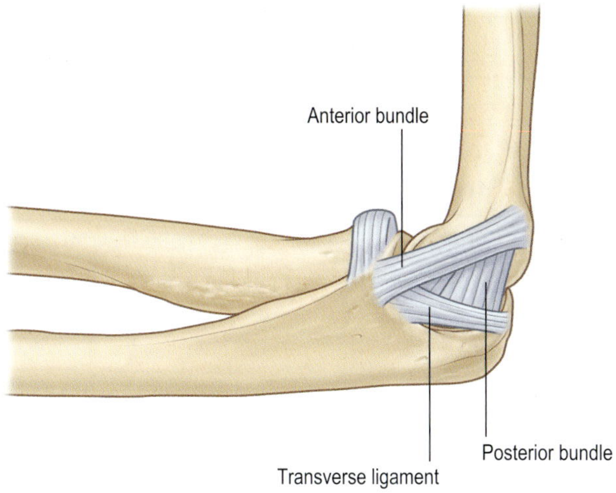

Figure 20.16 Medial complex of the elbow.

  - The musculocutaneous nerve is located deep to the brachioradialis muscle and medial to the biceps brachii tendon.
  - The brachial artery is palpable medial to the biceps brachii tendon.
  - The median nerve is located just medial to the brachial artery.
  - The ulnar nerve groove is palpable between the medial epicondyle and the ulna.
- Posterior:
  - The olecranon and olecranon fossa of the humerus are palpated.
  - The triceps brachii tendon is attached to the olecranon.
- Lateral ligament complex: consists of the following four ligaments ***(Fig. 20.15)***:
  1. Lateral ulnar collateral ligament: functions as a primary stabilizer of the joint when a varus stress is applied.
  2. Radial collateral ligament: located near the axis of the elbow joint and is uniformly taut during elbow motion.
  3. Annular ligament: originates from the anterior sigmoid notch and inserts on the posterior sigmoid notch of the ulna to connect the radial head to the ulna.
  4. Accessory collateral ligament: supports the annular ligament during varus stress.
- Medial collateral ligament complex: consists of three portions: the anterior bundle, the posterior bundle and the transverse ligament. The anterior bundle functions as the prime stabilizer of the elbow joint against valgus stress ***(Fig. 20.16)***.
- Instability of the elbow joint.
  - To assess collateral ligament integrity, the elbow should be flexed by about 15°. This position relaxes the anterior capsule and unlocks the olecranon from the fossa.
  - Varus instability of the elbow is assessed with the humerus in full internal rotation and varus stress is applied to the slightly flexed joint.
  - Valgus instability of the elbow is evaluated with the humerus in full external rotation while valgus stress is applied to the joint in slight flexion ***(Fig. 20.17)***.
- Posterolateral rotatory instability (PLRI).
  - Insufficiency (loosening, rupture or laceration) of the lateral ulnar collateral ligament causes posterolateral instability of the elbow joint. PLRI is evaluated using the pivot shift test maneuver ***(Fig. 20.18)***.

Physical examination of thoracic outlet syndrome

- Thoracic outlet syndrome (TOS): refers to compression of the neurovascular structures in the area just above the first rib and behind the clavicle resulting in upper extremity symptoms.
- Trauma to the neck, shoulder girdle, and upper extremity, particularly the lower trunk and C8–T1 spinal nerves, is thought to play an important role in developing the symptoms of thoracic outlet syndrome.
- TOS is usually classified into two groups:
- Neurogenic group:
  - Caused by compression or irritation of the brachial plexus trunks.
  - Comprises 90% of the TOS.
  - Divided into three types, depending on involvement of cervical nerve roots:
  - The upper type (C5, C6, C7 spinal nerve involvement).
  - Lower type (C8, T1 spinal nerve involvement).
  - Combined type.
  - The lower and combined types comprise 85–90% of all patients with TOS.
  - 40–50% of TOS is associated with distal compression neuropathies.
- Vascular group:
  - Subtyped into the venous type and arterial type.
  - The venous type comprises 70–80% of the vascular group of TOS.

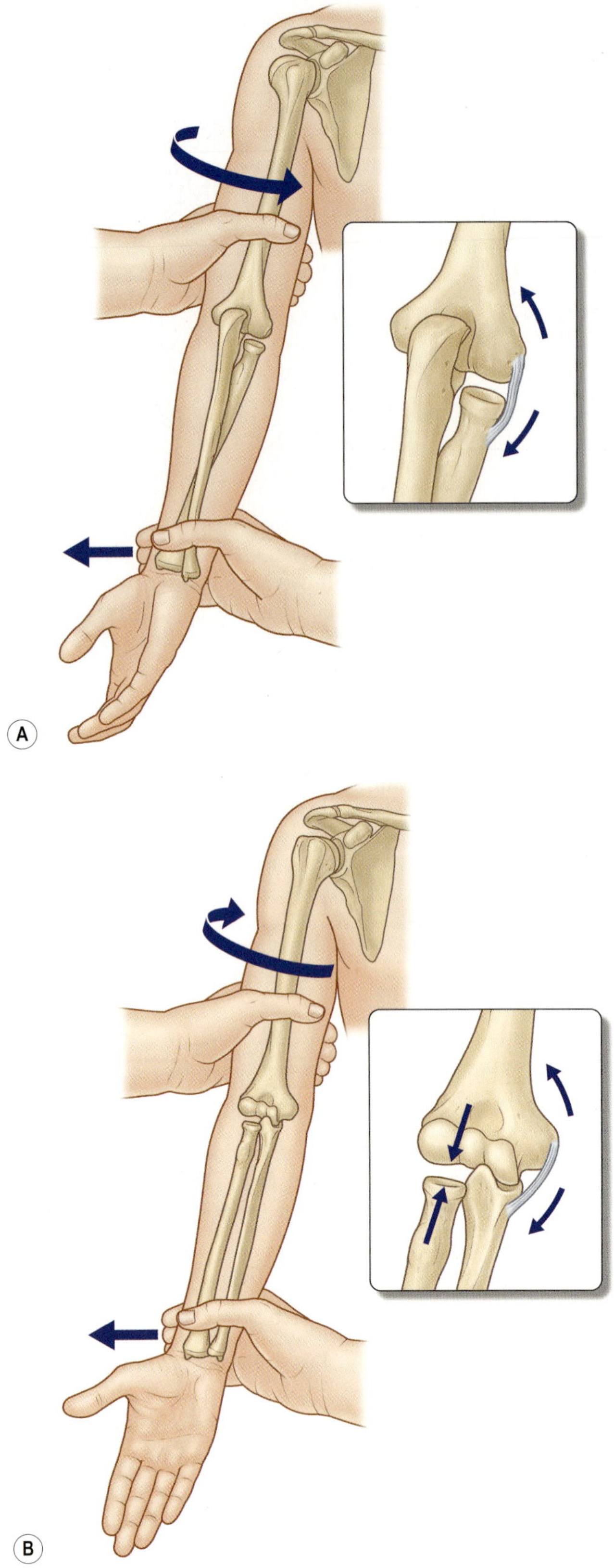

Figure 20.17 Assessment of the lateral instability of the elbow. **(A)** Varus instability of the elbow is examined with the humerus in full internal rotation. **(B)** Valgus instability is assessed with the humerus in full external rotation.

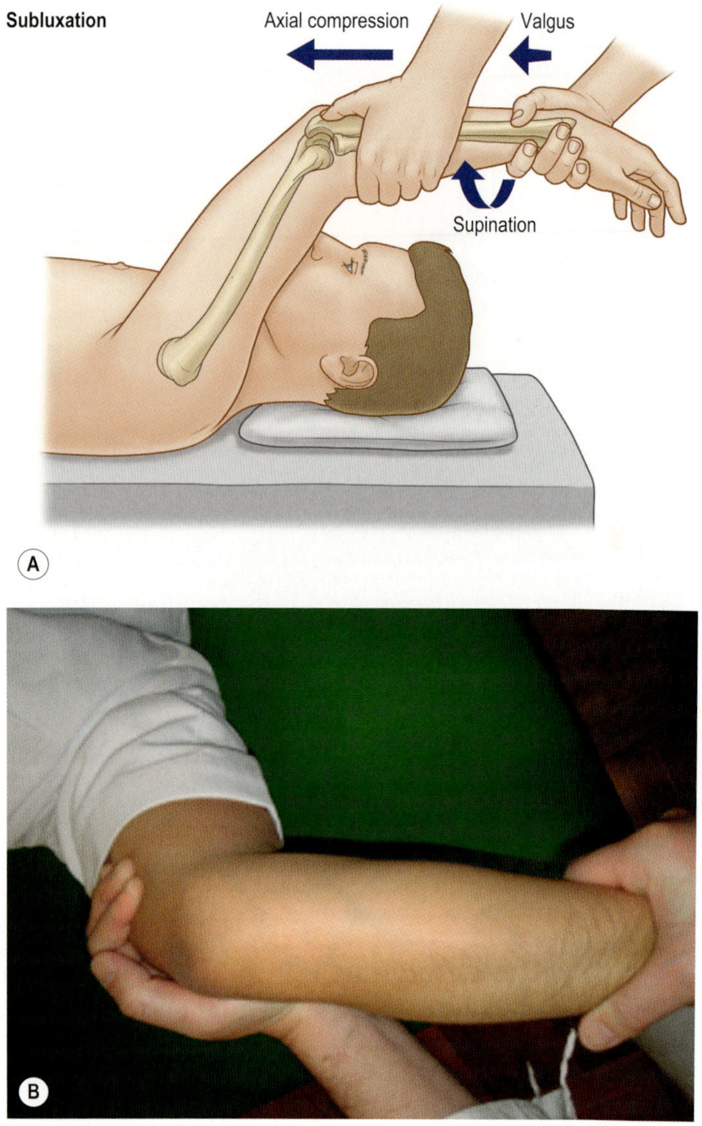

Figure 20.18 Pivotal shift test of the elbow.

- Symptoms include pain, swelling, distended vein, and discoloration of the affected upper limb.
- Compression of the subclavian vein usually occurs at the area between the anterior scalene insertion to the first rib and at the costcoracoid ligament and subclavius tendon insertion of the first rib.
- The arterial type comprises only 20–30% of the vascular group and occurs from direct pressure of the cervical rib, or an abnormal middle scalene muscle to the first rib, or anomalous band-like structure under the subclavian artery.

Important TOS anatomy

- The brachial plexus trunks and subclavian vessels are subject to compression or irritation in thee spaces at the thoracic outlet region:
  - Interscalene space (triangle).
  - The most important and most proximal site of compression.

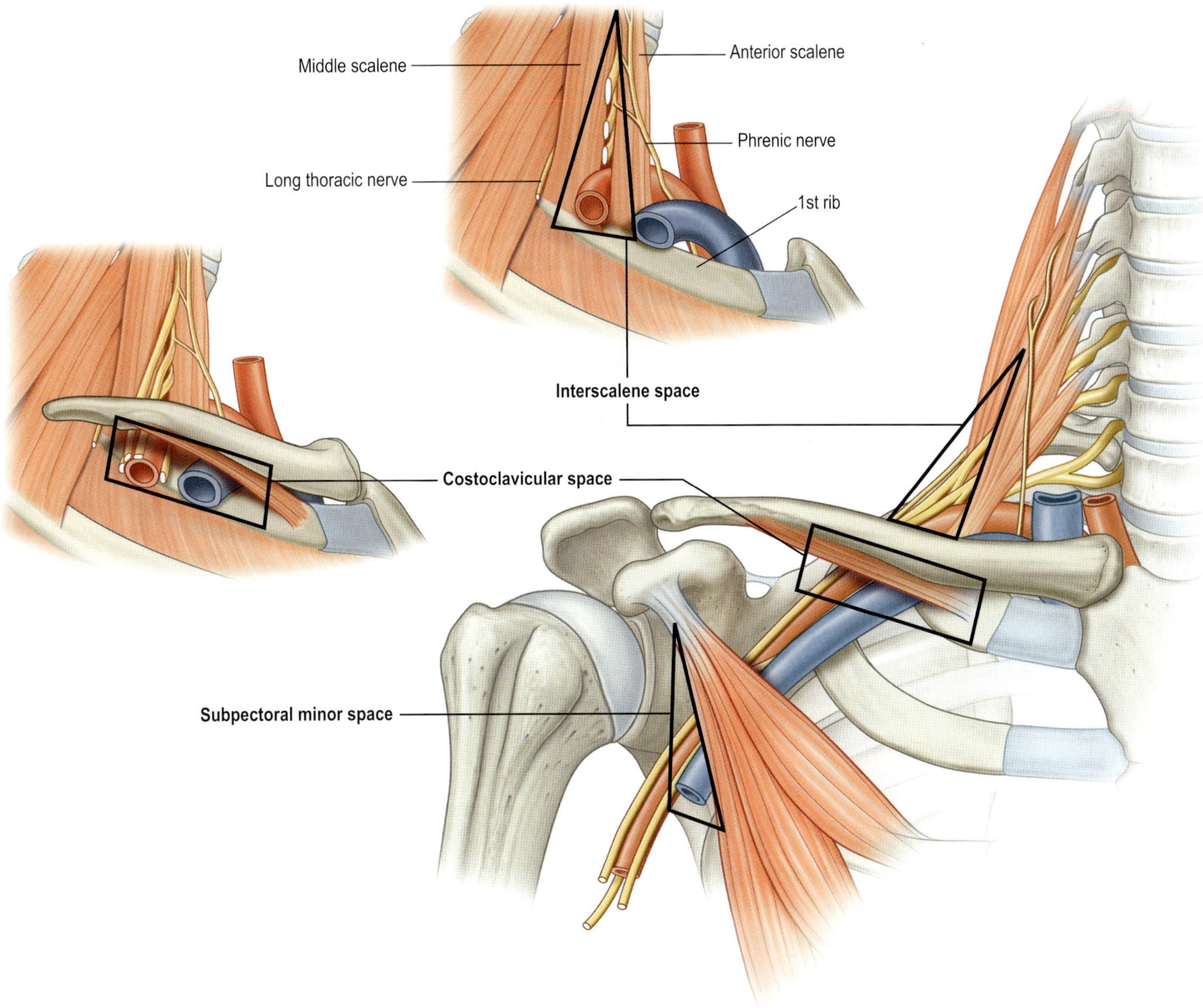

Figure 20.19 The three spaces that potentially entrap the neurovascular bundle in patients with thoracic outlet syndrome.

- Bordered by the anterior scalene muscle anteriorly, the middle scalene muscle posteriorly, and the medial surface of the first rib inferiorly. This area may be small at rest and may become even smaller with extremity motion or anomalous anatomy.
- Costoclavicular space.
- Bordered anteriorly by the middle third of the clavicle, posteromedially by the first rib, and posterolaterally by the upper border of the scapula.
- Subpectoralis minor space.
- Located beneath the coracoid process just deep to the pectoralis minor tendon ***(Fig. 20.19)***.

Provocative maneuvers

- These provocative tests should be performed on the bilateral upper limbs and the outcomes of the involved limb should be compared with those of the opposite one, because the tests can be positive in a normal person.

- Adson test: Patient is asked to inhale deeply with the chin up and tilt their neck towards the involved arm while holding their breath. If the radial artery pulsation disappears or is diminished, the test is positive (Video 20.16). This test is considered sensitive to compression in the interscalenus space ***(Fig. 20.20)***. Video 20.16
- The neck tilting test: Patient is asked to inhale deeply and tilt their neck to the opposite direction of the involved arm while holding their breath. In patients with TOS, this action produces arm heaviness, numbness, and tingling in the fingers or/and arm, with some pain.
- The costclavicular compression test: Patient is asked to inhale deeply and hold their breath. The examiner depresses the patient's shoulder of the involved limb. Patients with TOS complain of symptoms such as heaviness, pain, numbness or tingling in the limb, and the pulsation of the radial artery is often diminished. This maneuver calls attention to compression in the costclavicular space ***(Fig. 20.21)***.

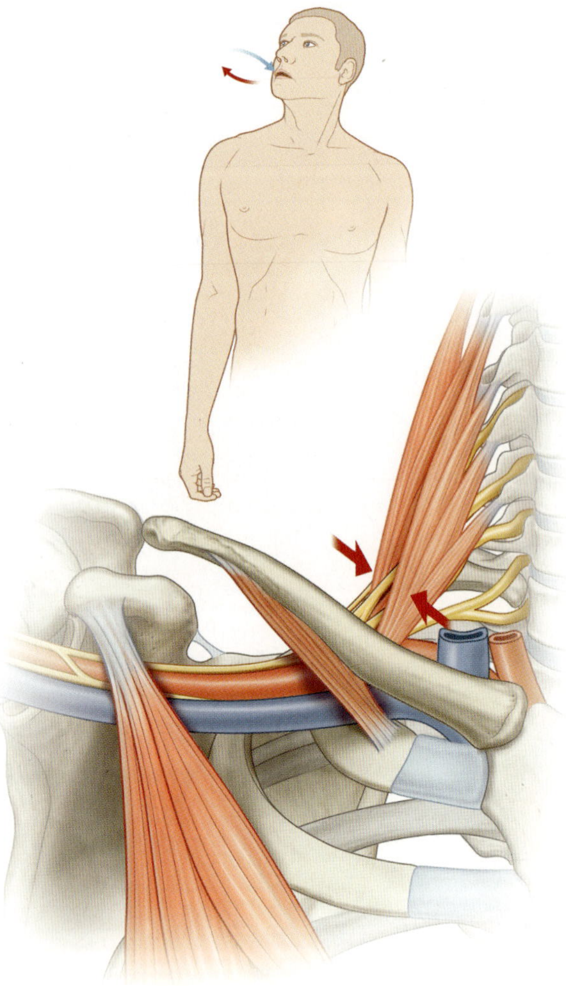

Figure 20.20 Adson test is sensitive to entrapment of the neurovascular bundle in the interscalene space (arrows).

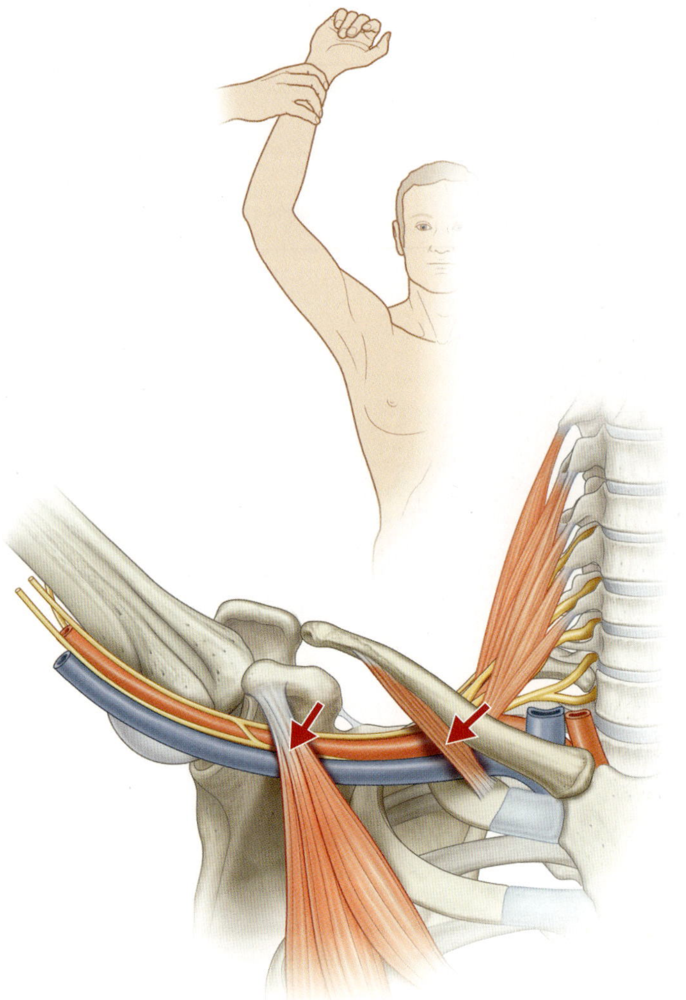

Figure 20.22 The neurovascular bundle can be potentially entrapped in the costclavicular space (red arrow) and the subpectoralis minor space by the Wright test.

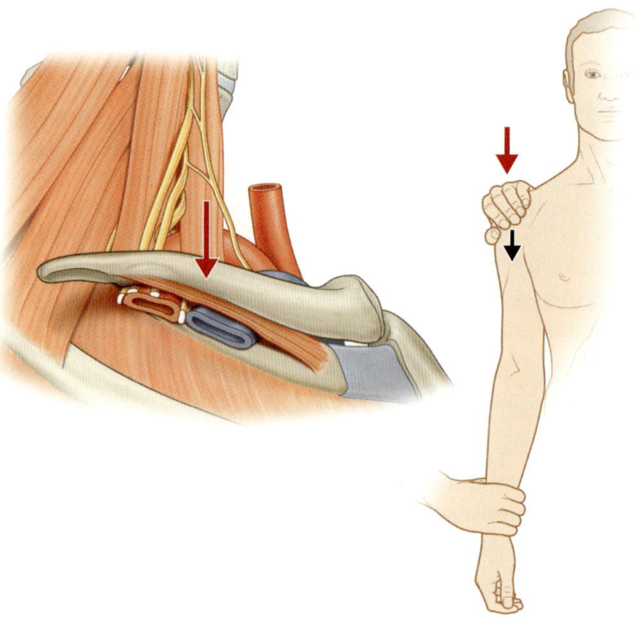

Figure 20.21 The costclavicular compression test is considered to detect the entrapment in the costclavicular space (arrow).

- Wright test: The examiner holds the patient's arm in 90° abduction with the elbow 90° flexed, and rotates the arm externally. If the pulsation is diminished and the symptoms are provoked by this maneuver, the test is positive. Entrapment of the neurovascular bundle at the subpectoralis minor space or the costclavicular space can make the test positive ***(Fig. 20.22)***.
- Roos extended arm stress test: The patient is asked to hold both arms with the shoulders in 90° abduction and 90° external rotation position and open and close the hands repetitively. If the patient develops any fatigue, pain, numbness or tingling in the hand or arm within 3 min, the test is positive (Video 20.17). Video **20.17**
- Morley's test: The patient complains of pain, numbness, tingling or uncomfortable feelings when the examiner pushes the patient's brachial plexus in the supraclavicular fossa.

Physical examination of the upper extremity in children

- Often difficult because of communication issues.
- Physical examination should include observing the child's activities when he or she is held by a parent or is playing.
- The affected limb should be examined from the tip of fingers to the hemithorax, which should be compared with the contralateral limb to confirm the anomaly.
- Primitive reflexes, including the Moro reflex, the systemic tonic neck response, the mouth lip reflex, and palmar grasp stimulation are used to assess neuromuscular function in newborns.

Video 20.1: Flexor profundus test in a normal long finger.

Video 20.2: Flexor sublimis test in a normal long finger.

Video 20.3: Test for the extensor pollicis longus (EPL) muscle in a normal hand.

Video 20.4: Test for the extensor digitorum communis (EDC) muscle in a normal hand.

Video 20.5: Test for assessing thenar muscle function.

Video 20.6: The "cross fingers" sign.

Video 20.7: Static two point discrimination test (s-2PD test).

Video 20.8: Moving 2PD test (m-2PD test) performed on the radial or ulnar aspect of the finger.

Video 20.9: Semmes–Weinstein monofilament test. The patient should sense the pressure produced by bending the filament.

Video 20.10: Allen's test in a normal patient.

Video 20.11: Digital Allen's test in a normal person.

Video 20.12: Scaphoid shift test.

Video 20.13: Dynamic tenodesis effect in a normal hand.

Video 20.14: The milking test of the fingers and thumb in a normal hand.

Video 20.15: Eichhoff test.

Video 20.16: Adson test.

Video 20.17: Roos test.

Further reading

Hotchkiss RN, An KN, Sowa DT, et al. An anatomic and mechanical study of the interosseous membrane of the forearm: pathomechanics of proximal migration of the radius. *J Hand Surg*. 1989;14A:256–261.

When the radial head was resected, 90% of the axial load applied to the wrist joint was transmitted to the ulna through the interosseous membrane. The central band of the interosseous membrane provided 71% of the overall mechanical stiffness of the forearm.

Kleinman WB. Stability of the distal radioulnar joint: Biomechanics, pathophysiology, physical diagnosis and restoration of function what we have learned in 25 years. *J Hand Surg*. 2007;32A:1086–1106.

The author describes detailed anatomy and biomechanics of the ulnar side of the wrist, including the TFCC. The deep layer of the distal radioulnar ligament plays an important role to stabilize the distal radioulnar joint. The dorsal deep layer of the ligament becomes tight in the supinated forearm and the palmar deep layer increases the strain in the pronated forearm.

O'Driscoll SW, Bell DF, Morrey BF. Posterolateral rotatory instability of the elbow. *J Bone Joint Surg*. 1991;73A:440–446.

The authors addressed grades of dislocation of the joint caused by lateral ligament insufficiency (from instability of the joint to complete dislocation) and described a maneuver of the pivot shift test that was provocative of the elbow dislocation due to the lateral ligament instability.

Ranade AV, Rai R, Prabhu LV, et al. Incidence of extensor digitorum brevis manus muscle. *Hand (NY)*. 2008;3:320–323.

Small vestigial extensor tendons are sometimes found in the long and ring fingers besides the extensor digitorum communis tendons, which are called the extensor digitorum brevis manus. This muscle is often found as a soft tissue mass and sometimes causes pain in the dorsum of the hand.

Watson HK, Ryu J, Akelman E. Limited triscaphoid intercarpal arthrodesis for rotatory subluxation of the scaphoid. *J Bone Joint Surg*. 1968;68:245–349.

Watson described his original maneuver of the so-called "scaphoid test" in this article. This maneuver has been modified by several authors and is now recognized as the "scaphoid shift test", which is a useful physiological examination to identify the instability of the scapholunate ligament complex.

21 Chapter

Flexor tendon injury and reconstruction

This chapter was created using content from Neligan & Chang, Plastic Surgery 3rd edition, Volume 6, Hand and Upper Extremity, Chapter 9, Flexor tendon injury and reconstruction, Jin Bo Tang.

SYNOPSIS

- Tendons transmit forces generated by muscles to move joints or to create action power. Flexor tendon injuries are common, but recovery of satisfactory function, particularly after injuries within the digital sheath, is sometimes difficult. Lacerated flexor tendons should be treated by primary surgical repair whenever possible.
- The current trend of end-to-end surgical tendon repairs is to use multistrand core sutures (four-strand repairs such as cruciate, double-Tsuge, Strickland, modified Savage, or six-strand repairs such as modified Savage, Tang).
- In tendon repairs in the digital sheath area, a number of surgeons advocate that the A2 pulley can be released up to two-thirds of its length, and the A4 pulley can be entirely released when necessary and tendon repair is in the proximity of the pulley, given the integrity of the other pulleys. The release may reduce the resistance to tendon motion and the chance of repair ruptures. This technique is somewhat controversial.
- Postoperatively, early tendon mobilization should always be employed, except in children or in some rare instances; motion protocols vary greatly among different treatment centers.
- Repair ruptures, adhesion formations, and finger joint stiffness are major complications of primary surgery.
- Combined use of multistrand core repairs, release of constricting pulley parts, and well-designed postoperative combined passive and active motion protocols – that do not overload, but sufficiently move the tendon – can help minimize adhesions, avoid repair ruptures, and restore optimal function.
- Secondary surgeries include tenolysis, free tendon grafting, and staged tendon reconstruction. Tenolysis is indicated when restricting adhesions hamper tendon gliding and soft tissues and joint conditions of the hand are favorable. Free tendon grafting is a salvage operation for failed primary repairs, delayed treatment (>1 month) of an acute cut, or lengthy tendon defects. Staged reconstruction is indicated in cases of extensive scar formation or multiple failed surgeries. Preservation or reconstruction of major annular pulleys is vital to restoring function of the digits during these secondary surgeries.
- Closed ruptures of flexor tendons usually require surgical repairs.
- The success of flexor tendon surgeries is very expertise-dependent. A thorough mastery of anatomy and meticulous surgical techniques are requirements for satisfactory restoration of function.

Brief introduction

- Tendons are composed of dense connective tissues that transmit forces generated by muscles to move the joints or to create action power. Functionally, the hand is dependent upon the integrity and ample gliding of the tendons.
- Difficulties in restoration of function of digital flexor tendons relate chiefly to the intricate anatomy of flexor tendon systems: the coexistence of superficialis and profundus tendons within a tight fibro-osseous tunnel.
- (Box 21.1)
- Whenever possible, acutely lacerated flexor tendons in the hand and forearm should be treated primarily or at the delayed primary stage.
  - Primary tendon repair is the end-to-end repair performed immediately after wound cleaning and debridement, usually within 24 h of trauma.
  - Delayed primary repair is defined as repair performed within 3 or even 4 weeks after tendon lacerations.
  - The tendon injured in critical areas (such as zone 2) should not be repaired by an inexperienced surgeon.

BOX 21.1 General tips for surgeons of flexor tendon repairs

- Repairing flexor tendons requires meticulous surgery built upon a thorough master of anatomy and biomechanics of the flexor tendon system. Surgeons should know the anatomy in detail, including the length of major pulleys, characteristic changes in the diameter of the sheath, and tendon gliding amplitude
- Primary repairs should be performed by experienced surgeons whenever possible, or if a less experienced surgeon has to be the operator, before surgery the surgeon must review the anatomy of the flexor tendon system, and understand every detail of the requirements of an optimal tendon repair
- The mastery of atraumatic techniques is essential for the operator. The outcome of the repair is very expertise-dependent: repair of tendons by an inexperienced surgeon is a frequent cause of tendon adhesions and poor function, thus should be avoided
- Conventional two-strand repairs are weak; stronger surgical repairs are preferable
- Complete closure of the tendon sheath is not a necessity. Venting of a part of sheath (<2.0 cm), including a critical portion of the pulleys, provides easy access to injured tendons, and may decrease resistance to tendon gliding after surgery; this procedure does not lead to loss of digital function, when other sheath parts are intact
- Surgeons should emphasize strengthening suture techniques and decreasing compression to the tendons, which facilitate increases in safety and expertise in hand therapy

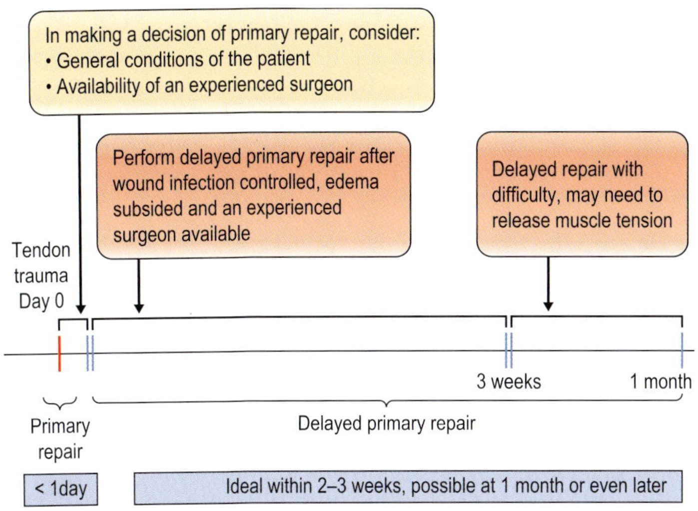

Figure 21.1 A decision-making flow chart of primary and delayed primary flexor tendon repairs.

Rather, tendon repair can be delayed until an experienced surgeon is available.

- My preferred period of deliberate delay is 4–7 days, when the risk of infection can be properly addressed and edema has reduced substantially.
- Delay of the repair beyond 3–4 weeks may cause myostatic shortening of the muscle–tendon unit; for these late cases, lengthening the tendon within the muscles in the forearm can ease the tension ***(Fig. 21.1)***.

- Rupture of the repaired flexor tendons after surgery can be re-repaired if the rupture occurs within a few weeks up to a month after surgery; secondary tendon grafts may be the only choice for ruptured cases in the presence of obvious retraction of the tendon end or extensive scarring in the intact flexor digitorum superficialis (FDS) tendon when the the flexor digitorum profundus (FDP) tendon ruptures.
- Traumatic FDP tendon avulsion from the tendon–bone junction accounts for a major portion of closed rupture cases. The tendon disrupts at its insertion to the distal phalanx.
  - The injury mechanism is hyperextension of the distal interphalangeal (DIP) joint, which subjects the FDP tendon to excessive load.
  - Athletic injuries can lead to this type of injury. When one player grabs another's jersey, a finger may be caught and pulled, resulting in disruption of flexor tendons. This injury ("jersey finger") is seen most commonly in the ring finger.
- Closed tendon ruptures at the wrist can be associated with fractures in carpal bones.
- Flexor pulleys are prone to sprains and ruptures during climbing. Rupture of the pulleys occurs in up to 20% of climbers. The A2 pulley of the ring finger is the most often injured. Closed pulley ruptures are treated conservatively or by surgical reconstruction.
- Closed tendon ruptures can be classified into the following types:
  - Class I: the FDP tendon is avulsed from the phalanx and retracts into the palm. The vincula of the FDP tendon are disrupted. There is no active flexion of the DIP joint. A tender mass is present in the palm.
  - Class II: the FDP tendon retracts to the level of the proximal interphalangeal (PIP) joint. This is the most common type. The sheath is not compromised, and muscle contracture does not develop easily.
  - Class III: a large bone fragment is attached to the FDP tendon. This bone fragment frequently prevents the tendon from retracting proximal to the A4 pulley.
  - Class IV: the FDP tendon avulses from the bony fragment and retracts beyond the middle phalanx and even into the palm.
- Early recognition of closed tendon ruptures is of paramount importance. In cases where there is late diagnosis, primary repair is difficult or even impossible. Chronic cases require free tendon grafting.
- Tendon grafting is indicated: (1) when the lacerated tendons are not treated during primary or delayed primary stage; (2) when the primary repairs have ruptured and cannot be re-repaired directly; and (3) in the cases not indicative of primary tendon repairs because of severe contamination, infection, lengthy loss of tendon substance, extensive destruction of the pulleys, or accompanying injuries.

Preoperative considerations

- Flexor tendon injuries are open in most cases, resulting from a sharp cut or a crush, but they can also present as closed injuries.
  - Open injuries due to extensive trauma are frequently associated with neurovascular deficits.

- Closed injuries often relate to forced extension during active flexion of the finger.
- Flexor tendon rupture can also occur as a result of chronic attrition in rheumatoid disease, Kienbock disease, scaphoid nonunion, or hamate or distal radius fracture.
- Careful attention to the patient's history and the mechanism of injury can alert the surgeon to the extent of the tendon trauma and associated injuries.
- The natural resting posture of the wounded digits is important for evaluation.
    - Complete lacerations of both FDP and FDS tendons are easily diagnosed when the affected fingers are seen in a relatively extended position with loss of active finger flexion at PIP and DIP joints.
    - If the patient can actively flex the DIP joint while the motion of the PIP joint is blocked, no injuries or only partial injuries to the FDP tendon can be diagnosed.
    - To assess the continuity of the FDS tendon, the adjacent fingers are held in full extension by the examiner. If the patient cannot actively flex the PIP joint, the FDS tendon is completely severed.
    - Variations in the FDS tendons in the little finger are frequent. The FDS in 30–35% of the little fingers is connected with the FDS in the ring or middle fingers. Some little fingers (10–15%) are missing an FDS tendon. These patients have limited or no PIP flexion of the little finger during testing.
    - Weakness during resisted finger flexion indicates a possible partial tendon cut.
    - To test the FPL tendon, the thumb metacarpophalangeal joint (MCP) is stabilized in a neutral position. The patient is asked to flex the IP joint. Loss of active flexion at the joint indicates complete severance of the FPL tendon.
- Nerve and vascular function should be assessed routinely, because accompanying injuries in the neurovascular bundles in one or both sides of the fingers or median and ulnar nerves at the carpal tunnel or distal forearm are common.
    - Loss of sensation in the finger pulps or loss of function of intrinsic muscles in the hand is indicative of such accompanying injuries; treatment of neurovascular injuries must be included when planning surgical strategies.
    - If fingers or hands are found to be hypovascular or avascular due to vascular lacerations, vascular anastomosis should be a surgical emergency.
    - Otherwise, after wound debridement, either the lacerated flexor tendons can be repaired (when experienced surgeons are readily available) or the skin can be closed to allow for delayed primary repairs within days by experienced surgeons.
- Radiographs should always be taken. Associated fractures are not infrequent and require treatment.
- CT or MRI should be prescribed for the cases suspicious of closed tendon ruptures. Ultrasonographic examination may also reveal rupture of the tendons.

BOX 21.2 **Primary flexor tendon repairs**

Indications

- Clean-cut tendon injuries
- Tendon cut with limited peritendinous damage, no defects in soft tissue coverage
- Regional loss of soft tissue coverage or fractures of phalangeal shafts are borderline indications
- Within several days or at most 3 or 4 weeks after tendon laceration

Contraindications

- Severe wound contamination
- Bony injuries involving joint components or extensive soft tissue loss
- Destruction of a series of annular pulleys and lengthy tendon defects
- Experienced surgeons are not available

- Primary or delayed primary end-to-end tendon repairs are mainly indicated in clean-cut tendon injuries with limited damage to peritendinous tissues.
- Serious crush injuries, severe wound contamination, loss of extensive soft tissues, or extensive destruction of pulleys and tendon structures are contraindications for primary tendon repairs.
- Fractures involving multiple bones, particularly at different levels or not yielding stable internal fixation, are contraindications for primary tendon repairs (Box 21.2).
- Flexor tendon repairs in children have a better prognosis than those in adults. As children may be less compliant with instructions to limit movement, the repaired digits are usually immobilized for 3–3.5 weeks after surgery. Either a two-strand or a four-strand repair can be used.

Anatomical/technical pearls

- There are 12 flexor tendons in the hand and forearm regions including finger and thumb flexors and wrist flexors.
    - Finger flexor tendons are: the flexor digitorum superficialis (FDS), the flexor digitorum profundus (FDP), and the flexor pollicis longus (FPL).
    - The FDS and FDP originate from muscles at about the midforearm, while the FPL tendon arises from the volar aspect of the midportion of the radial shaft and from its adjacent interosseous membrane.
    - The tendons of the FDP come from a common muscle belly while the tendons of the FDS originate from separate muscle bellies, which allows more independent finger flexion.
    - The wrist flexors are: the flexor carpi radialis (FCR) and ulnaris, and the palmaris longus.
    - The PL is absent in about 15–20% of the normal population and wrist flexion power is not affected by its absence.
- Within the carpal tunnel, nine tendons exist – four FDS, four FDP, and one FPL.
    - The relationship of these tendons within the carpal tunnel is fairly constant.

- The FDS tendons to the ring and middle fingers lie superficially, deeper are the FDS tendon to the index and small fingers, and deeper still are the FDP tendons.
- The FPL tendon is located deep and radially adjacent to the scaphoid and the trapezium.
- After emerging from the carpal tunnel, the tendons enter the palm. At about the level of the superficial palmar artery arch, the lumbrical tendons originate from the FDP tendons.

- The most intricate portions of the flexor tendons are within the fingers, where the tendons glide within a closed fibro-osseous sheath with segmental, semirigid, constrictive dense connective tissue bands present.
  - The digital sheath forms a closed synovial compartment extending from the distal palm to the middle of the distal phalange.
  - The FDS tendons lie superficial to the FDP tendons up to the bifurcation of the FDS tendon at the level of the MCP. There, in the A2 pulley area, the FDS tendons become two slips coursing laterally and then deeper to the FDP tendons.
  - Now deep to the FDP tendon, the FDS slips rejoin to form Camper's chiasm (a fibrous interweaved connection between two FDS slips), and distally insert on the proximal and middle parts of the middle phalanx as two separate slips.
  - The FDP tendon inserts into the volar aspect of the distal phalanx.
  - The FPL tendon is the only tendon inside the flexor sheath of the thumb and inserts at the distal phalanx.
- The synovial sheath is a thin layer of continuous smooth paratenon covering the inner surface of the fibrous sheath, providing a smooth surface for tendon gliding and nutrition to the tendons.
- The pulley system of the digital flexor tendon is unique; it consists of annular pulleys (condensed, rigid, and heavier annular bands) and cruciate pulleys (filmy cruciform bands) ***(Fig. 21.2)***. The annular pulleys maintain the anatomical paths of tendons close to bones and phalangeal joints, thus optimizing the mechanical efficiency of digital flexion. The more compressible cruciate pulleys allow for digital flexion to occur with condensation of the fibro-osseous sheath at the inner part of flexed fingers.
  - There are five annular pulleys (A1–A5), three cruciate pulleys (C1–C3), and one palmar aponeurosis pulley.
  - The A1, A3, and A5 pulleys originate from the palmar plates of the MCP, proximal (PIP) and distal interphalangeal (DIP) joints, and the A2 and A4 pulleys originate from the middle portion of the proximal and middle phalanges respectively.
  - The broadest annular pulley is the A2 pulley, which covers the proximal two-thirds of the proximal phalanx and encompasses the bifurcation of the FDS tendon at its middle part.
  - The A4 pulley is located at the middle third of the middle phalanx.
  - The A2 and A4 pulleys are the largest among five annular pulleys and have the most important function.

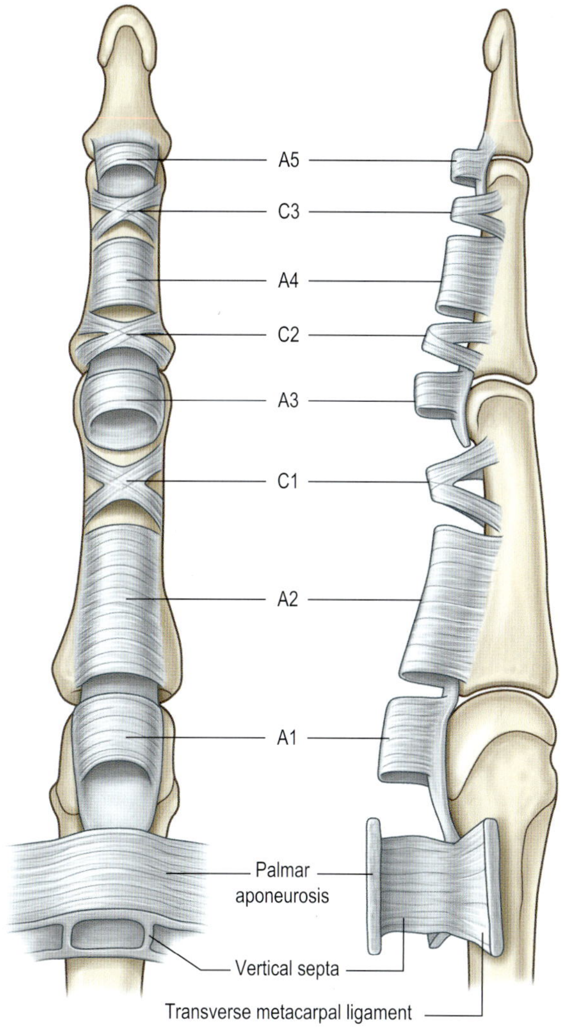

Figure 21.2 Annular pulleys (condensed, rigid, and heavier annular bands) and cruciate pulleys (filmy cruciform bands) are present in the fingers. There are five annular pulleys (A1–A5), three cruciate pulleys (C1–C3), and one palmar aponeurosis pulley.

- In the thumb, there are three pulleys (A1, oblique, and A2) with no cruciate pulleys ***(Fig. 21.3)***.
  - The A1 and oblique pulleys are functionally important.
  - The A1 pulley is located palmar to the MCP joint while the oblique pulley spans the middle and distal parts of the proximal phalanx.
  - The A2 pulley is near the site of insertion of the FPL tendon.
- The FDP tendon has two vincula: a fan-like short vinculum and a cord-like long vinculum. The short vinculum is located at the insertion of the FDP tendon ***(Fig. 21.4)***. The long vinculum connects the FDP tendon through the short vinculum of the FDS tendon to the floor of the palmar surface of the phalanges.
- The FDS tendon also has two vincula: one connecting to the proximal phalanx, and another at the insertion of the FDS tendon.
- Vincula carry blood vessels to the dorsum of these tendons, providing limited nutrition. Tendon insertion

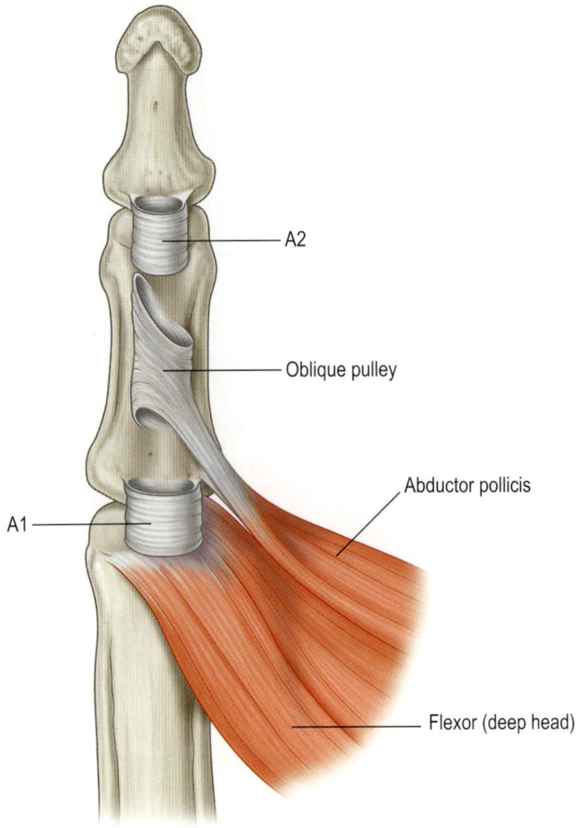

Figure 21.3 Locations of flexor pulleys of the thumb. There are three pulleys in the thumb: A1, oblique, and A2 pulley, from distal to proximal.

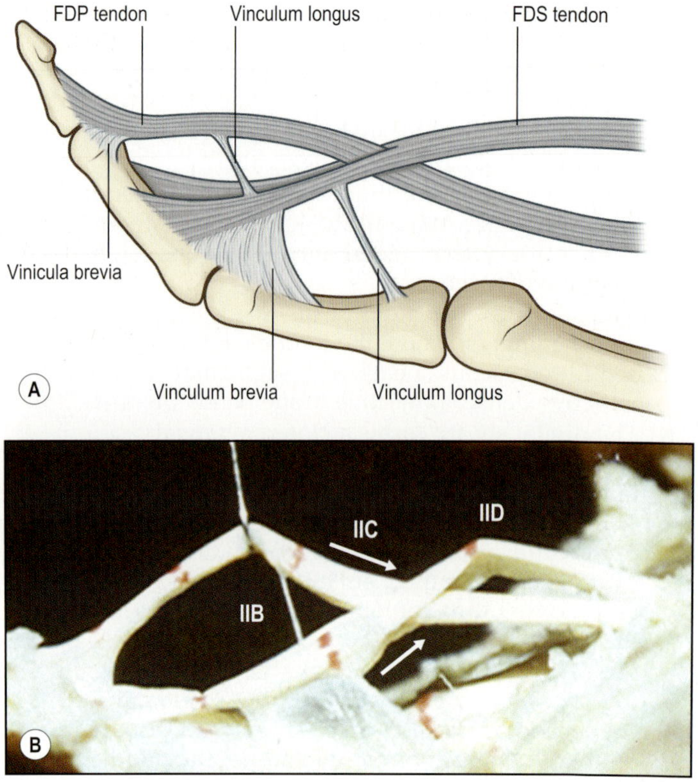

Figure 21.4 Insertions and relative positions of the flexor digitorum superficialis (FDS) and flexor digitorum profundus (FDP) tendons and vincula. Each of the FDS and FDP tendons has two vincula, one short and one long. The relations of the FDS and FDP tendons are complex in the middle part of the proximal phalanx under the A2 pulley (zone 2C).

sites to bones also carry vessels into tendons over a very short distance.

- According to anatomical features, the flexor tendons in the hand and forearm are divided into five zones, which offer the fundamental nomenclature for flexor tendon anatomy and surgical repairs ***(Figs 21.5, 21.6)***:
  - Zone 1: from the insertion of the FDS tendon to the terminal insertion of the FDP tendon.
  - Zone 2: from the proximal reflection of the digital synovial sheath to the FDS insertion.
  - Zone 3: from the distal margin of the transverse carpal ligament to the digital synovial sheath.
  - Zone 4: area covered by the transverse carpal ligament.
  - Zone 5: proximal to the transverse carpal ligament.
- In the thumb, zone 1 is distal to the interphalangeal (IP) joint, zone 2 is from the IP joint to the A1 pulley, and zone 3 is the area of the thenar eminance.

Flexor tendon healing

- Flexor tendons derive nutrition from both synovial and vascular sources. Tendons outside the synovial sheath are supplied with a segmental vascular network through paratenon; however, the tendons within the synovial sheath are mostly deprived of a vascular network with only limited dorsal regions around the vincular insertions being vascularized.

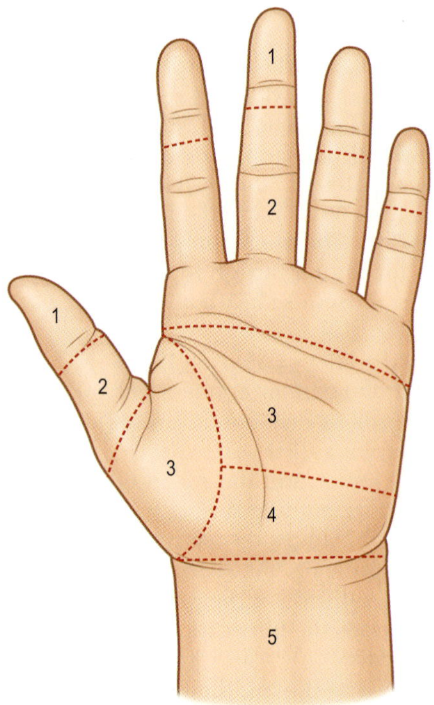

Figure 21.5 Division of the flexor tendons into five zones according to anatomical structures of the flexor tendons, presence of the synovial sheath, and the transverse carpal ligament.

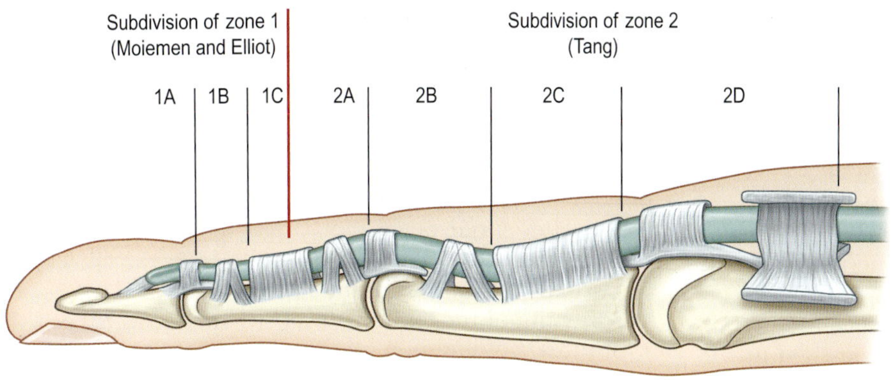

Figure 21.6 Subdivisions of zones 1 and 2 of flexor tendons in the fingers and their relations to the flexor pulleys.

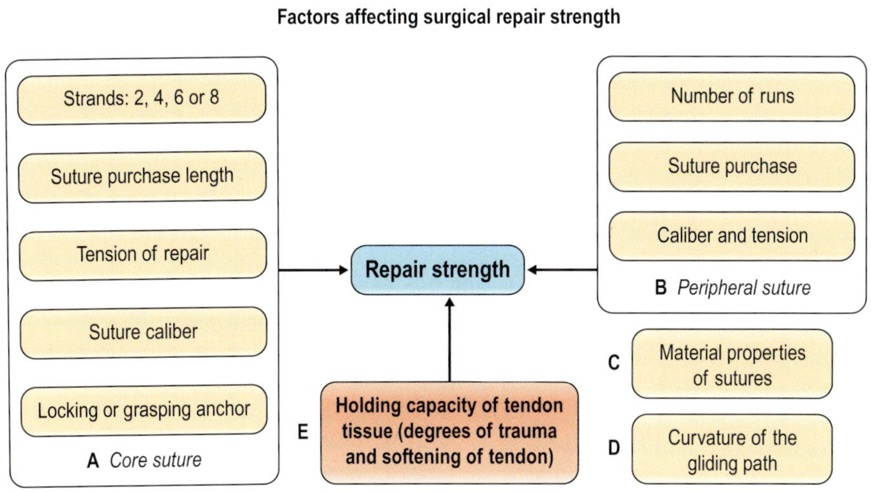

Figure 21.7 Factors affecting the surgical repair strength of the tendon.

- Intrasynovial flexor tendons can heal through two mechanisms – intrinsic and extrinsic.
  - Intrinsic healing takes place through the proliferation of tenocytes and production of extracellular matrix by intrinsic cells.
  - Intrinsic healing capacity is innately weak and healing exclusively through this mechanism does not occur *in vivo*.
  - Extrinsic healing is through the growth of tissues or cells seeding from outside the tendon.
  - Extrinsic healing becomes dominant when intrinsic healing capacity is disabled (such as in the case of severe trauma to the tendon or peritendinous tissues) or under conditions (such as postsurgical immobilization) favoring extrinsic healing.
  - Extrinsic healing may act on the tendon-healing process either by forming adhesions or seeding the extrinsic cells without adhesions to the laceration site.
  - Clinically, the lacerated tendon heals through a combination of both intrinsic and extrinsic mechanisms, whose balance depends upon the condition of the tendon and surrounding tissues.
- The following five variants (grades) of adhesions and their effects on tendon motion are seen clinically:
  1. No adhesions; no effect on motion.
  2. Filmy adhesions: formation of visible, filmy, and membranous tissue from tendon to outside tissues; no effect on motion.
  3. Loose adhesions: loose and largely movable; mildly affects motion.
  4. Moderately dense adhesions: of limited mobility; dramatically affects motion.
  5. Dense adhesions: dense, almost immovable, and invading deep into the tendon; dramatically affects motion.
- The most effective methods to prevent adhesions in clinic are meticulous surgery and early postoperative motion; the prime cause of adhesions is tendon repair by inexperienced surgeons.

Biomechanics of tendon repair and gliding

- Many factors affect the strength of a surgical repair ***(Fig. 21.7)***: (1) the number of suture strands across the repair sites – strength is roughly proportional to the number of core sutures; (2) the tension of repairs – this is most relevant to gap formation and stiffness of repairs; (3) the core suture purchase; (4) the types of tendon–suture junction – locking or grasping; (5) the diameter of suture locks in the tendons – a small-diameter lock diminishes anchor power; (6) the suture caliber (diameter); (7) the material properties of suture materials; (8) the peripheral sutures; (9) the curvature of tendon gliding paths – the repair strength decreases as tendon curvature increases; and (10) above all, the holding capacity of a tendon, affected by varying degrees of trauma and posttraumatic tissue softening, plays a vital role in repair strength.

- To achieve an optimal surgical repair, the factors outlined above must be considered and incorporated into repair design.
  - A core suture purchase of at least 0.7–1.0 cm is necessary to generate maximal holding power.
  - A locking tendon–suture junction is generally better than a grasping junction in terms of holding power ***(Fig. 21.8)***.
- Clinically, the caliber of suture used in adults is either 3-0 or 4-0; sutures of 2-0 or greater are too large and rigid in the hand.
- Annular pulleys are critical to the function of the digital flexor tendons. Lengthy loss of the sheath and pulleys causes anterior displacement – bowstringing – of the flexor tendon during finger flexion.
  - In fingers, the A2 and A4 pulleys are most critically located and functionally important.
  - Preservation or reconstruction of the two pulleys is necessary in the absence of other pulleys or sheath.
  - Nevertheless, given the presence of other pulleys and sheaths, the loss of any individual pulleys, including the A2 or A4 pulley, appears to result in few detrimental consequences.
  - Incision of the A2 pulley up to one-half or two-thirds of its length or of the entire A4 pulley has been shown to result in no tendon bowstringing and little loss of digital flexion.
- Flexor tendons in the digits glide in a fairly resistance-free synovial environment. Resistance to tendon motion is increased when the tendons are injured and repaired. The following create resistance to tendon gliding: (1) rough tendon gliding surface; (2) biological reactions of the wound, e.g., subcutaneous and tendon edema; (3) friction caused by exposure of suture materials; (4) increases in tendon bulkiness due to placement of sutures; (5) tight closure of sheath or pulleys that narrows the tendon gliding tunnel; (6) tendon-catching at pulley or sheath edges; (7) postsurgical extensor tethering and joint stiffness that burden the movement of the flexor tendon; and (8) adhesions that restrict tendon gliding.
- Biological healing strength is a central issue underlying all tendon repairs. After tendon repair, studies have demonstrated that the strength either remained consistent or actually decreased somewhat over the initial few weeks after surgery.
  - Decreases in strength, typically those in the second postsurgical week, are thought to be caused by softening of the tendon stumps, which lower the sutures' holding power.
  - Animal models have demonstrated that the strength of a healing tendon is steady during the initial 4 weeks, followed by a substantial increase (greater than threefold) in the fifth and sixth weeks; thereafter, the tendon heals strongly and is difficult to disrupt.
  - The fifth and sixth weeks after surgery appear crucial to regaining strength.

Operative techniques

- Brachial plexus block is usually sufficient; general anesthesia can also be used when associated injuries are severe.
- The tendons are exposed through zigzag skin incisions on the volar side of the fingers, e.g., Bruner's incision, or a lateral incision. When the wounds are in the palm or forearm, incision by extending the wound opening is often necessary ***(Fig. 21.9)***.

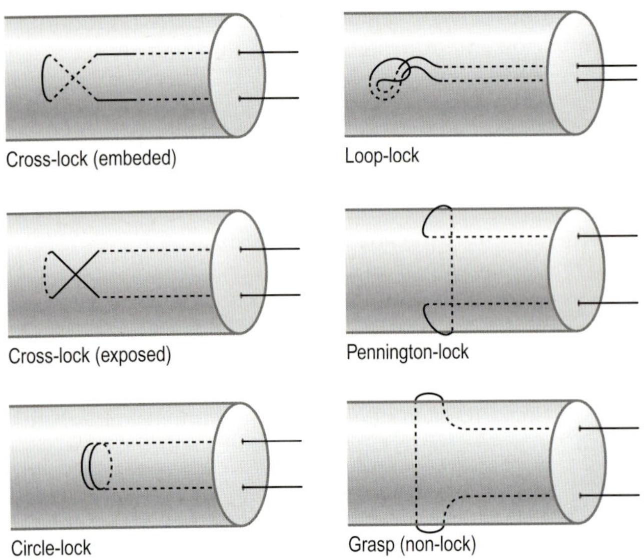

Figure 21.8 Different tendon–suture junctions in tendon repairs: locking and grasping junctions.

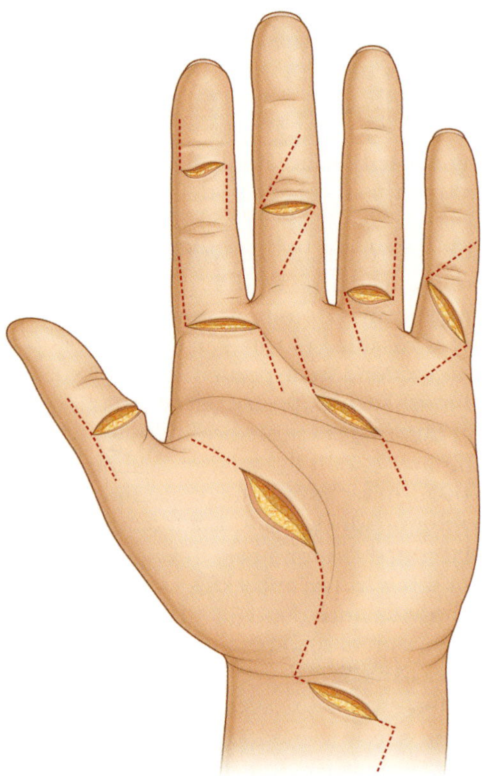

Figure 21.9 Skin incisions utilized to approach the tendons in the digits and palms.

Zone 1 injuries

- In this area, only the FDP tendon is located.
- When the tendon laceration is in the distal part of this zone, the distal stump is usually too short for direct end-to-end repair. In this instance, the proximal tendon end can be sutured with Bunnell or modified Becker suture with 3-0 polypropylene, and an osteoperiosteal flap is raised at the base of the distal phalanx *(Fig. 21.10)*. The suture is led through an oblique drill hole, brought out through the nail, and tied over a button above the nail.
- Injuries more proximal in this zone, usually create tendon stumps of sufficient length (~1 cm) for a direct surgical repair, which can be treated by methods similar to treatment in zone 2.
  - Core tendon sutures, such as the modified Kessler, cruciate, modified Becker, or double Kessler repair, can be placed to the proximal end through a window opening in the proximal sheath.

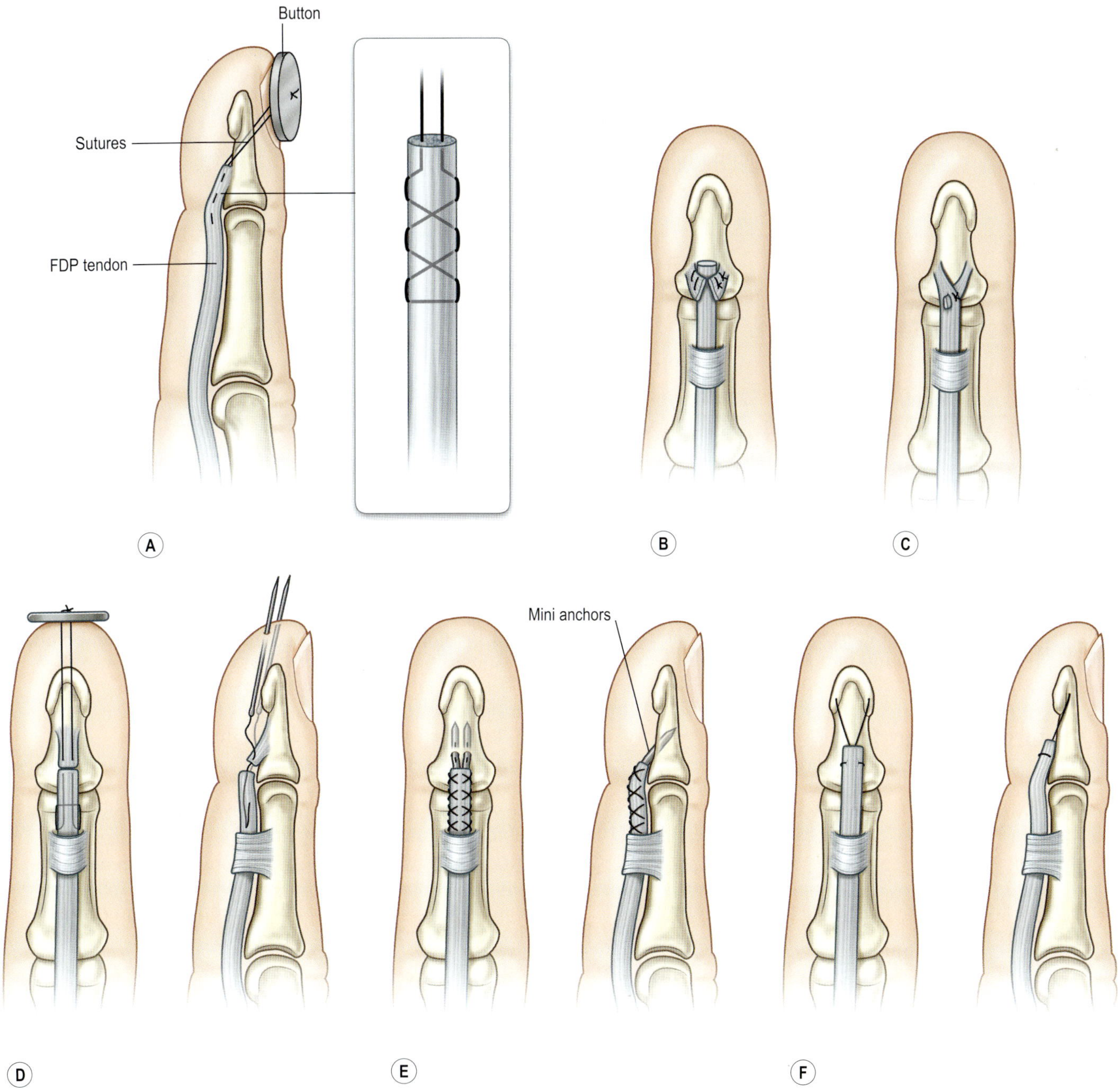

Figure 21.10 Methods of making a tendon-to-bone junction in zone 1. **(A)** A conventional method of anchoring the flexor digitorum profundus (FDP) tendon to the bone by pull-out sutures through the nail tied over a button. Alternative ways to anchor the distal tendon stump to the bone by: **(B)** directly suturing the stump to residual FDP tendon, **(C)** looping the tendon through the bone, **(D)** pull-out suture over the fingertip, **(E)** mini-anchors, and **(F)** looping the sutures through a transverse hole in the bone **(F)**.

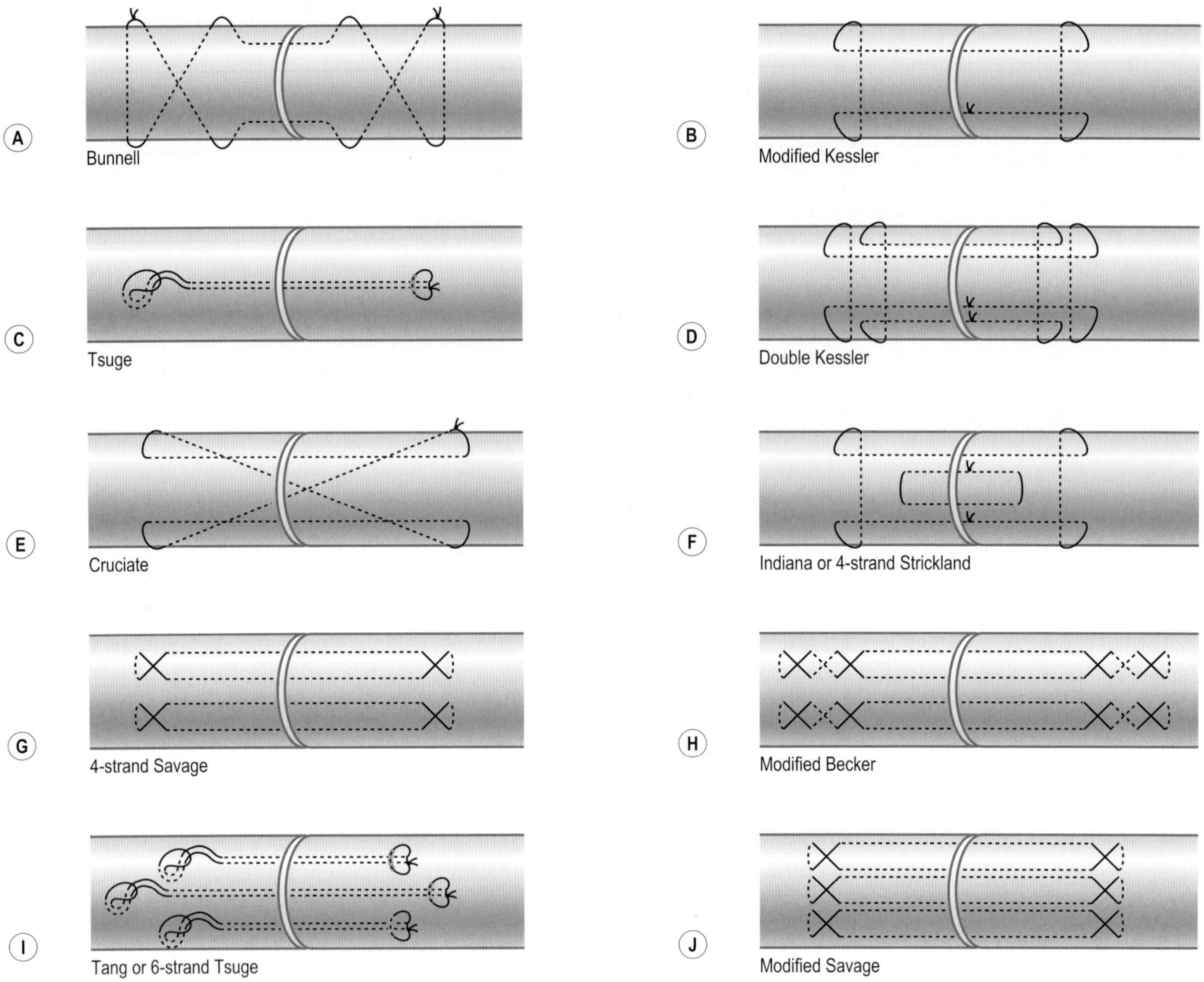

Figure 21.11 Summary of methods used to make core sutures in flexor tendon repairs.

- The proximal end is brought underneath the intact sheath between the wound and the proximal opening to approximate the distal end.

Video 21.1

Zone 2 injuries (Video 21.1)

- Tendon injuries in this area are often exposed through a Bruner skin incision and a window opening in the synovial sheath, a release, or local excision of a short part of the annular pulleys.
- If the tendon ends have not retracted far proximally, flexion of the MCP or PIP joint can effectively bring the proximal end into sight.
  - Sometimes the proximal tendon end is found retracted even to the middle of the palm. In this instance, an additional incision is made in the palm to expose the tendons, and the proximal tendon end is pulled distally within the synovial sheath by loosely suturing the tendon to a catheter.
  - The end is brought out of the distal opening in the sheath to approximate the distal end. While the finger is held in slight flexion, a 25 G needle is then inserted at the base of the finger through the proximal tendon to hold the tendon temporarily and to release the tension at the surgical suture site.
- Stronger suture materials are preferred: 3-0 or 4-0 sutures (nylon or coated nylon) are common choices.
- Basic requirements of a tendon repair are: (1) sufficient strength; (2) smooth tendon gliding surface, with minimal suture (and knot) exposure; (3) prevent gapping of the repair site under tension; and (4) easy to perform.
- Surgical suture techniques vary among surgeons. Some core suture methods are shown in ***(Figure 21.11)***. The modified Kessler and cruciate techniques are further shown in ***(Figures 21.12–21.14)***.
- Epitendinous stitches smooth the approximation of the tendon ends and resist gapping during tendon movement.
- Simple running peripheral, locking running peripheral, cross-stitch peripheral, and Halsted horizontal mattress sutures are among those most often used, with the first two more popular ***(Fig. 21.15)***. My preference is to use a simple running peripheral suture with 6-0 nylon after completion of a four- or six-strand core suture repair.

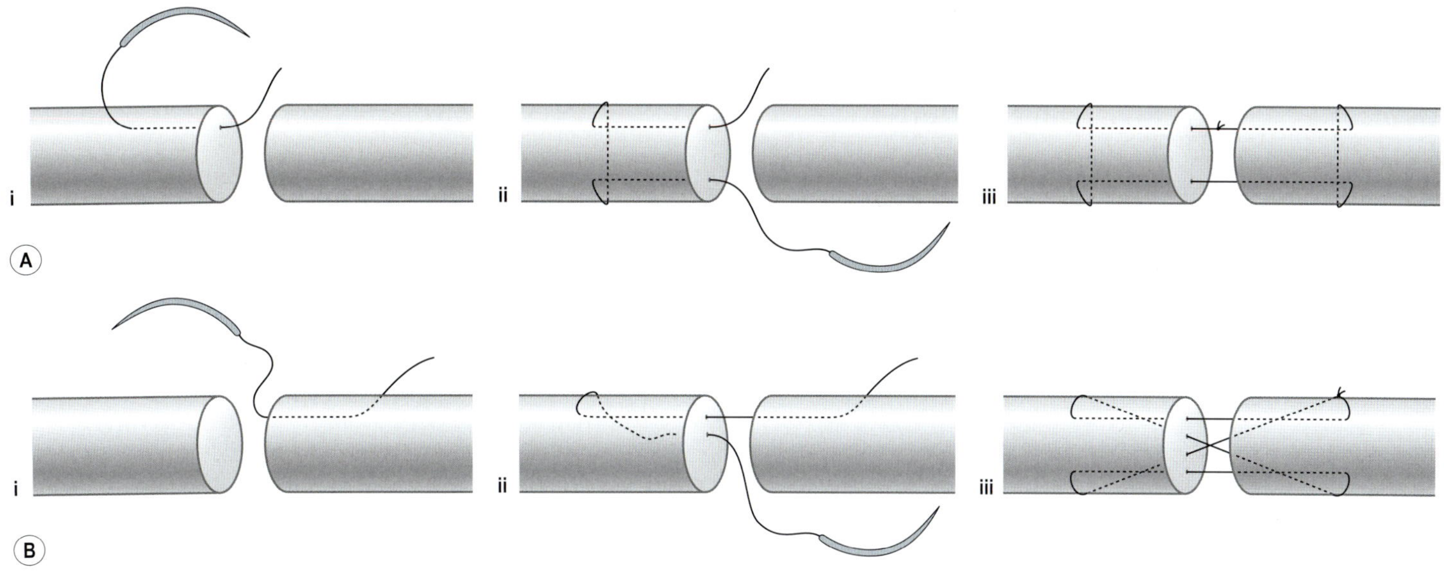

Figure 21.12 Two common techniques in flexor tendon repairs: **(A)** modified Kessler method; and **(B)** cruciate method.

- Technically, to make an optimal surgical repair, the length of core suture purchase in each tendon end should be at least 7 mm to 1 cm as surgical repair strength decreases as the length of the suture purchase decreases ***(Fig. 21.16)***.
- After completing the repair, the cut tendon ends should align well, and no gapping between the tendon ends should be observed (Box 21.3).
- Closure of the synovial sheath is no longer considered essential for tendon repairs after hot debate in the 1980s and early 1990s. Closure may be attempted in clean-cut injury when sheath defects or abrasions are absent. It is now agreed that avoiding compression or constriction to the edematous tendons by the sheath or annular pulleys after surgery is very important to tendon healing.
- With major pulleys and a majority of the sheath intact, leaving a part of the synovial sheath open has no significant adverse effect on tendon function and healing. On the other hand, incision of one single annular pulley (A1, A3, or A4) or a critical part (up to two-thirds of its length) of the A2 pulley does not significantly affect tendon gliding when all other pulleys or the synovial sheath are intact. Such a release can in fact be beneficial to tendon healing and gliding: as healing responses and adhesions arise, it releases constrictions on edematous tendons.
- Contrary to the practice of 10 or 20 years ago, releasing the A4 pulley entirely and releasing a part of the A2 has become accepted clinical practice in recent years ***(Fig. 21.17)***.
- Whether or how to repair the FDS tendon when both flexor tendons are injured is a subject of diverse opinions, particularly in the areas covered by the A2 pulley or distal to it. A few reports have discussed it specifically. Repair of one slip of the FDS is also feasible.
- Surgical options currently advised to deal with tendons and pulleys in the most complex areas of finger flexor tendons are summarized in Table 21.1.

BOX 21.3 **Recommended surgical tendon repairs**

- More than two strands as the core repair – four or six strands are recommended
- Certain tension across the repair site – 10% shortening of tendon segment after repair
- Core suture purchase: 7–10 cm
- Locking tendon–suture junctions in core suture
- Diameter of the locks: 2 mm or over
- Suture calibers: 3-0 or 4-0 for core suture
- A variety of nylon sutures, or a FiberWire suture
- A simple running or locking peripheral suture
- No peripheral suture if core repair is very strong
- Avoid extensive exposure of sutures over the tendon surface

Zone 3, 4, and 5 injuries

- The repair techniques for injured flexor tendons proximal to zone 2 are almost identical to those used in zone 2. These zones have a better prognosis because of richer vascularity around the tendon and lack of constricting pulleys over the tendons. Adhesions in these areas are less likely to impede tendon motion.
- Zone 4 tendon injuries are frequently accompanied by lacerations in the median nerve and arteries. The transverse carpal ligament may be partly opened to facilitate repairs and left partly open after tendon repairs.
- In most cases zone 5 tendon injuries are presented as multiple tendon lacerations with neurovascular injury.
- A wrist with transection of a majority of tendons, vessels, and nerves (at least 10 out of 15 of these structures, excluding palmaris longus) is called a "spaghetti" wrist. A "spaghetti" wrist was reported to have an adverse effect on the recovery of the independent FDS action but not on the recovery of the digital range of motion.

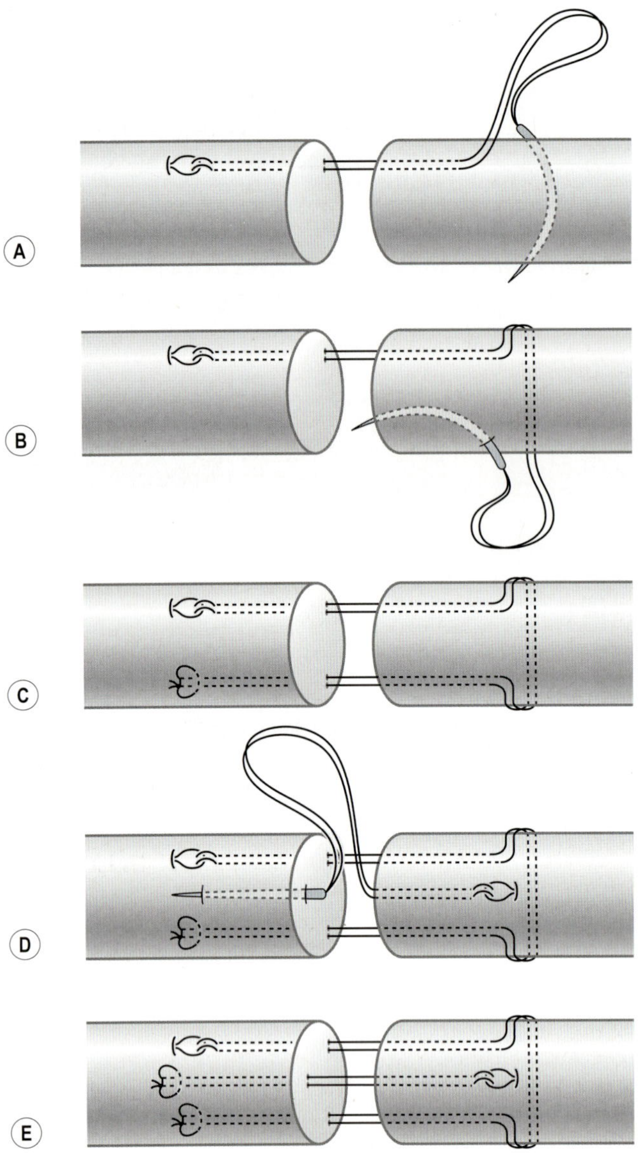

Figure 21.13 The technique for making a six-strand M-Tang tendon repair. Two separate looped sutures are used to make an M-shaped repair within the tendon. **(A–C)** A U-shaped four-strand repair is completed, which can be used alone for tendon repair. **(D and E)** An additional looped repair is added at the center, to complete the six-strand repair. In tendon cross-sections, three suture groups are placed at points of a triangle to avoid interference to the dorsal center of the tendon where the vascular networks converge. The dorsolateral sutures may act as tension bands to resist gapping of the tendon.

- In zone 5, repair of the FDS tendon is preferred, and early postoperative tendon motion is advised. This favors independent movement of the superficialis.

FPL injuries

- Repair of the injured FPL tendons in the thumb usually follows the same principles and methods of repair of the FDP tendon in fingers.
- In repairing the FPL tendon, the proximal cut end of the tendon frequently retracts into the thenar muscles. This end can be retrieved with the techniques described for retracted FDS and FDP tendons.
  - If the proximal stump of the FPL tendon has retracted proximal to the thenar muscles, a separate incision in the forearm is required to locate the stump. The FPL stump usually lies deep to the FCR tendon and the radial artery.

Partial tendon lacerations

- Laceration through less than 60% of the diameter of the tendon does not necessitate a repair by core sutures.
  - For lacerations less than 60%, the tendon wound can be trimmed to lessen the chance of entrapment by pulley edges and friction against the sheath. Alternatively, the cut portion of the tendon can be repaired with epitendinous stitches to smooth the tendon surface and to strengthen the tendon.
- An increased risk of triggering, entrapment, or ruptures is associated with partial laceration over 60%.
  - Laceration of 60–80% requires at least an epitendinous repair and is better repaired using a two-strand core suture through the cut portion.
  - Laceration of 80–90% is treated identically to a complete laceration.

Closed tendon rupture

- Class I: the FDP tendon is avulsed from the phalanx and retracts into the palm.
  - The tendon should be reinserted within 7–10 days before the sheath collapses, which may prevent advancing the tendon distally. Muscle contracture may also prevent tendon advancement.
- Class II: the FDP tendon retracts to the level of the PIP joint.
  - Repair may be attempted 1 month after injury.
- Class III: a large bone fragment is attached to the FDP tendon.
  - Bony fixation using a K-wire or a screw usually suffices.
- Class IV: the FDP tendon avulses from the bony fragment.
  - The bony fragment is attached into the distal phalanx first
  - The avulsed tendon is advanced.
  - The DIP joint is immobilized for 4–5 weeks, or a gentle motion regimen is prescribed.

Postoperative considerations

- With the exception of a few instances – such as tendon repairs in children, adults who are unable to follow through the protocol, or associated with fractures or particular health conditions – motion of repaired tendons should be initiated from the early postsurgical period.
- Several postoperative motion protocols have been described.

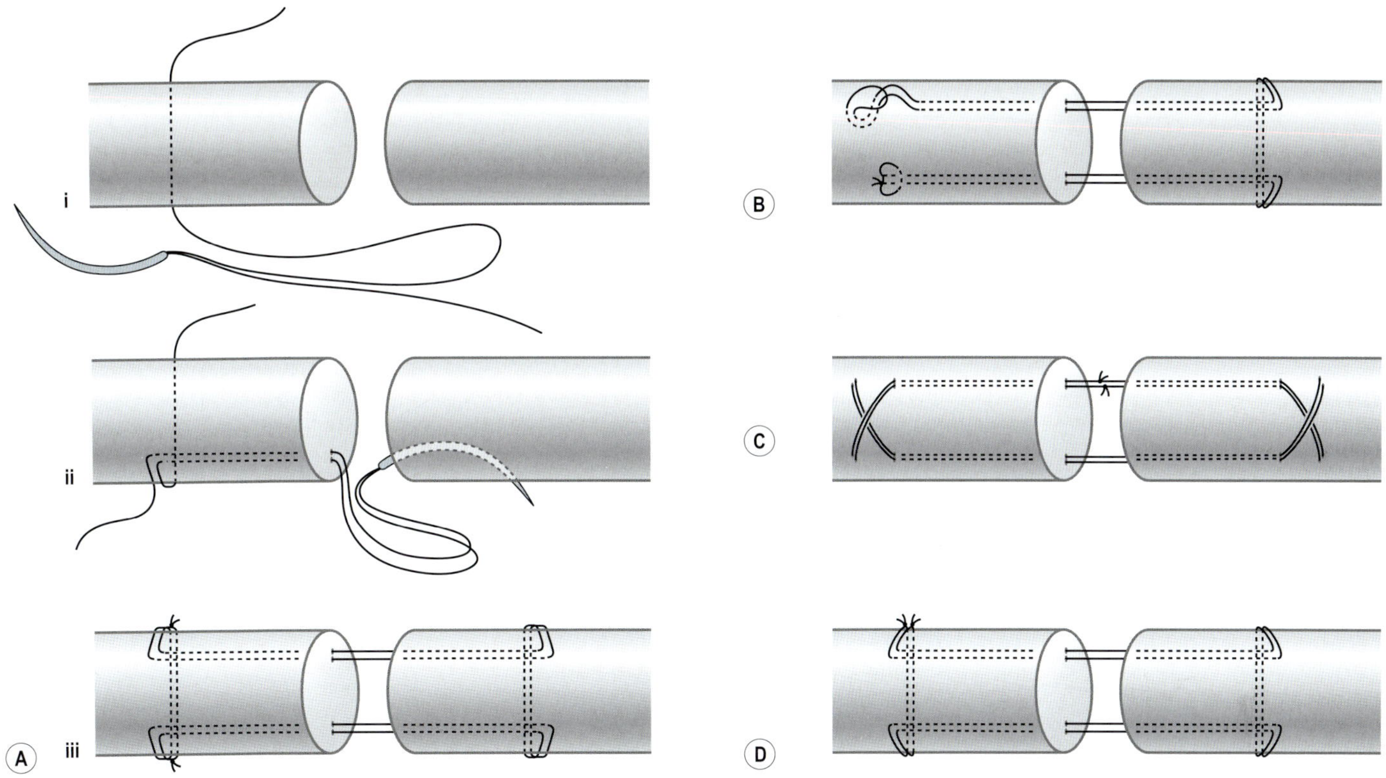

Figure 21.14 Other designs of four-strand repairs by two separate strands or one looped suture line led by a single needle. These repairs, with fewer needle passages within the tendon, have strengths identical to the double Kessler method. **(A)** A four-strand repair with knots on two lateral sides of the tendon. **(B)** A U-shaped four-strand repair made with one looped suture line. **(C and D)** Two separate strands carried by a single needle to make a four-strand cross-lock repair or a four-strand Kessler repair (knots on one side of the tendon).

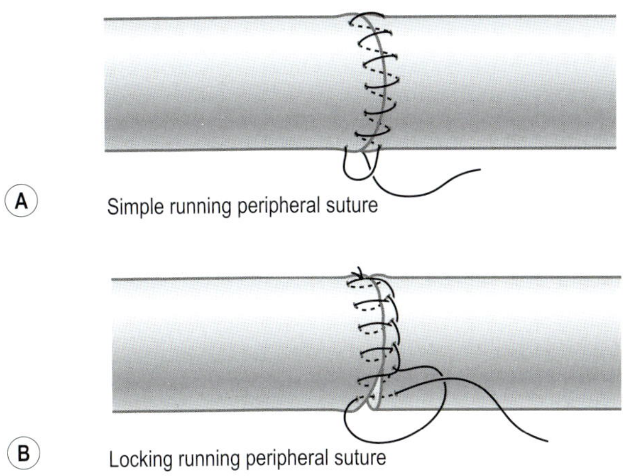

Figure 21.15 Two simple common methods of peripheral suture. **(A)** Simple running peripheral suture. **(B)** Running locking peripheral suture.

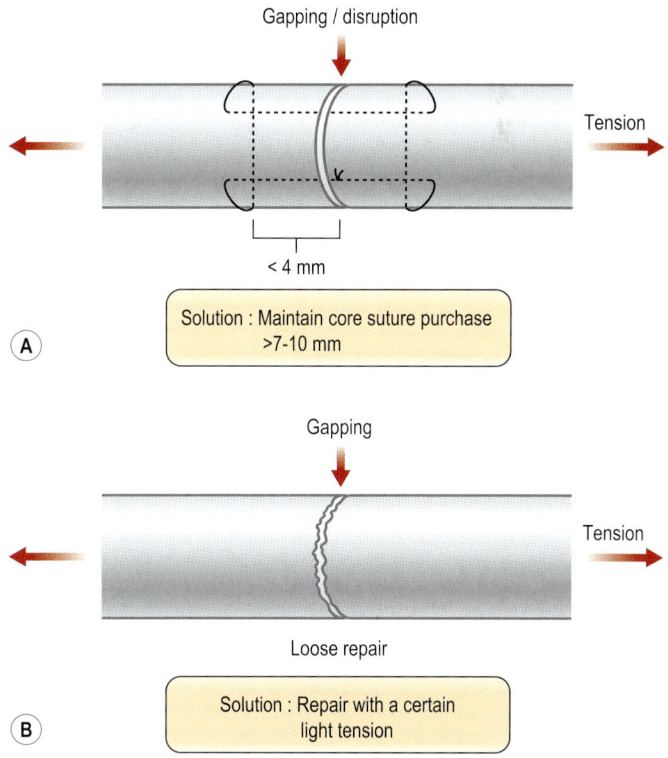

Figure 21.16 **(A)** Sufficient core suture purchase and **(B)** a certain pretension favor resisting gapping and decreases the chance of repair failure during tendon motion after surgery.

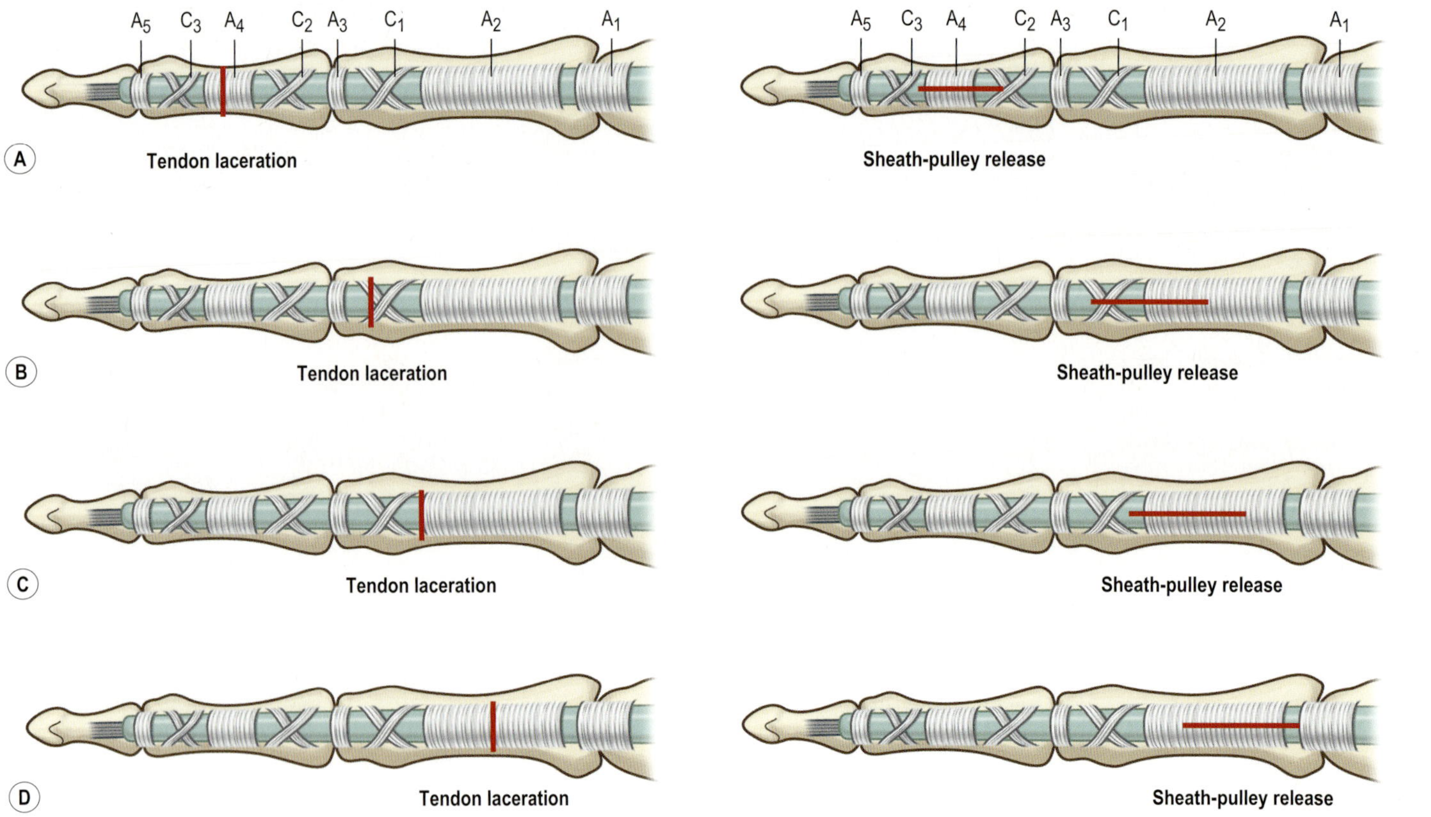

Figure 21.17 Drawings depicting the length and areas of release of the pulley–sheath complex to decompress the repaired tendons, without bowstringing or loss of tendon function. **(A)** Release of the entire A4 pulley when the flexor digitorum profundus tendon has been cut around the A4 pulley and the tendon cannot pass easily beneath this pulley during surgery. **(B)** Release of a part of the sheath distal to the A2 pulley and the distal half of the A2 pulley, when the tendons are cut slightly distal to the A2 pulley. **(C)** Release of a short part of the sheath distal to the A2 pulley and the distal two-thirds of the A2 pulley when repairing tendons cut at the edge of, or in the distal part of, the A2 pulley. **(D)** Release of the proximal two-thirds of the A2 pulley when repairing a cut in the middle, or proximal part of, the A2 pulley.

Table 21.1 Summary of mechanical basis and surgical options advised to deal with the flexor digitorum superficialis (FDS) tendon and pulleys in zone 2 of the finger

Investigations	Area of FDS insertion (2A)	Distal to A2 pulley (2B)	Beneath A2 pulley (2C)	Proximal to A2 pulley (2D)
Anatomic				
FDS tendon	Insertion	2 slips, dorsal to FDP, with vincula	Bifurcation	One single band, flattened palmar to FDP
Pulleys	A4, C2 narrow	A3, C1	A2, narrow	A1, PA
Biomechanical				
FDS tendon	No gliding	Not constricting FDP	Constricting FDP, as a moving and second "pulley"	Little constriction
Pulleys	A4 release is feasible	May incise one pulley	Partial release is feasible	
Clinical options				
FDS tendon		Repair	Resection or do not repair Resect one slip	Repair both tendons when possible
Pulleys	A4 venting		Partial release Pulley shortening or plasty	

FDP, flexor digitorum profundus; PA, palmar aponeurosis.

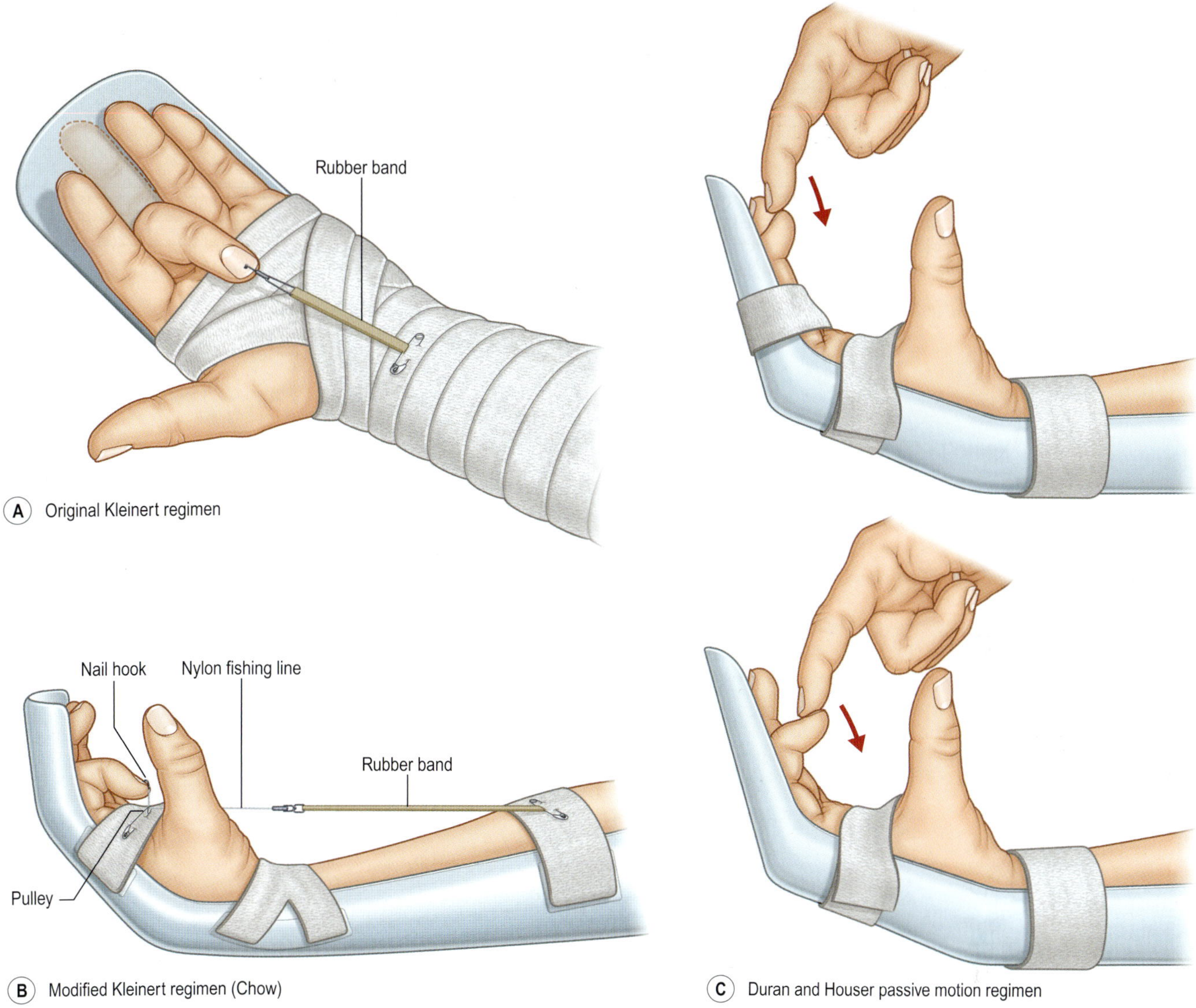

Figure 21.18 (A) Original and **(B)** modified Kleinert passive extension protocols, and **(C)** Duran passive tendon motion protocols. A volar bar was added to increase flexion of the interphalangeal joints in the modified Kleinert protocol.

The modified Kleinert method

- The wrist is palmarly flexed with a dorsal protective splint with 30–40° wrist flexion, 60–70° MCP joint flexion, and the IP joints are allowed full extension.
- Rubber bands are secured to the volar forearm and attached to the tip of the injured finger ***(Fig. 21.18)***.
- Patients are allowed to extend the fingers actively and the fingers are brought back to flexion passively by the tensed rubber bands. In recent years, some surgeons have advised abandoning rubber band traction.

Duran–Houser method

- A dorsal splint is applied with the wrist in 20° flexion, the MCP joint in 50° flexion, and the IP joints are allowed full extension (see Fig. 21.18).
- Within the first 4.5 weeks, the patients perform 10 passive DIP joint extensions with PIP and MCP joint flexions, and 10 passive PIP joint extensions with MCP and DIP joint flexions hourly within the splint (see Fig. 21.18).
- This protocol decreased the frequency of PIP joint contracture seen with Kleinert's rubber band traction.

Early active motion

- Postoperatively, a splint is applied from the elbow to the fingertips with the wrist in midflexion, the MCP joint at slightly less than 90° flexion, and the IP joints straight.
- The light dressing is removed from the digits and exercises are started 48 h after surgery.
- Under supervision, the exercises consist of two passive movements followed by two active movements and are performed at 2 h intervals.

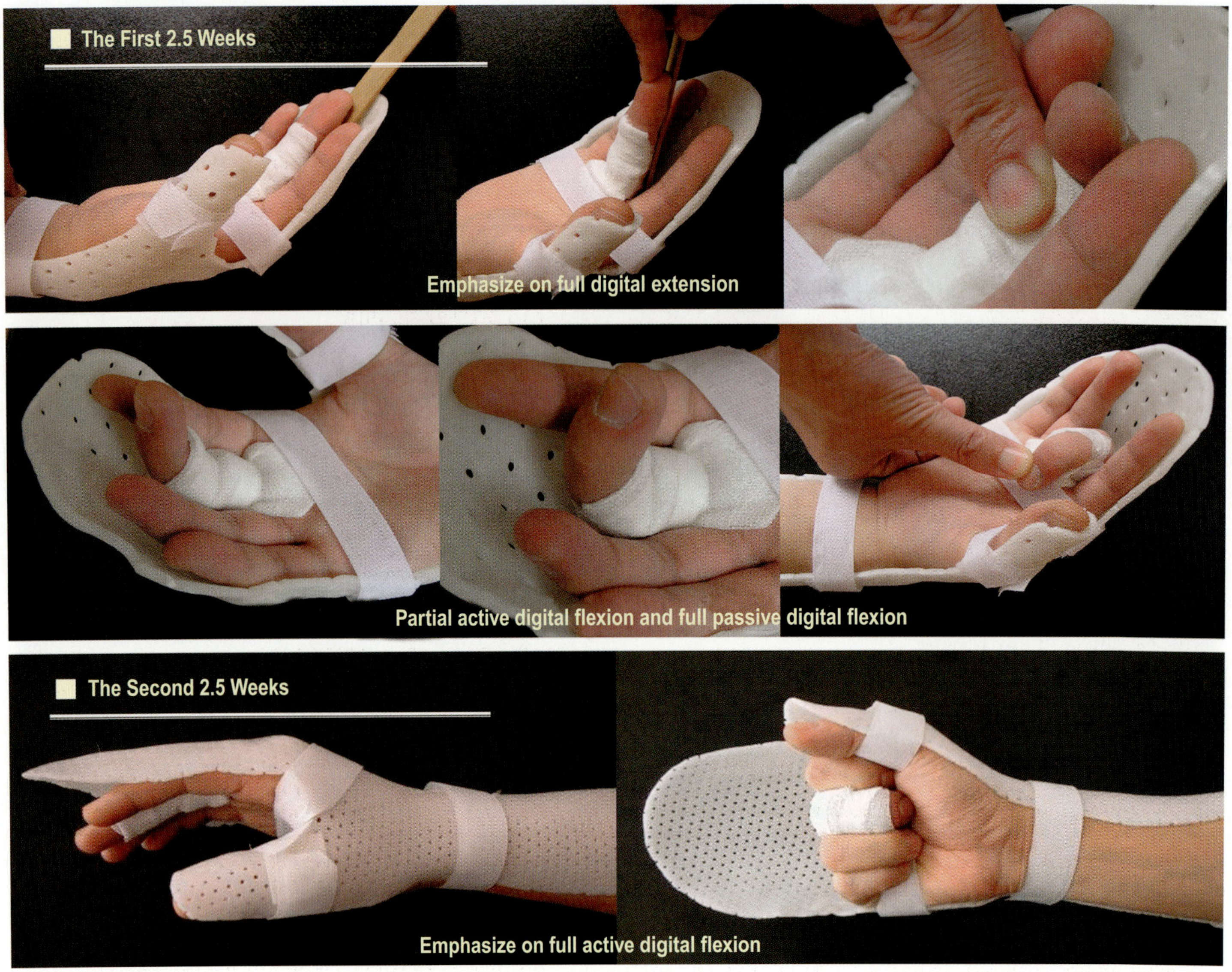

Figure 21.19 Author's combined passive–active tendon motion protocol. This protocol is divided into two 2.5-week periods. In the first 2.5 weeks, with wrist in slight flexion, finger extension is emphasized. Only partial active digital flexion is allowed, but full range of passive motion is implemented. In the second 2.5 weeks, with wrist in extension, full active finger flexion is encouraged. This protocol incorporates the concept of synergistic wrist and finger motion. When the wrist is flexed, finger extension is less tensed; when the wrist is extended, finger flexion is less tensed.

Author's preferred combined active–passive method (Nantong regimen)

- After surgery, the hand is protected in a dorsal thermoplastic splint, with the wrist at 20–30° flexion, MCP joint at slight flexion, and the IP joints in extension for the initial 2.5 weeks ***(Fig. 21.19)***.
  - We do not encourage patients to move the finger in the initial postoperative days.
  - Exercise starts at 3–5 days (in most cases, at 4 or 5 days) after surgery.
  - Patients are instructed to flex the finger actively with gentle force 20–30 times in the morning, noon, evening, and before sleep, up to the range they feel comfortable with.
  - In this 2.5-week period, full active extension is particularly encouraged, and prevention of extension deficits rather than achieving full range of active flexion is emphasized.

Complications and outcomes

- Review of outcomes reported over 20 years show excellent or good active range of finger motion in more than three-fourths of primary tendon repairs.
- Multistrand core sutures have dramatically reduced the incidence of repair ruptures.
- Adhesions remain one of the most common complications preventing satisfactory return of active joint motion.

BOX 21.4 **Secondary surgery: grafting and staged reconstruction**

Indications

- Tendon injuries not treated within about 1 month of injuries
- Rupture of the tendon repairs at primary or delayed primary stages
- Tendon injuries not indicated for primary repair
- Badly scarred digits are indicative for staged tendon reconstruction

Essential requirements

- Supple passive motion of the hand
- Soft tissue conditions: good
- Sufficient time passed after initial tendon injury: 3 months

Contraindications

- Joint motion is very limited (but may be suitable for staged reconstruction)
- Presence of soft tissue wounds or defects, and fractures not well healed

  - Tenolysis is indicated when the passive range of digital motion greatly exceeds the range of active flexion several months after direct end-to-end tendon repair or tendon grafting.
- Outcomes of flexor tendon repairs are affected by patient age, extent and zones of injuries, timing of the repairs, postoperative exercise, and the expertise of the surgeon.
  - Results of tendon repairs in children are generally better than those in adults.
  - Tendon repairs associated with extended soft tissue damage or accompanied by phalangeal fractures are likely to have worse outcomes.
- Secondary tendon repairs are achieved by free tendon grafting, or a staged reconstruction.
  - These procedures are reserved for severed tendons that could not be repaired primarily or for lengthy tendon defects.
  - These techniques, developed by the early masters of hand surgery, remain largely unchanged today (Box 21.4).
  - Patients who have serious scarring in the tendon bed or failed previous efforts at secondary flexor tendon procedures are appropriate for a staged tendon reconstruction, rather than one-stage tendon grafting.
  - Before surgery is attempted, the soft tissue wound should be well healed, with supple passive motion of the hand. Lack of passive range of joint motion is contraindicated for one-stage tendon grafting, but may be suitable for staged tendon reconstruction.
  - The timing of tendon grafting is usually 3 months after injury.

Further reading

Boyes JH, Stark HH. Flexor-tendon grafts in the fingers and thumb. A study of factors influencing results in 1000 cases. *J Bone Joint Surg (Am)*. 1971;53:1332–1342.

This classic article reported perhaps the largest case series of free tendon grafting in the fingers and thumbs. The authors analyzed the factors influencing the prognosis for free tendon grafting and showed that the tendon-grafting procedure used can produce clinically acceptable function. However, hand conditions are extremely important. Prognostic factors include conditions of the soft tissues and joints. Extensively scarred tendon bed and joint damage led to the worst prognosis after tendon graft surgeries.

Elliot D. Primary flexor tendon repair – operative repair, pulley management and rehabilitation. *J Hand Surg (Br)*. 2002;27:507–513.

This article summarized developments in surgical tendon repair techniques, methods of venting the annular pulleys, and active tendon motion regimes for primary flexor tendon repairs in the hand. Of particular clinical interest, the authors reviewed methods of early active or combined passive–active tendon motion (representing a current trend in digital flexor tendon rehabilitation) and the pulley venting procedure that the author and his colleagues have been using in their practice.

Giesen T, Sirotakova M, Copsey AJ, et al. Flexor pollicis longus primary repair: further experience with the Tang technique and controlled active mobilisation. *J Hand Surg (Eur)*. 2009;34:758–761.

This clinical study reported the most up-to-date clinical outcomes of repairs of lacerated fl exor pollicis longus (FPL) tendons from a renowned center dealing with flexor tendon injuries. These authors have made a series of reports of their results in treating FPL injuries over the past two decades; this most recent report documents their outcomes in 50 FPL injuries. With a six-strand core tendon repair alone (without peripheral repairs), they achieved good or excellent functional recovery in 80% of thumbs, with zero tendon rupture with an active motion regimen. These are the best clinical results of FPL tendon repairs reported thus far. It is worth noting that the authors did not elaborate peripheral sutures in these FPL tendon repairs, and the oblique pulley in the thumb was vented to accommodate tendon repairs.

Hunter JM, Salisbury RE. Flexor-tendon reconstruction in severely damaged hands. A two-stage procedure using a silicone-Dacron reinforced gliding prosthesis prior to tendon grafting. *J Bone Joint Surg (Am)*. 1971;53:829–852.

Kleinert HE, Schepel S, Gill T. Flexor tendon injuries. *Surg Clin North Am*. 1981;61: 267–286.

Savage R, Risitano G. Flexor tendon repair using a "six strand" method of repair and early active mobilization. *J Hand Surg (Br)*. 1989;14:396–399.

Strickland JW. Delayed treatment of flexor tendon injuries including grafting. *Hand Clin*. 2005;21:219–243.

This article provides an update on historical developments of surgical techniques, the author's personal approaches, and current practice of these secondary repair procedures, which are generally considered classic operations. Little has changed over recent decades.

Tang JB. Clinical outcomes associated with flexor tendon repair. *Hand Clin*. 2005;21:199–221.

Tang JB. Indications, methods, postoperative motion and outcome evaluation of primary flexor tendon repairs in zone 2. *J Hand Surg (Eur)*. 2007;32:118–129.

This article provides a comprehensive and updated review of the current indications for primary tendon repairs in zone 2. The author's techniques of multistrand repairs and rehabilitation are detailed. Most importantly, the author defines the needs, mechanical basis, and areas of releasing the critical parts of the major digital annular pulleys to facilitate tendon repairs. The author highlights the importance of releasing the critical pulley parts and strong surgical repairs in achieving predictable primary flexor tendon repairs in this most difficult area. Subdivision of zone 2 and novel criteria for outcome evaluation are also presented in this article.

Verdan CE. Primary repair of flexor tendons. *J Bone Joint Surg (Am)*. 1960;42:647–657.

Chapter 22

Nerve transfers

This chapter was created using content from Neligan & Chang, Plastic Surgery 3rd edition, Volume 6, Hand and Upper Extremity, Chapter 33, Nerve transfers, Kirsty U. Boyd, Ida K. Fox and Susan E. Mackinnon.

SYNOPSIS

- Nerve injuries are often devastating, with associated pain and impaired function.
- Motor nerve injuries must be managed expeditiously, because regenerating axons must reach target muscle prior to degeneration and fibrosis – "time is muscle".
- Nerve transfers offer an advantageous method of reconstruction by delivering regenerating nerve fibers to the target end organ more quickly, thus converting a proximal injury to a more distal injury.
- Nerve transfers allow for dissection outside the original zone of injury, providing a safer and more technically straightforward procedure.
- Unlike tendon transfers, the muscle–tendon biomechanical structure is preserved, thus excursion, origin, insertion, and length–tension relationships are undisturbed.
- Nerve transfers require time for the nerve to regenerate and extensive physical therapy for retraining.
- Intraneural dissection is technically demanding, and nerve transfers require intimate knowledge of nerve topography.

Brief introduction

- Nerve transfers can be performed to restore sensory or motor deficits and essentially convert a proximal injury to a distal injury, providing a source of regenerating axons in close proximity to the end target.
- Advantages of nerve transfers:
  - Bring regenerating motor fibers closer to the target end organ more rapidly, essentially converting a more proximal-level injury to a more distal-level injury.
  - Enable surgical reconstruction outside the zone of the original injury, avoiding complex dissections and limiting injury to critical neurovascular structures.
  - Allow for a very targeted intervention in cases of partial nerve.
  - Unlike tendon transfers, nerve transfers require only minimal immobilization (7–10 days), which is especially valuable in patients presenting with significant baseline stiffness.
  - Preserve the biomechanical properties of the musculotendinous unit.
  - Can restore unique function such as pronation, which is incredibly difficult to restore by traditional surgical techniques.
- Indications for nerve transfers (Table 22.1).
- Absolute contraindications:
  - End organ unresponsiveness.
  - Muscle that is in complete discontinuity with the nerve for greater than 1 year will not be reinnervated no matter the elaborate reinnervation strategy employed.
- Relative contraindications:
  - Extensive time required for regeneration
  - Surgeon inexperience: challenges of the surgery, the anatomic knowledge required, and problems of postoperative retraining and therapy.
  - Patients who may prefer the more rapid recovery associated with tendon transfer at the expense of the independent fine motor control that could be achieved through the use of nerve transfers.

Table 22.1 **Indications for nerve transfer**

- Proximal brachial plexus injuries where grafting is not possible
- Proximal peripheral nerve injuries requiring long distance for reinnervation of distal targets
- Severely scarred areas with risk of damage to critical structures
- Segmental nerve loss
- Major upper-extremity trauma
- Partial nerve injuries with functional loss
- Delayed presentation with inadequate time for reinnervation of distal targets with grafting
- Sensory nerve deficits in critical regions

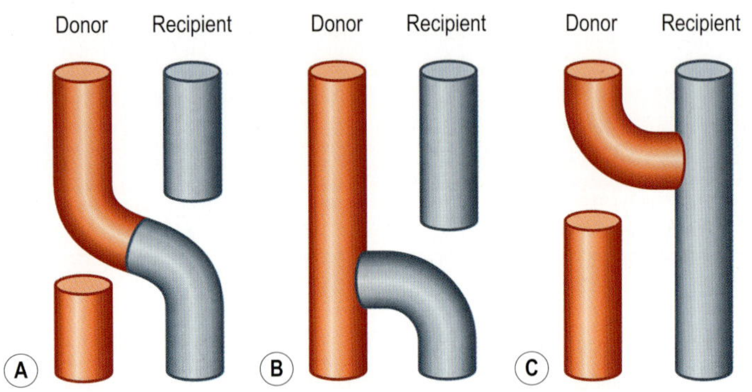

Figure 22.1 The various options for coaptation in nerve transfer. **(A)** End-to-end coaptation between the donor nerve (red) and the recipient nerve (blue). **(B)** End-to-side coaptation, where the distal end of the divided recipient nerve (blue) is transferred to the side of the intact donor nerve (red). In this transfer, fascicles from the donor will "sprout" into the distal donor nerve. The recipient nerve essentially "pulls" the donor fascicles into the distal nerve. **(C)** Reverse end-to-side coaptation. In this transfer, the donor nerve (red) has been divided and transferred to the side of the intact recipient nerve (blue). The donor essentially "pushes" regenerating fascicles into the distal donor nerve.

- The most relevant recent basic science advances pertaining to nerve transfers relate to end-to-side transfers ***(Fig. 22.1)***.
  - End-to-side neurorrhaphy involves the coaptation of the distal end of an injured recipient nerve into the lateral aspect of an intact nerve, which serves as a proximal source of axons to regenerate into the injured nerve.
  - Sensory recovery has typically been more impressive than motor recovery.
- Reverse end-to-side nerve transfers involve the complete transection of the donor nerve, which is then coapted into the side of the intact recipient nerve.
  - This maximizes the potential number of available motor axons from the donor nerve.
  - This procedure does not interrupt any recovery in the injured recipient nerve because the nerve remains in continuity; however, the additional axons recruited from the donor nerve improve distal target reinnervation, a concept known as "supercharging."
  - In a proximal nerve injury, with a long distance required for reinnervation, this technique can protect target muscles from denervation atrophy and fibrosis.

Hints and tips

The end-to-side transfer can be considered as the recipient nerve "pulling" regenerating axons out of the intact donor, whereas the reverse end-to-side transfer can be considered as the donor nerve "pushing" regenerating axons out into the intact recipient.

- The biggest challenge facing peripheral nerve surgeons is that with increasing time since injury, the ability to achieve good motor function becomes increasingly limited.
  - For any nerve injury where there is complete discontinuity with the motor end organ, no reinnervation procedure will be able to restore muscle once denervation and fibrosis have occurred, a process which occurs as early as 1 year.
- Direct nerve repair and nerve grafting also remain valuable tools for the peripheral nerve surgeon and should continue to be the treatment of choice in a variety of scenarios, including:
  - Multiple nerve injuries where there is a paucity of nerve donor material for nerve transfer.
  - Distal single-function nerve injuries where direct or graft repair is preferable to nerve transfer because one-to-one function is preserved, no retraining is necessary, no donor function is sacrificed, and the distance to the end target is short.
- In the event of a failed nerve transfer, and the necessity of further secondary procedures, there are several important considerations.
  - When planning nerve transfers, one must consider the possible salvage procedures required should the transfer fail.
  - Thus, when deciding on donor nerve, it is prudent to ensure that options are left for later.
  - A donor for tendon transfer requires MRC grade 5 of 5 strength because following transfer it will be downgraded by a minimum of one grade.

Hints and tips

Avoid using a donor nerve that may be required for a secondary procedure such as a tendon transfer down the road. Prior to cutting a donor nerve, make sure the rest of the nerve performs all essential functions with fastidious intraoperative nerve stimulation.

- Tendon transfers have the benefit of not being restricted by time, given that distal motor denervation and fibrosis do not affect the outcome. For this reason, there is no harm in attempting a nerve transfer as a primary procedure, and reserving the tendon transfer for a secondary procedure if the functional outcome is less than desired.
- Nerve transfers should not be attempted if there are not suitable, redundant, available donors, as in the setting of a multinerve injury. In this setting, nerve grafting combined with tendon transfer, or even arthrodesis, may be warranted.

Preoperative considerations

- On history, details of the mechanism and timing of injury are crucial. The mechanism of injury will determine timing of intervention, with prompt exploration of penetrating sharp trauma, and more expectant management of closed injuries and gunshot wounds.
- Specific patient symptoms such as loss of function, both sensory and motor, and pain should be precisely elicited, as this will help focus the subsequent physical examination.
- A complete physical examination of the upper extremity includes assessment of sensory and motor function, deep tendon reflexes, joint suppleness, and range of motion.
- Particularly in patients with late presentation, the presence of fixed joint contractures may preclude functional recovery.
- Sensation should be examined by both dermatome and peripheral nerve distribution, and can be helpful in distinguishing these injuries. The authors advocate the use of both two-point discrimination and the ten-test to evaluate sensory loss in the hand.
- A Tinel's sign, the tingling sensation elicited with percussion over a regenerating nerve, will help to localize the level of nerve injury, and may also be followed on serial clinical examination to check for signs of advancement, indicating spontaneous recovery.
- An advancing Tinel's sign quite often precedes actual motor recovery, which might be quite distal to the site of the initial injury.
- The scratch collapse test is useful primarily for patients with nerve compression pathology, but also has a role in evaluating the patient for potential nerve transfer procedures, as it can provide additional confirmation of the level of nerve injury (Video 22.1).

Video 22.1

- The test is performed by having the patient sit facing the examiner with their shoulders adducted, elbows held in 90° of flexion, neutral prosupination, and wrist and fingers extended. The examiner will then lightly scratch the area of the presumed nerve injury and exert force to the patient's arms in the direction of internal shoulder rotation as the patient resists. Nerve injury at the test site is indicated by the inward collapse of the arm on the side ipsilateral to the injury.
- One of the most important components of the physical examination is the simple determination of what is functioning, and what function has been lost.
- In the presence of an injury requiring surgical intervention, it is important to examine the patient for putative nerve donors, both intraplexal and extraplexal (spinal accessory, medial pectoral, and thoracodorsal).

Hints and tips

Remember to check not only for what muscles have lost function, but also for potential nerve transfer donors.

- Electrodiagnostic testing, performed by an experienced person, can be a useful adjunct to physical examination for serial assessment of reinnervation in closed nerve injuries.
- Initial electrodiagnostic testing should be deferred until a minimum of 6–8 weeks postinjury to assess for signs of both axonal injury and root-level avulsion.
- In patients with no evidence of recovery 3 months after a closed nerve injury, the balance should tilt towards consideration of surgical intervention.

Hints and tips

Order baseline electrodiagnostic studies at 6–8 weeks and subsequent testing as indicated by the injury. Fibrillations and positive sharp waves suggest denervation. Motor unit potentials and nascent units suggest reinnervation.

Anatomical/technical pearls for specific injury patterns

Hints and tips

- Avoid, or use short-term paralytics with anesthesia induction to allow for nerve stimulation
- Minimize or avoid tourniquet time to avoid interference with nerve stimulation
- Use plain epinephrine in proximal incisions to minimize blood loss without lidocaine paralysis
- Obtain wide surgical exposure to identify nerves and appropriate branches
- Choice of optimal nerve donor is based on quantity of motor axons, proximity to target muscles, synergy of muscle function, and donor expendability
- Conduct neurolysis with your "eyes" except at the site of actual transfer to avoid prolonged dissection and increased trauma to nerve branches
- Confirm no intraoperative stimulation in putative recipient before dividing donor
- Divide donor nerve distally and recipient nerve proximally
- Use 9-0 nylon and the operating microscope to perform tension-free epineurial repair
- Use bupivacaine block at end of case for postoperative pain control

Upper plexus injury

Specific patient exam findings

- Upper plexus injuries involve injuries at the C5, C6, and/or C7 root or upper trunk level.
- Commonly include deficits of:
  - The dorsal scapular n. innervates the rhomboid muscles and the levator scapulae muscles, which contribute to scapular adduction, retraction, and elevation.

- The long thoracic n. innervates the serratus anterior muscle, which abducts the scapula, permitting the full range of shoulder flexion past 90°.
- The suprascapular n. innervates the supraspinatus and infraspinatus muscles. These muscles are rotator cuff muscles. The supraspinatus contributes to shoulder abduction with the deltoid muscle. The infraspinatus contributes to shoulder external rotation with the teres minor.
- The axillary n. arises from the posterior cord, receiving innervation from C5 and C6. Supplies the deltoid and teres minor muscles, which provide shoulder abduction and external rotation respectively. Provides cutaneous innervation over the lateral shoulder.
- The musculocutaneous n. arises from the lateral cord and is primarily innervated by C5, C6, and occasionally C7. Innervates coracobrachialis, biceps brachii, and brachialis, which power elbow flexion. The biceps is also the primary forearm supinator. The lateral antebrachial cutaneous (LABC) nerve is a terminal branch and provides cutaneous innervation to the lateral forearm.

• Patients with upper plexus injuries present with glenohumeral joint subluxation, loss of shoulder abduction and external rotation, and absent or weakened elbow flexion depending on the involvement of C7. Numbness over the lateral shoulder and forearm is noted.

Specific operative techniques

Hints and tips

Priorities for upper plexus injuries include restoration of shoulder external rotation and abduction, as well as elbow flexion. Standard transfers include: (1) spinal accessory to suprascapular nerve; (2) medial triceps to axillary nerve; and (3) double fascicular nerve transfer.

Use of spinal accessory nerve (cranial nerve XI) to suprascapular nerve transfer (motor)

• Restoration of shoulder stability and external rotation are facilitated by transferring the spinal accessory nerve (cranial nerve XI) to the suprascapular nerve. This transfer can be conducted by either an anterior or a posterior approach *(Fig. 22.2)*.

• Posterior approach:
  - The spinal accessory nerve runs parallel to the border of trapezius and is localized 40% of the way along a line connecting the acromion to the dorsal midline at the level of the superior border of the scapula *(Fig. 22.3)*.
  - The suprascapular nerve is located midway between the medial border of the scapula and the acromion as it runs through the suprascapular notch.
  - The nerves are accessed through an incision located slightly obliquely just above the superior border of the spine of the scapula. Dissection is carried through the trapezius in a muscle-splitting fashion and an end-to-end coaptation, sparing the upper trapezius nerve branches, is performed.

• Anterior approach:
  - An incision is designed 2 cm superior to and parallel to the clavicle extending laterally from the posterior border of the sternocleidomastoid *(Fig. 22.4)*.
  - The upper trunk is identified between the anterior and middle scalene muscles.
  - The suprascapular nerve is a distinct branch of the upper trunk that sits on the superolateral aspect.
  - The spinal accessory nerve is located in the posterior aspect of the incision on the deep surface of the trapezius muscle.
  - Although an end-to-end transfer can be performed, the end-to-side approach with a partial neurectomy of the donor accessory nerve is preferred as this preserves some donor function.
  - In the end-to-side transfer, a short interpositional graft from the recipient suprascapular nerve to the donor spinal accessory nerve is required to avoid tension.

Use of triceps to axillary nerve transfer (motor component)

• Additional reduction of glenohumeral subluxation and abduction of the shoulder are provided by transferring a branch of the triceps, usually from the medial head, to the axillary nerve *(Fig. 22.5)*.

• Better results in upper plexus injury patients are achieved by reinnervating both the suprascapular and axillary nerves.

• Through a longitudinal incision on the posterior surface of the arm that extends in a curvilinear fashion above the posterior axillary fold *(Fig. 22.6)*, the axillary nerve is identified in the quadrangular space and dissected proximally to include the branch to teres minor, then divided proximally.

• The natural cleavage plane between the lateral and long heads of the triceps is identified and blunt dissection is conducted to expose the donor radial nerve running along the humerus.
  - The branch to the medial triceps sits superficially and medially on the surface of the radial nerve as a distinct branch.
  - The donor triceps nerve is dissected as far distally as possible and then coapted to the axillary nerve *(Fig. 22.7)*.

Use of the double fascicular (ulnar/median redundant branches to biceps brachii and brachialis branches of the musculocutaneous) nerve transfer (motor)

• Restoration of elbow flexion is achieved with the double fascicular nerve transfer *(Fig. 22.8)*.
  - This transfer reinnervates the biceps brachii and brachialis muscles using redundant fascicles from the ulnar and median nerves.

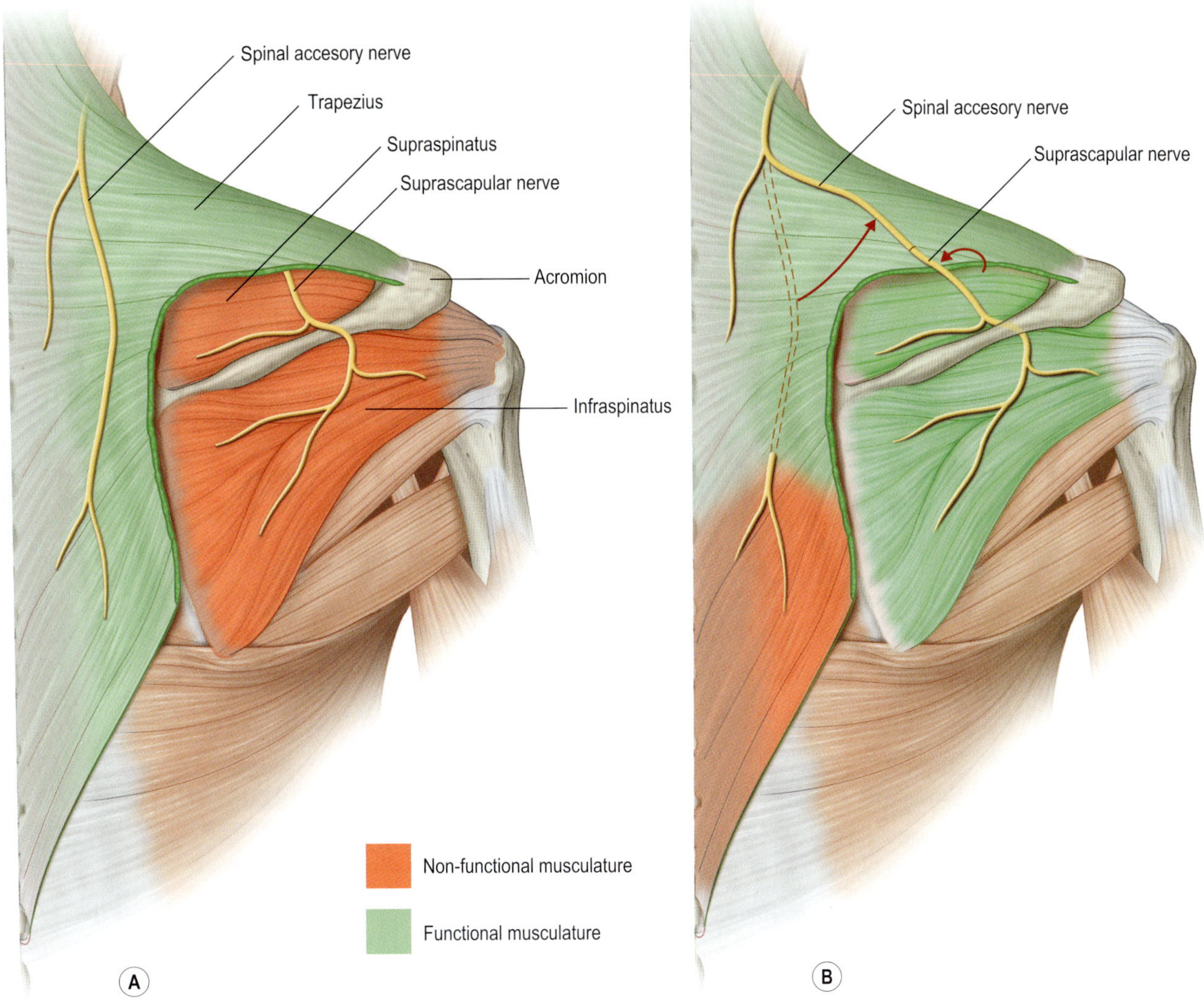

Figure 22.2 The posterior approach for spinal accessory to suprascapular nerve transfers. **(A)** The nerves can be seen in their original orientation. **(B)** The end-to-end transfer has been completed. The transfer includes the functional spinal accessory nerve (donor) being transposed and coapted to the non-functional suprascapular nerve (recipient).

- A longitudinal incision in the bicipital groove facilitates exposure of the musculocutaneous, median, and ulnar nerves.
- An intramuscular dissection at the underside of the biceps brachii muscle allows exposure of the musculocutaneous nerve.
  - The biceps brachii branch is the more proximal branch and is located about halfway between the shoulder and elbow exiting the nerve from the lateral side.
  - The brachialis branch exits the musculocutaneous branch on the medial side of the arm approximately 13 cm proximal to the medial epicondyle, usually under a leash of crossing vessels ***(Fig. 22.9)***.
  - These branches are divided and draped over to the median and ulnar nerves to determine best donor–recipient pairings.
  - Confirmation of a tension-free inset with elbow range of motion is mandatory.
  - The ulnar and median nerves are then neurolyzed at the appropriate level, and redundant fascicles to the flexor carpi ulnaris (FCU: ulnar), flexor carpi radialis (FCR), flexor digitorum superficialis (FDS), or palmaris longus (median) are identified.
  - The redundant fascicles are divided distally and coapted end to end. Reinnervation occurs at approximately 5–6 months postoperatively.

Other potential donors (medial pectoral nerve and thoracodorsal nerve)

- Other potential donors that can be used to restore elbow flexion include the medial pectoral nerves and the thoracodorsal nerve.
  - The medial pectoral nerves are identified by making an incision in the deltopectoral groove, dividing the pectoralis major tendon distally, and

elevating pectoralis minor from lateral to medial *(Fig. 22.10)*.

- The thoracodorsal nerve runs along the lateral chest wall and can be exposed through an incision running along the free border of latissimus dorsi.

Lower plexus injury

Specific patient exam findings

- Lower plexus injuries usually involve damage to C8 and T1 nerve roots or to the lower trunk.

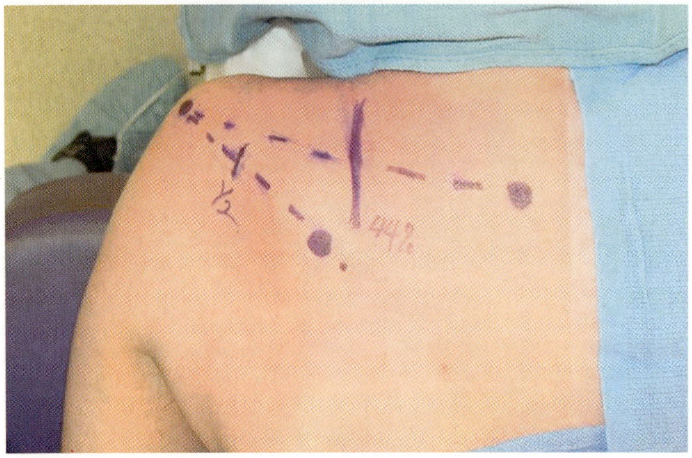

Figure 22.3 Surface markings for posterior approach to spinal accessory to suprascapular. The spinal accessory nerve is located 44% of the way along a line connecting the dorsal midline to the acromion. The suprascapular nerve is located at the halfway point between the medial border of the scapula and the acromion on an obliquely oriented line at the superior aspect of the scapular spine. It runs in the suprascapular notch.

- Often they are a result of a forceful pull on an adducted arm.
- The lower trunk contributes primarily to the ulnar nerve, and thus patients have a resultant loss of the intrinsic muscles of the hand, with weakened wrist and finger flexion.
- Contribution to the median and radial nerves may impact thumb and finger flexion and extension respectively.
- Involvement of C7 can dramatically influence available options for nerve transfer.

Hints and tips

Priorities for lower plexus injuries include restoration of hand extrinsic function. Restoration of hand intrinsic function is virtually unobtainable except in the very young pediatric patient.

Specific operative techniques

- There are few good options for lower plexus injury reconstruction. Recently, the authors have incorporated transferring the nerve to brachialis (a branch of the musculocutaneous nerve) to the anterior interosseous nerve to regain thumb and finger flexion.

Complete/near-complete plexus injury

Specific patient exam findings

- Often results from high-velocity, penetrating, or crush-type mechanisms and result in devastating loss of function.

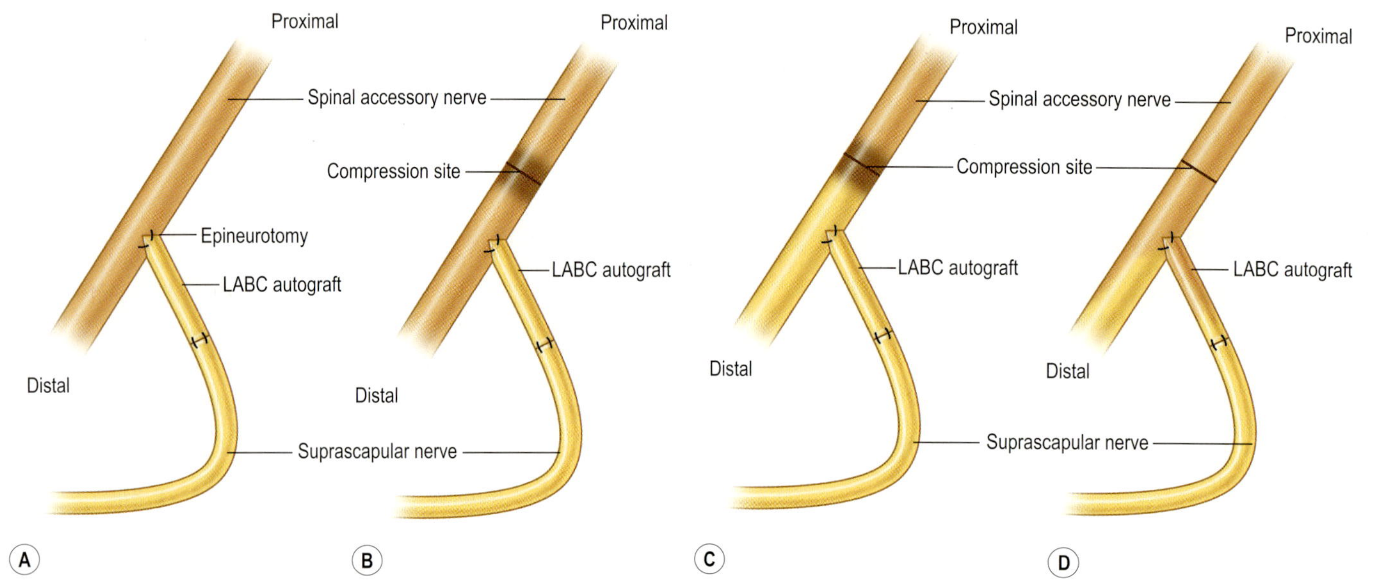

Figure 22.4 In the anterior approach to the spinal accessory to suprascapular nerve transfer, upper trapezius function is preserved by performing the nerve transfer in an end-to-side manner. **(A)** To inset this transfer with no tension, an interpositional lateral antebrachial cutaneous (LABC) nerve graft is used. **(B)** To facilitate regenerative sprouting, injury to the donor nerve is required proximally. This is accomplished by "crushing" the nerve with a hemostat to cause a second-degree nerve injury. **(C)** Wallerian degeneration occurs distal to the site of compression. **(D)** Axons regenerate from the level of the crush injury, with some axons following the donor nerve and restoring function to the upper trapezius muscle, and some axons diverting into the distal recipient nerve via the LABC graft.

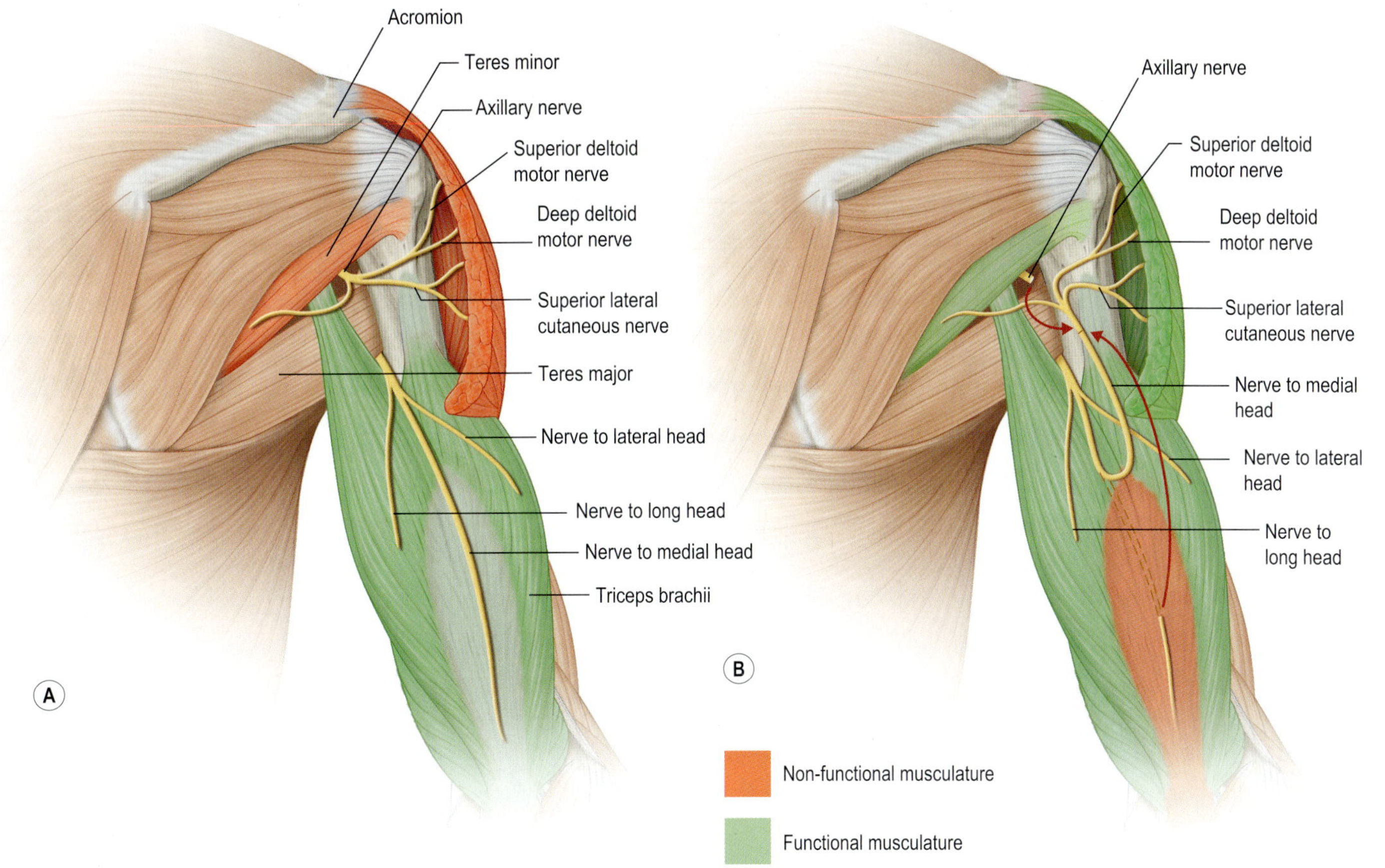

Figure 22.5 The triceps to axillary nerve transfer via a posterior approach to the upper arm. **(A)** The axillary and radial nerves in their normal anatomical position. **(B)** The branch to the medial head of the triceps (donor) is transposed to meet the divided end of the axillary nerve (recipient). The branch to the medial head is coapted end to end to the axillary nerve.

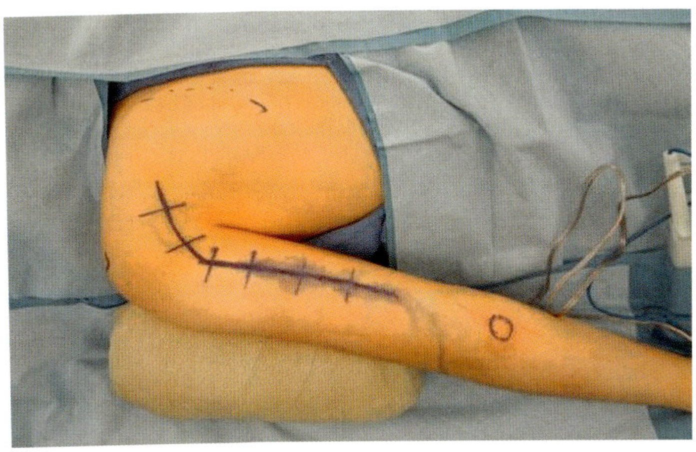

Figure 22.6 Set-up and incision for triceps to axillary. The patient is positioned in the prone position and draped with the entire extremity free and the medial border of the scapula exposed. A line connecting the olecranon and the acromion is drawn on the posterior aspect of the arm and then extended in a curvilinear fashion just above the posterior axillary fold. Positioning is facilitated by placing a "bump" beneath the anterior shoulder preventing internal rotation and anterior subluxation. The arm is draped free so that distal function can be assessed with intraoperative nerve stimulation.

- These patients will typically have an insensate, flail upper extremity with glenohumeral joint subluxation and a positive sulcus sign.
- Most will lack shoulder stability, abduction, rotation, flexion and extension, elbow flexion and extension, wrist flexion and extension, finger flexion, extension, and intrinsic function.

Specific operative techniques

Hints and tips

Priorities for complete plexus injuries are to restore function in the following order of priority: (1) elbow flexion; (2) shoulder stability/external rotation; and (3) hand extrinsic function/grasp. Techniques include extraplexal to intraplexal nerve transfers and free functional muscle flap reconstruction. Contralateral C7 and phrenic nerve transfers are also described with modest results.

Use of spinal accessory and intercostal nerves as donors (motor)

- Reconstruction in this scenario has very different goals and outcomes from less traumatic injuries. The extremity will often be a "helper" extremity at best. The severe

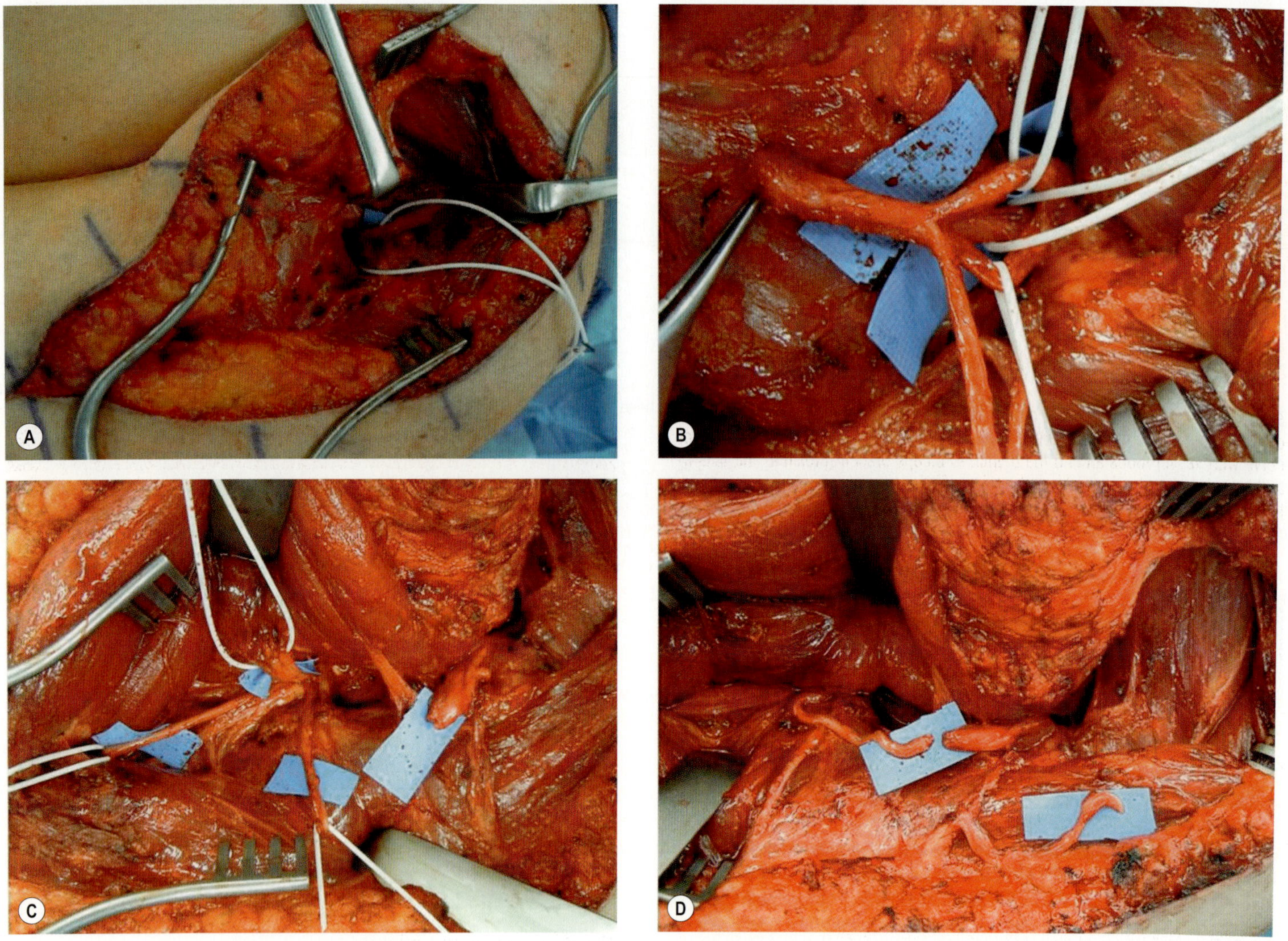

Figure 22.7 A clinical example of the triceps to axillary nerve transfer. The patient is positioned with their head to the top right. The cross-hatchings of the posterior midline incision in the upper arm are visible and the quadrangular space is exposed. **(A)** The intact nerve *in situ* prior to division. A white vessel loop surrounds the entire nerve at that level. **(B)** The divided nerve transposed caudally with the proximal-most aspect held by the forceps. The branches are clearly visible with vessel loops around motor branches. The superior-most branch is the branch to teres minor. The sensory branch is the most inferior branch (no vessel loop) and can be visualized heading more superficially than the other branches. **(C)** The cut end of the recipient axillary nerve is visible on the most proximal blue background. The radial nerve is visualized at the base of the wound, with vessel loops around branches to the medial, long, and lateral heads of triceps. **(D)** The divided branch to the medial head (donor) is transposed proximally and anastomosed to the recipient axillary nerve.

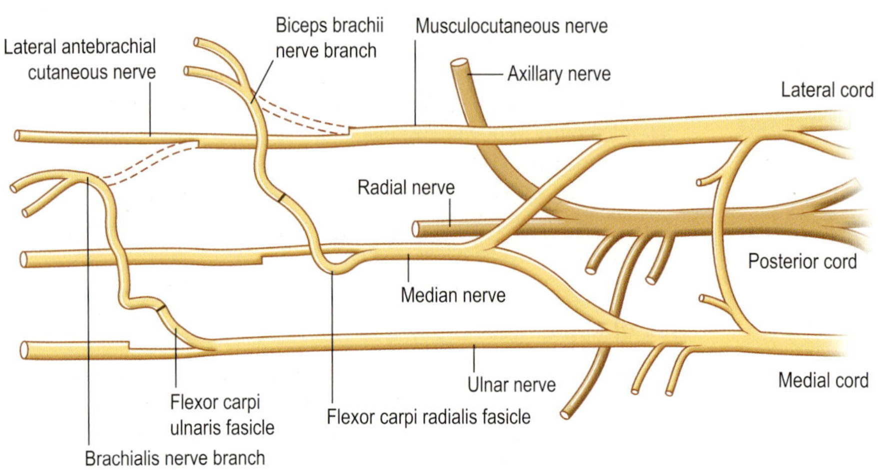

Figure 22.8 A schematic of the double fascicular nerve transfer. The divided recipient branches of the musculocutaneous nerve (biceps brachii laterally and brachialis medially) are transposed medially to the median and ulnar nerves. In this example, a redundant fascicle to flexor digitorum superficialis (median donor) is transferred to the biceps brachii branch and a redundant fascicle of the flexor carpi ulnaris (ulnar donor) is transferred to the brachialis branch.

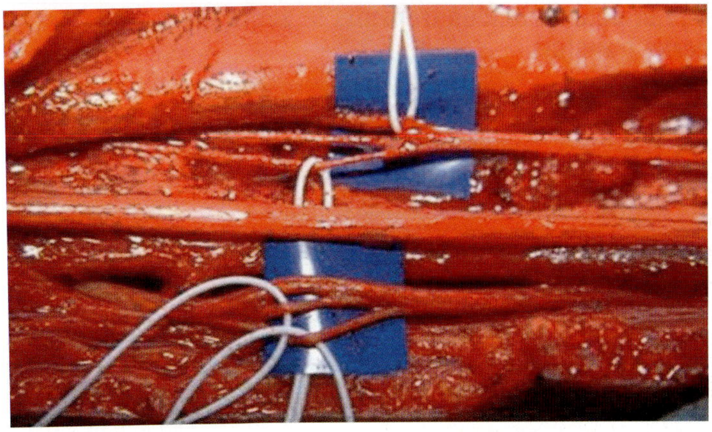

Figure 22.9 Operative photo of double fascicular nerve transfer. A clinical example of the double fascicular nerve transfer. The superior nerve is the musculocutaneous nerve with vessel loops around the branch to biceps brachii (proximal and lateral) and branch to brachialis (distal and medial). The ulnar nerve is also neurolyzed at the level appropriate for transfer. Redundant fascicles determined by intraoperative nerve stimulation that can serve as potential donors are marked with vessel loops.

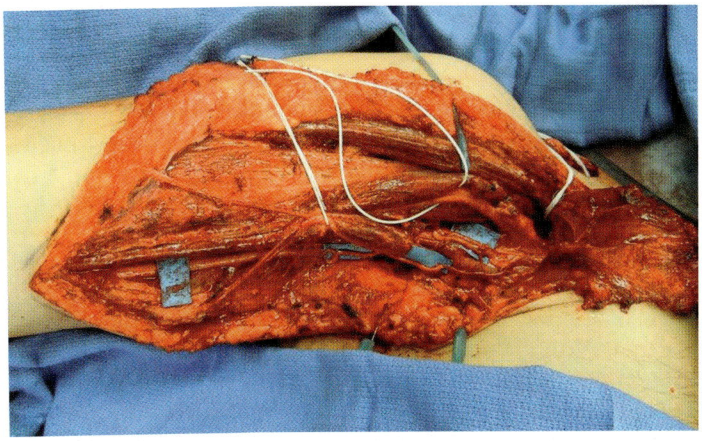

Figure 22.10 Harvesting medial pectoral nerve. Clinical photograph of a patient with medial pectoral nerve harvested as a donor. The divided pectoralis major muscle is flipped proximally and lying on the anterior chest wall. The medial pectoral nerves have been dissected from the deep surface of the pectoralis minor and divided distally. They have then been transposed towards the donor nerves in the arm and are lying on the most proximal blue background.

damage to the brachial plexus means that options for nerve transfers are limited, and that extraplexal donors must be considered. Specifically, available extraplexal nerve donors include the spinal accessory, medial pectoral, thoracodorsal, and intercostal nerves.

- The spinal accessory nerve is harvested as described previously.
- Intercostal nerves are harvested through an L-shaped incision extending from the anterior axillary fold and curving anteriorly below the nipple-areolar complex. Rib periosteum is incised and peeled down to expose the neurovascular bundles running along the posterior inferior surface of each rib ***(Fig. 22.11)***. The motor nerves are smaller and sit more superiorly than the sensory nerves. Often several are required. These are dissected as far medially as possible and then divided.

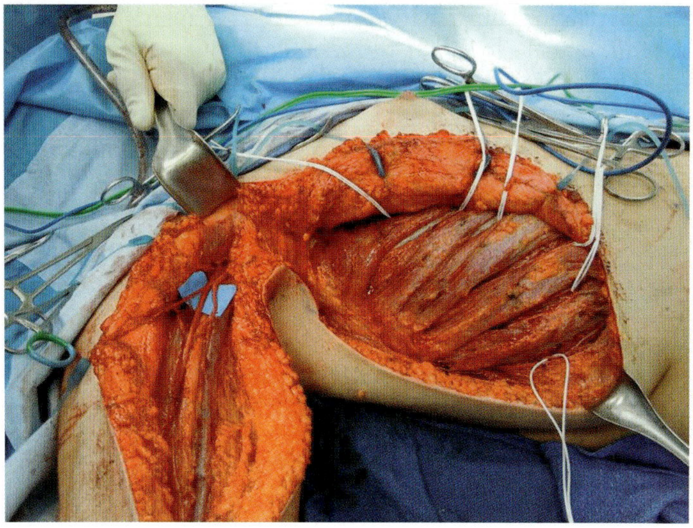

Figure 22.11 Harvesting intercostals. Clinical photograph of a female patient undergoing intercostal to musculocutaneous nerve transfer. The anterior subcutaneous flap has been turned over medially to expose the anterior chest wall. White vessel loops are around intercostal nerves at the inferior border of each rib. The recipient nerve is visualized in the upper arm on a blue background.

- These extraplexal donor nerves can be transferred to a variety of potential recipients, depending on surgical goals. They can be used to establish shoulder stability and external rotation (suprascapular and axillary nerves), elbow flexion (musculocutaneous), or even to recreate elbow extension or finger flexion by neurotizing one or two free-functioning gracilis flaps. This is often accomplished as a two-stage procedure.

Median nerve injury

Specific patient exam findings

- The median nerve is a mixed motor and sensory nerve that is derived from C5, C6, C7, C8, and T1.
- There are no branches in the arm as the nerve courses lateral to the brachial artery and then passes over brachialis in the antecubital fossa.
- In the forearm, the median nerve proper supplies pronator teres (PT), FCR, palmaris longus, and FDS. The nerve then divides.
  - The anterior interosseous nerve innervates flexor pollicus longus, flexor digitorum profundus (FDP) to the index finger and sometimes long finger, and pronator quadratus (PQ).
  - The remainder of the nerve is largely sensory, with a small motor component contributing to the recurrent motor branch, which innervates the thenar muscles (abductor pollicus brevis, opponens pollicus, and the superficial head of flexor pollicus brevis) and the two radial lumbricals.
  - The sensory contribution is to the volar surface of the thumb, index, long, and radial half of the ring and to the dorsal aspect of those digits distal to the distal interphalangeal joint.

- Patients presenting with a median nerve injury will have:
  - Numbness in the distribution of the median nerve and depending on the level of injury, motor deficits will vary.
  - Distal forearm injury: the primary deficits will be thumb abduction and opposition.
  - Proximal forearm injuries: the patient will also have loss of pronation, thumb flexion and index (and possibly long) finger flexion. Flexion of the wrist will be present with ulnar deviation, due to the intact FCU function provided by the ulnar nerve. Similarly, finger flexion to the ring and small fingers will be retained because of the ulnarly innervated preserved FDP function.

Hints and tips

Priorities with median nerve injury are to re-establish anterior interosseous nerve (AIN) function, thumb opposition, index and long finger flexion, and critical sensation to the first webspace. A combination of nerve and tendon transfers can be done. For reconstruction of proximal median nerve injuries, radial to median nerve transfers are used. For reconstruction of more distal median nerve or isolated AIN injuries, brachialis to AIN branch transfers can be done. This transfer is also useful for patients with lower plexus injuries.

Specific operative techniques

Use of radial to median branch nerve transfers (motor)

- Branches of the radial nerve may be used to restore median nerve function in a proximal median nerve injury.
  - Transfer of the extensor carpi radialis brevis branch (ECRB) of the radial nerve is used to restore PT function.
  - Transfer of the supinator branch is used to restore anterior interosseous nerve (AIN) function ***(Fig. 22.12)***.
  - Recovery of pronation occurs approximately 3–4 months postoperatively.

Use of brachialis branch to AIN branch nerve transfer

- The brachialis branch of the musculocutaneous nerve may be used to restore AIN function ***(Fig. 22.13)***.
- The LABC nerve is identified traveling with the cephalic vein, and a tug test is used to confirm the identity of this cutaneous nerve. The LABC is followed proximally to its branch point from the musculocutaneous nerve where the nerve to brachialis is identified medially approximately 13 cm proximal to the elbow crease ***(Fig. 22.14)***.
- Knowledge of the internal topography of the median nerve is crucial to performing this transfer.
  - The lateral aspect of the median nerve is all sensory and the medial aspect is motor.
  - The AIN portion of the nerve is located at the deep medial aspect of the nerve.

Use of adjunct tendon transfers to augment nerve transfers

- Tendon transfers can be utilized to augment nerve transfers in median nerve injury. The most commonly performed tendon transfer would be to restore thumb opposition, as this is innervated by the most distal branches of the median nerve and will be slowest to recover.
  - The authors' preference for restoration of thumb opposition is transfer of extensor indicis proprius tendon to abductor pollicis brevis. Another option is to use extensor digiti minimi.

Ulnar nerve injury

Specific patient exam findings

- The ulnar nerve is a mixed motor and sensory nerve that receives contribution from C7, C8, and T1.
- There are no branches in the arm as the nerve courses medial to the brachial artery, dorsal to the medial intermuscular septum, and then posteriorly around the medial epicondyle.
- Branches of the ulnar nerve proper in the forearm include FCU and FDP to the ring and small fingers.
- The nerve then courses through the forearm deep to FCU and gives off the dorsal cutaneous branch approximately 9 cm proximal to the wrist crease providing sensation to the dorsal ulnar aspect of the distal forearm and hand. A superficial motor branch provides innervation to palmaris brevis.
- As the nerve courses into the wrist through Guyon's canal, it divides into a superficial sensory branch and a deep motor branch.
  - Superficial sensory branch: provides sensation to the small finger and the ulnar aspect of the ring finger.
  - Deep motor branch, which courses around the hook of the hamate under the tendinous leading edge of the hypothenar muscles and innervates the hypothenar muscles (flexor digiti minimi, opponens digiti minimi, and abductor digiti minimi), the palmar and dorsal interossei, the lumbricals to the small and ring fingers, the deep head of flexor pollicis brevis, and the adductor pollicus.
- Patients presenting with an ulnar nerve injury will have:
  - Numbness in the sensory distribution of the ulnar nerve and depending on the level of injury, sensation to the dorsum of the hand and wrist may also be affected.
  - The motor deficits associated with ulnar nerve injury are particularly devastating.
  - The deep motor branch of the ulnar nerve innervates all of the intrinsic muscles of the hand, and injury results in the inability to pinch, abduct and adduct the fingers, and impairs power grasp.
  - More proximal injuries will also further impair grip, with added losses of FDP to the small and ring fingers and FCU.

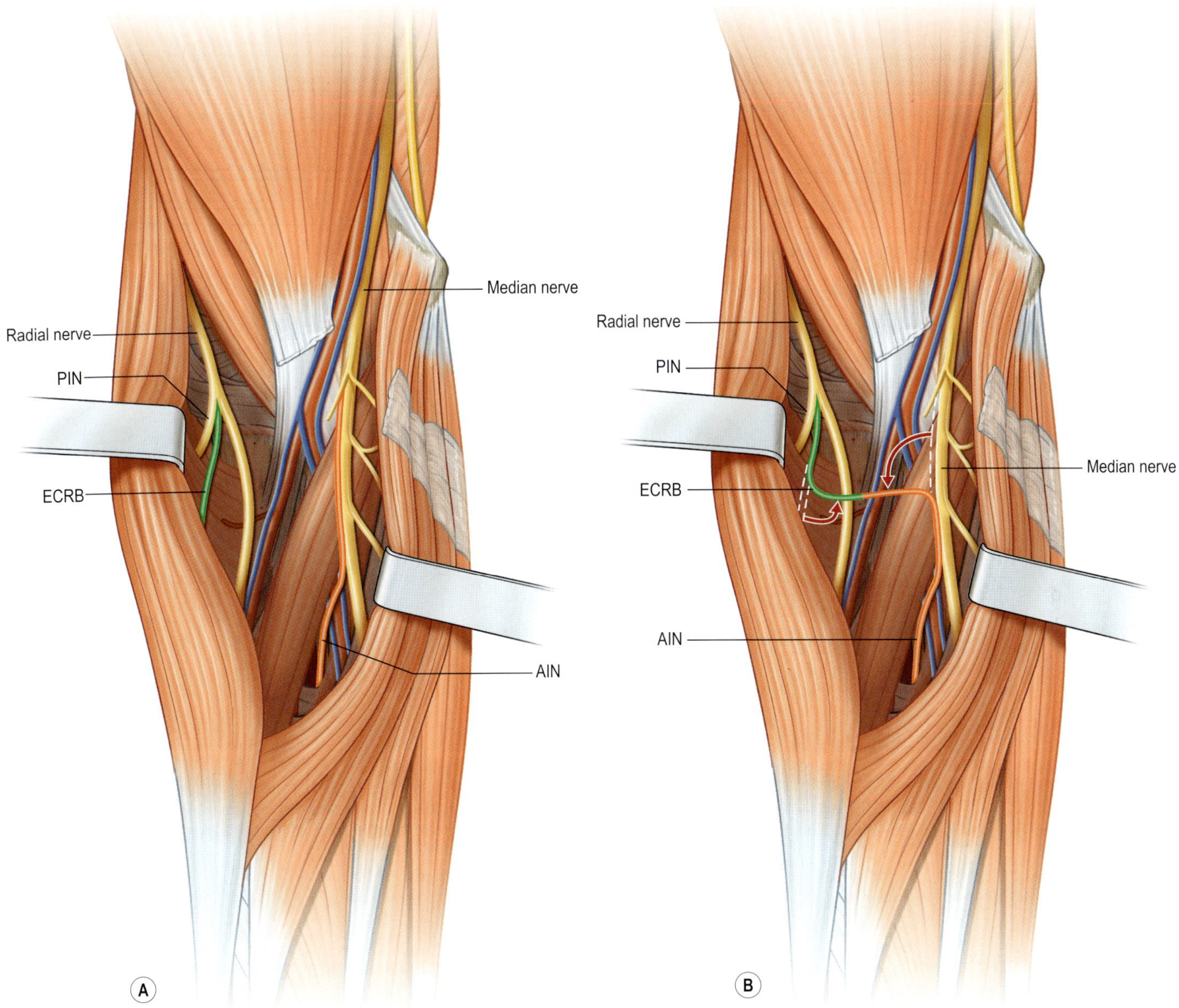

Figure 22.12 A schematic of radial to median nerve transfers. **(A)** The radial nerve is visualized superiorly as it branches into three branches, from lateral to medial: posterior interosseous nerve (PIN), extensor carpi radialis brevis (ECRB), and radial sensory. The donor ECRB nerve is green. The median nerve is visualized inferiorly, with the non-functioning anterior interosseous nerve (AIN) illustrated branching off the lateral aspect of the nerve (red). Note that the AIN is the only branch to exit radially. **(B)** The donor ECRB has been coapted end to end with the distal recipient AIN nerve.

> **Hints and tips**
>
> Priorities for ulnar nerve injury are to re-establish intrinsic muscle function, especially pinch, ring, and small finger flexion, and critical sensation to the ulnar border of the hand. A combination of nerve and tendon transfers can be done. For reconstruction of proximal nerve injuries, a direct end-to-end anterior interosseous nerve (AIN) to deep motor branch of ulnar nerve transfer is useful. For incomplete, or partial, nerve injuries where level of recovery is uncertain, reverse end-to-side AIN to deep motor branch "supercharging" should be considered.

Specific operative techniques

Use of median to ulnar branch nerve transfers (motor)

- The median nerve may be used to restore ulnar nerve function, especially following very proximal injuries where time to regenerate to motor end plate becomes an issue.
  - Both sensory and motor nerve transfers are utilized to restore optimal function.
  - For restoration of intrinsic muscle function, the distal AIN nerve is transferred to the deep motor branch of the ulnar nerve at the distal forearm level *(Fig. 22.15)*.

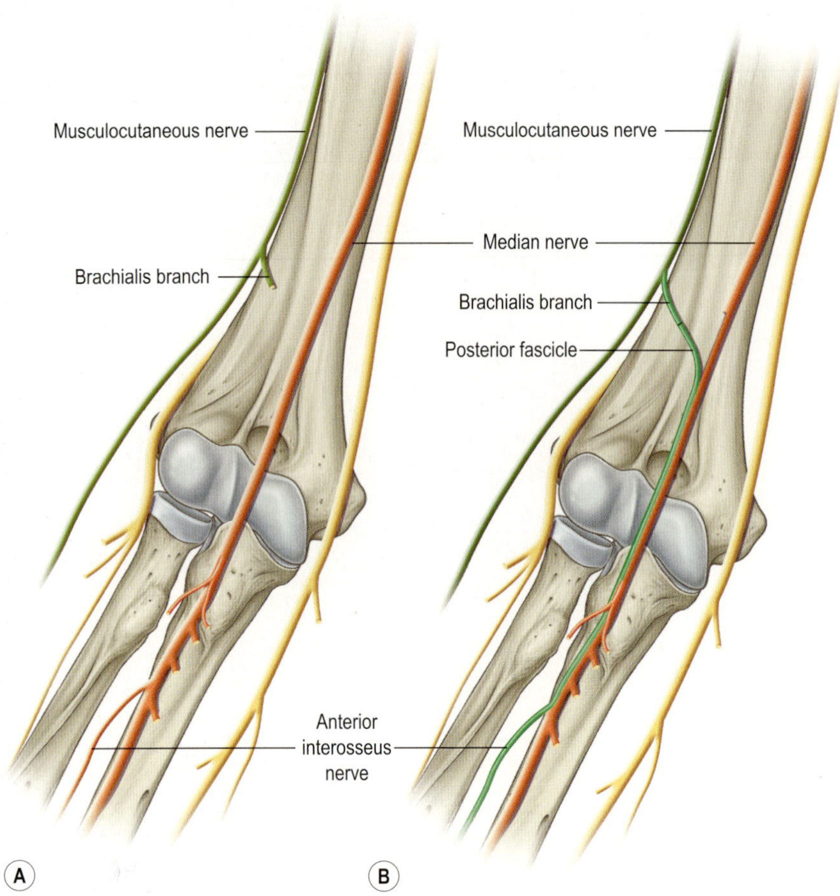

Figure 22.13 A schematic of the nerve to brachialis to anterior interosseous nerve transfer. **(A)** The median nerve (red) and musculocutaneous nerve (green) are shown in their normal anatomic position. Note that the branch to brachialis exits medially approximately 13 cm to the elbow crease. **(B)** The brachialis branch of the musculocutaneous nerve (donor) is coapted end to end with the divided distal end of the anterior interosseous nerve (recipient), which is located on the medial and deep aspect of the median nerve.

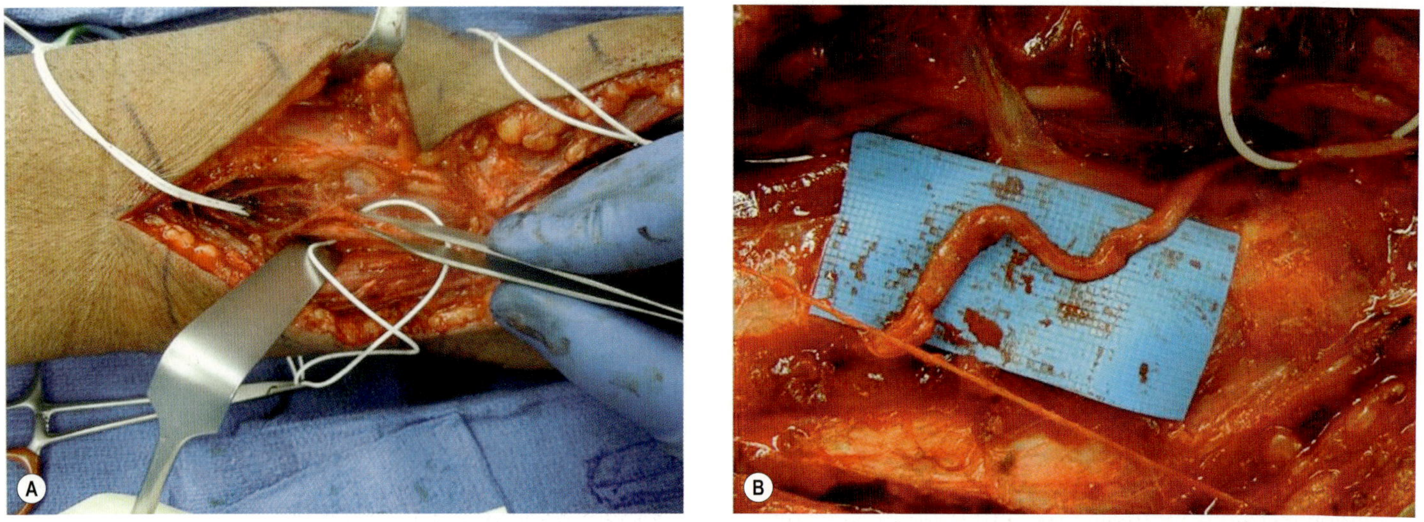

Figure 22.14 Clinical photos of nerve to brachialis to anterior interosseous nerve. A clinical example of a nerve to brachialis to anterior interosseous nerve (AIN) transfer. **(A)** The median nerve is isolated with a vessel loop. Forceps are used to reveal the AIN nerve branching off the radial aspect of the median nerve. **(B)** A magnified view illustrating the branch to brachialis (marked with a vessel loop) divided and transposed over, to be coapted end to end with the recipient distal AIN.

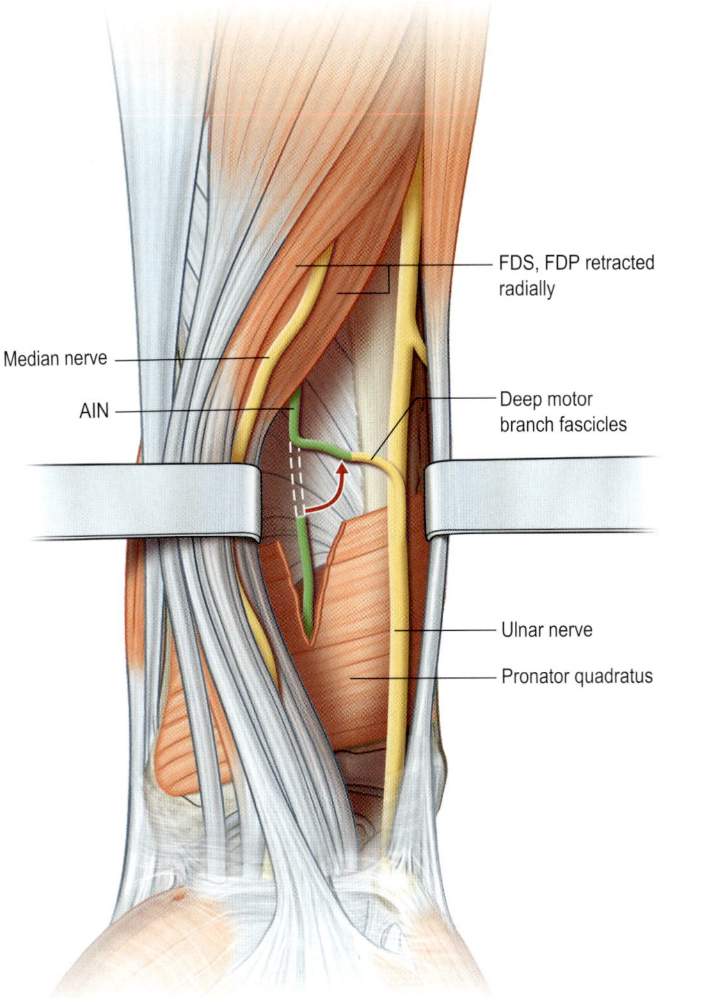

Figure 22.15 Anterior interosseous nerve (AIN) to deep motor branch of ulnar nerve. A schematic of the distal AIN to deep motor branch transfer. The donor AIN (green) is seen divided under the pronator quadratus muscle and transposed over to the recipient deep motor branch of the ulnar nerve. At this level, distal to the take off the dorsal cutaneous ulnar branch, the motor fascicles are ulnar and the main sensory component of the nerve is radial. The coaptation is performed in an end-to-end manner. FDS, flexor digitorum superficialis; FDP, flexor digitorum profundus.

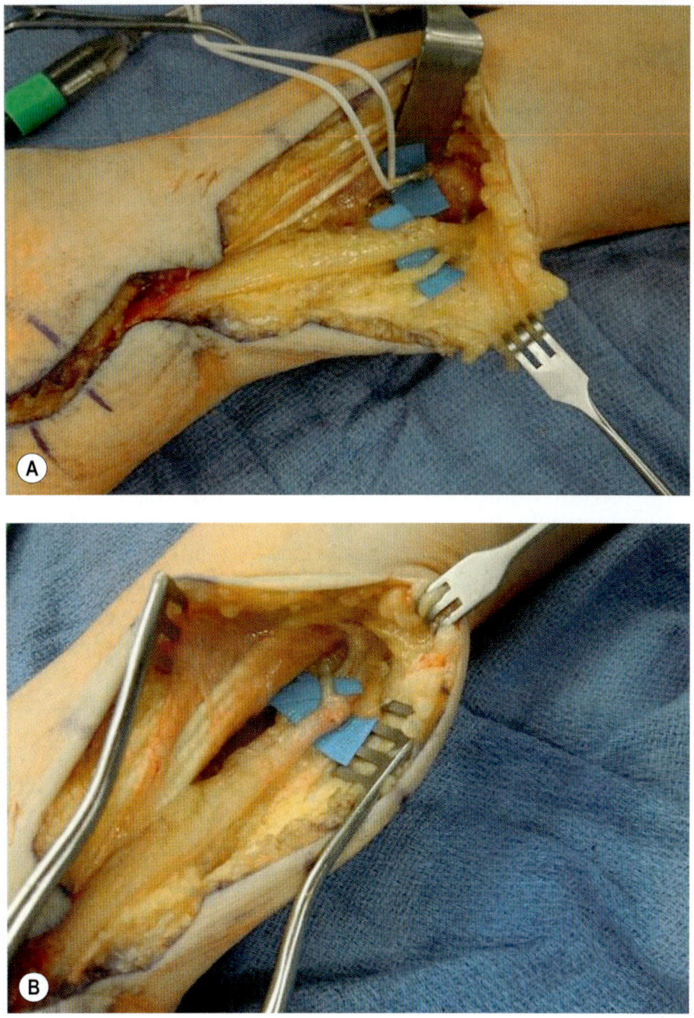

Figure 22.16 Clinical photos of anterior interosseous nerve (AIN) to deep motor branch of ulnar nerve. Clinical example of an AIN to deep motor branch nerve transfer. **(A)** A vessel loop surrounds the distal AIN. The ulnar nerve is exposed on a blue background. The dorsal cutaneous ulnar branch is illustrated branching off ulnarly. **(B)** The donor AIN is divided distally and transposed over to the ulnar nerve. The dorsal cutaneous branch of the ulnar nerve is now located beneath the blue background, and a motor fascicle from the ulnar aspect of the main nerve is divided as the recipient and coapted end to end to the AIN nerve.

- Release of the nerve through Guyon's canal, with particular attention to adequate release of the deep motor branch, is an essential component of this transfer *(Fig. 22.16)*.

Use of adjunct tendon transfers to augment nerve transfers

- Tendon transfers are frequently performed to augment median to ulnar nerve transfers. The intrinsic muscles are so distal and are so important for function that these tendon transfers are often performed at the same time as the nerve transfers, even though their use might be considered redundant.
  - Tenodesis of the ulnar nerve-powered ring and small FDP tendons to the median nerve-powered index and long FDP tendons is performed.
  - Thumb adduction is also augmented using extensor indicis proprius to adductor pollicus tendon transfer.
  - In patients with a prominent Wartenburg's sign, abductor digiti minimi is transferred to the extensor digitorum communis tendon of the small finger.

Radial nerve injury

Specific patient exam findings

- The radial nerve is a mixed motor and sensory nerve that receives contribution from C5, C6, C7, C8, and T1.
- In the axilla, the radial nerve gives off the posterior cutaneous nerve of the arm. It then provides innervation

to the three heads of the triceps muscle before piercing the lateral intermuscular septum and coursing through the spiral groove.

- In the distal arm, there are branches to anconeus epitrochlearis and brachioradialis as the nerve crosses the elbow between brachialis and brachioradialis.
- The extensor carpi radialis longus (ECRL) is the last branch of the radial nerve proper.
- The nerve then branches into the posterior interosseous nerve (PIN), which continues distally into the arm, passing between the superficial and deep heads of the supinator at the arcade of Froshe, and the radial sensory branch.
  - The radial sensory branch: innervates the dorsoradial aspect of the forearm and wrist, and the dorsal aspect of the thumb, index, long, and radial half of the ring finger.
  - The PIN: innervates the remainder of the muscles on the extensor aspect of the forearm, including ECRB, supinator, extensor carpi ulnaris, extensor indicis proprius, extensor digitorum communis, extensor digiti minimi, abductor pollicus longus, extensor pollicus longus, and extensor pollicus brevis.
- Patients presenting with radial nerve injuries will have:
  - Sensory defects in the distribution of the radial nerve, as described above and motor deficits will depend on the level of injury.
  - Injury at the level of the PIN: results in the inability to extend thumb and fingers, with weak, radially deviated wrist extension powered primarily by the ECRL.
  - More proximal injury: results in complete loss of wrist extension in addition to loss of thumb and finger extension.

Hints and tips

Priorities with radial nerve injury are to re-establish wrist, finger, and thumb extension. Unlike tendon transfers, use of median to radial nerve transfers allows for individual and separate finger extension in addition to wrist and thumb extension.

Specific operative techniques

Use of median to radial branch nerve transfers

- The deficit created by radial nerve injury can be corrected with median nerve transfers. Primary goals include restoration of wrist, finger, and thumb extension.
  - The most commonly performed transfers include using redundant fascicles to FDS or FCR as donors to provide innervation to PIN and ECRB *(Fig. 22.17)*.

Use of adjunct tendon transfers to augment nerve transfers

- The authors suggest augmenting median to radial nerve transfers with tendon transfer of PT to ECRB during the same procedure. This transfer provides earlier restoration of wrist extension, which is then enhanced once the nerve transfer becomes viable at 9–12 months.

Sensory nerve injury

Restoration of key sensory functions

- Restoration of discriminatory sensation in critical areas can be accomplished using non-critical area donors. One of the newer developments in nerve transfer surgery is to maintain some donor territory protective sensation by use of adjunct end-to-side transfers. A number of studies have demonstrated that "collateral sprouting" occurs with an end-to-side sensory repair, and novel axonal regeneration from the donor nerve occurs into the recipient stump.

Specific operative techniques

Use of ulnar to median branch nerve transfers (sensory)

- The first webspace is an area of critical sensation as it is primarily used for pinch.
- A fourth webspace (ulnar) to first webspace (median) nerve transfer can be performed to restore first webspace sensation only. Alternatively, a triad of nerve transfers from the ulnar nerve can restore more extensive sensation and minimize donor deficits *(Figs 22.18, 22.19)*.

Use of median to ulnar branch nerve transfers (sensory)

- A third webspace (median) to ulnar small-finger nerve transfer can be used to restore sensation to the ulnar border of the hand. Alternatively, restoration of ulnar nerve sensation can be provided by a triad of nerve transfers from the median nerve *(Figs 22.20, 22.21)*.

Use of median and ulnar nerve transfers to restore first webspace sensation in C5–C6 root level brachial plexus injury (sensory)

- In patients with an isolated upper-trunk injury, sensation to the first and second webspaces will be absent. A combination of distal transfers at the level of the median and ulnar nerve proper can be used to reconstruct this deficit *(Fig. 22.22)*. The third webspace nerve is dissected out from the median nerve, transected, and coapted end to end to the radial aspect of the median nerve to restore thumb and first webspace sensation. The distal end of the transected third webspace is coapted end to side to the ulnar nerve to restore protective sensation of the donor site. This effectively transfers intact sensation that originated from the C7 and C8 roots to the C5 and C6 level at a close-to-target end organ level.

Use of lateral antebrachial cutaneous nerve to radial nerve transfers (sensory)

- Coaptation of the expendable LABC to the denervated radial sensory nerve territory may not restore

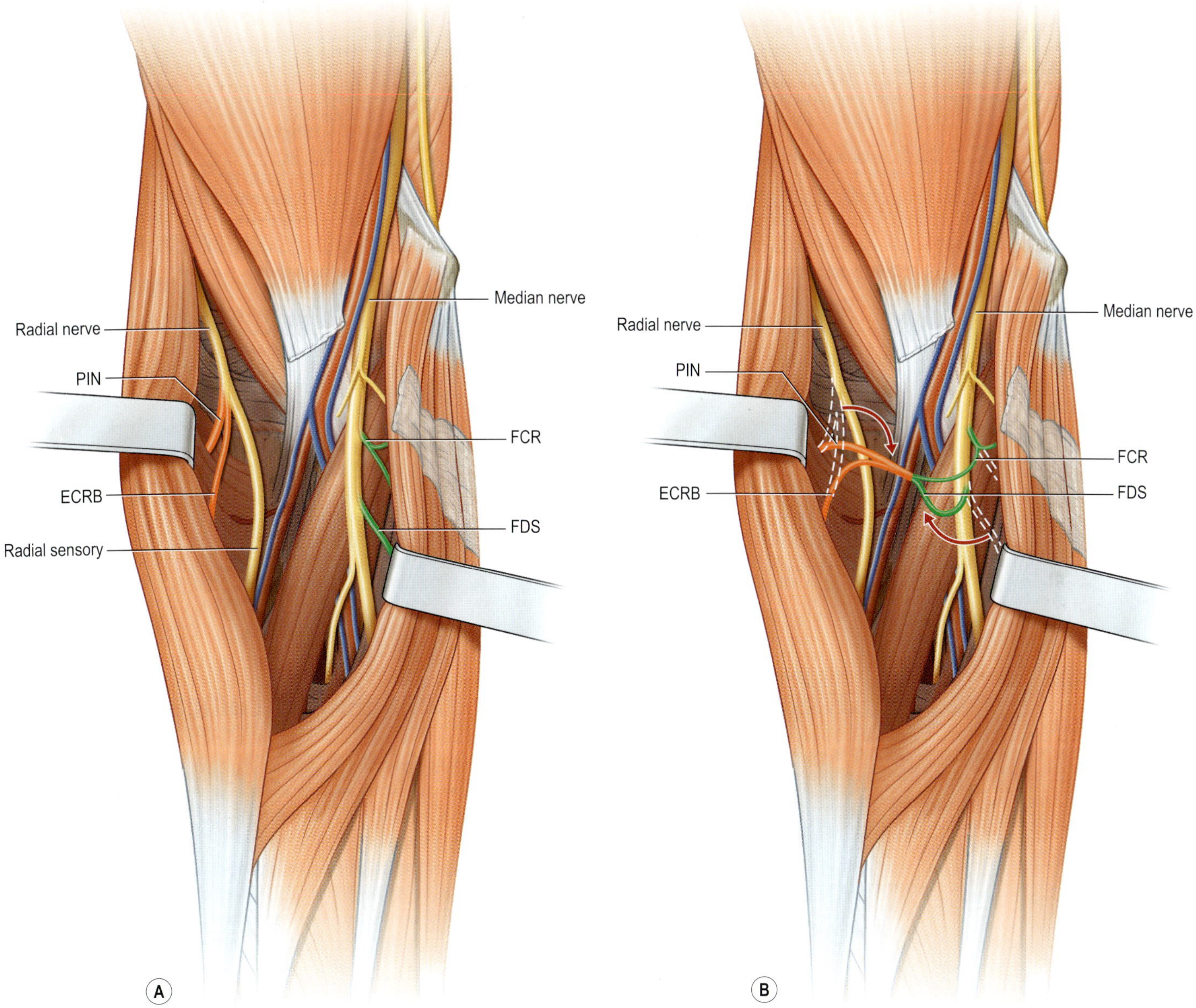

Figure 22.17 Median to radial nerve transfers. A schematic diagram of median to radial nerve transfers. The redundant fascicles to flexor carpi radialis (FCR) and flexor digitorum superficialis (FDS) (donors) are transferred to the extensor carpi radialis brevis (ECRB) and posterior interosseous nerve (PIN) respectively.

completely normal sensation, but can significantly interrupt the neuropathic pain cycle and reduce phantom pain.

Use of radial to axillary nerve transfers (sensory)

- Patients with axillary nerve injury have numbness on the lateral aspect of the shoulder. To re-establish sensation in this distribution, the axillary nerve can be transferred end to side to a functioning intact nerve such as the radial. At this level, the internal topography of the radial nerve is such that the lateral aspect is sensory.

Postoperative considerations

- Patients are encouraged to move their extremity early to promote nerve gliding, as all nerve transfers are performed under no tension.
- Protective splinting for distal nerve transfers is maintained for approximately 7–10 days, although patients come out of their splints for therapy.
- Concomitant tendon transfers may also dictate splinting and therapy regimens and will supersede

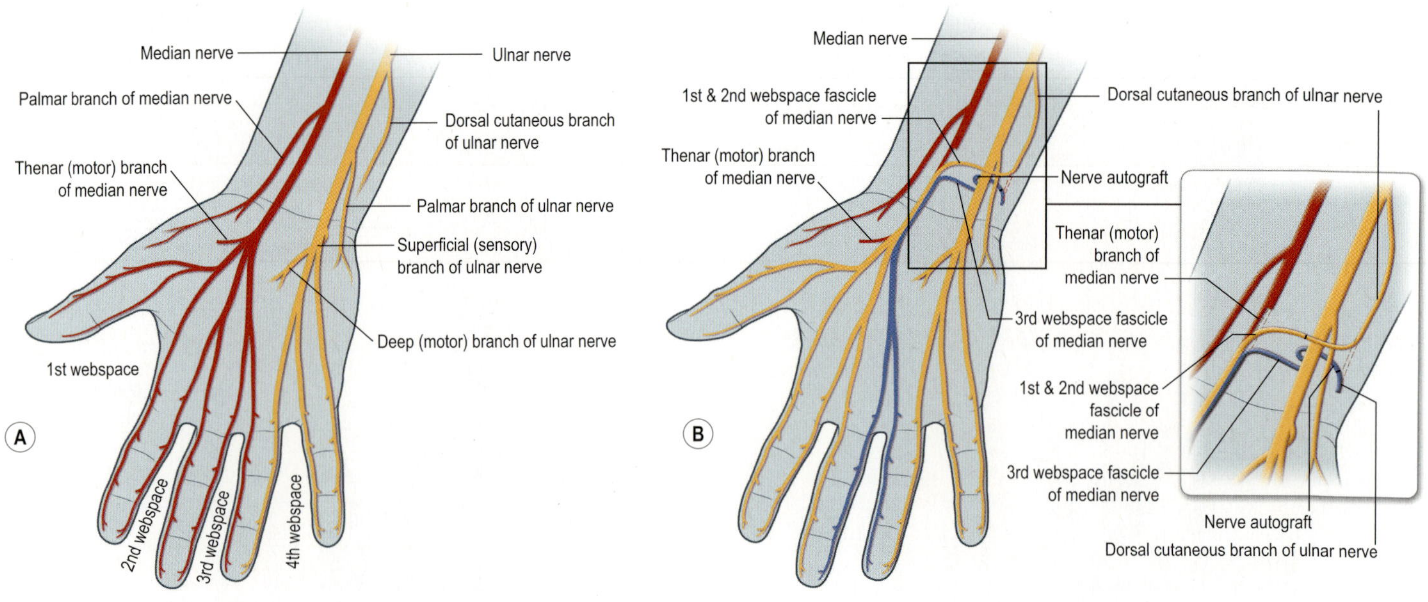

Figure 22.18 A schematic of the triad of transfers used to restore sensation in a median nerve deficit. **(A)** The non-functional median (red) and the functioning ulnar nerve (yellow). **(B)** The triad of nerve transfers from ulnar to median (inset) is a magnification of the transfers showing the dorsal cutaneous branch of the ulnar nerve (donor) coapted end to end to the radial side of the median (recipient) to restore first webspace sensation, the distal third webspace (recipient) end to side to the ulnar sensory (donor), and the distal dorsal cutaneous branch of the ulnar nerve end to side to restore sensation to the donor deficit. The third webspace fascicle is shown in blue.

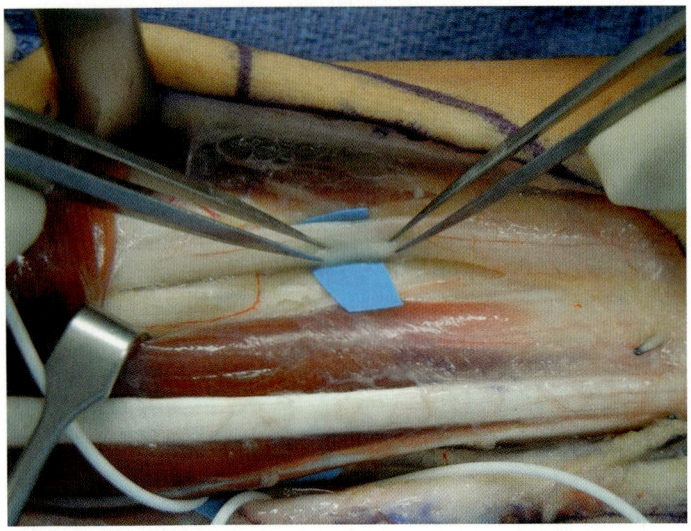

Figure 22.19 Identifying the fascicle to the third webspace. This clinical photograph demonstrates identifying the third webspace fascicle at the proximal wrist level. Microforceps were walked along the surface of the nerve until they plunged into the natural cleavage plane. The division is also marked with a prominent vessel on the surface of the nerve.

the minor restrictions required for postnerve transfer patients.

- If the insertion of the pectoralis major muscle was disinserted to allow access to the medial pectoral nerve, the tendon is reapproximated and the shoulder is immobilized for a full 4 weeks.

Complications and outcomes

- Complications specific to nerve surgery include temporary neurapraxia secondary to retraction or manipulation of nerves, neuroma, and inadequate functional recovery.
- The long-term focus of rehabilitation is on re-education, as the cortical command required to initiate target muscle function will differ from before. Hand therapists are critical for rehabilitation in these patients.
- The patient will "relearn" motor control of the reinnervated target muscle by activating the nerve to the donor muscle, similar to the re-education required following tendon transfer.
- For restoration of sensation, as patients perceive input stimulus from the reinnervated territory, cortical remapping occurs.
- Prior to reinnervation, the focus is on maintaining full active and passive range of motion and on prevention of pain syndromes related to musculoskeletal imbalances associated with lost or impaired muscle strength. Maintaining full passive range of motion throughout is paramount.
- Once reinnervation has occurred, therapy is focused on strengthening.
- It is difficult to compare different surgical approaches with regard to patient outcome and prognosis; however, there have been numerous articles reporting favorable outcomes on an increasing number of nerve transfer options.

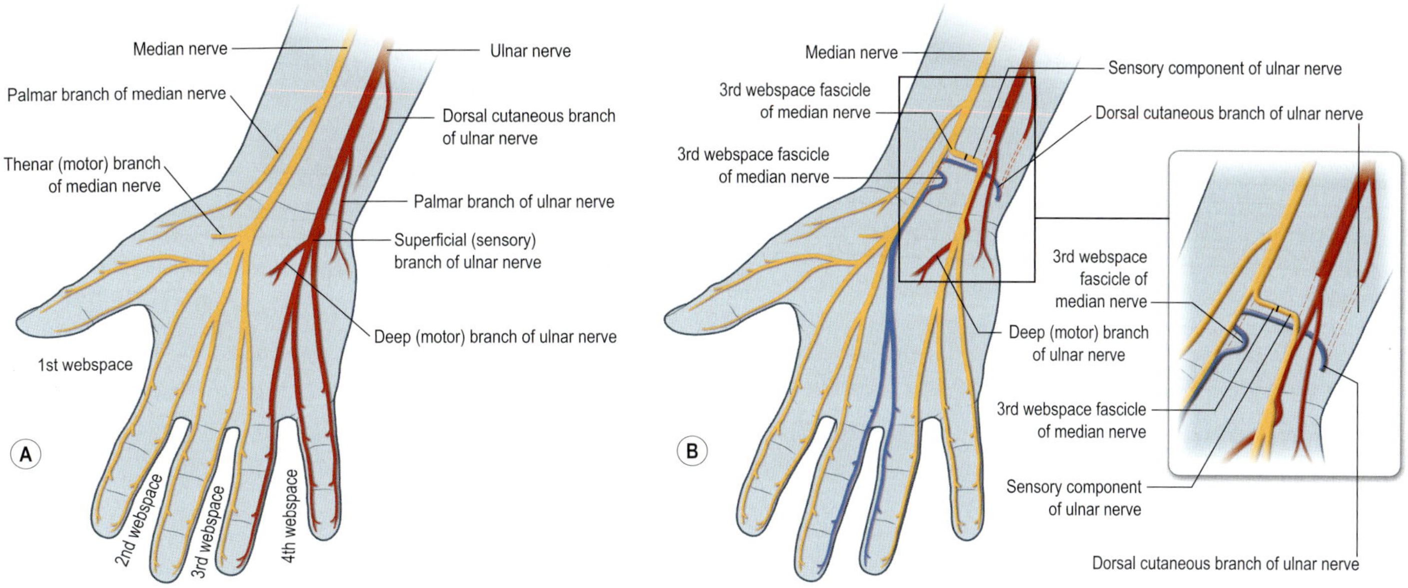

Figure 22.20 Sensory nerve transfers to restore ulnar nerve deficit. A schematic of the triad of nerve transfers used to restore ulnar nerve sensation. **(A)** The functioning median nerve is shown in yellow and the non-functioning ulnar nerve is shown in red. **(B)** The triad of nerve transfers to restore sensation. (Inset) A magnified view of the nerve transfers illustrating the third webspace fascicle (donor) coapted end to end with the ulnar sensory (recipient), the distal dorsal cutaneous branch of the ulnar nerve (recipient) coapted end to side to the sensory side of the intact median nerve (donor), and the distal third webspace nerve coapted end to side to the median sensory to restore donor sensory loss.

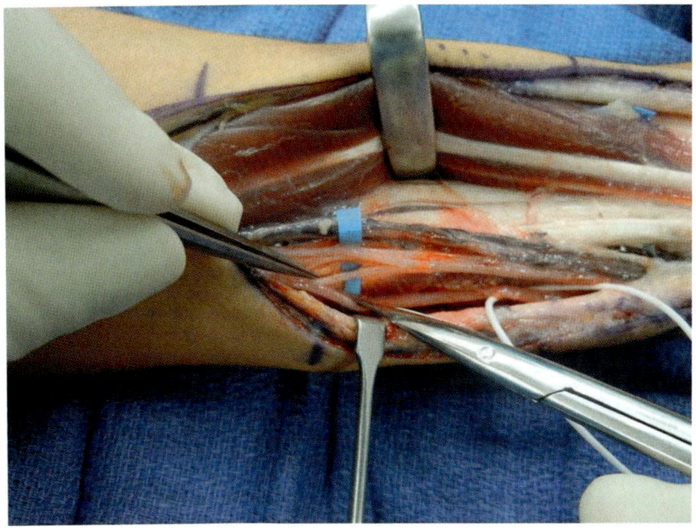

Figure 22.21 Internal topography of the ulnar nerve in the distal forearm. A clinical photograph illustrating the internal topography of a neurolyzed ulnar nerve at the wrist. The tenotomy scissors are displacing the dorsal cutaneous branch of the ulnar nerve ulnarly, the microforceps are separating the deep motor branch fascicles ulnarly, and the remainder of the radial portion of the nerve is sensory. At this level, the topography of the ulnar nerve is sensory–motor–sensory in a radial to ulnar direction.

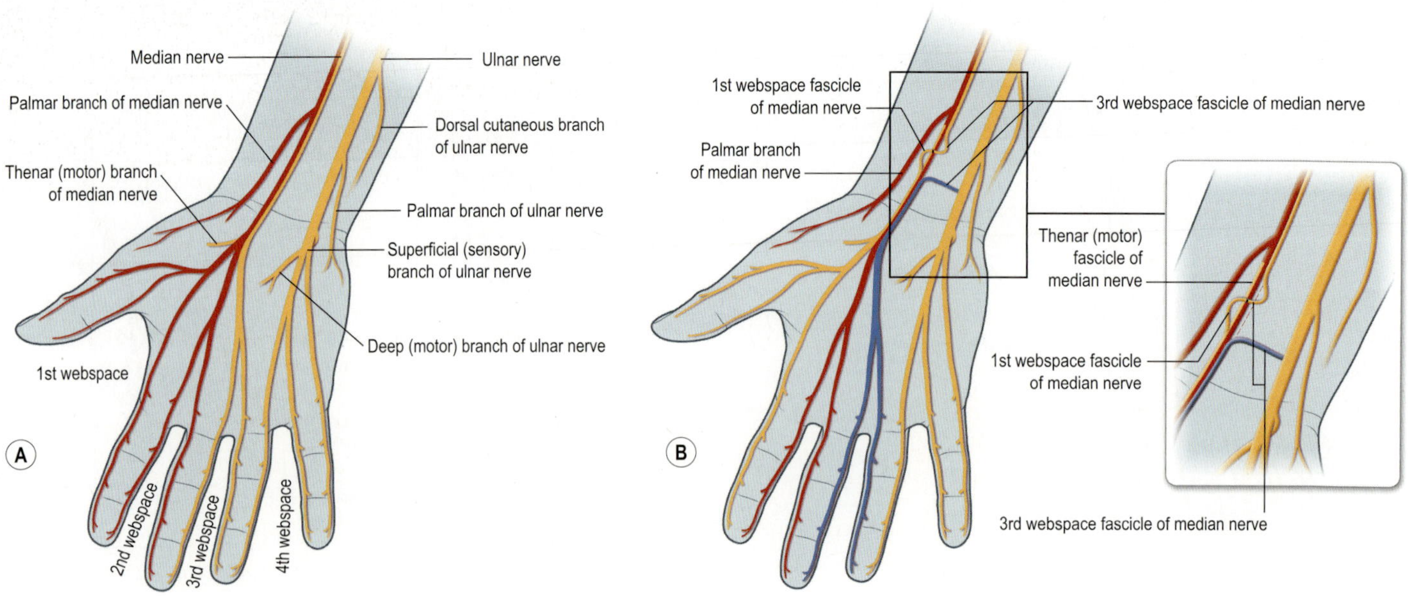

Figure 22.22 Sensory nerve transfers to restore C5/C6 deficit. A schematic of sensory nerve transfers used to restore sensation to the first webspace following C5/C6 root injuries of the brachial plexus. **(A)** The non-functional nerves are visualized in red and the functioning nerves are yellow. **(B)** The ulnar and median nerves are used to restore sensation to the first webspace and the radial border of the thumb. (Inset) A magnified view of the nerve transfers illustrating end-to-end coaptation of the third webspace nerve (donor) to the first webspace nerve (recipient). The distal third webspace nerve is then coapted end to side with the sensory portion of the ulnar nerve to restore sensation to the donor third webspace.

Further reading

Brown JM, Yee A, Mackinnon SE. Distal median to ulnar nerve transfers to restore ulnar motor and sensory function within the hand: technical nuances. *Neurosurgery*. 2009;65:966–977; discussion 977–978.

This is an up-to-date description of the technical nuances of transfer from the distal anterior interosseous nerve to the motor component of the ulnar nerve. This anterior interosseous nerve to deep motor branch of ulnar nerve was first done by the authors in 1991 and is generally accepted as a procedure of choice for high ulnar nerve problems.

Brown JM, Tung TH, Mackinnon SE. Median to radial nerve transfer to restore wrist and finger extension: technical nuances. *Neurosurgery*. 2010;66(3 Suppl):75–83; discussion 83.

Cheng CJ, Mackinnon-Patterson B, Beck JL, et al. Scratch collapse test for evaluation of carpal and cubital tunnel syndrome. *J Hand Surg Am*. 2008;33:1518–1524.

Hayashi A, Pannucci C, Moradzadeh A, et al. Axotomy or compression is required for axonal sprouting following end-to-side neurorrhaphy. *Exp Neurol* 2008;211:539–550.

This study demonstrated that sensory nerves would collaterally sprout from a normal nerve into a distal end-to side positioned nerve spontaneously. By contrast it showed that a motor nerve needed an injury in order to sprout (traumatic sprouting). This is a significant paper in that it shows that if you want to get some sensory recovery, then the end to side will work, but if you want motor, you need to injure the motor nerve traumatically in order to get it to sprout in an end-to-side fashion.

Kale SS, Glaus SW, Yee A, et al. Evaluation of the reverse end-to-side nerve transfer in an animal model. *J Hand Surg*. 2011 (in press).

Kozin SH. Injuries of the brachial plexus. In: Iannotti JP, Williams GR, eds. *Disorders of the Shoulder: Diagnosis and Management*. Philidelphia, PA: Lippincott Williams & Wilkins; 2007:1087–1130.

Mackinnon SE, Novak CB. Nerve transfers. *Hand Clin*. 2008;24:319–490.

This Hand Clinics is a multiauthored text covering all aspects of nerve transfers from surgical techniques to physical therapy.

Ray WZ, Mackinnon SE. Clinical outcomes following median to radial nerve transfers. *J Hand Surg Am*. 2010;36:201–208.

This manuscript describes the outcome of a number of patients undergoing median to radial nerve transfer and provides the technical nuances and the pearls and pitfalls of this nerve transfer.

Ray WZ, Mackinnon SE. Management of nerve gaps: autografts, allografts, nerve transfers, and end-to-side neurorrhaphy. *Exp Neurol*. 2010;223:77–85.

This summary review article outlines the key challenges in the reconstruction of nerve gaps, with critical points on the use of nerve autografts, allografts, nerve repairs, nerve transfers, and end-to-side repair.

Tung TH, Mackinnon SE. Nerve transfers: indications, techniques, and outcomes. *J Hand Surg Am*. 2010;35:332–334.

Chapter 23

Tendon transfers in the upper extremity

This chapter was created using content from Neligan & Chang, Plastic Surgery 3rd edition, Volume 6, Hand and Upper Extremity, Chapter 34, Tendon transfers in the upper extremity, Neil F. Jones.

SYNOPSIS

- Tendon transfers in the upper limb are indicated to restore function to paralyzed muscle and tendon following nerve injury, direct muscle or tendon injury, and to restore balance to hands affected by neurological disease.
- In selecting donor tissue, the surgeon has to consider expendability of the muscle–tendon unit, the native strength of donor and paralyzed muscle, and the direction of transfer and integrity of the muscle.
- The timing of tendon transfers can be classified as early, conventional or late.
- Upper extremity neurological injury can be subdivided into radial nerve palsy, low and high median nerve palsy, low and high ulnar nerve palsy, and combined nerve injuries.

Brief introduction

- There are three general indications for tendon transfers in the upper extremity:
  1. To restore function to a paralyzed muscle due to injuries of the peripheral nerves, the brachial plexus or the spinal cord
  2. To restore function following closed tendon ruptures or open injuries to the tendons or muscles
  3. To restore balance to a deformed hand due to various neurological diseases.

- Tendon transfers are best conceptualized as a means to restore a lost "function", rather than a means of substituting for a specific muscle, i.e., restoring strong pinch as opposed to restoring function of the flexor pollicis longus (FPL) (Table 23.1).
- Timing of tendon transfers may be classified as early, conventional or late.
- A conventional tendon transfer: usually performed after reinnervation of the paralyzed muscle fails to occur 3 months after the expected time of reinnervation based on the rate of nerve regeneration of 1 mm per day.
- Early tendon transfer: performed simultaneously with peripheral nerve repair or before the expected time of reinnervation of the muscle; serves as a temporary substitute for the paralyzed muscle until reinnervation occurs, by acting as an internal splint.

Preoperative considerations

- Before performing tendon transfers:
- All fractures should be healed.
  - Chronic scarred skin and subcutaneous tissues or skin grafts in the line of pull of a tendon transfer should be excised and the defect resurfaced with a flap that is itself allowed to heal with mature scars.
  - Full passive range of motion of the metacarpophalangeal (MCP) and proximal interphalangeal (PIP) joints should be achieved by physical therapy and dynamic splinting.
  - The donor muscle–tendon unit must be expendable. Its sacrifice must not create an important new deficit.
  - If multiple tendon transfers are required, a minimum of one wrist flexor, one wrist extensor, and one extrinsic flexor and extensor tendon to each digit should always be retained.

Table 23.1 Basic principles of tendon transfers
Soft tissue equilibrium
Full passive range of motion of involved joints
Adequate amplitude of donor muscle
Adequate excursion of donor muscle
Direct line of pull
Single function for each transferred tendon
Synergy of transfer

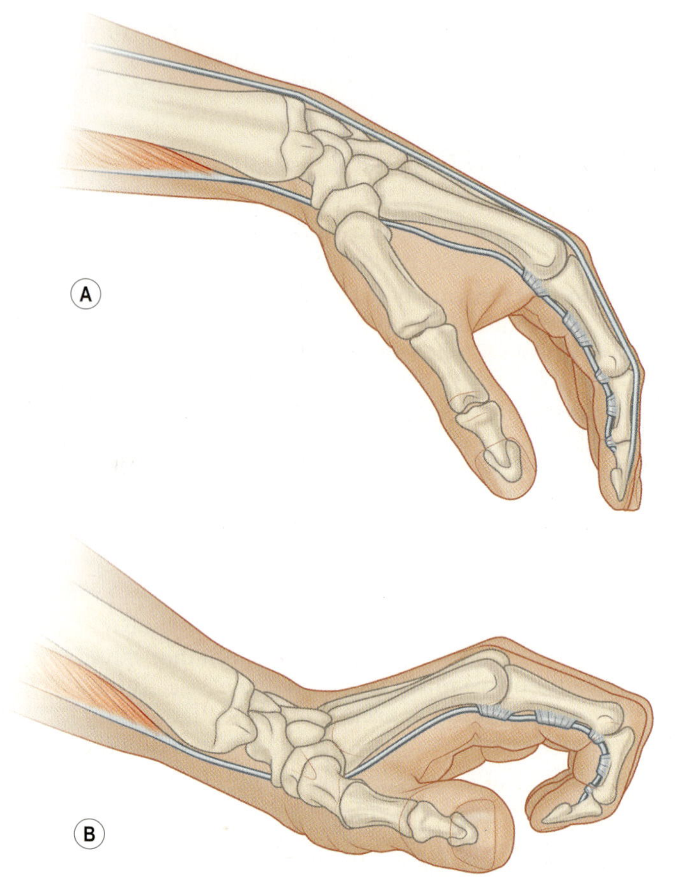

Figure 23.1 The wrist tenodesis effect: **(A)** Wrist flexion may increase the potential amplitude of a tendon transfer to restore finger extension by 25 mm. **(B)** Similarly wrist extension may increase the potential amplitude of a tendon transfer to restore finger flexion by 25 mm.

Anatomical/technical pearls

- The potential excursion of a donor muscle–tendon unit must be sufficient to restore the specific lost function.
- The finger flexors have an amplitude of 70 mm, the finger extensors 50 mm and the wrist flexors and extensors 33 mm (*Fig. 23.1*).
- The tenodesis effect of wrist flexion or extension may also increase the effective amplitude of a tendon transfer by 25 mm.
- Excursion of a donor muscle may also be increased by extensive release of its surrounding fascia.
- A tendon transfer should pass in a direct line from the origin of the donor muscle to its new insertion.
- Tendon transfers should only act across one joint and perform one single function.
- However, a transfer may be inserted into several recipient tendons as long as they each perform the same function in adjacent digits.
- The donor muscle selected should preferably be synergistic with the function of the muscle to be restored or at least be potentially retrainable.
- Every muscle in the forearm and hand should be tested by manual muscle testing to document which are functioning and their strength graded.
- From this list of functioning muscles, only those that are expendable are available as donor transfers.
- The specific functions of the hand that need to be restored are listed in order of priority.
- The final step is to match the available donor muscles with the functions that need to be restored, based on the force, amplitude and direction of the various muscles available.
- The success of any tendon transfer depends entirely on preventing scarring or adhesions along the path of the transferred tendon.
- Incisions should be carefully planned prior to elevation of the tourniquet so that the final tendon junctures lie transversely beneath skin flaps rather than lying immediately beneath and paralleling the incisions.
- The donor muscle should be carefully mobilized to prevent damage to its neurovascular bundle which usually enters in the proximal third of the muscle.
- The transferred tendon should glide in a tunnel through the subcutaneous tissues and not cross bone devoid of uninjured periosteum or through small fascial windows.
- Only the distal end of the tendon should be grasped with surgical instruments and care taken to prevent desiccation of the tendon.
- Tendon junctures are performed using a Pulvertaft weave technique where possible.

Operative techniques for specific nerve injuries

Radial nerve palsy

- Functional motor deficit: inability to extend the wrist, inability to extend the fingers at the MCP joints and inability to extend and radially abduct the thumb (*Fig. 23.2*), and inability to stabilize the wrist with grip resulting in marked weakness in grip strength.
- Tendon transfers are required to provide wrist extension, extension of the fingers at the MCP joints and extension and radial abduction of the thumb.

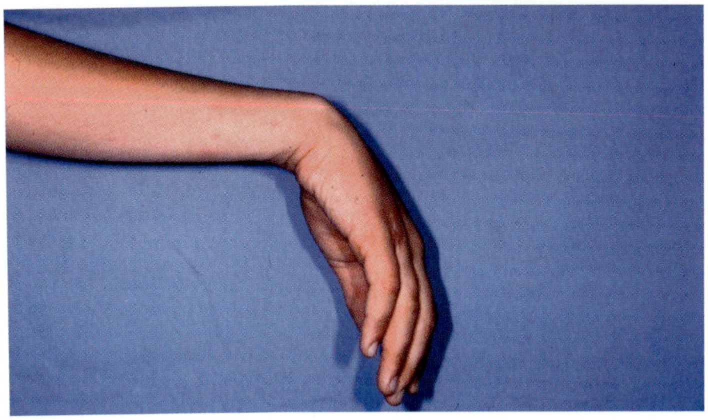

Figure 23.2 The typical posture of the hand and wrist of a patient with a high radial nerve palsy. The wrist cannot be extended. The fingers are extended through the tenodesis effect.

- Unlike the median and ulnar nerves, sensory loss following radial nerve injury is not functionally disabling unless the patient develops a painful neuroma.
- Timing of tendon transfers: remains controversial. Either "early" tendon transfer simultaneously with repair of the radial nerve to act as an internal splint to provide immediate restoration of power grip; or delay any tendon transfers until reinnervation of the most proximal muscles, brachioradialis and ECRL fails to occur within the calculated time limit.
- The more proximal the nerve injury, the less likely that functional muscle reinnervation will occur. If the nerve remains in-continuity, most surgeons would suggests that three months of observation are indicated to await spontaneous recovery in peripheral nerve palsies.

Specific operative techniques

- Several different tendon transfers have been reported for radial nerve palsy but three patterns of transfer have evolved.
- The use of pronator teres (PT) to provide wrist extension has become universally accepted, the only remaining controversy being whether to insert pronator teres into extensor carpi radialis brevis (ECRB) alone or into both extensor carpi radialis longus (ECRL) and brevis.
- The three patterns of tendon transfer differ therefore only in the technique of restoring finger extension and thumb extension and radial abduction (Table 23.2).

Standard flexor carpi ulnaris transfer

- This is the author's preferred technique for radial nerve palsy; in the patient with a PIN palsy, the FCR transfer is preferred *(Figs 22.3–22.7)*.

Flexor carpi radialis transfer

- See *(Fig. 22.8)*

Table 23.2 Tendon transfers for radial nerve palsy

Standard FCU transfer	FCR transfer	Boyes superficialis transfer
PT to ECRB	PT to ECRB	PT to ECRB
FCU to EDC	FCR to EDC	FDS of ring finger to EDC middle, ring, and small fingers
PL to EPL	PL to EPL	FDS middle finger to EIP and EPL
		FCR to APL & EPB

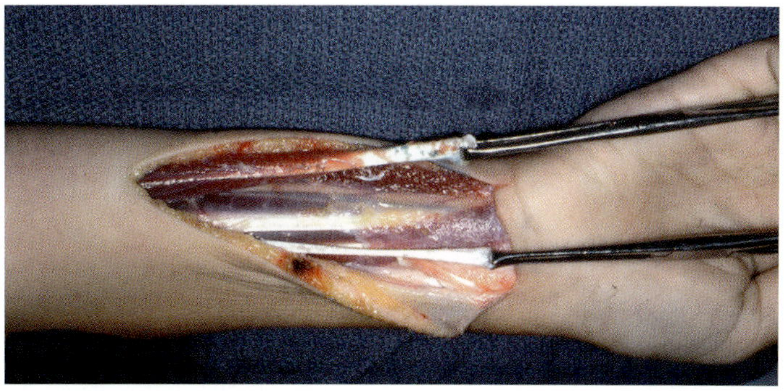

Figure 23.3 The FCU tendon and distal muscle are dissected. In this case, a palmaris longus was present and its tendon is dissected for later transfer to the EPL.

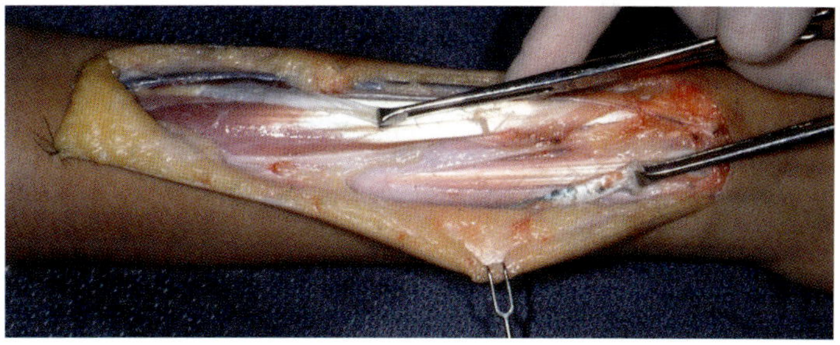

Figure 23.4 A dorsal incision exposes the wrist and finger extensors. The FCU tendon has been brought from palmar to dorsal, around the ulnar border of the forearm.

Boyes superficialis transfer

- Boyes advocated using the superficialis tendons to the long and ring fingers to act as donor tendons to restore finger extension.
- Advantages: potentially allow simultaneous wrist and finger extension, may allow independent thumb and index finger extension, does not weaken wrist flexion.
- Disadvantages: the long and ring fingers are deprived of superficialis function and this may result in weak grip, harvesting of the superficialis tendons may also lead to

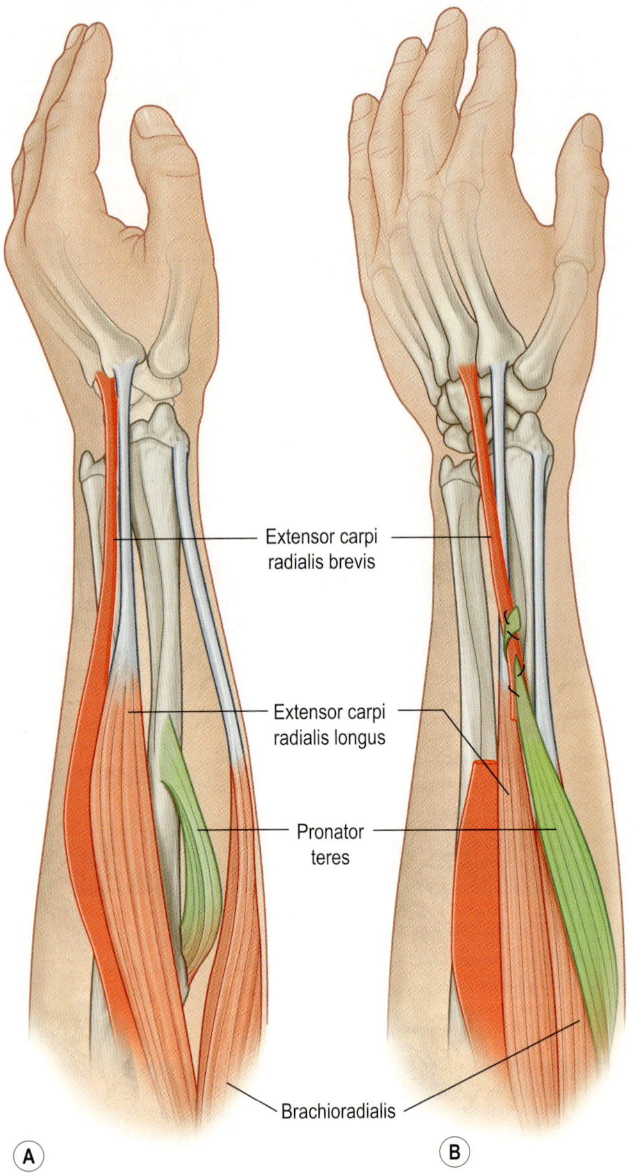

Figure 23.5 **(A)** The relatively short tendon of insertion of the PT can be extended by elevating a strip of periosteum. **(B)** The PT will be woven into the tendon of the ECRB.

the subsequent development of either a "swan neck" deformity or a flexion contracture at the PIP joint *(Fig. 22.9)*.

Low median nerve palsy (distal to innervations of the extrinsic forearm flexors)

- Functional deficit: loss of opposition of the thumb and absent sensation over the thumb, index, long and radial half of the ring finger.
- Opposition is a composite motion, which occurs at all three joints to position the thumb pad opposite the distal phalanx of the partially flexed long finger.
- Abduction, pronation and flexion occur at the carpometacarpal joint, abduction and flexion at the metacarpophalangeal joint and either flexion or extension at the interphalangeal joint.

Preoperative considerations

- Prior to any opposition transfer, patients with median nerve injuries should be instructed to prevent the development of an adduction or supination contracture of the thumb by a program of passive abduction exercises.
- If patients present with an established adduction or supination contracture of the thumb, release of the thumb-index finger web space skin, fascia over the first dorsal interosseous muscle or even the first dorsal interosseous and adductor muscles themselves may be required prior to any opposition tendon transfer.
- Opposition transfers that are directed along the radial aspect of the palm will produce a greater component of palmar abduction whereas transfers that pass from the pisiform will produce both abduction and pronation. The more distal the transfer passes across the palm, the greater the power of thumb flexion.
- Several methods of insertion of opposition transfers have been advocated; however, a biomechanical study has shown that opposition tendon transfers inserted into the APB tendon alone will produce full abduction and pronation. Therefore, the more complex dual insertions should probably be reserved for combined median and ulnar nerve palsies.
- Conventional timing of an opposition tendon transfer may only be required in those patients who fail to demonstrate signs of reinnervation within the usual calculated time interval.
- For older patients or those with poor prognostic co-morbid factors, early tendon transfers should be considered.
- Careful observation of thumb function following either a low or high median nerve palsy will reveal whether an "early" tendon transfer for thumb opposition is necessary.
- FPB remains innervated by the ulnar nerve in approximately 70% of median nerve injuries so that thumb function may not be significantly compromised. If the patient is able to pick up an object with the forearm in neutral or grasp an object with the forearm in supination, it is likely that FPB remains innervated by the ulnar nerve and consequently the decision for performing an "early" opposition tendon transfer can be delayed.
- If the surgeon or therapist observes the patient attempting to grasp objects by radial abduction of the thumb with the forearm in pronation, an "early" opposition tendon transfer should be strongly considered. Burkhalter extensor indicis proprius transfer.

Specific operative techniques

- The extensor indicis proprius (EIP) transfer is the author's preferred technique *(Fig. 23.10A,B*; Video 23.1), except in elderly patients with thenar atrophy secondary

Video 23.1

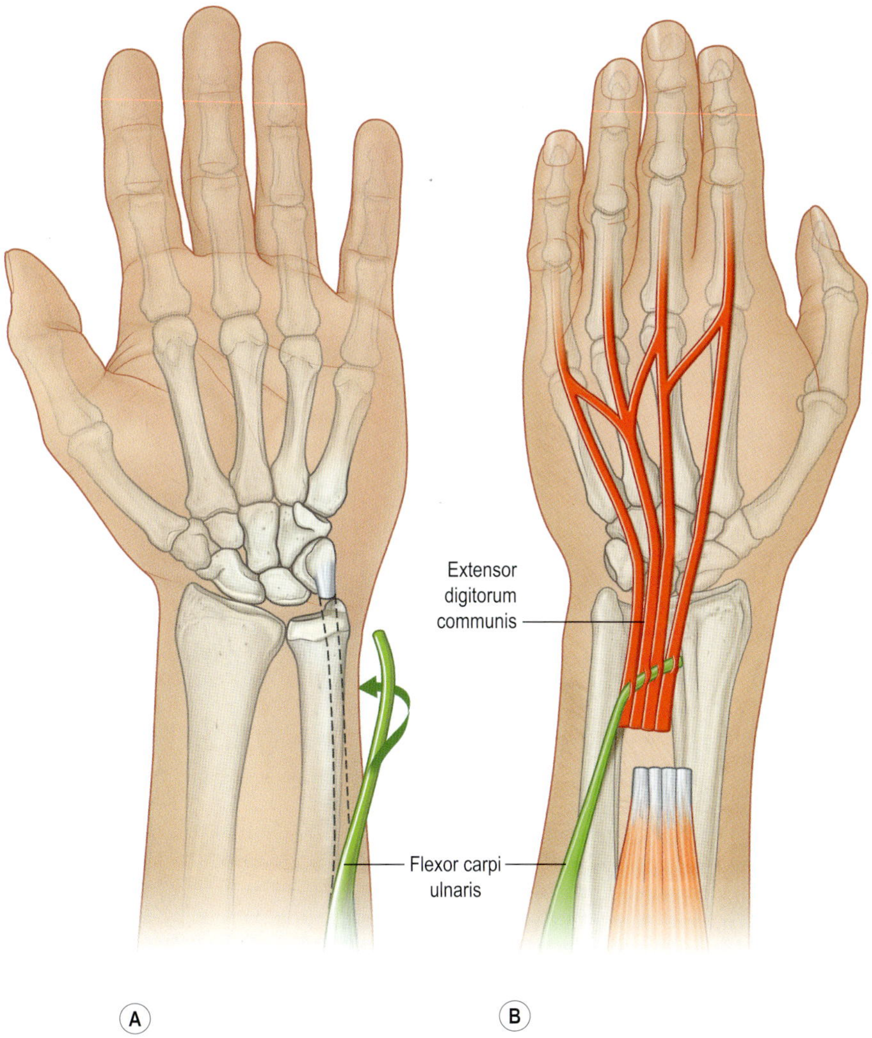

Figure 23.6 The FCU is brought around the ulnar border of the forearm **(A,B)** and woven into the combined tendons of the EDC.

to severe carpal tunnel syndrome *(Fig. 23.11)*. The only potential disadvantage with this tendon transfer is that the EIP tendon is only just long enough to reach the APB tendon. The postoperative results have been very predictable *(Fig. 23.12)*.

Bunnell ring finger flexor digitorum superficialis transfer

- Bunnell described using the ring finger superficialis tendon as the donor for opponensplasty *(Figs 22.13, 22.14)*.
- Compared with the EIP transfer, the ring finger superficialis is relatively stronger and has greater length.
- Contraindications:
  - High median nerve palsy or in low median nerve injuries in which there have been associated injuries to the flexor tendons.
  - Combined low median and high ulnar nerve palsies since the ring finger superficialis is the only remaining flexor tendon in the ring finger.
  - Low median–low ulnar nerve palsies as the ring finger superficialis may be required for correction of clawing.
  - Harvesting of the superficialis tendon may result in either a flexion contracture or a "swan-neck" deformity of the PIP joint of the donor finger.
- This is perhaps the strongest of the opposition transfers.

Camitz palmaris longus transfer

The PL tendon Camitz transfer is a simple transfer that will provide abduction of the thumb but little pronation or flexion and is particularly indicated in elderly patients with thenar atrophy due to long-standing carpal tunnel syndrome *(Figs 23.15, 23.16)*.

Other opposition tendon transfers

- Huber and Nicolaysen described transfer of the abductor digiti minimi (ADM) which may occasionally be indicated in patients with a combined median and radial nerve palsy and also in children with congenital anomalies affecting the thumb. Since the muscle originates at the pisiform, this transfer provides excellent flexion and pronation of the thumb but little palmar abduction.

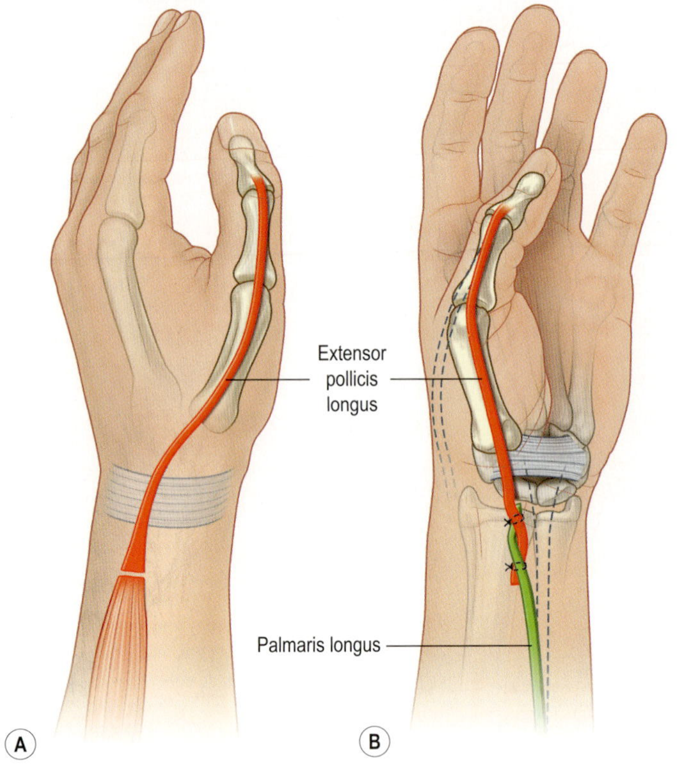

Figure 23.7 The PL, **(A)** if present, can **(B)** be attached to the rerouted EPL tendon to provide both thumb extension and some radial abduction.

- Phalen and Miller advocate the use of the EPB tendon graft activated by ECU.
- Taylor described the use of the extensor digiti minimi (EDM) which re-routes the EDM around the ulnar side of the hand to the thumb MCP joint.

High median nerve palsy (proximal to innervations of extrinsic forearm flexors)

- Functional deficit: inability to flex the index finger at the PIP and DIP joints and the thumb at the interphalangeal joint, loss of opposition *(Fig. 23.17)*.
  - Due to paralysis of all four FDS muscles, the FDP tendons to the index and long fingers and the FPL muscle.
- Patients are often still able to flex the long finger due to interconnections between the profundus tendons to the long, ring and small fingers in the distal forearm.
- The functions that need to be restored: flexion at the interphalangeal joint of the thumb and flexion of the PIP and DIP joints of the index and long fingers, and opponensplasty.

Specific operative techniques

- Flexion of the interphalangeal joint of the thumb may be restored by transfer of brachioradialis to FPL and flexion of the distal joint of the index and middle fingers by side-to-side tenodesis of the FDP II and III to IV and V *(Fig. 23.18)*.

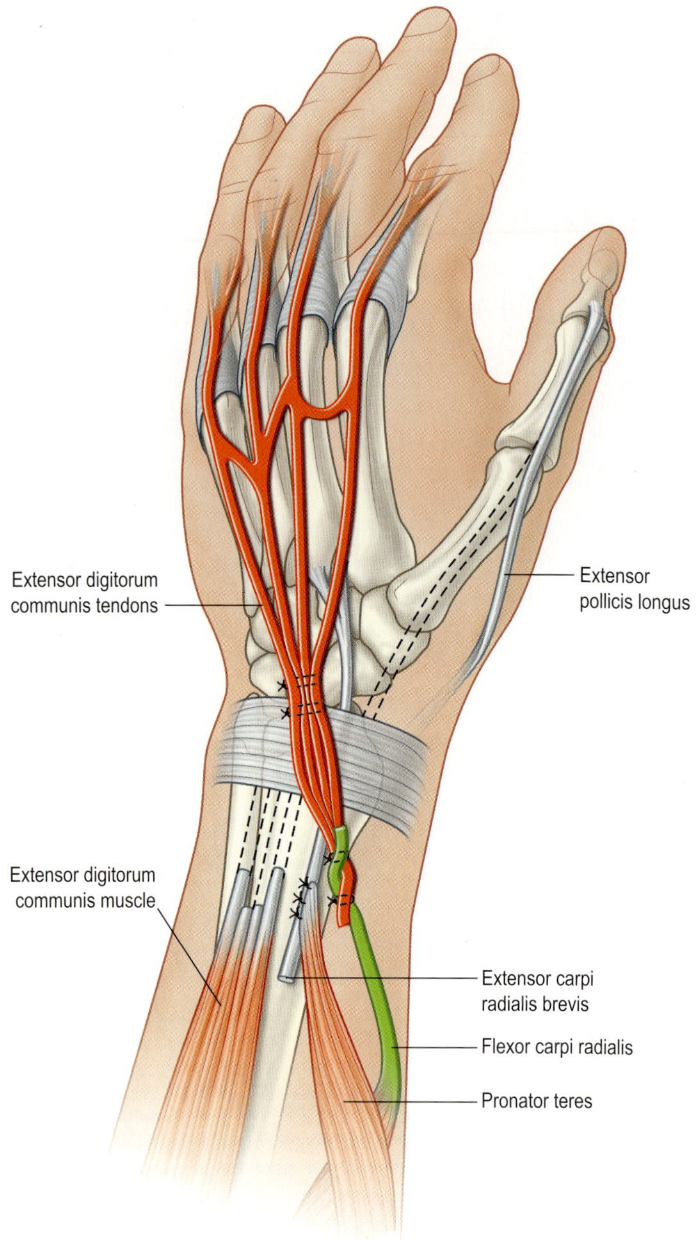

Figure 23.8 Transfer of the FCR to the combined tendons of the EDC.

- If reinnervation of the FPL muscle is not expected to occur following repair or grafting of the median nerve, the tendon can be divided at its musculotendinous junction and woven end-to-end into the brachioradialis tendon.
- However, if there is any possibility of reinnervation of FPL, the brachioradialis tendon should be woven end-to-side into the FPL tendon which remains in-continuity (see Fig. 23.18).
- If power flexion of the index and long fingers is required, then formal transfer of the ECRL tendon to the index and long finger profundus tendons may be performed *(Fig. 23.19)*.
- The timing of tendon transfers in a high median nerve palsy remains controversial.

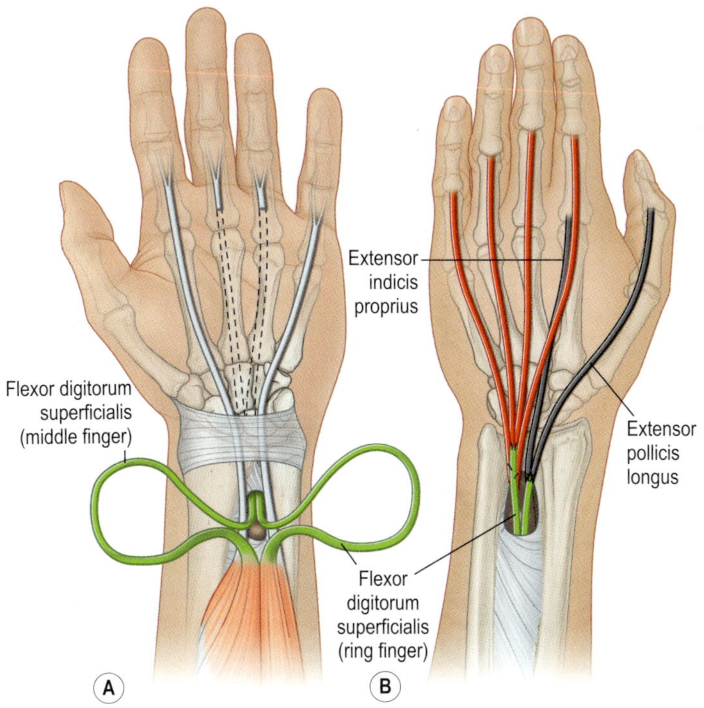

Figure 23.9 Transfer of the long and ring finger superficialis tendons (FDS_L, FDS_R) through a window in the interosseous membrane **(A)** to restore function to the extensor digitorum communis (EDC) tendons and extensor indicis proprius (EIP) and extensor pollicis longus (EPL) **(B)**.

- If a good primary or delayed primary nerve repair can be performed, there is a reasonable chance of reinnervation of the extrinsic flexor muscles in a young patient.
- If the patient is seen late and requires secondary nerve grafting of the median nerve, then tendon transfers for restoration of thumb flexion and index and long finger flexion should be performed simultaneously with the nerve graft.

Low ulnar nerve palsy (distal to the innervation of the ring and small finger FDP and FCU)

- Functional deficit: paralysis of all seven interossei, the ulnar two lumbricals, the hypothenar and the adductor pollicis (AP) and part of the flexor pollicis brevis (FPB) muscles.
- Results in an imbalance of the flexor and extensor forces at the MCP, PIP and DIP joints of the fingers to produce the claw hand appearance (hyperextension of the MCP joint and reciprocal flexion at the PIP/DIP joints – Duchenne sign).
- In a low ulnar nerve palsy, the clawing and loss of integrated MCP and interphalangeal joint flexion are confined to the ring and small fingers and to a lesser extent the long finger, since the lumbricals to the index and long fingers remain innervated by the median nerve.
- With a combined median and ulnar nerve palsy, all four fingers are affected.

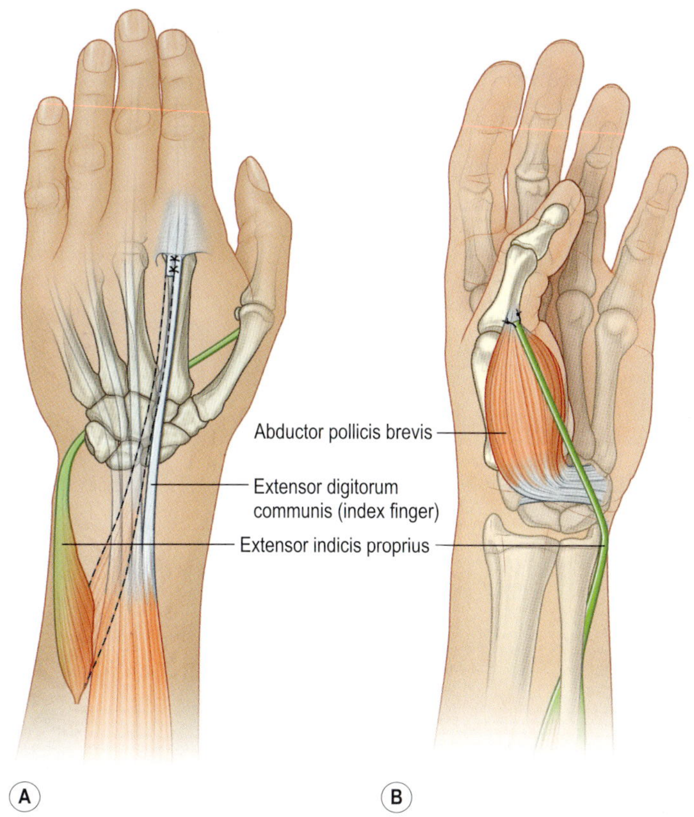

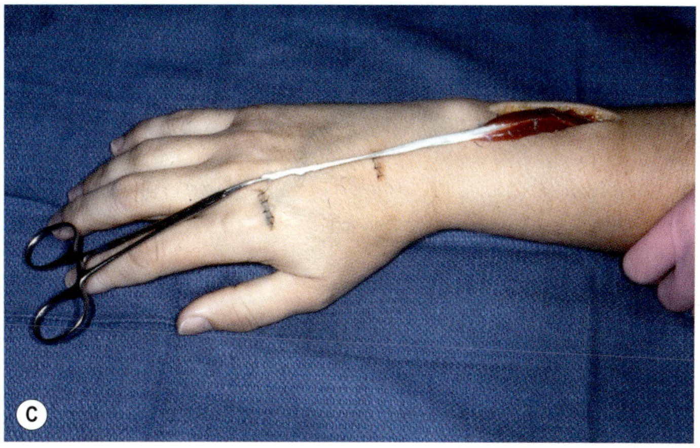

Figure 23.10 **(A,B)** The EIP transfer to restore opposition. **(C)** Incisions for harvesting the EIP tendon.

- Other significant impairment: weak thumb–index finger pinch, which may be only 20–25% of normal due to paralysis of the adductor pollicis, one half of the FPB and the first dorsal interosseous muscles.
- Loss of key pinch is usually manifest by compensatory activation of the FPL producing excessive flexion at the interphalangeal joint (Froment's sign) ***(Fig. 23.20)*** and occasionally hyperextension at the MCP joint (Jeanne's sign) as the patient attempts forceful pinch.
- In such patients with weak pinch, tendon transfers will be required to restore adduction of the thumb and abduction of the index finger.
- Patients may also develop an irritating ulnar deviation of the small finger in addition to clawing at the MCP joint

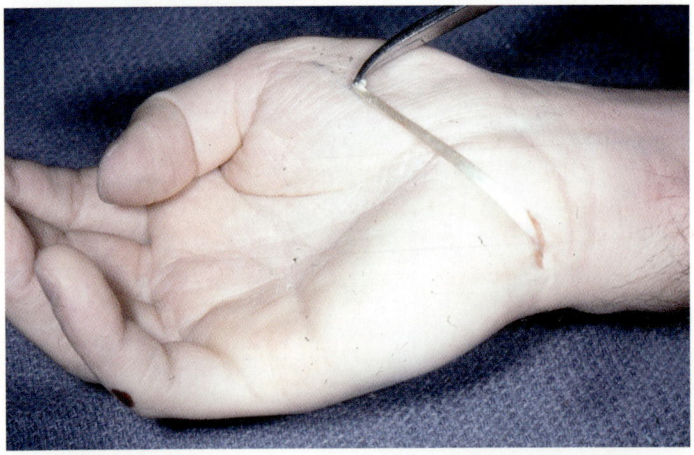

Figure 23.11 The palmar incision and the direction of the EIP transfer across the palm.

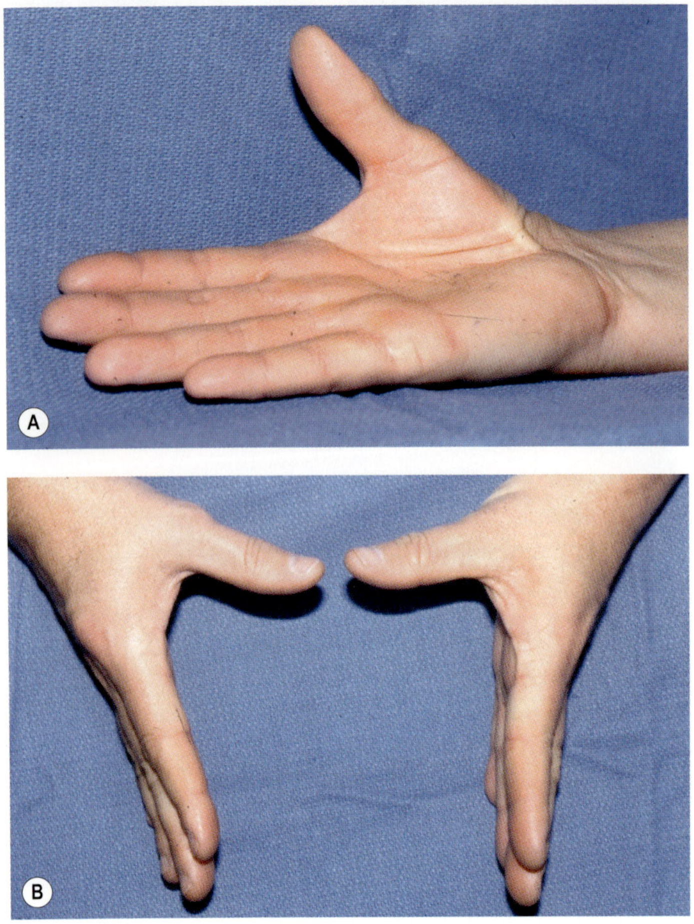

Figure 23.12 (A,B) Postoperative opposition restored by the EIP transfer.

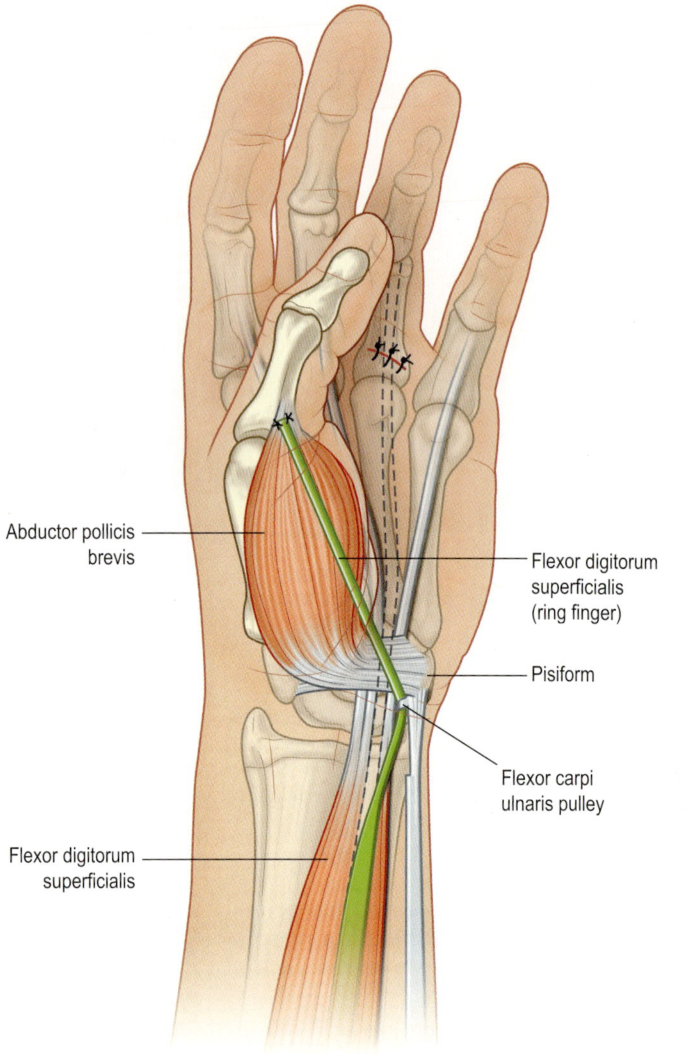

Figure 23.13 The FDS to APB transfer to restore thumb opposition is depicted schematically.

of the small finger (Wartenberg sign) caused by the unopposed action of the EDM tendon due to paralysis of the third palmar interosseous muscle.

- Occasionally, a tendon transfer may be required to correct this ulnar deviation of the small finger.
- Therefore, tendon transfers may be indicated in an ulnar nerve palsy (Table 23.3) to correct:
  - Clawing and asynchronous flexion of the fingers.
  - Weak thumb-index finger pinch.
  - Ulnar deviation deformity of the small finger.
  - Weak FDP flexion at the DIP joints of the ring and small fingers.
- Timing of tendon transfers for ulnar nerve palsy is primarily dependent on two factors: the probability of motor recovery and the severity of the functional deficit.
- Primary microsurgical repair of the ulnar nerve at the wrist can be expected to yield useful results in about 75% of patients.
- Secondary nerve grafting has been reported to provide some functional motor recovery in approximately 40–75% of cases, with a somewhat worse prognosis for sensory recovery.
- "Early" tendon transfers should be considered for those with a debilitating claw deformity.
- While clawing should be treated proactively using a lumbrical block splint, some patients may benefit from early static transfers to prevent MCP hyperextension and clawing.

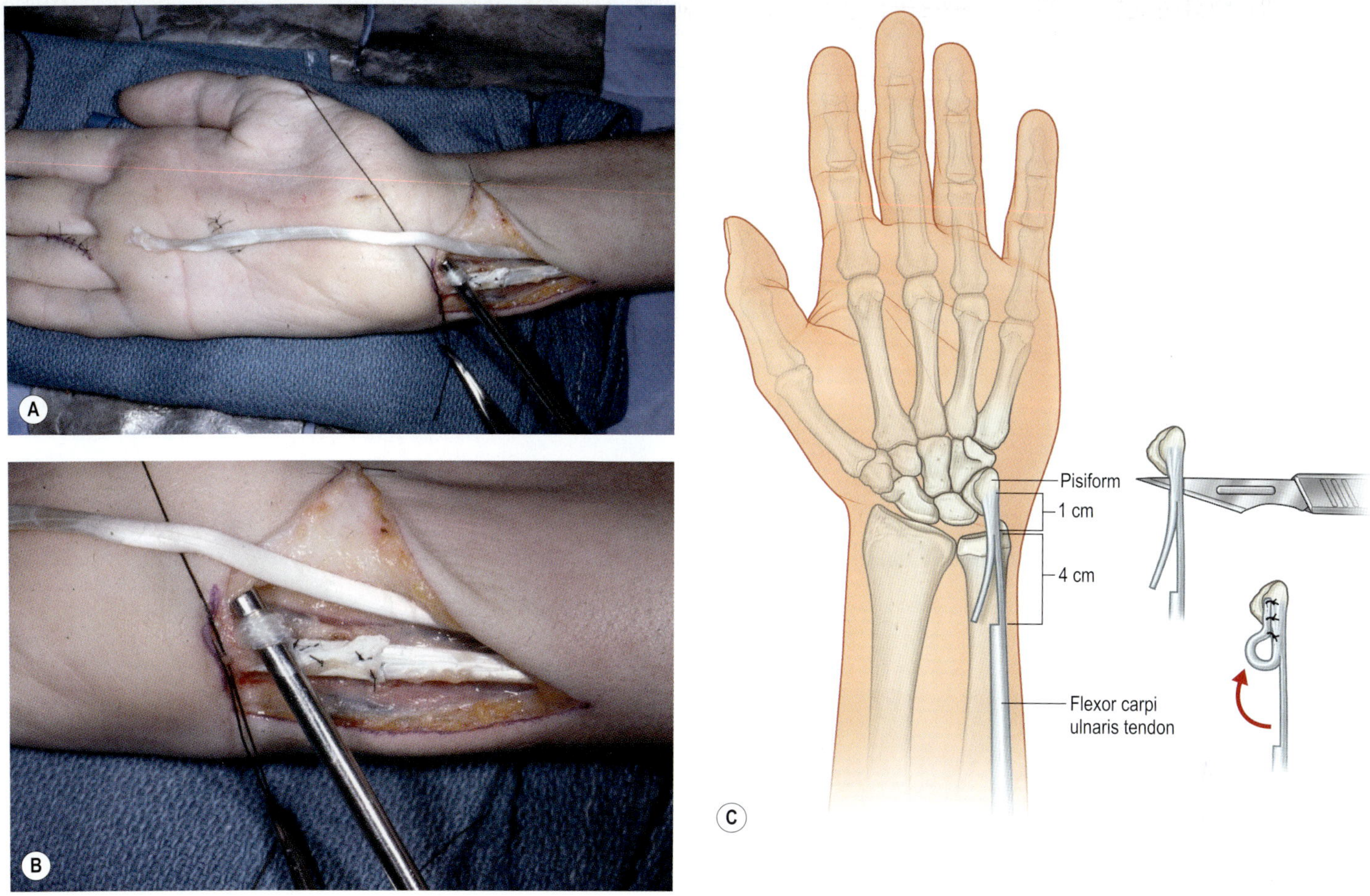

Figure 23.14 **(A)** Incisions used to transfer the ring finger FDS tendon. **(B,C)** The technique of using one half of the FCU sutured to itself as a pulley is demonstrated.

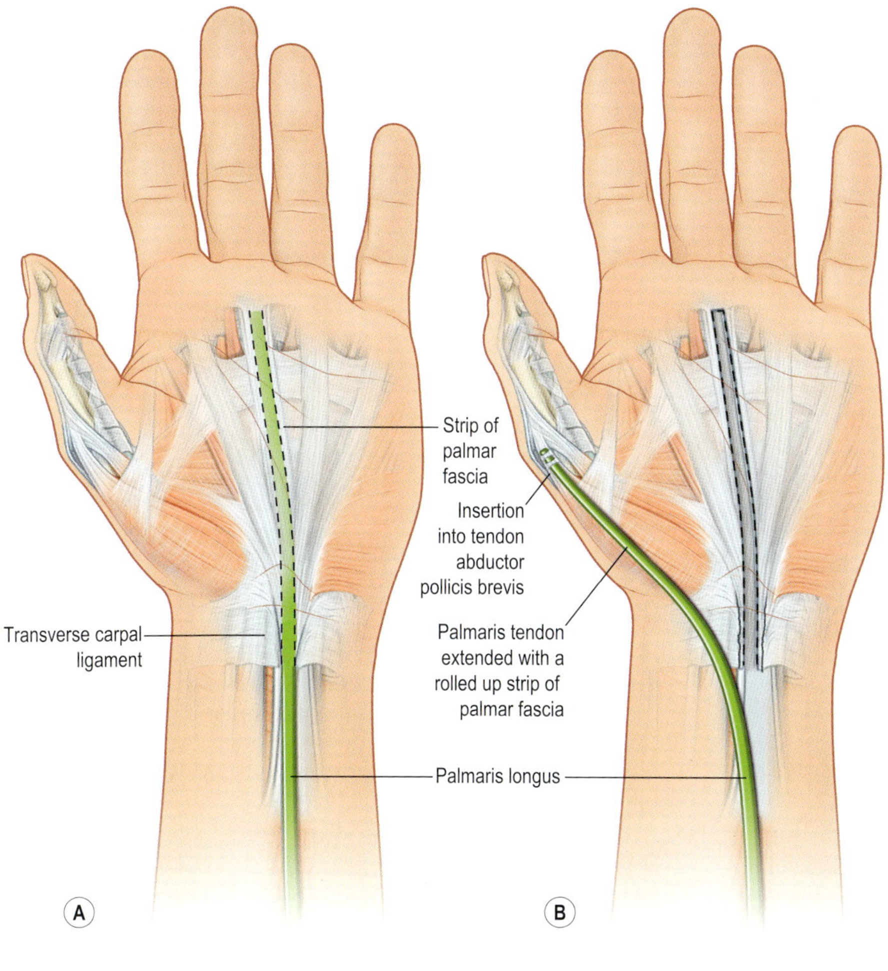

Figure 23.15 The Camitz transfer using the palmaris longus with its tendon extended by palmar fascia is depicted schematically.

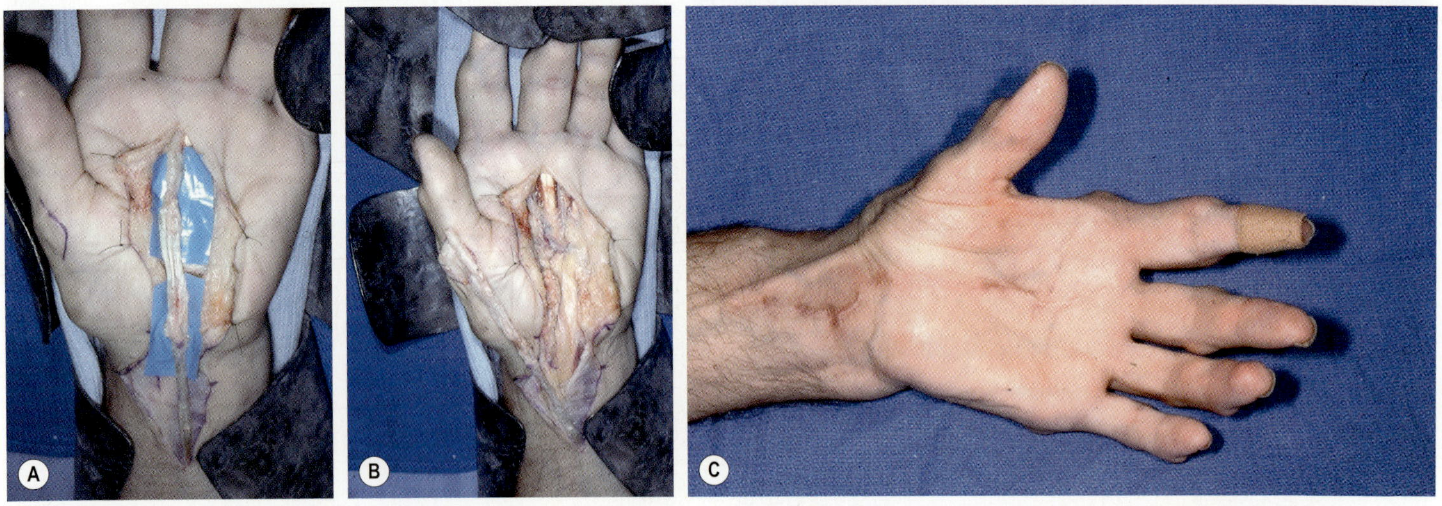

Figure 23.16 **(A)** A wide strip of palmar fascia is dissected in-continuity with the PL tendon. **(B)** This is transferred directly to be inserted into the tendon of APB. **(C)** Postoperative result of the Camitz transfer.

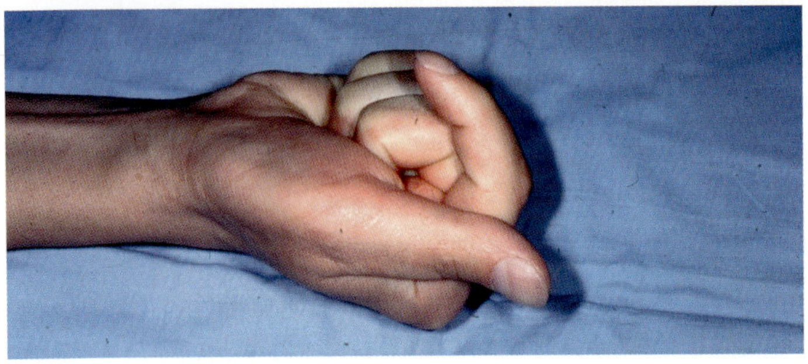

Figure 23.17 Inability to flex the interphalangeal joint of the thumb and the distal interphalangeal joint of the index finger as a consequence of a high median nerve palsy.

Specific operative techniques

- Static procedures to prevent hyperextension of the proximal phalanges at their MCP joints include A1 pulley release, fasciodermadesis at the MCP joint level, capsulodesis and various tenodeses.
- Capsulodesis of the MCP joint, described by Zancolli, is a very simple technique in which the A1 pulley is first released, the volar plate is incised longitudinally and detached from the metacarpal to create two distally-based flaps, which are then advanced proximally and attached to the metacarpal neck to maintain the MCP joint in approximately 20° of flexion ***(Fig. 23.21)***. Recurrence of clawing has been demonstrated in long-term follow-up studies.
- Parkes described an effective tenodesis by using tendon grafts sutured to the transverse carpal ligament and passed volar to the deep transverse intermetacarpal (intervolar plate) ligaments to insert into the radial lateral band of each finger.
- The various dynamic tendon transfers that have been described to correct clawing differ primarily as to whether they provide only MP joint flexion or whether they provide both MP joint flexion and interphalangeal joint extension. The surgeon can determine which general type of transfer is most appropriate by preoperative testing of PIP and DIP joint extension with the MCP joints held passively flexed – the Bouvier maneuver.
- If, with the MCP joints flexed, the extrinsic extensor tendons can produce full extension at the PIP and DIP joints ***(Fig. 23.22)*** the transfer may only need to produce strong MCP joint flexion by insertion of the transfer either into the A1 pulley (see Fig. 23.20), the A2 pulley ***(Fig. 23.23)***, the A1 and proximal half of the A2 pulley, or through a drill hole in the proximal phalanx (Fig. 23.23B).
- If the patient cannot actively extend the PIP joints using the extrinsic extensor tendons, then the transfer should be inserted into one of the lateral bands; or into the dorsal base of the middle phalanx; or into the combined interosseous tendons so that both MCP joint flexion and PIP joint extension can potentially be restored.

Tendon transfers to correct clawing

- All of the following have been described as the donor muscle–tendon unit in tendon transfers to correct asynchronous finger flexion and clawing in ulnar nerve palsy:
  - Flexor digitorum superficialis.
  - Extensor carpi radialis brevis.
  - Extensor indicis proprius and extensor digiti minimi.
  - Flexor carpi radialis.
  - Extensor carpi radialis longus.
  - Palmaris longus.

  (Fig. 23.24).
- In patients with a high ulnar palsy, the ring and small finger superficialis tendons cannot be used and therefore the middle finger superficialis tendon is divided into two slips and each slip is passed under the A1 pulleys of the ring and small fingers and sutured to itself (see Fig. 23.20).
- In combined high median-ulnar nerve palsy, all the superficialis tendons are paralyzed and consequently an "indirect lasso" procedure is required. After passing the

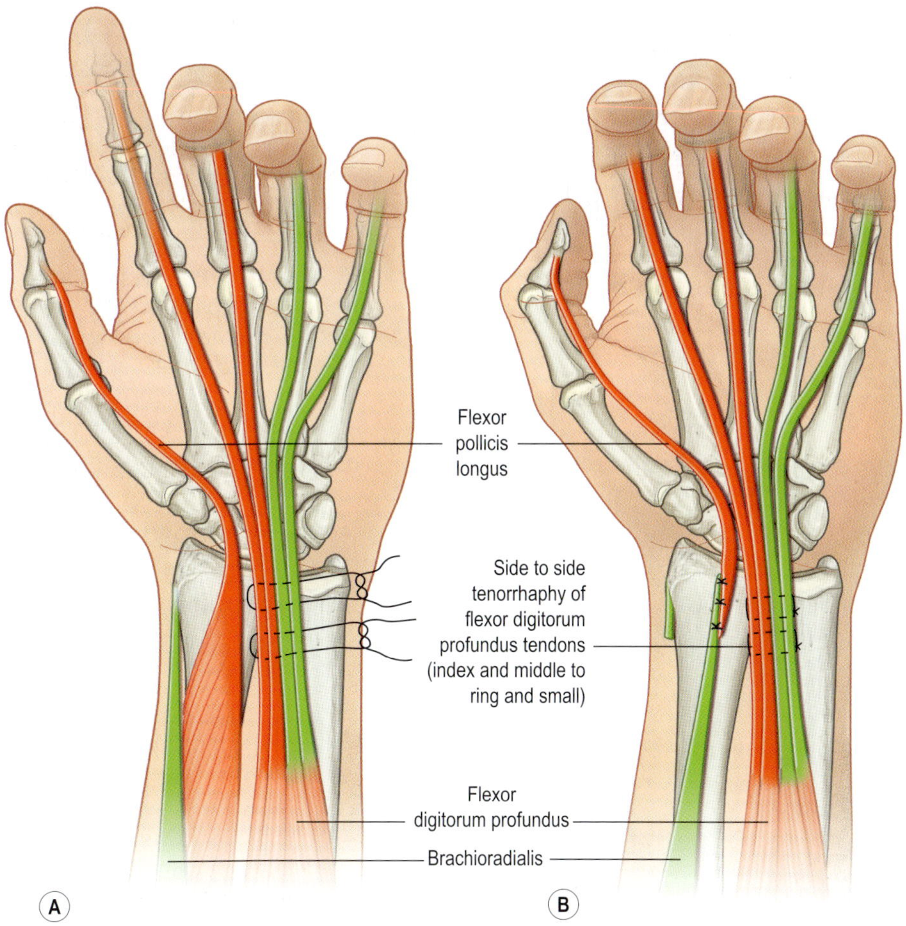

Figure 23.18 Transfer of the brachioradialis to FPL and side-to-side FDP tenorrhaphy.

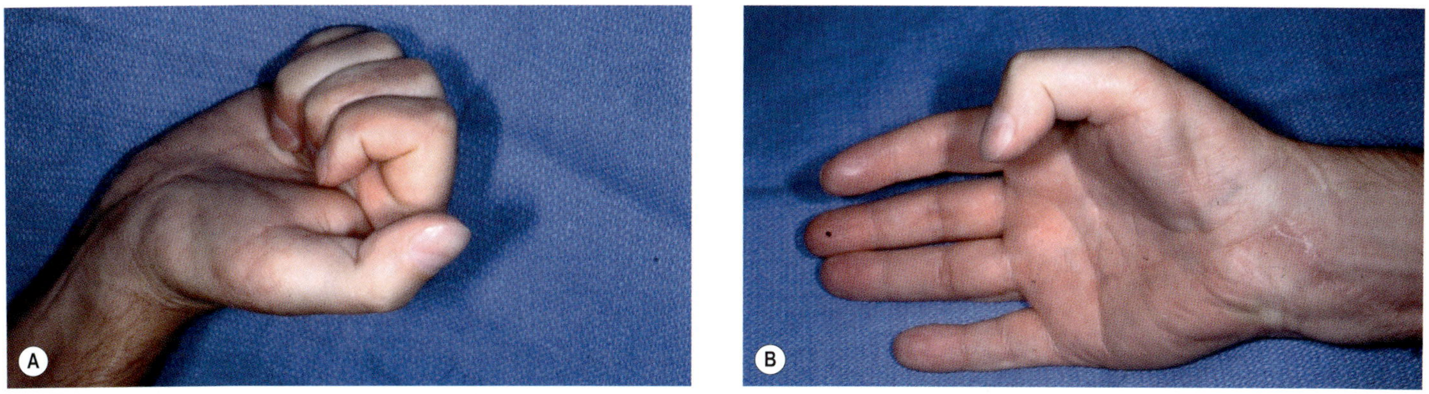

Figure 23.19 **(A)** The postoperative finger flexion cascade has been restored by side-to-side tenorrhaphy of the FDP tendons. **(B)** Semi-independent flexion of the IP joint of the thumb following Br to FPL transfer.

superficialis tendons around the A1 pulleys, the proximal ends of the superficialis tendons are activated either by ECRL or FCR.

Modified Stiles–Bunnell transfer

- The ring finger FDS tendon is divided just proximal to the PIP joint, withdrawn through a transverse distal palmar crease incision and split longitudinally into two slips which are sutured to the radial lateral bands with the MCP joints in 45–55° of flexion and the interphalangeal joints fully extended.
- In a high ulnar nerve palsy, the ring finger superficialis tendon is the only extrinsic flexor tendon in the ring finger and therefore the long finger FDS tendon is used (see Fig. 23.24).
- With a total intrinsic palsy, the superficialis tendons to both the long and ring fingers are each divided into two slips and passed down the lumbrical canals to the

radial lateral bands of the index, long, ring and small fingers.

- Disadvantages:
  - The ring finger superficialis is not expendable in a high ulnar nerve palsy or in a combined high median–high ulnar nerve palsy.
  - The transfer may eventually result in a "swan-neck" hyperextension deformity at the PIP joints.
  - The donor middle or ring finger may develop a flexion contracture at the PIP joint or loss of extension at the DIP joint.
- This should therefore only be used in patients with mild PIP joint flexion contractures or stable fingers without passive hyperextension at the PIP joints.

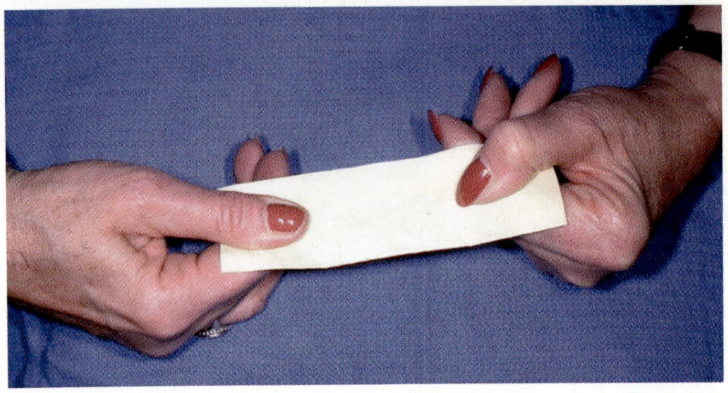

Figure 23.20 The thumb in ulnar nerve palsy. In the absence of the AP and FPB, the FPL must provide all the power of thumb flexion. As the prime flexor of the IP joint, it preferentially flexes this joint, leading to IP hyperflexion (Froment's sign) and occasionally hyperextension at the MCP joint (Jeanne's sign).

Table 23.3 **Tendon transfers for ulnar nerve palsy**

Function to be restored	Preferred tendon transfer
Clawing of the ring and small fingers	Ring finger or middle finger FDS, 2 slips to the radial lateral bands, proximal phalanges or A2 or A1 and A2 pulleys of the ring and small fingers
Clawing of all 4 fingers	EF4T or PL4T transfers to the radial lateral bands of the middle, ring and small fingers and the ulnar lateral band of the index finger; or to the combined interosseous tendon insertion
Thumb adduction	ECRB + tendon graft to adductor pollicis
Index finger abduction	Accessory APL to first dorsal interosseous
Severe thumb MCP joint hyperextension	MCP joint fusion
Fixed thumb IP joint contracture	IP joint fusion
Weak DIP joint flexion of ring and small fingers	Side-to-side tenorrhaphy of the ring and small finger FDP tendons to the middle finger FDP tendon

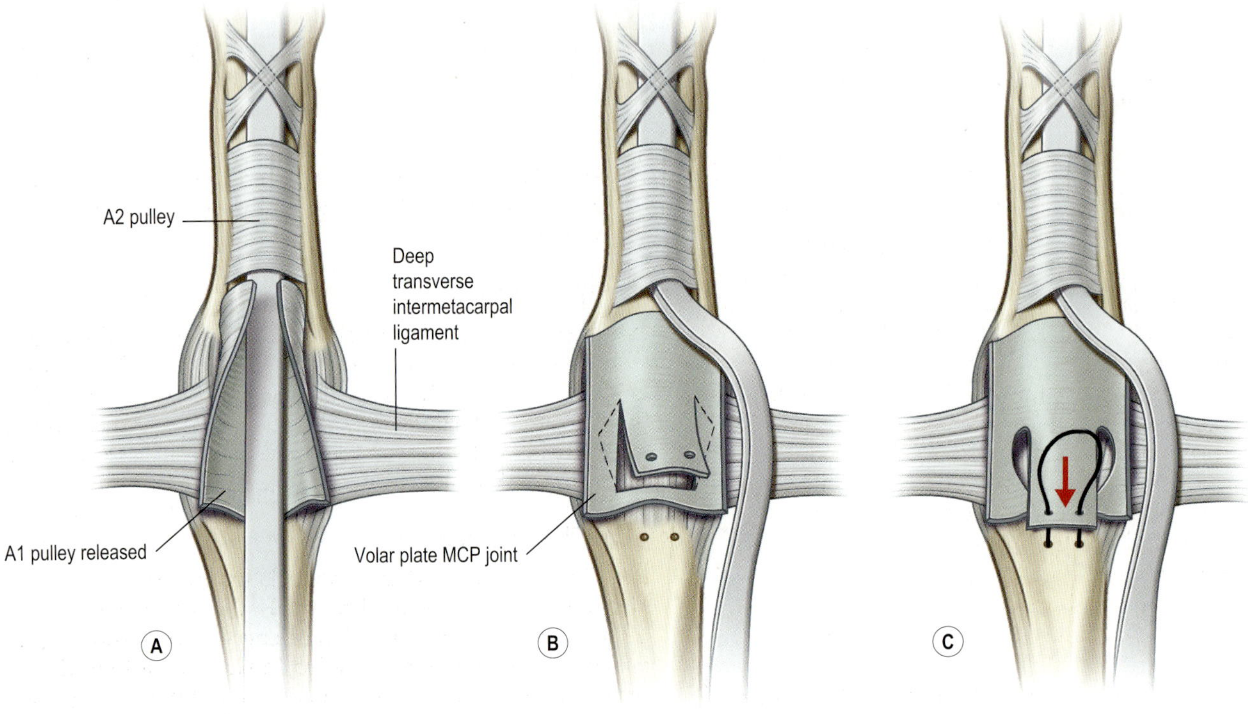

Figure 23.21 The Omer modification of the Zancolli capsulodesis. **(A)** The A1 pulley is released. **(B)** A distal-based flap is created in the volar plate. **(C)** The distal-based flap of the volar plate is advanced proximally and fixed to the metacarpal neck.

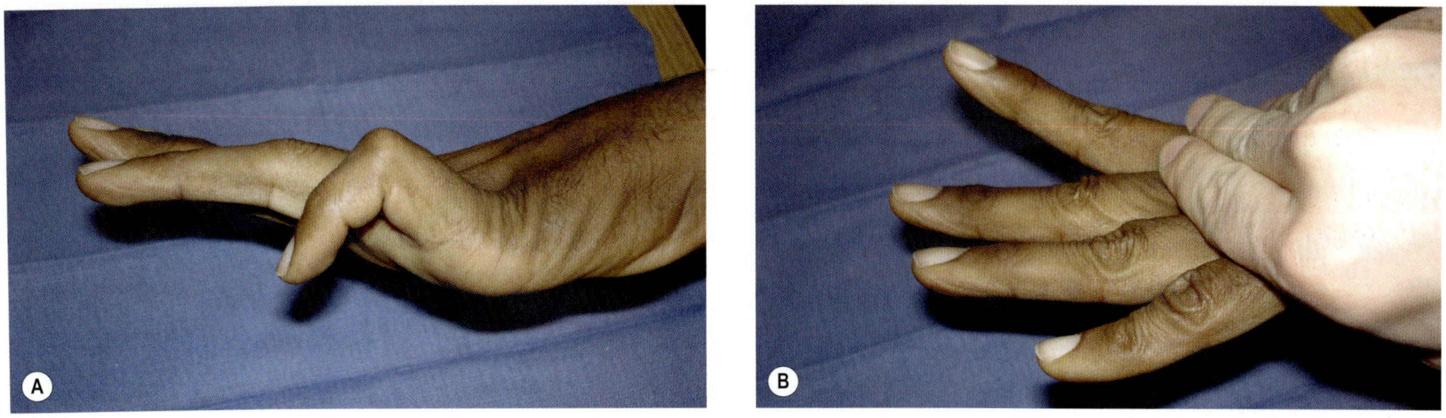

Figure 23.22 The Bouvier maneuver. **(A)** Typical claw deformity of the small finger and to a lesser extent the ring finger with hyperextension at the MCP joint and flexion at the PIP and DIP joints. **(B)** By preventing hyperextension at the MCP joints, the extrinsic extensor tendons are able to produce full extension at the PIP and DIP joints.

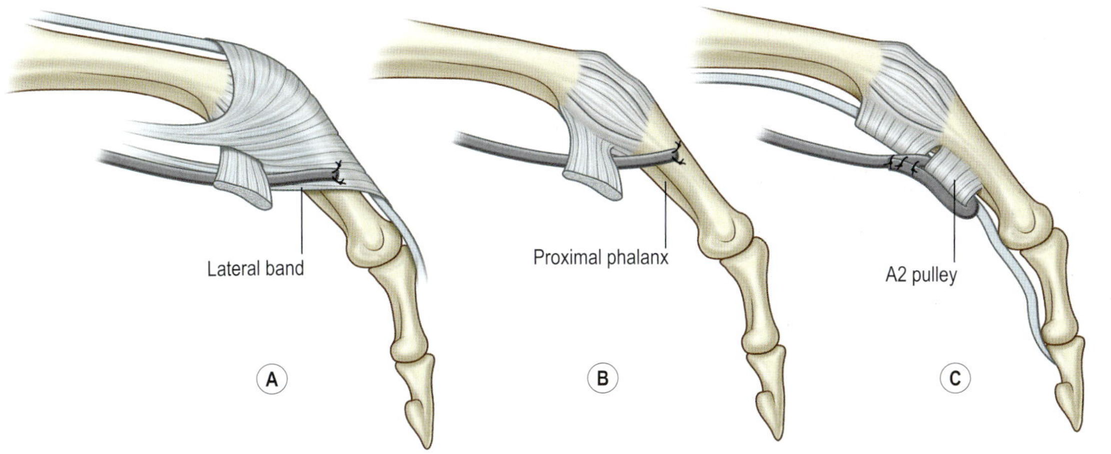

Figure 23.23 Alternative insertions for tendon transfers to prevent clawing. **(A)** Insertion into the lateral band. **(B)** Burkhalter insertion through a drill hole in the proximal phalanx. **(C)** "Lasso" procedure either into the A1 pulley (Zancolli), the A2 pulley (Brooks–Jones) or the A1 and proximal half of the A2 pulley (Anderson).

Brand EE4T transfer

- Transfer of the extensor carpi radialis brevis (ECRB), extended with three or four tendon grafts, passed from dorsal to palmar to be attached to the radial lateral bands of the middle, ring and small fingers *(Fig. 23.25)* and to the ulnar lateral band of the index finger (EE4T: extensor tendon, extensor route, four-tailed graft).
- However, during wrist extension, the ECRB and tendon grafts relax which is a relative disadvantage of this dorsal routing of the original Brand transfer.
- So, Burkhalter and Strai modified the Brand EE4T transfer, by using ECRL instead of ECRB and by only correcting the ring and small fingers.
- Only produces MCP joint flexion, but is an alternative transfer for a combined high median–high ulnar nerve palsy when the modified Stiles–Bunnell FDS transfer is not available.
- The Fowler transfer uses both the EIP and EDM tendons. The EIP tendon controls the index and middle fingers and the EDM tendon controls the ring and small fingers. This is rarely used.
- Disadvantage of the Fowler transfer: the EIP and EDM tendons are only just long enough to reach the radial lateral bands.

Brand EF4T transfer

- Brand modified his original dorsal transfer of ECRB by extending ECRL with a four tailed tendon graft or fascia lata graft through the carpal tunnel to the radial lateral bands of the middle, ring and small fingers and the ulnar lateral band of the ring finger (EF4T: extensor tendon, flexor route, four-tailed graft) *(Figs 23.26, 23.27)*.

Fritschi PF4T transfer

- Fritschi has described the palmaris longus as an alternative motor for the Brand EF4T transfer. The palmaris longus tendon is lengthened with a tendon graft or fascia lata graft and tunneled in similar route to the Brand EF4T procedure. However, the palmaris longus is a much weaker donor muscle than the ECRL.
- Two alternative insertions have been described for the Brand EF4T and Lennox–Fritschi PL4T transfers, either

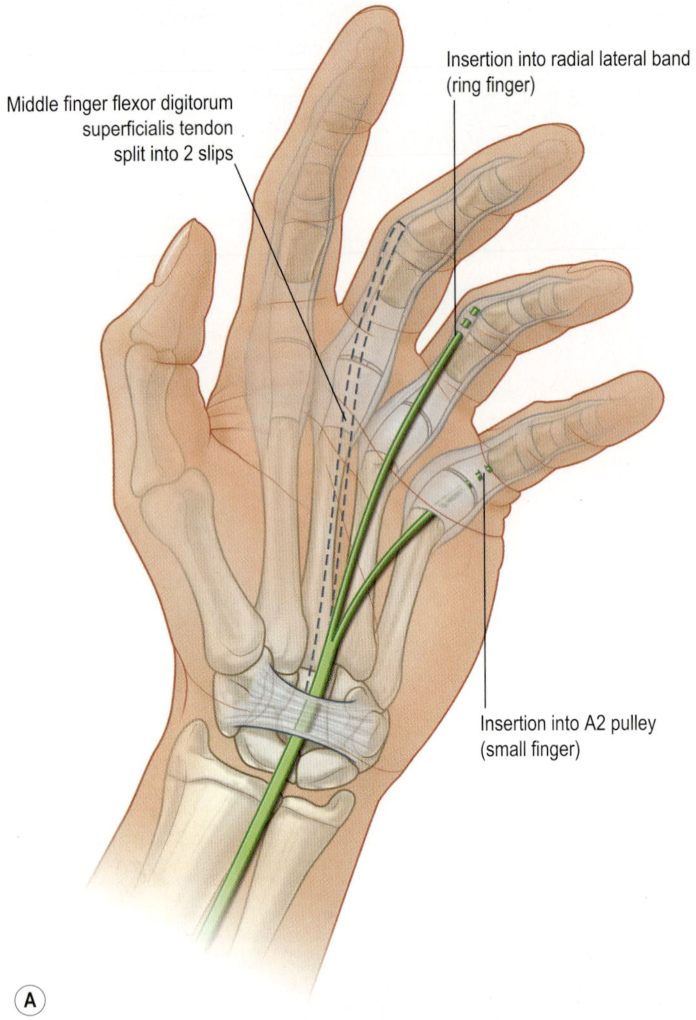

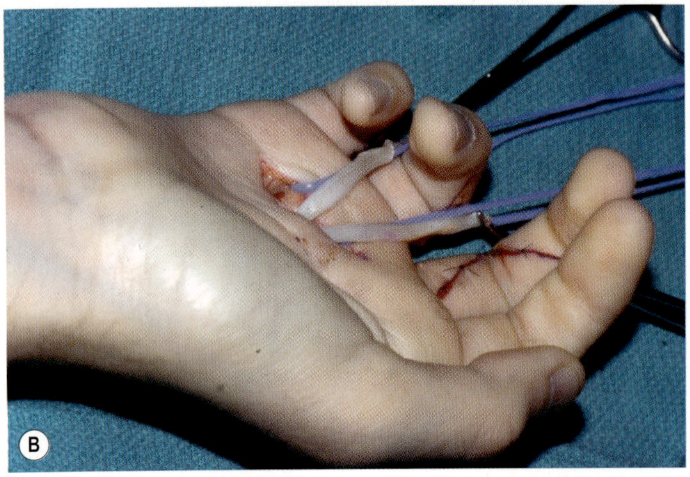

Figure 23.24 (A,B) Transfer of the long finger FDS to the radial lateral band of the ring finger or the A2 pulley of the small finger.

the common interosseous tendon insertion or the A2 pulley.

- Brooks and Jones described elongating the ECRL or FCR with plantaris or toe extensor tendon grafts which are tunneled and looped around the A2 pulleys of each finger.

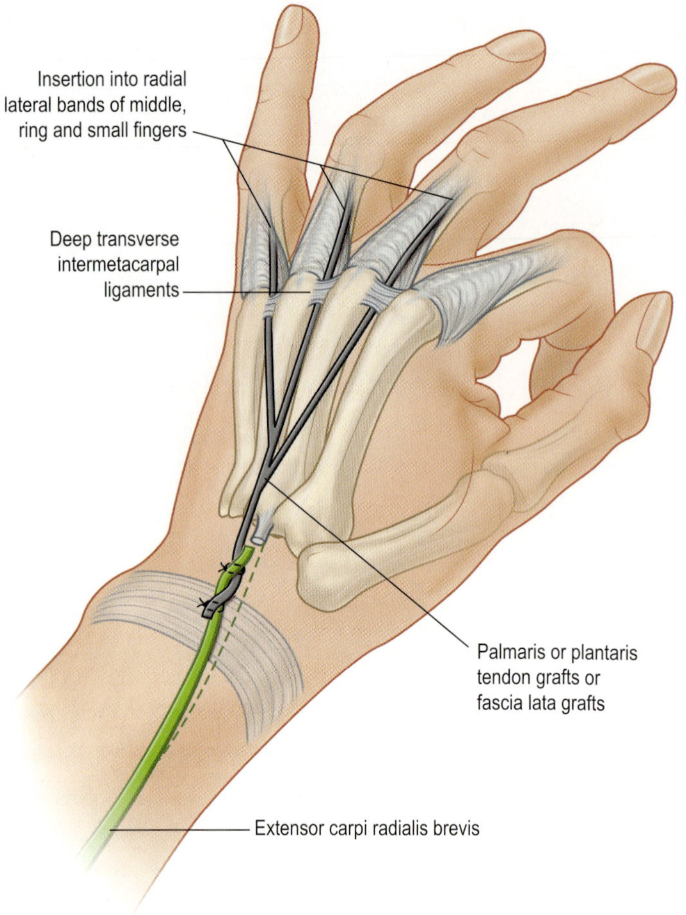

Figure 23.25 Brand EE4T transfer of ECRB extended by three tendon grafts into the three ulnar fingers.

Tendon transfer to correct ulnar deviation of the small finger

- A variant of the Fowler transfer has been advocated by Blacker et al. to correct the ulnar deviation deformity of the small finger (Wartenberg's sign).
- The ulnar half of EDM is detached, passed volar and sutured into the insertion of the radial collateral ligament of the MCP joint at the base of the proximal phalanx, or if there is associated clawing of the small finger, it is looped under the A2 pulley and sutured back to itself (Brooks insertion).
- Chung et al. described transferring EIP to the distal radial aspect of the extensor hood of the small finger to correct the persistent abduction deformity of the small finger in an ulnar nerve palsy.

Tendon transfers to provide adduction of the thumb

- The most successful tendon transfers to restore adduction of the thumb have a transverse direction of pull across the palm deep to the flexor tendons to insert into the tendon of adductor pollicis.
- Littler advocated transfer of the ring finger superficialis inserted into a drill hole just distal to the adductor insertion.

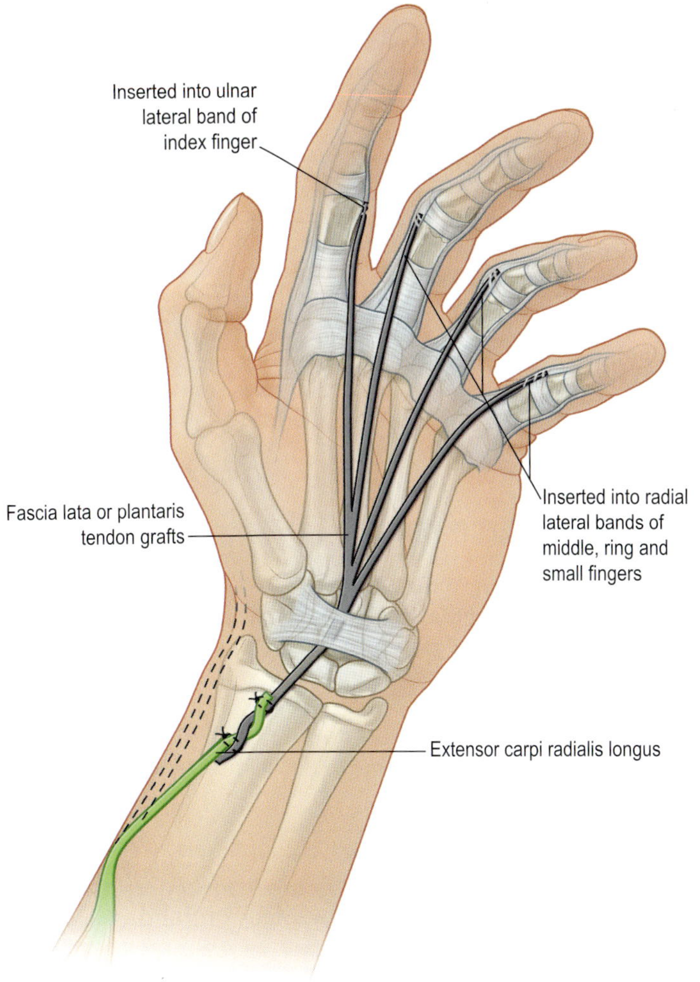

Figure 23.26 Brand EF4T transfer of the ECRL extended by four tendon grafts into all four lateral bands in a patient with clawing of all four fingers.

- Smith described using ECRB extended by a free tendon graft passed through the second intermetacarpal space and tunneled deep to the flexor tendons but superficial to the adductor pollicis to an insertion into the adductor tendon *(Fig. 23.28)*.
- Other tendon transfers to restore adduction of the thumb have included either the brachioradialis or ECRL elongated with a tendon graft and passed through the third intermetacarpal space to the thumb MCP joint, and the EIP passed through the second intermetacarpal space.
- If there is a severe collapse Z-deformity of the thumb with hyperextension at the MCP joint and flexion at the IP joint, or an exaggerated Jeanne's sign when attempting to pinch, arthrodesis of the MCP joint may be necessary.
- For mild collapse deformities of the thumb without a fixed contracture, a split FPL to EPL transfer may be indicated.

Ring finger flexor digitorum superficialis transfer

- The ring finger FDS tendon is transected between the A1 and A2 pulleys, passed transversely across the palm deep to the index and long finger flexor tendons to the ulnar aspect of the thumb MCP joint, and either sutured into the adductor pollicis tendon or passed through a drill hole in the proximal phalanx just distal to the adductor insertion, and tied over a button.
- Cannot be used as an adductor transfer in patients with a high ulnar nerve palsy since this would deprive the ring finger of its only remaining flexor tendon.

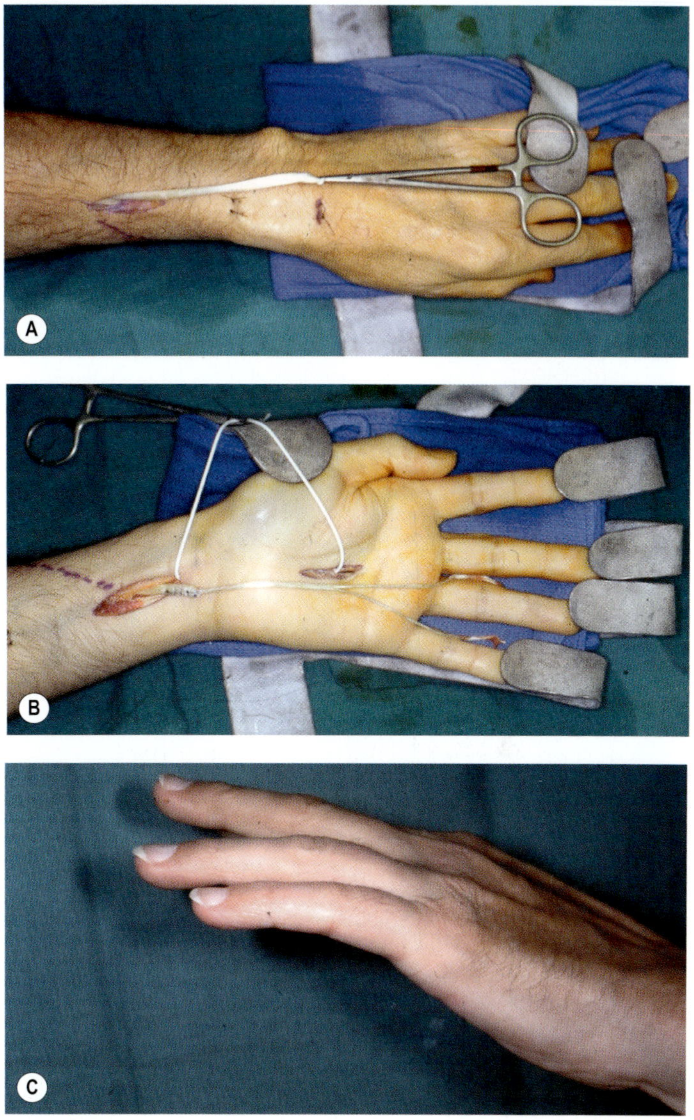

Figure 23.27 Brand EF4T transfer to correct clawing of the ring and small fingers. **(A)** The ECRL is detached from its insertion into the base of the second metacarpal. **(B)** A palmaris longus graft is attached to the ECRL which has been brought volarly around the radial side of the forearm (or through the interosseous membrane). **(C)** Postoperatively, this has corrected the preoperative claw deformity of the 4th and 5th fingers.

Smith extensor carpi radialis brevis transfer

- ECRB is used to power the APL tendon with assistance from a Palmaris or plantaris interposition tendon graft *(Fig. 23.29)*.

Tendon transfers to provide index finger abduction

- Restoration of strong abduction of the index finger is the second component required for powerful pinch.

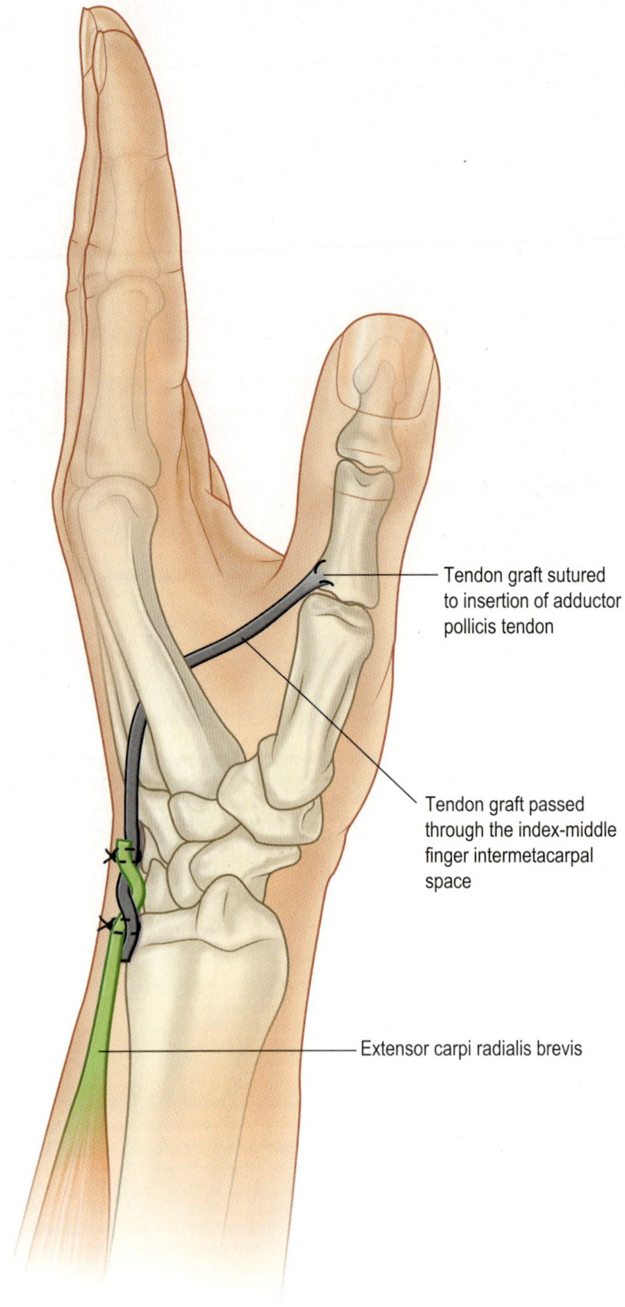

Figure 23.28 Schematic representation of the Smith transfer for restoration of thumb adduction. The extensor carpi radialis brevis is extended by a tendon graft through the second intermetacarpal space to the adductor tubercle on the ulnar base of the proximal phalanx of the thumb.

- Bunnell described the transfer of extensor indicis proprius (EIP) extended with a short tendon graft and inserted into the first dorsal interosseous tendon.
- Bruner divided the extensor pollicis brevis (EPB) tendon, tunneled it subcutaneously beneath the EPL tendon and into the first dorsal interosseous tendon.
- Hirayama lengthened the palmaris longus tendon with a strip of palmar fascia (similar to the Camitz transfer) and tunneled it subcutaneously around the radial border of the forearm over the dorsum of the wrist and hand to insert into the first dorsal interosseous tendon.
- Graham and Riordan transferred the FDS of the ring finger
- One of the accessory tendons of APL extended with a free tendon graft, or attached to the rerouted EDC tendon of the index finger, may be the best choice to restore abduction of the index finger ***(Fig. 23.30)***.

Neviaser accessory abductor pollicis longus and free tendon graft

- Neviaser et al. described an accessory APL tendon elongated with a palmaris or plantaris tendon graft transferred to the insertion of the first dorsal interosseous tendon (see Figs 23.29, 23.30).

High ulnar nerve palsy

- Functional deficit: paralysis of the FCU and FDP tendons to the ring and small fingers, paralysis of all seven interossei, the ulnar two lumbricals, the hypothenar and the adductor pollicis (AP) and part of the flexor pollicis brevis (FPB) muscles.
- The only remaining tendons on the ulnar side of the hand are the superficialis tendon to the ring finger and the usually diminutive superficialis tendon to the small finger.
- Paralysis of the profundus tendons to the ring and small fingers will often be masked by interconnections between these two tendons and the long finger profundus tendon at the wrist.

Specific operative techniques

- If there is significant weakness of DIP joint flexion of the ring and small fingers (Pollock's sign), power grip can be restored by side-to-side tenorrhaphy of the ring and small finger FDP tendons to the median-innervated middle finger FDP tendon.
- This should be performed before tendon transfers to correct clawing are performed, but patients should be warned that this will temporarily exaggerate their clawing and that they should use a lumbrical block splint.
- To restore independent flexion of the ring and small fingers, the FDS tendon of the middle finger may be used as a donor tendon to activate the FDP tendons of the ring and small fingers.
- Patients requiring strong ulnar deviation and flexion of the wrist may occasionally need to be considered for transfer of the FCR tendon to FCU.

Tendon transfers for combined nerve injuries

- As a general rule, the results of tendon transfers for combined nerve injuries are inferior to those for a single nerve injury.
- Adding to the complexity of these problems, the number of donor tendons is limited, more joints need to be mobilized, there is a more profound sensory loss, and the

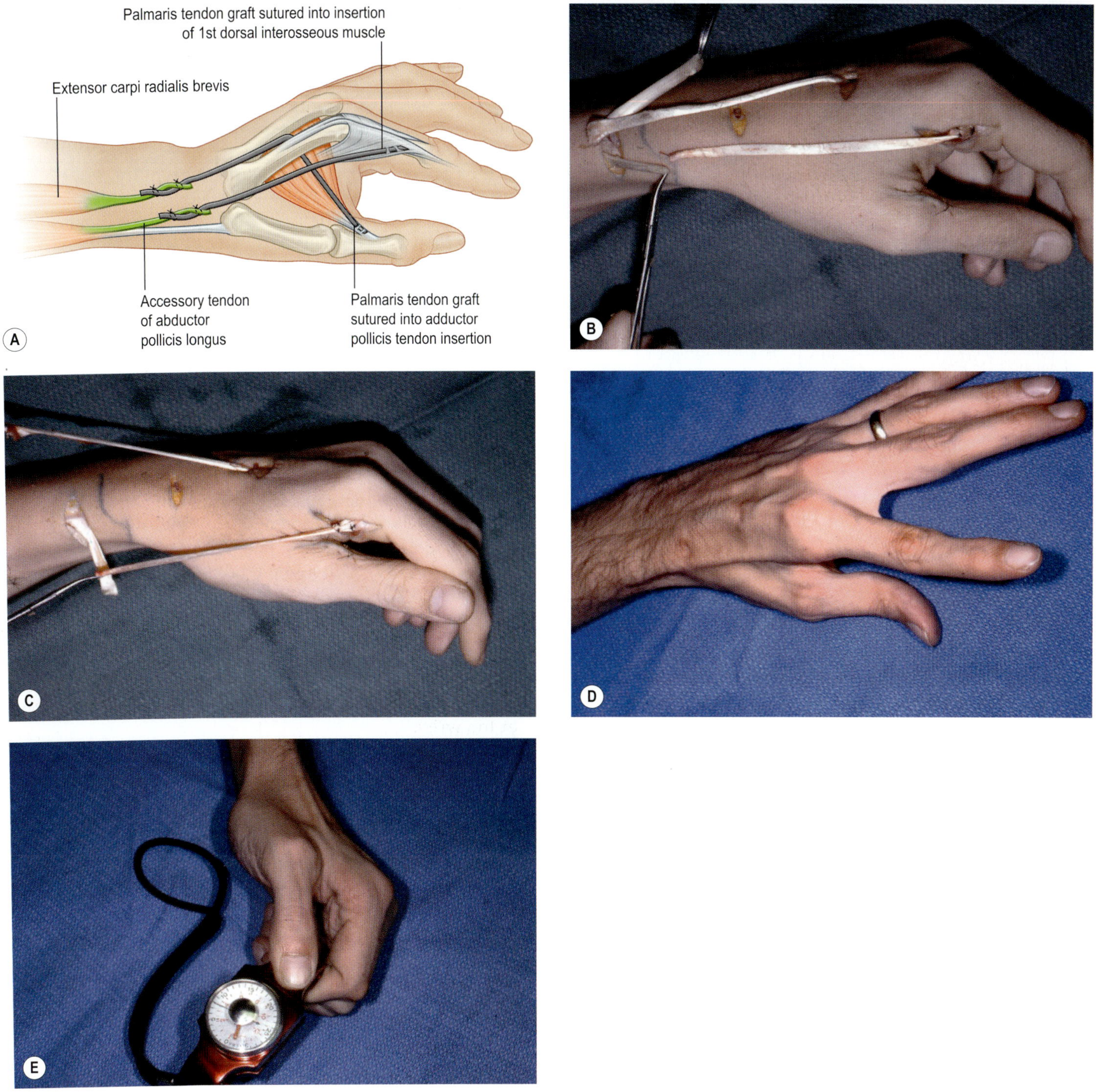

Figure 23.29 **(A)** Transfers to restore thumb adduction and abduction of the index finger. **(B)** A tendon graft has been anchored to the tendon of the adductor pollicis. It is passed dorsal to the flexor tendons and neurovascular bundles and then from palmar to dorsal through the second intermetacarpal space. A tendon graft has been sutured into the tendon of the first dorsal interosseous. **(C)** Traction on these two grafts flexes and adducts the thumb and abducts the index finger at its MCP joint. **(D)** Postoperative function following these two transfers. **(E)** Pinch force is significantly improved.

soft tissues may be more scarred in this patient population.

- Dynamic tenodesis is an important concept in reconstruction of these combined nerve injuries. Wrist flexion or extension can be used to augment the excursion of any tendon transfer that crosses the wrist.

Tendon transfers for low median–low ulnar nerve palsy

- The most common combined nerve injury in the upper extremity and is usually the result of a "spaghetti-wrist" laceration. This leads to complete loss of sensation on the palmar surface of the hand and a complete intrinsic motor paralysis that results in a claw hand deformity.

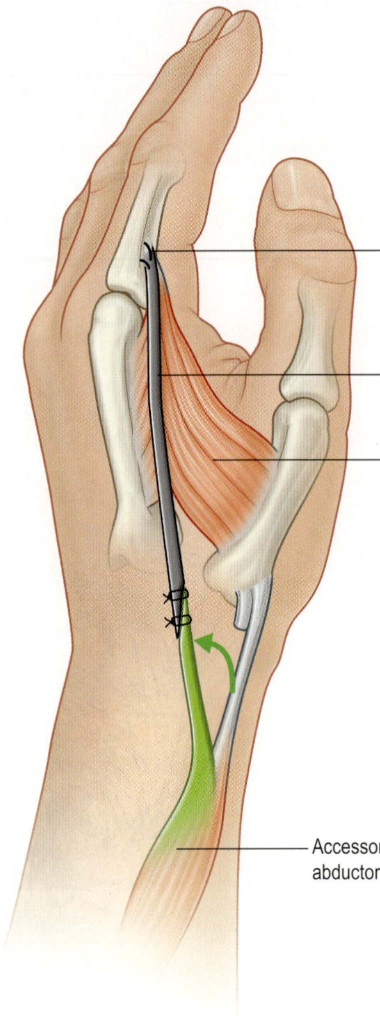

Figure 23.30 The Neviaser transfer to restore abduction of the index finger. One of the accessory tendons of the abductor pollicis longus is extended by a palmaris tendon graft and sutured to the insertion of the first dorsal interosseous muscle on the base of the proximal phalanx of the index finger.

- A flat transverse metacarpal arch with hyperextension at the MP joints and hyperflexion of the PIP joints accompanied by an abducted small finger are the hallmark of this injury.
- The goals of reconstruction: to restore thumb adduction, thumb abduction and opposition, abduction of the index finger and improved extension of the PIP joints of the fingers.
- Thumb adduction for key pinch can be restored by transfer of the ECRB extended by a tendon graft and inserted into the adductor tubercle of the thumb metacarpal or alternatively by transfer of the superficialis tendon from the ring finger to the adductor insertion.
- The best option for reconstruction of thumb opposition is the EIP transfer rerouted around the ulnar border of the hand and inserted into the APB tendon. This transfer can be combined with arthrodesis of the MCP joint of the thumb to allow for maximum stability.
- Index finger abduction for strong pinch can be restored by transfer of one of the APL tendon slips extended by a tendon graft to the first dorsal interosseous insertion.
- Finally, clawing of the fingers can be corrected by using ECRL or palmaris longus extended by four tendon grafts and inserted either into the radial lateral bands or the A2 pulleys as previously discussed.
- If the patient still has poor palmar sensibility despite nerve repair or nerve grafting, consideration should be given to transfer of a superficial radial nerve innervated flap to the thumb or nerve transfer of the superficial radial nerve to the distal median nerve.

Tendon transfers for high median–high ulnar nerve palsy

- Very severe injury in which there is no active flexion of the fingers and thumb and loss of thumb opposition and key pinch in addition to the loss of palmar sensibility.
- Tendon transfers for reconstruction of a high median–high ulnar nerve palsy have to be performed in two or three stages.
- Goals: restore finger and thumb flexion, thumb-index finger pinch, abduction and opposition of the thumb and correct the later development of clawing of the fingers.
- Thumb adduction and key pinch can be achieved by transfer of ECRB with a free tendon graft to the adductor pollicis insertion.
- Finger flexion can be restored by transfer of ECRL to the four FDP tendons. This can be combined with tenodesis of the DIP joints of the three ulnar fingers.
- Flexion of the thumb can be restored by transfer of the brachioradialis to FPL through the same palmar incision.
- As in a low median–low ulnar nerve palsy, the most reliable procedure for thumb opposition is transfer of the EIP to the APB insertion.
- If the IP joint of the thumb tends to assume a flexed position, the EIP transfer should be inserted both into the APB insertion and then into the EPL tendon just proximal to the IP joint.
- If after finger flexion has been restored, the fingers begin to adopt a clawed position, there are no expendable wrist extensors (ECRL and ECRB) remaining to provide integration of MP flexion and IP joint extension, static tenodesis techniques may be necessary.
- The importance of restoring sensibility to the radial side of the hand in a high median–high ulnar nerve palsy cannot be overstated, either by secondary nerve repair or nerve grafting.

Tendon transfers for reconstruction after trauma

- Tendon transfers are an excellent method of restoring active motion to the hand and wrist following traumatic injuries of the muscles and tendons of the forearm, wrist and hand.
- If there has been segmental loss of tendon, a tendon graft is often used instead of a tendon transfer.
- With more severe trauma (industrial or motor vehicle accidents, blast, missile and explosion injuries), associated damage to the soft tissues will leave a scarred bed which is unsuitable for tendon grafts, since a tendon graft is

more likely to become adherent to the scarred surrounding tissue than a tendon transfer.

- Myostatic contracture and atrophy are the unavoidable fate of injured muscle if there has been a long delay between the traumatic event and the reconstructive procedure, again making a tendon transfer a more suitable option for reconstruction.

Tendon transfers to restore thumb extension

- Rupture of the EPL tendon occurs in approximately 1 in 200 distal radius fractures, classically at Lister's tubercle and may happen at any time from several weeks to several months after the fracture. Ischemia of the tendon due to swelling and edema of the tenosynovium and attrition over the roughened dorsal radial cortex have been postulated as the etiology for this tendon rupture.
- Patients present with weakness or loss of extension at the interphalangeal joint or paradoxically with incomplete extension at the MP joint as well as inability to raise the thumb dorsal to the plane of the hand ***(Fig. 23.31A)***.
- The optimal choice for restoration of thumb extension is the EIP to EPL transfer which can be performed under local anesthesia (see Fig. 23.31B–D).

Tendon transfers to restore finger extension

- Restoration of finger extension after trauma can be accomplished by tendon transfers similar to those used for radial nerve palsy. Those transfers were discussed in detail earlier in this chapter and include transfer of either of the wrist flexors (FCU or FCR) to the EDC or the Boyes transfer of the FDS of the long and ring fingers to the EDC.

Tendon transfers to restore thumb flexion

- Acute lacerations or ruptures of the flexor pollicis longus (FPL) tendon can be treated by primary or delayed primary repair or tendon grafting. However, with missed diagnosis, the muscle fibers undergo significant shortening, atrophy and fibrosis within 6 months to a year from injury. In these situations, it is preferable to restore thumb flexion using a tendon transfer, usually the FDS of the ring finger.

Tendon transfers to restore finger flexion

- Occasionally, patients may present with severe crushing or avulsion injuries involving the forearm flexor muscles. The options for secondary reconstruction of finger flexion are either a tendon transfer of the ECRL to all four FDP tendons or a functioning free gracilis muscle transfer ***(Fig. 23.32)***.

Postoperative considerations

- Postoperatively, the hand is immobilized in the desired position for 3–4 weeks, at which time gentle active range of motion exercises are started, usually under the supervision of a therapist, but the hand is protected for a further 3 weeks in a light-weight protective splint.
- In general active flexion and extension of the fingers and thumb are started at 3.5–4 weeks and active exercises of the wrist at 5 weeks. Protective splinting is continued until 6–8 weeks' postoperatively.

Complications and outcomes

- Several factors influence the likelihood of useful motor and sensory return following median nerve injury including patient age, level of injury, length of nerve defect and interposition graft and period of preoperative delay.
  - Best results are in distal injuries in young patients requiring only primary repair.
  - Associated injuries (vascular damage, tendon injury, and concomitant ulnar nerve transaction) portend a worse prognosis.
  - The chances of reinnervation of the thenar muscles following group fascicular repair of a distal median nerve laceration should be reasonably optimistic.
- The FDS of the ring finger and the ECU are the best transfers at replacing thenar strength, abduction and pronation. Reports indicate that the ECU and FDS transfers restore 60% and 40%, respectively, of required thenar muscle strength (Table 23.4).

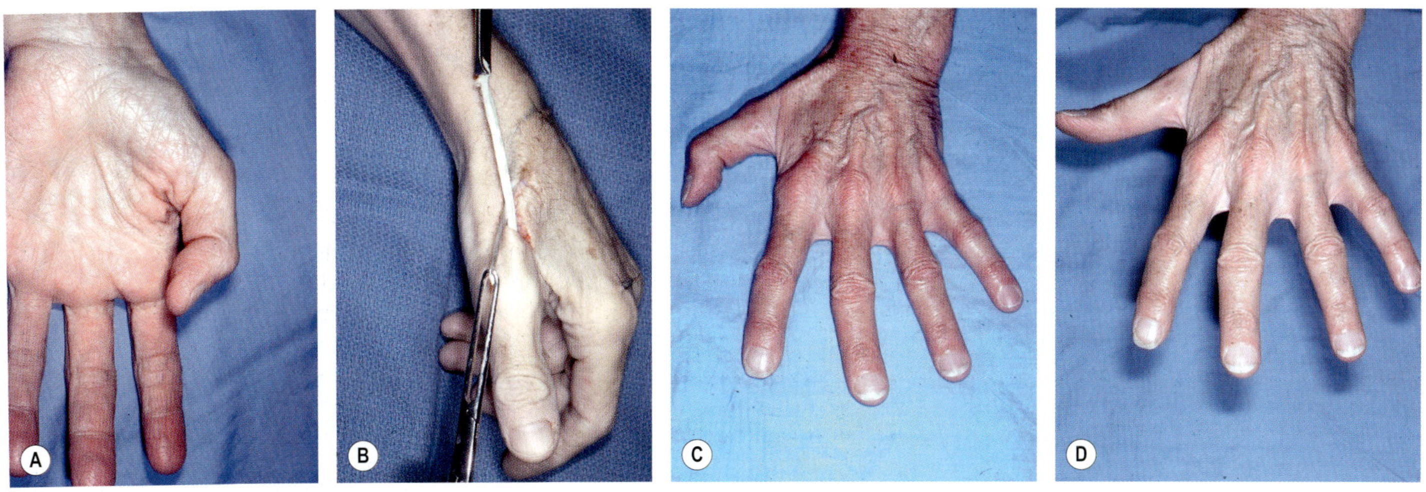

Figure 23.31 **(A)** Rupture of the EPL. **(B)** Transfer of the EIP to the EPL. **(C)** Preoperative thumb extension. **(D)** Postoperative thumb extension.

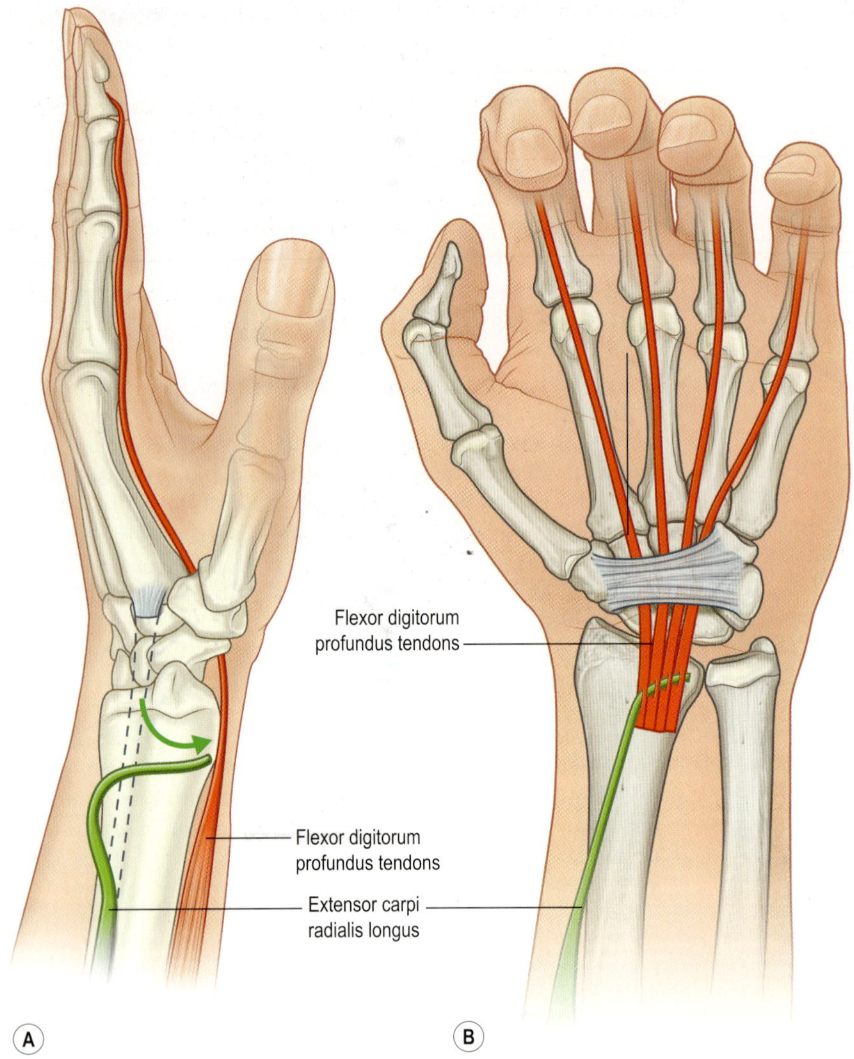

Figure 23.32 Tendon transfer to restore flexion of the fingers. The extensor carpi radialis longus tendon is transected from the base of the index finger metacarpal, transferred subcutaneously around the radial border of the forearm and sutured to the flexor digitorum profundus tendons to the index, middle, ring and small fingers in the distal forearm proximal to the carpal tunnel.

Table 23.4 **Opposition tendon transfers for median nerve palsy**

Technique	Etiology	Author	Success rate (%)
Huber	Trauma	Wissinger (1977)	80
	Neurologic disease		
Camitz	Nerve compression	Terrono et al. (1993)	94
		Foucher et al. (1991)	91
EIP	Trauma	Anderson et al. (1991)	88
		Burkhalter et al. (1973)	88
Bunnell	Leprosy	Brandsma et al. (1992)	83
	Leprosy	Palande (1975)	94
	Trauma	Kirklin (1948)	85
	Trauma	Groves and Goldner (1975)	75
EDQ	Trauma	Schneider (1969)	80

- Tendon transfers for radial nerve palsy are generally predictable. Recent results reported that wrist extension averaged 73% of the opposite side, finger extension 32% and thumb extension 80%. Grip strength was reduced to 49% and pinch strength to 28% of the opposite hand.
- The author's preferred technique is to use pronator teres to restore wrist extension, FCR to restore finger extension and palmaris longus to restore thumb extension with tenodesis of the APL to brachioradialis to restore thumb abduction.

Further reading

Boyes JH. Tendon transfers for radial palsy. *Bull Hosp Joint Dis*. 1960;21:97.

The original description of the Boyes transfer for radial nerve palsy, using the flexor digitorum superficialis tendons from the middle and ring fingers transferred through the interosseous membrane to restore independent index finger and thumb extension.

Brand PW. *Clinical mechanics of the hand*. St Louis: Mosby; 1985.

This is the definitive reference book detailing the biomechanics of tendon transfers.

Brand PW. Tendon transfers for median and ulnar nerve paralysis. *Orthop Clin North Am*. 1970;1: 447–454.

Brand PW. Tendon grafting illustrated by a new operation for intrinsic paralysis of the fingers. *J Bone Joint Surg*. 1961;43B:444–453.

This paper describes the dorsal route of the extensor carpi radialis brevis tendon extended with free tendon grafts and the palmar route of the extensor carpi radialis longus tendon extended with free tendon grafts to correct the clawing in ulnar nerve palsy due to leprosy.

Bunnell S. Opposition of the thumb. *J Bone Joint Surg*. 1938;20:725–732.

The original description of the Burkhalter transfer to restore thumb opposition in a low median nerve palsy using the extensor indicis proprius tendon.

Bunnell S. Surgery of the intrinsic muscles of the hand other than those producing opposition of the thumb. *J Bone Joint Surg*. 1942;24:1.

Kirklin JW, Thomas CG. Opponents transplant: an analysis of the methods employed and results obtained in 75 cases. *Surg Gynecol Obstet*. 1948;86:213.

Palande DD. Correction of intrinsic minus hands with reversal of transverse metacarpal arch. *J Bone Joint Surg Am*. 1983;65:514–521.

Smith RJ. Extensor carpi radialis brevis tendon transfer for thumb adduction – a study of power pinch. *J Hand Surg Am*. 1983;8:4–15.

Smith RJ. *Tendon transfers of the hand and forearm*. Boston: Little Brown; 1987.

This classic monograph, unfortunately out of print, is an excellent reference source describing tendon transfers for nerve injuries, trauma, rheumatoid arthritis, congenital anomalies, cerebral palsy and spinal cord injuries.

Wissinger HA, Singsen EG. Abductor digiti quinti opponensplasty. *J Bone Joint Surg Am*. 1977;2:22–23.

24 Chapter

Extensor tendon injuries

This chapter was created using content from Neligan & Chang, Plastic Surgery 3rd edition, Volume 6, Hand and Upper Extremity, Chapter 10, Extensor tendon injuries, Kai Megerle and Günter Germann.

SYNOPSIS

- A thorough understanding of the complex anatomy is crucial for successful treatment of extensor tendon injuries.
- Injuries are classified into nine anatomic zones. Treatment strategies vary considerably according to the location of the lesion, ranging from splinting to tendon grafting.
- Minimal variations in tendon length may result in considerable alteration in range of motion.
- As in flexor tendon injuries, postoperative care is an essential part of the treatment concept.
- Closed ruptures of the extensor tendon at the level of the distal interphalangeal (DIP) and proximal interphalangeal (PIP) joints are typically treated conservatively.
- Lacerations at the level of the metacarpophalangeal (MP) joint (zone V) are not infrequently caused by human bites and are prone to infection unless thoroughly debrided.
- Ruptures of the sagittal bands may result in subluxation of the extensor tendon at the level of the MP joint.
- The swan-neck deformity is characterized by DIP joint flexion and PIP joint hyperextension. It can be caused by an untreated mallet injury or palmar plate laxity.
- The boutonnière deformity is characterized by hyperextension of the DIP joint and PIP joint flexion. It can be caused by rupture of the central slip of the extensor tendon or palmar subluxation of the lateral bands.
- Complex injuries to the dorsum of the hand can involve skin, tendon, and bone. Adequate debridement is of paramount importance. Before reconstructing tendons, fractures must be stabilized and stable soft tissue coverage must be provided.

Brief introduction

- In contrast to common belief, injuries to the extensor tendon apparatus are often more difficult to treat than those of flexor tendons.
- A thorough understanding of the complex interactions between the long extensor tendons and the intrinsic muscles of the hand is necessary to achieve good postoperative results.
- The extensor apparatus consists of superficial, thin structures that are very close to the underlying bones, which makes them prone to develop severe adhesions.
- Their excursion amplitude is limited, so that even subtle lengthening or shortening will result in severe restrictions of range of motion.
- Postoperative regimens vary considerably in respect to the exact location of the lesion and have to be selected carefully.

Preoperative considerations

- The diagnosis of extensor tendon injuries is often evident. However, partial lesions can be missed if the remaining tendon is strong enough to create some extension force.
- As a general rule, open lesions should therefore be surgically explored to identify the extent of the injury and prevent secondary ruptures.
- The function of the EDC tendon should be assessed by extension of the MP joint of the affected digit against resistance.
- If there is a questionable rupture of the EPL tendon, it should not be tested by extension of the IP joint as the EPB tendon inserts into the extensor tendon apparatus of the thumb at varying levels and may be able to extend the IP joint.

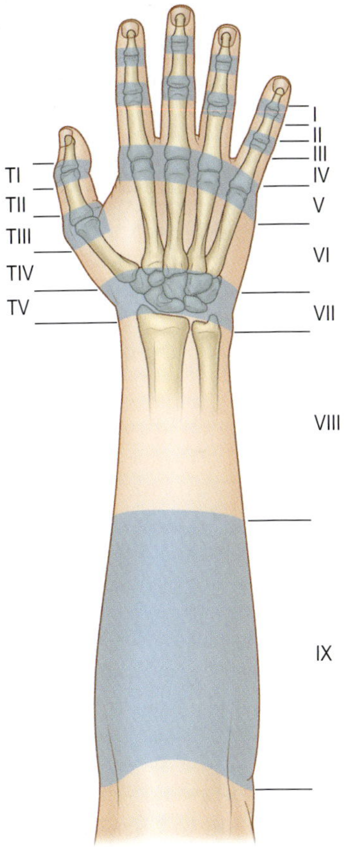

Figure 24.1 The zones of extensor tendon injuries.

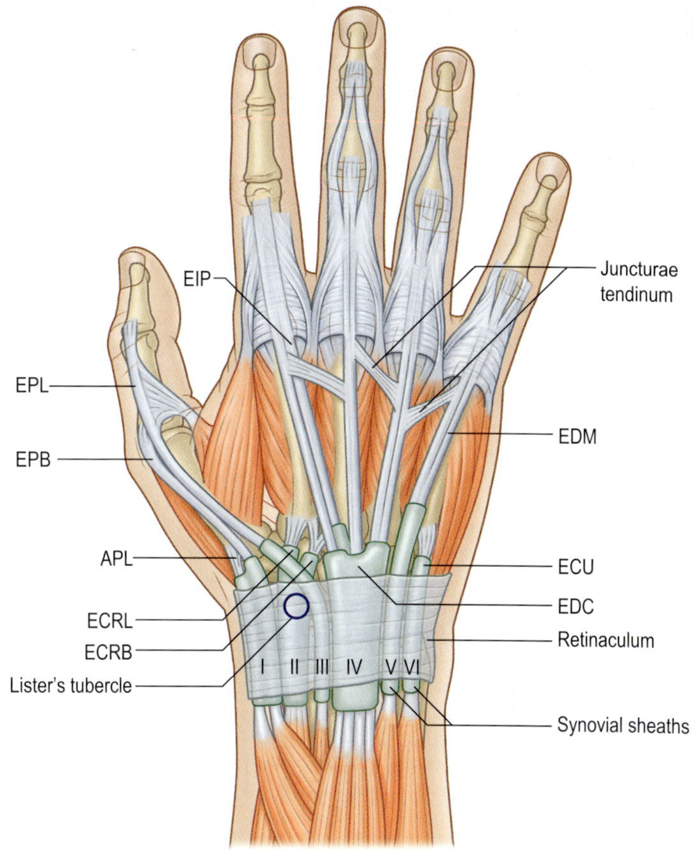

Figure 24.2 Extensor compartments. EIP, extensor indicis propius; EPL, extensor pollicis longus; EPB, extensor pollicis brevis; EDM, extensor digiti minimi; APL, abductor pollicis longus; ECU, extensor carpi ulnaris; ECRL, extensor carpi radialis longus; ECRB, extensor carpi radialis brevis; EDC, extensor digitorum communis.

- Instead, the patient should be asked to lift the thumb off the table, which will be impossible without an intact EPL tendon.
- The extensor tendon apparatus is classified into nine zones according to the level of the lesion ***(Fig. 24.1)***.
- The repair of simple lacerations of the extensor tendon can be safely performed in the emergency room.
- Lesions proximal to zone VI should be treated in the operating room.

Anatomical pearls

- The extensor mechanism consists of extrinsic muscles, which are located on the forearm (extensor communis, extensor indicis, extensor digiti minimi (EDM)), intrinsic muscles, which are located at the level of the metacarpals (interosseous and lumbrical muscles), and fibrous structures.

Extrinsic muscles

- All extrinsic tendons pass through the six compartments of the extensor retinaculum on the back of the wrist ***(Fig. 24.2)***:
  - 1st Compartment: attached to the outer rim of the radius and contains the tendons of the abductor pollicis longus (APL) and extensor pollicis brevis (EPB) muscles.
  - In 34% of patients the compartment is further divided by an additional septum, which has implications for the etiology and treatment of de Quervain's disease.
  - 2nd Compartment: bordered by Lister's tubercle on the ulnar side and contains the extensor carpi radialis longus (ECRL) and extensor carpi radialis brevis (ECRB).
  - 3rd Compartment: crosses the wrist in a diagonal fashion above the second compartment, while Lister's tubercle acts as a pivot point for the extensor pollicis longus (EPL) tendon.
  - While passing through the compartment, the tendon is quite vulnerable to ruptures, e.g., in fractures of the distal radius.
  - 4th Compartment: contains both the extensor digitorum communis (EDC) and extensor indicis propius (EIP) tendons.
  - 5th Compartment: contains the EDM tendon.
  - 6th Compartment: contains the extensor carpi ulnaris (ECU) tendon.
  - The ECU not only functions as an extensor for the wrist, but is also part of the triangular fibrocartilage

complex (TFCC) and thus a major stabilizer for the distal radioulnar joint.

- The two extensor proprii tendons of the index and the little finger are located on the ulnar sides of the corresponding communis tendons and allow for individual movements of the peripheral fingers.
- On the dorsum of the hand, the EDC tendons are interconnected by the juncturae tendinum which facilitate combined extension of the fingers.
- Lacerations of the extensor tendons proximal to the juncturae may be masked by the function of these bands.
- At the level of the proximal phalanges, the extensor tendons split up into three parts: the central band and two lateral bands ***(Fig. 24.3)***.

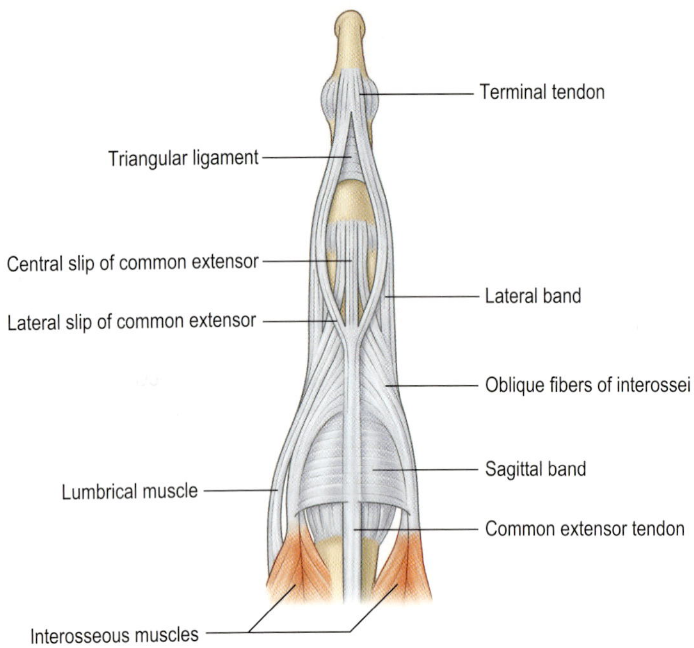

Figure 24.3 Extensor apparatus.

- These merge with the intrinsic extensor system to form the complex extensor apparatus of the digits.
- The extrinsic extensor tendons themselves have three insertion sites on the phalanges.
- Proximally, the tendon is fixed at the level of the metacarpal heads to the palmar plate by the sagittal bands.
- This attachment centers the tendon of the MP joint and prevents hyperextension.
- The most important insertion is located at the base of the middle phalanx.
- Distally, the terminal tendon is attached to the distal phalanx.

Intrinsic muscles

- The intrinsic muscular system of the hand consists of seven interosseous and four lumbrical muscles.
- The three palmar interosseous muscles arise from the medial sides of the second, fourth, and fifth metacarpal bones and join the extensor apparatus of the digits at the level of the proximal phalanx after crossing palmar to the axis of the MP joint.
- They function to adduct the fingers, and flex the MP joint, and extend the IP joints.
- The four dorsal interosseous muscles originate with two heads each from the adjacent sides of the five metacarpal bones. The first two interosseous muscles approach the index and middle finger from the radial side; the third and fourth approach the middle and ring finger from the ulnar side. They insert at the proximal phalanges and the interosseous hood of the extensor apparatus before joining the lateral bands.
- They function to abduct the fingers, flex the MP joint, and extend the IP joints.
- The lumbrical muscles arise from the radial sides of the flexor digitorum profundus tendons at the level of the metacarpals and join the extensor apparatus from the radial side ***(Fig. 24.4)***.

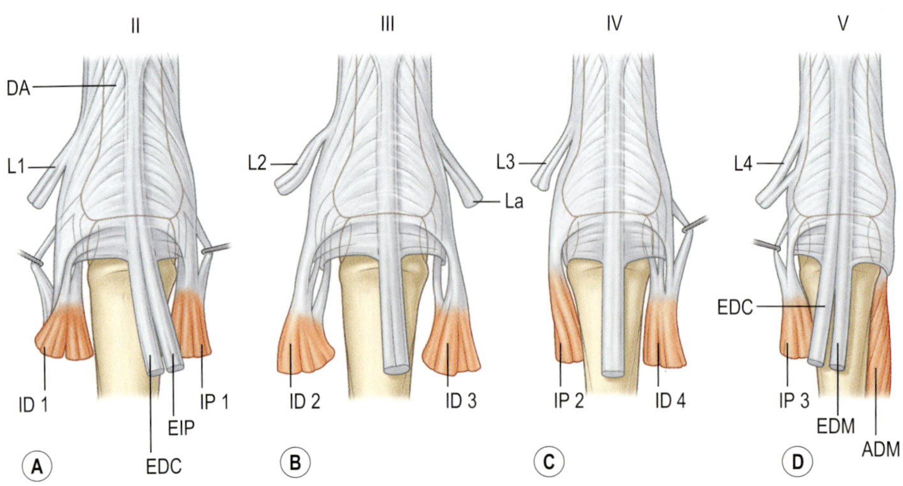

Figure 24.4 The distribution of intrinsic muscles in the fingers. Roman numbers indicate finger numbers. DA, dorsal aponeurosis; L, lumbrical muscles, numbered from radial to ulnar; La, accessory lumbrical muscle (variation); EDC, extensor digitorum communis; EIP, extensor indicis proprius; EDM, extensor digiti minimi; ADM, abductor digiti minimi; ID, dorsal interosseous muscles; IP, palmar interosseous muscles, numbered from radial to ulnar.

- They function primarily as IP joint extenders.
- The thumb also has three short muscles that join the extensor apparatus: the flexor pollicis brevis (FPB) and abductor pollicis brevis (APB) muscles on the radial side and the adductor pollicis (ADP) muscle on the ulnar side.

Functional anatomy

- The movement of the fingers is dependent upon a delicate equilibrium between the extrinsic extensor and flexor muscles and the intrinsic muscles.
- The extrinsic flexor and extensor muscles have a component that acts as an extensor on the proximal phalanx, which is counteracted under physiologic conditions by the intrinsic muscles.
- Paralysis of these muscles (as in ulnar nerve palsy) therefore results in hyperextension of the MP joints.
- Without intrinsic muscle function the long extensors exhaust their potential at the level of the proximal phalanx. Thus, for complete extension of the interphalangeal joints, intrinsic muscle function is therefore mandatory.

Mechanisms of joint extension

- The MP joint is extended by the extrinsic extensor tendon.
- Extension of the PIP joint is mediated by the central slip of the extensor tendon.
- However, as stated above, intrinsic muscle function is necessary in order to enable the extrinsic extensor tendon to act on the PIP joint.
- At the level of the PIP joint, the extensor tendon is centered by the transverse retinacular ligaments.
- Extension of the DIP joint is a combination of terminal lateral bands and a tenodesis effect mediated by the oblique retinacular ligaments.

Operative techniques

Suturing techniques

- Suturing techniques have to be adapted specifically to the location of the lesion because the size of the tendon varies along its length.
- Whatever technique is chosen, it should provide the best stability with the least shortening possible.
- In zones VI and proximally, the extensor tendon resembles a flexor tendon and as such can be repaired with a core suture and an epitendinous running suture.
- Commonly used suture strengths include 3-0 and 4-0 for core sutures and 5-0 for epitendinous sutures *(Fig. 24.5)*.
- In order to achieve maximum core suture strength, locking stitches should be preferred over grasping stitches in order to prevent suture pull-out and reduce gapping.

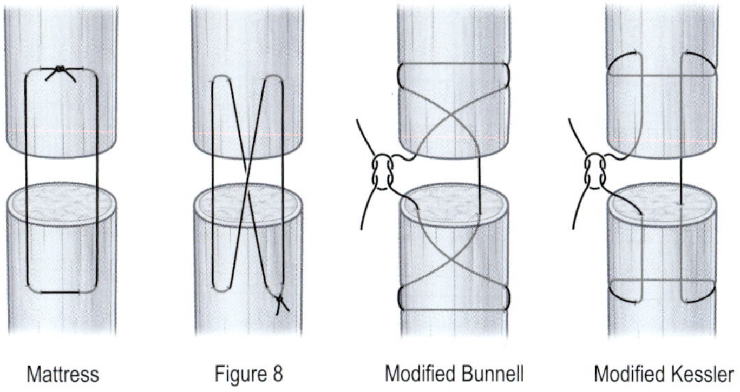

Figure 24.5 Different types of core sutures.

- In the more distal zones of injury, locking or grasping core stitches become increasingly difficult due to flattening of the tendon.
- Grasping stitches in zone IV injuries are strong enough to enable postoperative early active motion.
- Simple running stitches should be avoided due to the low pull-out strength in favor of more complex locking suture techniques.

Clinical tip

Always check the stability of the sutured tendon intraoperatively by gentle movements of the finger. If possible, use locking core stitches in preference to other techniques. Soft tissue coverage can be very thin in fingers, so patients may be able to make out dyed suture material through the skin.

Zone I

The mallet finger

- Characterized by persistent flexion of the distal phalanx due to a lesion of the extensor apparatus at the level of the DIP joint.
- Represents a classic closed injury that is usually treated conservatively, although open injuries may occur as well.
- The flat terminal extensor tendon inserts at the base of the distal phalanx where it blends with the joint capsule.
- Mallet fingers can be classified by the degree of osseous involvement.
- Isolated tendinous ruptures are differentiated from injuries that involve bony avulsions.
- Most surgeons prefer conservative treatment with splints over operative therapy for uncomplicated injuries, although the scientific evidence is limited.
- Conservative treatment usually implies immobilization of the DIP joint in extension while sparing the PIP joint.
- By extension or slight hyperextension of the joint the two ruptured ends of the tendon are approximated.
- The fibrous tissue of the resulting scar is thought to be strong enough to restore extension of the joint.
- The type of splint is not nearly as important as patient compliance *(Figs 24.6, 24.7)*.

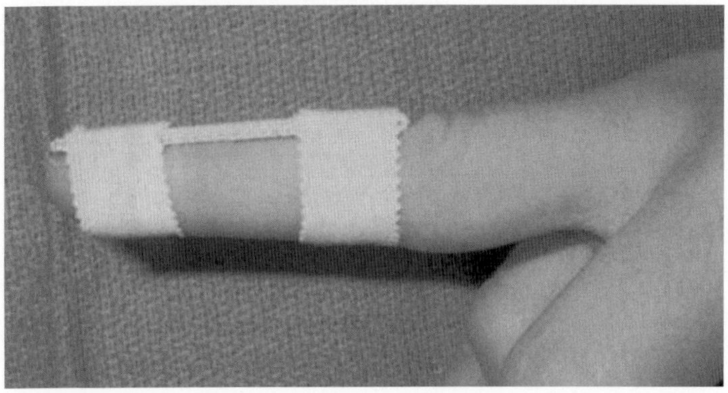

Figure 24.6 Aluminum splint.

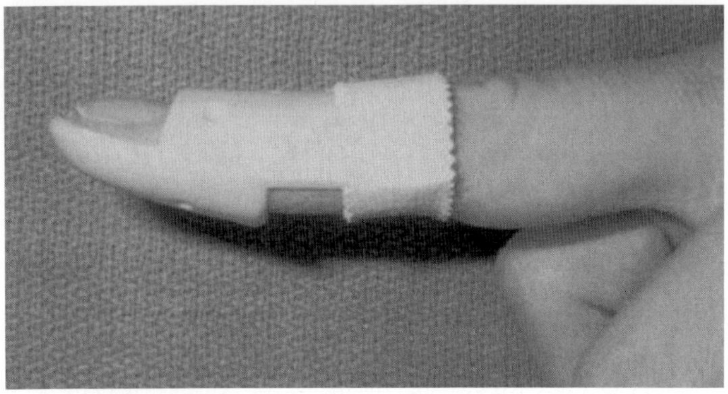

Figure 24.7 Stack splint.

- Most authors recommend full-time splinting for at least 6–8 weeks followed by a period of 2–6 weeks of splinting at night to enable further shrinking of the immature scar.
- By thorough splinting, a residual lack of extension of 10° or less can be expected.
- Surgical treatment for closed injuries should only be considered in fragment sizes greater than one-third of the joint surface.
- Transfixation of the DIP joint with a Kirschner wire has been suggested for sole treatment of the mallet injury in addition to other surgical interventions.
- To avoid scarring of the finger pulp, Tubiana has suggested an oblique angle when crossing the DIP joint.
- In case of a rather small fragment, indirect reduction by extension block pin fixation should be preferred ("doorstop osteosynthesis").
- In this technique, the distal phalanx is maximally flexed and a 1 mm Kirschner wire is advanced into the middle phalanx dorsal to the avulsed fragment at a 45° angle, creating the extension block against which the fragment is reduced. The joint is then extended, reducing the fragment. This position is secured by a second Kirschner wire inserted longitudinally across the DIP joint for transfixation. The wires are cut and a splint is applied for at least 6 weeks ***(Figs 24.8, 24.9)***.
- If the avulsed fragment seems large enough, it may either be pinned directly percutaneously or reduced in an open fashion through a zigzag incision of the distal and middle phalanges.

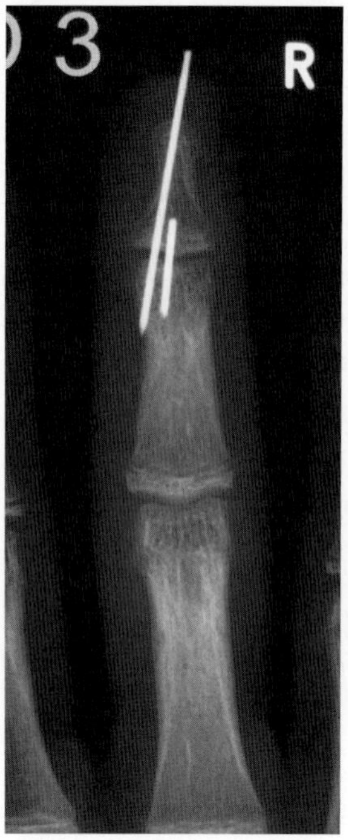

Figure 24.8 Postoperative doorstop: posteroanterior view.

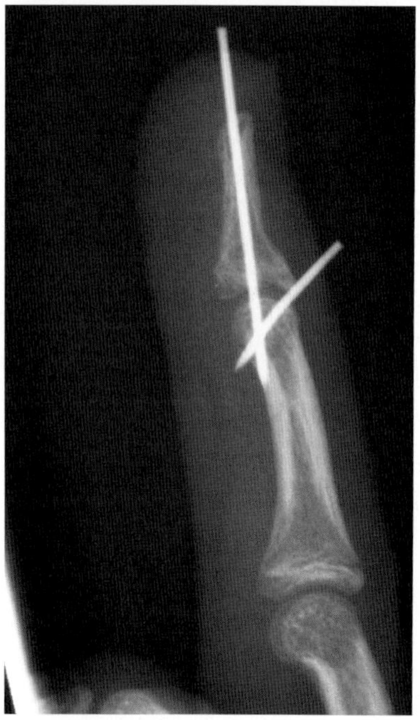

Figure 24.9 Postoperative doorstop: lateral view 6 weeks after doorstop osteosynthesis.

- In case of open reduction, screw fixation seems preferable. Alternatively, a pull-out suture may be applied, as described by Doyle.
- Most authors agree to operative treatment for open injuries.
- In some cases, suturing of the skin alone and supporting the joint in extension or slight hyperextension is enough to approximate the ends of the ruptured tendon and allow direct healing.

- When sutures are needed to approximate the tendon ends, a suture that incorporates both skin and tendon may be superior to individual suturing of the tendon, because further tendon dissection may decrease the blood supply and compromise healing.

Zone II

- Injuries to the extensor tendon over the middle phalanx usually result from sharp, direct lacerations or crush injuries.
- Acute lacerations should be explored to determine the extent of the tendon injury.
- If less than 50% of the tendon substance is injured, the tendon is considered stable and no further treatment is necessary.
- If more than half of the tendon is involved, additional suturing is necessary.
- Care should be taken to avoid considerable shortening of the tendon which will result in lack of flexion of the DIP joint.

Zone III

- Injuries to the extensor tendon at the level of the PIP joint (zone III) occur as both closed and open injuries, ranging from minor strains to complete ruptures or lacerations.
- Injuries at this level can give rise to the characteristic boutonnière deformity when the proximal phalanx herniates through the central slip defect.
- The deformity will not develop immediately after the injury.
- Disruption of the tendon first leads to an inability to extend the PIP joint actively while passive extension is possible.
- Only after the lateral bands migrate palmarly and retraction of the central slip occurs will hyperextension of the DIP joint develop.
- A closed avulsion injury of the central slip may not be immediately evident and extension may be retained by means of the lateral bands.
- The central slip may be restored without surgical intervention by extension splinting.
- The DIP joint should not be included in immobilization. Instead, patients should be encouraged to move the DIP joint actively and passively while wearing the PIP splint ***(Fig. 24.10)***.
- Several authors have proposed pinning the PIP joint in extension by a Kirschner wire.
- Most authors suggest keeping the joint in extension for 5–6 weeks.
- Surgical treatment has been suggested for avulsion injuries with large bony fragments or unstable transarticular fractures.
- If the fragment is too small to be pinned directly, it may be excised and the tendon reinserted into the middle fragment with a bone anchor.
- Open injuries should always be thoroughly explored. Care should be taken specifically to include the lateral bands and the triangular ligament in the inspection.

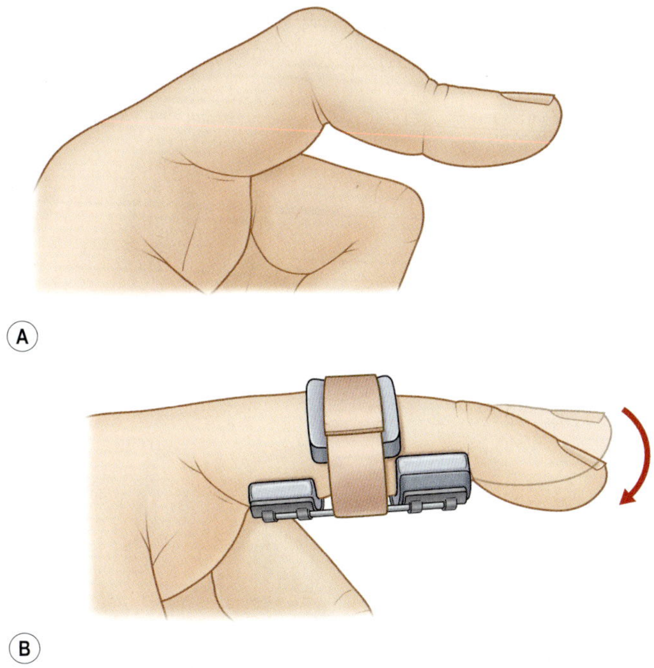

Figure 24.10 (A, B) Splinting for closed extensor tendon ruptures in zone III.

- In clean and sharp lacerations, the wound can be easily enlarged and the injured tendon should be sutured directly or reinserted into the middle phalanx.
- In contrast, contaminated defect wounds, e.g., after saw injuries, are a lot more difficult to deal with.
- If there is considerable loss of tendon, an immediate reconstruction should be attempted.
- Snow described a retrograde tendinous flap created from the proximal tendon that is flipped over to bridge the defect over the joint ***(Fig. 24.11)***.
- Aiache et al. proposed a longitudinal split of the two lateral bands that are joined in the midline to reconstruct the tendinous insertion and to cover the joint ***(Fig. 24.12)***.
- Any loss of covering skin should be replaced immediately as well.
- Options include local random pattern flaps, reversed cross-finger flaps, or flaps from the dorsal metacarpal artery system.

Zone IV

- As the extensor becomes very broad over the proximal phalanx, partial lacerations are more commonly observed than complete injuries of the tendons.
- Extensor tendon injuries in zone IV are often associated with fractures of the proximal phalanx.
- Due to the close relationship between tendon and bone, adhesions frequently occur and tenolysis is often necessary.
- Some form of a postoperative early active motion regimen is therefore advisable to reduce loss of range of motion.
- Maintenance of the wrist in an extended position will "unload" the tendon and allow early range of motion of the finger.

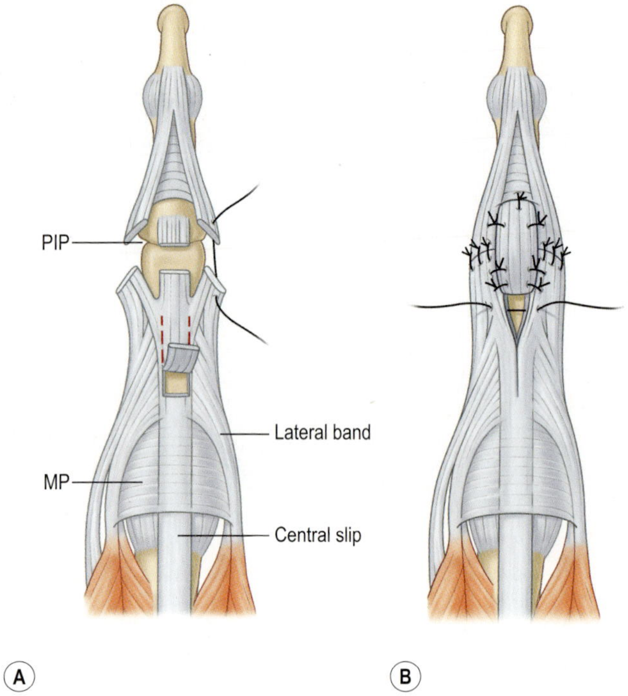

Figure 24.11 (A, B) Snow's technique of reconstructing the central slip. PIP, proximal interphalangeal; MP, metacarpophalangeal.

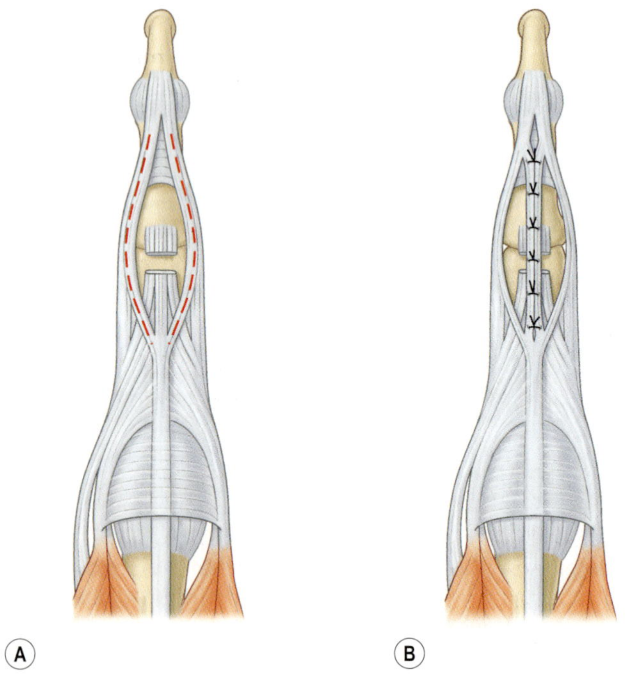

Figure 24.12 (A, B) Reconstruction of the central slip involving splitting of the lateral bands (Aiache's technique).

Zone V

- At the level of the MP joints, the extensor tendon consists of the central extensor tendon and the sagittal bands. Due to its broad width, complete lacerations are uncommon.
- Surgical exploration is warranted and it should be taken into account that the injury to the tendon may be located more proximally than the skin laceration if the tendon was injured in flexion.
- If possible, a core suture with an epitendinous running stitch should be performed.

Human bite injuries

- A common mechanism of injuries to the extensor tendon in zone V caused by a punch to the opponent's face (fight bites).
- Bite wounds are heavily contaminated and prone to serious infection.
- As skin damage is often minimal, these injuries are frequently underestimated by the patient and treatment is delayed until infection has developed.
- Primary inspection is mandatory in fresh injuries, as are X-ray studies to detect avulsed bony fragments or teeth.
- During exploration, the tendon should be split longitudinally and the MCP joint irrigated with antibiotic solution.
- Partial lacerations of the tendon often do not require suturing.
- A number of authors suggest delayed primary treatment after the occurrence of infection has been ruled out.

Sagittal band injuries

- The central tendon is centered over the MP joint by the lateral bands which attach to the palmar plate of the joint.
- Open or closed injuries to the sagittal bands may result in subluxation of the tendon to the unaffected side during flexion.
- Partial lacerations will not result in subluxation unless two-thirds of the sagittal band is affected.
- Stable lacerations can be treated by buddy-taping of the affected finger to an adjacent finger for 3 weeks.
- In case of an unstable tendon, the laceration should be sutured.
- Closed ruptures of the sagittal bands are much more common than open injuries and usually occur in the course of a primary disease of the joints such as rheumatoid arthritis.
- Traumatic and spontaneous ruptures of the sagittal bands may be treated by splinting within 10–14 days.
- In older injuries, direct suturing of the bands should be attempted.

Zone VI

- Extensor tendon lesions at the level of the metacarpal bones can usually be sutured by a 3-0 core stitch and an epitendinous running suture.
- Postoperatively, early mobilization with a dynamic splinting regimen is indicated to reduce tendon adhesions.
- Loss of flexion has been reported to be more common than loss of extension.

Zone VII

- Injuries to the extensor tendons at the level of the extensor retinaculum are due to either open lacerations that often affect multiple tendons or closed ruptures, most often after distal radius fractures.
- To repair open lacerations at this level, at least a part of the retinaculum has to be opened.
- The tendon repair itself should be performed with a stable core suture and an epitendinous running stitch.
- Special attention should also be paid to concomitant injuries of sensory branches of the radial and ulnar nerves.
- Primary coaptation of the nerve ends should be performed in order to prevent the development of painful and difficult-to-manage neuromas.
- As the tendons are arranged very close to each other, injuries of multiple tendons through one laceration occur frequently.
- Identification of the tendons can be quite difficult, because they tend to retract into the forearm. A thorough knowledge of the surgical anatomy is therefore mandatory.
- Ruptures of the EPL tendon are most often associated with fractures of the distal radius or rheumatoid arthritis.
- Because of the degenerative nature of the process, an end-to-end repair of the tendon is usually not possible without unacceptable shortening of the tendon.
- Instead, reconstruction of the tendon can be performed by EIP to EPL tendon transfers or interposing tendon grafts.

Zones VIII/IX

- Lesions of the extensor tendons at levels VIII and IX include injuries of the musculotendinous junctions and muscle bellies.
- As in zone VII injuries, the recovery and identification of retracted tendons can be quite challenging.
- Combined injuries to muscles and/or nerves are possible and knowledge of the sequence of motor innervation helps to distinguish a motor nerve injury from a tendon injury.
- The motor branches of the wrist and fingers have been divided into two groups, a proximal superficial group and a distal deep group.
- The proximal superficial group consists of the ECRL, ECRB, EDC, EDM, and ECU muscles.
- The entry of nerve fibers into the muscles is near the lateral epicondyle.
- When exposing the posterior interosseous nerve, the interval between the wrist ECRB and ECRL tendon (proximal to the supinator muscle) and the EDC, EDM, and ECU (distal to the supinator) should be chosen to avoid injury to motor branches.
- The distal deep group consists of the APL, EPB, EPL, and EIP.
- They originate in the distal half of the forearm, close to the skeletal plane.
- Sutures of muscle fibers alone have virtually no tensile strength. Therefore an effort should be made to suture tendons or fascial layers instead of muscle fibers alone.
- These sutures are usually not strong enough for dynamic postoperative treatment protocols and immobilization for 3–4 weeks should be initiated postoperatively.

Secondary procedures

Clinical tip

Secondary correction of established finger deformities is exceedingly difficult. Patients should be aware that restoration of "normal" finger movement is rare.

The hanging fingertip

- Even a minimal increase in tendon length will result in an extensor lag after a mallet injury.
- In many patients, therefore, some residual deformity will occur, although it is rarely of any relevance.
- With the extension lag exceeding 40–50°, however, a considerable number of patients will desire correction.
- In this case, additional immobilization should be considered for up to 6 months after the injury, especially if there is any doubt about the adequacy of the primary treatment.
- If conservative treatment fails, surgical treatment should be discussed with the patient.
- If surgical correction is indicated, a simple combined excision of callus and skin may be the procedure of choice, referred to as the Brooks–Garner procedure.
- An elliptical wedge of skin and underlying soft tissues, including the scarred extensor tendon, is excised from the dorsum of the involved DIP joint ***(Figs 24.13–24.15)***.
- The wound edges are closed by en bloc sutures, resulting in a slight hyperextension of the joint.
- The DIP joint is then transfixed with a Kirschner wire to keep the joint in the desired position for 6 weeks.

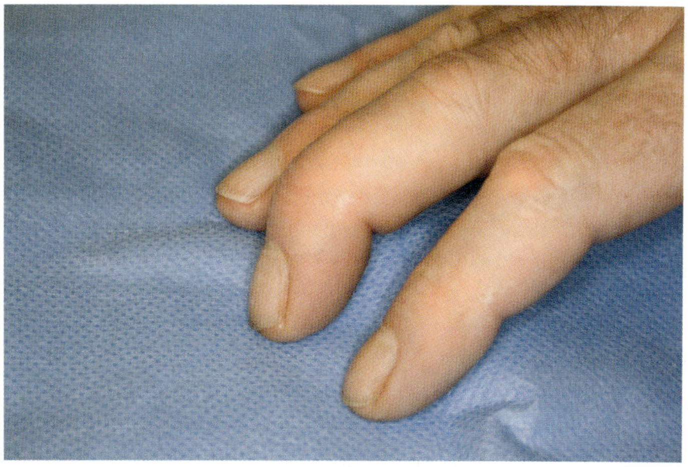

Figure 24.13 Hanging fingertip (Mallet Finger).

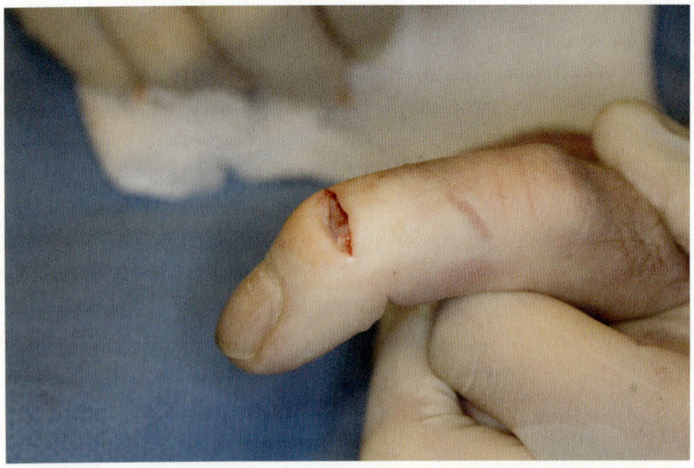

Figure 24.14 Resection of skin and tendon.

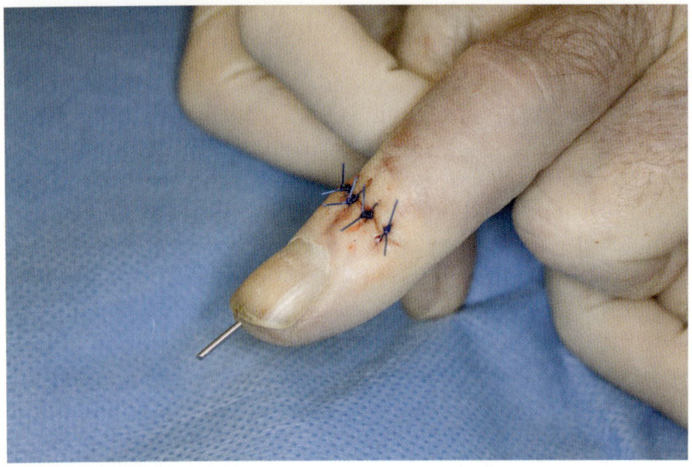

Figure 24.15 Transfixation of the distal interphalangeal joint.

- Alternatively, a Fowler release (central slip tenotomy) or even a reconstruction of the spiral oblique retinacular ligament may be performed.
- Both procedures are primarily used to correct swan-neck deformities and require a supple PIP joint.

The swan-neck deformity

- A classic finger deformity that can be caused by many reasons, including congenital PIP palmar plate laxity and intrinsic tightness.
- Often it is associated with some form of arthritis; however, it can also result from a mallet injury.
- In the mallet finger, the disrupted extensor tendon results in a concentration of extensor force at the PIP joint ***(Fig. 24.16)***.
- If the palmar plate of the joint is lax, the swan-neck deformity will occur immediately. However, even if it is not lax to begin with, it will stretch over time due to increased extensor pull. Once the PIP hyperextension exceeds a critical point, snapping of the joint will occur.
- A Fowler tenotomy (tenotomy of the central slip) has been used to address the swan-neck deformity in patients with a chronic mallet deformity in which the terminal extensor tendon cannot be repaired.

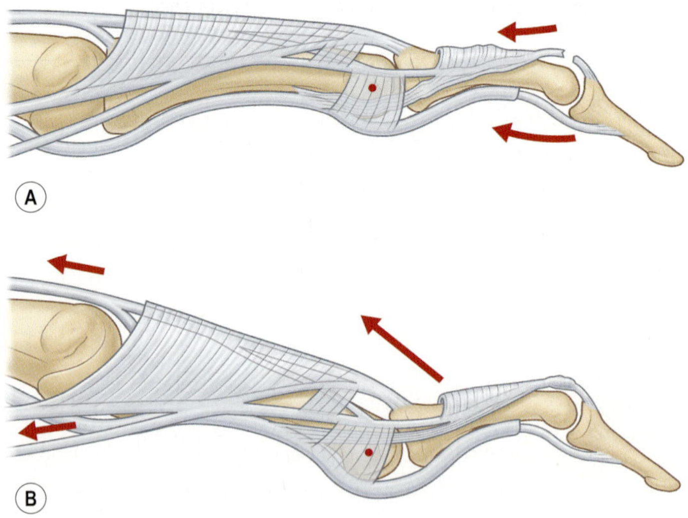

Figure 24.16 (A, B) Pathophysiology of the swan-neck deformity. The deformity persists when the tendon heals with lengthening.

- By transection of the central slip, rebalancing of the extensor mechanism should occur in order to increase the extension force on the DIP joint.
- Alternatively, the extensor tendon may be reconstructed by a tendon graft (spiral oblique retinacular ligament or SORL reconstruction: ***Fig. 24.17***).
- In this technically demanding operation, a palmaris tendon graft is fixed to the distal phalanx by a pull-out suture. It is then passed between the flexor tendon and the palmar plate of the PIP joint into an osseous tunnel in the proximal phalanx ***(Fig. 24.18)***.
- Swan-neck deformities which are not primarily related to injuries of the distal extensor tendon should be approached differently as these deformities are frequently caused by hyperlax palmar plates at the level of the PIP joint.
- In these cases, correction of the laxity can be indicated, e.g., by a tenodesis of the flexor digitorum superficialis tendon.

The boutonnière deformity

- Acute injury to the central band of the extensor tendon will result in an acute boutonnière deformity as both lateral bands shift palmarly due to the accompanied disruption of the triangular ligament.
- In the acute phase, the deformity should be easily reducible and may be treated as described above.
- However, if left untreated, a chronic contracture results from shortening of the oblique retinacular ligament ***(Fig. 24.19)***.
- This condition has long been recognized as one of the most challenging problems in hand surgery.
- Any surgical correction of the deformity should only be performed if the PIP joint can be extended passively.

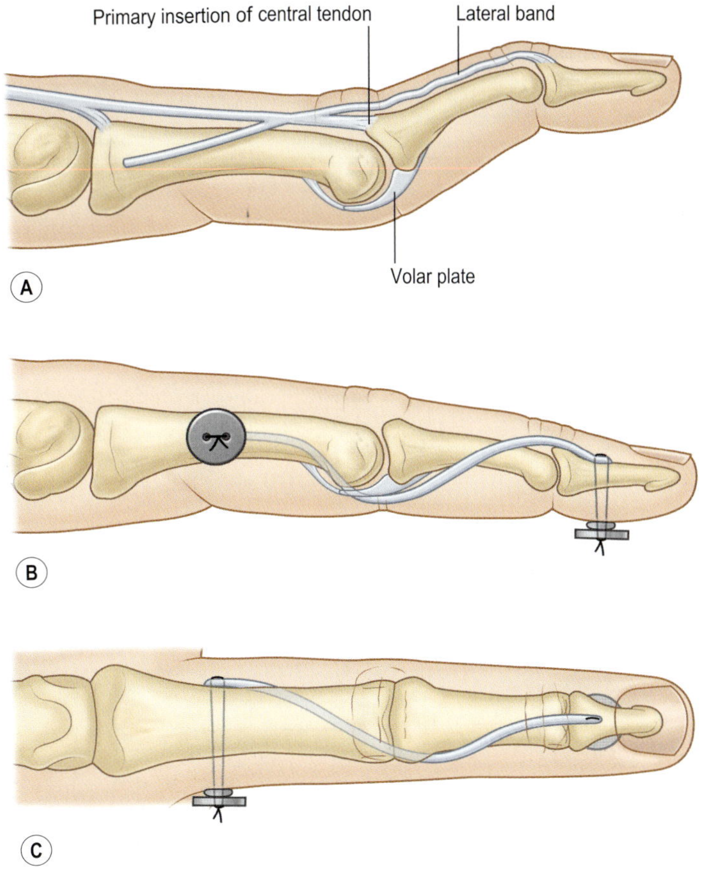

Figure 24.17 (A–C) Spiral oblique retinacular ligament. A palmaris longus tendon graft is passed between the flexor tendon and the palmar plate and fixed to the distal phalanx by a pull-out suture.

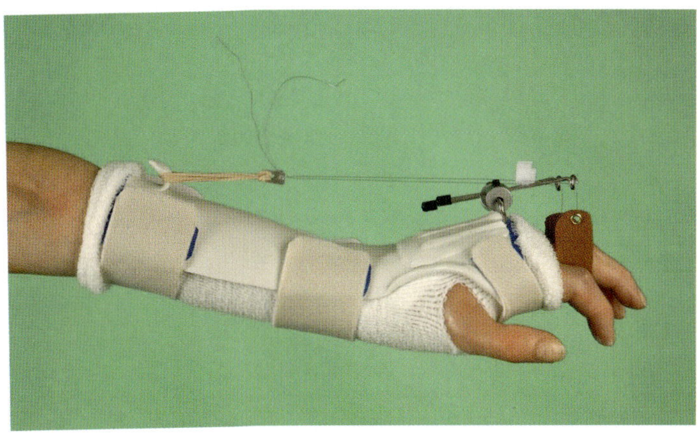

Figure 24.18 Dynamic extension splint.

- Patients should be aware that postoperative splinting is an essential part of the treatment strategy and may be necessary for months after surgery.
- An increase in extension of the joint should not be traded for a stiff finger or loss of grip strength.
- There are two main categories of procedure to address the boutonnière deformity: tenotomy or reconstruction of the extensor tendon by tendon relocation or tendon grafting.

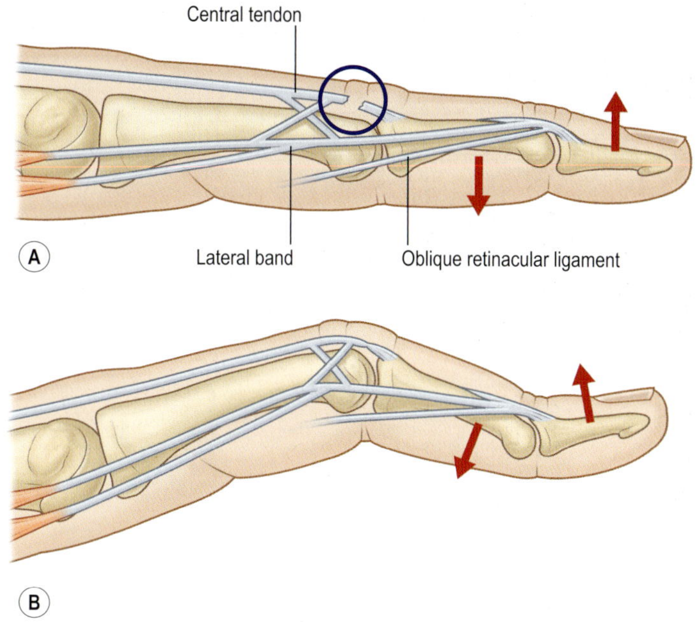

Figure 24.19 (A, B) Pathophysiology of the boutonnière deformity. Subluxation of the lateral bands results in redistribution of forces and an extensor lag in the proximal interphalangeal joint. Retraction of the oblique retinacular ligament prohibits reduction in chronic deformities.

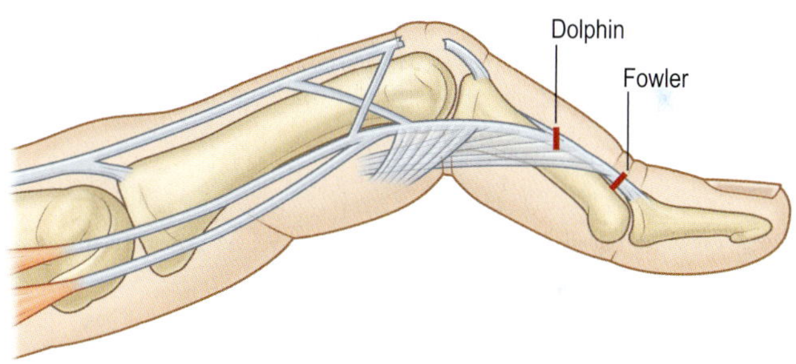

Figure 24.20 Treatment of the boutonnière deformity by tenotomy as described by Dolphin and Fowler. Dolphin's tenotomy preserves the insertions of the oblique retinacular ligament.

- Tenotomy of the extensor tendon on the middle phalanx is referred as the Dolphin or Fowler procedure.
- It may be the procedure of choice when patients mainly complain about hyperextension of the DIP joint.
- The incision should be performed just distally to the insertion of the central slip.
- In Dolphin's description, the tendon is divided more proximally in order to preserve the distal insertions of the oblique retinacular ligament ***(Fig. 24.20)***.
- The lateral bands should be able to slide proximally in order to increase the tone on the PIP joint to allow improved extension and reduce tension on the DIP joint.
- Postoperatively, the PIP joint should be splinted in extension for 6–8 weeks, allowing free range of motion of the DIP joint.
- If the main patient complaint is the lack of extensive function, secondary reconstruction of the extensor should be considered.

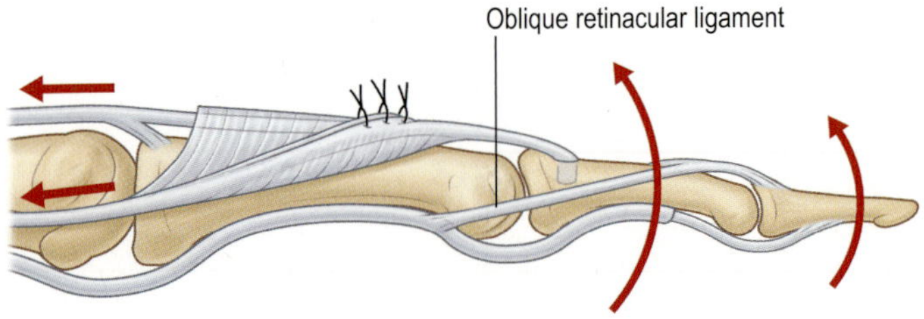

Figure 24.21 Littler operation. The lateral bands are resected and relocated to the central tendon.

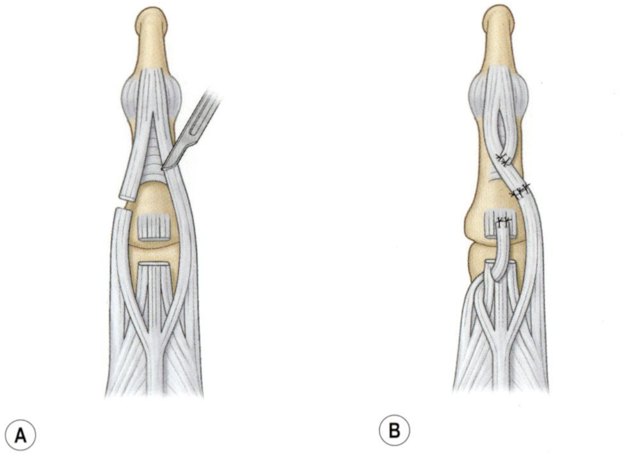

Figure 24.22 (A, B) Matev's technique for reconstruction of the central slip. Both lateral bands are cut at different heights and relocated to reconstruct the central slip.

- This goal can be achieved by either tendon relocation or tendon grafting.
- The central slip can be reconstructed as described by Snow (see Fig. 24.11). The end of the reconstructed tendon is either sutured to the remaining insertion on the middle phalanx or reinserted directly into the phalanx.
- A large number of techniques have been described to reconstruct the central slip using the lateral bands *(Figs 24.21, 24.22)*.
- In extensive defects of the central slip, the lateral bands may be insufficient for reconstruction and, in these cases, free tendon grafts may be indicated.

Delayed sagittal band reconstruction

- If the sagittal band is ruptured, the tendon may subluxate to the unaffected side.
- Tendon dislocation rarely occurs in patients not suffering from rheumatoid arthritis.
- If conservative treatment fails, surgical reconstruction of the sagittal band is indicated.
- In addition to the reconstruction, a release of the contracted contralateral sagittal band may be necessary in long-standing cases.
- Several techniques have been described for reconstruction, if direct repair is not possible because of missing soft tissue or severe scarring *(Fig. 24.23)*.

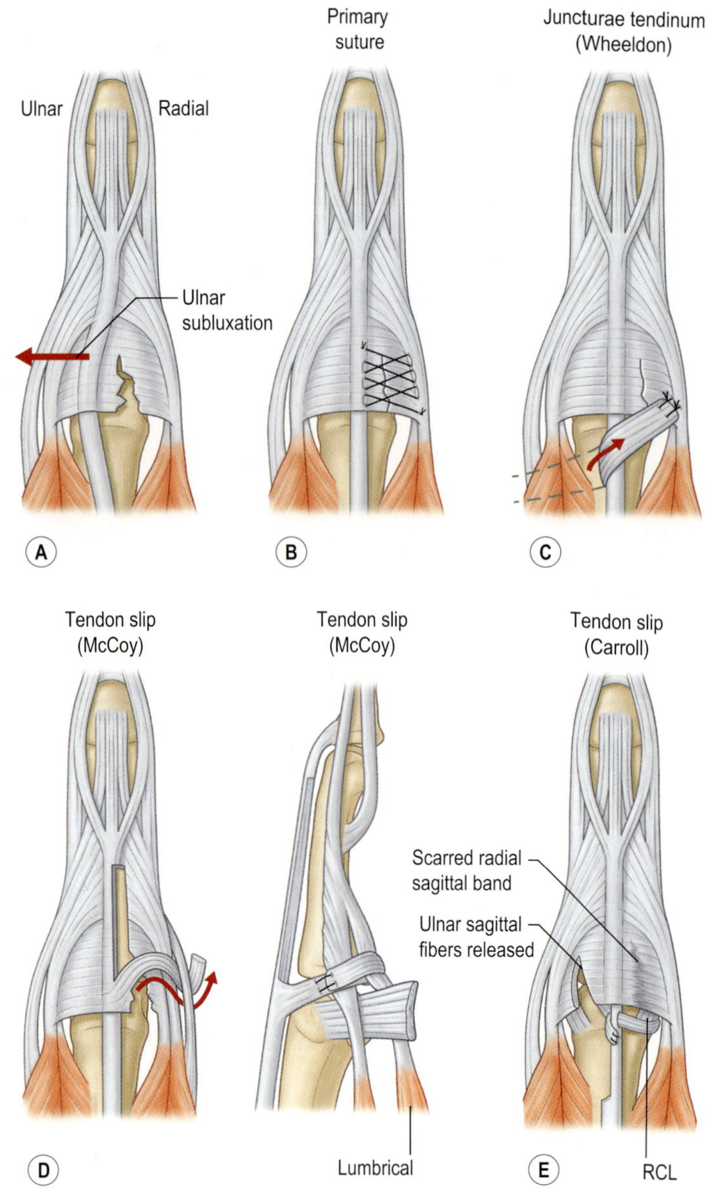

Figure 24.23 Different techniques for reconstruction of the sagittal band. **(A)** Disruption of the radial sagittal band results in ulnar subluxation of the extensor tendon. **(B)** Primary suturing. **(C)** Wheeldon's technique: the ulnar junctura tendinum is relocated to the deep intercarpal ligament. **(D)** McCoy's technique: the tendon is split distally and wrapped around the lumbricalis muscle. **(E)** Carroll's technique: an ulnarly distal-based slip of the extensor digitorum communis tendon is wrapped around the radial collateral ligament (RCL).

The missing tendon: tendon transfers versus tendon grafting

- In cases of degenerative rupture of an extensor tendon, direct suturing is not usually possible because of an existing gap or extensive degeneration of the tendon ends.
- To reconstruct extensor function two options exist.
- First, the tendon can be reconstructed with the use of a tendon graft, e.g., derived from the palmaris longus tendon.

- Second, reconstruction is possible by transfer of another tendon.

Soft tissue management and staged reconstruction in combined injuries

- Lesions of the extensor tendons are often complicated by lesions of the bones and joints and by loss of skin.
- As in other mutilating injuries, basic reconstructive principles apply.
- Before attempting reconstruction of the tendons, several requirements must be fulfilled:
- Radical debridement of all devitalized tissue is mandatory.
- Before closure, the wound should not contain any contamination or tissue of compromised blood supply in order to prevent infection.
- Primary radical debridement has been shown to be superior to several serial debridement steps, because of the formation of edema and infected granulation tissue, which is only poorly penetrated by antibiotic treatment.
- Osseous structures must be stabilized before turning to soft tissues.
- This can be achieved by internal or external fixation as appropriate.
- Stable soft tissue coverage for tendons and bony structures must be provided.
- In case of combined lesions of the dorsum of the hand, often pedicled or free tissue transfer is necessary.
- The pedicled radial forearm flap is a classic pedicled workhorse flap for coverage of the dorsum of the hand.
- Another classic pedicled flap is the posterior interosseous artery flap.
- With the advancement of microsurgical techniques, free tissue transfers are now more frequently performed.
- The timing of combined reconstructive procedures has been subject to discussions.
- Traditionally, these injuries have been addressed by multistage procedures.
- Today, most surgeons probably aim for achieving soft tissue coverage within 72 h.
- Several authors have reported excellent results after one-stage procedures for defects involving the dorsum of the hand with the use of emergency free flaps.
- Reconstruction of missing tendons is usually performed at the time of soft tissue coverage by primary grafting or tendon transfers.
- Because the creation of a secondary tendon sheath is not necessary, staged reconstruction of extensor tendons utilizing silicone rods is rare.

Postoperative considerations

- As with flexor tendon injuries, the importance of an adequate postoperative treatment cannot be overestimated.
- In recent years, dynamic postoperative treatment protocols have been developed that reduce postoperative adhesion formation without jeopardizing the stability of the sutured tendon.
- Strict immobilization is the treatment of choice for some indications.
- Mallet injuries should be treated by full-time static splinting for 8 weeks.
- The same is true for closed ruptures of the central slip (zone III injuries).
- Immobilization should also be considered for injuries proximal to the extensor retinaculum (zones VIII and IX) because it may not be possible to achieve adequate tensile strength by suturing fascial layers around the muscle.
- Postoperative immobilization of open injuries in zones III–V will inevitably result in severe adhesions, because the tendon is very broad and in close relationship to the adjacent bone in this area.
- To overcome this problem, Evans described a postoperative treatment protocol that reduces adhesions by limited early active motion ("short arc motion").
- Dynamic mobilization for injuries in zones V–VII can be achieved by passive extension with a rubber band system combined with active flexion of the affected digit (see Fig. 24.18).
- Early dynamic motion is also superior to immobilization after transfer of the EIP tendon for EPL reconstruction.
- After performing a Pulvertaft weave, the tendon is more stable and splinting can be discontinued after 3 weeks.

Complications and outcomes

- Outcomes vary considerably with the location of the lesion, the extent of concomitant injuries to the bone or surrounding soft tissues, timing of the repair, and adequate postoperative care.
- Lesions distal to the MP joints lead to less favorable results than more proximal lesions.
- The most common complication after extensor tendon injuries is the formation of adhesions between the tendon and surrounding tissues.
- Adhesion formation should be addressed first by hand therapy and splinting of the affected joints in order to improve tendon gliding. If there is not adequate improvement in range of motion after 4–6 months, extensor tendon tenolysis can be considered.
- A stable skin envelope is a prerequisite before performing any additional procedures.
- Tenolysis can be elegantly performed utilizing the wide-awake technique with no sedation and no tourniquet, with the use of tumescent lidocaine and epinephrine.
- Tenolysis alone may not be sufficient to achieve an improvement in range of motion. An additional capsulotomy, collateral ligament release, or even flexor tendon tenolysis may be necessary.

Further reading

Bowers WH, Hurst LC. Chronic mallet finger: The use of Fowler's central slip release. *J Hand Surg Am.* 1978;3:373–376.

Dolphin JA. Extensor tenotomy for chronic boutonnière deformity of the finger; report of two cases. *J Bone Joint Surg Am.* 1965;47:161–164.

Description of the classic technique to address the problem of the boutonnière deformity.

Duran RJ, Houser RG, Stover MG. Management of flexor tendon lacerations in Zone 2 using controlled passive motion postoperatively. In: Hunter JM, Schneider LH, Mackin EJ, et al, eds. *Rehabilitation of the Hand.* St Louis: CV Mosby; 1978:217–224.

Evans RB. Early active short arc motion for the repaired central slip. *J Hand Surg Am.* 1994;19:991–997.

Based on several anatomical studies, Evans introduces a new early active motion protocol for extensor tendon injuries in zones III and IV. Sixty-four digits in 55 patients were investigated. Patients who were treated by early active motion demonstrated better functional results than those who were treated by immobilization.

Harris CJ, Rutledge GLJ. The functional anatomy of the extensor mechanism of the finger. *J Bone Joint Surg Am.* 1972;54:713–726.

Handoll HH, Vaghela MV. Interventions for treating mallet finger injuries. *Cochrane Database Syst Rev.* 2004;CD004574.

Landsmeer JM. The anatomy of the dorsal aponeurosis of the human finger and its functional significance. *Anat Rec.* 1949;104:31–44.

Classic description of the function of the oblique retinacular ligaments which is the anatomical foundation for numerous reconstructive procedures of the distal extensor tendon.

Littler JW, Eaton RG. Redistribution of forces in the correction of boutonnière deformity. *J Bone Joint Surg Am.* 1967;49:1267–1274.

Littler and Eaton describe the pathophysiology of the boutonnière deformity and the results of 8 patients who were treated by detachment and proximal reinsertion of the lateral bands.

Mowlavi A, Burns M, Brown RE. Dynamic versus static splinting of simple zone V and zone VI extensor tendon repairs: a prospective, randomized, controlled study. *Plast Reconstr Surg.* 2005;115:482–487.

Newport ML, Williams CD. Biomechanical characteristics of extensor tendon suture techniques. *J Hand Surg Am.* 1992;17:1117–1123.

Snow JW. Use of a retrograde tendon flap in repairing a severed extensor in the PIP joint area. *Plast Reconstr Surg.* 1973;51:555–558.

Although only 6 cases in 3 years are reported, this is the classic description of one of the most commonly used techniques to reconstruct defects of the central slip.

Index

Page numbers followed by "f" indicate figures, "t" indicate tables, and "b" indicate boxes.

Page numbers followed by "f" indicate figures, "t" indicate tables, and "b" indicate boxes.

D

E

Page numbers followed by "f" indicate figures, "t" indicate tables, and "b" indicate boxes.

Page numbers followed by "f" indicate figures, "t" indicate tables, and "b" indicate boxes.

Page numbers followed by "f" indicate figures, "t" indicate tables, and "b" indicate boxes.

Page numbers followed by "f" indicate figures, "t" indicate tables, and "b" indicate boxes.

Page numbers followed by "f" indicate figures, "t" indicate tables, and "b" indicate boxes.